THE 5-MINUTE VETERINARY CONSULT EQUINE

THE 5-MINUTE VETERINARY CONSULT

Equine

Christopher M Brown, BVSc, PhD, Diplomate ACVIM
Professor
Department Executive Officer, Veterinary Clinical Sciences
Director, Veterinary Teaching Hospital
College of Veterinary Medicine
Iowa State University
Ames, Iowa

Joseph Bertone, DVM, MS, Diplomate ACVIM
Alpine Animal Hospital
Carbondale, Colorado

Lippincott Williams & Wilkins
A Wolters Kluwer Company

LIPPINCOTT WILLIAMS & WILKINS
A Wolters Kluwer Company

Editor: David Troy
Managing Editor: Dana Battaglia
Marketing Manager: Christine Kushner
Production Editor: Jennifer Ajello
Compositor: TechBooks
Printer: RR Donnelley & Sons–Willard

351 West Camden Street
Baltimore, MD 21201

530 Walnut Street
Philadelphia, PA 19106

Printed in the United States of America

Library of Congress Cataloging-in-Publication Data

Bertone, Joseph.
The 5-minute veterinary consult : equine / Joseph Bertone, Christopher Brown.
p. cm.
ISBN 0-683-30605-7
1. Horses—Diseases—Handbooks, manuals, etc. I. Title: Five-minute veterinary consult. II. Brown, Christopher (Christopher Miles). III. Title.
SF951 .B47 2001
636.1′0896—dc21 2001050328

01 02 03 04 05
1 2 3 4 5 6 7 8 9 10

PREFACE

Information in the area of equine medicine and related disciplines has grown at an extraordinary rate over the last 25 years. This poses a major challenge to the busy equine practitioner who may not have enough time to read all of the relevant journals and to attend the major meetings. Often he or she requires a concise reliable resource to answer a very specific question, or a brief, but thorough, overview of a more generalized topic. From these needs the concept of the 5-*Minute Consult* was born. Following the success of the concept in human medicine, Drs. Tilley and Smith applied it with great success to the dog and cat. We have followed the same formula in this volume on the horse. We have tried to ensure that all of the major topics have been covered, with the deliberate exception of a detailed consideration of the vast area of equine lameness.

This work reflects the contributions of a large number of equine experts who, together with their topic editors, have produced hundreds of articles on a wide range of issues. They have all been prepared in one of four different formats to ensure consistency and ease of use. These have been arranged in alphabetical order so that the index will not usually be needed to locate a topic. We are very grateful to all of the authors for their contributions, and for their patience. This was a complex process, and the writing, editing, and compiling of so many articles was a major challenge.

We believe that we have produced a very comprehensive, highly usable and useful text. Undoubtedly we may have overlooked a specific point, and we hope that readers will not hesitate to let us know if they find such omissions. During the production of the text, we became aware that some topics in dermatology and cardiology had been overlooked, but to ensure that the other material would be available in a timely fashion, we went forward. We will correct these and any other problems that are identified in the next edition.

Chris Brown
Joe Bertone

CONSULTING EDITORS

JOSEPH BERTONE, DVM, MS,
Diplomate ACVIM
Alpine Animal Hospital
Carbondale, Colorado
Neurology

CHRISTOPHER M BROWN, BVSc, PhD
Diplomate ACVIM,
Professor
Department Executive Officer
Veterinary Clinical Sciences
Director, Veterinary Teaching Hospital
College of Veterinary Medicine
Iowa State University
Ames, Iowa

VIRGINIA B. REEF, DVM,
Diplomate ACVIM
Professor of Medicine in the Widener Hospital
Director of Large Animal Cardiology and Ultrasonography
Chief, Section of Sports Medicine and Imaging
University of Pennsylvania
New Bolton Center
Kennett Square, Pennsylvania
Cardiovascular

MICHAEL LEVY, DVM,
Diplomate ACVIM
Associate Professor
Large Animal Internal Medicine
School of Veterinary Medicine
Purdue University
West Lafayette, Indiana
Endocrine/Metabolic

HENRY STÄMPFLI, DVM, PhD, Vet.,
Diplomate ACVIM
Associate Professor
Large Animal Medicine, Clinical Studies
Ontario Veterinary College
University of Guelph
Guelph, Ontario
Canada
Gastrointestinal

DEBRA C. SELLON, DVM, PhD
Diplomate, ACVIM
Associate Professor, Equine Medicine
College of Veterinary Medicine
Washington State University
Pullman, WA
Hematopetic

MARY ROSE PARADIS, DVM, MS
Department of Clinical Sciences
Tufts University School of Veterinary Medicine
North Grafton, Massachusetts
Neonates

DENNIS E. BROOKS, DVM, PhD,
Diplomate American College of Veterinary Ophthalmologists
Professor of Ophthalmology
University of Florida
College of Veterinary Medicine
Gainesville, Florida
Ophthalmology

JEAN-PIERRE LAVOIE, DMV,
Diplomate ACVIM (Internal Medicine)
Professor
Department of Clinical Sciences
Faculty of Veterinary Medicine
University of Montreal
St-Hyacinthe, Quebec
Respiratory

CARLA L. CARLETON, DVM, MS,
Diplomate American College of Theriogenologists
Michigan State University
College of Veterinary Medicine
East Lansing, Michigan
Reproductive

HAL SCHOTT, II, DVM, PhD,
Diplomate ACVIM
Associate Professor
Department of Large Animal Clinical Sciences
College of Veterinary Medicine
Michigan State University
East Lansing, MI 48824
Urinary

CORINNE SWEENEY, DVM
New Bolton Center
University of Pennsylvania
Kennett Square, Pennsylvania
Infectious Diseases

ROBERT H. POPPENGA, DVM, PhD,
Diplomate American Board of Veterinary Toxicology
University of Pennsylvania
School of Veterinary Medicine
New Bolton Center
Kennett Square, Pennsylvania
Toxicology

CLAIRE B. ANDREASEN, DVM, PhD,
Diplomate ACVP
Interim Chair
Department of Veterinary Pathology
College of Veterinary Medicine
Iowa State University
Ames, Iowa
Laboratory Medicine

ANTHONY YU, DVM, MS,
Diplomate ACVD
Animal Allergy & Skin Clinic
Beaverton, Oregon
Integumentary

DANIEL Q. ESTEP, PhD, Certified Applied Animal Behaviorist (Animal Behavior Society)
Animal Behavior Associates, Inc.
Littleton, Colorado
Behavior

CONTRIBUTORS

JENNIFER G. ADAMS, DVM,
Diplomate ACVIM
Winder, Georgia

V.J. AMMANN, Dr Med Vet,
Diplomate ACVIM
Mossens, France

CLAIRE B. ANDREASEN, DVM, PhD,
Diplomate ACVP
Interim Chair
Department of Veterinary Pathology
College of Veterinary Medicine
Iowa State University
Ames, Iowa

DINA ANDREWS, DVM, PhD,
Diplomate ACVP
Assistant Professor of Veterinary Pathobiology
School of Veterinary Medicine
Purdue University
West Lafayette, Indiana

JANE E. AXON, BVSc
Adelaide, South Australia, Australia

JOHN D. BAIRD, BVSc, PhD
Professor, Large Animal Medicine
Ontario Veterinary College
University of Guelph
Guelph, Ontario

JANE A. BARBER
Lake Norman Animal Hospital
Mooresville, North Carolina

BONNIE S. BARR, VMD
Rood and Riddle Equine Hospital
Lexington, Kentucky

MICHELLE H. BARTON, DVM, PhD
Department of Large Animal Medicine
College of Veterinary Medicine
University of Georgia
Athens, Georgia

RALPH E. BEADLE, DVM, PhD
Baton Rouge, Louisiana

DANIELA BEDENICE, DVM
Department of Clinical Sciences
Tufts University School of Veterinary Medicine
North Grafton, Massachusetts

RODNEY BELGRAVE, DVM
Department of Veterinary Clinical Sciences
Washington State University
Pullman, Washington

JOSEPH BERTONE, DVM, MS,
Diplomate ACVIM
Alpine Animal Hospital
Carbondale, Colorado

R. JAY BICKERS, DVM
Emergency Clinician
Large Animal Teaching Hospital
University of Tennessee
Knoxville, Tennessee

DANIEL BIROS, DVM, Diplomate, ACVO
Postdoctoral Fellow
Schepens Eye Research Institute
Department of Ophthalmology
Harvard Medical School
Boston, Massachusetts

DENNIS J. BLODGETT, DVM, PhD
Department of Biomedical Sciences and Pathobiology
Virginia-Maryland Regional College of Veterinary Medicine
Virginia Tech
Blacksburg, Virginia

G. DANIEL BOON†

LAURA BOONE, DVM, PhD
Lilly Research Laboratories
Greenfield, Indiana

DENISE BOUNOUS, DVM, PhD
Department of Veterinary Pathology
College of Veterinary Medicine
University of Georgia
Athens, Georgia

LUDOVIC BOURÉ, Med Vet, MSc,
Diplomate ACVS, Diplomate ECVS
Assistant Professor
Large Animal Surgery
Department of Clinical Studies
Ontario Veterinary College
Guelph, Ontario
Canada

CHRISTOPHER P. BOUTROS, DVM, DVSc,
Diplomate ACVS
Waller Equine Hospital
Waller, Texas

E. RICARDO BRIDGES, DVM,
Diplomate ACT
Tuskegee University
School of Veteterinary Medicine
Tuskegee University, Alabama

JOHAN T. BRÖJER, DVM, MSc
Department of Large Animal Clinical Sciences
Faculty of Veterinary Medicine
Swedish University of Agricultural Sciences
Uppsala, Sweden

DENNIS E. BROOKS, DVM, PhD,
Diplomate American College of Veterinary Ophthalmologists
Professor of Ophthalmology
University of Florida
College of Veterinary Medicine
Gainesville, Florida

CHRISTOPHER BROWN, BVSc, PhD
Director, Veterinary
Iowa State University
Department of Veterinary Clinical Sciences
Ames, Iowa

GORDON BRUMBAUGH, DVM,
Diplomate ACVIM
Texas A&M University
College of Veterinary Medicine
Department of Physiology and Pharmacology
College Station, Texas

MARIE E. CADARIO, DVM, MS,
Diplomate ACT
Department of Theriogenology
College of Veterinary Medicine
University of Florida
Gainesville, Florida

CARLA L. CARLETON, DVM, MS,
Diplomate American College of Theriogenologists
Michigan State University
College of Veterinary Medicine
East Lansing, Michigan

THOMAS L. CARSON, DVM, PhD,
Diplomate ABVT
Toxicology Section Leader
Department of Veterinary Diagnostic and Production Animal Medicine
College of Veterinary Medicine
Iowa State University
Ames, Iowa

STAN W. CASTEEL, DVM, PhD,
Diplomate ABVT
Director, Veterinary Medical Diagnostic Laboratory
College of Veterinary Medicine
University of Missouri
Columbia, Missouri

JOHN CHRISTIAN, DVM, PhD
Professor, Emeritus
Department of Veterinary Pathobiology
Purdue University School of Veterinary Medicine
West Lafayette, Indiana

NOAH D. COHEN, DVM, PhD,
Diplomate ACVIM
Large Animal Medicine and Surgery
College of Veterinary Medicine
Texas A&M University
College Station, Texas

CHRYSANN COLLATOS, VMD, PhD,
Diplomate ACVIM
Reno, Nevada

NATHALIE COTE, DMV, DVSc,
Diplomate ACVS
Large Animal Clinic
Veterinary Teaching Hospital
University of Guelph
Guelph, Ontario
Canada

LAURENT COETIL
Assistant Professor of Large Animal Medicine
Purdue University
School of Veterinary Medicine
West Lafayette, Indiana

RICK L. COWELL, DVM, MS,
Diplomate ACVP
Professor, Veterinary Clinical Pathology
Director, Clinical Pathology Laboratory
Oklahoma State University
Department of Veterinary Pathobiology
Stillwater, Oklahoma

SHARON CROWELL-DAVIS, DVM, PhD, DACVB
Professor of Veterinary Medicine
Department of Anatomy and Radiology
College of Veterinary Medicine
University of Georgia
Athens, Georgia

EDNA CURRID, DVM
New England
Horse Care Center
N. Smithfield, Rhode Island

THOMAS J. DIVERS, DVM, ACVIM, ACVECC
Professor of Medicine
Cornell Large Animal Hospital
Ithaca, New York

BRETT A. DOLENTE, VMD
Lecturer, Section of Medicine
New Bolton Center
University of Pennsylvania
Kennett Square, Pennsylvania

MARK T. DONALDSON, VMD,
Diplomate ACVIM
Assistant Professor of Medicine
University of Pennsylvania
School of Veterinary Medicine
New Bolton Center
Kennett Square, Pennsylvania

WENDY DUCKETT, DVM, MSc,
Diplomate ACVIM
Associate Professor
Department of Health Management
Atlantic Veterinary College
University of Prince Edward Island
Charlottetown, Prince Edward Island
Canada

NORM G. DUCHARME, DVM, MSc.
Diplomate American College of Veterinary Surgeons
Professor of Surgery
Medical Director of Equine and Farm Animal Hospital
Department of Clinical Sciences
College of Veterinary Medicine
Cornell University
Ithaca, New York

G. BARRIE EDWARDS, BVSc, DVetMet, FRCVS
University of Liverpool
Veterinary Field Station
Leahurst, Neston, Cheshire
England

DANIEL Q. ESTEP, PhD
Certified Applied Animal Behaviorist (Animal Behavior Society)
Animal Behavior Associates, Inc.
Littleton, Colorado

ELLEN EVANS, DVM, PhD
Schering-Plough Research Institute
Lafayette, New Jersey

TIM J. EVANS, DVM, MS, DABVT, DACT
Veterinary Medical Diagnosis Laboratory
Columbia, Missouri

MOLLIE C. M. FERRIS
Lakeland Veterinary Clinic
British Columbia, Canada

JENNIFER JACOBS FOWLER, DVM
New Jersey Department of Agriculture
Division of Animal Health
Trenton, New Jersey

NICHOLAS FRANK, DVM, DACVIM
Department of Veterinary Clinical Sciences
Purdue University
West Lafayette, Indiana

LISA FREEMAN, DVM, PhD, DACVN
Department of Clinical Sciences
Tufts University School of Veterinary Medicine
North Grafton, Massachusetts

MARTIN FURR, DVM
Associate Professor of Medicine
Marion duPont Scott Equine Medical Center
Virginia-Maryland Regional College of Veterinary Medicine
Leesburg, Virginia

TAM GARLAND, DVM, PhD
Department of Veterinary Physiology and Pharmacology
College of Veterinary Medicine
Texas A&M University
College Station, Texas

RAYMOND J. GEOR BVSc, MVSc, PhD
Kentucky Equine Research, Inc.
Versailles, Kentucky

TERRY GERROS, DVM, MS,
Diplomate ACVIM
Santiam Equine
Salem, Oregon

DAVID E. GRANSTROM, DVM, PhD
Assistant Director
Education and Research Division
American Veterinary Medical Association
Schaumburg, Illinois

STEVEN T. GRUBBS, DVM, PhD,
Diplomate ACVIM
Fort Dodge Animal Health
Division of American Home Products
Princeton, New Jersey

VALERIE O. GUILPIN, DMV, MSBM
Clinical Pathology
Department of Pathology and Biomedical Sciences
College of Veterinary Medicine
Colorado State University
Fort Collins, Colorado

RICHARD P. HACKETT, DVM, MS,
Diplomate ACVS
Professor of Surgery
Section of Large Animal Surgery
Chair, Department of Clinical Sciences
Cornell University
College of Veterinary Medicine
Ithaca, New York

JEFFERY O. HALL, DVM, PhD,
Diplomate ABVT
Assistant Professor
Diagnostic Veterinary Toxicologist
Department of Animal, Dairy, and Veterinary Sciences
Utah State University
Logan, Utah

WILLIAM HARE, DVM, PhD
Williamston, Michigan

DIANA M. HASSEL, DVM, Diplomate ACVS
Associate Veterinarian, Equine Surgery
Department of Surgical and Radiological Sciences
Graduate Student, Comparative Gastroenterology Laboratory
University of California, Davis
Davis, California

JOANNE HEWSON, DVM, Diplomate ACVIM
Department of Pathobiology
Ontario Veterinary College
University of Guelph
Guelph, Ontario
Canada

MELISSA T. HINES, DVM, PhD
Department of Veterinary Clinical Sciences
Washington State University
Pullman, Washington

SUSAN J. HOLCOMBE,
Veterinary Clinical Center
Michigan State University
East Lansing, Michigan

STEPHEN B. HOOSER, DVM, PhD,
Diplomate American Board of Veterinary Toxicology
Head, Toxicology Section & Assistant Director
Animal Disease Diagnostic Laboratory
Purdue University
West Lafayette, Indiana

KATHERINE A. HOUPT, VMD, PhD, DACVB
Animal Behavior Clinic
College of Veterinary Medicine
Cornell University
Ithaca, New York

JEREMY D. HUBERT
Veterinary Clinical Sciences
College of Veterinary Medicine
Louisiana State University
Baton Rouge, Louisiana

KENT HUMBER, DVM, MS,
Diplomate ACVIM
Rancho Santa Fe, California

ARMADO R. IRIZARRY-ROVIRA, DVM
Department of Veterinary Pathobiology
Purdue University School of Veterinary Medicine
West Lafayette, Indiana

DANIEL JEAN
Ecole Nationale Veterinaire d'Alfort
Cedex, France

SORAYA V. JUARBE-DIAZ, DVM, PhD, DACVB
Department of Comparative Medicine
College of Veterinary Medicine
University of Tennessee
Knoxville, Tennessee

MARIA KALLBERG, DVM
University of Florida
College of Veterinary Medicine
Gainesville, Florida

DANIEL G. KENNEY, VMD, Diplomate ACVIM
Staff Veterinarian
Ontario Veterinary College
Guelph, Ontario
Canada

JANENE K. KINGSTON, BVSc, DVSc
Department of Veterinary Clinical Sciences
Washington State University
Pullman, Washington

DONALD P. KNOWLES, DVM, PhD
Research Leader
Animal Disease Research Unit
ARS-USDA
Washington State University
Pullman, Washington

CATHERINE W. KOHN, VMD, Diplomate ACVIM
Department of Veterinary Clinical Sciences
Ohio State University
Columbus, Ohio

ANDRAS KOMAROMY
University of Florida
College of Veterinary Medicine
Gainesville, Florida

ANITA M. KORE, DVM, PhD,
Diplomate ABVT
3M Corporate Toxicology
St. Paul, Minnesota

JEFFREY LAKRITZ, DVM, PhD,
Diplomate ACVIM Large Animal
Assistant Professor Veterinary Medicine and Surgery
College of Veterinary Medicine
University of Missouri-Columbia
Columbia, Missouri

ANNE LANEVSCHI, DVM, MS
Faculty of Medicine
Department of Pathology and Microbiology
College of Veterinary Medicine
University of Montreal
St. Hyacinthe, Quebec Canada

E. DUANE LASSEN, DVM, PhD
Professor
Department of Pathology
College of Veterinary Medicine and Biomedical Sciences
Colorado State University
Fort Collins, Colorado

JEAN-SEBASTIEN LATOUCHE, BSc, DMV
Department of Pathology and Microbiology
Faculte de Medecine Veterinaire
Universite of Montreal
St. Hyacinthe, Quebec Canada

SHEILA LAVERTY, MVB, Diplomate ACVS,
Diplomate ECVS
Professor
Department of Clinical Sciences
Faculty of Veterinary Medicine
University of Montreal
St. Hyacinthe, Quebec
Canada

JEAN-PIERRE LAVOIE, DMV,
Diplomate ACVIM (Internal Medicine)
Professor
Department of Clinical Sciences
Faculty of Veterinary Medicine
University of Montreal
St. Hyacinthe, Quebec
Canada

GUY D. LESTER BVMS, PhD
College of Veterinary Medicine
University of Florida
Gainesville, Florida

MICHEL LEVY, DVM, Diplomate ACVIM
Associate Professor
Large Animal Internal Medicine
Purdue University
West Lafayette, Indiana

JEANNE LOFSTEDT, BVSc, MS,
Diplomate ACVIM
Associate Dean, Academic Affairs
Atlantic Veterinary College
University of Prince Edward Island
Charlottetown, Prince Edward Island
Canada

MAUREEN T. LONG, DVM, PhD
College of Veterinary Medicine
University of Florida
Gainesville, Florida

JOSE GARCIA-LOPEZ, VMD
Department of Clinical Sciences
Tufts University School of Veterinary Medicine
North Grafton, Massachusetts

CHARLES G. MacALLISTER, DVM,
Diplomate ACVIM
Department of Clinical Sciences
College of Veterinary Medicine
Oklahoma State University
Stillwater, Oklahoma

MARGO L. MACPHERSON, DVM, MS,
Diplomate ACT
Assistant Professor, Reproduction
College of Veterinary Medicine
University of Florida
Gainesville, Florida

JOHN E. MADIGAN, DVM, Diplomate ACVIM
Department of Medicine & Epidemiology
School of Veterinary Medicine
University of California, Davis
Davis, California

K. GARY MAGDESIAN, DVM,
Diplomate ACVIM and ACVECC
Veterinary Medical Teaching Hospital
University of California, Davis
Davis, California

PEGGY S. MARSH, DVM, Diplomate ACVIM
Equine Medicine Lecturer
Department of Large Animal Medicine and Surgery
Texas A&M University
College Station, Texas

HILARY K. MATTHEWS, DVM, PhD, DACVIM
Capital Veterinary Referral Center
Columbus, Ohio

MELISSA MAZAN, DVM, Diplomate ACVM
Assistant Professor, Large Animal Medicine
Department of Clinical Sciences
Tufts University School of Veterinary Medicine
North Grafton, Massachusetts

CYNTHIA A. McCALL, PhD, DACAABS
Department of Animal and Dairy Sciences
Auburn University
Auburn, Alabama

J. TRENTON McCLURE, DVM, Diplomate ACVIM
Department of Health Management
Atlantic Veterinary College
University of Prince Edward Island
Charlottetown, Prince Edward Island
Canada

JILL JOHNSON McCLURE, DVM, MS, Diplomate ACVIM and ABVP
Professor of Equine Medicine
Department of Veterinary Clinical Sciences
School of Veterinary Medicine
Louisiana State University
Baton Rouge, Louisiana

REBECCA S. McCONNICO, DVM, PhD, Diplomate ACVIM
Assistant Professor of Equine Medicine
Equine Health Studies Program
Department of Veterinary Clinical Sciences
Louisiana State University
School of Veterinary Medicine
Baton Rouge, Louisiana

JESSIE McCOY, DVM
Department of Laboratory Animals
Tufts University School of Veterinary Medicine
North Grafton, Massachusetts

SUE M. McDONNELL, PhD
University of Pennsylvania School of Veterinary Medicine
New Bolton Center
Kennett Square, Pennsylvania

ROBERT H. MEALEY, DVM
Department of Veterinary Microbiology & Pathology
Washington State University
Pullman, Washington

JAMES MEINKOTH, DVM, PhD
Department of Veterinary Anatomy, Pathology, and Pharmacology
College of Veterinary Medicine
Oklahoma State University
Stillwater, Oklahoma

STUART A. MEYERS, DVM, PhD, Diplomate, American College of Theriogenologists
Department of Anatomy, Physiology & Cell Biology
School of Veterinary Medicine
University of California, Davis
Davis, California

CAROLE C. MILLER, DVM, PhD, Diplomate ACT
Program Director, Veterinary Technology
Athens Technical College
Athens, Georgia

PETER R. MORRESEY, BVSc, MACVSc, Diplomate ACT, Diplomate ACVIM
University of Pennsylvania
New Bolton Center
Kennett Square, Pennsylvania

MICHAEL J. MURRAY, DVM, MS, Diplomate ACVIM
Professor and Adelaide C. Riggs Chair in Equine Medicine
Marion duPont Scott Equine Medical Center
Virgina-Maryland Regional College of Veterinary Medicine
Virginia Tech
Leesburg, Virginia

OLIMPO OLIVER E., DVM, MSc, DVSc
Associate Professor
Head of Large Animal Clinic
Department of Animal Health
Facultad de Medicina Veterinaria y de Zootecnia
Universidad Nacional de Colombia
Bogota, Colombia

JOHN E. PALMER, DVM, Diplomate ACVIM
Associate Professor of Medicine
Director of Neonatology Programs
Graham French Neonatal Section
Connelly Intensive Care Unit
New Bolton Center
University of Pennsylvania
Kennett Square, Pennsylvania

MARY ROSE PARADIS, DVM, MS
Department of Clinical Sciences
Tufts University School of Veterinary Medicine
North Grafton, Massachusetts

ERIC J. PARENTE, DVM, Diplomate ACVS
Assistant Professor of Surgery
New Bolton Center
University of Pennsylvania
Kennett Square, Pennsylvania

JILL PARKER, VMD, Diplomate ACVS
Assistant Professor of Large Animal Surgery
College of Veterinary Medicine
Oregon State University
Corvallis, Oregon

JOHN R. PASCOE, BVSc Diplomate ACVS
Professor
Department of Surgical and Radiological Sciences
University of California, Davis
School of Veterinary Medicine
Davis, California

DEBORAH A. PARSONS, DVM, DACVIM
Waterloo, Ontario
Canada

SIMON PEARCE, BVSc, PhD, Diplomate ACVS
Large Animal Surgeon
Department of Clinical Studies
Ontario Veterinary College
University of Guelph
Canada

MICHAEL E. PETERSON, DVM
Reid Veterinary Hospital
Albany, Oregon

RICHARD J. PIERCY, DVM
Imperial College School of Medicine
Hammersmith Hospital
London, United Kingdom

KONSTANZE PLUMLEE, DVM, MS
ASPCA NAPCC
1717 S. Philo Road
Suite 36
Urbana, IL 61802

ROBERT H. POPPENGA, DVM, PhD, Diplomate American Board of Veterinary Toxicology
University of Pennsylvania
School of Veterinary Medicine
New Bolton Center
Kennett Square, Pennsylvania

MERL F. RAISBECK, DVM, PhD, MS, Diplomate ABVT
Professor of Veterinary Toxicology
University of Wyoming
Department of Veterinary Sciences
Laramie, Wyoming

GABRIEL RAMIREZ, DVM
Department of Clinical Sciences
Tufts University School of Veterinary Medicine
North Grafton, Massachusetts

VIRGINIA B. REEF, DVM, Diplomate ACVIM
Professor of Medicine in the Widener Hospital
Director of Large Animal Cardiology and Ultrasonography
Chief, Section of Sports Medicine and Imaging
University of Pennsylvania
New Bolton Center
Kennett Square, Pennsylvania

LAURA K. REILLY, VMD, DACVIM
University of Pennsylvania
New Bolton Center
Kennett Square, Pennsylvania

N. EDWARD ROBINSON, B.Vet. Med, MRCVS, PhD
Doctor Honoris Causa (Liege)
Matilda R. Wilson Professor
Department of Large Animal Clinical Sciences
College of Veterinary Medicine
Michigan State University
East Lansing, Michigan

MARIE-FRANCE ROY, DMV,
Diplomate ACVIM
Equine Internal Medicine
Faculté de Médecine Vétérinaire,
Université de Montréal
St-Hyacinthe, Quebec
Canada

KAREN RUSSELL, DVM, PhD
Department of Veterinary Pathobiology
Texas A&M University
College Station, Texas

JIM SCHUMACHER, DVM, MS,
Diplomate ACVS, MRCVS
Auburn University, Alabama

HAROLD C. SCHOTT, II, DVM, PhD,
Diplomate ACVIM
Large Animal Clinical Sciences
College of Veterinary Medicine
Michigan State University
East Lansing, Michigan

DEBRA C. SELLON, DVM, PhD
Diplomate, ACVIM
Associate Professor, Equine Medicine
College of Veterinary Medicine
Washington State University
Pullman, WA

BARBARA SHERMAN SIMPSON, PhD, DVM, DACVB
Adjunct Professor, North Carolina State University
College of Veterinary Medicine
The Veterinary Behavior Clinic
Southern Pines, North Carolina

JANICE SOJKA, DVM, Diplomate ACVIM
Associate Professor of Large Animal Medicine
Purdue University
West Lafayette, Indiana

WENDY S. SPRAGUE, DVM
Department of Pathology and Biomedical Sciences
College of Veterinary Medicine
Colorado State University
Fort Collins, Colorado

ERIC STAIR, DVM
Department of Anatomy, Pathology, Pharmacology
College of Veterinary Medicine
Oklahoma State University
Stillwater, Oklahoma

HENRY STÄMPFLI, DVM, Dr.Med.Vet.,
Diplomate ACVIM
Associate Professor
Large Animal Medicine, Clinical Studies
Ontario Veterinary College
University of Guelph
Guelph, Ontario
Canada

D. TODD STRUBBE, DVM, Diplomate ACVO
Veterinary Opthalmologist
Animal Eye Specialty Clinic
Stuart, Florida

NUALA SUMMERFIELD, BSc, BVMS, MRCVS
University of Pennsylvania
School of Veterinary Medicine
Veterinary Hospital
Philadelphia, Pennsylvania

G. ABELLS SUTTON, DVM, MS
Koret School of Veterinary Medicine
Hebrew University of Jerusalem
Rehovot, Israel

CORINNE SWEENEY, DVM,
Diplomate ACVIM
University of Pennsylvania
School of Veterinary Medicine
New Bolton Center
Kennett Square, Pennsylvania

RAYMOND W. SWEENEY, VMD,
Diplomate ACVIM
Associate Professor of Medicine
University of Pennsylvania
School of Veterinary Medicine
New Bolton Center
Kennett Square, Pennsylvania

CYPRIANNA E. SWIDERSKI, DVM, PhD
Arkansas Diagnostic Lab of the Livestock and Poultry Commission
One Natural Resources Drive
Little Rock, Arkansas

ANNETTE SYSEL

PATRICIA TALCOTT, MS, DVM, PhD
Certified Diplomate ABVT
Associate Professor
Department of Food Science and Toxicology
University of Idaho
Moscow, Idaho
Washington Animal Disease Diagnostic Laboratory
College of Veterinary Medicine
Pullman, Washington

JENNIFER THOMAS, DVM, PhD
Department of Veterinary Pathobiology
College of Veterinary Medicine
Texas A&M University
College Station, Texas

LARRY J. THOMPSON, DVM, PhD,
Diplomate ABVT
Clinical Toxicologist
University of Georgia College of Veterinary Medicine
Veterinary Diagnostic and Investigational Lab
Tifton, Georgia

WALTER R. THRELFALL, DVM, MS, PhD, ACT
Professor and Head
Theriogenology Area
The Ohio State University,
College of Veterinary Medicine
Columbus, Ohio

PETER J. TIMONEY, MVB, PhD, MSc FRCVS
University of Kentucky
Veterinary Science
Lexington, Kentucky

SUSAN J. TORNQUIST, DVM, PhD,
Diplomate American College of Veterinary Pathologists (Clinical Pathology)
Assistant Professor
Department of Biomedical Sciences
College of Veterinary Medicine
Oregon State University
Corvallis, Oregon

SUSAN C. TROCK, DVM, Diplomate ACVPM
Subspecialty, Epidemiology
Epidemiologist
Cornell University and NYS Agriculture & Markets
Albany, New York

ERIC TULLENERS†

WENDY E. VAALA, VMD
Mid-Atlantic Equine Medical Center
PO Box 188, 40 Frontage Road
Ringoes, NJ 08551

LAURENT VIEL, DVM, PhD
Department of Clinical Sciences
University of Guelph
Guelph, Ontario

VICTORIA L. VOITH, DVM, PhD, DACVB
Applied Animal Behavior Consultants
Dayton, Ohio

K. JANE WARDROP, DVM, MS,
Diplomate ACVP
Associate Professor
Clinical Pathology
Department of Veterinary Clinical Sciences
College of Veterinary Medicine
Washington State University
Pullman, Washington

JOHANNA L. WATSON, DVM, PhD,
Diplomate ACVIM
Department of Medicine and Epidemiology
University of California, Davis
School of Veterinary Medicine
Davis, California

J. SCOTT WEESE, DVM, DVSc,
Diplomate ACVIM
Department of Clinical Studies
Ontarioa Veterinary College
University of Guelph
Guelph, Ontario
Canada

ELIZABETH G. WELLES, DVM, PhD
Department of Pathobiology
College of Veterinary Medicine
Auburn University, Alabama

HEIDI WHIGHAM, DVM
University of Florida
College of Veterinary Medicine
Gainesville, Florida

SUSAN L. WHITE, DVM, MS,
Diplomate ACVIM
Professor
Department of Large Animal Medicine
University of Georgia
Athens, Georgia

ROBERT H. WHITLOCK, DVM, PhD
Associate Professor of Medicine
University of Pennsylvania
School of Veterinary Medicine
New Bolton Center
Kennett Square, Pennsylvania

MARLYN S. WHITNEY, DVM, PhD
Texas Veterinary Medical Diagnostic
Laboratory
Amarillo, Texas

PAMELA A. WILKINS, DVM, MS, PhD,
Diplomate ACVIM
School of Veterinary Medicine
New Bolton Center
University of Pennsylvania
Kennett Square, Pennsylvania

JULIA WILSON, DVM, Diplomate ACVIM
Associate Professor
School of Veterinary Medicine
University of Minnesota
St. Paul, Minnesota

W. DAVID WILSON, BVMS, MS
Professor
Department of Medicine and
Epidemiology
Associate Director, Large Animal Clinic
Veterinary Medical Teaching Hospital
University of California, Davis
Davis, California

SHARON WITONSKY, DVM, PhD
Phase II, Duck Pond Drive
Dept. LACS, VMRCVM
Virginia Tech
Blacksburg, Virginia

ANTHONY YU, DVM, MS, Diplomate ACVD
Animal Allergy & Skin Clinic
Beaverton, Oregon

†deceased

CONTENTS

CONTENTS

BEHAVIOR

CARDIAC

DERMATOLOGY

ENDOCRINE/METABOLIC

GASTROENTEROLOGY

HEMATOPOIETIC

INFECTIOUS DISEASES

LABORATORY TESTS

MISCELLANEOUS

NEONATES

NEUROLOGY

Ophthalmology

Respiratory

THERIOGENOLOGY

TOXICOLOGY

URINARY

ABDOMINAL DISTENTION IN THE ADULT

BASICS

DEFINITION

Enlargement of the abdominal contour, which produces a perceptible change in abdominal shape.

PATHOPHYSIOLOGY

Changes in the contour of the abdomen may occur as a result of increased intra-abdominal pressure by gas, fluid, or solid masses, or due to abnormalities associated with the abdominal wall itself.

SYSTEMS AFFECTED

- Gastrointestinal—Strangulating lesions cause ischemia and necrosis of the affected bowel and can potentiate ileus. Hypovolemia may contribute to impaction of the large or small colon.
- Cardiovascular—Collapse from hypovolemic or endotoxemic shock may occur secondary to fluid accumulation, intra-abdominal blood loss (hemoperitoneum), intra-organ hemorrhage (rupture of the spleen or liver), ascites secondary to heart failure. Cardiac arrhythmias can develop as a result of hyperkalemia, as seen in foals with ruptured bladder.
- Behavioral—Conditions causing bowel obstruction or ileus will produce signs of abdominal pain. Mares with rupture of the prepubic tendon may be reluctant to walk, or may display a sawhorse stance. Conditions such as hydrops, peritonitis and advanced neoplasia may cause the horse to assume recumbency.
- Respiratory—Gastrointestinal lesions or the presence of hydrops may increase pressure on the diaphragm and make respiration difficult. Hypoventilation may occur as a voluntary response to abdominal pain, or may develop to compensate for metabolic alkalosis. Aspiration pneumonia is possible with gastric reflux.
- Musculoskeletal/Nervous/Ophthalmologic/Skin—These systems may be injured through self-inflicted trauma secondary to abdominal pain.
- Reproductive—Hypovolemia contributes to uterine hypoperfusion and fetal hypoxemia. Rupture of the prepubic tendon and hydrops may necessitate induction of parturition.

SIGNALMENT

- Horses of any age, sex, or breed may develop abdominal distention.
- Uroperitoneum may be observed occasionally in mares shortly after parturition.
- Hydrops usually develops in mares in at least the seventh month of gestation. Rupture of the prepubic tendon occurs in older, sedentary mares in late pregnancy. Colonic displacements or strangulating lesions are seen in older postpartum mares.
- Miniature horses are predisposed to development of fecaliths and enteroliths.

SIGNS

Historical Findings

Chronicity of clinical signs may help to distinguish between acute conditions, such as bloat from carbohydrate overload, and chronic ones, such as ascites due to heart or liver failure.

Physical Findings

Findings on rectal examination may be very valuable in determining the possible cause of abdominal distention.

CAUSES

Accumulation of Gas

- Ileus—carbohydrate overload, electrolyte disturbances, peritonitis, surgery, diarrhea, drugs
- Large colon obstruction—displacement, impaction, intussusception, tympany, torsion/volvulus, foreign body, enterolith
- Cecal obstruction
- Small intestinal obstruction
- Aerophagia (cribbers)
- Free gas within the abdominal cavity may occur secondary to trauma or anaerobic infections

Accumulation of Fluid

- Hemoperitoneum—ruptured spleen or liver, tumor
- Uroperitoneum—ruptured bladder secondary to obstructive urolithiasis or stressful parturition
- Hydrops amnion or allantois
- Ascites—peritonitis, neoplasia, hypoproteinemia, right-sided heart failure

Solid Mass

- Abscess
- Neoplasia—lymphosarcoma, squamous cell carcinoma, mammary adenocarcinoma, mesothelioma, hemangiosarcoma

Body Wall Abnormality

- Hernia*
- Prepubic tendon rupture

RISK FACTORS

- Horses with vices such as cribbing are predisposed to tympany of the colon.
- Sudden exposure to large amounts of carbohydrate-rich feed or diets consisting of increased proportions of concentrate (especially whole-grain corn) and decreased amounts of roughage can predispose to gastric tympany and large colon displacement or volvulus.
- Colonic impactions often occur in horses that are old or debilitated or that have poor dentition.
- Enterolithiasis occurs frequently in the states of California, Florida, and Indiana.
- Sand impactions are seen frequently in the southern states, including Florida and Arizona, and the coastal states, including California and New Jersey.

DIAGNOSIS

DIFFERENTIAL DIAGNOSIS

Differentiating Similar Signs

Other conditions that can give the appearance of abdominal distention include:

- Marked subcutaneous edema along the ventral abdomen and thorax—If edema is warm and painful, a localized wound or abscess may be identified; if cool, pitting edema is present, swelling may be secondary to hypoproteinemia, disturbed regional lymphatic drainage (e.g., pleuropneumonia), or cardiac failure.
- Pregnancy—Diagnosis may be made via rectal palpation with or without ultrasonography.
- "Hay belly"—May be diagnosed on history (malnourished or severely parasitized horses, diets high in poor-quality roughage) and by fecal examination.
- Pendulous abdomen secondary to pituitary adenoma—Usually accompanied by other distinctive signs, such as hirsutism.
- Extreme obesity—Ribs not palpable, fat deposits evident along crest of neck, over tailhead, etc.

Differentiating Causes

Signalment, history, physical examination, and rectal palpation findings often provide sufficient information to permit a tentative diagnosis. Some conditions are associated with characteristic findings:

- Gastrointestinal gas accumulation (bloat)—On auscultation of the abdomen, few to no gastrointestinal sounds may be heard, and increased gaseous distention may be identified on percussion as a hyperresonant "ping"; depending on the inciting cause and the degree of distention present, various degrees of abdominal pain are usually present.
- Ascites from right-sided heart failure—Tricuspid insufficiency results in findings including heart murmur, exercise intolerance, jugular distention and pulse, and edema of the ventral abdomen, pectoral muscles, and distal limbs.
- Ascites from intra-abdominal mesothelioma—Because this tumor originates from the fluid-producing cells of the peritoneum, several liters of peritoneal fluid may be produced within a 24-hr period; ascites may be more dramatic than is noted with other conditions.
- Body wall defect from prepubic tendon rupture—One of the only causes of unilateral abdominal distention in the horse; also results in cranioventral positioning of the mammary gland, cranial tilting of the pelvis, and severe ventral abdominal swelling.

ABDOMINAL DISTENTION IN THE ADULT

CBC/BIOCHEMISTRY/URINALYSIS

Results are dependent on the cause.

OTHER LABORATORY TESTS

Abdominocentesis should be performed carefully in pregnant mares with intestinal distention, where the bowel may be torn easily by inadvertent penetration with a needle or teat cannula despite proper restraint. WBC count, TP level, and SG of the peritoneal fluid should be measured, and the fluid should be assessed cytologically for evidence of degenerate neutrophils, neoplastic cells, bacteria, or plant material. Other parameters such as creatinine (Cr) may also be measured. An increase in WBC count and TP levels and the appearance of degenerate neutrophils are indicative of increasing inflammation within the abdomen. With hemoperitoneum, free-flowing blood may be evident from the needle or teat cannula during the centesis procedure. In cases of uroperitoneum, Cr in the peritoneal fluid exceeds serum Cr levels by a ratio of >2 to 1.

IMAGING

Abdominal radiography may be of benefit in the diagnosis of gas accumulation within bowel segments in small horses and ponies. Enteroliths or sand impactions may be evident in adult horses in the mid- to ventral abdomen on the lateral view. Standing radiographs of these regions in a 500-kg horse require approximately 450 mA and 100 kvp.

Ultrasonography of the abdomen can be used to identify the location, amount, character, and echogenicity of peritoneal fluid. It can also provide information on the condition of the heart, small intestine, large colon, liver, spleen, kidney, and bladder, and can help identify the presence of intra-abdominal adhesions or masses.

DIAGNOSTIC PROCEDURES

Laparoscopy permits direct visualization of the abdominal cavity in the standing horse, and can be used to provide a definitive diagnosis of the cause of abdominal distention. It can also be used to direct appropriate therapy and treatment.

Exploratory laparotomy may be performed through a flank incision in the standing horse, or through a ventral midline incision in the anesthetized horse. Although a flank incision provides limited access to the abdomen, visualization may be sufficient to permit a diagnosis.

TREATMENT

Specific treatment is largely dependent on the cause of abdominal distention. Stabilization through rehydration and correction of electrolyte and acid/base abnormalities should be initiated prior to treatment of the primary disease process.

In horses with severe gaseous distention, trocarization of the cecum and/or large colon may be necessary to improve ventilation. Any horse that is trocarized should be treated preemptively with anti-inflammatory drugs and broad-spectrum antibiotic therapy to reduce the inherent risk of peritonitis. The site for trocarization is situated within the paralumbar fossa and can be delineated through auscultation and percussion of the distended viscus. Because the distended viscus shrinks down and away from the trocarization needle as it becomes decompressed, the trocarization site should ideally be situated in the mid-proximal region of the most tympanitic area. Following clipping and aseptic preparation of the site, a small bleb of local anesthetic should be injected into the skin and muscle layers. A 6-in. (15-cm) 16-gauge spinal needle or a 5.25-in. (13.3-cm) 14-gauge stiff intravenous catheter may be used for trocarization. The needle/catheter should be inserted through the skin, muscle layers, and distended viscus with a gentle thrust. The stylette should be left in place at all times to avoid inadvertent bending, breakage, and intra-abdominal loss secondary to movement of the bowel or of the horse. The audible escape of gas, combined with fogging of the end of needle/catheter, confirms correct placement within the lumen of the distended viscus. In order to prevent laceration of the bowel wall, the needle/catheter should be held carefully during the decompression phase and the hand should follow gently in the direction that gastrointestinal motility dictates. As the bowel becomes decompressed, the needle/catheter may require further advancement into the lumen of the viscus. In order to prevent leakage of intestinal contents from the tip of the needle/catheter into the peritoneal cavity, the needle should not be withdrawn until the decompression process is complete. The needle and stylette are then withdrawn together in one swift motion. The trocarization site should be wiped clean with alcohol.

Mares with hydrops or rupture of the prepubic tendon may require induction of parturition.

Horses with abdominal distention should be confined to a stall until a diagnosis has been made and appropriate treatment initiated. Feed should be withheld from horses showing any signs of abdominal discomfort. Referral to a hospital facility may be required in cases requiring surgical intervention or prolonged nursing care.

MEDICATIONS

Drug therapy is dictated by the inciting cause.

FOLLOW-UP

Plans for monitoring are based on cause and treatment.

MISCELLANEOUS

ASSOCIATED CONDITIONS

N/A

AGE-RELATED FACTORS

N/A

PREGNANCY

- Termination of pregnancy may be indicated in mares with hydrops. If these mares are bred in the future, a different stallion should be selected.
- Induction of parturition may be necessary in mares close to term that have experienced rupture of the prepubic tendon. These mares should be monitored carefully, as they may require assistance with delivery due to their inability to perform effective abdominal press for fetal expulsion.

SYNONYMS

Bloat

SEE ALSO

See inciting causes

ABBREVIATIONS

- Cr = creatinine
- SG = specific gravity
- TP = total protein
- WBC = white blood cell

Suggested Reading

Foreman JH. Abdominal distention. In: Reed SM, Bayly WM (eds). Equine internal medicine. Philadelphia: WB Saunders Co., 1998.

Author Annette M. Sysel

Consulting Editor Henry Stämpfli

ABDOMINAL HERNIA IN ADULT HORSES

BASICS

OVERVIEW

An abdominal hernia is the exteriorization of internal organs through a defect or an anatomic opening in the abdominal wall. In adult horses, abdominal hernias include ventral hernias, incisional hernias, acquired inguinal/scrotal hernias, and (rarely) diphragmatic hernias. Diaphragmatic hernias are not considered further in this chapter.

SIGNALMENT

Ventral Hernia

Most frequently seen in older, late-term pregnant mares.

Incisional Hernia

An incisional hernia is a complication of ventral celiotomy that occurs in up to 15% of the horses that undergo this procedure. Dehiscence (acute incisional disruption) usually develops within 8 days after surgery. Incisional herniation can develop up to 3 months after ventral celiotomy.

Acquired Inguinal Hernia

An acquired inguinal hernia occurs almost exclusively in the intact male horse. Standardbreds, Tennessee Walking Horses, American Saddlebreds, and the draft breeds are reported to be predisposed.

SIGNS

Ventral Hernia

A large swelling over the flank or caudal ventral abdomen develops that is associated with progressive abdominal wall edema. Mares with ventral hernia walk slowly and often lie down. Commonly, they are distressed and have increased heart and respiratory rates. Signs of abdominal pain may be present if the herniated contents are compromised.

Incisional Hernia

In acute incisional dehiscence, brown serosanguinous fluid discharges from the incision and progressively increases prior to dehiscence. Ventral swelling develops over the abdominal incision site. Gaps in the abdominal wall between sutures may also be palpated.

Acquired Inguinal/Scrotal Hernia

Scrotal swelling may be mild in acute acquired inguinal hernias, but is usually marked in horses with scrotal hernia. The testicle on the herniated side is usually cooler and firmer to the touch compared with the opposite normal testicle. Abdominal pain may vary from mild to severe, depending on the degree of intestinal strangulation.

CAUSES AND RISK FACTORS

Ventral Hernia

Ventral hernia occurs in pregnant mares and is associated with degenerative change in the body wall in old broodmares and twin gestations as well as in hydroallantois and trauma.

Incisional Hernia

Incisional infection and swelling, postoperative endotoxemia and pain, repeated celiotomy and use of chromic gut suture to close the abdominal wall predispose to incisional hernia.

Acquired Inguinal/Scrotal Hernia

Inguinal/scrotal hernia often follows breeding activity or strenuous athletic exercise. Large vaginal rings may predispose to herniation.

DIAGNOSIS

DIFFERENTIAL DIAGNOSIS

Ventral Hernia

Ventral hernia should be differentiated from prepubic tendon rupture because the latter is generally not surgically correctable. However, in prepubic tendon rupture there is cranioventral orientation of the pelvis because tension is lost from the cranial aspect of the pelvis. Lordosis may be present because the pelvis and vertebral column cannot maintain normal alignment. Cranioventral displacement of the udder as a result of the tipping of the pelvis can lead to rupture of blood supply, and blood can be observed in the milk.

ABDOMINAL HERNIA IN ADULT HORSES

Incisional Hernia
Postoperative wound infection, severe peri-incisional edema, seroma, and sinus formation are easily differentiated from incisional hernias with the abdomen being intact on palpation.

Acquired Inguinal/Scrotal Hernia
Torsion of the spermatic cord, infectious epididymitis or orchitis, thrombosis of the testicular artery, hydrocele, hematocele, and testicular neoplasia should be included in the differential diagnosis.

CBC/BIOCHEMISTRY/URINALYSIS
N/A

OTHER LABORATORY TESTS
N/A

IMAGING
Abdominal Ultrasonography
Transcutaneous ultrasonographic examination with a 3.5 or 5 MHz transducer is helpful to rule in herniation and evaluate the extent of the abdominal wall defect. Ultrasonographic examination of the scrotum and the inguinal region may reveal the presence of the herniated intestine.

DIAGNOSTIC PROCEDURES
External Palpation
In ventral and incisional hernia, external palpation of the abdominal wall may define the hernia ring and hernia contents. When there is extensive abdominal edema, this procedure is difficult. External palpation of both the inguinal region and the scrotum is mandatory in every stallion with signs of colic. Scrotal swelling and the presence of a painful, cooler, and firmer testicle is highly suggestive of acquired inguinal/scrotal hernia.

Rectal Palpation
In ventral hernia, rectal palpation may help to differentiate the condition from prepubic tendon rupture. However, palpation of the abdominal wall defect per rectum can be difficult depending on the defect's location and the size of the fetus. Rectal palpation of stallions with acquired inguinal/scrotal hernia reveals the presence of a loop of intestine entering the vaginal ring on the affected side.

TREATMENT
Ventral Hernia
Surgical herniorrhaphy is advocated. If the mare is close to term (at least 330 days pregnant), parturition should be induced prior to surgery. Delivery should be assisted because the abdominal push is often insufficient.
When acute herniation occurs without clinical evidence of intestinal obstruction, the surgical treatment should be delayed to allow formation of fibrosis within the hernia ring. In this case, management consists in the application of an abdominal support bandage, the use of anti-inflammatory drugs to decrease swelling, and feeding with low-residue pelleted ration to decrease intestinal bulk volume.
Suture or mesh herniorrhaphy is performed depending on the diameter of the hernia ring.

Incisional Hernia
In general, surgical herniorrhaphy is postponed for 4–6 months to allow resolution of the wound infection and the development of hernia ring fibrosis. Initially, an abdominal support bandage is applied and antimicrobials are administered based on culture and sensitivity. Suture or mesh herniorrhaphy is performed when incisional infection has resolved.

Acquired Inguinal/Scrotal Hernia
Once an acute intestinal obstruction occurs, the intestine herniated through the vaginal ring becomes strangulated within hours. Rapid surgical correction of the hernia is thus mandatory.

MEDICATION
Ventral Hernia
Pending surgical correction, the use of non-steroidal anti-inflammatory drugs is advocated to decrease abdominal edema.

Incisional Hernia
Administration of both non-steroidal anti-inflammatory drugs and parenteral broad-spectrum antibiotics is required.

FOLLOW-UP
The prognosis for successful correction of ventral hernia is guarded. Incisional and inguinal/scrotal herniations warrant a favorable prognosis. After surgical correction of both ventral and incisional hernia, 3–5 months of rest are required.

Suggested Reading

Auer JA. Equine surgery. WB Saunders Co., 1992:415-422.

Kawcak CE, Stashak TS. Predisposing factors, diagnosis, and management of large abdominal wall defects in horses and cattle. J Am Vet Med Assoc. 1995:206;607-611.

Author Ludovic Bouré
Consulting Editor Henry Stämpfli

ABDOMINOCENTESIS

BASICS

DEFINITION

- A procedure for sampling peritoneal fluid by collection through the abdominal wall
- Fluid is collected into EDTA and into a sterile clot tube for bacterial culture or biochemical tests.
- Equine abdominal fluid normally is present in a relatively small volume and appears clear and colorless to slightly yellow.
- Total protein commonly is assessed by refractometer and normally is <2.5 g/dL.
- Fibrinogen, as measured using heat precipitation, normally is undetectable at <100 mg/dL, and normal peritoneal fluid does not clot.
- Nucleated cell count in fluid from normal horses is <10,000 cells/μL, with a predominance of nondegenerate neutrophils (22%–98%) and large mononuclear cells (1%–68%), which include mesothelial cells, nonreactive macrophages, and reactive macrophages. Small lymphocytes may comprise 0%–36% of the total and eosinophils up to 7%; mast cells and basophils rarely are seen. Normally, few erythrocytes are present in abdominal fluid.
- Biochemical measurements other than total protein generally are not performed on peritoneal fluid, except in certain circumstances—suspected uroabdomen

PATHOPHYSIOLOGY

- Normal peritoneal fluid is a dialysate of plasma; therefore, many of the low-molecular-weight substances in blood are present in the peritoneal fluid at similar concentrations.
- High-molecular-weight molecules (e.g., proteins) normally are not present in abdominal fluid.
- Cells in normal peritoneal fluid—mesothelial cells; small numbers of cells from the blood and lymphatics
- Fluid circulates constantly through the abdominal cavity and normally is drained via lymphatic vessels. When fluid production exceeds drainage, an effusion develops. This may occur with some systemic disorders (e.g., cardiovascular disease) or with local disorders of abdominal organs or mesothelium. Changes in peritoneal fluid constituents (e.g., protein, cell numbers and types) may reflect those disorders.

SYSTEMS AFFECTED

- GI
- Hepatobiliary
- Hemic/lymphatic/immune
- Renal/urologic
- Cardiovascular
- Reproductive

SIGNALMENT

Any breed or sex

SIGNS

- Colic
- Chronic weight loss
- Abdominal distention
- Diarrhea

CAUSES

- Peritonitis caused by compromised gut wall—ischemia, infarction, volvulus, impaction, or rupture
- Hemorrhage—from trauma or granulosa/thecal cell tumor
- Neoplasia—lymphoma, gastric squamous cell carcinoma, mesothelioma, hemangiosarcoma, metastatic adenocarcinoma, and melanoma
- Intestinal parasitism and thromboembolism secondary to parasitism
- Inflammation of abdominal organs—liver; pancreas
- Breeding and foaling injuries—vaginal perforation during breeding; uterine torsion or rupture
- Bile or urine leakage
- Postsurgical inflammation, including postcastration
- Abdominal abscess—localized or ruptured
- Decreased oncotic pressure—protein-losing enteropathy; chronic hepatopathy
- Congestive heart failure

RISK FACTORS

N/A

DIAGNOSIS

DIFFERENTIAL DIAGNOSIS

Peritonitis

- Fluid typically is an exudate, with increased nucleated cell count and a predominance of neutrophils, which may appear degenerate.
- Total protein usually is >2.5 g/dL because of inflammation.
- Bacteria are present in septic peritonitis and may be intracellular or extracellular.
- With gut rupture, cells often are very degenerate, and mixed bacterial types as well as ciliated protozoa and plant material are seen.
- Postsurgical peritonitis also produces an exudate with increased cell numbers and total protein within 24 hours. Neutrophils generally are not degenerate, however, and no bacteria are seen. This fluid also may contain increased RBCs.

Hemorrhage

- With a splenic tap, PCV is higher in abdominal fluid than in the circulation, and small lymphocyte numbers may be increased.
- With hemorrhage into the abdomen, PCV of fluid is lower than that of blood. Platelets are absent, and erythrophagocytosis may be present.
- With blood contamination at the time of sampling, fluid initially may look clear, with bloody streaks appearing during sampling. Phagocytosis of RBCs is not seen, and platelets may be present.

Neoplasia

- Diagnosis may be established on finding neoplastic cells in fluid.
- Absence of neoplastic cells does not rule out neoplasia, because cells from a tumor may not exfoliate into fluid or associated inflammation may mask the presence of neoplastic cells.

Parasitism

Migration of parasitic larvae may be associated with increased eosinophils, but this does not occur often and is not diagnostic for parasitism.

Uroabdomen

- Typically, increased creatinine in peritoneal fluid as compared to serum creatinine
- Urea nitrogen is high in urine. Levels equilibrate rapidly between the serum and peritoneum, however, because this molecule readily diffuses across the peritoneum.
- Hyperkalemia, marked hyponatremia, and hypochloremia are typical but are not present in all cases.

Ascites

- A transudate with low cell numbers, low protein content, and normal cytologic findings may be present with hypoalbuminemia or lymphatic or vascular obstruction or stasis.
- Serum biochemical profile and history contribute to establishing this diagnosis.

ABDOMINOCENTESIS

Congestive Heart Failure

• Increased hydrostatic pressure within vessels may result in a modified transudate with a higher cell count and protein level than a transudate, but these values may remain within normal limits for equine abdominal fluid.
• Diagnosis is established by increased fluid volume and absence of other significant findings.

LABORATORY FINDINGS

Drugs That May Alter Lab Results

N/A

Disorders That May Alter Lab Results

N/A

Valid If Run in Human Lab?

Cell count and protein determination may be done in any lab, but interpretation of equine cytology requires special training.

CBC/BIOCHEMISTRY/URINALYSIS

• Inflammatory causes of abdominal effusion may be reflected by leukocytosis or hyperfibrinogenemia if they cause systemic disease.
• Left shift or toxic changes in neutrophils indicate systemic inflammation.
• Serum biochemistries help to assess causes of transudates—panhypoproteinemia is consistent with GI protein loss; elevated liver enzymes suggest hepatic disease.
• Serum electrolytes and comparison of serum and fluid creatinine are important in establishing the diagnosis of uroperitoneum.

OTHER LABORATORY TESTS

Bacterial culture is helpful in some cases—abdominal abscess

IMAGING

Ultrasonography

• May be used to look for intestinal entrapment, intussusception, masses, adhesions, enlarged liver, and enteroliths.
• Ultrasonographic location of peritoneal fluid sometimes helps in performing abdominocentesis.

Abdominal Radiography

In adult horses, may aid in establishing the diagnosis of diaphragmatic hernia, sand, and enteroliths.

DIAGNOSTIC PROCEDURES

• Laparoscopy may be used to establish the diagnosis in cases of chronic colic or weight loss.
• Gastroscopy can be useful in establishing the diagnosis of gastric ulcers, impaction, and neoplasia.
• Exploratory laparotomy is necessary for definitive diagnosis in some cases.

TREATMENT

Directed at the underlying cause of the abnormal abdominal fluid.

MEDICATIONS

DRUGS OF CHOICE

N/A

CONTRAINDICATIONS

N/A

PRECAUTIONS

N/A

POSSIBLE INTERACTIONS

N/A

ALTERNATIVE DRUGS

N/A

FOLLOW-UP

PATIENT MONITORING

N/A

POSSIBLE COMPLICATIONS

Accidental enterocentesis (rarely associated with clinical disease) causes increased nucleated cell count in abdominal fluid within 4 hours.

MISCELLANEOUS

ASSOCIATED CONDITIONS

N/A

AGE-RELATED FACTORS

Foals normally have protein levels similar to but peritoneal fluid cell counts (<1500 cells/μL) lower than adults.

ZOONOTIC POTENTIAL

N/A

PREGNANCY

No significant differences in fluid from mares that are pregnant or have recently foaled compared with fluid from nonperipartum mares.

SYNONYMS

Abdominal paracentesis

SEE ALSO

N/A

ABBREVIATIONS

• GI = gastrointestinal
• PCV = packed cell volume

Suggested Reading

Garma-Avina A. Cytology of 100 samples of abdominal fluid from 100 horses with abdominal disease. Equine Vet J 1998;30:435–444.

Hoogmoed LV, Snyder JR, Christopher M, Vastistas N. Peritoneal fluid analysis in peripartum mares. J Am Vet Med Assoc 1996;209:1280–1282.

Parry BW, Brownlow MA. Peritoneal fluid. In: Cowell RL, Tyler RD, eds. Cytology and hematology of the horse. Goleta, CA: American Veterinary Publications, 1992:121–151.

Author Susan J. Tornquist
Consulting Editor Claire B. Andreasen

ABNORMAL ESTRUS INTERVALS

BASICS

DEFINITION

Estrus is the period of sexual receptivity by the mare for the stallion. Estrus is abnormal when overt sexual behavior is displayed for longer or shorter periods than considered normal for the species or the individual. Abnormal interestrus intervals can result from short or long estrus or diestrus intervals.

PATHOPHYSIOLOGY

The mare is seasonally polyestrus, with estrous cycles in spring and summer months. Length of the average estrous cycle is 21 days (range: 19–22 days) and is defined as the period of time between ovulations that coincides with progesterone levels of <1 ng/mL. Estrus and estrous cycle lengths are quite repeatable by individual mare from cycle to cycle.

Key Hormonal Events/Sequence of the Equine Estrous Cycle

- FSH (pituitary-origin) causes ovarian follicular growth.
- Estradiol (follicular origin) stimulates LH (pituitary-origin) secretion as a result of the increasing GnRH pulse frequency.
- LH surge causes ovulation, after which estradiol returns to basal levels.
- Progesterone (CL origin) rises from basal levels (<1 ng/mL) at ovulation to >4 ng/mL by 4–7 days post-ovulation.
- Natural prostaglandin ($PGF_2\alpha$), of endometrial origin, is released 14–15 days post-ovulation, causing luteolysis and a concurrent decline in progesterone levels.

Length of Estrus

In normal, cycling mares averages from 5 to 7 days, but can range from 2 to 12 days.

Length of Diestrus

Less variation, averaging 15 ± 2 days.

Sexual Behavior

A reflection of serum progesterone and estrogen levels.

- The absence of progesterone allows the onset of estrus behavior even if estrogens are present in very small quantities.
- Conditions that eliminate progesterone and/or increase estrogen concentrations are likely to induce estrus behavior. Persistence of these conditions results in abnormal estrus periods or interestrus intervals. The converse is also true.

SYSTEMS AFFECTED

- Reproductive
- Behavioral
- Endocrine

SIGNALMENT

- Mares of any breed may be affected.
- Geriatric mares (>20 years) tend to have prolonged transition periods, longer estrus duration, and fewer estrous cycles per year.
- Ponies may regularly have longer estrous cycles than horses (average = 25 days).

SIGNS

General Comments

- Complete teasing records (methods used, frequency, type of stallion [pony, horse, or gelding], stallion behavior [aggressive/passive, vocal, proximity], and handler experience) are essential to investigate suspected estrus abnormalities.
- Understand seasonal influences on reproduction. Individual variation in the onset/duration/termination of cyclicity can be mistaken for estrus irregularity.
- Individual reproductive history: estrous cycle length, response to teasing, foaling data, and injuries or infections of the genital tract may relate to current clinical abnormalities.
- Current and past history of drugs administered to a mare and their relationship to abnormal estrous cycles.

Historical Findings

Mare managers may report infertility, failure to show estrus, prolonged estrus, split estrus, or frequent estrus behavior.

Physical Examination Findings

- Mares in poor body condition are less likely to have regular estrous cycles.
- Poor perineal conformation can be related to pneumovagina, ascending infections, and urine pooling.
- Clitoral enlargement may be related to past treatment with anabolic steroids.
- Vaginal examination to identify inflammation, urine pooling, cervical competency or conformational abnormalities. One method to identify the stage of the estrous cycle (appearance, degree of relaxation, of external cervical os).
- Transrectal palpation by skilled individual: essential in evaluation of mare with abnormal cycles; should include uterine size and tone, ovarian size, shape and location, and cervical relaxation. Serial examination over the course of several weeks may be necessary to completely define the patient's cycle.
- Ultrasonography of the genital tract, an adjunct to define normal vs abnormal features of the uterus or ovaries.

CAUSES

Shortened Estrus Duration

- Seasonal influence—Duration of estrus shortens in the height of the breeding season; may relate to more efficient folliculogenesis.
- Silent estrus—Normal cyclic ovarian activity without overt signs of sexual receptivity. Often a behavior-based problem associated with nervousness, foal at side, or a maiden mare; may be associated with prior anabolic steroid use.

ABNORMAL ESTRUS INTERVALS

Lengthened Estrus Duration

• Erratic estrus behavior associated with the transition period. Receptivity can be short or long during vernal transition, but protracted estrus behavior is most common.
• Ovarian neoplasia, GCT, GTCT—Affected mare may be in chronic anestrus, exhibit persistent or frequent estrus behavior, or develop stallion-like (increased aggression) behavior.
• Persistent estrus—Older mares may fail to ovulate and exhibit prolonged estrus, presumably due to ineffective LH release.

Shortened Interestrus Interval

• Early luteolysis—Uterine inflammation (endometritis, pyometra) can result in early endometrial $PGF_2\alpha$ release, regression of the corpus luteum, and return to estrus.
• Systemic illness—Endotoxin-induced $PGF_2\alpha$ release can lead to premature luteolysis and a shortened interestrus period.
• Iatrogenic—$PGF_2\alpha$ administration, intrauterine infusions, and uterine biopsy procedures can also result in early regression of the CL and subsequent estrus induction.

Lengthened Interestrus Interval

• Prolonged luteal activity—Can occur with a normal diestrus ovulation, severe uterine disease (pyometra) that prevents release of luteolytic factors, EED after maternal recognition of pregnancy has occurred, persistent corpus luteum function, or luteinization of an ovarian hematoma. Persistent CLs have been associated with fescue consumption.
• Estrus behavior during pregnancy is a normal occurrence and can be confused with abnormal interestrus intervals.
• Pregnancy—Luteal function persists in the presence of a conceptus.
• Iatrogenic, pharmaceutical:
  • Parenteral administration of progestin compounds to suppress behavioral estrus.
  • NSAIDs can interfere with endometrial $PGF_2\alpha$ release and result in prolonged luteal activity.

RISK FACTORS

N/A

DIAGNOSIS

DIFFERENTIAL DIAGNOSIS

Differentiating Similar Signs

• Frequent urination caused by cystitis, bladder atony, or pneumovagina may mimic submissive urination, a response to teasing.
• Defensive or aggressive behavior can be confused with anestrus.
  • Alter teasing method, clarify relationship of response to actual estrus events.
  • Alter approach of stallion to mare, or mare to stallion, or use a different stallion.

Differentiating Causes

• Minimum data-base—Complete history, teasing records/response, vaginal examination, transrectal palpation and ultrasound to distinguish pregnancy and pyometra, and identify abnormalities that warrant further investigation.
• Additional diagnostic samples (uterine cytology, culture, biopsy) may aid early diagnosis.
• Transition period in the northern hemisphere typically extends from February through April, the period in which anestrus mares begin to develop follicles, but do not have regular estrous cycles. Mares may exhibit persistent estrus behavior, irregular estrus periods, or irregular diestrus intervals. Diagnostic—season, combined with results of transrectal palpation and ultrasonography confirming the presence of numerous small to larger follicles on both ovaries that fail to progress to ovulatory size.
• Silent heat is often due to poor estrus detection (teasing). Transrectal palpation at least three times per week or frequent serum progesterone assays may allow detection of a short estrus period.
• Ovulations can occur in diestrus. The CL that forms from a diestrus ovulation may or may not be sufficiently mature ($\geq$5 days post-ovulation) to be lysed by endogenous $PGF_2\alpha$ at the end of the normal 21-day cycle. Therefore, ovulations after day 10 of the estrous cycle result in persistence of CL activity. Diagnosis can be established by demonstration of a normal reproductive tract with failure of clinical estrus for $>$2 weeks post-ovulation and progesterone levels of $>$4 ng/mL for $>$2 weeks.

ABNORMAL ESTRUS INTERVALS

• GCT/GTCT can occur at any age, but are more typically seen in the middle-age to older mare. The affected ovary is usually enlarged and often the ovulation fossa is obliterated. The contralateral ovary is usually small and inactive. Ultrasonography of the affected ovary often reveals a multilocular "honeycomb" appearance. Endocrine analyses are useful in diagnosing GCT/GTCT, i.e., elevations of serum testosterone in at least 50% and serum inhibin in 90% of all cases, with a progesterone <1ng/mL.
• The diagnosis of pregnancy, pyometra, endometritis, abortion, and EED are discussed elsewhere.

OTHER LABORATORY TESTS

• Serum progesterone concentrations. Basal levels of <1 ng/mL indicate there is no ovarian luteal tissue. Active CL function is associated with progesterone levels of <4 ng/mL.
• Serum inhibin, testosterone, and progesterone concentrations. Mares typically have testosterone values <50–60 pg/mL and inhibin <0.7 ng/mL.
• Hormone levels suggestive of a granulosa theca cell tumor (in a non-pregnant mare) are: testosterone of >50–100 pg/mL (produced if theca cells are a significant component of her tumor), inhibin levels >0.7 ng/mL, and progesterone levels of <1 ng/mL.

IMAGING

Transrectal ultrasonography is routinely used to evaluate the equine reproductive tract. The reader is referred to other texts for a comprehensive discussion on this technique.

DIAGNOSTIC PROCEDURES

• Uterine endoscopy can be useful to diagnose intrauterine adhesions, glandular or lymphatic cysts, and polyps.
• Uterine cytology, culture, and biopsy techniques are discussed elsewhere.

TREATMENT

• Vary teasing methods; silent estrus may be a reflection of poor teasing management.
• Monitor the problem mare, including transrectal palpation and/or ultrasonography, three times weekly to allow better definition of her reproductive cycle.
• Artificial lighting (photostimulation) is a management tool used to initiate ovarian activity earlier in the year. When successful, mares bred earlier in the season foal earlier the next year, to accommodate breed registries that use the January 1 "universal birth date." Photostimulation does not eliminate vernal transition; it merely shifts it to an earlier time of onset. Photostimulation should begin no less than 90 days prior to the onset of early season breeding.
• GCT/GTCT: ovariectomy.
• Poor vulvar conformation—Vulvoplasty, aka episioplasty, (a "'Caslick'") of a portion of the dorsal vulvar commissure to control pneumovagina.
• Surgical correction for urine pooling, rectovaginal fistulas, and cervical tears.

MEDICATIONS

DRUG(S) OF CHOICE

• $PGF_2\alpha$ (Lutalyse, 10 mg, IM, Upjohn, Kalamazoo, MI) to lyse a persistent CL.
• Ovulation can be stimulated, if a follicle is ≥35 mm, by hCG, 2500 IU, IV.
• Progesterone (altrenogest, 0.044 mg/kg, P/O, SID, minimum 15 days) can be used to shorten the duration of vernal transition, providing a mare has follicles that are >20 mm in diameter and she is teasing-in. $PGF_2\alpha$, 10 mg, IM, on day 15 of the altrenogest treatment increases the reliability of this transition management regimen. Medical management of endometritis and pyometra are discussed elsewhere.

PRECAUTIONS

- $PGF_2\alpha$ causes sweating and colic-like symptoms due to its stimulatory effect on smooth muscle cells. If cramping has not subsided within 1–2 h, symptomatic treatment can be instituted.
- $PGF_2\alpha$ should not be handled by pregnant women.
- Altrenogest can be absorbed across skin. Wear latex gloves when administering oral progesterone to mares.
- Antibodies to hCG can develop after treatment. It is desirable to limit its use to no more than two times during one breeding season. The half-life of these antibodies ranges from 30 days to several months, i.e., no persistence from one season to the next.

POSSIBLE INTERACTIONS

N/A

ALTERNATIVE DRUGS

N/A

FOLLOW-UP

PATIENT MONITORING

Until normal cyclicity is established or pregnancy has been confirmed, regular reproductive examinations are recommended.

POSSIBLE COMPLICATIONS

Unless corrected, abnormalities in estrus behavior frequently result in infertility.

MISCELLANEOUS

PREGNANCY

Prostaglandin administration to pregnant mares can cause CL lysis and abortion. Carefully rule out pregnancy before administering this drug.

SEE ALSO

- Anestrus
- Large ovary syndrome
- Endometritis/pyometra
- Uterine disease
- Ovarian hypoplasia
- Vulvar conformation

ABBREVIATIONS

- $PGF_2\alpha$ = PGF, natural prostaglandin ($F_2\alpha$)
- CL = corpus luteum
- EED = early embryonic death
- FSH = follicle stimulating hormone
- GCT = granulosa cell tumor
- GnRH = gonadotropin releasing hormone
- GTCT = granulosa theca cell tumor
- hCG = human chorionic gonadotropin
- LH = luteinizing hormone
- NSAIDs = non-steroidal anti-inflammatory drugs
- teasing in = exhibiting estrus behavior

Suggested Readings

Daels PF and Hughes JP. The abnormal estrous cycle. In: Equine reproduction. McKinnon AO and Voss JL, eds. Philadelphia: Lea & Febiger 1993;144-160.

Ginther OJ. Reproductive biology of the mare: Basic and applied aspects. 2nd ed. Cross Plains, WI: Equiservices 1992.

Ginther OJ. Ultrasonic imaging and animal reproduction: Horses. Cross Plains, WI: Equiservices 1995.

Hinrichs K. Irregularities of the estrous cycle and ovulation in mares. In: Current therapy in large animal theriogenology. Youngquist RS, ed. Philadelphia: WB Saunders 1997;166-171.

Author Carole C. Miller

Consulting Editor Carla L. Carleton

ABNORMAL SCROTAL ENLARGEMENT

BASICS

DEFINITION

A condition causing the gross appearance of the scrotum to deviate from normal size and texture—scrotal enlargement or asymmetry

PATHOPHYSIOLOGY

- The equine scrotum and associated contents are positioned on a horizontal axis between the hind limbs and are protected relatively well from external insult.
- The scrotal skin is thin and pliable, and the contents are freely movable within the scrotum.
- Blunt trauma (e.g., breeding accident, jumping) is the most common cause of scrotal abnormality.
- Trauma can result in scrotal hemorrhage, edema, tunica albuginea rupture, hematocele, hydrocele, and inflammation. Similar signs can occur with inguinal/scrotal herniation, torsion of the spermatic cord, or neoplasia.

SYSTEM AFFECTED

Reproductive

GENETICS

N/A

INCIDENCE/PREVALENCE

N/A

SIGNALMENT

Intact male horses of any age

SIGNS

Historical Findings

- Gross changes in scrotal size—usually acute
- Pain—generally colic-like symptoms
- Reluctance to breed, jump, or walk
- Environmental temperature extremes

Physical Examination Findings

- Increased scrotal size—unilateral or bilateral
- Abnormal testicular position
- Abnormal scrotal temperature—too warm or cold
- Edema/engorgement of scrotum, contents, or both
- Scrotal laceration
- Derangements in systemic parameters—elevated heart rate, respiratory rate, inappetence, and CBC abnormalities
- **NOTE:** Not all signs are present in every animal; any combination may occur.

CAUSES

- Trauma
- May include testicular hematoma/rupture.
- Inguinal/scrotal hernia
- Torsion of the spermatic cord
- Inflammatory/infectious causes
- EIA
- EVA
- Orchitis/epididymitis
- Neoplasia
- Primary scrotal—melanoma; sarcoid
- Testicular neoplasia—seminoma, teratoma, interstitial cell tumor, and Sertoli cell tumor
- See also *Abnormal Testicular Size.*
- Noninflammatory scrotal edema
- Hydrocele/hematocele
- Varicocele

RISK FACTORS

- Breeding activity
- Large internal inguinal rings
- Systemic illness
- Extremes of ambient temperature—hot or cold

DIAGNOSIS

DIFFERENTIAL DIAGNOSIS

- Acute—traumatic injury, torsion of spermatic cord, herniation, and infection
- Chronic—neoplasia, temperature-induced hydrocele/edema, varicocele, and infection
- History of recent breeding, semen collection, or trauma
- Palpation of the caudal ligament of the epididymis—attaches epididymal tail to caudal testis and aids in determination of testicular orientation.
- Palpation of the inguinal rings
- Ultrasonography (see *Imaging*).

CBC/BIOCHEMISTRY/URINALYSIS

- Inflammatory or stress leukocyte response—increased fibrinogen
- Results of serum biochemistry profile and urinalysis usually are normal.

OTHER LABORATORY TESTS

EVA

- Serum neutralization or complement fixation (i.e., acute and convalescent serum samples)
- If a stallion is seropositive, carrier state is determined with virus isolation from serum or seminal plasma—semen is the best route to establish a diagnosis.
- Send sample to an approved laboratory.

EIA

AGID or Coggins test

IMAGING

Scrotal ultrasonography may reveal:

- Bowel with inguinal/scrotal herniation
- Testicular/tunica albuginea rupture—accumulation of hypoechoic fluid in scrotum with loss of discrete hyperechoic tunica albuginea around testicular parenchyma; hypoechoic appearance of contents will gradually contain echogenic densities with the formation of fibrin clots.
- Engorgement of the pampiniform plexus or testicular congestion with torsion of the spermatic cord—Doppler can verify loss of blood flow to the testis.
- Hypoechoic dilation of venous plexus of spermatic cord with varicocele
- Hypoechoic accumulation of fluid within the vaginal cavity—hydrocele
- Loss of homogeneity in testicular parenchyma with neoplasia—may have areas of increased or decreased echogenicity.

DIAGNOSTIC PROCEDURES

- Needle aspiration and cytology may be used to differentiate hydrocele from recent hemorrhage.
- Neoplasia is diagnosed using fine-needle aspiration or biopsy.

PATHOLOGIC FINDINGS

N/A

TREATMENT

APPROPRIATE HEALTH CARE

- Directed at the cause of scrotal enlargement.
- Management of inflammation is a primary concern.
- Sexual rest for all causes
- Acute causes warrant hospitalization for treatment and care.
- Chronic causes may or may not warrant hospitalization.

ABNORMAL SCROTAL ENLARGEMENT

NURSING CARE

- Implement cold therapy (cold packs or ice water baths) for acute scrotal trauma (without testicular rupture). Such sessions should not exceed 20 minutes and can be repeated every 2 hours.
- Scrotal massage with emollient salve is useful for reducing scrotal edema and ischemic injury.
- With hydrocele, consider fluid removal using an aseptically placed needle or an IV catheter; excess fluid accumulation may cause thermal damage to the testes.
- IV fluids, depending on the systemic status of the horse.

ACTIVITY

Activity restriction depends on the cause.

DIET

Modification is necessary only with secondary ileus or as a preoperative consideration.

CLIENT EDUCATION

- Fertility may be irreversibly impaired with acute scrotal trauma.
- Perform semen evaluation 90 days after nonsurgical resolution of scrotal enlargement.
- Compensatory semen production may occur in the remaining testis of horses undergoing hemicastration.
- Carefully examine horses with neoplasia for metastatic tumor growth.

SURGICAL CONSIDERATIONS

Hemicastration

Treatment of choice for:

- Torsion of the spermatic cord, if the duration of vascular compromise has caused irreversible damage or gonadal necrosis
- Unilateral inguinal/scrotal herniation
- Testicular rupture
- Unilateral neoplasia
- Varicocele
- Nonresponsive hydrocele/hematocele

Primary Repair of Scrotal Laceration

- Required to protect scrotal contents.
- Generally fails because of extensive scrotal edema associated with traumatic injury.

MEDICATIONS

DRUGS OF CHOICE

- Anti-inflammatory therapy in all cases—phenylbutazone (2–4 mg/kg PO or IV BID) or flunixin meglumine (1 mg/kg IV BID)
- Diuretics may be useful in managing scrotal edema—furosemide (0.5–1 mg/kg IV)
- Consider antibiotic therapy for scrotal laceration or hemorrhage.
- Administer tetanus toxoid for scrotal trauma or before surgery.

CONTRAINDICATIONS

N/A

PRECAUTIONS

N/A

POSSIBLE INTERACTIONS

N/A

ALTERNATIVE DRUGS

N/A

FOLLOW-UP

PATIENT MONITORING

Semen collection and evaluation 90 days after complete resolution of the cause or surgery

PREVENTION/AVOIDANCE

N/A

POSSIBLE COMPLICATIONS

- Infertility
- Endotoxemia
- Laminitis
- Scrotal adhesions
- Death

EXPECTED COURSE AND PROGNOSIS

N/A

MISCELLANEOUS

ASSOCIATED CONDITIONS

N/A

AGE-RELATED FACTORS

N/A

ZOONOTIC POTENTIAL

N/A

PREGNANCY

N/A

SYNONYMS

N/A

SEE ALSO

- Abnormal Stallion Semen
- Abnormal Testicular Size
- Normal Stallion Semen

ABBREVIATIONS

- AGID = agar-gel immunodiffusion
- EIA = equine infectious anemia
- EVA = equine viral arteritis

Suggested Reading

Love CC. Ultrasonographic evaluation of the testis, epididymis and spermatic cord of the stallion. Vet Clin North Am Equine Pract 1992;8:167–182.

Varner DD, Schumacher J, Blanchard T, Johnson L. Diseases and management of breeding stallions. Goleta, CA: American Veterinary Publications, 1991.

Author Margo L. Macpherson

Contributing Editor Carla L. Carleton

ABNORMAL TESTICULAR SIZE

BASICS

DEFINITION

A condition causing the gross appearance of a testis to deviate from normal size and texture—testicular enlargement, reduction, or asymmetry.

PATHOPHYSIOLOGY

- The testes and epididymides are positioned in a horizontal orientation between the hind limbs and are freely movable within the scrotum.
- The scrotum and its contents, though relatively protected from external insult, are at increased risk for injury during breeding or athletic activity.
- Acute enlargement of a testis occurs after trauma, torsion of the spermatic cord, or orchitis/epididymitis—bacterial, viral, autoimmune, or parasitic.
- Testicular neoplasia (i.e., seminoma, teratoma, Sertoli cell tumor, interstitial cell tumor) is uncommon in horses. Seminoma is the most frequently reported testicular tumor. Most equine testicular tumors arise from germ cells. The effect of neoplasia on testicular size (increase or decrease) may be insidious.
- Hypoplastic and degenerative testes are smaller than normal. Testicular degeneration can be transient or permanent, but hypoplasia is irreversible.
- Hypoplastic testes are incompletely developed, and the condition usually is congenital. Suspected causes of testicular hypoplasia include genetic aberrations, teratogens, cryptorchidism, and postnatal insult.
- Testicular degeneration is an acquired condition that may arise from thermal injury, infection, vascular insult, hormonal disturbances, toxins, and age.

SYSTEMS AFFECTED

- Reproductive
- Other systems (e.g., respiratory, GI, lymphatic) may be affected subsequent to metastasis of primary testicular neoplasia.

GENETICS

N/A

INCIDENCE/PREVALENCE

N/A

SIGNALMENT

Intact male horses of any age.

SIGNS

Historical Findings

- Recent history of breeding or semen collection.
- Gross changes in size of a testis.
- Reduced fertility
- Pain—generally colic-like symptoms.
- Reluctance to breed, jump, or walk.

Physical Examination Findings

- Increased or decreased scrotal size.
- Increased or decreased testicular size.
- Abnormal testicular texture—too soft or firm.
- Abnormal testicular position.
- Abnormal scrotal temperature—too warm or cold.
- Edema/engorged scrotum or contents.
- Derangements in systemic parameters—elevated heart rate, respiratory rate, inappetence, and CBC abnormalities.

CAUSES

- Trauma
- Cryptorchidism
- Torsion of the spermatic cord.
- Testicular degeneration, hypoplasia, or hematoma/rupture.
- Neoplasia
- Seminoma
- Teratoma
- Interstitial cell or Sertoli cell tumor.
- Orchitis/epididymitis.
- Bacterial infection.
- EIA
- EVA
- *Strongylus edentatus* infection.
- Autoimmune disorders.

RISK FACTORS

- Breeding activity
- Systemic illness
- Temperature extremes
- Anabolic steroid use

DIAGNOSIS

DIFFERENTIAL DIAGNOSIS

Differentiating Similar Signs

- Scrotal enlargement caused by scrotal hydrocele/hematocele and scrotal or inguinal hernia may be confused with testicular enlargement.
- Testicular ultrasonography and measurement is the best means of differentiating pathologies.

Differentiating Causes

- Acute—traumatic injury, torsion of spermatic cord, and infection.
- Chronic—cryptorchidism, neoplasia, infection, or testicular degeneration/hypoplasia.
- History of recent breeding or trauma.
- Palpation of the *caudal ligament* of the epididymis—attaches epididymal tail to caudal testis and aids in the determination of testicular orientation.
- Testicular hypoplasia usually is congenital, whereas testicular degeneration is acquired.
- Ultrasonography (see *Imaging*).

CBC/BIOCHEMISTRY/URINALYSIS

- Inflammatory or stress leukocyte response
- Indication of parasitic infection may be eosinophilia.
- Increased fibrinogen.
- Results of serum biochemistry profile and urinalysis usually are normal.

OTHER LABORATORY TESTS

EVA

- SN or CF—acute and convalescent serum samples.
- If seropositive, carrier state is determined with virus isolation from serum or seminal plasma.
- Semen is the best sample to submit for diagnostics.
- Send samples to an approved laboratory.

EIA

- AGID or Coggins test.
- Testicular degeneration—endocrine profile (e.g., LH, FSH, testosterone, estrogen) from pooled samples obtained hourly for a minimum of four samples (because of pulsatile release of hormones); abnormal elevation of FSH and low total estrogen concentration indicate testicular degeneration.

IMAGING

On scrotal/testicular ultrasonography, testicular parenchyma should appear uniformly echogenic. Aberrations that may be identified include:

- Rupture of the testis/tunica albuginea—hypoechoic fluid accumulates in the scrotum with loss of discrete hyperechoic tunica albuginea around testicular parenchyma; *hypoechoic* appearance of contents will gradually be replaced with echogenic densities as fibrin clots form.
- Engorged pampiniform plexus or testicular congestion with torsion of the spermatic cord—Doppler can verify loss of blood flow to the testis.
- Heterogeneity (usually a circumscribed area) in testicular parenchyma with neoplasia.
- Sometimes areas of increased or decreased echogenicity.

DIAGNOSTIC PROCEDURES

- Needle aspiration and cytology may be used to establish the diagnosis of recent hemorrhage or neoplasia.
- Testicular histopathology can be used to establish the diagnosis of neoplasia and testicular degeneration/hypoplasia.
- Semen evaluation is useful to establish the diagnosis of testicular degeneration or hypoplasia—oligospermia, azoospermia, or premature release of spermatids.

PATHOLOGIC FINDINGS

N/A

ABNORMAL TESTICULAR SIZE

TREATMENT

APPROPRIATE HEALTH CARE

- Treatment is directed at the cause of the testicular abnormality.
- Most causes require hospitalization for treatment/resolution.
- Horses with testicular degeneration that are not systemically ill may be treated on the farm.
- Horses with hypoplastic testes can be treated on an outpatient basis.

NURSING CARE

- Cold therapy (cold packs or ice water baths) or hydrotherapy may be useful with acute orchitis/epididymitis. Sessions should not exceed 20 minutes and can be repeated every 2 hours.
- Sexual rest is indicated in most cases until the problem resolves.
- IV fluids depending on the systemic status of the horse.

ACTIVITY

Restriction depends on the cause of the testicular aberration.

DIET

Modification is necessary only in cases of secondary ileus or as a preoperative consideration.

CLIENT EDUCATION

- Fertility may be permanently lowered.
- Testicular degeneration and subsequent reduction in semen quality can be transient or permanent, depending on the inciting cause.
- Testicular hypoplasia is permanent.
- Carefully examine horses with neoplasia for metastatic tumor growth.
- Compensatory sperm production may occur in the remaining testis of a horse undergoing hemicastration.
- Serial semen evaluations are beneficial in monitoring the fertility status of horses after testicular insult and treatment.
- Evaluate semen 75–90 days after complete resolution of the testicular insult.

SURGICAL CONSIDERATIONS

Hemicastration is the treatment of choice for:

- Torsion of the spermatic cord, if the duration of vascular compromise has caused irreversible damage or gonadal necrosis.
- Testicular rupture.
- Unilateral neoplasia or any condition causing irreparable damage.

MEDICATIONS

DRUGS OF CHOICE

- Anti-inflammatory therapy is indicated in most cases—phenylbutazone (2–4 mg/kg PO or IV BID) or flunixin meglumine (1 mg/kg IV BID).
- Consider antibiotic therapy with orchitis/epididymitis and testicular trauma.
- Administer tetanus toxoid after testicular trauma or before surgery.
- Antiparasitic therapy for *S. edentatus* infection—ivermectin (0.2 mg/kg PO q30d until resolution of lesions).

CONTRAINDICATIONS

N/A

PRECAUTIONS

N/A

POSSIBLE INTERACTIONS

N/A

ALTERNATIVE DRUGS

N/A

FOLLOW-UP

PATIENT MONITORING

Semen collection and evaluation 90 days after complete resolution of the testicular problem or surgery.

PREVENTION/AVOIDANCE

N/A

POSSIBLE COMPLICATIONS

- Infertility/subfertility
- Endotoxemia
- Laminitis
- Scrotal adhesions
- Death

EXPECTED COURSE AND PROGNOSIS

N/A

MISCELLANEOUS

ASSOCIATED CONDITIONS

- Cryptorchidism commonly is associated with testicular hypoplasia.
- Male equine hybrids (e.g., mules, *hinnies*) often have hypoplastic testes.

AGE-RELATED FACTORS

- Prepubertal testes are small and can be misdiagnosed as pathologically hypoplastic.
- Testicular growth increases rapidly from 12–24 months of age in horses.
- Testes may take 4–5 years to reach full size and maturity.

ZOONOTIC POTENTIAL

N/A

PREGNANCY

N/A

SYNONYMS

N/A

SEE ALSO

- Abnormal Scrotal Enlargement
- Cryptorchidism

ABBREVIATIONS

- AGID = agar-gel immunodiffusion
- CF = complement fixation
- EIA = equine infectious anemia
- EVA = equine viral arteritis
- FSH = follicle stimulating hormone
- GI = gastrointestinal
- LH = luteinizing hormone
- SN = serum neutralization

Suggested Reading

Brinsko SP. Neoplasia of the male reproductive tract. Vet Clin North Am Equine Pract 1998;14:517–533.

Love CC. Ultrasonographic evaluation of the testis, epididymis and spermatic cord of the stallion. Vet Clin North Am Equine Pract 1992;8:167–182.

Varner DD, Schumacher J, Blanchard T, Johnson L. Diseases and management of breeding stallions. Goleta, CA: American Veterinary Publications, 1991.

Author Margo L. Macpherson
Consulting Editor Carla L. Carleton

ABORTION, SPONTANEOUS, INFECTIOUS

BASICS

DEFINITION

Fetal loss after day 40 of gestation caused by maternal, placental, or fetal invasion of microorganisms—viruses, bacteria, rickettsiae, fungi, and protozoa.

PATHOPHYSIOLOGY

- Fetal death from invasion of microorganisms
- Fetal expulsion subsequent to placental infection, insufficiency, or separation.
- Premature parturition from microbial toxins, fetal "stress," or a combination of mechanisms.
- Ends in fetal reabsorption, maceration, autolysis, or live fetus incapable of extrauterine survival.

SYSTEMS AFFECTED

- Reproductive
- Other organ systems depending on the maternal systemic disease.

GENETICS

N/A

INCIDENCE/PREVALENCE

- Rate of infectious abortion may be 5%–15%.
- Infectious abortion "storms" can occur, especially in the case of EHV-1.

SIGNALMENT

Nonspecific, but may be associated with specific risk factors.

SIGNS

General Comments

- Early pregnancy loss can occur completely unobserved and be termed "asymptomatic."
- Unless complications (e.g., dystocia, RFM) develop, abortion may occur rapidly, and the only clinical sign may be that of a relatively normal, previously diagnosed pregnant mare found open at a subsequent check.
- Range of signs—none to multisystemic and life-threatening.
- May involve multiple animals.
- Most "symptomatic" spontaneous infectious abortions occur during the second half of gestation (see signs in specific conditions).

Historical Findings

One or more of the following:

- Vaginal discharge—mucoid, hemorrhagic, or serosanguinous.
- Premature udder development; dripping of milk.
- Anorexia or colic; GI disease.
- Failure to deliver a foal on the expected due date.
- "Recent" (i.e., 1–16 weeks before presentation) systemic infectious disease.
- Recent abortions in other mares.
- Absence of or inadequate EHV-1 prophylaxis.
- History of placentitis.
- Previous endometrial biopsy results indicating moderate to severe endometritis or fibrosis.
- No, or excessive, abdominal distention consistent with the stage of pregnancy.
- Behavioral estrus in a pregnant mare—may be normal depending on stage of pregnancy, the time of year, and stage of pregnancy at time of loss.

Physical Examination Findings

- Fetal parts or placental structures protruding from between the vulvar lips; abdominal straining or discomfort.
- Vulvar discharge (appearance can be variable); premature udder development and dripping of milk.
- A previously documented pregnancy is not apparent at subsequent examination; evidence of fetal death as determined by palpation or by transrectal or transabdominal ultrasonography.
- Anorexia, fever, or signs of concurrent systemic disease, especially with endotoxemia or in cases of dystocia or RFM.
- Evidence of placental separation during transrectal or transabdominal ultrasonography.

CAUSES

Viruses

- EHV-1 (1P and 1B strains, >7 months of gestation); rarely EHV-4 (>7 months of gestation).
- EVA (>3 months of gestation).
- EIA—direct causal relationship not yet established.

Bacteria

- Placentitis and possible, subsequent fetal infection caused by *Streptococcus* sp., *Escherichia coli, Pseudomonas* sp., *Klebsiella* sp., *Staphylococcus* sp., *Nocardioform actinomycete* (reported in one study of 3000 abortions), *Taylorella equigenitalis* (rare and reportable), and *Leptospira* serovars (most commonly *pomona* and *grippotyphosa*; sporadically *hardjo, bratislava,* and *icterohemorrhagiae*).
- Endotoxemia and septicemia by Gram-negative bacteria cause release of $PGF_2\alpha$ (especially <80 days of gestation [day 60 in many mares]; may be factor later in gestation, with repeated exposure).

Rickettsiae

Ehrlichia risticii—PHF

Fungi

Placentitis caused by *Aspergillus* sp., *Candida* sp., or *Histoplasma capsulatum.*

Protozoa

Sarcocystis neurona or, possibly, *Neospora* sp. have been identified histopathologically in fetuses aborted from mares affected with EPM.

RISK FACTORS

- Pregnant mares intermixed with young horses or horses-in-training are susceptible to EHV-1, EVA, or *Ehrlichia risticii.*
- Immunologically naïve mares brought to premises with enzootic EHV-1, EVA, *Ehrlichia risticii,* or *Leptospira* infections.
- Pregnant mares traveling to horse shows or competitions.
- Poor perineal conformation, which predisposes mares to bacterial or fungal placentitis and, possibly, to subsequent fetal infection.
- Concurrent maternal GI disease or EPM (possibly).

ABORTION, SPONTANEOUS, INFECTIOUS

DIAGNOSIS

• Except for placentitis and abortion secondary to endotoxemia, most abortions present as "asymptomatic," and the expelled fetus and fetal membranes vary in condition from intact to autolytic.
• Definitive causative diagnosis of equine abortion in $\cong$50–60% of all cases.
• Excluding twins and EHV-1, the diagnostic rate may approach only 30% when a limited number of samples are submitted and accompanied by moderate to severe fetal and placental autolysis.

DIFFERENTIAL DIAGNOSIS

Other Causes of Abortion

Abortion, spontaneous, noninfectious:
• Twinning
• Fetal abnormalities—teratogenesis.
• Umbilical cord abnormalities—excessive twisting; thrombosis.
• Placental pathology.
• Maternal malnutrition or other noninfectious systemic disease.
• Old mare with history of EED or abortion.
• Old mare with poor endometrial biopsy—inflammation, fibrosis.
• Endophyte-infected tall fescue pasture during the last month of gestation with no mammary development (agalactia if term is reached); phytoestrogens; xenobiotics.

Other Causes of Signs of Labor or Abdominal Discomfort

• Normal parturition.
• Dystocia unassociated with abortion.
• Prepartum uterine artery rupture.
• Colic associated with uterine torsion.
• Discomfort associated with hydrops of fetal membranes or prepubic tendon rupture.
• Colic unassociated with reproductive disease.

Other Causes of Vulvar Discharge

• Normal parturition
• Dystocia unassociated with abortion.
• Normal estrus
• Endometritis
• Metritis or partial RFM
• Mucometra or pyometra

CBC/BIOCHEMISTRY/URINALYSIS

Indicated to determine inflammatory or stress leukocyte response or other organ system involvement.

OTHER LABORATORY TESTS

Maternal Progesterone

• Indicated with questionable pregnancy outcome (before diagnosis of an infectious cause of impending abortion) or with suspected endotoxemia.
• ELISA or RIA for progesterone may be useful at <80 days of gestation (normal levels vary from >1 to >4 ng/mL, depending on the reference lab).
• At >100 days, RIA will detect both progesterone (may be very low after day 150) and cross-reacting 5α-pregnanes of uterofeto-placental origin. Acceptable levels of 5α-pregnanes vary with the stage of gestation and the laboratory used.

Maternal Serology

• Take serum samples in all cases of abortion in which the cause is unknown. A paired sample, taken 21 days later, also may be indicated.
• May be diagnostic in abortions caused by *Leptospira* serovars.
• Confirms abortion caused by EVA.

IMAGING

Transrectal and transabdominal ultrasonography to evaluate fetal viability, placentitis, and other gestational abnormalities.

DIAGNOSTIC PROCEDURES

Pathology, Serology, and Culture

If entire fetus and membranes are unavailable, appropriate samples include:
• Fresh/chilled fetal thoracic or abdominal fluid or fetal serum from fetal heart or cord blood (if available).
• Fetal stomach contents.
• 10% Formalin-fixed and chilled/frozen samples of fetal heart, lung, thymus, liver, kidney, lymph nodes, thymus, spleen, adrenal, skeletal muscle, and brain.
• 10% Formalin-fixed and chilled/frozen fetal membranes—allantochorion; allantoamnion.

Maternal Uterine Swabs

May aid in establishing the diagnosis of abortions caused by placentitis.

PATHOLOGIC FINDINGS

Viruses

EHV-1:
• Gross—increased amounts of thoracic and abdominal fluid, fetal icterus, pulmonary congestion and edema, and 1-mm, yellowish-white spots on an enlarged liver, fetus is fresh.
• Histopathologic (also for EHV-4)—areas of necrosis with prominent, eosinophilic, intranuclear inclusion bodies in lymphoid tissue, liver, adrenal cortex, and lung as well as a hyperplastic, necrotizing bronchiolitis; FA staining of fetal tissues; virus isolation from aborted fetus.

EVA:
• Few gross lesions.
• *Autolyzed fetus.*
• Placental and fetal vascular lesions.

Bacteria and Fungi

Fetal Infection and Placentitis:
• Gross—increased amounts of fetal thoracic and abdominal fluid, enlarged liver, rare plaques of mycotic dermatitis, and placental edema and thickening with fibronecrotic exudate (chorionic surface), especially at the "cervical star" (particularly fungal).
• Histopathologic—consistent with inflammatory disease; autolysis may make interpretation difficult.

Leptospirosis:
• Gross—fetal icterus and autolysis
• Histopathologic—nonspecific; mild, diffuse placentitis.

Endotoxemia

Fetus minimally autolyzed.

Rickettsiae

Ehrlichia risticii:
• Gross—placentitis.
• Histopathologic—typical fetal lesions include colitis, periportal hepatitis, lymphoid hyperplasia, and necrosis.

Protozoa

Sarcocystis neurona—anecdotal reporting of organisms seen histopathologically in aborted fetuses from mares diagnosed with EPM.

ABORTION, SPONTANEOUS, INFECTIOUS

TREATMENT

APPROPRIATE HEALTH CARE

- Except possibly for late-gestational placentitis (>270 days) and endotoxemia, no therapy is indicated to preserve fetal viability in cases of spontaneous, infectious abortion.
- Aborting mares generally require only "prophylactic" therapy for metritis or endometritis. Therapy may be limited to intrauterine or include a systemic component.
- Pre-existing GI disease and complications (e.g., dystocia and RFM and their sequelae) may warrant hospitalization and intensive care.
- See specific topics for additional details.

NURSING CARE

Most affected horses require limited nursing care, except those with endotoxemia and Gram-negative septicemia, dystocia, RFM, metritis, and laminitis.

ACTIVITY

Free exercise in an area sufficiently small to permit supervision may be beneficial.

DIET

N/A

CLIENT EDUCATION

Inform owners regarding the possible complications of abortion.

SURGICAL CONSIDERATIONS

N/A

MEDICATIONS

DRUG(S) OF CHOICE

- Altrenogest 0.044–0.088 mg/kg PO SID may be started later during gestation, continued longer, or used for only short periods of time depending on serum progesterone levels during the first 80 days of gestation, clinical circumstances, risk factors, and clinician preference. **NOTE**: serum levels reflect only endogenous progesterone, not the exogenous/oral product.
- If used near term, altrenogest frequently is discontinued 7–14 days before the expected foaling date unless indicated otherwise by fetal maturity/viability or questions arise regarding correct gestational age.
- See specific topics for details.

CONTRAINDICATIONS

Only use altrenogest to prevent abortion in cases of endotoxemia or placentitis (>270 days of gestation) with a viable fetus.

PRECAUTIONS

Altrenogest is absorbed through the skin; persons handling it should wear gloves and wash their hands.

POSSIBLE INTERACTIONS

N/A

ALTERNATIVE DRUGS

Injectable progesterone (150–500 mg, oil base) can be administered IM.

FOLLOW-UP

PATIENT MONITORING

- At 7–10 days after abortion, transrectal palpation and ultrasonography to monitor uterine involution.
- Further assessment of genital tract health may be indicated—vaginal speculum examination, uterine cytology, culture, and endometrial biopsy.
- Base treatment on clinical results, but recognize that uterine cultures performed <14 days postpartum or postabortion will be affected by contaminants introduced at parturition.

PREVENTION/AVOIDANCE

Vaccines

- A killed-virus vaccine for EHV-1 administered at 5, 7, and 9 months of gestation is approved for prevention of EHV-1 abortion in pregnant mares. Revaccination at the 2-month interval addresses the relatively short-lived (8 week) immunity provided by the vaccine.
- Vaccine for EVA is available but is not specifically labeled for abortion prevention. A modified-live product, it should be administered only to nonpregnant mares 3 weeks before anticipated exposure to infected semen or in enzootic conditions. Isolation of first-time vaccinated mares is recommended for 3 weeks after exposure to infected semen. Some countries forbid importation of horses with positive titers to EVA.

ABORTION, SPONTANEOUS, INFECTIOUS

Additional Prophylactic Steps

- Segregate pregnant mares from other horses susceptible to and exposed to infections.
- Isolate immunologically naïve individuals until their immunity to enzootic infections can be established or enhanced; depending on the infectious agent, protection may only be accomplished postpartum.
- Limit transport of pregnant mares to exhibitions or competitions.
- Isolate aborting mares, and dispose of contaminated fetal tissues properly.
- Practice proper diagnostic evaluation to identify infectious causes.
- Correct perineal conformation, if poor, to prevent placentitis.

POSSIBLE COMPLICATIONS

Future fertility and reproductive value can be impaired by dystocia, RFM, endometritis, laminitis, septicemia, and trauma to the genital tract.

EXPECTED COURSE AND PROGNOSIS

- The majority of patients recover uneventfully with appropriate treatment.
- Complications can have a significant impact on the survivability and future fertility of the mare.
- Prognosis is guarded for pregnancy maintenance in mares with endotoxemia and placentitis.

MISCELLANEOUS

ASSOCIATED CONDITIONS

- Abortion, spontaneous, noninfectious
- Dystocia
- EHV-1
- Endometritis
- EPM
- EVA
- Metritis
- Placental insufficiency
- Placentitis
- Potomac horse fever
- Premature placental separation
- Retained fetal membranes

AGE-RELATED FACTORS

None, other than risk of previous exposure and immunologic status of young mares.

ZOONOTIC POTENTIAL

N/A

PREGNANCY

N/A

SYNONYMS

N/A

SEE ALSO

- Abortion, spontaneous, noninfectious.
- Dystocia
- Endometrial biopsy
- Endometritis
- Fetal stress/viability
- High-risk pregnancy
- Metritis
- Placental insufficiency
- Placentitis
- Premature placental separation.
- RFM

ABBREVIATIONS

- EED = early embryonic death
- EHV = equine herpes virus
- EIA = equine infectious anemia
- ELISA = enzyme-linked immunoadsorbent assay
- EPM = equine protozoal encephalomyelitis
- EVA = equine viral arteritis
- FA = fluorescent antibody
- GI = gastrointestinal
- PHF = Potomac horse fever
- RIA = radioimmunoassay
- RFM = retained fetal membranes/placenta

Suggested Reading

Ball BA, Daels PF. Early pregnancy loss in mares: application for progestin therapy. In: Robinson NE, ed. Current therapy in equine medicine 4. Philadelphia: WB Saunders 1997:531–533.

Giles PC, Donahue JM, Hong CB, et al. Causes of abortion, stillbirth, and perinatal death in 3,527 cases (1986–1991). J Am Vet Med Assoc 1993;208:1170–1175.

LeBlanc MM. Abortion. In: Colahan PT, Mayhew IG, Merritt AM, Moore JM, eds. Equine medicine and surgery. 5th ed. St. Louis: Mosby 1999;2:1202–1207.

Troedsson MHT. Abortion. In: Robinson NE, ed. Current therapy in equine medicine 4. Philadelphia: WB Saunders 1997:534–540.

Author Tim J. Evans

Consulting Editor Carla L. Carleton

ABORTION, SPONTANEOUS, NONINFECTIOUS

BASICS

DEFINITION

Fetal loss after day 40 of gestation (the term *stillbirth* may apply after day 300) associated with a variety of noninfectious conditions.

PATHOPHYSIOLOGY

- Fetal death or premature parturition from some intrinsic structural or functional defect or from exposure to xenobiotics.
- Fetal expulsion at <80 days of gestation caused by regression of CL as a result of endometritis or other factors.
- Fetal death or expulsion caused by placental insufficiency or separation
- Fetal "stress,"dead twin fetus, maternal "stress," or some combination of these.
- May be fetal reabsorption, maceration, mummification, autolysis, or a live fetus incapable of extrauterine survival.

SYSTEM AFFECTED

Reproductive

GENETICS

N/A

INCIDENCE/PREVALENCE

- Rate of spontaneous abortion ranges from 5%–15%, depending on a variety of risk factors.
- Some breeds predisposed to twinning.

SIGNALMENT

- May be nonspecific.
- Breeds—Thoroughbred, draft mares, Standardbreds, and related breeds (for twinning).
- Mares older than 15 years.
- Maiden American Miniature Horse mares—anecdotal placental insufficiency.

SIGNS

General Comments

- Depending on the cause, time of fetal death, stage of gestation, duration of condition, and whether the pregnancy ended in dystocia or with RFM, the dam may show few signs or, in extreme cases, suffer life-threatening multiple-organ-system disease.
- Most occur during the second half of gestation.

Historical Findings

One or more of the following:

- Signs consistent with labor at an unexpected stage of gestation.
- Dystocia with birth of a nonviable foal.
- Vaginal discharge—mucoid, hemorrhagic, or serosanguinous.
- Premature udder development; dripping of milk.
- Anorexia or colic.
- "Recent" systemic disease.
- Previous endometrial biopsy results indicating moderate to severe endometritis or fibrosis.
- Failure to deliver a foal on the expected due date.
- No, or excessive, abdominal distention consistent with the stage of pregnancy.
- Behavioral estrus in a pregnant mare—may be normal depending on the stage of pregnancy; dependent on the time of year and stage of pregnancy at time of loss.

Physical Examination Findings

- Fetal parts or placental structures protruding from and/or between the vulvar lips; abdominal straining or discomfort.
- Vulvar discharge (appearance can be variable), premature udder development, and dripping of milk.
- A previously documented pregnancy not apparent at subsequent examination; evidence of fetal death as determined by palpation or by transrectal or transabdominal ultrasonography.
- Twin fetuses identified by transrectal or transabdominal ultrasonography.
- Evidence of placental separation or hydrops of fetal membranes during transrectal or transabdominal ultrasonography.
- Signs of concurrent, systemic disease, dystocia, or RFM.
- **NOTE:** Signs are variable. Mares pregnant at an early check can remain "asymptomatic" but abort, unobserved, early during gestation. Abortion may occur rapidly and with no warning signs.

CAUSES

Twins

- Of twin pregnancies that persist beyond 40 days, ≅70% end in abortion or stillbirth.
- Placental insufficiency.

Luteal Insufficiency/Early CL Regression

- Anecdotal
- Caused by decreased levels of luteal progesterone at <80 days of gestation.

Placental Abnormalities

- Umbilical cord torsion—twisting of the equine cord is normal, so there must be evidence of vascular compromise (e.g., cord thrombus) to confirm the diagnosis.
- Confirmed body pregnancy.
- Placental separation.
- Villous atrophy or hypoplasia.
- Hydrops

ABORTION, SPONTANEOUS, NONINFECTIOUS

Fetal Abnormalities

- Developmental abnormalities—hydrocephalus; anencephaly.
- Fetal trauma.
- Chromosomal abnormalities.

Maternal Abnormalities

- Concurrent maternal disease.
- Trauma
- Malnutrition—starvation; selenium deficiency.
- Severe maternal anxiety—anecdotal.
- Moderate to severe endometritis or fibrosis.
- Maternal chromosomal abnormalities.

Xenobiotics

- Ergopeptine alkaloids associated with equine fescue toxicosis (although prolonged gestation is more common).
- Phytoestrogens—anecdotal.
- Xenobiotics causing maternal disease—organophosphates.
- Possible deleterious effects of medications on pregnancy—EPM therapies (anecdotal).
- Repeated large doses of corticosteroids during late gestation.

Iatrogenic Causes

- Administration of $PGF_2\alpha$—may require repeated injections if >40 days of gestation.
- Procedures mistakenly done on a pregnant mare—AI; intrauterine infusions; samples taken for cytology, culture, or biopsy.

RISK FACTORS

- Family history of twinning or noninfectious, spontaneous abortion.
- Breeds—Thoroughbred, draft mares, and Standardbreds.
- Higher spontaneous abortion rate in American Miniature Horse mares because of placental insufficiency and hyperlipemia.
- Age of >15 years.
- Systemic maternal disease.
- Grazing endophyte-infected fescue pastures or plants producing phytoestrogens (anecdotal) during late gestation.
- Exposure to xenobiotics.

DIAGNOSIS

- Most mares are "asymptomatic" before aborting.
- Fetus(es) in various states—fresh to autolytic
- Definitive diagnosis possible in ≅50%–60% of cases.
- Excluding twins and EHV-1, the diagnostic rate is only 30% if few samples are submitted and moderate to severe autolysis of fetal and placental tissues is present.

DIFFERENTIAL DIAGNOSIS

Other Causes of Abortion

- Infectious, spontaneous abortion—see specific topic.
- Evidence of an infectious cause of abortion in diagnostic workup.
- Placentitis on physical examination or laboratory diagnostic workup.

Other Causes of Signs of Labor or Abdominal Discomfort

- Normal parturition.
- Dystocia unassociated with abortion.
- Prepartum uterine artery rupture.
- Colic associated with uterine torsion.
- Discomfort associated with hydrops of fetal membranes or prepubic tendon rupture.
- Colic unassociated with reproductive disease.
- For details, refer to specific topics.

Other Causes of Vulvar Discharge

- Normal parturition
- Dystocia unassociated with abortion
- Normal estrus
- Endometritis
- Metritis or RFM
- Mucometra or pyometra
- For details, refer to specific topics.

CBC/BIOCHEMISTRY/URINALYSIS

May be indicated to determine presence of an inflammatory or stress leukocyte response or other organ system involvement.

OTHER LABORATORY TESTS

Maternal Progesterone

- Indicated with history of abortion or in an old mare with previous biopsy—endometritis or fibrosis.
- ELISA or RIA is useful <80 days of gestation; acceptable levels are >1 to >4 ng/mL, depending on the reference lab.
- After 100 days of gestation, RIA will detect both progesterone (may be very low after day 150) and cross-reacting 5α-pregnanes of uterofetoplacental origin.
- Decreased maternal levels of 5α-pregnanes are seen in cases of equine fescue toxicosis.

Maternal Estrogens

Reflections of fetal estrogen production and viability, especially conjugated estrogens—estrone sulfate.

Maternal T_3/T_4

- Anecdotal reports of lower levels in mares with history of conception failure, EED, or abortion.
- Significance of low T_4 levels is unknown at present.

Cytogenetic Studies

- If maternal chromosomal abnormalities are suspected.
- Difficult if fetus is autolyzed.

Maternal and Fetal Assays for Xenobiotics

- Indicated in cases of specific intoxications.
- Sample dam's whole-blood, plasma, or urine samples.
- Sample fetal serum from heart blood, thoracic or abdominal fluid, liver, and kidney.

Feed Analysis

Indicated for specific xenobiotics—ergopeptine alkaloids, phytoestrogens, heavy metals, or endophyte (*Neotyphodium coenophialum*).

ABORTION, SPONTANEOUS, NONINFECTIOUS

IMAGING

Transrectal and transabdominal ultrasonography to confirm pregnancy, diagnose twins, evaluate fetal viability and development, assess placental health, and diagnose other gestational abnormalities—hydrops of fetal membranes.

DIAGNOSTIC PROCEDURES

- If entire fetus and placenta are unavailable, collect appropriate samples for pathology, histology, culture, and serology.
- Samples—fresh/chilled fetal thoracic or abdominal fluid or fetal serum from fetal heart or cord blood (if available); fetal stomach contents; 10% formalin-fixed and chilled/frozen samples of fetal heart, lung, thymus, liver, kidney, lymph nodes, thymus, spleen, adrenal gland, skeletal muscle, and brain; 10% formalin-fixed and chilled/frozen fetal membranes (i.e., allantochorion and allantoamnion).
- Uterine swabs from dam may be useful to establish the diagnosis of placentitis.
- Unless the cause is obvious (e.g., twins, iatrogenic), rule out infectious causes of abortion, especially if multiple mares are at risk.

PATHOLOGIC FINDINGS

Twins

- Two fetuses, often dissimilar in size, with one generally mummified or severely autolyzed
- Avillous chorionic membrane at point of contact of two placentae.

Placental Abnormalities

- Umbilical cord torsion—evidence of vascular compromise must be present to confirm the diagnosis.
- Villous atrophy or hypoplasia may suggest endometrial fibrosis.
- Placental edema, gross and histopathologic, is consistent with equine fescue toxicosis.
- Hydrops allantois and amnion—gross diagnosis if dam suffers prepartum death.

Fetal Abnormalities

Developmental abnormalities—hydrocephalus; anencephaly; gross and histopathologic confirmation.

TREATMENT

APPROPRIATE HEALTH CARE

- Treatment is only recommended with early diagnosis of the pathologic process, before irreversible fetal or placental compromise occurs.
- Main therapeutic approach to twinning should be early selective reduction.
- Late-gestation diagnosis of twins—pregnancy may be maintained until term, in some instances, with progestin and antibiotic therapy.
- Mares with a history of abortion—evaluate and treat before rebreeding; progestin supplementation may be appropriate, especially with suspected luteal insufficiency (anecdotal) or early luteal regression, but this therapy is controversial and is contraindicated in some circumstances; ET may be indicated for mares with a history of repeated abortion.
- Signs of fescue toxicosis can be treated with D_2-dopamine receptor antagonists, but cases of abortion (i.e. stillbirth) frequently occur before commencement of therapy.
- Aborting mares generally only require "prophylactic" therapy for metritis or endometritis.
- Most patients can be dealt with on an ambulatory basis.
- Systemic maternal disease may warrant hospitalization and intensive care.

NURSING CARE

Most noninfectious abortions require limited nursing care, unless systemic disease develops.

ACTIVITY

Permit exercise in an area small enough to allow supervision.

DIET

N/A

CLIENT EDUCATION

Problem mares are likely to have future reproductive problems.

SURGICAL CONSIDERATIONS

N/A

MEDICATIONS

DRUGS OF CHOICE

See specific topics for recommendations.

History of Abortion, Endometritis, or Fibrosis

- These mares may be treated with altrenogest (0.044–0.088 mg/kg PO SID).
- Begin administration 2–3 days after ovulation or at diagnosis of pregnancy, and continue until at least 100 days of gestation.
- Taper the dose gradually during a 14-day period at end of treatment.

Altrenogest

- Administration may be started later during gestation, continued longer, or used for only short periods of time depending on serum progesterone levels during the first 80 days of gestation (>1 to >4 ng/mL), clinical circumstances, risk factors, and clinician preference.
- If used near term, altrenogest frequently is discontinued 7–14 days before the expected foaling date, unless otherwise indicated by assessment of fetal maturity/viability or if questions arise challenging the accuracy of the gestational age.

Domperidone

Begin (1.1 mg/kg PO SID) at the earliest recognition of signs of equine fescue toxicosis, and continue until parturition and development of normal mammary gland.

CONTRAINDICATIONS

- Limit use of altrenogest for prevention of abortion of a viable fetus and for noninfectious placentitis and endotoxemia.
- Monitor fetal viability at least weekly at first to avoid retaining a dead fetus in utero or aid in the development of pyometra.
- Altrenogest is absorbed through the skin; persons handling it should wear gloves and wash their hands.
- Success of supplemental progestin to maintain equine pregnancy is anecdotal.

ABORTION, SPONTANEOUS, NONINFECTIOUS

ALTERNATIVE DRUGS

- Injectable progesterone (150–500 mg, oil base) can be administered IM SID instead of the oral preparation.
- T_4 supplementation has been anecdotally successful in treating subfertile mares. Its use remains controversial, however, and some clinicians consider it to be deleterious.

FOLLOW-UP

PATIENT MONITORING

- At 7–10 days after abortion, use palpation, ultrasonography, or both to evaluate uterine involution.
- Rate of involution depends on the therapy used, presence of systemic disease, and secondary complications.
- Further examination may be appropriate—vaginal speculum, uterine cytology and culture, or endometrial biopsy

PREVENTION/AVOIDANCE

- Early recognition of at-risk mares
- Records of double ovulations
- Early twin diagnosis (<25 days, and as early as day 14 or 15) may be useful.
- Selective embryonic or fetal reduction
- Managing pre-existing endometritis before the next breeding
- Removal of mares from fescue pasture during last third of gestation (minimum of 30 days)
- Careful use of medications in pregnant mares
- Avoiding exposure to known toxicants

POSSIBLE COMPLICATIONS

- Uneventful recovery after many "asymptomatic" abortions
- Dystocia, RFM, metritis, laminitis, septicemia, endometritis, and reproductive tract trauma may impact the mare's future well-being and reproductive value.

EXPECTED COURSE AND PROGNOSIS

Uneventful recovery in most cases with appropriate treatment.

MISCELLANEOUS

ASSOCIATED CONDITIONS

- Abortion, spontaneous, infectious
- Dystocia
- Endometritis
- Fetal stress/distress/viability
- Placental insufficiency
- Placentitis
- Premature placental separation
- RFM
- Metritis

AGE-RELATED FACTORS

- Development of chronic endometritis and endometrial fibrosis
- Maiden American Miniature Horse mares

ZOONOTIC POTENTIAL

N/A

PREGNANCY

Condition is pregnancy-associated by definition.

SYNONYMS

N/A

SEE ALSO

- Abortion, spontaneous, infectious
- Dystocia
- Endometrial biopsy
- Endometritis
- Fetal stress/distress/viability
- High-risk pregnancy
- Hydrops amnion/allantois
- Metritis, postpartum
- Multiple ovulations
- Placental insufficiency
- Placentitis
- Premature placental separation
- Prepubic tendon rupture
- RFM
- Twin pregnancy

ABBREVIATIONS

- AI =
- CL = corpus luteum
- EED = early embryonic death
- EHV = equine herpes virus
- ELISA = enzyme-linked immunoadsorbent assay
- EPM = equine protozoal encephalomyelitis
- ET =
- RIA = radioimmunoassay
- RFM = retained fetal membranes/placenta
- T_3 = triiodothyronine
- T_4 = thyroxine

Suggested Reading

Ball BA, Daels PF. Early pregnancy loss in mares: application for progestin therapy. In: Robinson NE, ed. Current therapy in equine medicine 4. Philadelphia: WB Saunders, 1997:531–533.

Brendemuehl JP. Reproductive aspects of fescue toxicosis. In: Robinson NE, ed. Current therapy in equine medicine 4. Philadelphia: WB Saunders, 1997:571–573.

Giles RC, Donahue JM, Hong CG, et al. Causes of abortion, stillbirth, and perinatal death in 3,527 cases (1986–1991). J Am Vet Med Assoc 1993;208:1170–1175.

LeBlanc MM. Abortion. In: Colahan PT, Mayhew IG, Merritt AM, Moore JM, eds. Equine medicine and surgery. 5th ed. St. Louis: Mosby, 1999;2:1202–1207.

Author Tim J. Evans

Consulting Editor Carla L. Carleton

ACER RUBRUM (RED MAPLE) TOXICOSIS

BASICS

DEFINITION

An equine disease that follows ingestion of wilted or dried *Acer rubrum* (red maple) leaves and is characterized by methemoglobinemia, hemolytic anemia, and Heinz-body formation.

PATHOPHYSIOLOGY

- Clinical findings are consistent with oxidative injury to RBCs.
- The specific toxin has not been identified but, apparently, is found only in wilted or dried leaves, because the disease has not been induced using fresh leaves.
- The unknown oxidizing agent causes formation of methemoglobin (i.e., oxidation of iron in hemoglobin from ferrous to ferric form) and Heinz bodies (i.e., precipitated oxidized hemoglobin).

SYSTEMS AFFECTED

- Hematologic—methemoglobinemia, hemolytic anemia, and Heinz bodies.
- Renal—pigmenturia, hematuria, and proteinuria; renal failure secondary to hemoglobin deposition in the kidney.
- Cardiovascular—tachycardia secondary to anemia.
- Respiratory—polypnea secondary to anemia.
- Reproductive—abortion secondary to fetal hypoxia.

GENETICS

N/A

INCIDENCE/PREVALENCE

- Usually occurs during the summer and fall months.
- Most frequently reported in the eastern half of North America, where trees are more prevalent.

SIGNALMENT

Species

Horses and ponies

Breed Predilections

N/A

Mean Age and Range

N/A

Predominant Sex

N/A

SIGNS

General Comments

- Acute death can result from rapid formation of methemoglobin.
- Alternatively, hemolytic crisis can develop over several days as the hemolysis and methemoglobinemia progressively worsen.

Historical Findings

- Weakness
- Lethargy
- Anorexia
- Colic
- Fever

Physical Examination Findings

- Yellow or brown mucous membranes
- Red or brown urine
- Tachycardia
- Polypnea
- Dehydration

CAUSES

Ingestion of dried or wilted red maple leaves

RISK FACTORS

Toxicosis occurs after an event that results in leaf wilting—tree pruning, fallen branches after a storm, or autumn leaves falling.

DIAGNOSIS

DIFFERENTIAL DIAGNOSIS

- Hemolytic anemia accompanied by Heinz bodies or methemoglobinemia indicates oxidant toxicosis, the most common causes of which in horses are onions, red maple, and phenothiazine anthelmintics, which can only be differentiated by a history of ingestion.
- Without Heinz body or methemoglobin formation, consider all causes of equine hemolytic anemia—oxidants, EIA, immune-mediated, piroplasmosis, and liver failure.

CBC/BIOCHEMISTRY/URINALYSIS

- Interpretation of laboratory findings is difficult because of the hemolysis, with resultant discoloration of the serum and urine.
- Decreased PCV, hemoglobin, and erythrocyte count confirm anemia, whereas increased MCHC and MCH support intravascular hemolysis with hemoglobinemia.
- Heinz bodies are not present in all cases. They may be seen on routinely stained blood smears but are more apparent in new methylene blue–stained smears.
- Eccentrocytes and ghost cells have been reported.
- BUN and creatinine increase if acute renal failure results from pigment nephropathy.
- Increased albumin and total protein result from dehydration.
- Elevated liver enzymes and creatine phosphokinase probably result secondary to cell damage caused by anemia-induced hypoxia.
- Serum bilirubin, especially unconjugated bilirubin, is increased because of hemolytic anemia and inappetence.
- Urinalysis results include hemoglobinuria, with few or no intact erythrocytes, and proteinuria.

OTHER LABORATORY TESTS

The percentage of methemoglobin in the blood often is elevated.

IMAGING

N/A

DIAGNOSTIC PROCEDURES

N/A

PATHOLOGIC FINDINGS

Gross Findings

- Generalized icterus, enlarged spleen, and discolored kidneys.
- Petechiae and ecchymoses may be present on serosal surfaces.

Histopathologic Findings

- Erythrophagocytosis by macrophages, renal pigment casts and sloughed epithelial cells, splenic and hepatic hemosiderin, and centrilobular hepatic lipidosis.
- Pulmonary thrombosis has been reported in one horse.

ACER RUBRUM (RED MAPLE) TOXICOSIS

TREATMENT

APPROPRIATE HEALTH CARE
- The decision regarding inpatient or outpatient treatment depends on severity of the clinical signs and ability of the owner to care for the animal.
- Frequently monitor progression of the methemoglobinemia and anemia.

NURSING CARE
- IV fluids to replace fluid deficits and to maintain adequate renal perfusion.
- Blood transfusion may be needed with severe anemia.
- Continuous nasal oxygen administration may be helpful.

ACTIVITY
Limit physical activity of anemic animals.

DIET
Offer a high-quality diet, especially because affected horses often lack an appetite.

CLIENT EDUCATION
N/A

SURGICAL CONSIDERATIONS
N/A

MEDICATIONS

DRUGS OF CHOICE
Ascorbic acid has been used for its antioxidant effects (30–50 mg/kg BID added to IV fluids). It also can be given orally but may take several doses to achieve adequate tissue levels.

CONTRAINDICATIONS
Do not treat methemoglobinemia with methylene blue because of its poor efficacy in horses and reports that it may increase Heinz-body formation.

PRECAUTIONS
NSAIDs may be necessary to control pain but can compromise renal function.

POSSIBLE INTERACTIONS
N/A

ALTERNATIVE DRUGS
N/A

FOLLOW-UP

PATIENT MONITORING
Monitor methemoglobinemia and anemia, and adjust therapy based on the severity and speed of progression.

PREVENTION/AVOIDANCE
- Instruct owners not to plant red maples.
- Prune or remove existing trees only when no leaves are on the trees.
- Owners should check for fallen branches immediately after storms.

POSSIBLE COMPLICATIONS
N/A

EXPECTED COURSE AND PROGNOSIS
- Prognosis depends on the quantity of leaves ingested and how soon veterinary care is sought after ingestion.
- Death is attributed to severe methemoglobinemia or anemia or to renal failure after pigment nephropathy.

MISCELLANEOUS

ASSOCIATED CONDITIONS
Laminitis can occur during or after the course of the disease.

AGE-RELATED FACTORS
N/A

ZOONOTIC POTENTIAL
N/A

PREGNANCY
Anemia and methemoglobinemia can result in fetal hypoxia, followed by abortion.

SYNONYMS
N/A

SEE ALSO
N/A

ABBREVIATIONS
- EIA = equine infectious anemia
- MCH = mean corpuscular hemoglobin
- MCHC = mean corpuscular hemoglobin concentration
- PCV = packed cell volume

Suggested Reading

Semrad SD. Acute hemolytic anemia from ingestion of red maple leaves. Compend Contin Educ Pract Vet 1993;15:261–264.

Author Konstanze H. Plumlee
Consulting Editor Robert H. Poppenga

ACIDOSIS, METABOLIC

BASICS

DEFINITION

- A disruption of acid–base homeostasis producing increased H^+ concentration, which is reflected by acidemia—decreased pH and low plasma HCO_3^-.
- Normal equine plasma bicarbonate level is ≅24 mEq/L.
- Normal equine pH of arterial blood ranges from 7.35–7.45.
- Hyperventilation should lower CO_2 levels to increase pH; however, respiratory compensation is often incomplete.

PATHOPHYSIOLOGY

- Fixed acid is produced via normal metabolic processes in large quantities daily.
- The H^+ concentration is regulated by intracellular and extracellular buffering, respiratory buffering (i.e., regulation of CO_2 levels in blood via changes in ventilation), and regulation of HCO_3^- concentration in the blood via renal excretion of H^+.
- Renal H^+ excretion is accomplished by direct secretion of limited amounts of H^+, increased generation of ammonium ions, and titration to phosphates and urates (titratable acidity).
- Bicarbonate is reabsorbed when H^+ is secreted—90% occurs in the proximal tubule, with the rest in the distal nephron.
- Secretion of H^+ is limited by the minimum pH (4.5) of the tubular fluid.
- Titratable acidity increases minimally in acidotic patients.
- In most species, production of ammonia with subsequent excretion of ammonium ion is the major mechanism by which the kidney handles an acid load.
- Intracellular and extracellular buffering of H^+ occurs immediately or within minutes and is accomplished by proteins (primarily albumin and hemoglobin), phosphates, and bicarbonate.
- Carbonate storage in bone also is a significant site of intracellular buffering.
- The most important buffer is HCO_3^-, because it is present in high concentrations and the end product of its activity, CO_2, is readily eliminated by the lungs.
- Respiratory compensation responds within minutes and is effective for mild and moderate acidemia.
- Definitive regulation of H^+ and HCO_3^- levels is controlled by the kidney.
- Renal processing of an acid load begins within hours but may take days to normalize pH.
- Inability to excrete H^+, loss of bicarbonate, increased production of H^+ (i.e., lactic acidosis), and accumulation of acids are the major mechanisms producing equine metabolic acidosis.
- Hyperproteinemia (i.e., weak acids) and overhydration (i.e., dilutional acidosis) also produce metabolic acidosis via alterations of the balance between strong cations and anions in body fluids.

SYSTEMS AFFECTED

Respiratory

- Peripheral and central chemoreceptors sense low pH in blood or CSF and stimulate hyperventilation to increase elimination of CO_2 and increase pH.
- Decreased respiratory muscle strength can lead to muscle fatigue and worsening metabolic status, especially in neonates.

Cardiovascular

- Decreased cardiac contractility.
- May predispose to arrhythmias.
- Vasodilation of arterioles; constriction of veins.
- Vascular effects may be offset by catecholamine effects.

Neuroendocrine

- Catecholamine release
- CNS depression
- CSF acidosis in acute situations
- Vasodilation of cerebral vessels, resulting in increased cerebral blood flow and CSF pressure

Renal

- The kidney responds to low arterial pH by increasing H^+ excretion and generating increased levels of HCO_3^- to bring the systemic pH back to normal.
- This response begins within hours, but it may take days to be effective.

Metabolic

- Inhibition of anaerobic glycolysis
- Insulin resistance
- Decreased affinity of oxygen–hemoglobin binding
- Increased protein catabolism

SIGNALMENT

Equine of any type

SIGNS

- Historical and physical examination findings vary primarily with the underlying cause.
- Weakness, depression, and tachypnea are clinical signs specific to acidosis.

CAUSES

- Many diseases result in metabolic acidosis via more than one mechanism.
- Loss of bicarbonate most commonly is seen in horses with colitis; RTA results in HCO_3^- loss both directly and indirectly, depending on the type of tubular dysfunction.
- Renal failure produces inability to excrete H^+ and accumulation of uremic acids.
- Increased H^+ production (i.e., lactic acidosis) is seen with diseases producing decreased effective circulating blood volume—hypotension or hypovolemia caused by inadequate intake, hemorrhage, isotonic or hypotonic fluid loss or sequestration (e.g., uroperitoneum, peritonitis, pleuritis, ascites, nonstrangulating types of colic), strangulating lesions of the GI tract, endotoxemia, or cardiac failure.
- Chronic causes of hypoxemia also produce lactic acidosis.

ACIDOSIS, METABOLIC

- Grain overload produces metabolic acidosis via production of lactic acid, fluid sequestration in the GI tract, secretion into the GI tract, and endotoxemia.
- High-intensity anaerobic exercise results in short-term production of lactate, which can affect fluid balance/SID and result in metabolic acidosis.
- Severe exertional rhabdomyolysis associated with anaerobic exercise also produces lactic acidosis.
- Acute or end-stage hepatic failure may result in metabolic acidosis because of a variety of mechanisms, including failure by the detoxification systems of the liver.
- Asphyxial damage at parturition causes multiorgan damage or failure, which often results in metabolic acidosis in neonates.
- Accumulation of exogenous acids is uncommon in horses, because this usually is caused by ingestion of toxic substances but may be seen with salicylates, propylene or ethylene glycol, paraldehyde, and methanol.
- Malignant hyperthermia is uncommon but has occurred in anesthetized horses and results in lactic acidosis.
- Proteins are weak acids; conditions producing significant hyperproteinemia (e.g., chronic infection, immune-mediated disease, plasma cell myeloma, lymphoma) produce metabolic acidosis.
- Excessive or inappropriate fluid therapy, especially in neonates, produces free-water excess and dilutional acidosis.
- TPN can lead to metabolic acidosis when cationic (i.e., lysine, arginine) or sulfur-containing amino acids are metabolized, because H^+ is formed.
- Endotoxemia produces acidosis via several mechanisms—hypotension, decreased cardiac contractility, tissue ischemia, fluid shifts, hypoxemia, hepatic damage, and so on

RISK FACTORS

- Patients with chronic renal failure or chronic hypoxemia (i.e., COPD) may be at greater risk for acidosis with progression of their primary problem or if acid load develops for other reasons.
- Horses with HYPP on acetazolamide therapy may develop acidosis more readily, because acetazolamide is a carbonic anhydrase inhibitor causing increased HCO_3^- excretion.
- Highly anionic diets have been suggested to induce equine metabolic acidosis.

DIAGNOSIS

DIFFERENTIAL DIAGNOSIS

- Decreased bicarbonate levels also are seen in conditions involving chronic respiratory alkalosis.
- PCO_2 also is low in such conditions, but pH is close to normal or high.

LABORATORY FINDINGS

Drugs That May Alter Lab Results

- Excessive anticoagulant may falsely decrease results via dilution.
- Excessive sodium heparin may alter HCO_3^- levels, because it is an acidic compound.

Disorders That May Alter Lab Results

With poor peripheral perfusion or cardiovascular shunt, results of blood gas analysis on samples taken from peripheral vessels may differ from those taken elsewhere or not reflect the overall systemic condition.

Valid If Run in Human Lab?

Yes, if properly submitted.

CBC/BIOCHEMISTRY/URINALYSIS

- Measurement of serum electrolytes and protein levels is important to determine the cause and to guide treatment.
- Calculation of the anion gap also may be useful, especially in mixed acid–base disorders.
- Proportionate changes in sodium and chloride levels occur with alterations of fluid balance.
- Normal sodium levels with hypo- or hyperchloremia indicate acid–base imbalance.
- Disproportionate changes in Na^+/Cl^- usually are associated with simultaneous acid–base imbalance and hydration abnormalities.
- Albumin/protein levels are not considered when calculating the anion gap; however, because proteins are weak acids, hyperproteinemia can produce the condition—dehydration, chronic infection, and neoplasia.
- Many causes of acidosis can be distinguished on physical examination; urinalysis and fractional excretion of electrolytes are useful in cases of renal failure and RTA.

Affected Horses with Hyperchloremia and Normal AG

- Loss of HCO_3^-—diarrhea, type II RTA, and primary respiratory alkalosis; however, severely affected equine colitis patients often are acidotic and low in Na^+, K^+, Cl^-, and HCO_3^- because of water intake after isotonic fluid loss.
- Addition of Cl^-—fluid therapy with Cl^-–containing fluids (i.e., 0.9% NaCl, KCl), salt poisoning, TPN, NH_4Cl, or KCl supplementation.
- Cl^- retention—renal failure, type I or IV RTA, and acetazolamide therapy.

ACIDOSIS, METABOLIC

Affected Horses with Increased AG

Accumulation of unmeasured anions:

- Lactate—conditions producing hypovolemia or hypotension (e.g., shock, sepsis, cardiac failure, ischemic/inflammatory types of colic); conditions with inflammation or fluid sequestration (e.g., pleuritis, peritonitis, uroperitoneum, grain overload); conditions utilizing anaerobic glycolysis (e.g., anaerobic exercise, severe exertional rhabdomyolysis, malignant hyperthermia).
- Phosphates, sulfates, and organic acids—renal failure, toxic ingestion.

OTHER LABORATORY TESTS

Total CO_2:

- Measured by many labs using the same sample submitted for electrolytes.
- Closely approximates HCO_3^-, because most CO_2 is carried in the blood as bicarbonate.
- Low with metabolic acidosis; can be used in place of HCO_3^- or base excess/deficit.
- Respiratory alkalosis also decreases this measure; differentiation can only be made based on complete blood gas analysis.
- Analyze rapidly and with minimal room-air exposure within the sample tube, because CO_2 can dissipate from the sample.

IMAGING

Diagnosis of cardiac, renal, and hepatic failure can be facilitated via ultrasonography.

DIAGNOSTIC PROCEDURES

Biopsy for suspected organ failure and cytology and microbiology of exudates or effusions may be useful with inflammation or infection.

TREATMENT

- Directed at the primary cause.
- Replacement of fluid losses with balanced isotonic fluids may be all that is needed to restore acid–base status in mild cases.
- With hypovolemia caused by hemorrhage, hypertonic saline, colloids, or blood transfusion may be necessary to restore effective circulating volume.
- Address specific electrolyte losses; massive volumes may be needed in some cases with colitis.

MEDICATIONS

DRUGS OF CHOICE

- Treatment with alkalinizing agents is reserved for patients with severe bicarbonate loss, severe lactic acidosis, or organic acidoses with a pH <7.2.
- Sodium bicarbonate is most frequently utilized.
- The deficit can be calculated as follows: Base deficit × body weight (kg) × 0.3 (ECF space [0.5 in foals]) = HCO_3^- (mEq).
- A negative BE (or 24 − (total CO_2 or HCO_3^-]) can be used for the base deficit.
- In acute cases, half this deficit can be given safely over 30–45 minutes, either in fluids or as a 5% solution to adults.
- Isotonic bicarbonate (1.3%) is a good choice in neonates or severely affected adults with colitis.
- Correction to a pH >7.2 and BE better than -5 usually is all that is necessary, especially with organic acidoses, because these are metabolized (resulting in increased HCO_3^-) once the primary problem improves.

CONTRAINDICATIONS

Sodium bicarbonate cannot be mixed with calcium.

PRECAUTIONS

- Use bicarbonate therapy very cautiously in patients with respiratory compromise, because the increased CO_2 that is generated may not be eliminated, causing a further decrease in pH.
- Hyperosmolar solutions may cause vascular irritation and affect tonicity of the CSF.
- Sodium load may affect blood volume in neonates and patients with compromised renal or cardiac function.
- Rebound alkalosis or cerebral acidosis may result from overdose or too-rapid administration of bicarbonate.

POSSIBLE INTERACTIONS

Sodium bicarbonate may combine with Ca^{2+} in calcium-containing solutions and form a potentially harmful precipitate.

ALTERNATIVE DRUGS

• Replacement IV fluid solutions containing other alkalinizing agents (e.g., lactate, citrate) can be used, because these are metabolized to HCO_3^-. Adequate hepatic function must be present, however, so these may not be useful in severely acidotic, hypoxemic, or septic patients.
• Oral rehydration solutions (1–2 gallons PO q3–h in adults without ileus) have been used as primary therapy or an adjunct to IV fluid therapy.

FOLLOW-UP

PATIENT MONITORING

Serial blood gas analysis is very important in evaluating efficacy of therapy and should be repeated within a few hours of initial treatment and thereafter according to patient response.

POSSIBLE COMPLICATONS

• Electrolyte abnormalities—hyperkalemia
• Cardiac arrhythmias
• Severe, untreated metabolic acidosis with a pH <7.0 may result in death.

MISCELLANEOUS

ASSOCIATED CONDITIONS

• Hyperchloremia
• Hyperkalemia
• Respiratory alkalosis

AGE-RELATED CONDITIONS

• Asphyxia during parturition in neonates of any gestational age
• Conditions associated with premature neonates.

ZOONOTIC POTENTIAL

N/A

PREGNANCY

Severe metabolic acidosis may decrease uterine blood flow and result in placental insufficiency.

SYNONYMS

Nonrespiratory acidosis

SEE ALSO

• Causes of colitis
• RTA

ABBREVIATIONS

• AG = anion gap
• BE = base excess
• COPD = chronic obstructive pulmonary disease
• CSF = cerebrospinal fluid
• ECF = extracellular fluid
• GI = gastrointestinal
• HYPP = hyperkalemic periodic paraparalysis
• RTA = renal tubular acidosis
• SID = strongion difference
• TPN = total parenteral nutrition

Suggested Reading

Carlson GP. Fluid, electrolyte, and acid–base balance. In: Kaneko JJ, Harvey JW, Bruss ML, eds. Clinical biochemistry of domestic animals. 5th ed. San Diego: Academic Press, 1997:485–516.

McGinness GS, Mansmann RA, Breuhaus BA. Nasogastric electrolyte replacement in horses. Compend Contin Educ Pract Vet 1996;18:942–951.

Muir WW, de Morais HSA. Acid–base balance: traditional and modified approaches. In: Thurmon JC, Tranquilli WJ, Benson GJ, eds. Lumb & Jones' veterinary anesthesia. 3rd ed. Baltimore: Williams & Wilkins, 1996:558–571.

Author Jennifer G. Adams
Consulting Editor Claire B. Andreasen

ACIDOSIS, RESPIRATORY

BASICS

DEFINITION

- Increase in blood P_{CO_2}.
- Homeostatic mechanisms maintain normal blood levels within a narrow range.
- Arterial levels range from 35–42 mm Hg.
- Venous levels range from 43–49 mm Hg.

PATHOPHYSIOLOGY

- CO_2 is formed in all tissues during metabolic energy production and diffuses passively out of cells and into the blood in gaseous form.
- Most of this CO_2 (65–70%) combines with water almost instantaneously to form carbonic acid, which then dissociates into bicarbonate ion and hydrogen.
- Most CO_2 is transported in the blood as bicarbonate. Some is bound to proteins, especially deoxygenated hemoglobin, and a small amount is dissolved directly into plasma.
- In the lungs, the reverse occurs, and CO_2 passively diffuses out of capillaries into the alveoli.
- The three forms of CO_2 exist in equilibrium in the blood, but the P_{CO_2} as measured by blood gases depends on the dissolved portion.
- The chemical components of the carbonic acid equilibrium are:
$CO_2 + H_2O = H_2CO_3 = H^+ + HCO_{3-}$
- Alveolar CO_2 then is removed mechanically by ventilation as air moves in and out of the lungs.
- Hypercapnia is present only when tissue production exceeds the capacity of normal lungs to eliminate CO_2 or when components of the respiratory system are abnormal.
- Hypercapnia is uncommon in conscious patients, because the respiratory center responds to even minor abnormalities by increasing minute ventilation.
- Respiratory acidosis results from disease or alteration of the respiratory center in the medulla and peripheral chemoreceptors that control respiration, the mechanical components (i.e., chest wall, respiratory muscles), or the conducting airways, alveoli, and pulmonary vasculature, which are directly involved in gas exchange, by causing hypoventilation, barriers to diffusion, or V/Q mismatching.
- Because CO_2 diffuses very readily across the respiratory membrane in direct proportion to ventilation, hypoventilation usually has the most significant effect on blood levels.
- Hypermetabolism, as seen with malignant hyperthermia, may produce CO_2 in greater amounts than the lung can eliminate.
- Increased CO_2 also develops as a compensatory response of the lungs to metabolic alkalosis.

SYSTEM AFFECTED

Respiratory—see *Pathophysiology.*

SIGNALMENT

- Any horse.
- Almost every anesthetized patient develops some degree of hypercapnia when breathing spontaneously.
- Because of their size, equine are especially predisposed to hypoventilation under anesthesia.

SIGNS

Historical Findings

- Respiratory noise may heard, especially with exercise, in cases of upper airway obstruction.
- Exercise intolerance may be reported with many causes.

Physical Examination Findings

- None if minute ventilation is increased via increased tidal volume; if not, tachypnea may be present.
- Anesthetized animals with very high levels of CO_2 may have increased rate or depth of respiration.
- Decrease or absence of airway sounds may be found at auscultation in cases with damage or disease of the chest wall or thorax.
- Abnormal sounds may be present with pulmonary disease.

CAUSES

- Nasal edema, cysts, mass lesions, or infection of the paranasal sinuses; laryngeal or pharyngeal paralysis; soft-palate displacement; pharyngeal or epiglottal cysts; and tracheal masses or collapse all cause upper airway obstruction and impede airflow into the lungs.
- Injury or disease of the thorax, diaphragm, or pleura may restrict movement of the chest wall or respiratory muscles or lead to atelectasis because of fluid, blood, air, or intestinal organs in the pleural space.
- Uroperitoneum, diseases producing portal hypertension (e.g., cardiac or liver failure), and other diseases that result in large volumes of peritoneal fluid also may restrict diaphragmatic movement. Some may lead to pleural effusion as well.
- Displacement or distention of the intestine can restrict diaphragmatic movement.
- Weakness or paralysis of the respiratory muscles can be seen with neurologic dysfunction—encephalitis, botulism, tetanus, cranial or spinal trauma, and so on.
- Severe cases of pulmonary disease (e.g., viral, bacterial, or interstitial pneumonias), allergic small airway disease, and COPD affect gas exchange, ventilation, and diffusion.

ACIDOSIS, RESPIRATORY

• Hypoventilation caused by lung collapse, muscle relaxation, and decreased sensitivity of the respiratory centers to CO_2 occurs in all anesthetized horses. Heavy sedation also may produce temporary hypercapnia via muscle relaxation and respiratory center insensitivity.
• Exhaustion of the CO_2 absorbent, improper ventilator settings, or improper set up of the breathing system can lead to hypercapnia under anesthesia as well.
• Pregnant animals are more prone to hypoventilation under anesthesia because of abdominal distention from the pregnant uterus.
• Defective cellular metabolism of muscle is seen with malignant hyperthermia. This syndrome is very rare but has been seen in horses with inhalant anesthesia or succinyl choline administration. Abnormal metabolic processes in muscle cells are triggered, resulting in tremendous production of heat and CO_2, such that elimination mechanisms are overwhelmed and respiratory acidosis results.
• Anaerobic exercise produces temporary respiratory acidosis, because ventilation is limited when chest wall movement is linked to stride at high speeds.

RISK FACTORS

• General anesthesia; heavy sedation.
• Pregnancy, which increases the volume of abdominal contents and may predispose to hypercapnia under anesthesia.
• Prolonged recumbency.
• History of malignant hyperthermia in related individuals.
• Prematurity, dystocia, asphyxia or sepsis, persistent fetal circulation, or pulmonary hypertension in neonates.

DIAGNOSIS

DIFFERENTIAL DIAGNOSIS

• Physiologic states or disease processes that present with tachypnea—fever, hyperthermia, excitement, anxiety, painful conditions, hypoxemia, metabolic acidosis, and CNS derangements.
• Under anesthesia, tachypnea also may result from a light plane of anesthesia, hypoxemia, metabolic acidosis, or faulty anesthetic rebreathing systems.
• Diseases resulting in metabolic alkalosis may have a compensatory hypercapnia—upper GI obstruction, early large colon impactions or simple obstructions, supplementation with bicarbonate or other alkalinizing agents. Measurements of pH in these cases often are still higher than normal, because compensatory hypoventilation is limited once hypoxemia develops.

LABORATORY FINDINGS

Drugs That May Alter Lab Results

N/A

Disorders That May Alter Lab Results

• With poor peripheral perfusion or cardiovascular shunt, results of blood gas analysis on samples taken from peripheral vessels may differ from those taken elsewhere or not reflect the overall systemic condition.
• Exposure to room air via air bubbles in the sample may change the P_{CO_2} level, because the sample equilibrates with the air.
• Cellular metabolism of RBCs continues after sampling; if not measured quickly, CO_2 levels may be falsely elevated.

Valid If Run in Human Lab?

Yes, if properly submitted.

CBC/BIOCHEMISTRY/URINALYSIS

N/A

OTHER LABORATORY TESTS

• Arterial blood gas analysis is necessary to evaluate adequacy of ventilation and gas exchange and to document hypercapnia.
• Handheld analyzers are available and easy to use, and some require only small amounts of whole blood. Otherwise, syringes should be heparinized before sampling.
• Perform sampling anaerobically. Immediately evacuate any air bubbles, and cap the needle with a rubber stopper.
• Perform analysis within 15–20 minutes. If not possible, samples can be stored on ice, and results will be valid for 3–4 hours.

IMAGING

N/A

DIAGNOSTIC PROCEDURES

• Capnography or capnometry to measure CO_2 indirectly from expired gases.
• Samples of end-tidal gases reflect arterial P_{CO_2} levels, because this gas is essentially alveolar gas.
• Continuous monitoring on anesthetized or ventilated patients.
• V/Q mismatch is always present in anesthetized or recumbent patients, and end-tidal levels may underestimate arterial levels by ≅10–15 mm Hg.

ACIDOSIS, RESPIRATORY

TREATMENT

• Emergency therapy occasionally may be necessary for upper airway obstructions—passage of a nasotracheal tube or tracheotomy.
• Definitive therapy for hypercapnia involves resolution of the primary disease process affecting ventilation, diffusion, or gas exchange; improvement of ventilation usually is most effective.
• Avoid excessive anesthetic depth. Lightening of anesthesia may improve ventilation and decrease PCO_2 levels. If depth is adequate, controlled ventilation is necessary when hypoventilation is severe (i.e., >60 mm Hg).
• In neonates, postural therapy and coupage may improve gas exchange. Improvement of overall status, especially cardiovascular and neurologic, may improve respiratory function dramatically.
• With severe lung disease, treat hypercapnia with controlled ventilation. This generally is not feasible in adults, but neonates respond well. Heavy sedation or muscle relaxant therapy may be necessary in some individuals; however, most relax once respiratory function improves.

MEDICATIONS

DRUGS OF CHOICE

Doxapram

• A respiratory stimulant that may be a useful adjunct (0.5–1 mg/kg IV or an infusion of 0.02–0.05 mg/kg per minute) in emergency resuscitation and some patients, especially foals with neurologic or muscular weakness.
• Anesthetized patients who are breathing poorly may respond temporarily to its effects, but controlled ventilation, decreasing depth, and anesthetic reversal are more specific and appropriate therapies.
• Not indicated for healthy patients being weaned from controlled ventilation.

Other Drugs

Anti-inflammatory therapy with corticosteroids or bronchodilator therapy with α_2-agonists or xanthine derivatives may be useful in patients with allergic airway disease and COPD once environmental factors are controlled.

CONTRAINDICATIONS

• Controlled ventilation may cause barotrauma in foals with meconium aspiration.
• Partial obstruction of the small airways may lead to air-trapping in alveoli, which may rupture.

PRECAUTIONS

• Monitor ventilated patients continuously for airway obstruction caused by accumulation of secretions, kinking of tubing, hoses, and so on.
• Oxygen toxicity can develop with inspired PO_2 >50% or if PaO_2 >100 mm Hg is maintained for prolonged periods (10–12 hours).

POSSIBLE INTERACTIONS

N/A

ALTERNATIVE DRUGS

N/A

FOLLOW-UP

PATIENT MONITORING

• Decreased respiratory effort should be seen quickly after improvement of ventilation.
• Use serial arterial blood gas analysis or capnometry to assess adequacy of ventilation and monitor progress, especially during weaning.

ACIDOSIS, RESPIRATORY

POSSIBLE COMPLICATIONS

- Respiratory acidosis lowers systemic pH and may affect ionization of protein-bound drugs.
- Acidosis decreases heart contractility and may cause or contribute to CNS depression.
- Hypercapnia and the resultant acidosis predispose patients to cardiac arrhythmias, especially under anesthesia.
- The $PaCO_2$ level greatly affects cerebral blood flow and CSF pressure.
- Severe or prolonged hypercapnia may contribute to brain damage or herniation in cases with head trauma.

MISCELLANEOUS

ASSOCIATED CONDITIONS

Disorders that result in metabolic alkalosis

AGE-RELATED FACTORS

Neonates, especially premature foals, may be more prone to hypercapnia because of decreased compliance of the lungs and lack of strength (i.e., immaturity) of the chest wall.

ZOONOTIC POTENTIAL

N/A

PREGNANCY

See *Risk Factors.*

SYNONYM

- Hypercapnia
- Hypercarbia
- Hypoventilation

SEE ALSO

See specific diseases in *Causes.*

ABBREVIATIONS

- COPD = chronic obstructive pulmonary disease
- CSF = cerebrospinal fluid
- GI = gastrointestinal
- V/Q = ventilation/perfusion

Suggested Reading

Coons TJ, Kosch PC, Cudd TA. Respiratory care. In: Koterba AM, Drummond WA, Kosch PC, eds. Equine clinical neonatology. Philadelphia: Lea & Febiger, 1990:200–239.

Section VII: Respiration. In: Guyton AC, ed. Medical physiology. 9th ed. Philadelphia: WB Saunders, 1992:465–526.

Palmer JE. Ventilatory support of the neonatal foal. Vet Clin North Am Equine Pract 1994;10:167–186.

Weinberger SE, Schwartzstein RM, Weiss JW. Hypercapnia. N Engl J Med 1989;321:1223–1231.

West JB. Respiratory physiology—the essentials. 5th ed. Baltimore: Williams & Wilkins, 1995.

Soma LR. Equine anesthesia: causes of reduced oxygen tension and increased carbon dioxide tensions. Compend Contin Educ Pract Vet 1980;2:S57–S63.

Author Jennifer G. Adams
Consulting Editor Claire B. Andreasen

ACTINOBACILLOSIS

BASICS

OVERVIEW

• Acute rapidly progressive septicemia due to *Actinobacillus equuli* or *A. suis*-like organisms in neonatal foals.
• *Actinobacillus equuli* is a gram-negative coccobacillary to rod-shaped pleomorphic organism that produces flat gray 1–3 mm colonies after 24-hr incubation on blood agar. *Actinobacillus equuli* is a normal inhabitant of the mucous membranes of the alimentary tract.
• Fetal infection may follow transplacental infection. The kidneys are a frequent site of neonatal infection.
• In adults, infection is frequently endogenous and results from fecal contamination or spread from oral mucous membranes. Adults have soft tissue abscesses, respiratory infections, and rarely conjunctival, urinary tract, joint, guttural pouch, skin, and genital tract infections.

SIGNALMENT

• Foals less than 2 days of age.
• Adults of any age and use.

SIGNS

Foals

• Acute onset, depression, diarrhea, recumbency, distended painful joints, sudden death.
• Fever may not be present and foals may be hypothermic. If left untreated, foals may progress rapidly to septic shock.
• Bone and joint infections in neonates may not be obvious for days to weeks and may be unaccompanied by signs of systemic disease.

Adults

Signs are generally referable to the affected organ system.

CAUSES AND RISK FACTORS

Foals

• Commonly seen associated with failure of passive transfer of immunoglobulins. Perinatal stress, prematurity, and/or unsanitary environmental conditions may predispose the foal.
• Portals of entry include respiratory tract, gastrointestinal tract, placenta, and umbilical remnant.

Adults

• Pneumonia and pleuropneumonia may develop secondary to viral infection or stressful events including but not limited to general anesthesia, athletic events, transport over prolonged distance, and other environmental stressors and concurrent illnesses.
• Trauma may predispose to abscess formation.

DIAGNOSIS

DIFFERENTIAL DIAGNOSIS

Foals

• Any other cause of neonatal sepsis including bacterial, viral, and fungal causes.
• Gram-negative organisms are the most common bacterial agents isolated in cases of neonatal sepsis, although infections with only gram-positive pathogens have been reported.
• Foals with equine herpes virus type-1 and equine viral arteritis infections may appear identical to foals with bacterial infection.
• Foals suffering perinatal hypoxic ischemic anoxic insult may present with nearly identical clinical signs, depending on severity.

Adults

• Any other bacterial, viral, or fungal agent causing pneumonia or pleuropneumonia.
• Other causes of respiratory distress, fever, coughing, and nasal discharge should be considered, including:
  • sinusitis
  • guttural pouch empyema
  • chronic obstructive pulmonary disease
  • small airway inflammatory disease
  • interstitial pneumonia
  • mycoplasma infections
  • neoplasia
  • dysphagia

CBC/BIOCHEMISTRY/URINALYSIS

Foals

• Leukocytosis or leukopenia.
• Hyperfibrinogenemia is occasionally present with *in utero* infections.
• Increased creatinine and/or blood urea nitrogen with renal involvement.
• Metabolic acidosis, hypoxemia, and hypercapnia may be observed with foals in septic shock.
• Hypoglycemia may be present.
• Frequent complete or partial failure of passive transfer (serum IgG < 800 mg/dL).
• Urinalysis may be abnormal with renal involvement.

Adults

• Leukocytosis and hyperfibrinogenemia possible.
• Low PCV in longstanding infection due to anemia of chronic disease.
• Other abnormalities, depending on body system involved.

OTHER LABORATORY TESTS

N/A

IMAGING

Foals

- Thoracic radiographs may demonstrate pulmonary involvement. Radiographs of affected joints.
- Ultrasonographic examination of the umbilical remnant may demonstrate focal infection. Ultrasonographic examination of kidneys may be abnormal.

Adults

Radiographic and ultrasonographic evaluation of affected body system may be beneficial.

OTHER DIAGNOSTIC PROCEDURES

Foals

- Blood culture may be diagnostic.
- Kidneys frequently have multifocal microabscesses at post-mortem examination.

Adults

- Culture of affected body system may be diagnostic.
- Culture and cytology of trans-tracheal aspirates and thoracocentesis fluids may be diagnostic. Because *A. equuli* is normal inhabitant of equine gastointestinal mucosa, results should be interpreted cautiously.

TREATMENT

Foals

Affected foals are quite ill and are best managed in a hospital. Intranasal oxygen supplementation as needed.

MEDICATIONS

DRUG(S) OF CHOICE

Foals

- Administer isotonic polyionic balanced fluids or 0.9% NaCl to maintain adequate hydration and fluid balance. Intravenous plasma as required based on serum IgG levels.
- Intravenous dextrose or TPN as needed for nutritional management.
- Broad spectrum antimicrobial therapy, gentamicin 8 mg/kg IV SID or amikacin 25–30 mg/kg IV SID and potassium penicillin 10,000 IV/kg IV QID or ceftiofur sodium 10 mg/kg IV QID.
- Foals with SIRS or MODS may require more intensive fluid management and pressor therapy.
- Foals with severe respiratory disturbance may require assisted ventilation.

Adults

Antimicrobial therapy based on culture and sensitivity results.

CONTRAINDICATIONS/POSSIBLE INTERACTIONS

N/A

MISCELLANEOUS

Antimicrobial therapy should be modified based on response and culture/sensitivity results. Therapeutic monitoring of aminoglycoside levels should be performed. Continue treatment until white blood count, differential, and fibrinogen are within normal limits for 48 hr.

ABBREVIATIONS

- SIRS = systemic inflammatory response
- MODS = multiple organ dysfunction syndrome
- TPN = total parenteral nutrition

Suggested Reading

Sternberg S. Isolation of *Actinobacillus equuli* from the oral cavity of healthy horses and comparison of isolates by restriction enzyme digestion and pulsed field electrophoresis. Vet Microbiol 1998, 59(2-3):147-156.

Carr EA, Carlson GP, Wilson WD, Read DH. Acute hemorrhagic pulmonary infarction and necrotizing pneumonia in horses:21 cases (1967–1993). J Am Vet Med Assoc, 1997, 210(12):1774-1778.

Raisis AL, Hodgson JL, Hodgson DR. Equine neonatal septicemia: 24 cases. Aust Vet J, 1996, 73(4):137-140.

Nelso KM, Darien BJ, Konkle DM, Hartmann FA. *Actinobacillus suis* septicaemia in two foals. Vet Rec, 1996, 138(2):39-40.

Author Pamela A. Wilkins

Consulting Editor Corinne R. Sweeney

ACUTE ABDOMINAL PAIN

BASICS

DEFINITION

- Discomfort or pain that can be localized to the abdominal cavity, often manifesting as anorexia, lying down frequently, pawing, rolling in dorsal recumbency, grunting, grinding teeth, abdominal distention, and salivation.
- Also known as *colic.*

PATHOPHYSIOLOGY

- Events leading to colic in foals—enteritis and enterocolitis resulting from specific GI pathogens; ileus and GI dysmotility resulting from hypoxic ischemic asphyxia syndrome; septicemia; meconium impaction; intestinal accidents, including intussusception and small intestinal volvulus; intestinal incarceration in inguinal or umbilical hernia; ruptured bladder; and gastroduodenal ulceration.
- Certain causes in foals are fairly well restricted to specific are groups—meconium impaction in newborns; ascarid impaction in weanlings.

SYSTEMS AFFECTED

- Usually the GI system.
- The urinary tract may be involved in certain specific causes—uroperitoneum associated with ruptured bladder or urachus.

SIGNALMENT

- Foals <1 year.
- Any breed or sex.
- Some diseases (e.g., ruptured bladder) more commonly occur in certain age and sex groups.

SIGNS

General Comments

- Foals are not stoic and react strongly even to low-grade pain; therefore, unlike adults, degree of pain cannot be used reliably to distinguish medical from surgical causes of colic.
- Depression and unwillingness to stand also may be primary presenting complaints for foals with serious abdominal disease.

Historical Findings

- History varies with the underlying disease.
- A complete history aids in establishing an accurate diagnosis and ensuring proper treatment.
- Foals with impending enteritis may have histories of fever, anorexia, and depression.
- Foals with a ruptured urinary bladder generally present at 2–5 days of age with a history of apparent straining to urinate and slow, mild to moderate abdominal distention.
- Foals with meconium impaction present at <5 days of age, and generally at <2 days of age, with a history of straining to defecate, progressive abdominal distention, and increasing pain. Owners may confuse such foals with those suffering from urinary bladder rupture.

Physical Examination Findings

- Examination of the dam may reveal udder engorgement, and the dam may stream milk, indicating the foal has not been eating.
- Foals frequently may stand and lie down, roll, paw, lie in dorsal recumbency, and strain to defecate or urinate.
- Tachycardia frequently is present, as is tachypnea.
- Dyspnea may be observed in foals with severe abdominal distention.
- Some foals may grunt audibly.
- A few foals may spontaneously reflux; others may have diarrhea.
- Foals with gastric ulceration may demonstrate bruxism and ptyalism.
- Fever is variable.
- Abdominal distention frequently is observed.
- Borborygmi may be absent, decreased, or increased, depending on the cause.
- Foals may be depressed.
- Dehydration is variable but usually present.
- Intestine may be palpable within scrotal, inguinal, or umbilical hernias.

CAUSES

Infectious Causes

- Viral—rotavirus, coronavirus, equine herpes virus 1, equine viral arteritis, and adenovirus
- Bacterial—salmonellosis, *Clostridium perfringes, Clostridium difficile, Escherichia coli, Actinobacillus equlli, Rhodococcus equi, Streptococcus equi* var *zooepidemicus* or var *equi*, or any bacteria resulting in neonatal septicemia.
- Parasitic—*Stongyloides westerii, Parasacaris equorum*, and small strongyles.

Noninfectious Causes

- Rupture of the urinary bladder
- Hypoxic ischemic asphyxial insult to the intestine
- Lethal white syndrome—GI aganglionosis in the progeny of overo parents carrying the recessive gene
- Gastroduodenal ulceration
- Right dorsal colitis
- Pyloric stenosis
- Small intestinal obstruction—feed impaction, ascarid impaction, duodenal stricture, intussusception, ileocecal intussusception, segmental volvulus, and scrotal, inguinal, or umbilical hernia
- Large intestinal obstruction—meconium impaction, feed impaction, fecalith impaction, displacement, and strangulation of the large colon
- Small colon impaction

RISK FACTORS

Dystocia, high-risk pregnancy, maternal illness, poor management, unsanitary conditions, overcrowding, concurrent illness, antimicrobial treatment, and treatment with NSAIDs may increase the incidence of different types of colic—enteritis; gastric ulcers.

DIAGNOSIS

DIFFERENTIAL DIAGNOSIS

- Other causes of depression or anorexia—CNS depression resulting from hypoxic ischemic asphyxia syndrome, bacterial meningitis, sepsis, or trauma.
- Other causes of increased recumbency—CNS depression resulting from hypoxic ischemic asphyxia syndrome, bacterial meningitis, sepsis, trauma, white muscle disease, spinal cord trauma, vertebral body abscess, joint sepsis, or botulism.
- Other causes of ptyalism and bruxism—dysphagia associated with white muscle disease, sepsis, botulism, cranial nerve dysfunction resulting from trauma, sepsis, hypoxic ischemic asphyxia syndrome, or cleft palate.
- Oral candidiasis; oral foreign body.
- Other causes of abdominal distention—ileus associated with botulism, abdominal mass, especially abscess resulting from *R. equi*, parasitism, or high-roughage diet.
- Other causes of tachypnea—pneumonia, pain from extra-abdominal sources, "idiopathic" tachypnea, anxiety, high ambient temperature, or centrally driven tachypnea.

CBC/SERUM BIOCHEMISTRY/ URINALYSIS

- Inflammatory or stress leukogram is usual—foals with sepsis (i.e., bacterial/viral) may be leukopenic; diarrheic foals may be leukopenic.
- Hyperfibrinogenemia with infectious causes of >2 days of duration; hypofibrinogenemia with protein-losing enteropathy or DIC.
- Increased creatinine/BUN in foals with ruptured urinary bladder, dehydration, or acute renal failure.
- Hyponatremia, hypochloremia, and hyperkalemia in foals with ruptured urinary bladder, acute renal failure, or profound enterocolitis.
- Increased GGT is possible in foals with gastroduodenal ulceration and enteritis.

OTHER LABORATORY TESTS

Infectious Causes

- Fecal culture to identify GI pathogens—*Salmonella* sp. and *Clostridia* sp.; testing for toxins of *C. difficile* and *C. perfringen* is recommended.
- Fecal examination for parasites—interpret with caution, because many foals with parasitic problems are in the prepatent period for the parasite and not shedding oocysts; a negative result does not necessarily rule out parasitism.

Noninfectious Causes

Creatinine measured in abdominal fluid—foals with ruptured urinary bladder have significantly higher creatinine values in peritoneal fluid than in peripheral blood.

IMAGING

Abdominal Radiography

- May demonstrate gas-distended large or small intestine.
- Visualization of large quantities of meconium in large and small colon in cases of meconium impaction.
- Loss of radiographic detail in cases of excess fluid with uroperitoneum.
- Mass may be seen with abdominal abscessation.
- Pneumotosis intestinalis may be observed with intestinal clostridiosis and hypoxic ischemic asphyxia syndrome; this change is seen most easily in a horizontal-beam, ventrodorsal view obtained with the foal in lateral recumbency.
- Free gas in the abdomen sometimes can be visualized and indicates a ruptured viscus, most often a gastric perforation secondary to gastric ulcers.
- Decreased gastric emptying time (>1 hour) during barium studies in foals with duodenal obstruction resulting from gastroduodenal ulceration.

Abdominal Ultrasonography

Particularly useful in cases of ruptured urinary bladder, intussusception, and abdominal abscessation.

DIAGNOSTIC PROCEDURES

- Nasogastric intubation—significant gastric reflux supports anatomic or functional obstruction; character of obtained fluid may support gastroduodenal ulceration (e.g., acidic, hemorrhagic, "coffee ground–like" sediment) or lower small intestinal obstruction (e.g., alkaline, bile tinged).
- Digital rectal examination—may confirm hard meconium in the distal rectum, thus supporting a diagnosis of meconium impaction.
- Abdominocentesis—increased protein and cell numbers indicate an inflammatory process. Serosanguinuous fluid is consistent with a strangulating lesion, and creatinine in the fluid is increased with urinary bladder rupture. Culture of abdominocentesis fluid is indicated with suspected sepsis or abdominal abscess.
- Abdominal palpation—may reveal a mass (i.e., abscess) or meconium-filled colon.

ACUTE ABDOMINAL PAIN

TREATMENT

- Based on the inciting cause.
- Refer foals with severe disease that do not respond readily to conservative medical management to a hospital prepared to provide 24-hour nursing care and surgical intervention if necessary.
- Surgical correction is required for ruptured urinary bladder, intussusception, intestine incarcerated within a hernia, displacement of large and small intestine, and duodenal stricture. Meconium impactions that do not respond to medical management also may require surgery.
- Intranasal oxygen insufflation is beneficial in almost all cases; administer if available.
- IV fluid support is necessary in many cases; balanced polyionic fluids generally are useful. Most foals with acute abdominal pain are poorly hydrated and may have metabolic acidosis secondary to poor perfusion. Shock boluses of fluids (20 mL/kg over 20 minutes, then re-evaluate) may be necessary.
- Acid–base and electrolyte values may be deranged. Monitor closely, and correct abnormalities judiciously through respiratory support if necessary and fluid therapy.
- Neonatal foals that are held off feed or have not been sucking may require dextrose supplementation (4–8 mg/kg per min). Monitor glucose levels. Foals requiring long periods of GI rest should receive TPN.
- Consider drainage of abdominal urine by catheter or teat cannula in cases of ruptured urinary bladder.

MEDICATIONS

DRUGS OF CHOICE

- Torbugesic (0.1 mg/kg IV or IM) is useful for analgesia in foals. Xylazine also may be used but decreases GI motility.
- Consider broad-spectrum antimicrobials in all cases—amikacin (20–25 mg/kg IV SID) and ampicillin (15–20 mg/kg IV or IM QID) or ceftiofur (4 mg/kg IV or IM BID) are good choices. Consider renal function when making antimicrobial choices.
- Consider metronidazole (10–15 mg/kg PO or IV TID) in foals with suspected intestinal clostridiosis.
- Sucralfate (1–2 g per 100 kg PO BID or TID), cimetidine (6–20 mg/kg PO TID), ranitidine (6.6 mg/kg PO TID), and omeprazole (0.7 mg/kg PO SID) may be used in foals with gastroduodenal ulceration.

CONTRAINDICATIONS

N/A

PRECAUTIONS

- NSAIDs are implicated in the pathogenesis of gastroduodenal ulceration, potentially nephrotoxic, and should be avoided. They also are effective analgesics and, therefore, may hide signs of pain indicating a surgical problem.
- Aminoglycoside antimicrobials are nephrotoxic and should be used judiciously. Obtain peak and trough values and use to monitor drug therapy. Creatinine also should be closely monitored.

POSSIBLE INTERACTIONS

N/A

ALTERNATIVE DRUGS

N/A

FOLLOW-UP

PATIENT MONITORING

- Monitor patients closely for pain.
- Evaluate hydration frequently, and adjust fluid rate accordingly. Evidence of edema in the axilla, proximal limbs, and dorsum suggests fluid overload or poor kidney function.
- Evaluate caloric intake frequently. Foals on IV dextrose or TPN should have blood glucose values monitored several times daily. If possible, foals should be weighed daily to ensure proper weight gain—a large jump in weight over 12–24 hours suggests renal problems or fluid overload.
- Monitor foals sucking their dams for aspiration pneumonia.
- Monitor fecal production, quality, and consistency, particularly in foals with diarrhea or meconium impaction.

POSSIBLE COMPLICATIONS

- Sepsis, septic shock, death from ruptured viscus or severe electrolyte abnormalities, small or large bowel stricture, perforation of ulcers, septic peritonitis, adhesion formation, anesthetic death, aspiration pneumonia, and chronic poor body condition are possible complications of severe colic.
- Foals are predisposed to developing adhesions after abdominal surgery and are at higher risks than adults.

MISCELLANEOUS

ASSOCIATED CONDITIONS
N/A

AGE-RELATED FACTORS
- Ruptured urinary bladder, meconium impaction, hypoxic ischemic asphyxia syndrome, and sepsis are primarily neonatal problems occurring in the first few days of life.
- Parasitism, abdominal abscessation, and duodenal stricture are primarily problems of weanling foals.

ZOONOTIC POTENTIAL
Salmonella sp.

PREGNANCY
N/A

SYNONYMS
N/A

SEE ALSO
- Gastric ulceration
- Meconium retention
- Shock
- Uroperitoneum

ABBREVIATIONS
- DIC = disseminated intravascular coagulation
- GGT = γ-glutamyltransferase
- GI = gastrointestinal
- TPN = total parenteral nutrition

Suggested Reading

Common digestive tract problems. In: Koterba A, Drummond WH, Kosch PC, eds. Equine clinical neonatology. Malvern: Lea & Febiger, 1990:414–446.

Fenger CK. Neonatal and perinatal disease. In: Reed SM, Bayley WM, eds. Equine internal medicine. Philadelphia: WB Saunders, 1998:959–966.

Rakestraw PC. Surgical treatment of acute abdominal crisis in foals. Proc Int Vet Emerg Crit Care Symp 1998;6:742–746.

Author Pamela A. Wilkins

Consulting Editor Mary Rose Paradis

ACUTE ADULT ABDOMINAL PAIN–ACUTE COLIC

BASICS

DEFINITION

Adult abdominal pain is defined by clinical signs associated with discomfort originating within the abdominal cavity. The abdominal pain may develop acutely or progressively. If the signs of discomfort persist for more than 3–4 days, the abdominal pain is considered chronic.

PATHOPHYSIOLOGY

Most acute abdominal pain originates from the gastrointestinal tract but it may also arise from other abdominal structures such as liver, spleen, kidneys, uterus, or peritoneum. In those cases where the intestinal tract is involved, pain may originate from increased intramural tension, tension on a mesentery, regional or generalized ischemia, mucosal inflammation, and smooth muscle spasms associated with hypermotility or a combination of any of these. Causes can be divided into strangulated and non-strangulated lesions. Non-strangulated lesions have no compromise to the local blood supply. Intraluminal lesions (impaction, foreign body, concretions), extraluminal lesions (adhesions, strictures), mural lesion (thickening), as well as spasmodic colic, intestinal displacement, ileus and inflammatory bowel disease are usually considered non-strangulated lesions. Strangulating lesions are usually associated with a compromise of local blood supply and result in intestinal necrosis and release of inflammatory mediators and endotoxin followed by cardiovascular shock.

SYSTEMS AFFECTED

- Gastrointestinal—disorders of the types cited previously; anywhere from the stomach to the small colon can be involved.
- Cardiovascular system—dehydration and endotoxemia may lead to shock and result in organ failure.
- Other systems can be the source of abdominal pain (e.g., urinary system, reproductive tract, hepatobiliary, the peritoneum).

SIGNALMENT

Nonspecific. There may be an age, breed, or sex predisposition for a specific problem (e.g. intussusception of the small intestine is more commonly seen in young horses; pedunculated lipomas are commoner on older horses; fecalliths are more common in the miniature horse; pain from the reproductive tract is seen in pregnant or post-partum mares and in stallions of breeding age).

SIGNS

General Comments

Signs of abdominal pain may be subtle initially and are often easily missed. In the early course of the disease the source of the abdominal pain may be difficult to identify. As the disease progresses, changes in clinical parameters, rectal examination findings, and laboratory data may allow a more accurate localization of the problem.

Historical Findings

The signs of abdominal pain can appear acutely or following an episode of anorexia, depression, and/or decrease in fecal output. History of change in the exercise regimen, the diet, or the availability of drinking water may also precede the signs of abdominal pain, which can be of different intensity:

- Mild abdominal pain—decrease in appetite, mild depression, decrease in fecal output, yawning, extended neck and rolling of the upper lip in Flehmen-like response, teeth grinding.
- Moderate abdominal pain—pawing at the ground, flank watching, groaning, posture for urinating but only a small quantity of urine is passed, leaning against the wall, kicking the abdomen with the hind legs, ears pinned backward, lying down more frequently, may attempt to roll.
- Severe abdominal pain—walking in a tight circle, constantly getting up and down, rolling, traumatizing self and handlers, sweating, labored breathing.

Physical Examination Findings

Signs may vary, depending on stage of the disease:

- General findings—abdominal distention, sweating, increase in respiratory rate, elevated or subnormal body temperature, decrease or absence of feces.
- Cardiovascular findings—abnormal color of the mucous membrane, increase in capillary refill time, increase in heart rate, signs of dehydration, cold extremities. In those cases where endotoxemic shock is present, the cause of the abdominal pain is probably related to a strangulated lesion or to a severe inflammatory process such as colitis or peritonitis. The cardiovascular status of horses with a non-strangulated obstructive lesion is usually better in comparison to horses with strangulating obstructive lesions.

• Gastrointestinal findings—decrease or increase in gut motility, gas-filled resonant viscus on percussion, presence of gastric reflux on passage of the nasogastric tube. If gastric reflux is present, lesion is most likely located at the level of the stomach or small intestine. The pH of the gastric reflux may also be helpful in identifying the origin of the reflux.
• Abnormalities on rectal examination—distension of a viscus by gas, liquid, or food; displacement of a viscus; uterine or renal abnormalities; findings will assist in the differentiation among problems involving the small intestine, large colon, cecum, small colon, or non-gastrointestinal lesions.

CAUSES

Gastrointestinal

• Gastric—gastric ulcers, gastric distention or impaction, gastric rupture
• Small intestine—nonstrangulated obstructive lesion: duodenal ulcer, duodenojejunal enteritis, ascarid impaction, ileal impaction, ileal hypertrophy, stricture. Strangulated obstructive lesion: incarceration of a segment of the small intestine into the epiploic foramen, a space/rent in the mesentery/inguinal ring/gastrosplenic ligament, strangulation by a lipoma, volvulus, adhesions, etc.
• Large intestine—nonstrangulated obstructive lesion: ulceration, colitis, impaction, idiopathic gas distention, mild displacement, nephrosplenic entrapment, enterolith, adhesions, sand impactions. Strangulated obstructive lesion: volvulus, herniation, incarceration, thromboembolic infarction
• Cecum—nonstrangulated obstructive lesion: impaction, adhesions. Strangulated obstructive lesion: torsion, cecal-cecal, ceco-colic-intussusception, thromboembolic infarction, torsion, incarceration
• Small colon—nonstrangulated obstructive lesion: impaction, enterolith. Strangulated obstructive lesion: incarceration, strangulating lipoma, submucosal hematoma, thromboembolic infarction
• Reproductive—uterine torsion, abortion, parturition, testicular torsion, hematoma in the broad ligament, trauma
• Renal/urologic—renal/ureteral/bladder/urethral calculi, cystitis, renal inflammatory processes
• Hepatobiliary—hepatitis, hepatobiliary calculi
• Others—peritonitis

RISK FACTORS

• No access to water
• Sudden change in diet
• Poor enteric parasite control
• Pregnancy
• Previous abdominal surgery
• Congenital abnormalities

DIFFERENTIAL DIAGNOSIS

Other causes of pain that might mimic pain originating from the abdominal cavity include myositis, pleuropneumonia, neurologic diseases such as rabies, and musculoskeletal injuries.

CBC/BIOCHEMISTRY/URINALYSIS

Increase in PCV and TP may be present in face of dehydration. Possible hypoproteinemia secondary to protein loss in the intestinal lumen and/or in the abdominal cavity. Leukopenia in acute inflammatory process and endotoxemia or leukocytosis in chronic inflammatory process. Possible metabolic acidosis related to cardiovascular shock and release of lactic acid and/or loss of bicarbonate and electrolytes (colitis) or metabolic alkalosis if a large amount of gastric reflux is present, resulting in loss of chloride. Hypokalemia and hypocalcemia can be present, especially if the horse has been anorexic or is a lactating mare. Hypochloremia and hyponatremia may be present in colitis. Alkaline phosphatase may be increased. Azotemia is found in horses with severe dehydration or urinary tract disease. The presence of an increase in some or all of the following enzymes is suggestive of liver disease: SDH (IDH), AST, GGT, conjugated bilirubin, and LDH-5.

OTHER LABORATORY TESTS

Abdominal Paracentesis

Normal fluid has a pale, clear yellow color. Turbidity of the sample indicates an elevation of WBC, RBC, or contamination with intestinal contents. Increase of the protein level and WBC is indicative of primary peritonitis or secondary to morphologic change of the viscera. A sanguineous fluid is probably indicative of intra-abdominal bleeding or a strangulated obstructive lesion. A foul-smelling reddish-brown fluid with an increase in the RBC, WBC, and protein is indicative of presence of necrotic bowel. Presence of plant materials in the absence of an enterocentesis suggests intestinal rupture. Few leukocytes or cells should be present if an enterocentesis was performed.

Urinalysis

A change in specific gravity, increase in leukocyte content, RBC, and pH may be noticed in cases with renal disease.

ACUTE ADULT ABDOMINAL PAIN-ACUTE COLIC

IMAGING

Radiographs

May be useful in the identification of sand impactions or enteroliths in adults.

Ultrasonography

Evaluation of the amount, quality, and characteristics of abdominal fluid; evaluation of wall thickness and diameter of small intestine; evaluation of the nephrosplenic space; abnormal findings, such as intussusceptions, abscesses, or adhesions. Also useful in evaluating the kidneys, liver, spleen, uterus, etc.

Endoscopy

- Gastroscopy—evaluation of the stomach for ulcers or impaction. In small horses, the duodenum may also be observed.
- Cystoscopy—evaluation of the urethra, bladder, and opening of the ureters for inflammation or calculi.
- Laparoscopy—visualization of abdominal viscera

DIAGNOSTIC PROCEDURES

Exploratory laparotomy

TREATMENT

Horses presenting signs of abdominal pain should be taken off feed until diagnosis of the underlying problem. The history, physical examination, and laboratory results should assist in identifying horses requiring surgical exploration versus horses requiring medical treatment. Indication for an exploratory laparotomy includes: signs of severe abdominal pain, unresponsiveness to medical treatment, moderate to severe abdominal distention, ileus or progressive reduction in gut motility, progressive increase in heart rate or heart rates above 60–70 per minute, cardiovascular compromise or deterioration, presence of moderate to severe gas distension or of a displacement of the large colon on rectal examination, gas distension of small intestine on rectal examination, gastric reflux, abnormal paracentesis findings, or presence of severe impaction of the large colon or the cecum. Animals presenting with these signs should be referred to a surgical facility. Supportive treatment includes intravenous fluids, gastric decompression if necessary, electrolyte replenishment, and control of the abdominal pain.

MEDICATIONS

DRUG(S) OF CHOICE

- Analgesics—control the abdominal pain
- Non-steroidal anti-inflammatory drugs (NSAIDs) —flunixin meglumine) (0.5–1.1 mg/kg IV, IM q8hr), phenylbutazone (2.2–4.4 mg/kg IV q12–24 hr) alpha-2-blockers such as xylazine (0.25–0.5 mg/kg IV or IM), detomidine (5–10 μg/kg IV or IM), or romifidine (0.02–0.05 mg/kg IV or IM) can also be given if the pain is not controlled by NSAIDs. The narcotic analgesics such as butorphanol (0.02–0.04 mg/kg IV) or meperidine (pethidine) can be given alone or in conjunction with xylazine. These two drugs potentiate each other. Any drugs should be used judiciously as they may mask clinical signs and may lead to postponement of surgery, thereby decreasing the chance of survival.
- Spasmolytics (indicated in spasmodic colic)—hyoscine (20–30 mL IV)
- Laxatives—to soften ingesta; mainly used for treatment of pelvic flexure and other impactions
- Mineral oil—10 mL/kg via nasogastric tube.
- Osmotic laxative—diluted di-sodium (0.5 g/kg) or magnesium sulfate (0.5–1 g/kg) in 4 L of warm water via nasogastric tube. Dioctyl sodium succinate (DSS) (10–30 mg/kg of a 10% solution). Water, via an indwelling nasogastric tube, is often beneficial in the management of impactions, and can be given at 4–5 L/hr. Alternatively, if there is gastric reflux, fluids can be given intravenously.
- Parenteral fluid treatments—In cases of dehydration or moderate to severe impaction problems, intravenous fluid (100–200 mL/kg/day). If cardiovascular shock is present, hypertonic saline (2 L of 7% NaCl in an adult horse) prior to balanced electrolyte solutions. Electrolyte imbalances should be corrected, especially hypokalemia and hypocalcemia, which are important for intestinal motility
- Treatment of endotoxemia—flunixin meglumine 0.25 mg/kg q6 hr. Other anti-endotoxemic treatments include hyperimmune plasma (see Endotoxemia).
- Intestinal motility stimulants—post-operative ileus is the most common indication. Metoclopramide acts on the stomach and proximal small intestine (0.1 mg/kg/hr in a constant drip infusion over several hours); erythromycin lactobionate (1g QID intravenously in 1 L saline).
- Antimicrobial therapy if peritonitis is suspected or if surgery is performed

CONTRAINDICATIONS

Acepromazine is contraindicated due to its peripheral vasodilatory effect.

PRECAUTIONS

Repeat use of alpha-2-blockers and butorphanol causes prolonged ileus. Repeat dose of NSAIDs, especially in presence of dehydration, can result in gastric or large colon ulceration as well as renal damage.

ACUTE ADULT ABDOMINAL PAIN–ACUTE COLIC

FOLLOW-UP

PATIENT MONITORING

The patient should be monitored closely for deterioration of clinical signs and cardiovascular status until resolution of the abdominal pain. Following resolution of these signs, reintroduction to feed should be done gradually.

POSSIBLE COMPLICATIONS

- Endotoxemia
- Circulatory shock
- Adhesions
- Gastrointestinal rupture
- Peritonitis

ASSOCIATED CONDITIONS

N/A

AGE-RELATED FACTORS

Older horses are more predisposed to strangulated lipoma and epiploic foramen entrapment; pregnant mares are more predisposed to large colon torsion; and younger horses are more predisposed to ulcer problems, intussusception, and ascarid impactions.

ZOONOTIC POTENTIAL

N/A

PREGNANCY

Mares in late gestation or in the post-partum period are predisposed to large colon torsion. Parturition can present clinical signs similar to a gastrointestinal accident.

SYNONYMS

Colic

ABBREVIATIONS

- PCV = packed cell volume
- TP = total protein

Suggested Reading

White NA. Epidemiology and etiology of colic. In: NA White. The equine acute abdomen. Pennsylvania: Lea & Febiger, 1990:50-60.

Allen D Jr, Tyler, DE. Pathophysiology of acute abdominal disease. In: NA White. The equine acute abdomen. Pennsylvania: Lea & Febiger, 1990:66-85.

White NA. Examination and diagnosis of the acute abdomen. In: NA White. The equine acute abdomen. Pennsylvania: Lea & Febiger, 1990:102-147.

Edwards GB. Gastroenterology. 1. Colic. In: Mair, Love, Schumacher, Watson, ed. Equine medicine, surgery and reproduction. Philadelphia: WB Saunders, 1998:20-54.

Author Nathalie Coté

Consulting Editor Henry Stämpfli

ACUTE EPIGLOTTIDITIS

BASICS

OVERVIEW
Epiglottiditis is a non-specific inflammatory disease which affects the epiglottis.

SIGNALMENT
- Primarily affects racehorses (2–10 years) in active race training or other horses undergoing repeated, strenuous exercise.
- No known breed or sex predilection.

SIGNS
- Chief complaints—variable amount of abnormal respiratory tract noise and exercise intolerance.
- Coughing during eating is fairly common.
- Some horses act mildly pained when swallowing.

CAUSES AND RISK FACTORS
- Cause—unknown
- Repeated, strenuous exercise may induce inflammatory changes on the lingual (ventral) mucosal epiglottic surface between this tissue and the dorsal surface of the free edge of the soft palate.
- The role of inhaled particulate matter during galloping, abrasive feed or bedding material during swallowing, and bacterial or viral infections is unknown.

DIAGNOSIS

DIFFERENTIAL DIAGNOSIS
- The diagnosis is established based on endoscopy of the upper respiratory tract.
- Occasionally, the endoscopic appearance is misinterpreted as epiglottic entrapment by the aryepiglottic folds.

CBC/BIOCHEMISTRY/URINALYSIS
These tests are not typically performed.

OTHER LABORATORY TESTS
Additional laboratory tests are not typically performed.

IMAGING
Imaging is not usually performed.

DIAGNOSTIC PROCEDURES
- During routine endoscopy, the epiglottis may appear swollen and discolored (reddish-purplish), primarily along the lateral margins and ventral (lingual) mucosal surfaces. This swelling may obscure the normal, serrated margins and cause the epiglottis to appear more rounded and bulbous. The ventral mucosal surfaces often are ulcerated, and in more chronic, untreated cases, granulation tissue surrounded by fibrous connective tissue is seen. The cartilage tip of the epiglottis may be visible, projecting out where the mucosa has eroded. The epiglottis looks thicker and may be elevated a variable amount into an abnormal axis above the soft palate.
- Introduction of the endoscope into the nasal pharynx may induce repeated swallowing, chewing movements, or collapse of the pharyngeal walls because of irritation or apparent pain.
- Horses with epiglottiditis often intermittently displace the soft palate dorsally and may experience difficulty replacing the soft palate into a normal position underneath the epiglottis.
- The caudal free margin of the soft palate may have a variable amount of inflammation, ulceration, or thickening. If the inflammatory insult is more diffuse, then inflammation of adjacent structures characterized by reddening, thickening, edema, and ulceration may occur in the corniculate processes of the arytenoids and adjacent nasal pharyngeal mucosa.

TREATMENT
- Outpatient (stall-side) basis
- Discontinue exercise for a minimum of 7–14 days, depending on the extent of the problem.
- If swallowing is difficult or stimulates coughing, hay may need to be eliminated from the diet or, at least, made wet until the inflammation resolves; a complete ration or gruel made from pellets may be easier to swallow.

ACUTE EPIGLOTTITIS

MEDICATIONS

DRUGS

• Epiglottiditis usually responds to medical therapy consisting of NSAIDs, parenteral corticosteroids, and topical pharyngeal sprays that contain anti-inflammatory and antimicrobial medication.
• With evidence of infection or a fever, antimicrobial therapy may be indicated—IM procaine penicillin G, PO trimethoprim sulfamethoxazole, or IM or IV ceftiofur at normal recommended dosages for 5–7 days.
• Horses are initially treated with phenylbutazone (4.4 mg/kg IV) or flunixin meglumine (1.1 mg/kg IV) and dexamethasone (0.044 mg/kg IV). Ten milliliters of a pharyngeal spray (750 mL of Furacin, 250 mL of DMSO, 1000 mL of glycerin, and 2.0 g of prednisolone) is sprayed slowly, while watching for swallowing, into the pharynx twice daily for 7–14 days through a 10-F catheter introduced into the nasal pharynx through the nasal passages. After the initial IV dose of either phenylbutazone or flunixin meglumine and dexamethasone, oral therapy is continued with phenylbutazone (2.2 mg/kg PO twice daily for 7–14 days) and prednisone (0.9 mg/kg PO once daily for 7 days). The same dose is then administered orally every other day for three treatments. Subsequently, a dose of 0.45 mg/kg is given orally every other day for three treatments.

CONTRAINDICATIONS/POSSIBLE INTERACTIONS

No contraindications

FOLLOW-UP

• Substantial improvement in the overall appearance of the epiglottis and adjacent tissue and in pharyngeal function usually is seen at follow-up endoscopy after $\cong$1 week of therapy with acute inflammation. Continue rest and therapy until healing is judged complete based on repeated endoscopy performed at $\cong$1-week intervals.
• Horses with more chronic-appearing inflammation may require more protracted therapy (2–4 weeks), and complete resolution of thickening and cartilage deformity may not occur. Occasionally, epiglottic entrapment may develop, but this usually can be corrected using axial midline division with a curved bistoury or a contact laser. Extremely bulbous or fibrotic-appearing entrapping membranes may need to be excised through a laryngotomy.
• Advise owners that healing may result in fibrosis or cicatrix on the lingual epiglottic surface sufficient to interfere with normal soft-palate function. Endoscopy may reveal intermittent or persistent dorsal displacement of the soft palate, which may need surgical treatment—bilateral sternothyroideus tenectomy, soft-palate trim, or excision of fibrous connective tissue on the lingual epiglottic surface.
• Epiglottiditis is a serious, potentially career-limiting or -ending problem in racehorses. Prognosis depends primarily on severity of the condition during the initial examination. Resolution of acute inflammation results in complete return to normal exercise tolerance and elimination of abnormal respiratory tract noise. Horses with more chronic or extensive lesions may suffer from intermittent to persistent dorsal displacement of the soft palate despite appropriate medical or surgical therapy.

MISCELLANEOUS

ASSOCIATED CONDITIONS

N/A

AGE-RELATED FACTORS

N/A

ZOONOTIC POTENTIAL

N/A

PREGNANCY

SEE ALSO

• Dorsal displacement of the soft palate
• Inspiratory dyspnea

ABBREVIATION

DMSO = dimethyl sulfoxide

Suggested Reading

Hawkins JF, Tulleners EP. Epiglottitis in horses: 20 cases (1988–1993). J Am Vet Med Assoc 1994; 205:1577–1580.

Author Eric Tulleners
Consulting Editor Jean-Pierre Lavoie

ACUTE HEPATITIS IN ADULT HORSES (THEILER'S DISEASE)

BASICS

OVERVIEW

- Many conditions can potentially lead to acute liver failure in adult horses, with the most common being a syndrome occurring 4–10 weeks after animals have received an equine biologic. This is usually tetanus antitoxin, but other agents have been implicated—equine serum and encephalitis vaccine.
- The liver has multiple functions—protein, carbohydrate and lipid metabolism; excretion of bile; biotransformation of both endogenous and exogenous toxins.
- Acute failure of liver functions leads to various biochemical derangements, with accumulation of some agents, lack of some, and imbalances in others. These biochemical imbalances are responsible for many of the clinical signs seen in this disease.

SIGNALMENT

Predominantly in adult horses

SIGNS

- Usually sudden in onset and rapidly progressive, with death occurring 2–6 days after onset of signs in some cases.
- Horses often are very icteric and pass dark urine caused by the presence of bilirubin.
- As many as 80% show signs of hepatic encephalopathy, which can manifest in various ways that may change during the course of the disease.
- Initially, there may be subtle changes in behavior, progressing to excitement or depression with head pressing.
- Some may wander aimlessly around the stall or paddock.
- Frequent yawning has been reported in some cases.
- If animals live long enough and are outside in the sun, they may develop photodermatitis on white parts of the body.
- Possible hemorrhagic diathesis.

CAUSES AND RISK FACTORS

- Most commonly associated with administration of an equine biologic 4–6 weeks before the onset of signs; however, not all cases have been exposed to an equine biologic.
- Some epidemiologic evidence suggests that some cases may result from an infectious agent, probably a virus. None has been isolated as yet, however, and attempts to reproduce the disease with material from affected horses have failed.
- Occasional cases caused by *Clostridium novyi* type B have been described.

DIAGNOSIS

DIFFERENTIAL DIAGNOSIS

- Acute onset of icterus in adult horses has multiple causes—prehepatic, hepatic, or posthepatic; serum biochemistries and CBC assist in differentiating these causes.
- Prehepatic—red-maple leaf toxicity, wild onion toxicity, phenothiazine toxicity, and nitrate poisoning.
- Hepatic—anorexia, Theiler's disease, *C. novyi,* bacterial cholangiohepatitis, EIA, EVA, *Strongyle* sp. migration, arsenic toxicity, and halogenated hydrocarbons.
- Posthepatic—cholelithiasis and other causes of biliary obstruction.
- Signs of hepatic encephalopathy can be very similar to several acute neurologic diseases—rabies, EEE, WEE, and acute protozoal myeloencephalitis; icterus and serum biochemical changes help in differentiating these problems.
- Hematuria, hemoglobinuria, myoglobinuria, and bilirubinuria may cause pigmenturia; urinalysis and serum biochemistries aid in differentiation.

CBC/BIOCHEMISTRY/URINALYSIS

- Bilirubin—moderate increase in unconjugated and conjugated levels
- Liver enzymes—increases in SDH (IDH), AST, GGT and ALP
- Some may assay LDH, particularly isoenzyme 5.
- Glucose—normal to low
- Urea—normal to low
- Bilirubinuria
- CBC—usually normal

OTHER LABORATORY TESTS

Bromsulphalein clearance—2.2 mg/kg IV. Half-life is determined by sampling at 3, 6, and 9 minutes after injection; normal half-life is 2.8 ± 0.5 min. Half-life is prolonged when $>50\%$ of liver function lost.

IMAGING

Ultrasonography may suggest the liver is smaller than normal, with a loss of normal parenchymal structure.

DIAGNOSTIC PROCEDURES

- Liver biopsy performed on the right side between the twelfth and fourteenth intercostal space, where a line drawn from the tuber coxae to the elbow intersects the selected intercostal space. Ultrasound guidance may ensure accurate placement of the biopsy needle.
- Coagulation profile recommended by some before biopsy.
- Histopathology defines the nature and severity of the lesions.

PATHOLOGIC FINDINGS

- The liver usually is smaller than normal, but it may be enlarged in peracute cases.
- Generalized icterus.
- Histologically, centrolubular to midzonal hepatocellular necrosis, with mononuclear cell accumulation in the portal triads.
- Possibly mild bile ductule proliferation in more chronic cases.

ACUTE HEPATITIS IN ADULT HORSES (THEILER'S DISEASE)

TREATMENT

• Restrict activity, and avoid sunlight.
• In cases with hepatoencephalopathy, house the horse in a quiet place, preferably padded to avoid injury.
• If the horse is still eating, a high-carbohydrate, low-protein diet is recommended. The protein should be high in BCAAs—two parts beet pulp with one part cracked corn and added molasses. Oat or grass hay is preferred over alfalfa, and the diet should be fed in small amounts five or six times daily.

MEDICATIONS

DRUGS

• Xylazine (0.5–1.0 mg/kg) or detomidine (0.05–0.4 mg/kg) can be used to control the signs of hepatoencephalopathy.
• In hypoglycemic animals, 10% glucose solution at 0.2 mL/kg may be given, followed by continuous drip of 5% glucose solution at 2 mL/kg per hour, reducing after 24 hour to half this rate.
• If the animal is not drinking, administer IV polyionic fluids at maintenance rates.
• Reduced production and absorption of toxic metabolites can be achieved with mineral oil and neomycin (20–30 mg/kg QID), both via stomach tube.

CONTRAINDICATONS/POSSIBLE INTERACTIONS

• Neomycin should not be given for more than 24–36 hours, because it may induce severe diarrhea.
• Because the liver metabolizes many drugs, their duration of action may be increased in acute hepatic disease.

FOLLOW-UP

PATIENT MONITORING

Monitor liver enzymes and bilirubin every 2–3 days.

PREVENTION/AVOIDANCE

N/A

POSSIBLE COMPLICATIONS

N/A

EXPECTED COURSE AND PROGNOSIS

• Horses with severe hepatoencephalopathy have a poor prognosis, but if the animal survives for a week after the onset of clinical signs, recovery is possible.
• If the SDH (IDH) continues to fall, then the prognosis improves.

MISCELLANEOUS

ASSOCIATED CONDITIONS

N/A

AGE-RELATED FACTORS

N/A

ZOONOTIC POTENTIAL

N/A

PREGNANCY

N/A

SEE ALSO

N/A

ABBREVIATIONS

• ALP = alkaline phosphatase
• AST = aspartate aminotransferase
• BCAAs = branched-chain amino acids
• EEE = eastern equine encephalomyelitis
• EIA = equine infectious anemia
• EVA =
• GGT = γ-glutamyltranspeptidase
• IDH = iditol dehydrogenase (SDH)
• LDH = lactate dehydrogenase
• SDH = sorbitol dehydrogenase (IDH)
• WEE =

Suggested Reading

Divers TJ. Liver disease and liver failure in horses. Proc Am Assoc Equine Pract 1983;29:213–223.

Author Christopher M Brown
Consulting Editor Michel Levy

ACUTE RENAL FAILURE (ARF)

BASICS

DEFINITION

A consequence of an abrupt, sustained decrease in GFR, resulting in azotemia and disturbances in fluid, electrolyte, and acid–base homeostasis.

PATHOPHYSIOLOGY

- Usually prerenal or renal; most commonly due to hemodynamic or nephrotoxic insults.
- Except for neonatal bladder rupture, postrenal failure is uncommon in horses.
- Perpetuated by decreased GFR from damaged glomeruli and tubular obstruction with desquamated tubular epithelial cells and debris.
- Continued use of NSAIDs can further perpetuate ARF by compromising renal blood flow.

SYSTEMS AFFECTED

- Renal/urologic—failure.
- Endocrine/metabolic—disturbances in electrolyte and acid–base homeostasis.
- GI—inappetance, possible diarrhea, and increased risk of ulcers.
- Nervous/neuromuscular—occasional ataxia or dementia in severe cases; tremors or muscle fasciculations may accompany metabolic disturbances.
- Hemic/lymphatic/immune—altered hemostasis and increased susceptibility to infection.
- Musculoskeletal—acute laminitis in severe cases; often refractory to treatment.

GENETICS

N/A

INCIDENCE/PREVALENCE

- Low
- 0.5%–1.0% of hospitalized horses have serum Cr > 5.0 mg/dL at admission

SIGNALMENT

Breed Predilections

N/A

Mean Age and Range

- Foals <30 days of age (especially when receiving nephrotoxic medications) may be at greater risk, but all ages may be affected.
- Ureteral and bladder rupture—more common in neonates and postpartum mares.

Predominant Sex

Bladder rupture—more likely in male neonates.

SIGNS

Historical Findings

- Often secondary to other problems leading to hypovolemia and renal ischemia—colic, diarrhea, or prolonged exercise.
- When a primary disease process is not apparent, question progressive abdominal distension (consistent with uroperitoneum), repeated positioning to urinate without passage of urine (consistent with urethral obstruction), and exposure to potential nephrotoxins.
- Polyuric cases may manifest by more substantial depression and anorexia than would be expected with the primary disease.

Physical Examination Findings

- Depression, lethargy, anorexia, dehydration, edema, injected oral membranes with petechiae, ulcers, or uremic odor in the oral cavity.
- Severity of depression and anorexia often are greater than would be expected with the primary disease process.
- Rectal examination may reveal an enlarged, painful left kidney.
- Laminitis, often rapidly progressive.
- Markedly azotemic patients may have neurologic deficits—ataxia, hypermetria, and mental obtundation.
- Colic and repeated positioning to urinate, with passage of a few drops of blood-tinged fluid, may be seen with urethral obstruction; rectal examination reveals a markedly enlarged, turgid bladder.

CAUSES

Prerenal Failure

- Hemorrhagic, hypovolemic, or endotoxic shock
- Prolonged, exhaustive exercise
- Severe rhabdomyolysis, vasculitis, or hemolytic diseases
- Disseminated intravascular coagulation

Intrinsic Renal Failure

- Prolonged duration of above disorders, lack of adequate fluid support, or concurrent use of normal dosages of nephrotoxic medications—gentamicin; NSAIDs.
- Excessive doses of NSAIDs or prolonged use of gentamicin, particularly in dehydrated horses.
- Other nephrotoxins include heavy metals (e.g., mercury [in counterirritants or blisters], lead, cadmium), endogenous pigments (e.g., hemoglobin, myoglobin), vitamins D and K_3, and high doses of oxytetracycline administered to neonates with flexural deformities.
- In occasional cases, infectious agents—*Actinobaccillus equiili* in neonates; *Leptospira* sp. in all age groups.

Postrenal Failure

- Uroperitoneum during the first few days of life is most common with bladder rupture in male neonates.
- A slightly later development of uroperitoneum occurs in sick neonates of both sexes with urachal leakage or in foals with ruptured ureters.
- Uroperitoneum occasionally may develop in postpartum mares with bladder rupture.

RISK FACTORS

- Renal hypoperfusion.
- Exposure to nephrotoxins, particularly in patients with dehydration or primary renal disease.
- Dystocia may increase the risk of bladder or ureteral rupture in neonates.

DIAGNOSIS

DIFFERENTIAL DIAGNOSIS

- All conditions leading to hemorrhagic, hypovolemic, or endotoxic shock; severe rhabdomyolysis; vasculitis and hemolytic diseases; or disseminated intravascular coagulation.
- Prerenal failure—supported by oliguria with concentrated urine (specific gravity > 1.035) and rapid correction of azotemia with rehydration.
- Postrenal failure—supported by stranguria, anuria, or uroperitoneum.
- CRF—history of weight loss, poor body condition, ventral edema, polyuria and polydipsia, hypercalcemia, and poor correction of azotemia with fluid therapy.
- Acute-onset CRF—history of compromised renal function or early CRF complicated by another disease primary process (as above); incomplete correction with fluid therapy.

ACUTE RENAL FAILURE (ARF)

CBC/BIOCHEMISTRY/URINALYSIS

• Normal to high PCV, variable leukopenia to leukocytosis, lymphopenia, normal to decreased platelets, CBC changes more often reflect underlying primary disease process.
• Progressive (moderate to severe) increases in BUN (50–150 mg/dL) and Cr (2.0–20 mg/dL).
• Variable hyponatremia, hypochloremia, hyperkalemia, hypocalcemia, and hyperphosphatemia—hyperkalemia and hyperphosphatemia more common with intrinsic cases.
• Mild to moderate metabolic acidosis, severity varying with the underlying disease process; development of renal tubular acidosis may complicate recovery.
• Mild to moderate hyperglycemia.
• Urine specific gravity—high (>1.035) with prerenal failure, low (<1.020) with intrinsic ARF; specific gravity best assessed in urine collected during initial patient evaluation (before rehydration) or while the horse is not receiving fluids.
• Intrinsic cases may be accompanied by mild to moderate proteinuria, glucosuria, pigmenturia, and increased RBCs and casts on sediment examination.
• Urine pH—normal to acidic, especially with concurrent depletion of body potassium stores.

OTHER LABORATORY TESTS

• Increased fractional clearances (i.e., excretions) of sodium and phosphorous; decreased fractional clearance of potassium
• Enzymuria—urinary GGT:Cr ratio > 25
• Rising titers to *Leptospira* sp. may be found in horses with ARF attributable to leptospinosis.

IMAGING

Transabdominal Ultrasonography

• Kidneys may be enlarged (diameter, >8 cm; length, >15 cm), with loss of detail of corticomedullary junction.
• Variable subcapsular/perirenal edema or hemorrhage.
• Variable dilation of renal pelves—may be marked in obstructive postrenal failure).
• Bilateral nephrolithiasis/ureterolithiasis with acute-onset CRF may be further detected by imaging ureters and left kidney via transrectal ultrasonography.

Urethroscopy/Cystoscopy

Useful in suspected obstructive disease.

DIAGNOSTIC PROCEDURES

• Urine collection—collect initial urine produced by all at-risk horses.
• Percutaneous renal biopsy with routine histopathologic, immunohistochemical, and electron-microscopic evaluation of the sample may provide information regarding cause, severity, and prognosis. Pursued with caution, however, because life-threatening hemorrhage can be a complication.

PATHOLOGIC FINDINGS

• Gross findings—enlargement of kidneys due to nephrosis and subcapsular and interstitial edema, causing tissue to bulge on cut surfaces.
• Histopathologic findings—glomeruli may be congested and have a cellular infiltrate; tubules have denuded or flattened epithelium and varying amounts of accumulated debris.

TREATMENT

APPROPRIATE HEALTH CARE

• Proper recognition and treatment of all underlying primary disease processes, usually on an inpatient basis for continuous fluid therapy.
• Possible emergency surgical treatment of urinary obstruction or uroperitoneum after initial stabilization of electrolyte (e.g., hyperkalemia) and acid–base alterations.
• Reassess dosage schedule of, and possibly discontinue, potentially nephrotoxic medications.

NURSING CARE

Fluid Therapy

• After initial measurement of body weight, correct estimated dehydration with normal (0.9%) saline or another potassium-poor electrolyte solution over 6–12 hours.
• Fluids may be supplemented with calcium gluconate or sodium bicarbonate if hyperkalemia or acidosis requires specific correction.
• Monitor for SC and pulmonary edema—increased respiratory rate and effort.
• Conjunctival edema may develop rapidly in cases of intrinsic oliguric to anuric ARF.
• Use maintenance fluid therapy judiciously in animals not clinically dehydrated.
• If hemorrhage is a contributing cause to hypovolemia and decreased renal perfusion, initial treatment with hypertonic saline may have value.

ACUTE RENAL FAILURE (ARF)

Oral Electrolyte Supplementation

• Sodium chloride (30 g) can be administered in concentrate feed or as an oral slurry/paste BID–QID to encourage increased drinking and urine output.
• Potassium chloride can be supplemented in nonhyperkalemic patients with total body potassium depletion—common with anorexia of ≥2 days.

ACTIVITY

Stall rest, with limited hand-walking for grazing grass if appetite is poor.

DIET

• Encourage intake by offering a variety of concentrate feeds, bran mash, and hay types.
• Hand-walking or short periods of turn-out to graze grass may be the most effective way to encourage feed intake.

CLIENT EDUCATION

• Prognosis is most dependent on progression of the underlying primary disease process.
• ARF may complicate recovery, prolong hospitalization and treatment, and increase cost.

SURGICAL CONSIDERATIONS

• Surgery generally is required for postrenal failure due to urethral obstruction or development of uroperitoneum consequent to bladder rupture.
• Surgery may be required for obstructive ureteroliths (e.g., electrohydraulic lithotripsy) or ureteral tears (e.g., stent placement).

MEDICATIONS

DRUGS OF CHOICE

• Judicious fluid therapy is the mainstay of treatment—see *Nursing Care.*
• Severe hyperkalemia (>7.0 mEq/L) or cardiac arrhythmias—treat with agents that decrease serum potassium concentration (e.g., sodium bicarbonate [1–2 mEq/kg IV over 5–15 minutes) or counteract the effects of hyperkalemia on cardiac conduction (e.g., calcium gluconate [0.5 mL/kg of a 10% solution by slow IV injection).
• Furosemide—for oliguria/anuria (i.e., lack of urination during first 6 hours of fluid therapy), this diuretic may be administered two times (1–2 mg/kg IV) at 1–2-hour intervals; if effective, urination should be observed within 1 hour after the second dose; if ineffective, discontinue treatment.
• Mannitol—for oliguria/anuria unresponsive to furosemide, hypertonic mannitol (10%–20% solution) can be administered (0.5–1.0 g/kg IV over 30–60 minutes); if effective, treatment can be repeated 4–6 hours later.
• Dopamine–for persistent oliguria/anuria, an infusion (3–5 μg/kg per minute IV in a 5% dextrose solution) can be given for 3–6 hours; monitor heart rate and rhythm regularly during infusion; may be combined with furosemide for potential synergistic effects.
• Antiulcer drugs (e.g., omeprazole [2–4 mg/kg PO q24h], cimetidine [5–10 mg/kg IV q8h in anorexic horses]) may be useful in decreasing the associated risk of gastric ulcer disease.

CONTRAINDICATIONS

• Dopamine—use cautiously, may induce cardiac arrhythmias.
• Avoid all nephrotoxic medications unless specifically indicated for the underlying disease process, and then modify dosage accordingly.

PRECAUTIONS

• Monitor response to fluid therapy—as little as 40 mL/kg of IV fluids (20 L per 500-kg horse) may produce significant pulmonary edema in oliguric/anuric patients.
• Reassess dosage schedule of drugs eliminated by urinary excretion; consider discontinuing all potentially nephrotoxic medications—gentamicin, tetracycline, and NSAIDs.

POSSIBLE INTERACTIONS

Use of multiple anti-inflammatory drugs (e.g., corticosteroids and one or more NSAIDs) will have additive negative effects on renal blood flow; avoid combined administration in azotemic patients.

ALTERNATIVE DRUGS

Consider peritoneal dialysis or hemodialysis (foals only) in refractory cases.

FOLLOW-UP

PATIENT MONITORING

• Assess clinical status (emphasizing hydration), urine output, and body weight at least twice daily during the initial 24 hours of treatment and at least daily thereafter.
• Assess magnitude of azotemia and electrolyte and acid–basis status at least daily for the initial 3 days of treatment.
• Consider placing a central venous line to maintain central venous pressure <8 cm H_2O in more critical patients and neonates.

PREVENTION/AVOIDANCE

• Anticipate compromised renal function in patients with other diseases or undergoing prolonged anesthesia and surgery; institute appropriate treatment to minimize dehydration and potential renal damage.
• Ensure adequate hydration status in patients receiving nephrotoxic medications.
• Avoid concurrent use of multiple anti-inflammatory drugs—NSAIDs.

POSSIBLE COMPLICATIONS

• Pulmonary and peripheral edema; conjunctival edema may be dramatic.
• Severe hyperkalemia accompanied by cardiac arrhythmias, cardiac arrest, and death.
• Laminitis—often refractory to supportive care.
• Signs of neurologic impairment—ataxia; mental obtundation.
• GI ulceration or bleeding.
• Coagulopathy
• Sepsis

ACUTE RENAL FAILURE (ARF)

EXPECTED COURSE AND PROGNOSIS

- Prognosis for recovery varies with the underlying primary disease process.
- Prognosis for recovery from prerenal failure and nonoliguric intrinsic ARF usually is favorable if azotemia decreases by 25%–50% after the initial 24 hours of treatment; extent of recovery of renal function in patients with intrinsic failure may require 3–6 weeks to fully assess.
- Guarded prognosis for patients with Cr > 10 mg/dL at initial evaluation and when azotemia remains unchanged after the initial 24 hours of treatment.
- Poor prognosis for patients with Cr > 15 mg/dL at initial evaluation, that have increased magnitude of azotemia after the initial 24 hours of treatment, that rapidly develop edema, or that remain oliguric/anuric >72 hours.
- Prognosis for recovery from postrenal failure depends on successful surgical correction of the cause of the obstruction or uroperitoneum.

MISCELLANEOUS

ASSOCIATED CONDITIONS

- Colic; enterocolitis
- Pleuritis; peritonitis; septicemia
- Laminitis
- Exhausted horse syndrome—multiple-organ failure

AGE-RELATED FACTORS

- Neonates with hypoxic-ischemic multiple-organ damage or septicemia may have increased risk of intrinsic ARF.
- Neonates, especially premature or dysmature foals, may have markedly elevated Cr concentrations (approaching 25 mg/dL) due to placental insufficiency; this azotemia typically resolves in 2–3 days and should not be confused with intrinsic ARF or uroperitoneum.

ZOONOTIC POTENTIAL

Leptospirosis has infectious and zoonotic potential; avoid direct contact with infective urine.

PREGNANCY

Postpartum mares are at risk of hemorrhagic shock and prerenal failure or intrinsic ARF consequent to rupture of a uterine artery.

SYNONYMS

- Acute nephrosis
- Acute tubular necrosis
- Vasomotor nephropathy

SEE ALSO

- Anuria/oliguria
- Aminoglycoside toxicity
- NSAID toxicity
- CRF

ABBREVIATIONS

- Cr = creatinine
- CRF = chronic renal failure
- GGT = γ-glutamyltransferase
- GI = gastrointestinal
- GFR = glomerular filtration rate

Suggested Reading

Bayly WM. Acute renal failure. In: Reed SM, Bayly WM, eds. Equine internal medicine. Philadelphia: WB Saunders, 1998:848–856.

Divers TJ, Whitlock RH, Byars TD, Leitch M, Crowell WA. Acute renal failure in six horses resulting from hemodynamic causes. Equine Vet J 1987;19:178–184.

Schmitz DG. Toxic nephropathy in horses. Compend Contin Educ Pract Vet 1988;10:104–111.

Author Harold C. Schott II

Consulting Editor Harold C. Schott II

ACUTE RESPIRATORY DISTRESS SYNDROME (ARDS) IN FOALS

BASICS

DEFINITION
Ventilatory efforts in excess of the metabolic demands of the animal.

PATHOPHYSIOLOGY
- Cause unknown
- Several inflammatory stimuli are likely to initiate the events leading to clinical signs of respiratory failure—aspiration pneumonia; viral, bacterial or fungal infections; thermal injury (i.e., heat stroke), sepsis/endotoxemia, and inhalation of irritant gases/smoke.
- Immunosuppression is thought to be a factor associated with development of ARDS/interstitial lung disease in foals infected with *Pneumocystis carinii,* but the nature of proposed immune deficits has not been defined.
- Clinical signs reflect diffuse injury to pulmonary capillary endothelium and alveolar epithelium.
- The causative disease processes may progress to multiple organ dysfunction, resulting in azotemia, liver dysfunction, ileus, or bleeding.

SYSTEMS AFFECTED
- Primarily respiratory.
- Often accompanied by dysfunction of the renal, hepatic, and cardiovascular systems and by clotting cascades as disease progresses—multiple organ dysfunction syndrome.

GENETICS
N/A

INCIDENCE/PREVALENCE
- Not established, but relatively uncommon.
- Worldwide, with most cases in areas with hot summer weather.

SIGNALMENT
- All ages, but foals 1–8 months of age are predisposed (mean age, 3.5 ± 1.0 months).
- No sex or breed predilections.

SIGNS
- Acute or peracute onset of depression, lethargy, fever, labored breathing, tachypnea, nostril flaring, extended head and neck position, increased abdominal and intercostal effort (i.e., "double expiratory lift" or "heave line"), and cyanosis.
- Nasal discharge and cough are frequent but inconsistent findings.
- Thoracic auscultation—often reveals loud bronchial sounds over central airways, with increased peripheral airway sounds; crackles and polyphonic wheezes become more prominent as the foal responds to therapy.

CAUSES
- The initial event leading to pulmonary lesions is unknown.
- During hot weather, heat stress may play a role. Foals with subclinical respiratory disease are disadvantaged regarding dissipation of body heat; therefore, take care to prevent extreme temperatures. Use of erythromycin in some foals during hot weather appears to be associated with increased susceptibility to environmental temperatures.
- Viral and bacterial pneumonia have been suggested to produce respiratory distress in foals with widespread infections throughout the lungs. *Rhodococcus equi* has been cultured from approximately 25% of foals with respiratory distress in one study, and opportunistic pathogens (e.g., enteric bacteria, *Pseudomonas aeruginosa, Pneumocystis carinii*) have been incriminated as causative agents of ARDS in foals. Some also suggest that infections with these agents are markers of underlying immune suppression.
- Lesions in affected foals are similar to those in ruminants with atypical interstitial pneumonia, suggesting this syndrome results, in part, from ingestion of toxicants.

RISK FACTORS
- Unknown
- Risk factors that may prove to be significant—pre-existing subclinical respiratory tract disease; treatment with antimicrobial agents or bronchodilators, which may produce significant interactions in some patients when used in combination; viral, bacterial, or fungal respiratory tract infections; heat stress; inhaled irritant gases and pneumotoxicants; and immunosuppression.

DIAGNOSIS

DIFFERENTIAL DIAGNOSIS
- Viral pneumonia—equine influenza, equine viral arteritis, equine herpes viruses 1 and 4, equine paramyxovirus, and equine adenovirus.
- Bacterial pneumonia—*P. carinii* infection
- Pulmonary abscessation or granuloma.
- Upper airway dysfunction, with aspiration of oropharyngeal fluids.
- Ingestion or exposure to xenobiotics, resulting in pulmonary injury.

CBC/BIOCHEMISTRY/URINALYSIS
Common abnormalities—neutrophilic leukocytosis with a left shift, elevated fibrinogen, and anemia

OTHER LABORATORY TESTS
- Arterial blood gas reveals arterial hypoxemia, hypercapnia, and respiratory acidosis.
- Blood culture may help to identify bacterial agents.
- Other laboratory abnormalities reflecting dehydration, disseminated intravascular coagulation, and injury to other organs may be seen.

ACUTE RESPIRATORY DISTRESS SYNDROME (ARDS) IN FOALS

IMAGING

Thoracic Radiography

- Findings vary, depending on the stage of injury.
- Lesions include prominent interstitial patterns, coalescing to alveolar infiltrates, with superimposed, mixed bronchial patterns of varying severity throughout all lung fields.
- A prominent miliary reticulonodular pattern is observed commonly, but not exclusively, in foals with *P. carinii* infection.
- Other changes sometimes include consolidating anteroventral pneumonia or diffusely distributed pyogranuloma in foals with *R. equi* infection.

Transthoracic Ultrasonography

Consolidation, abscesses, or other lesionszin some foals.

DIAGNOSTIC PROCEDURES

- Because many affected foals are near death, antemortem culture of respiratory secretions before initiation of treatment may not be practical; however, culture of transtracheal washes or bronchoalveolar lavages may provide invaluable information, especially when Gram-negative sepsis is suspected.
- Routine culture of lower airway secretions should be accompanied by cytologic evaluation using routine Romanowsky-type stains (i.e., Diff-Quick) and Gram stains.
- In affected foals, examination of fluid usually reveals acute inflammation reactions, with large numbers of macrophages that may have phagocytized bacteria.
- Recognition of *P. carinii* is difficult with any stain.
- Transthoracic lung biopsy may provide useful diagnostic information but should not be performed in foals that demonstrate a tendency to bleed.

PATHLOGIC FINDINGS

Gross Findings

- Lungs are diffusely red, wet, heavy, firm, and fail to collapse when the chest is opened.
- In many instances, lungs have a lobulated appearance, with dark, reddened areas interspersed between areas of more normal-appearing tissue.
- Airway lumina usually contain pink, foamy fluid, and cut surfaces of the lungs exude fluid from edematous separation of lobules.
- A substantial number of foals also have other lung lesions (e.g., *R. equi* pyogranuloma) representing pre-existing pulmonary disease.
- Many foals demonstrate hypoxemia- or sepsis-induced lesions in other organs.

Histopathologic Findings

- Pulmonary lesions—diffuse, necrotizing bronchiolitis; alveolar septal necrosis; and filling of alveolar spaces with large numbers of mononuclear cells, desquamated pneumocytes, and epithelioid-like cells in an eosinophilic, proteinaceous material (i.e., hyaline membranes).
- Other prominent lesions—congestion and edema of the interstitium, hyperplasia of the type II alveolar pneumocytes, and in more chronic cases, interstitial fibrosis.
- Multinucleate syncytial cells are in the alveoli of some, but not all, affected foals and appear to be consistent in foals with *P. carinii* infection.

TREATMENT

APPROPRIATE HEALTH CARE

- Do not transport these patients before relief of clinical signs. Transportation of foals in extreme temperatures may be responsible for their demise.
- If performing an examination at a farm with a high environmental temperature, consider moving the mare and foal to a controlled environment on the premises or awaiting stabilization and the cooler period of the day before loading and transport.

NURSING CARE

- These cases are respiratory emergencies and require immediate stabilization.
- Reduce core body temperature using alcohol baths, fans, misters, or by carefully moving the mare and foal to an air-conditioned stall.
- Cold water enemas provide significant relief, especially when used in conjunction with the above-mentioned treatments.
- Judicious use of chilled IV fluids lowers core temperature; however, rapid infusion of a large volume may exacerbate pulmonary edema. Preferably, fluid solution should be selected by acid–base status and blood electrolyte values. A balanced electrolyte solution (e.g., lactated Ringer solution) is appropriate for initial therapy.
- Nasal oxygen insufflation (2–5 L/min) is facilitated by placement of a nasal or transtracheal catheter.

ACUTE RESPIRATORY DISTRESS SYNDROME (ARDS) IN FOALS

ACTIVITY

Reduce the patient's activity, including confinement to a clean, cool stall with appropriate environmental temperature and humidity control—fans, misters, or swamp coolers.

DIET

- Lowering body temperature may provide substantial relief and allow improved intake.
- Allow nursing foals adequate time with the mare, and provide high-quality feed.

CLIENT EDUCATION

- Education is aimed at prevention.
- Proper management of the neonate is imperative, because early handling and training of foals to accept physical examination and daily rectal temperature (preferably in the morning, when ambient environmental temperatures are low) allow early detection of subclinical cases.
- Clients should observe the mare and foal carefully on a daily basis and consult a veterinarian when a foal has a fever or appears to be unthrifty or depressed.
- Removing foals from extremes of heat while maintaining excellent stall hygiene and providing shade or fans to lower stall temperature may be beneficial.
- Exercise care when treating foals with antimicrobial agents (especially erythromycin) not to expose these animals to high environmental temperatures.

MEDICATIONS

DRUGS OF CHOICE

- The treatment protocol should specifically address inflammation and hyperthermia. Modulation of the pulmonary inflammatory response and appropriate antimicrobial therapy and supportive care are mandatory.
- Use of corticosteroids in stressed foals demonstrating clinical signs of sepsis is controversial; however, single or multiple doses of short-acting corticosteroids (e.g., dexamethasone sodium phosphate [20–60 mg IV], prednisolone sodium succinate [100–300 mg IV]) provide potent, short-duration relief of pulmonary inflammation in many cases.
- NSAIDs (e.g., flunixin meglumine [0.25 mg/kg q8h], phenylbutazone [4.4 mg/kg q12h]) may be useful in lowering body temperature, decreasing the effects of mediators produced in association with sepsis or endotoxinemia, and reducing discomfort associated with the underlying respiratory disease.
- Appropriate antibiotic therapy should be guided by bacteriologic culture, if possible, but minimizing stress also is critical. Use of oral antibiotics (e.g., trimethoprim-potentiated sulfonamides [30 mg/kg q12h]), parenteral antibiotics (e.g., procaine penicillin G [10,000 IU/lb IM q12h]), or cephalosporins (e.g., ceftiofur [2–5 mg/lb IM q12h]) may be substituted for other antimicrobial agents used before the onset of respiratory distress.

CONTRAINDICATIONS

- Discontinue any medications (especially erythromycin/rifampin) and drugs with an effect that may be altered by concurrent therapy with drugs undergoing metabolism by the liver—theophylline, aminophylline.

PRECAUTIONS

- Because sepsis may represent the underlying cause in some foals, overuse of corticosteroids is discouraged.
- Employ NSAIDs with caution, because they may be associated with gastrointestinal ulceration.

ACUTE RESPIRATORY DISTRESS SYNDROME (ARDS) IN FOALS

FOLLOW-UP

PATIENT MONITORING

- Arterial blood gases are the most sensitive indicator of progress.
- Frequent, careful thoracic auscultation may reveal increased bronchovesicular sounds in foals with positive response to therapy (as ventilation of the peripheral airways improves).
- Reduction in respiratory rate and effort and improvement in mucous membrane color also indicate clinical improvement.
- Repeated thoracic radiography is useful, but the overall radiographic appearance of the lungs may lag behind the clinical appearance of the animal by several days.

PREVENTION/AVOIDANCE

- Careful client education regarding prevention and early recognition of respiratory tract disease in foals is beneficial—minimizing heat stress, control of dust, manure dispersal, and plasma therapy on farms with endemic *R. equi.*
- Client education regarding use of anthelmintics and vaccination of foals for respiratory pathogens, as well as proper management of the foal at birth, is necessary.

POSSIBLE COMPLICATIONS

N/A

EXPECTED COURSE AND PROGNOSIS

- The initial prognosis is guarded to poor in most affected foals.
- The mortality rate is high without intensive therapeutic intervention.
- Long-term outcomes vary, but cases that are recognized and treated early respond well to therapy. In some instances, full recovery appears to be possible.

MISCELLANEOUS

ASSOCIATED CONDITIONS

N/A

AGE-RELATED FACTORS

- Can occur at all ages.
- In 1–8-month foals, the lack of a fully developed immune system and being born and developing during the warmer months of the year may predispose to respiratory tract disease.

ZOONOTIC POTENTIAL

N/A

PREGNANCY

N/A

SYNONYMS

- Bronchointerstitial pneumonia
- Interstitial pneumonia
- Respiratory distress

SEE ALSO

- Expiratory dyspnea
- Inspiratory dyspnea

Suggested Reading

Ainsworth DM, Biller DS. Respiratory system. In: Reed SM, Bayly WM, eds. Equine internal medicine. Philadelphia: WB Saunders, 1998:282–283.

Derksen FJ. Interstitial pneumonia in foals. In: Colahan PT, Mayhew IG, Merritt AM, Moore JN, eds. Equine medicine and surgery. 5th ed. St. Louis: Mosby, 1999:552.

Traub-Dargatz J, Wilson WD, Conboy HS, et al. Hyperthermia in foals treated with erythromycin alone or in combination with rifampin for respiratory disease during hot environmental conditions. Proc Am Assoc Equine Pract 1996;42:243–244.

Wilson WD, Lakritz J. Bronchointerstitial pneumonia and acute respiratory distress in foals. In: Robinson NE, ed. Current therapy: equine medicine 4. Philadelphia: WB Saunders, 1996.

Authors Jeffrey Lakritz and W. David Wilson

Consulting Editor Jean-Pierre Lavoie

ADENOVIRUS

BASICS

OVERVIEW

• Causes fatal respiratory disease in Arabian foals with severe combined immunodeficiency syndrome (SCID).
• Other breeds may be affected as foals, but seldom succumb.
• Approximately 25% of affected foals also have diarrhea.
• A role for adenovirus in the development of respiratory disease in adult horses has been suggested.

SIGNALMENT

• Foals are usually older than 8–10 weeks of age when clinical signs become present.
• Adenovirus affects primarily Arabians, although other breeds are affected sporadically.
• SCID affected foals are frequently clinically normal at birth.

SIGNS

• Signs are essentially identical to other causes of foal pneumonia and include fever, tachypnea, dyspnea, depression, and abnormalities on thoracic auscultation.
• Mild to moderate diarrhea may also be present.

CAUSES AND RISK FACTORS

Foals with SCID have a defect in lymphoid stem cells that may result from altered purine metabolism. The absence of an adaptive immune response causes these foals to be susceptible to even minor pathogens, such as adenovirus. Due to maternally derived immunity reaching a nadir at between 1 and 2 months of age, these foals become unable to mount an appropriate immune response and deteriorate after 2 months of age. Foals that are immunosuppressed for other reasons are also susceptible. It has been suggested that adenovirus may predispose foals to bacterial pneumonia and may play a significant role in the pathogenesis of bacterial pneumonia in non-SCID foals. An antigenically distinct adenovirus has been identified in non-SCID foals with diarrhea, usually associated with concurrent rotavirus infection. The role of adenovirus in foal diarrhea is not clear.

DIAGNOSIS

DIFFERENTIAL DIAGNOSIS

Other viral and bacterial causes of pneumonia in immunocompromised foals include, but are not limited to:
• equine herpes virus type 1
• equine influenza virus
• equine arteritis virus
• *Streptococcus equi* var *zooepidemicus*
• *Actinobacillus equuli*
• *Pasturella* spp.
• *Klebsiella pneumoniae*
• *Salmonella* spp.
• *Bordatella bronchiseptica*
• *Rhodococcus equi*

Other causes of diarrhea in foals include, but are not limited to, bacterial, viral, and parasitic causes.

CBC/BIOCHEMISTRY/URINALYSIS

Ante-mortem diagnosis of SCID is supported by finding appropriate clinical signs in an Arabian foal of the appropriate age with persistent severe lymphopenia, $\leq$ 500 cells/μL and the absence of IgM on SRID.

OTHER LABORATORY TESTS

• Antibody titers—SCID foals do not demonstrate a 4-fold rise in antibody titer to adenovirus, whereas non-SCID affected foals develop a rise in antibody titer in 10 days.
• Virus isolation—Adenovirus may be isolated from normal and infected foals.
• Histopathology—Intranuclear inclusions can be detected in tissues. Ante-mortem testing may demonstrate intranuclear inclusions in conjunctival and nasal epithelial cells. At post-mortem examination there is gross and histologic evidence of lymphoid hypoplasia of the thymus, spleen, and lymph nodes.
• SRID—Precolostral testing of SCID foals also demonstrates an absence of IgM, but as IgM is absorbed by the foal from colostrum, foals with adequate transfer of maternal antibody cannot be tested until IgM levels have waned, usually at $\geq$3 weeks of age.

IMAGING

• Radiographs are consistent with pneumonia.
• Ultrasonographic imaging of lymphoid tissues may be suggestive of, but not diagnostic for, SCID.

TREATMENT

• There currently is no treatment specifically for adenovirus.
• In non-SCID foals treatment is primarily supportive, with broad-spectrum antimicrobial coverage provided.
• Foals with SCID eventually die, and treatment is not productive. There has been some investigation into immunologic reconstitution of SCID patients by transplantation of bone marrow stem cells. This treatment remains experimental as of the time of this writing.

MEDICATIONS

DRUG(S) OF CHOICE

- Non-SCID foals should be treated for concurrent bacterial infection based on culture and sensitivity results.
- Foals with adenovirus associated with rotavirus should be treated with supportive therapy, including intravenous isotonic polyionic fluid replacement of deficits and nutritional support as warranted.

CONTRAINDICATIONS/POSSIBLE INTERACTIONS

N/A

FOLLOW-UP

CLIENT EDUCATION

- Prevention of SCID requires identification of carriers and removal of them from breeding programs.
- Approximately 1 of 4 foals resulting from the mating of two heterozygotes results in a SCID foal.
- Arabian foals should be tested at birth for IgM levels (presuckle) and lymphocyte count. Those foals with an absolute lymphopenia should be closely monitored until 5 months of age. Alternatively, there are genetic tests available now to identify carriers of the genetic defect.

MISCELLANEOUS

ABBREVIATION

- SRID = serial radial immunodiffusion

Suggested Reading

Bernoco D, Bailey E. Frequency of the SCID gene among Arabian horses in the USA. Anim Genet, 1998, 29(1):41-42.

Burrell M, Wood JL, Whitwell KE, Chanter N, Mackintosh ME, Mumford JA. Respiratory disease in thoroughbred horses in training: The relationship between disease and viruses, bacteria and environment. Vet Rec, 1996, 139(13):308-313.

Campbell TM, Studdert MJ, Ellis WM, Paton CM. Attempted reconstitution of a foal with severe combined immunodeficiency. Equine Vet J, 1983, 15(3):233-237.

Perryman L, McGuire TC, Crawford TB. Maintenance of foals with combined immunodeficiency: causes and control of secondary infections. Am J Vet Res, 1978, 39(6):1043-1047.

Studdert MJ, Blackney MH. Isolation of adenovirus antigenically distinct from equine adenovirus type 1 from diarrheic foal feces. Am J Vet Res, 1982, 43(3):543-544.

Author Pamela A. Wilkins

Consulting Editor Corinne R. Sweeney

ADRENAL INSUFFICIENCY (AI)

BASICS

OVERVIEW

- Synonymous with hypoadrenocorticism and "steroid let-down syndrome"
- Characterized by glucocorticoid and mineralocorticoid deficiency caused by adrenal cortex destruction (i.e., primary AI or Addison's disease) or ACTH deficiency (i.e., secondary AI)
- Primary AI—both glucocorticoid and mineralocorticoid are deficient.
- Secondary AI—mineralocorticoid secretion usually is normal.
- Organ systems—endocrine, cardiovascular, renal, musculoskeletal, GI, and behavioral

SIGNALMENT

Any age, sex, and breed

SIGNS

- Acute cases—muscular weakness, hypotension, anorexia, hemoconcentration, hypothermia, polyuria, cardiovascular collapse, and death.
- Chronic cases—depression, anorexia, weight loss, poor hair coat, exercise intolerance, polyuria/polydipsia, mild abdominal pain, salt craving, and diarrhea.

CAUSES AND RISK FACTORS

- Chronic administration of glucocorticoids, exogenous ACTH, or anabolic steroids
- Pituitary-adrenal axis immaturity attributable to prematurity
- Adrenal hemorrhage and necrosis subsequent to septicemia or severe bouts of endotoxemia

DIAGNOSIS

DIFFERENTIAL DIAGNOSIS

- Acute cases—endotoxemia, septicemia, renal failure, and colitis
- A normal ACTH stimulation test rules out adrenal insufficiency.

CBC/BIOCHEMISTRY/URINALYSIS

- Acute AI is characterized by hemoconcentration, hyponatremia, hypochloremia, hyperkalemia, decreased sodium:potassium ratio (reference range, >27), and hypoglycemia.
- Additional abnormalities—metabolic acidosis and azotemia
- Chronic cases, including secondary AI—mineralocorticoid secretion (i.e., aldosterone) generally is maintained; therefore, serum electrolytes are within normal limits.

OTHER LABORATORY TESTS

- With insufficient aldosterone secretion, fractional excretion of sodium (reference range, <1%) is increased despite a normal or low serum sodium concentration.
- Administration of exogenous ACTH (1 U/kg IM) resulting in less than a doubling of the cortisol baseline 6–8 hours later is consistent with AI. Because acute AI is life-threatening, dexamethasone (0.044 mg/kg IV) should be administered simultaneously with exogenous ACTH. Serum cortisol is measured 2 hours later, and horses with AI exhibit a negligible increase in cortisol. This eliminates any delay in treatment while diagnostic tests are being performed.

IMAGING

N/A

DIAGNOSTIC PROCEDURES

N/A

TREATMENT

- Complete rest and avoidance of stress, particularly surgery, infection, and trauma.
- Treat the underlying primary cause.
- Provide sodium supplementation (e.g., salt) to horses with increased sodium losses.

ADRENAL INSUFFICIENCY (AI)

MEDICATIONS

DRUGS

- Glucocorticoid and, if necessary, mineralocorticoid replacement—the maintenance dose of prednisone, which is equivalent to daily corticosteroid secretion in normal adult horses, is ≅25 mg/day, but exposure to stress dramatically increases corticosteroid requirements. During periods of stress, increase the dose by 2- to 10-fold, and divide into 2–3 daily doses.
- Acute AI—dexamethasone in conjunction with IV crystalloid solutions (i.e., normal saline) and dextrose in cases of hypoglycemia. Although dexamethasone has minimal mineralocorticoid activity, 20 mg administered daily is sufficient to maintain live adrenalectomized horses.
- Mineralocorticoid replacement with fludrocortisone may be considered.

CONTRAINDICATIONS/POSSIBLE INTERACTIONS

N/A

FOLLOW-UP

PATIENT MONITORING

- Monitor electrolytes, renal function, and acid-base and hydration status.
- Once the animal is stable, adrenal recovery can be documented by repeating ACTH-stimulation tests.

PREVENTION/AVOIDANCE

Avoid excessive use of exogenous glucocorticoids, ACTH, and anabolic steroids.

POSSIBLE COMPLICATIONS

Excessive glucocorticoid administration, especially with long-acting forms (e.g., triamcinolone), increases susceptibility to infections and may result in laminitis.

EXPECTED COURSE AND PROGNOSIS

N/A

MISCELLANEOUS

ASSOCIATED CONDITIONS

N/A

AGE-RELATED FACTORS

N/A

ZOONOTIC POTENTIAL

N/A

PREGNANCY

N/A

SEE ALSO

N/A

ABBREVIATION

- GI = gastrointestinal

Suggested Reading

Dybdal NO. Endocrine disorders. In: Smith BP, ed. Large animal internal medicine. 2nd ed. St Louis: Mosby, 1996:1449–1450.

Author Laurent Couëtil
Consulting Editor Michel Levy

AFLATOXICOSIS

BASICS

OVERVIEW

- Intoxication by the *Aspergillus* fungal metabolite, aflatoxin.
- Diffuse liver disease is the hallmark, with acute and chronic forms dictated by dose and duration of exposure.
- Aflatoxin-contaminated feed grains, especially corn, are the sources of toxin.
- Aflatoxin usually is produced on grain that is grown during drought conditions.

SIGNALMENT

Younger horses are more susceptible.

SIGNS

- Ponies given single, lethal doses of aflatoxin (2 mg/kg) have had increased temperatures, elevated heart and respiratory rates, tenesmus, bloody feces, and tetanic convulsions.
- Elevations of prothrombin time and serum AST, ALT, and GGT were consistent with the severe liver necrosis and biliary hyperplasia seen at postmortem examination.
- Some ponies died within 3 days; others lived for 32 days after dosing.
- Ponies administered high doses PO (0.4 mg/kg for 5 days; the equivalent of several ppm in the feed) were lethargic, anorectic, and slightly icteric on the fifth day.
- Serum liver enzymes were elevated on the fourth day of dosing.
- Signs of hepatic encephalopathy (e.g., belligerence, somnolence, circling, blindness, head pressing) may occur when serum ammonia levels are sufficiently elevated.
- Chronic, low-level exposure may manifest as an ill-defined loss of condition.

CAUSES AND RISK FACTORS

- The most likely contaminated diets are corn based, whereas less likely exposure comes from diets containing peanut and cottonseed meals.
- Forage is an unproven source of aflatoxin.

DIAGNOSIS

DIFFERENTIAL DIAGNOSIS

- Signs and lesions of aflatoxicosis reflect liver disease; none are pathognomonic for either acute or chronic aflatoxin poisoning.
- Feed concentrations of several hundred ppb aflatoxin in grain rations, together with appropriate clinical findings, are supportive of the diagnosis.
- Ill thrift is associated with lower levels of aflatoxin intake.
- Elevated serum hepatic enzyme levels can occur in association with many multisystemic diseases.
- Specific causes of hepatic disease—fumonisin-induced mycotoxicosis, alsike clover or kleingrass toxicoses, hepatic neoplasia or abscessation, biliary obstruction, and Theiler's disease.
- Pyrrolizidine alkaloid–containing plants such as *Amsinckia, Crotalaria,* and *Senecio* sp. cause chronic, progressive liver disease.

CBC/BIOCHEMISTRY/URINALYSIS

- WBC count, especially lymphocytes, is decreased, as is serum glucose.
- Total serum lipid and cholesterol are increased.

OTHER LABORATORY TESTS

- Chemical analysis of feed samples is necessary to confirm the presence of aflatoxin.
- Inability to obtain samples at the time of exposure often precludes detection of aflatoxin levels consistent with acute intoxication.
- Feed concentrations necessary to induce acute intoxication typically approach the ppm range, whereas chronic exposure to several hundred ppb is sufficient to induce subclinical liver damage and associated ill thrift.

IMAGING

N/A

DIAGNOSTIC PROCEDURES

- Necropsy findings—fatty liver, hemorrhagic enteritis, and pale, swollen kidneys.
- Histopathologic findings—liver changes include fatty degeneration, centrilobular necrosis, periportal fibrosis, and bile-duct hyperplasia.

AFLATOXICOSIS

TREATMENT

- Specific antidotes are unavailable.
- Horses suffering only moderate liver damage benefit from supplementation with high-quality protein, fat-soluble vitamins, and selenium.
- Management for liver failure includes high-carbohydrate, low protein diets.

MEDICATIONS

DRUGS AND FLUIDS

- Give 5% dextrose slowly IV to hypoglycemic animals.
- Balanced electrolyte solutions for maintenance.

CONTRAINDICATIONS/POSSIBLE INTERACTIONS

Use drugs subject to hepatic clearance with caution.

FOLLOW-UP

PATIENT MONITORING

Monitor liver enzymes to evaluate liver function.

PREVENTION/AVOIDANCE

Reliable feed sources are critical when grains are produced during drought conditions; test grain before feeding.

EXPECTED COURSE AND PROGNOSIS

Survival of acute intoxication does not guarantee complete recovery; ponies have died from liver failure as long as 30 days after a single toxic dose of aflatoxin.

MISCELLANEOUS

ASSOCIATED CONDITIONS

N/A

AGE-RELATED FACTORS

N/A

ZOONOTIC POTENTIAL

N/A

PREGNANCY

N/A

SEE ALSO

N/A

ABBREVIATION

- ALT = alanine aminotransferase
- AST = aspartate aminotransferase
- GGT = γ-glutamyltransferase

Suggested Reading

Raisbeck MF. Feed-associated poisoning. In: Robinson NE, ed. Current therapy in equine medicine 3. Philadelphia: WB Saunders, 1992:366–372.

Author Stan W. Casteel
Consulting Editor Robert H. Poppenga

AFRICAN HORSE SICKNESS

BASICS

OVERVIEW

• Infectious disease affecting the cardiovascular and respiratory systems, characterized by fever and edema.
• Not reported in the United States. Most commonly found on the African continent, with recent outbreaks investigated in South Africa, Zimbabwe, and Mozambique. India, Turkey, Iraq, Syria, Lebanon, Jordan, and Spain have reported outbreaks in the past.
• Geographic range of the disease is limited by that of its principal vector, *Culicoides* spp. The disease is most prevalent in low-lying, moist, warm areas.

SIGNALMENT

• All breeds of horses as well as other equids, such as donkeys and mules, are susceptible.
• There is no apparent breed, age, or sex predilection.
• Angora goats are also susceptible. Zebras and elephants may serve as natural reservoirs of the virus that causes AHS. Dogs fed uncooked infected horse-meat have developed AHS.

SIGNS

• Fever (but not accompanied by inappetence)
• Pulmonary edema with coughing, frothy nasal discharge, dyspnea
• Subcutaneous edema of head and neck, edema of supraorbital fossa
• Colic

CAUSES AND RISK FACTORS

• Caused by the African horse sickness virus, a viscerotropic RNA virus of the genus *Orbivirus.*
• Transmitted by arthropod vectors, primarily *Culicoides* spp., but also mosquitoes and ticks.
• Spread of the disease to uninfected countries can occur through travel of infected horses or movement of infected insect vectors in aircraft or heavy wind.
• Virus affects vascular endothelium, resulting in the clinical sign of edema that predominates.
• Disease occurs seasonally, during warm wet periods.

DIAGNOSIS

DIFFERENTIAL DIAGNOSIS

• Equine infectious anemia, equine viral arteritis, purpura hemorrhagica, equine ehrlichiosis, and equine piroplasmosis may have similar clinical presentation to AHS and may require laboratory testing to differentiate.
• Index of suspicion for AHS should be raised when there is a history of travel to countries known to harbor the disease.
• Congestive heart failure may result in pulmonary and subcutaneous edema, but heart murmurs and/or venous distention should be present, and fever may not be present.

CBC/BIOCHEMISTRY/URINALYSIS

N/A

OTHER LABORATORY TESTS

• Definitive diagnosis depends on isolation of virus from whole blood or tissues, or antibodies to AHS virus in serum.
• In the United States, if AHS is suspected, the federal area veterinarian-in-charge should be notified immediately so that appropriate samples can be forwarded for testing.

IMAGING

• Thoracic radiography may reveal evidence of pulmonary edema.
• Thoracic ultrasound may reveal pleural effusion or pericardial effusion.

PATHOLOGIC FINDINGS

• Pulmonary edema, with frothy fluid in the bronchi and trachea
• Pleural effusion
• Pericardial effusion
• Yellow-gelatinous edema fluid in the musculature of the neck and jugular groove
• Petechial hemorrhages on endocardium, epicardium, and oral mucous membranes and tongue

TREATMENT

There is no specific treatment for AHS. Supportive nursing care and symptomatic treatment may improve outcome in some cases, but usually the course of the disease is not altered by treatment.

AFRICAN HORSE SICKNESS

MEDICATIONS

DRUG(S) OF CHOICE

N/A

CONTRAINDICATIONS/POSSIBLE INTERACTIONS

N/A

FOLLOW-UP

PREVENTION/AVOIDANCE

- Vaccination is effective. However, 42 antigenic strains of the virus exist, and vaccination with one strain does not result in immunity to heterologous strains, so polyvalent strains of vaccine should be used.
- Vaccination should be combined with other measures aimed at limiting exposure to insect vectors, such as fly-proof stabling, pasturing only during daylight, use of insect repellents, and keeping horses on high ground away from low-lying, swampy, insect-infested areas.
- Countries free of the disease restrict importation of horses from countries known to harbor the disease, or impose quarantine of at least 30 days in insect-proof housing.

EXPECTED COURSE AND PROGNOSIS

- Mortality in horses generally is high, up to 90%. In mules and donkeys, mortality may be lower (50%).
- The incubation period ranges from 7 to 21 days. Once clinical signs are observed, the clinical progression is rapid. Death usually occurs within 4 to 5 days after the onset of fever.
- Survivors do not harbor the virus.

MISCELLANEOUS

ZOONOTIC POTENTIAL

The disease does not affect humans.

Suggested Reading

Dardiri AH. African Horsesickness. In: Ferris DH, ed. Foreign Animal Disease Reference Manual. 4th ed. Ames: USDA, APHIS, NVSL, 1984.

Author Raymond W. Sweeney

Consulting Editor Corinne R. Sweeney

AGALACTIA/HYPOGALACTIA

BASICS

DEFINITION

Agalactia is the failure of lactation after parturition. Hypogalactia is milk production at volumes less than what is considered normal.

PATHOPHYSIOLOGY

Estrogens produced by the fetoplacental unit in late pregnancy induce the development of mammary ducts while progesterone stimulates lobuloalveolar growth. Lactogenesis is triggered when progesterone sharply decreases and prolactin sharply increases just prior to parturition. The increase in prolactin production by the anterior pituitary gland is made possible by suppression of a prolactin inhibitory factor (presumed to be dopamine) and possibly the release of a prolactin releasing factor (proposed to be serotonin) from the hypothalamus. Agalactia/hypogalactia can be the result of interference with these hormonal events (primary endocrinologic disease), a defect in the mammary tissue itself (primary mammary gland disease), or as a result of systemic illness or disease.

SYSTEMS AFFECTED

- Reproductive, primary
- Endocrine/metabolic, secondary

SIGNALMENT

No age or breed predisposition.

SIGNS

General Comments

Widespread use of tall fescue grass in pasture management in the central and southeastern United States has led to the recognition of "fescue syndrome." The most frequently reported clinical finding in this syndrome is agalactia at the time of parturition. Currently, the grazing of endophyte-infected fescue pastures is considered the most likely cause of lactation failure in mares.

Historical Findings

- Agalactia/hypogalactia or mammary gland disease at previous parturition.
- Prolonged gestation, dystocia, thickened fetal membranes, retained placenta.
- Clinical manifestations of systemic disease or a history of exposure to infectious disease.
- Grazing of endophyte-infected tall fescue pastures by pregnant mares.

Physical Examination Findings

- Weak and/or septicemic foals due to FPT and/or inadequate nutrition.
- A flaccid udder and secretion of a clear or thick, yellow-tinged fluid from the teats.
- Mastitis results in a swollen, painful udder that is warm to the touch, and secretion of visibly or microscopically abnormal milk.
- In the case of mammary abscessation or neoplasia, distinct masses may be palpable.

CAUSES

Primary Endocrinologic Disorders

- Ingestion of tall fescue grass infected with *Acremonium coenophialum**, an ergot alkaloid–producing fungus. Ergot alkaloids depress prolactin secretion because they are dopamine D2 receptor agonists and serotonin antagonists.
- Ingestion of feedstuffs contaminated with *Claviceps purpurea* (ergot) *sclerotia.*
- Abortion/premature birth affects the normal progesterone, estrogen, and prolactin fluctuations necessary for the onset of lactation.

Primary Mammary Gland Disease

- Mastitis
- Mammary gland abscessation or fibrosis
- Mammary gland neoplasia
- Mammary gland trauma

Systemic Disease

- Any debilitating systemic disease or stress-producing disorder
- Malnutrition/nutritional deficiency

RISK FACTORS

N/A

DIAGNOSIS

DIFFERENTIAL DIAGNOSIS

Differentiating Similar Signs

- Agalactia must be differentiated from the refusal of nursing associated with mare anxiety, pain, or udder edema. Direct physical examination of the udder and its secretions and observation of the interaction between mare and foal during attempts at nursing should allow differentiation.
- Failure of milk letdown can occur in mares. Parenteral oxytocin can stimulate milk letdown, but does not stimulate milk secretion.

Differentiating Causes

- A history of fescue ingestion, prolonged gestation, dystocia, RFM, thickened fetal membranes, and a weak, dysmature foal with agalactia is indicative of fescue syndrome.
- Mastitis; mammary fibrosis, neoplasia, abscessation, or traumatic injury; and systemic illness should be apparent upon physical examination.

CBC/BIOCHEMISTRY/URINALYSIS

N/A

OTHER LABORATORY TESTS

Serum prolactin levels are decreased in fescue-induced agalactia.

IMAGING

N/A

DIAGNOSTIC PROCEDURES

- If mastitis is suspected—Cytology or microbiologic culture of udder secretion.
- If neoplasia is suspected—Fine-needle aspirate (cytology evaluation) or biopsy (histopathology).

TREATMENT

- Remove mares from endophyte-infected fescue pastures at least 30 days, preferably 90 days, prior to the expected date of parturition.
- Mastitis (equine)—Bovine intramammary infusion products; systemic antibiotics—trimethoprim-sulfa, 5 mg/kg (based on the trimethoprim portion), P/O, BID; frequent stripping of mammary gland/'milk out'; hot-packs or hydrotherapy.
- Correct nutritional deficiencies.
- Foals—Provide nutritional supplementation during period of agalactia and plasma transfusions if FPT.

AGALACTIA/HYPOGALACTIA

MEDICATIONS

DRUG(S) OF CHOICE

• Domperidone (1.1 mg/kg, P/O, SID), a selective D2 dopamine receptor antagonist, to reverse the effects of fescue ingestion. This drug has not yet received approval from the FDA, and is available only as an experimental product. There are no side effects associated with treating pregnant mares. Ideal: Begin treatment at least 15 days prepartum and discontinue when/if lactation is observed at foaling. However, if mares are agalactic at foaling and were not treated prior to parturition, initiate treatment at foaling and continue for 5 days or until lactation ensues.
• Thyrotropin-releasing hormone (TRH), 2.0 mg, SQ, BID, for 5 days beginning on day 1 postpartum. Increases serum prolactin levels in agalactic mares, presumably due to its action as a prolactin releasing factor.

CONTRAINDICATIONS

Evidence for perphenazine as an effective dopamine receptor antagonist has been published. Severe side effects when used in horses (sweating, colic, hyperesthesia, ataxia, posterior paresis) preclude its use in this manner.

PRECAUTIONS

N/A

POSSIBLE INTERACTIONS

N/A

ALTERNATIVE DRUGS

Acepromazine maleate (20 mg, IM, TID) has some dopamine antagonistic properties, suggested for use in fescue agalactia.
• At least one study where phenothiazine tranquilizer had no effect on lactation.
• Sedation is the primary side effect

Reserpine (0.5–2.0 mg, IM, q48 h) has been used to treat agalactia.
• Tranquilizers
• GI motility greatly increased, sometimes results in profuse diarrhea

Sulpiride (3.3 mg/kg, P/O, SID), also a dopamine antagonist
• Positive effects in reversing fescue-induced agalactia
• Lesser degree than domperidone
• Not FDA approved for this use

FOLLOW-UP

PATIENT MONITORING

Most treatments stimulate milk production in 2–5 days if they are going to have an effect. In the absence of other related systemic signs, agalactia is not life-threatening. The foal may require intensive medical and nutritional management in cases of prolonged agalactia.

POSSIBLE COMPLICATIONS

N/A

MISCELLANEOUS

ASSOCIATED CONDITIONS

Mare

Fescue agalactia is associated with prolonged gestation, abortion, dystocia, uterine rupture, thickened placental membranes, retained placentae, infertility, prolonged luteal function, EED, and weak and dysmature foals.

Neonate

• FPT
• Neonatal malnutrition

AGE-RELATED FACTORS

N/A

ZOONOTIC POTENTIAL

N/A

PREGNANCY

N/A

SYNONYMS

N/A

SEE ALSO

• Dystocia
• Prolonged pregnancy
• Retained fetal membranes
• Failure of passive transfer

ABBREVIATIONS

• EED = early embryonic death
• FPT = failure of passive transfer
• RFM = retained fetal membranes, retained placenta
• TRH = thyrotropin releasing hormone

Suggested Reading

Cross DL. Fescue toxicosis in horses. In: Neotyphodium/grass interactions. Bacon CW, Hill NS, ed. New York: Plenum Press 1997;289-309.

Lothrop CD, Henton JE, Cole BB, Nolan HL. Prolactin response to thyrotropin-releasing hormone stimulation in normal and agalactic mares. J Reprod Fert Suppl 1987;35,277-280.

McCue PM. Lactation. In: Equine reproduction. McKinnon AO, Voss JL, ed. Philadelphia, Lea & Febiger 1993;588-595.

Redmond LM, Cross DL, Strickland JR, Kennedy SW. Efficacy of domperidone and sulpiride as treatments for fescue toxicosis in horses. Am J Vet Res 1994;55,722-729.

Van Camp SD. Abnormalities of lactation. In: Current therapy in large animal theriogenology. Youngquist RS, ed. Philadelphia: WB Saunders 1997;154-156.

Author Carole C. Miller
Consulting Editor Carla L. Carleton

AGAMMAGLOBULINEMIA

BASICS

OVERVIEW

- A rare, primary immunodeficiency disorder characterized by complete absence of mature B lymphocytes resulting in the lack of endogenous immunoglobulin production.
- Normal cell-mediated response and T lymphocyte numbers.

SIGNALMENT

- Reported in Thoroughbreds, Standardbreds, and Quarter Horses. • Affected foals are 2–6 months of age but may survive for 1–2 years. • Reported only in males.

SIGNS

- Affected foals appear physically normal at birth. • Most owners seek veterinary attention because of signs attributable to secondary infectious disease. • Recurrent episodes of pyrexia and clinical signs of pneumonia, enteritis, dermatitis, arthritis, and laminitis are most common.

CAUSES AND RISK FACTORS

With only four reports in the literature, the cause is uncertain. However, all affected foals reported have been males, suggesting an X-linked genetic disorder similar to agammaglobulinemia in humans.

DIAGNOSIS

DIFFERENTIAL DIAGNOSIS

- Determining if infectious disease is the primary problem in the foal or secondary to an immunodeficient state is the major challenge.
- Transient hypogammaglobulinemic foals tend to have low but detectable serum concentrations of IgM and IgA, whereas agammaglobulinemic foals lack IgM and IgA. Both disorders may have decreased to absent IgG depending on the state of waning maternal antibodies. Serially measuring serum immunoglobulin concentrations over time demonstrates increased concentrations in foals with transient hypogammaglobulinemia.
- SCID affects only Arabian foals, usually at a young age (<2 months old). SCID foals have persistent lymphopenia and fail to respond to an intradermal PHA test. A DNA test can be used to identify SCID foals. • Failure of passive transfer occurs in foals 1–14 days old. Such foals should be producing endogenous immunoglobulins by 2 months of age.
- Foals with selective IgM deficiency have a low or absent IgM concentration but normal concentrations of other immunoglobulins.

CBC/BIOCHEMISTRY/URINALYSIS

- Normal absolute lymphocyte counts.
- Total WBC and neutrophil counts may be low, normal, or high depending on secondary infections. • Usually unremarkable biochemistry and urinalysis.

OTHER LABORATORY TESTS

- Low and declining serum IgG concentrations
- Absent serum IgA and IgM concentrations
- Negative flow cytometry of lymphocytes using specific monoclonal antibodies to B lymphocyte surface antigens

IMAGING

N/A

OTHER DIAGNOSTIC PROCEDURES

- Normal PHA intradermal test • Lack of antibody production after vaccination.

PATHOLOGIC FINDINGS

Hypoplasia of B lymphocyte–dependent regions of the lymph nodes and spleen.

AGAMMAGLOBULINEMIA

TREATMENT

• Therapy is supportive and directed at treating acquired secondary infections. • Plasma therapy for temporary replacement of immunoglobulins

MEDICATIONS

DRUGS

Antimicrobials for treatment of acquired secondary infections.

CONTRAINDICATIONS/POSSIBLE INTERACTIONS

Anaphylactic or hemolytic reaction may occur with plasma transfusions, especially if multiple transfusions are administered.

FOLLOW-UP

• The prognosis is grave, even with intensive conventional therapy. Foals will die from acquired infections but may survive until 2–3 years of age. • Owners of a mare that has given birth to a foal with agammaglobulinemia should be informed about the possibility of an X-linked genetic defect. • Only four reports are in the literature, with the last published in 1980, indicating a very rare occurrence of this disorder.

MISCELLANEOUS

ASSOCIATED CONDITIONS

N/A

AGE-RELATED FACTORS

N/A

ZOONOTIC POTENTIAL

N/A

PREGNANCY

N/A

ABBREVIATIONS

• PHA = phytohemagglutinin
• SCID = severe combined immunodeficiency

Suggested Reading

McClure JJ. Equine immunodeficiency disease. In: Smith BP, ed, Large animal internal medicine. 2nd ed. St. Louis: Mosby, 1996.

Author J. Trenton McClure
Consulting Editor Debra C. Sellon

AGGRESSION

BASICS

DEFINITION

• Those behaviors that do, or attempt to do, injury to another with the apparent motivation of causing harm.
• Aggression is part of a larger complex of related behaviors termed *agonistic behaviors*, which are acts that relate to conflicts among animals or between animals and people.
• In addition to aggression, agonism includes threats (i.e., behaviors signaling the imminent likelihood of aggression), appeasement (i.e., behaviors functioning to end the aggression or threats of another), and flight (i.e., behaviors taking the animal away from the conflict).
• When people discuss aggression, they often mean to include both aggressive acts as well as threats.
• Aggression can be directed toward people, other horses, or other animals.
• Aggression may occur in one or several different circumstances, and different kinds of aggression often are delineated, which are thought to reflect different motivations of the aggressor.

PATHOPHYSIOLOGY

• Not necessarily a pathologic condition, but rather a normal part of the agonistic behavior horses use in resolving conflicts.
• When extreme in frequency or intensity, it could be a sign of an underlying pathologic condition.
• Always carefully evaluate medical causes (though this chapter focuses on nonmedical causes).

SYSTEMS AFFECTED

• Behavioral—may lead to changes in normal social behavior, deficits in learning, or inadequate performance of learned acts.
• CNS—specific changes remain unknown, unless a specific pathology has been identified.
• Others—if aggression leads to injury, several systems may be affected depending on the nature and extent of the injury, including the skin, musculoskeletal, cardiovascular, and others.

SIGNALMENT

• Any age, sex, or breed, though some forms are more likely in some age and sex classes.
• Sex-related aggression—more common among intact stallions and mares of breeding age.
• Maternal aggression—more common among mares with unweaned foals.
• Playful aggression—more common in foals <1 year.

SIGNS

General Comments

• Shown by specific behavioral acts and postures.
• Threats—lying back of the ears against the head, lowering and extending the head forward, vigorous swishing of the tail, the tail extended horizontally, turning the body to orient the back legs toward the target, lifting a hindleg or foreleg to strike, stamping the ground with a foreleg or rear leg, swinging the head to orient toward the target with the mouth open, and snapping with the teeth toward the target or squealing.
• Aggression—biting, kicking with the forelegs or hindlegs, and pushing with the head or hindquarters.

Historical Findings

• Vary with the circumstances and kind of aggression shown.
• Ask questions to identify exactly what behaviors are shown; when, where, and how often they occur; the targets of the aggression; when it first began; the situations that tend to make it worse (and better); and what has been done thus far to deal with the problem. These answers form the basis for treatment and risk assessment.

Common Forms

• Pain-induced—occurs in response to stimuli that induce pain (e.g., hitting the horse, handling an injured leg, giving an injection).
• Fear-motivated—occurs in response to specific stimuli that produce a reaction of alarm, agitation or flight. Aggression may occur in response to particular people, horses or other animals (e.g., a snake), or inanimate objects (e.g., hair clippers) or situations (e.g., a horse stall).
• Protective—occurs as defense of other animals or people to whom the aggressor has a relationship and that are perceived to be under threat.
• Maternal—a special form of protective aggression that occurs in response to perceived threats to the mare's foal or to one she has adopted.
• Sex-related—occurs as part of courtship, copulation, or intrasexual competition. A mare may attack a stallion attempting to mate, or a stallion may attack a mare that he is attempting to mate. Stallions may fight with each other in the presence or absence of mares, and mares may attack each other for access to stallions or to block access to a stallion.

AGGRESSION

• Dominance—occurs in groups where horses fight over resources (e.g., food, water) or status displays (e.g., threats, appeasement). Can also be directed to people who have regular interactions with the horse.
• Possessive—occurs over resources (e.g., food, water, resting sites) and can be directed toward horses, people, or other animals. Among horses living together, this form most often occurs as a part of dominance aggression.
• Redirected—occurs during conflict situations in which a horse attacks another animal or person when access to the original target is blocked.
• Play—foals <1 year can injure horses or people as a part of play. The intent to do harm is not present, but injuries can be severe. Thus, it often is classified with other forms of aggression.

Physical Examination Findings

• Should be unremarkable, unless some underlying pathology is present.
• Take great care in examining any aggressive animal, and consider use of appropriate restraints during the examination.

CAUSES

• Genetics probably are involved, but the mechanisms are unknown.
• Poor socialization to people and animals early during life can influence aggression.
• Painful or frightening experiences at any age can predispose to some kinds of aggression, as can positive or negative reinforcement of aggressive responses (whether intentional or unintentional).

RISK FACTORS

Poor socialization, harsh training or handling, and painful or frightening experiences may predispose to aggression.

DIAGNOSIS

DIFFERENTIAL DIAGNOSIS

Rule out pathologic conditions that may lead to aggression before establishing a behavioral diagnosis.

CBC/BIOCHEMISTRY/URINALYSIS

N/A

OTHER LABORATORY TESTS

N/A

IMAGING

N/A

DIAGNOSTIC PROCEDURES

N/A

TREATMENT

RISK ASSESSMENT

• Always realistically assess the risks involved with keeping the animal before considering any treatment.
• Base the assessment on historical questions, direct observations, veterinary medical records, legal records, and other documents of relevance. Specific information includes how long the problem has been occurring, the severity of any injuries produced, whether the aggression occurs in one or many different situations, how predictable the aggression is, how easy it is to interrupt or stop the aggression, whether the aggression is directed toward one or many different targets, and whether elderly people or small children may be likely targets of aggression.
• Animals are more dangerous and the risk greater if the problem has been going on for a while, severe injuries have resulted, the aggression occurs in many different situations, is unpredictable or difficult to stop or interrupt, is directed toward many different targets, or if likely targets include elderly people or small children.

GENERAL COMMENTS

• Most treatments of nonmedical conditions involve changing the physical or social environment of the horse or using behavior modification techniques to change the motivational state of the animal.
• Consider surgical castration for all aggressive horses given the potential for inheritance of these traits; castration also may reduce some kinds of aggression in the horse itself.
• The primary goal always is to reduce the risk of injury to people and animals.
• If treatment cannot be undertaken or fails, consider euthanasia, which is the only option that guarantees the animal will not be aggressive in the future.
• Behavior modification most often involves systematic desensitization and counter-conditioning.
• Desensitization—gradual exposure to aggression-provoking stimuli in a way that does not elicit threatening or aggressive behavior; the animal is then rewarded for displaying calm, relaxed, and nonthreatening behavior.
• Counter-conditioning—eliciting an emotional and behavioral state that is incompatible with aggression and threat; gentle massage or feeding a preferred treat generally creates such incompatible states.

AGGRESSION

• Behavior modification must be done carefully and precisely if it is to be safe and effective. Referral to an experienced veterinary behaviorist, applied animal behaviorist, or trainer usually is necessary to help the client implement the plan.
• Punishment of any sort usually should be avoided, because it can lead the animal to become fearful or even more aggressive.
• Specific treatments may vary with the kind of aggression.

SPECIFIC TREATMENTS

Pain-Elicited

• Identify the cause of the pain. If medical, treat it; if related to management or handling, remove or avoid the source of pain.
• If neither is possible, consider medications to control pain; however, pain medication should not be considered an alternative to inadequate, poor, or harsh management or handling practices.

Fear-Motivated

Identify and remove or avoid the source of the fear; if removal or avoidance is not possible, use behavior modification.

Protective

Separate animals that are being protective, avoid protective situations, or use behavior modification.

Maternal

Separate the mare and foal from other animals or people, avoid situations leading to aggression, or use behavior modification.

Sex-Related

Separate animals that are fighting, use restraint devices to reduce injury to other animals or people in breeding situations, or use behavior modification.

Dominance

• Separate animals that are fighting.
• Introduce new animals gradually, and keep social situations as stable as possible.
• Spread out resources—food, water, and shade
• Use behavior modification.

Possessive

• Separate animals that are fighting.
• Spread out resources (e.g., food, water and shade), or remove them.
• Use behavior modification.

Redirected

Identify and remove or avoid the original stimulus leading to the aggression, or use behavior modification.

Play

Avoid situations in which foals can play with people.

MEDICATIONS

DRUGS OF CHOICE

• No drugs approved by the U.S. FDA for use with aggressive problems in horses.
• Pain medications may help to reduce or eliminate pain-elicited aggression.
• Anxiolytics or antidepressants may help with fear-motivated aggression.
• For other forms or for horses with mixed aggression (e.g., fear and dominance), these drugs actually may increase aggression; thus, drugs may be dangerous to use for aggression and should be prescribed only after careful evaluation.

CONTRAINDICATIONS

N/A

PRECAUTIONS

• Inform clients that use of psychoactive drugs for aggression problems constitutes off-label and experimental use.
• Inform clients regarding possible benefits, dangers, and side effects.
• Obtain written informed consent before prescribing medication.

POSSIBLE INTERACTIONS

N/A

ALTERNATIVE DRUGS

N/A

FOLLOW-UP

PATIENT MONITORING

- Contact clients on a regular basis to check compliance with recommendations and to provide additional support.
- Behavioral problems generally require intensive follow-up.

POSSIBLE COMPLICATIONS

Clients should be fully aware that an aggressive animal can deliver serious injury or even cause death, and that keeping an aggressive animal places the client at risk of criminal and civil legal actions.

MISCELLANEOUS

ASSOCIATED CONDITIONS

N/A

AGE-RELATED FACTORS

N/A

ZOONOTIC POTENTIAL

N/A

PREGNANCY

N/A

SYNONYMS

N/A

SEE ALSO

- Excessive maternal behavior/foal stealing
- Fears and phobias
- Maternal foal rejection
- Psychogenic sexual behavior dysfunction

Suggested Reading

Borchelt PL, Voith VL. Aggressive behavior in dogs and cats. In: Voith VL, Borchelt PL, eds. Readings in companion animal behavior. Trenton: Veterinary Learning Systems, 1996:217–229.

Crowell-Davis SL. Normal behavior and behavior problems. In: Kobluk CN, Ames TR, Geor RJ, eds. The horse: diseases and clinical management. Philadelphia: WB Saunders, 1995:1–21.

Houpt KA. Domestic animal behavior for veterinarians and animal scientists. 3rd ed. Ames: Iowa State University Press, 1998.

Waring GH. Horse behavior. The behavioral traits and adaptations of domestic and wild horses, including ponies. Park Ridge: Noyes Publications, 1983.

Author Daniel Q. Estep

Consulting Editor Daniel Q. Estep

ALBUMIN, HYPOALBUMINEMIA

BASICS

DEFINITION

A lower-than-normal concentration of plasma albumin.

PATHOPHYSIOLOGY

- May be accompanied by normal total plasma proteins.
- Most commonly results from increased loss (primarily in the GI and renal tracts), but decreased production may contribute.
- Albumin is produced in the liver, has the lowest molecular weight of all proteins, and is the most abundant protein, accounting for 75% of the osmotic pressure.
- Albumin binds and transports plasma components that have no specific transport protein.
- Decreased intake, decreased synthesis, excessive breakdown, and increased loss may result in hypoalbuminemia.
- Protein production depends on adequate nutrition. Starvation, malnutrition, and chronic GI disorders interfering with digestion and absorption may result in a lack of amino acid substrate for general protein production. In dietary deficiencies, hypoalbuminemia often precedes panhypoproteinemia.
- Acute liver disease usually does not result in decreased albumin synthesis. However, chronic, diffuse liver disease (e.g., chronic hepatitis, fibrosis, hepatic neoplasia) may cause hypoalbuminemia.
- Because the half-life of albumin is longer in horses and cattle than in companion animals, hypoalbuminemia rarely occurs with hepatic disease in equine and bovine species. When it does β- and γ-globulins often are increased. These changes only occur late in the disease process and, thus, may have more prognostic than diagnostic value.
- Excessive albumin breakdown can occur during negative nitrogen balance caused by increased metabolic demands—fever, trauma, surgery, and neoplasia.
- Albumin is broken down to provide amino acids as substrates for energy production.
- Chronic antigenic stimulation can increase albumin catabolism to provide amino acids for immunoglobulin production, but this increased catabolism typically does not produce a change in total plasma protein concentration.
- Urinary protein loss is determined by glomerular filtration rate, glomerular membrane permeability, and tubular resorption of proteins.
- Urine typically contains little or no protein, but transient physiologic proteinuria occurs with exercise, stress, convulsions, and excessive protein intake. This transient proteinuria does not result in hypoproteinemia.
- Neonates may demonstrate proteinuria for several days after nonspecific absorption of various colostral proteins that are not retained—lactalbumin.
- Because of its small size, albumin is readily filtered through glomerular basement membrane defects; therefore, glomerulonephritis is a common cause of albuminuria.
- Pyelonephritis and amyloidosis also can result in albuminuria and subsequent hypoproteinemia.
- Protein-losing enteropathy is the excessive loss of plasma proteins into the GI tract. Clinically important mechanisms of GI protein loss consist of ulceration, defective lymphatic drainage, increased mucosal permeability, and exudation resulting from inflammation.
- Protein-losing enteropathies result in loss of relatively more albumin than globulins, although panhypoproteinemia eventually develops, particularly with inflammation.
- Salmonellosis, NSAID toxicity, and other causes of acute colitis/enteritis may result only in hypoalbuminemia, although a general loss of all plasma proteins usually occurs.
- In cases involving acute diarrhea, assess the patient's hydration status when interpreting total plasma proteins, because dehydration may mask an actual hypoproteinemic state. A falling plasma protein with an elevated PCV indicates acute protein loss.

SYSTEMS AFFECTED

Most often is associated with GI or renal disorders resulting in protein loss and with cases of chronic hepatic disease.

SIGNALMENT

N/A

SIGNS

General Comments

- Clinical signs—edema of the distal extremities, ventral body wall, and face.
- Generally, albumin levels must fall to <1.5 g/dL before signs develop.
- Occasionally, pharyngeal and laryngeal edema can develop and result in upper airway obstruction, necessitating tracheotomy.
- Pulmonary edema can occur in hypoalbuminemic patients those undergoing intravascular fluid therapy.

Historical Findings

- Fever
- Decreased appetite
- Cough
- Nasal discharge
- Respiratory distress
- Exercise intolerance
- Poor performance
- Diarrhea
- GI dysfunction
- Dysuria
- Weight loss
- Prolonged NSAID administration

Physical Examination Findings

- Findings reflect the underlying cause and contributing factors.
- Edema of the distal extremities, ventral body wall, or face may be present.

CAUSES

- Salmonellosis
- Clostridiosis
- Colitis X
- Equine ehrlichial enterocolitis—Potomac horse fever
- NSAID toxicity
- Idiopathic granulomatous enteritis/enterocolitis
- Chronic eosinophilic gastroenteritis
- Intestinal malabsorption
- Malnutrition
- Parasitism
- Glomerulonephritis
- Pyelonephritis
- Chronic hepatic fibrosis—pyrrolizidine alkaloid toxicity
- Intestinal lymphosarcoma
- Hepatic neoplasia
- Amyloidosis
- Tuberculosis
- Histoplasmosis

RISK FACTORS

- Associated with a variety of diseases.
- May be exacerbated by aggressive IV fluid therapy.

ALBUMIN, HYPOALBUMINEMIA

DIAGNOSIS

DIFFERENTIAL DIAGNOSIS

Sources of albumin loss (e.g., GI or renal disease) and decreased production (e.g., inadequate nutrition, liver disease) must be explored as causes.

LABORATORY FINDINGS

Drugs That May Alter Lab Results

N/A

Disorders That May Alter Lab Results

N/A

Valid If Run in Human Lab?

Albumin determination is not valid if run in a human lab.

CBC/BIOCHEMISTRY/URINALYSIS

- Compensatory increase in globulin occasionally is present.
- Interpret PCV and protein values simultaneously to determine if hemoconcentration (i.e., dehydration) or concurrent anemia is present.
- Proteinuria is an abnormal finding and warrants further investigation of renal status.

OTHER LABORATORY TESTS

- Appropriate tests for infectious or inflammatory diseases may be necessary to establish a definitive diagnosis.
- Urinary fractional electrolyte excretion and GGT:creatinine ratio may help to define renal tubular disease.
- Fecal cultures or rectal biopsy may provide useful information regarding the cause of enterocolitis.

IMAGING

Ultrasonography and radiography of the thorax, abdomen, or soft tissue may help to identify a cause or direct further diagnostics necessary to establish a definitive diagnosis.

DIAGNOSTIC PROCEDURES

Abdominocentesis, thoracocentesis, transtracheal aspiration or bronchoalveolar lavage, endoscopy, laparoscopy, bone marrow aspiration, CSF evaluation, biopsy, and histopathology are available for establishing a definitive diagnosis and should be selected based on physical examination and laboratory findings.

TREATMENT

- Address sources of protein loss (e.g., hemorrhage, GI and renal disease) with appropriate medical or surgical treatment.
- Equine plasma administered IV may be warranted with marked hypoalbuminemia.
- Development of pulmonary edema requires aggressive therapy.

MEDICATIONS

DRUGS OF CHOICE

N/A

CONTRAINDICATIONS

N/A

PRECAUTIONS

Anaphylactic reactions can occur during IV plasma administration—give an IV test dose slowly, and monitor the patient closely during treatment.

POSSIBLE INTERACTIONS

N/A

ALTERNATIVE DRUGS

N/A

FOLLOW-UP

PATIENT MONITORING

- Perform clinical evaluation 3–4 times daily in critical cases.
- Perform laboratory evaluation with PCV and total protein determination twice daily.
- Adjust the frequency of monitoring based on severity of the case and clinical response to therapy.

POSSIBLE COMPLICATIONS

- Complications relate directly to the cause of the hypoalbuminemia.
- Dependent and pulmonary edema are possible in severe cases and may require diuretics.

MISCELLANEOUS

ASSOCIATED CONDITIONS

- Hypoproteinemia often is associated.
- A compensatory, relative hyperglobulinemia may exist.

AGE-RELATED FACTORS

N/A

ZOONOTIC POTENTIAL

In cases of enterocolitis, include salmonellosis on the differential list, which necessitates proper handling to avoid potential contamination and zoonosis.

PREGNANCY

N/A

SYNONYMS

N/A

SEE ALSO

Refer to individual conditions and diseases causing hypoalbuminemia.

ABBREVIATIONS

- CSF = cerebrospinal fluid
- GGT = γ-glutamyltransferase
- GI = gastrointestinal
- PCV = packed cell volume

Suggested Reading

Kobluk CN, Ames TR, Geor RJ, eds. The horse: diseases and clinical management. Philadelphia: WB Saunders, 1995.

Meyer DJ, Coles EH, Rich LJ. Veterinary laboratory medicine. Philadelphia: WB Saunders, 1992.

Smith BP. Large animal internal medicine. St. Louis: CV Mosby, 1990.

Author Kent A. Humber

Consulting Editor Claire B. Andreasen

ALKALINE PHOSPHATASE (ALP)

BASICS

DEFINITION

• Serum ALP mainly is used as a marker for cholestasis.
• Routine chemistry panels report total ALP, but nonhepatic tissues (especially bone) may contribute to total ALP.
• Only infrequently is used as a marker for changes in other tissues, which requires fairly complex isoenzyme separation techniques.
• For routine interpretations, the potential contributions by nonhepatic tissues must be understood to avoid misinterpreting increased ALP from these tissues as evidence for cholestasis.
• Reference intervals vary depending on the assay substrate employed; thus, comparisons across labs may not be valid.

PATHOPHYSIOLOGY

• Two genes produce distinct ALP. isoenzymes—intestinal ALP, and tissue-unspecific ALP.
• Generally, the intestinal ALP gene is expressed only in the intestine and the tissue-unspecific ALP gene elsewhere; however, the equine kidney expresses both.
• Posttranslational modification (especially glycosylation) produces additional tissue-specific isoforms of ALP (e.g., bone, liver) and affects biological behavior (e.g., circulating half-life).
• Various ALP forms can be quantified based on use of specific inhibitors—wheat germ lectin inhibits only bone ALP activity; levamisole inhibits both bone and liver ALP activity but not intestinal ALP.
• High tissue concentrations occur in kidney, intestine, liver, and bone; lower concentrations occur in placenta and other tissues.
• Although intestine and kidney have much higher tissue concentrations than liver and bone, renal ALP usually is not released into blood, and intestinal ALP has a very short half-life of ≅8 minutes. Thus, serum concentrations normally consist mostly of liver and, to a lesser extent, bone ALP.
• Liver ALP activity generally is greatest at the biliary canalicular surface of hepatocytes (i.e., membrane bound). Increased blood activity results from increased synthesis (i.e., induction) or membrane release. The mechanism of release into the blood is unclear but is proposed to involve membrane solubilization by bile salts, release of membrane fragments, or biliary regurgitation. A serum phospholipase may contribute to cleavage of the enzyme from the membrane.
• Cholestasis leads to increased serum ALP concentrations. Hepatocellular injury alone (e.g., carbon tetrachloride toxicity) has little effect, but bile duct ligation leads to nearly 3-fold elevations within 10 days. Presumably, much higher increases would require considerable chronicity.
• No evidence that blood concentrations rise in conjunction with cellular proliferation, as seen with GGT.
• Because increased ALP involves enzyme induction, serum ALP increases in acute obstructive jaundice are preceded by other markers such as conjugated bilirubin; bile salts.

SYSTEMS AFFECTED

• Hepatobiliary—increases are associated with cholestasis.
• Musculoskeletal—increases are associated with increased osteoblastic activity.
• GI—severe GI disease can be associated with mild increases, the source of which (i.e., mucosal cells vs. secondary liver changes) often is unclear.
• Reproductive—placental increases during pregnancy; impact on serum concentrations is equivocal.

SIGNALMENT

• Neonates and foals—very high ALP occurs in neonates; foals during the first year have higher ALP than adults.
• Pregnancy—equivocal impact on serum ALP; some diseases associated with cholestasis and increased ALP are seen with higher frequency in pregnant mares (e.g., hyperlipemia, Theiler's disease associated with receiving tetanus toxoid).
• Ponies and donkeys—particularly susceptible to hyperlipemia and hepatic lipidosis if subjected to negative nitrogen balance.
• Other factors—depend on the underlying cause.

SIGNS

General Comments

Signs do not result directly from increased serum ALP activity but from the underlying disease process.

Historical Findings

• Owners may report icterus, dark yellow/orange urine, anorexia, weight loss, listlessness, and behavioral changes associated with hepatic failure in conditions associated with cholestasis.
• Abdominal pain (e.g., sweating, rolling) may occur with acute hepatopathies (i.e., capsular swelling) or biliary obstructions.

Physical Examination Findings

• Icterus frequently is observed.
• Increased pulse and respiratory rates, fever, photosensitization, weight loss, or obesity vary with the type and severity of the underlying disease process.

ALKALINE PHOSPHATASE (ALP)

CAUSES

Hepatobiliary System

- Metabolic—secondary to severe anemia (see *Hematopoietic System*), hyperlipemia, or fasting (ALP may increase by <50% with a 2–3-day fast)
- Immune-mediated, infectious—chronic active hepatitis, Theiler's disease (i.e., serum hepatitis), amyloidosis, endotoxemia, viral (e.g., EIA, EVA, EHV in perinatal foals), bacterial (e.g., Tyzzer's disease, salmonellosis), fungal, protozoal, and parasitic (e.g., liver flukes, strongyle larval migrans)
- Nutritional—hepatic lipidosis
- Degenerative—cirrhosis; cholelithiasis
- Toxic—pyrrolizidine alkaloid–containing plants (e.g., senecio, crotolaria), alsike clover, aflatoxin, rubratoxin; chemical toxins (e.g., arsenic, chlorinated hydrocarbons, phenol, paraquat) typically cause primarily hepatocellular injury; some cholestasis may be secondary to hepatocellular swelling or, if lesions progress to end-stage liver disease, fibrosing effects on bile flow; some anesthetics (e.g., halothane) are associated with mild, transient increases.
- Anomaly—biliary atresia; portovascular shunts
- Neoplastic—primary liver tumors (rare); metastatic neoplasia (uncommon)

Musculoskeletal System

- Rapid bone growth—juveniles
- Severe bony lesions

GI System

Severe GI disease—diarrhea

Reproductive System

Pregnancy increases placental ALP, with mild increases in total serum ALP.

Hematopoietic System

- Severe anemia (e.g., acute EIA, red maple leaf toxicity, onion toxicity, postparturient hemorrhage) leads to hypoxic injury and hepatocellular swelling, with subsequent cholestasis
- Hepatic lymphosarcoma, leukemias, and so on

RISK FACTORS

Those associated with any disease leading to cholestasis—exposure to serum products in periparturient mares may increase risk for serum hepatitis with associated cholestasis.

DIAGNOSIS

DIFFERENTIAL DIAGNOSIS

- Increases caused by bone ALP mostly are seen in growing animals. In adults, increased bone ALP likely involves lameness or obvious bony lesions. Increases from bone ALP are relatively mild.
- Highest elevations generally are associated with long-standing conditions involving severe cholestasis—chronic active hepatitis, cirrhosis, cholelithiasis, and lipidosis.
- Concurrent obesity and high enzyme levels suggest hyperlipemia/lipidosis, whereas anorexia and weight loss are typical of most other differentials.

LABORATORY FINDINGS

Drugs that May Alter Lab Results

- Arsenate, beryllium, cyanide, fluoride, manganese, phosphate, sulfhydryl compounds, and zinc may cause falsely low values.
- Complexing anticoagulants (e.g., citrate, EDTA, oxalate) inhibit the enzyme and should not be used for sample collection.

Disorders that May Alter Lab Results

- Very high bilirubin values, severe lipemia, and marked hemolysis may cause falsely elevated values.
- Activity tends to increase with storage.

Valid If Run in Human Lab?

- Valid, but concentrations vary with the methodology employed.
- Each lab should have in house–generated reference intervals or, minimally, species-specific reference intervals based on the same methodology.

CBC/BIOCHEMISTRY/URINALYSIS

- No routine laboratory tests provide a causative or specific diagnosis for increases.
- Most suggest a type of injury (e.g., injury, cholestasis, insufficiency) rather than a cause.
- Others confirming the presence of cholestasis support a suspected hepatic origin for the increase.

Erythrocytes

- Nonregenerative anemia may be seen with liver disease.
- Morphologic changes may be reported—poikilocytosis, acanthocytosis, and target cells.
- Some morphologic changes induced by liver disease (e.g., acanthocytes, schistocytes from microvascular disease in the liver) are associated with decreased RBC survival and may contribute to mild hemolytic (i.e., regenerative) anemia.
- Severe hemolytic anemia from any cause (e.g., oxidation injuries manifested by Heinz bodies or eccentrocytes, immune-mediated anemia) can cause hypoxic injury, leading to hepatocellular swelling and secondary cholestasis.

Leukocytes

- Neutrophilia or neutropenia and monocytosis may occur with inflammatory liver disease—bacterial cholangiohepatitis.
- Evidence of antigenic stimulation (e.g., lymphocytosis, reactive lymphoid cells) may be seen.

Glucose

- Postprandial hyperglycemia or fasting hypoglycemia may occur with hepatic insufficiency/shunts.
- Hypoglycemia with liver disease carries a guarded prognosis.

ALKALINE PHOSPHATASE (ALP)

Albumin
• Decreased production with hepatic insufficiency may decrease serum levels.
• Albumin is a negative acute-phase reactant—mild decreases may occur during inflammatory liver disease.

BUN
Decreased (especially relative to creatinine) levels occur with hepatic insufficiency/shunts caused by decreased conversion of ammonia to urea.

SDH
• Increases with hepatocellular injury.
• May occur concurrent with or independent of cholestasis.

AST
Increases with hepatocellular or muscle injury.

GGT
Increases with either injury or cholestasis.

Bilirubin
• Conjugated—increases with cholestasis; seen with hepatocellular injury, presumably related to cell swelling and secondary cholestasis.
• Unconjugated—increases with increased RBC destruction (i.e., hemolysis) and with fasting.

Cholesterol
• May decrease with hepatic insufficiency/shunts.
• Sometimes increases with cholestasis and lipid metabolic disorders—hyperlipemia.

Triglycerides
Increased with hyperlipemia.

Urinalysis
• Bilirubinuria supports the presence of cholestasis.
• Ammonia urates may be observed with hepatic insufficiency/shunt.

OTHER LABORATORY TESTS

Bile Acids
• Sensitive indicator of hepatic disease, but not specific for the type of process—injury, cholestasis, or insufficiency.
• Assesses enterohepatic circulation, adequate hepatocellular perfusion, and hepatobiliary function.
• Often more sensitive than ALP for equine cholestasis.

Ammonia
Serum concentrations are affected by hepatic uptake and correlate inversely with hepatic functional mass.

Clearance Tests (BSP, ICG)
• Prolonged clearance intervals with decreased functional mass or cholestasis
• Accelerated clearance (possibly masking insufficiency) with hypoalbuminemia

Serology
Depends on the degree of suspicion for specific diseases—viral, fungal, and so on.

Coagulation Tests
May be prolonged with hepatic insufficiency/shunting—prothrombin time; activated partial thromboplastin time.

IMAGING
Ultrasonography—useful for assessing liver size, shape, position, and parenchymal texture; may help to detect focal parenchymal lesions (e.g., abscesses, neoplasms) and abnormalities in the biliary tree (e.g., dilatations, obstructions) or large vessels (e.g., shunts, thrombosis).

DIAGNOSTIC PROCEDURES
Aspiration cytology or biopsy for microbiologic testing, cytologic imprints, and histopathologic evaluation may provide specific diagnostic information.

TREATMENT
• Decision regarding outpatient vs. inpatient treatment depends on the severity of disease, intensity of supportive care required, need for isolation of infectious conditions, and so on.
• Fluid and nutritional support may be needed.
• Anorexic and hypoglycemic cases may benefit from IV 5% dextrose (2 mL/kg per hour); otherwise, fluid support depends on specific electrolyte and acid–base abnormalities.
• Avoid negative energy balance, especially in ponies and donkeys, by treating hyperlipemia and hepatic lipidosis.
• Toxicities or hepatic insufficiency may warrant efforts to reduce production/absorption of toxins.
• Mineral oil by nasogastric tube helps to reduce toxin absorption.
• Lactulose (0.3 mL/kg q6h) by nasogastric tube is suggested to combat GI ammonia production/absorption but also causes diarrhea.
• A high-carbohydrate, low-protein diet reduces ammonia production.
• Specific therapy, including surgery, depends on the specific underlying cause.

ALKALINE PHOSPHATASE (ALP)

MEDICATIONS

DRUGS OF CHOICE

Depend on the suspected cause and observed complications.

CONTRAINDICATIONS

Depend on the suspected cause and observed complications.

PRECAUTIONS

- Depend on the suspected cause.
- With suspected hepatic insufficiency, assess coagulation profiles before invasive procedures.

POSSIBLE INTERACTIONS

Depend on the underlying cause.

ALTERNATIVE DRUGS

Depend on the underlying cause.

FOLLOW UP

PATIENT MONITORING

Serial chemistries can help to establish a prognosis by characterizing disease progression and identifying evidence of improvement—initial evaluation at 1–2-day intervals helps to establish the disease course; subsequent testing can be at increasing intervals, depending on signs and severity.

POSSIBLE COMPLICATIONS

Depend on the underlying cause.

MISCELLANEOUS

ASSOCIATED CONDITIONS

Depend on the underlying cause.

AGE-RELATED FACTORS

- Healthy foals may have markedly higher ALP than adults.
- Highest activity is seen during the first 3 days of life (≤20-fold greater). These levels decrease to <5–10-fold over adult levels by 2 weeks, and then gradually decrease during the first year before approximating adult levels.
- High neonatal ALP activity may reflect a combination of intestinal pinocytosis, high osteoblastic activity, and liver ALP.
- High postneonatal (age, 1–12 months) ALP activity largely results from osteoblastic activity.

ZOONOTIC POTENTIAL

Depends on the underlying cause.

PREGNANCY

See *Signalment.*

SYNONYMS

N/A

SEE ALSO

See *Causes.*

ABBREVIATIONS

- AST = aspartate aminotransferase
- BSP = sulfobromophthalein
- EHV = equine herpes virus
- EIA = equine infectious anemia
- EVA = equine viral arteritis
- GGT = γ-glutamyltransferase
- GI = gastrointestinal
- ICG = indocyanine green
- SDH = sorbitol dehydrogenase

Suggested Reading

Barton MH, Morris DD. Diseases of the liver. In: Reed S, Bayly W, eds. Equine internal medicine. Philadelphia: WB Saunders, 1998.

Hoffmann W, Baker G, Rieser S, Dorner J. Alterations in selected biochemical constituents in equids after induced hepatic disease. Am J Vet Res 1987;48:1343–1347.

West HJ. Clinical and pathological studies in horses with hepatic disease. Equine Vet J 1996;28:146–156.

Authors John A. Christian and Armando Irizarry-Rovira

Consulting Editor Claire B. Andreasen

ALKALOSIS, METABOLIC

BASICS

DEFINITION

• A disruption of acid–base homeostasis producing decreased H^+ concentration reflected by alkalemia—increased pH and high plasma HCO_3^-, TCO_2, or BE.
• Normal plasma bicarbonate level in horses is ≅24 mEq/L.
• Normal pH of arterial blood ranges from 7.35–7.45.
• Hypoventilation should increase CO_2 levels to lower pH; however, respiratory compensation is limited once hypoxemia develops.

PATHOPHYSIOLOGY

• The kidney normally is extremely capable of responding to a high pH, correcting MAK via excretion of HCO_3^- into the urine. Even with daily administration of high bicarbonate levels, the alkalosis is short lived in normal horses. Therefore, MAK persists only when an initiating factor develops simultaneously with conditions in which renal excretion of HCO_3^- is impaired or reabsorption is enhanced.
• Excessive loss of H^+, retention of HCO_3^-, and contraction of ECF volume without loss of HCO_3^- (i.e., contraction alkalosis) are the common mechanisms thought to initiate MAK.
• HCO_3^- is retained by the kidney when inadequate filtration results from hypovolemia or renal failure or when reabsorption mechanisms are enhanced from volume depletion or K^+ or Cl^- depletion.
• Na^+ reabsorption occurs primarily in the proximal tubule and must be accompanied by a negative anion. Cl^- most is often utilized. When Cl^- is unavailable, Na resorption occurs in the distal tubule in exchange for H^+ or, sometimes, K^+. If K^+ is depleted, the kidney excretes H^+, because correction of volume deficits has priority over pH.
• Secretion of H^+ results in generation of HCO_3^- in the distal tubule. This HCO_3^- then is reabsorbed, maintaining the extracellular alkalemia.
• Secretion of H^+ results in production of acidic urine, considered paradoxic in the face of systemic alkalosis.
• Hypokalemia results as K^+ moves intracellularly to balance the loss of H^+ moving extracellularly.

SYSTEMS AFFECTED

Respiratory

Peripheral and central chemoreceptors sense high pH in blood or CSF and depress ventilation to decrease removal of CO_2; hypercapnia and hypoxemia may follow.

Cardiovascular

• Cardiac arrhythmias
• Arteriolar vasoconstriction
• Decreased coronary blood flow

Neuroendocrine

• Decreased cerebral blood flow caused by vasoconstriction.
• Neurologic signs (e.g., delirium, seizures, lethargy, stupor) are rare but can be seen with severe alkalemia.
• Neuromuscular excitability and tetany may occur.

Metabolic

• Increased affinity of oxygen-hemoglobin binding, which inhibits release of oxygen to the tissues
• Decreased ionized calcium concentration

Renal

The kidney responds to high pH by very effective HCO_3^- excretion under otherwise normal conditions. This response develops within hours, but it may take days to complete.

SIGNALMENT

• All breeds, ages, and sexes
• Horses used for endurance exercise may be more likely to be affected.

SIGNS

• Recent participation in endurance events or other exercise of long duration and moderate intensity may be included in the history.
• Physical examination findings vary with the primary cause.
• Respiratory rate or volume may be decreased, but tachypnea may be present.
• Hyperthermia, sweating, colic, ileus, synchronous diaphragmatic flutter (i.e., "thumps"), muscle fasciculations, weakness, anorexia, and depression may be present, especially in horses recently exercised.

CAUSES

• Some causes may include both an initiating factor(s) and condition(s) that encourage maintenance of alkalosis.
• GI loss of H^+ is seen with gastric reflux that occurs with anterior enteritis, ileus, or early small intestinal obstruction.
• Salivary loss of Cl^- occurs with dysphagia, esophageal trauma or obstruction, and esophagostomy.
• Cl^- loss is seen with gastric reflux, excessive sweating (especially in endurance horses), and diuretic therapy (especially with furosemide).
• K^+ depletion is associated with anorexia, restriction of GI intake, polyuric renal failure, and diuretic therapy (especially with acetazolamide).
• Endurance horses with exertional rhabdomyolysis present with MAK, likely associated with the loss of fluid and electrolytes via sweating.
• Sweating is the primary means of heat dissipation during exercise in horses. Equine sweat contains large amounts of chloride and potassium relative to serum levels. Fluid loss can be extreme with moderate-intensity exercise over long periods, especially in warm, humid conditions. Therefore, fluid and electrolyte losses can be very significant—even life-threatening—in sweating horses.
• Most of the mentioned conditions involve contraction alkalosis—fluid loss/shifts involving Na and Cl but not HCO_3^-.
• Contraction alkalosis also can occur with alterations of fluid balance seen with body-cavity effusions and cardiac failure.
• Bicarbonate therapy may result in MAK in race horses, especially if also given diuretics.
• Because proteins are weak acids, hypoproteinemia (especially albumin) produces MAK.
• Early large-colon obstructions and ileus may present with MAK caused by alteration of electrolyte, fluid, and HCO_3^- exchange in the large intestine.

RISK FACTORS

• Bicarbonate or diuretic therapy in horses before exercise
• Endurance or long-duration, moderate-intensity exercise
• Hot or humid weather/climates

DIAGNOSIS

DIFFERENTIAL DIAGNOSIS

• Increased bicarbonate levels also are seen in conditions with respiratory acidosis. PCO_2 is high but the pH close to normal or high on blood gas analysis.
• Compensation may be very effective in chronic respiratory acidosis.

LABORATORY FINDINGS

Drugs That May Alter Lab Results

• Excessive anticoagulant may falsely decrease results via dilution.
• Excessive sodium heparin may alter HCO_3^- levels.

Disorders That May Alter Lab Results

With poor peripheral perfusion or cardiovascular shunt, results of blood gas analysis on samples taken from peripheral vessels may differ from those taken elsewhere or may not reflect the patient's overall systemic condition.

Valid If Run in Human Lab?

Yes, if properly submitted.

CBC/BIOCHEMISTRY/URINALYSIS

- Measurements of serum electrolytes, protein levels, and serum chemistries are important to determine the cause and to guide treatment.
- Proportionate changes in sodium and chloride levels occur with alterations of fluid balance. Normal sodium levels with hypo- or hyperchloremia indicate acid–base imbalance, whereas disproportionate changes usually are associated with simultaneous acid–base imbalance and hydration abnormalities.
- Potassium and chloride are decreased in horses that sweat excessively. Potassium may be low because of the primary cause or as a response to the extracellular shift of H^+.
- Ionized calcium is decreased.
- Magnesium may be decreased, especially with sweat loss and colic.
- Urinalysis may reveal decreased urine pH.

OTHER LABORATORY TESTS

- Many labs measure TCO_2 using the same sample submitted for electrolytes.
- The TCO_2 closely approximates HCO_3^-, because most CO_2 is carried in the blood as bicarbonate.
- Like MAK, respiratory alkalosis also results in high TCO_2. These conditions can be differentiated only by complete blood gas analysis.
- The TCO_2 must be analyzed rapidly and with minimal room-air exposure within the sample tube, because CO_2 can dissipate from the sample.

IMAGING

N/A

DIAGNOSTIC PROCEDURES

N/A

TREATMENT

- Treatment of the primary cause is essential.
- Replacement of fluid losses with isotonic fluids may be all that is needed to restore acid–base status in mild cases.
- Address specific electrolyte losses.
- Large volumes may be needed in some endurance athletes with excessive fluid losses from sweating or hyperthermia.

MEDICATIONS

DRUGS OF CHOICE

- With hypochloremia, give fluids containing chloride, or the alkalosis will not be corrected even if hydration is restored.
- Saline or Ringer's solution with added calcium and KCl is the fluid of choice.
- IV administration is necessary with severe fluid losses; however, PO administration of rehydration fluid has been very successful in horses.
- From 1–2 gallons of electrolyte solutions without alkali can be given every 3–4 hours.
- With excessive potassium loss, PO supplementation is necessary if the horse remains anorexic.

CONTRAINDICATIONS

Lactated Ringer solution can worsen the alkalosis.

PRECAUTIONS

- Give calcium-containing solutions slowly to avoid arrhythmias.
- Monitor cardiac rhythm during administration.

POSSIBLE INTERACTIONS

N/A

ALTERNATIVE DRUGS

Oral rehydration solutions have achieved good results in horses, being very effective in mild cases and an excellent adjunct to IV therapy. From 1–2 gallons can be given PO every few hours to adults without ileus.

FOLLOW-UP

PATIENT MONITORING

Serial blood gas analysis and measurement of electrolytes and calcium are very important in evaluating efficacy of therapy; repeat within a few hours of initial treatment and thereafter according to patient response.

POSSIBLE COMPLICATIONS

- Hypokalemia
- Hypocalcemia
- Other, rare complications—cardiac arrhythmias, colic, synchronous diaphragmatic flutter, tetany, and neurologic signs

MISCELLANEOUS

ASSOCIATED CONDITIONS

- Hypochloremia
- Hypokalemia
- Respiratory acidosis

AGE-RELATED CONDITIONS

N/A

ZOONOTIC POTENTIAL

N/A

PREGNANCY

N/A

SYNONYMS

Nonrespiratory alkalosis

SEE ALSO

- Exertional rhabdomyolysis
- Exhausted horse syndrome
- Heat exhaustion
- Hyperthermia

ABBREVIATIONS

- BE = base excess
- CSF = cerebrospinal fluid
- ECF = extracellular fluid
- GI = gastrointestinal
- MAK = metabolic alkalosis

Suggested Reading

Androgue HJ, Madias NE. Management of life-threatening acid-base disorders. Part 2. N Engl J Med 1998;338:107–111.

Carlson GP. Fluid, electrolyte, and acid–base balance. In: Kaneko JJ, Harvey JW, Bruss ML, eds. Clinical biochemistry of domestic animals. 5th ed. San Diego: Academic Press, 1997:485–516.

Hinchcliff KW, ed. Fluids and electrolytes in athletic horses. Vet Clin North Am Equine Pract 1998;14:1–225.

Johnson PJ. Electrolyte and acid–base disturbances in the horse. Vet Clin North Am Equine Pract Clin Pathol 1995;11:491–514.

McGinness GS, Mansmann RA, Breuhaus BA. Nasogastric electrolyte replacement in horses. Compend Contin Educ Pract Vet 1996;18:942–951.

Rose BD. Acid–base physiology, regulation of acid–base balance, and metabolic acidosis. In: Rose BD, ed. Clinical physiology of acid–base and electrolyte disorders. 2nd ed. New York: McGraw Hill, 1984:202–224,225–247,374–393.

Author Jennifer G. Adams

Consulting Editor Claire B. Andreasen

ALKALOSIS, RESPIRATORY

BASICS

DEFINITION
- A decrease in blood P_{CO_2}
- Arterial levels range from 35–42 mm Hg.
- Venous levels usually range from 43–49 mm Hg.

PATHOPHYSIOLOGY
- CO_2 is formed in all tissues during metabolic energy production and diffuses passively out of cells and into the blood in gaseous form.
- Most (65%–70%) of this CO_2 combines with water almost instantaneously to form carbonic acid, which then dissociates into bicarbonate ion and hydrogen. Therefore, most CO_2 is transported in the blood as bicarbonate, with some bound to proteins (especially deoxygenated hemoglobin) and a small amount dissolved directly into plasma.
- In the lungs, the reverse occurs, and CO_2 passively diffuses out of capillaries and into the alveoli.
- These three forms of CO_2 exist in equilibrium in the blood, but P_{CO_2} as measured by blood gases depends on the dissolved portion.
- Chemical components of the carbonic acid equilibrium:

$$CO_2 + H_2O \rightleftharpoons H_2CO_3 \rightleftharpoons H^+ + HCO_3^-$$

- Alveolar CO_2 then is removed mechanically by ventilation as inspired air displaces alveolar gas, which is expired.
- Respiratory alkalosis is present with hyperventilation or when tissue production of CO_2 drops but ventilation remains unchanged.
- Metabolic acidosis develops in response to chronic respiratory alkalosis as the kidney generates increased H^+ and excretes HCO_3^- to return the pH to normal.

SYSTEMS AFFECTED
- The brain is most affected by CO_2 levels, because hypocapnia decreases cerebral blood flow.
- Low pH affects acid–base balance, protein binding, and electrolyte levels directly in the blood and via effects on the kidney.
- The kidney responds to low pH by generating more H^+ and excreting more HCO_3^-. It also reabsorbs Cl^- to maintain electroneutrality. Alkalosis decreases serum potassium and ionized calcium levels.
- Severe alkalemia can cause venoconstriction and predispose to arrhythmias, and it may result in hyperexcitability of muscle and nervous tissue.

SIGNALMENT
Any horse

SIGNS
- Respiratory rate, volume, or both usually are increased.
- Abnormal lung sounds are variable but may be present if hyperventilation is in response to hypoxemia caused by pulmonary disease.

CAUSES

Acute
- Usually is a temporary change in response to a stimulus causing hyperventilation.
- Physiologic causes of hyperventilation—exercise, fever, and hyperthermia
- Psychologic causes—pain, anxiety, excitement, and fear
- Stimulation of medullary respiratory centers by CNS disorders, early septicemia, acidosis, or endotoxemia may result in hyperventilation.
- Anemia, hypovolemia, and hypoxemia of any cause increase respiration in response to tissue hypoxia.

Chronic
- May result from chronic respiratory disease (e.g. pleuropneumonia, COPD) or chronic, painful conditions (e.g., laminitis, septic arthritis).
- Overventilation with mechanical ventilators produces low P_{CO_2} in anesthetized patients and sick neonates.
- Hypothermia or decreased metabolic rates seen with prolonged general anesthesia may lower tissue CO_2 production and produce respiratory alkalosis in patients ventilated at appropriate settings.
- Also seen as a compensatory response to primary metabolic acidosis.

RISK FACTORS
N/A

DIAGNOSIS

DIFFERENTIAL DIAGNOSIS
- Physiologic states or disease processes that present with tachypnea–fever, hyperthermia, excitement, anxiety, painful conditions, hypoxemia, metabolic acidosis, and CNS derangements; most of these can be differentiated with history and physical examination findings.
- Most acute problems have low pH and low P_{CO_2}; bicarbonate levels are.
- Chronic respiratory alkalosis results in compensatory metabolic acidosis, in which bicarbonate is low and pH should be normal, because compensation is very effective in this circumstance.
- Acute metabolic acidosis has low bicarbonate. Often, pH remains low in severe cases, because respiratory compensation rarely is complete.

LABORATORY FINDINGS

Drugs That May Alter Lab Results
N/A

Disorders That May Alter Lab Results
- With poor peripheral perfusion or cardiovascular shunt, results of blood gas analysis on samples taken from peripheral arteries may differ from those taken elsewhere or may not reflect the patient's overall systemic condition.
- Prolonged exposure to air may alter CO_2 levels, because RBC metabolism continues and equilibration with room air may occur.

Valid If Run in Human Lab?
Yes, if properly submitted.

CBC/BIOCHEMISTRY/URINALYSIS
N/A

OTHER LABORATORY TESTS

- Blood gas analysis is the definitive laboratory test.
- Venous samples may be adequate to identify the condition, but arterial samples are necessary to evaluate adequacy of pulmonary function as a cause.
- Handheld analyzers are now available and easy to use. Some require only small amounts of whole blood; otherwise, heparinize syringes before sampling.
- Perform sampling anaerobically. Immediately evacuate any air bubbles present, and cap the needle with a rubber stopper.
- Analysis should be performed within 15–20 minutes. If not, samples can be stored on ice, and results will be valid for 3–4 hours.

IMAGING

N/A

DIAGNOSTIC PROCEDURES

- Capnography is an indirect method of measuring CO_2 levels.
- Samples of ET gases reflect arterial P_{CO_2}, because ET gas is essentially the same as alveolar gas.
- Continous monitoring can be performed on anesthetized or ventilated patients via a gas-sampling port incorporated into the endotracheal tube or attached to an adapter.
- Because some V/Q mismatch usually is present, ET levels may underestimate arterial levels by 10–15 mm Hg.
- Periodically compare values obtained via capnography with those via blood gas analysis.

TREATMENT

- Most often, treatment of the primary problem resolves the need for hyperventilation, or metabolic rate will increase and normal P_{CO_2} levels return.
- Prevention of hypothermia in anesthetized patients is much more effective than treatment after the fact.
- Alteration of ventilator settings in anesthetized patients is necessary to return CO_2 and pH to normal; however, this may decrease oxygen levels.
- For prolonged procedures, the CO_2 level should be maintained at >20 mm Hg to ensure adequate cerebral blood flow.

MEDICATIONS

DRUGS OF CHOICE

N/A

CONTRAINDICATIONS

Alkali therapy is not indicated for compensatory metabolic acidosis, if present, because it may acutely destabilize an acid–base and electrolyte status that has responded to chronic respiratory alkalosis.

PRECAUTIONS

- Monitor ventilated patients continuously for airway obstruction caused by accumulation of secretions, movement of endotracheal tube, kinking of tubing or hoses, and so on.
- Inspiratory pressure should range from 20–30 cm H_2O in normal patients.
- Pressures of ≤ 40 cm H_2O may be utilized in patients with abdominal distention—those anesthetized for colic surgery.
- Pressures of >40 cm H_2O compromise venous return and cardiac output.
- Oxygen toxicity can develop if $>50\%$ oxygen is administered for prolonged periods.

POSSIBLE INTERACTIONS

N/A

ALTERNATIVE DRUGS

N/A

FOLLOW-UP

PATIENT MONITORING

- Decreased respiratory effort should be seen quickly after resolution of the primary problem.
- Evaluate repeat blood gases analyses soon after institution of mechanical ventilation to ensure appropriate settings have been selected. Further evaluation thereafter is dictated by the patient's condition.

POSSIBLE COMPLICATIONS

Severe alkalemia can result in neurologic signs from decreased cerebral blood flow, muscular excitability, and cardiac arrhythmias.

MISCELLANEOUS

ASSOCIATED CONDITIONS

- Hyperchloremia
- Hypokalemia
- Metabolic acidosis

AGE-RELATED FACTORS

N/A

ZOONOTIC POTENTIAL

N/A

PREGNANCY

Pregnant females often hyperventilate because of decreased lung volume caused by abdominal distention from the gravid uterus.

SYNONYMS

- Hypocapnia
- Hypocarbia

SEE ALSO

See specific diseases mentioned in *Causes.*

ABBREVIATIONS

- COPD = chronic obstructive pulmonary disease
- ET = end-tidal, refers to gas expired at the end of expiration, which should be the alveolar gas most recently involved in gas exchange
- V/Q = ventilation-perfusion ratio

Suggested Reading

Adrogue JG, Madias NE. Management of life-threatening acid-base disorders. Second of two parts. N Engl J Med 1998;338:107–111.

Carlson GP. Fluid, electrolyte and acid–base balance. In: Kaneko JJ, Harvey JW, Bruss ML, eds. Clinical biochemistry of domestic animals. San Diego: Academic Press, 1997:490–498.

Guyton AC, ed. Medical physiology. Section VII: Respiration. 9th ed. Philadelphia: WB Saunders, 1992:465–526.

Krapf R, Beeler I, Hertner D, Hulter HN. Chronic respiratory alkalosis: the effect of sustained hyperventilation on renal regulation of acid–base equilibrium. N Engl J Med 1991;324:1394–1401.

West JB. Respiratory physiology—the essentials. 5th ed. Baltimore: Williams & Wilkins, 1995.

Author Jennifer G. Adams

Consulting Editor Claire B. Andreasen

ALOPECIA AREATA (AA)

BASICS

OVERVIEW

AA is a common cause of hair loss that affects humans, non-human primates, rodents, dogs, cattle and horses. The pathology involves anagen hair follicles, and is characterized, histologically, as a classical "swarm of bees" (lymphocytes) around the inferior segment/bulb region, resulting in patchy to total hair loss (alopecia areata to alopecia universalis, respectively). While not life threatening, AA is disfiguring and can result in secondary bacterial infections and solar damage.

ORGAN SYSTEM

• Dermatologic

SIGNALMENT

• Currently no known age, breed, or sex predilection

SIGNS

• Diffuse thinning or complete alopecia of one or multiple areas
• Typically, clinically non-inflammatory and non-pruritic
• Occurs anywhere on the body or trunk
• May also be responsible for many of the mane, tail, and/or hoof dystrophies
• Clinical course is variable with possible episodes of spontaneous remission

CAUSES AND RISK FACTORS

• Currently, AA is thought to be a rare autoimmune condition.
• Anti-trichohyalin(ATHAb) antibodies have consistently been detected in sera of affected humans. Recently, ATHAb have been indentified in animal species.
• Also, the depletion of CD8+ cells allows regrowth of hair in rats within 29 days, emphasizing the importance of CD8+ T cells in the pathogenesis.
• The majority of intra-lesional T cells in a recent case of equine alopecia universalis expressed CD3+ and CD8+ T cells and had follicular keratinocytes unregulated with expression of MHC II (Affolter V, Cannon A, ACVD 1998).

DIAGNOSIS

DIFFERENTIAL DIAGNOSES

• Telogen effluvium
• Linear alopecia
• Dermatophytosis
• Occult sarcoid

CBC/BIOCHEMISTRY/URINALYSIS

N/A

OTHER LABORATORY TESTS

N/A

IMAGING

N/A

DIAGNOSTIC PROCEDURES

• Multiple biopsies from early lesions exhibit some or all of the following features:
  —Lymphocytic bulbitis (swarm of bees) of anagen follicles (early)
  —Malacic hair shafts within follicles indicating previous damage to the hair matrix cells
  —Diminutive to atrophic follicles with irregular bulbs and focal fibrosis (chronic)
• Immunohistochemistry usually shows
  —large number of CD3+, CD8+ T cells
  —many of which express MCH II (dendritic antigen presenting cells)

ALOPECIA AREATA (AA)

TREATMENT

MEDICATIONS

DRUGS

- Many horses do respond to systemic corticosteroids
  - —immunosuppressive dosages
  - —prednisone at 1.5–2.5 mg/kg/d for 7–14 days
  - —taper to 0.5–1 mg/kg every other day for maintenance

CONTRAINDICATIONS/POSSIBLE INTERACTIONS

Since longterm immunosuppressive therapy is required for control in most cases, the use of steroids for purely a cosmetic and uncertain outcome must be balanced with the potential for adverse reactions.

FOLLOW-UP

EXPECTED COURSE AND PROGNOSIS

- Guarded to poor for complete remission
- Difficult entity to treat in humans
- In some cases the condition can be self-limiting

MISCELLANEOUS

SEE ALSO

N/A

ABBREVIATIONS

N/A

Suggested Reading

Pascoe R, Knottenbelt D. Manual of Equine Dermatology. WB Saunders, London, England,1999.

Stannard A. Alopecia in the horse—an overview. Vet Derm 2000 Vol 11 (3):195–198.

Author Anthony A. Yu

AMINOGLYCOSIDE TOXICOSIS

BASICS

OVERVIEW

• Aminoglycoside antibiotics are used to treat Gram-negative bacterial infections in horses and include neomycin, gentamicin, kanamycin, amikacin, and streptomycin.
• Aminoglycoside-induced renal toxicity results from accumulation of these antibiotics within the renal cortex.
• Aminoglycoside nephrotoxicity is encountered more frequently than ototoxicity or neuromuscular blockade.
• Nephrotoxicosis results from cumulative sequestration of aminoglycosides in proximal renal tubular cells.
• Active reabsorption of aminoglycosides from tubular filtrate occurs by pinocytosis along the midconvoluted and straight portions of the proximal tubule by a cationic pump or electrostatic attraction of the cationic aminoglycoside for anionic phospholipids of cellular membranes. The greater the positive charge on the aminoglycoside, the greater the affinity of the pump for the drug.
• Intracellular accumulation of aminoglycosides causes lysosomal exocytosis, damage to the apical plasma membrane, and necrosis of the renal tubular cells.
• Mitochondrial respiration decreases roughly in relation to the net positive charge of the specific aminoglycoside.
• Aminoglycosides inhibit the activities of the cytoplasmic phospholipase and membranous enzyme systems.

SIGNALMENT

• Foals appear more susceptible than adults.
• Duration of drug administration before clinically significant nephrotoxicosis occurs—generally 3–5 days
• No breed or sex predispositions
• Disposition of aminoglycosides can be altered by diet.

SIGNS

• Clinical signs of toxicosis usually are apparent only after considerable renal injury.
• Signs include depression, anorexia, polyuria, or oliguria.
• Laboratory evaluation is important.

CAUSES AND RISK FACTORS

• Toxicity depends on the particular aminoglycoside (e.g., neomycin is more toxic than gentamicin or amikacin) and relates to its cationic charge.
• Predisposing factors—extremes of age, dose, cumulative dose, duration of administration, concurrent disease or sepsis, contraction of plasma volume, acidosis (e.g., acidemia, acidic tubular fluid), and concurrently administered medications (e.g., loop diuretics, NSAIDs, cephalosporin antimicrobials, nephrotoxic drugs)

DIAGNOSIS

DIFFERENTIAL DIAGNOSIS

• Renal intoxication by other toxicants—heavy metals, NSAIDs, vitamin K_3, and cantharidin
• Ischemic damage secondary to hypovolemia, sepsis, endotoxemia, or renal infarction
• Immune-mediated or postinfectious glomerulonephritis
• Acute interstitial nephritis secondary to Gram-negative sepsis

CBC/BIOCHEMISTRY/URINALYSIS

• Elevated BUN or creatinine occurs after 75% of nephrons are nonfunctional.
• Increased GGT concentrations in urine and presence of urinary casts are nonspecific, early indicators of renal tubular insult.

OTHER LABORATORY TESTS

N/A

IMAGING

N/A

DIAGNOSTIC PROCEDURES

TDM—plasma concentrations >1 μg/mL for gentamicin or 2.5 μg/mL for amikacin before subsequent dose of the respective drug increases risk of nephrotoxicosis; concurrent alterations in other variables also support the diagnosis.

PATHOLOGIC FINDINGS

Variable degrees of proximal tubular epithelial cellular necrosis are noted histologically.

TREATMENT

• Adjust dosage regimen as indicated by TDM results.
• Healing of damaged renal tubules can occur during continued, appropriate administration of the aminoglycoside, but consider discontinuing the aminoglycoside or other concurrently administered nephrotoxic drugs.
• Enhance elimination (see *Medications*).
• Peritoneal dialysis may be an option for horses, but data from other species suggest it is ineffective.
• Supportive care as indicated.

AMINOGLYCOSIDE TOXICOSIS

MEDICATIONS

DRUGS

- Polyionic, alkalinizing fluids
- Alkalinization of tubular fluid decreases cationic charge on the aminoglycoside and uptake by tubular cells, thus enhancing drug elimination in urine.
- Expansion of plasma volume and apparent volume of distribution may reduce circulating concentrations by dilution and create volume diuresis.
- Inactivation in vivo by interaction of some aminoglycosides (e.g., tobramycin) with penicillins (e.g., ticarcillin)
- Tobramycin generally is not toxic to horses.

CONTRAINDICATIONS/POSSIBLE INTERACTIONS

See *Causes and Risk Factors.*

FOLLOW-UP

PATIENT MONITORING

- Monitor circulating drug concentrations and time-course by TDM to adjust dosage regimen for each patient; many factors (e.g., diet, dosage regimen, concurrent disease, medication administration) introduce unpredictable variables that dictate TDM for monitoring and adjustments to treatment.
- Conduct a benefit/risk assessment for use of aminoglycosides, or make alternative choices.
- Once-daily administration may be appropriate for some patients.

PREVENTION/AVOIDANCE

- Using TDM, adjust the dosage regimen to maximize therapeutic efficacy and to reduce risks of toxicosis.
- Prolonged elimination or clearance with elevated trough concentrations increase the potential for toxicosis.

MISCELLANEOUS

ASSOCIATED CONDITIONS

N/A

AGE-RELATED FACTORS

N/A

ZOONOTIC POTENTIAL

N/A

PREGNANCY

N/A

SEE ALSO

N/A

ABBREVIATIONS

- GGT = γ-glutamyltransaminase
- TDM = therapeutic drug monitoring

Suggested Reading

Riviere JE, Spoo JW. Aminoglycoside antibiotics. In: Adams HR, ed. Veterinary pharmacology and therapeutics. 7th ed. Ames: Iowa State University Press, 1995:797–819.

Author Gordon W. Brumbaugh

Consulting Editor Robert H. Poppenga

AMMONIA, HYPERAMMONEMIA

BASICS

DEFINITION

Free ammonia (NH_3) is a nonprotein nitrogen compound that can permeate cells and result in hyperammonemia. At physiologic pH, almost all blood ammonia is the ammonium ion (NH_4^+), which is less permeable for cells. In order to eliminate waste nitrogen as ammonia, the mammalian body converts it to an excretable form, urea. To a lesser extent, ammonia is eliminated by conversion to glutamine. Reference intervals for plasma ammonia are 7.6-63.4 μmol/L, but are very dependent on the type of assay and reported units. Hyperammonemia occurs when concentrations exceed the established laboratory reference intervals.

Pathophysiology

Blood ammonia is derived primarily from dietary nitrogen with the gastrointestinal tract action of bacterial proteases, ureases, and amine oxidases resulting in the major source of blood ammonia. Ammonia is also derived from catabolism of glutamine and protein, and skeletal muscle exertion. Ammonia is delivered to the liver via the portal vein or hepatic artery, where functional hepatocytes remove ammonia to form urea by means of the Krebs-Henseleit urea cycle. If functional liver mass is inadequate, ammonia is not converted to urea, and plasma ammonia concentrations increase. Serum urea concentrations also rise when glomerular filtration is inadequate. Acid-base status affects the absorption of ammonia. As blood pH increases, free ammonia (NH_3) increases and can permeate cells via nonionic diffusion to produce toxicity. Ammonia is one of the compounds responsible for clinical signs of hepatic encephalopathy. Other described neurotoxins in hepatic encephalopathy are: alterations in monoamine neurotransmitters due to altered aromatic amino acids, alterations in gamma aminobutyric acid (GABA) and/or glutamate, and increased endogenous benzodiazepine-like substances.

Systems Affected

Nervous-ammonia is neurotoxic and the brain is affected by high plasma concentrations. The degree of hyperammonemia does not necessarily correlate to the severity of hepatic encephalopathy signs because other compounds are involved. Ammonia interferes with the blood-brain barrier, cerebral blood flow, cellular excitability, neurotransmitter metabolism, and ratios of neurotransmitter precursor amino acids. Degenerative changes of the neurons and supporting cells have been observed in chronically affected animals.

SIGNALMENT

- Portal-caval shunts have been reported in foals (rare).
- The presence of hyperammonemia is most often associated with diseases of the liver.

SIGNS

General Comments

- Clinical signs of hyperammonemia are primarily those of hepatic encephalopathy, although this is not the only substance responsible for all of the clinical signs.
- Signs may be sporadic and progressive and worsen after feeding.

Historical Findings

Ptyalism, behavior changes, visual deficits (blindness), compulsive circling, pacing, anxiety, head pressing, stupor, coma, unusual positions/posture, sudden falling to the ground, violent thrashing.

Physical Examination Findings

Stunted growth, loss of body condition, poor hair coat, mentation changes and aberrant behavior. Similar findings as discussed in liver disease, e.g., icterus may be observed, especially in horses with acute hepatitis. In animals affected chronically, neuronal degeneration occurs and signs become persistent.

CAUSES

- Liver disease: Hepatic encephalopathy is a prominent clinical feature of hepatic failure in the horse, and is associated with acute hepatitis and hepatic cirrhosis. Abnormalities of the urea cycle, abnormal portal blood flow, or any disorder that results in markedly impaired liver function can cause hyperammonemia. Decreased functional hepatic mass can result from pyrrolizidine alkaloid toxicity, acute hepatitis, chronic active hepatitis, hepatotoxic drugs or chemicals, Tyzzer's disease in foals, and hyperlipidemia in ponies with associated hepatic dysfunction.
- Portosystemic shunts: acquired or congenital.
- Toxicities: urea toxicity/poisoning, ammonium salt fertilizer toxicity.

RISK FACTORS

- Horses in known areas with hepatotoxic plants would be prone to develop hepatopathies.
- Administration of equine-derived biologics may induce hepatopathies.
- Feedstuffs contaminated with high levels of urea, nitrogen, or ammonium salts.

DIAGNOSIS

DIFFERENTIAL DIAGNOSIS

- Hepatic encephalopathy must be differentiated from primary neurologic diseases such as inflammatory, degenerative, infectious, or neoplastic CNS diseases. Rabies should be a differential diagnosis for abnormal behavior in the horse. Behavior-based alterations or problems should be ruled out.
- Differentiation consists of evaluating the history, signalment, and results of serum biochemistry, hematology, urinalysis, and hepatic biopsy.
- Possible intestinal bacterial overgrowth resulting in transient hyperammonemia (proposed).

LABORATORY FINDINGS

Nonammonium heparin salts should be used as the anticoagulant for ammonia assays.

Drugs That May Alter Lab Results

The following drugs alter blood ammonia concentration without affecting validity of test results:

- Antibiotics that reduce bacterial intestinal flora may decrease plasma ammonia concentration.
- Lactulose decreases the ammonia concentration.
- Enemas decrease the ammonia concentration.
- High concentrations of ammonia have been reported after blood transfusion and administration of parenteral amino acids, narcotics, and diuretics.

Disorders That May Alter Lab Results

- Prolonged occlusion of a vein during sampling may cause elevated concentrations, especially if there is muscle exertion during restraint.
- Entry of air into samples will increase ammonia concentrations.
- Laboratory atmosphere/environment and glassware can be a source of ammonia contamination.
- Use of serum results in variable and significantly higher ammonia concentrations than plasma concentrations.

Valid If Run in Human Lab?

This test can be performed in human labs. Samples should be kept on ice and analysis performed within 30 minutes. In-house dry chemistry analysis accounts for a resurgence of interest in plasma ammonia. This requires adequate controls, paired samples, and proper sample handling.

CBC/BIOCHEMISTRY/URINALYSIS

Findings vary with the nature of the liver disease.

- CBC—microcytosis may occur in animals with portosystemic shunts, but may be difficult to determine in the horse; RBC histograms may be useful.
- Biochemistry—liver enzymes may be normal in animals with portosystemic shunts, but bile acid concentrations as well as ammonia concentrations will be elevated. Usually, other biochemical abnormalities are present, indicating hepatic dysfunction if the liver disease is severe enough to produce hepatic encephalopathy. Finding elevated liver enzymes (SDH, GDH, ALP, GGT, or AST) and hyperbilirubinemia, hypoglycemia (not common), hyper- or hypocholesterolemia, or late in hepatic failure, hypoalbuminemia and low BUN support a diagnosis of liver disease.
- Urinalysis—ammonia biurate crystals and low urine specific gravity due to underlying liver disease in some animals.

OTHER LABORATORY TESTS

- Measurement of serum bile acid concentrations has largely replaced ammonia assays due to convenience of sampling.
- Coagulation factor production may be decreased in liver failure resulting in prolonged PT and PTT.

IMAGING

Ultrasound evaluation of the liver and portal vessels is advised.

DIAGNOSTIC PROCEDURES

- Hepatic biopsy is often necessary.
- The ammonia tolerance test has been used in companion animals when measurement of bile acids is not available, but caution should be used when conducting this test because it can precipitate hepatic encephalopathy. Bile acid concentrations or ammonia concentrations are more practical.

TREATMENT

- Restrict activity.
- Feed a very low protein diet, or fast the patient initially, and then institute a protein-restricted diet when the patient is stable.
- Fluid administration is needed to correct dehydration and maintain tissue perfusion. It is important to maintain normal plasma potassium concentrations because low plasma potassium may increase the intracellular movement of ammonia.

MEDICATIONS

DRUG(S) OF CHOICE

- Lactulose is an acidifying agent used to decrease ammonia absorption from the intestine and lower plasma ammonia concentration in equine hyperammonemia. Lactulose acts as a cathartic laxative and maintains ammonia in its nonabsorbable ammonium ion form.
- Antibiotics with a broad spectrum against intestinal flora have been used orally, such as a nonabsorbable aminoglycoside (e.g., neomycin). Metronidazole has been used in companion animals and in horses with acute colitis, but caution should be used with this drug because decreased hepatic clearance also can result in neurologic signs.

CONTRAINDICATIONS

Any drugs that affect the CNS must be used with caution because of the common association of hyperammonemia with hepatic encephalopathy and possibly impaired hepatic metabolism. Barbiturates and benzodiazepam-like drugs are of particular concern.

PRECAUTIONS

Sodium bicarbonate in fluids should be administered slowly, because rapid correction of acidosis may favor intracellular ammonia movement.

POSSIBLE INTERACTIONS

Because of impaired hepatic metabolism, any drugs that inhibit metabolism by the liver or are metabolized by the liver should be used with caution or the dosage should be adjusted.

ALTERNATIVE DRUGS

N/A

FOLLOW-UP

PATIENT MONITORING

Repeated assessment of plasma ammonia can be helpful. Monitoring of serum potassium and glucose is advised in critical patients.

POSSIBLE COMPLICATIONS

Inaccuracy is the biggest problem because of the labile nature of ammonia in blood samples. Delay in processing results in false readings of high ammonia concentration.

MISCELLANEOUS

ASSOCIATED CONDITIONS

N/A

AGE-RELATED FACTORS

N/A

ZOONOTIC POTENTIAL

N/A

PREGNANCY

N/A

SYNONYMS

N/A

SEE ALSO

- Hepatic encephalopathy
- Liver/hepatic disease
- Hepatic enzyme
- Bile acids

ABBREVIATIONS

- ALP = alkaline phosphatase
- BUN = blood urea nitrogen
- CNS = central nervous system
- GDH = glutamate dehydrogenase
- GGT = gamma glutamyltransferase
- PT = prothrombin time
- PTT = partial thromboplastin time
- SDH = sorbitol dehydrogenase

Suggested Reading

Peek SF, Divers TJ, Jackson CJ. Hyperammonaemia associated with encephalopathy and abdominal pain without evidence of liver disease in four mature horses. Equine Vet J 1997; 29:70-74.

Tennent BC. Hepatic function. In: Kaneko JJ, Harvey JW, Bruss ML eds., Clinical biochemistry of domestic animals. 5th ed San Diego: Academic Press, 1997:332-334.

Barton MH, Morris DD. Diseases of the liver. In: Reed SM, Bayly WM, eds. Equine internal medicine. Philadelphia: WB Saunders, 1998:713-716.

McGorum BC, Murphy D, Love S, Milne EM. Clinicopathological features of equine primary hepatic disease: A review of 50 cases. Vet Rec 1999; 145:134-139.

Author Claire B. Andreasen

Consulting Editor Claire B. Andreasen

AMYLASE AND LIPASE

BASICS

DEFINITION

Serum amylase or lipase concentrations above laboratory reference interval. In general, this would be >35 IU/L for amylase and >87 IU/L for lipase. Because pancreatitis is thought to be uncommon in the horse, most laboratories do not routinely analyze for serum amylase or lipase.

PATHOPHYSIOLOGY

Amylase in the blood comes from a number of sources, including the intestinal mucosa, liver, and pancreas. It is cleared from the blood by the kidneys, so renal dysfunction could lead to higher concentrations remaining in the blood. Damage to pancreatic cells can cause leakage of amylase into the blood or peritoneal fluid, but this is not common in the horse. Lipase is derived from the pancreas, gastrointestinal mucosa, and other tissues. Clinical serum assays detect all forms of lipase. In most species, it is cleared from the blood by the kidneys, so renal dysfunction could lead to higher concentrations remaining in the blood. Although uncommon in the horse, damage to pancreatic cells can cause release of lipase into the blood or peritoneal cavity.

Systems Affected

Serum amylase and lipase have little effect on other organ systems, but leakage into the peritoneal cavity can cause inflammation and colic.

SIGNALMENT

N/A

SIGNS

Varies with underlying cause.

- Pancreatitis: colic, gastric reflux, tachycardia, and signs of hypovolemic shock.
- Hyperlipemia: depression, anorexia, and lipemia serum.
- Other intestinal diseases: colic, gastric reflux, and tachycardia.

CAUSES

- Proximal enteritis
- High intestinal obstructions
- Intestinal mucosal damage
- Hyperlipemia
- Cortisol administration
- Heparin-induced lipoprotein lipase activity
- Obstruction to common bile and pancreatic duct
- Renal disease with renal failure
- Pancreatitis

RISK FACTORS

Unknown; negative energy balance increases risk of hyperlipemia.

DIAGNOSIS

DIFFERENTIAL DIAGNOSIS

- Colic with small bowel distention should lead a clinician to suspect inflammation or obstruction of the small intestine rather than pancreatic inflammation, although colic and ileus can be caused by peritonitis secondary to pancreatitis.
- In a pony or miniature horse, hyperlipemia should be considered.

LABORATORY FINDINGS

Drugs That May Alter Lab Results

N/A

Disorders That May Alter Lab Results

- Hemolysis inhibits lipase activity
- Lipemia falsely decreases serum lipase activity measured by kinetic assays

Valid if Run in Human Lab?

Not unless horse reference intervals are available.

CBC/BIOCHEMISTRY/URINALYSIS

- CBC may reflect an inflammatory leukogram during pancreatitis/peritonitis.
- Peritoneal fluid amylase and lipase activities are usually less than that in blood except in pancreatitis.
- Elevated BUN and creatinine may indicate inability of the kidney to excrete amylase or lipase.
- GGT is concentrated in the pancreas as well as the liver, so increased serum activity could mean pancreatitis as well as hepatitis or cholestasis, or elevations of GGT could be secondary to the proximity of the bile duct to an inflamed pancreatic duct.

OTHER LABORATORY TESTS

- Serum triglycerides above 500 mg/dl would mean hyperlipemia and expected increases in serum lipase or lipoprotein lipase activity.
- Nonesterified fatty acid (NEFA) concentrations above 0.5 mEq/L could mean hyperlipemia due to fat mobilization and expected increases in serum lipase activity.
- Urine GGT:Creatinine ratio above 25-50 would indicate renal tubular damage and possible impairment of renal excretion of amylase or lipase.

AMYLASE AND LIPASE

• Urinary fractional clearance of increased amylase would indicate high serum concentrations with a functional kidney, whereas inappropriate decreased fractional clearance of amylase in the face of hyperamylasemia would indicate renal failure. However, normal values for these clearances in the horse are not known.
• Abdominocentesis has been used for cytology to define inflammation and for chemical comparisons of peritoneal amylase and lipase concentrations to serum concentrations. Finding peritoneal fluid concentrations above serum concentrations can be indicative of pancreatitis, but this also can be a nonspecific finding in peritonitis/serositis.

DIAGNOSTIC PROCEDURES

Exploratory celiotomy may be indicated in cases of colic with undiagnosed causes of continued pain or indications of small intestinal obstruction. Abdominal fluid analysis should precede this invasive procedure.

TREATMENT

Treatment varies with the underlying cause. If the stomach is distended, continuous refluxing may be needed to prevent rupture.

MEDICATIONS

Medications vary with the underlying cause. The laboratory changes of increased blood amylase and lipase do not need treatment. Analgesics are needed in cases showing signs of colic. For pancreatitis, NPO and parenteral nutrition along with analgesics and anti-inflammatories may be helpful. Intravenous fluids are needed if there are signs of hypovolemic shock.

FOLLOW-UP

PATIENT MONITORING

• Repeat blood and peritoneal fluid activity of amylase and lipase.
• Observe every hour for signs of colic.

POSSIBLE COMPLICATIONS

• Small intestinal obstruction, pancreatitis, and hyperlipemia can cause death.
• Distention of the stomach may cause rupture and death due to peritonitis.
• Leakage of amylase and lipase into the peritoneal cavity can induce non-septic peritonitis.

MISCELLANEOUS

SEE ALSO

• Colic
• Gastric reflux

ABBREVIATIONS

• GGT = gamma glutamyltransferase
• BUN = blood urea nitrogen
• NPO = nothing per OS
• NEFA = nonesterified fatty acid

Suggested Reading

Kramer JW, Hoffman WE. Clinical enzymology. In: Kaneko JJ, Harvey JW, Brass ML eds., Clinical biochemistry of domestic animals. 5th ed. San Diego: Academic Press, 1997:320-321.

Brobst DF. Pancreatic function. In: Kaneko JJ, Harvey JW, Bruss ML, eds., Clinical biochemistry of domestic animals. 5th ed. San Diego: Academic Press, 1997: 359-361.

Gerros TG. Pancreatic disease. In: Smith BP ed., Large animal internal medicine. St Louis: Mosby, 1996:950-951.

Parry BW, Crisman MV. Serum and peritoneal fluid amylase and lipase reference values in horses. Equine Vet J 1991; 23:390-391.

Author Erwin G. Pearson
Consulting Editor Claire B. Andreasen

ANAEROBIC BACTERIAL INFECTIONS

BASICS

DEFINITION

Anaerobic bacterial infections are caused by organisms that do not use molecular oxygen for metabolic activity and require a reduced oxygen tension for growth. These organisms are widely distributed in the horse's environment and are major constituents of the normal microbial flora. They can be classified as either facultative or obligate, depending on their response to oxygen. The anaerobic infections being discussed in this section are the obligate anaerobes, which do not use oxygen for growth.

PATHOPHYSIOLOGY

A break in the horse's primary defense barriers, particularly the skin and mucous membranes, allows the normal flora to penetrate tissues and establish infection. In other cases contamination of a wound or injection site by organisms found in the soil or fecal material may lead to an infection. Once anaerobic organisms have infected they release a variety of toxins, enzymes, and virulence factors that result in tissue destruction and provide protection from the host's defenses. Primarily, body sites with a low oxygen tension, a low redox potential, or both are more likely to develop an infection.

SYSTEMS AFFECTED

Upper Respiratory Tract
- Tooth root abscesses
- Sinusitis
- Pharyngeal abscesses

Lower Respiratory Tract
- Pneumonia
- Pulmonary abscess
- Pleuropneumonia
- Pleuritis

Gastrointestinal Tract
- Peritonitis
- Abdominal abscess
- Enteritis
- Colitis

Musculoskeletal System
- Soft-tissue abscesses
- Osteomyelitis
- Sequestrums
- Septic arthritis
- Tenosynovitis
- Clostridial myonecrosis

Reproductive Tract

Metritis

Umbilical Cord
- Omphalophlebitis
- Omphalitis

Septicemia

GENETICS

N/A

INCIDENCE/PREVALENCE

Worldwide distribution

SIGNALMENT

Any age, breed, or sex can be affected.

SIGNS

Signs are variable depending on the organ system involved.

Upper Respiratory Tract
- Nasal discharge
- Facial swelling and crepitance
- Foul-smelling exudate

Lower Respiratory Tract
- Cough
- Nasal discharge
- Foul smelling breath, sputum, or pleural fluid
- Fever
- Lethargy
- Inappetance
- Abnormal lung sounds

Gastrointestinal Tract
- Abdominal discomfort
- Fever
- Diarrhea
- Inappetance
- Reflux

Musculoskeletal System
- Swollen and painful muscles or joints
- Lameness
- Fever
- Crepitance over swollen muscles

Reproductive Tract
- Vaginal discharge, possibly with a fetid odor
- Fever
- Lethargy
- Endotoxemia

Umbilical Cord
- Swollen and painful umbilicus
- Fever
- Lethargy
- Inappetance

Septicemia
- Fever
- Depression
- Tachycardia
- Tachypnea
- Labored respiratory effort
- Mucous membrane alterations
- Abdominal discomfort
- Laminitis abortion

CAUSES

Upper Respiratory Tract
- *Bacteroides* spp.
- *Fusobacterium* spp.
- *Peptostreptococcus* spp.

Lower Respiratory Tract
- *Bacteroides* spp.
- *Clostridium* spp.
- *Eubacterium lentum*
- *Peptostreptococcus* spp.

ANAEROBIC BACTERIAL INFECTIONS

Gastrointestinal Tract
- Peritonitis—*Bacteroides* spp. *Fusobacterium necrophorum*, and *Peptostreptococcus* spp.
- Enteritis/colitis—*Clostridium* spp. and *Bacteroides fragilis*

Musculoskeletal System
- Soft-tissue abscesses—*Bacteroides* spp. and *Fusobacterium necrophorum*
- Osteomyelitis/sequestrums—*Clostridium* spp.
- Septic arthritis/tenosynovitis—*Clostridium* and *Bacteroides* spp.
- Myonecrosis—*Clostridium* spp.

Reproductive Tract
Bacteroides fragilis, Peptococcus, Peptostreptococcus, and *Fusobacterium* spp.

Umbilical Cord
Bacteroides fragilis, Propionibacterium acnes, Peptostreptococcus magnus, and *Clostridium septicum.*

Septicemia
Clostridium septicum

RISK FACTORS
There may be a predisposition to developing anaerobic infections if there is a break in the host's primary defense mechanism, particularly the skin and mucous membrane surface. Other diseases, corticosteroid therapy, immunosuppression, leukopenia, tissue anoxia, prior or concurrent aerobic infections, or the presence of a foreign body may also predispose the horse to anaerobic infections.

DIAGNOSIS

DIFFERENTIAL DIAGNOSIS
Upper Respiratory Tract
- Neoplasia (fibroma, squamous cell carcinoma, osteogenic sarcoids, lymphosarcoma)
- Aerobic infection (*Streptococcus* spp., *Staphylococcus* spp.)
- Fungal infection (*Cryptococcus neoformans, Coccidioides immitis*)
- Granuloma

Lower Respiratory Tract
- Aerobic infection (*Streptococcus* spp., *Staphylococcus* spp., *Escherichia coli, Klebsiella, Pasturella, Bordetella* spp.)
- Fungal infection (*Coccidioides, Cryptococcus, Histoplasma, Aspergillus, Candida* spp.)
- *Mycoplasma* infection, neoplasia (primary neoplasia rare—granular cell tumor, bronchial myxoma, pulmonary carcinoma; metastatic neoplasia more common—adenocarcinoma, hemangiosarcoma)
- Thoracic trauma
- Esophageal rupture

Gastrointestinal Tract
- Peritonitis—aerobic infection (*Streptococcus* spp., *Escherichia coli*), neoplasia (primary neoplasia—lymphosarcoma; metastatic neoplasia—squamous cell carcinoma)
- Abdominal abscess—aerobic infection (*Streptococcus* spp., *Rhodococcus equi, Corynebacterium pseudotuberculosis*), neoplasia (squamous cell carcinoma, lymphosarcoma, leiomyosarcoma, adenocarcinoma, melanoma, ganglioneuroma, intestinal carcinoid), granuloma
- Enteritis/colitis—*Salmonella,* Potomac horse fever, idiopathic, parasitic (strongylosis, cyanthostomiasis), antibiotic-associated, NSAID drug toxicity, fungal infection

Musculoskeletal System
- Aerobic infection (*Staphylococcus aureus, Corynebacterium pseudotuberculosis*)
- Neoplasia (rhabdomyoma, osteochondroma)
- Fungal infection

Reproductive Tract
- Aerobic infection (*Streptococcus zooepidemicus, Escherichia coli, Klebsiella, Staphylococcus* spp., *Proteus, Pseudomonas, Corynebacterium* spp.)
- Neoplasia (leiomyoma, rhabdomyosarcoma, carcinomas), fungal infection (*Candida*)

Umbilical Cord
Aerobic infection (*Streptococcus* spp., *Escherichia coli, Proteus*)

Septicemia
Aerobic infections (*Streptococcus* spp., *Staphylococcus* spp., *Escherichia coli, Actinobacillus, Salmonella, Klebsiella*)

CBC/BIOCHEMISTRY/URINALYSIS
CBC
- Inflammatory leukocyte response
- Hyperfibrinogenemia
- Elevated total protein
- Anemia if chronic

Clinical Chemistry
Usually normal unless secondary systemic involvement.

Urinalysis
Normal

OTHER LABORATORY TESTS
- Clotting profile
- Potomac horse fever titers

IMAGING
Upper Respiratory Tract
- Skull radiographs revealing fluid line in sinus
- Sonogram revealing gas echos

Lower Respiratory Tract
- Thoracic radiographs revealing fluid line or consolidation
- Thoracic sonogram revealing fluid line, consolidation

Gastrointestinal Tract
Abdominal sonogram revealing character and amount of peritoneal fluid and presence and character of mass

Musculoskeletal System
- Limb radiographs revealing lytic bone changes
- Sonogram of muscles revealing gas echos

Reproductive Tract
Sonographic evaluation revealing gas or fluid within uterus

Umbilical Cord
Sonographic evaluation revealing gas or fluid

ANAEROBIC BACTERIAL INFECTIONS

DIAGNOSTIC PROCEDURES

Upper Respiratory Tract

- Sinus aspirates
- Surgical tissue samples obtained from deep infections during debridement
- Aspirations from loculated accumulations of purulent material

Lower Respiratory Tract

- Transtracheal wash aspirates
- Pleural fluid aspirates
- Percutaneous lung aspirates

Gastrointestinal Tract

- Peritoneal fluid aspirates
- Aspirates from loculated accumulations of purulent material via ultrasound guidance or surgery
- Fecal culture

Musculoskeletal

Surgical tissue specimens obtained from deep infections during debridement, sequestrums, or bone biopsies.

Reproductive Tract

Aspirates from purulent material obtained from uterine infections.

The aspirated fluid can be gram stained for each body system. Gram-positive cocci are suggestive of *Peptococcus* or *Peptostreptococcus* spp. Gram-positive rods are suggestive of *Clostridium* (spore forming), *Propionibacterium,* or *Eubacterium* spp. (non-spore forming), whereas gram-negative rods are suggestive of *Bacteroides* or *Fusobacterium* spp.

The specimen must be placed in the appropriate anaerobic bacterial transport medium and stored at room temperature with minimal exposure to oxygen.

PATHOLOGIC FINDINGS

Lesions are characterized by necrotic, edematous, gas-filled, and hyperemic tissue. Neutrophils, monocytes, and macrophages may accumulate in the tissue architecture, with bacteria interspersed among them.

TREATMENT

APPROPRIATE HEALTH CARE

Initially, the patient should be hospitalized for intensive treatment, then may return home for continued treatment once stabilized.

NURSING CARE

Nursing care depends on the severity of the infection and the body system affected. Care may include bandaging or hot packing, or extensive care, such as indwelling tubes for constant drainage of a body cavity. The appropriate supportive care may need to be provided, including intravenous fluids with supplementation or total/partial parenteral nutrition.

ACTIVITY

The amount of activity permitted varies depending on the body system affected, although most likely will be decreased or restricted.

DIET

The diet will most likely remain unchanged.

CLIENT EDUCATION

Some cases may be life-threatening depending on the extent of the illness. Complications may arise.

SURGICAL CONSIDERATIONS

Surgery may be necessary to debride necrotic tissue or for the placement of an indwelling catheter to allow for lavage and flushing.

MEDICATIONS

DRUG(S) OF CHOICE

Penicillin

Penicillin is the first line of defense against anaerobic infections and provides excellent activity against anaerobes except for beta-lactamase producing *Bacteroides.* Dose: 22,000–44,000 IU/kg q6h IV for aqueous or q12h IM for procaine.

Metronidazole

Metronidazole is effective only against obligate anaerobes, not facultative or aerobes. It is rapidly absorbed after oral administration and distributes well to synovial fluid, peritoneal fluid, cerebrospinal fluid, and urine, but poor endometrial concentrations. Orally it has a poor taste and the horse may become anorexic, which resolves with discontinuation. Dose: 15–25 mg/kg PO, IV, or per-rectum q6–8h.

Trimethoprim–Sulfa

Trimethoprim–sulfa is effective against some obligate anaerobes. Dose: 15–30 mg/kg PO q12h.

Choramphenicol

All obligate anaerobes are susceptible to chloramphenicol, but it may affect the metabolism of other drugs. Also, it is a human health hazard because it causes aplastic anemia; thus, it is not routinely used. It has good tissue penetration into peritoneal fluid, pleural fluid, synovial fluid, and cerebrospinal fluid. Dose: 50 mg/kg of the base form PO q6h.

Cephalosporins

All generations of cephalosporins are active against most anaerobic organisms except for *Bacteroides fragilis,* although generally they are too expensive to use. Cefoxitin does kill *B. fragilis.*

Ampicillin

Ampicillin provides activity against anaerobes and is comparable to penicillin, but is expensive. Dose: 25–100 mg/kg IV q6h.

ANAEROBIC BACTERIAL INFECTIONS

Rifampin

Rifampin is not necessary in most anaerobic infections but may be useful in polymicrobial infections in walled-off abscesses. Most strains of *Bacteroides* and *Clostridium* are sensitive to rifampin.

CONTRAINDICATIONS
N/A

PRECAUTIONS
N/A

POSSIBLE INTERACTIONS
Chloramphenicol may affect the metabolism of other drugs and is a human health hazard.

ALTERNATIVE DRUGS
N/A

FOLLOW-UP

PATIENT MONITORING
Response to therapy can be noted by monitoring changes in clinical signs. Hematologic changes and sonographic evaluations also help to establish the patient's response to therapy.

PREVENTION/AVOIDANCE
The proper treatment of wounds will help to prevent anerobic infection.

POSSIBLE COMPLICATIONS
The possibility of complications depends on the body system affected and the severity of the disease. Severe infections may result in laminitis, endotoxemia, or death.

EXPECTED COURSE AND PROGNOSIS
Depends on the body system affected and the severity of the disease.

MISCELLANEOUS

ASSOCIATED CONDITIONS
Depends on the body system affected and the severity of the disease.

AGE-RELATED FACTORS
N/A

ZOONOTIC POTENTIAL
N/A

PREGNANCY
Infection of the reproductive tract may result in breeding and conception problems.

SYNONYMS
N/A

SEE ALSO
N/A

ABBREVIATIONS
N/A

Suggested Reading

Kowalski, JJ. Bacterial and mycotic infections. In: Reed SM, Bayly WM, ed. Equine internal medicine. Philadelphia: WB Saunders, 1998:61-93.

Moore RM. Pathogenesis of obligate anaerobic bacterial infections in horses. Compend Contin Educ Pract Vet 1993;15(2):278-286.

Moore RM. Diagnosis and treatment of obligate anaerobic bacterial infections in horses. Compend Contin Educ Pract Vet 1993;15(7):989-994.

Author Bonnie S. Barr, VMD

Consulting Editor Corinne R. Sweeney, DVM

ANAPHYLAXIS

BASICS

OVERVIEW

• Classically, anaphylactic reactions occur when antigen binds to antigen-specific IgE on the surface of mast cells or basophils. This requires previous antigen exposure to stimulate antigen-specific IgE synthesis, which sensitizes the basophils and mast cells. Other antibody isotypes may mediate some reactions.
• Rare reactions may occur during initial exposure to highly charged or osmotically active agents (e.g., iodinated radiocontrast media, dextran) that can stimulate degranulation by perturbing the basophil or mast-cell membrane.
• Many mediators, including histamine, kinins, prostaglandins, and leukotrienes, are released from basophils, mast cells, and inflammatory cells. Mediators increase vascular permeability and dilate blood vessels, causing erythema and edema. Lung and GI smooth muscle constriction results in dyspnea and abdominal pain. Mediators alter platelet function; attract WBCs; activate complement and coagulation pathways; stimulate secretions of airway mucus, gastric acid, and catecholamines; and stimulate exocytosis of leukocyte lysosomes and granules.

SIGNALMENT

N/A

SIGNS

• Any combination of restlessness, excitement, pruritus at the site of antigen exposure, urticaria, erythema, edema, sweating, salivation, lacrimation, abdominal pain, diarrhea, laminitis, dyspnea, hypotension, or cardiac arrhythmia.
• Acute onset within seconds to minutes of antigen re-exposure is the hallmark; rare reactions may follow initial antigen exposure. Onset may be protracted if the inciting antigen is a metabolite.
• Reactions may be localized (e.g., urticaria) or systemic (e.g., anaphylactic shock). Localized reactions can progress to fatal systemic shock. The lung and GI tract are the primary shock organs; signs related to these systems warrant intensive monitoring.
• Dyspnea and systemic hypotension may lead to collapse and death from asphyxia, shock, or cardiac arrest.

CAUSES AND RISK FACTORS

• Reactions may occur in response to any foreign substance administered by any route. If medications are the cause, reactions can occur at any time in the course of therapy. Reactions generally are not dose dependent, but the chances of a reaction increase with parenteral dosing and with long-term, high-dose therapy.
• Agents implicated include, but are not limited to, insect venom, vaccines, food, blood products, and a variety of drugs, including thiamine, vitamin E/selenium, anthelmintics, penicillin, trimethoprim-sulfa, halothane, thiamylal, guaifenesin, chloramphenicol, aminoglycosides, and tetracycline.

DIAGNOSIS

DIFFERENTIAL DIAGNOSIS

• Presumptive diagnosis is based on an acute onset of clinical signs after re-exposure to a foreign antigen. Rare reactions may occur after a first exposure to some compounds.
• Rule out drug overdose, accentuation of a normal physiologic drug effect, or a drug interaction.
• Consider an inappropriate route of drug administration. Intra-arterial injections generally precipitate collapse associated with neurologic deficits (e.g., blindness, seizures).
• Manifestations of local reactions can be quite varied; differential diagnoses should address similar signs of the affected organ.

CBC/BIOCHEMISTRY/URINALYSIS

Abnormalities may include hemoconcentration, leukopenia, thrombocytopenia, hyperkalemia, increases in hepatic and myocardial enzyme activities, and coagulation deficits.

OTHER LABORATORY TESTS

Provocative dermal challenge testing with the suspected antigen may be confirmatory, but its value should be weighed against the risk of inducing severe systemic anaphylaxis.

IMAGING
N/A

OTHER DIAGNOSTIC PROCEDURES
ECG may reveal atrial and ventricular arrhythmias, ST-segment depression, or spiked T waves.

PATHOLOGIC FINDINGS
- Lesions—diffuse pulmonary edema and congestion, multifocal congestion and edema of the large colon, and congestion of the kidney, spleen, and liver
- Histopathologic lesions—alveolar hemorrhage and emphysema, and neutrophilic and mononuclear peribronchiolar infiltrate

TREATMENT
- Identify and remove inciting antigen.
- Not all reactions require therapy. Less severe reactions warrant monitoring for worsening of signs that might require therapy.
- Sudden dyspnea, hypotension, rapidly progressive and severe urticaria, and collapse suggest anaphylactic shock and warrant aggressive therapy.
- Therapeutic goals—prevent or reverse the effects of mediator release, and maintain respiratory and cardiovascular integrity.
- Upper airway obstruction secondary to mediator-induced edema may warrant tracheostomy. Administer oxygen if dyspnea or collapse occur.
- Large-volume fluid therapy is indicated in hypotensive patients.

MEDICATIONS

DRUGS
- Rapid-acting glucocorticoids (prednisolone sodium succinate, 0.25–1.0 mg/kg IV) in cases of local and systemic anaphylaxis; longer-acting glucocorticoids (dexamethasone, 0.05–0.1 mg/kg IV) are less desirable for systemic reactions.
- Systemic anaphylaxis—if dyspnea or hypotension are mild, administer epinephrine (1:1000) IM at 0.01–0.02 mg/kg (5–10 mL per 450-kg horse); if dyspnea or hypotension are severe, administer intravenous epinephrine at 0.005–0.01 mg/kg (2.25–4.5 mL per 450-kg horse).
- Antihistamines (tripelennamine hydrochloride, 1 mg/kg IM) have little benefit as the sole therapeutic agent and should be used only as adjunctive therapy.
- Hypotension refractory to IV fluid and epinephrine therapy may be treated with a dilute dobutamine solution (50 mg in 500 mL of 5% dextrose). Administer 1-3 μg/kg per min to effect. Dobutamine should be limited to instances when blood pressure and ECG monitoring are available.

CONTRAINDICATIONS/POSSIBLE INTERACTONS
- Epinephrine may cause profound excitement and potentiate myocardial ischemia, increasing the danger of arrhythmia.
- Glucocorticoid administration has been associated with laminitis.
- Dobutamine potentiates hypoxemia-induced cardiac arrhythmias.

FOLLOW-UP
- Continuous blood pressure and cardiac monitoring, via blood pressure manometer and ECG, are warranted during anaphylactic shock to determine effectiveness of therapy and to facilitate detection and correction of hypotension, cardiac conduction abnormalities, and cardiac arrhythmias.
- Anaphylactic shock warrants intense monitoring, as do patients with less severe reactions of a progressive nature.
- To prevent recurrence, identify and avoid the inciting antigen.
- Report adverse drug and biologic reactions to the manufacturer and the U.S. Pharmacopeia (800-487-7776, http://www.usp.org/prn/vprp.htm).

MISCELLANEOUS

ABBREVIATION
- GI = gastrointestinal

Suggested Reading

Swiderski C. Hypersensitivity. In: Kobluk C, Ames T, Geor R, eds. The horse: diseases and clinical management. Philadelphia: WB Saunders, 1995;1065–1072.

Author Cyprianna E. Swiderski
Consulting Editor Debra C. Sellon

ANEMIA

BASICS

DEFINITION

A decrease in the circulating RBC mass as evidenced by a decreased PCV, hematocrit, RBC count, or hemoglobin concentration.

PATHOPHYSIOLOGY

• Decreased RBC production in the bone marrow, decreased RBC life span (i.e., hemolysis), or loss of RBCs from the circulation (i.e., hemorrhage).
• Equine bone marrow regenerative responses cannot be assessed by evaluation of peripheral blood, because horses do not release reticulocytes into the circulation in response to severe hemorrhage or hemolysis. Regeneration can only be assessed by bone marrow evaluation or serial monitoring of RBC parameters in the circulation.
• Nonregenerative anemia may be caused by a general bone marrow insult that decreases production of all marrow precursors (i.e., leukocytes, erythrocytes, and platelets), which usually results from an infiltrative process, toxin, immune-mediated phenomena, or infection.
• Selective erythroid suppression may occur with disturbances in specific steps of RBC synthesis, unavailability of specific precursors for RBC synthesis, alterations in the hormonal and cytokine stimuli needed for RBC production, or specific destruction of RBC precursors.

SYSTEMS AFFECTED

• Hemic/lymphatic/immune—decreased blood viscosity and oxygen-carrying capacity; with regenerative anemia (e.g., hemolysis or hemorrhage), marked RBC hyperplasia in the bone marrow; with nonregenerative anemia, decreased bone marrow erythrocyte precursors. Splenomegaly may occur with extravascular hemolysis.
• Cardiovascular—low blood viscosity may result in a holosystolic heart murmur; tissue hypoxia stimulates tachycardia.
• Hepatobiliary—tissue hypoxia can result in centrilobular degeneration; hemolytic anemia can result in hyperbilirubinemia and icterus.

SIGNALMENT

No general breed, sex, or age predilections, though some specific diseases may be more likely in some types of horses.

SIGNS

General Comments

Usually secondary to another underlying disease; clinical signs referable to the primary disease process often are more apparent than signs directly related to anemia.

Historical Findings

• Vary depending on the primary disease process
• Lack of energy; exercise intolerance

Physical Examination Findings

• Tachycardia, tachypnea, and holosystolic heart murmur
• Pale mucous membranes
• Weakness, lethargy, and depression
• Other signs vary depending on the primary disease process—icterus with hemolysis; uremic breath, weight loss, polyuria, and polydipsia with chronic renal failure; weight loss and lymphadenopathy with lymphosarcoma; colic with GI disease; and fever with infectious, inflammatory, or immune-mediated disease

CAUSES

Hemorrhage

• External hemorrhage—trauma, surgery, coagulopathy, and parasites
• Epistaxis—guttural pouch mycosis, pulmonary abscess, EIPH, ethmoid hematoma, sinusitis, trauma, neoplasia, coagulopathy, and pneumonia
• Hemothorax—trauma (e.g., fractured rib and lacerated heart or great vessels), ruptured pulmonary abscess, ruptured great vessel, aneurysm, neoplasia, and coagulopathy
• Hematuria—pyelonephritis, cystitis/urolithiasis, neoplasia, trauma, urethral ulceration, and coagulopathy
• Hemoperitoneum—trauma (e.g., splenic or hepatic rupture), ovarian hemorrhage, mesenteric vessel rupture (i.e., verminous arteritis), aneurysm, abdominal abscess, neoplasia, and coagulopathy
• GI—ulceration, parasites, granulomatous inflammatory disease, neoplasia, coagulopathy, and foreign bodies

Hemolysis

• Infectious diseases—babesiosis (i.e., piroplasmosis) and EIA
• Immune-mediated disease—autoimmune hemolytic anemia, secondary immune mediated anemia (e.g., infection, neoplasia, or drugs), and neonatal isoerythrolysis
• Oxidative damage to RBCs—red-maple leaf, phenothiazine, onion, and familial methemoglobinemia
• Iatrogenic—hypotonic or hypertonic solutions administered IV
• Other toxicities—intravenous DMSO, bacterial toxins (*Clostridium* sp.), snake venom, and oak
• Miscellaneous—end-stage hepatic disease, hemolytic uremic syndrome, and DIC*

Nonregenerative Anemia

- Iron deficiency—chronic hemorrhage and nutritional deficiency
- Anemia of chronic disease—chronic infection or inflammation, neoplasia, and endocrine disorders
- Bone marrow failure—myelophthisis, myeloproliferative disease, bone marrow toxins (e.g., phenylbutazone and chloramphenicol), radiation, immune-mediated, and idiopathic
- Miscellaneous—chronc renal disease, chronic hepatic disease, and recent hemorrhage or hemolysis

RISK FACTORS

- Vary depending on the primary disease process
- Any infectious or inflammatory disease
- Foals nursing incompatible colostrum are at risk for neonatal isoerythrolysis.
- Trauma
- Chronic blood loss
- Renal failure
- Neoplasia
- Coagulopathy

DIAGNOSIS

DIFFERENTIAL DIAGNOSIS

- Sudden onset of clinical signs is more consistent with hemorrhage or hemolysis than with nonregenerative anemia; however, chronic nonregenerative anemia can appear to have a sudden onset as the anemia becomes severe or an underlying disease condition exacerbates.
- History of trauma suggests hemorrhage.
- Fever suggests anemia secondary to infectious, inflammatory, or immune-mediated conditions.
- Significant weight loss suggests infectious, inflammatory, neoplastic, or end-stage organ disease.

CBC/BIOCHEMISTRY/URINALYSIS

- Decreased PCV, hematocrit, hemoglobin, and total RBC count
- Reticulocytes are not observed in the peripheral blood of horses with regenerative anemia.
- MCV may increase slightly with regenerative anemia, but this is uncommon—RBC indices usually remain within normal limits.
- Heinz bodies in erythrocytes with hemolysis due to oxidative injury
- Spherocytosis or RBC autoagglutination with immune-mediated anemia.
- Insufficient mixing of the sample may result in a falsely low RBC or PCV.
- In vitro hemolysis from delays in sample processing or excessive heat can result in falsely low PCV and total RBC count and falsely high MCH and MCHC.
- Plasma protein concentration usually is normal with hemolysis and nonregenerative anemia, unless altered by the primary disease process, but usually decreased with hemorrhage.
- Decreased MCH, MCHC, and MCV with iron deficiency anemia
- Inflammatory leukogram and hyperfibrinogenemia with chronic infectious or inflammatory disease
- Abnormal, neoplastic cells in the circulation of some horses with myeloproliferative disorders
- Severe neutropenia and thrombocytopenia, with generalized bone marrow failure
- Hyperbilirubinemia, especially direct bilirubin, with hemolysis
- Biochemical alterations may reflect the underlying disease process—increased BUN and creatinine with renal failure; increased hepatocellular or cholestatic enzyme activities with hepatic disease
- Increased globulin concentration and decreased albumin:globulin ratio with chronic infectious or inflammatory disease
- Bilirubinuria or hemoglobinuria with some hemolytic disorders
- Isosthenuria with chronic renal failure

OTHER LABORATORY TESTS

- Direct Coombs' test often is positive with immune-mediated hemolysis.
- Autoagglutination of erythrocytes may be observed with immune-mediated hemolysis; this must be differentiated from normal rouleaux formation.
- Anemia of chronic disease—serum iron concentration usually increased and total iron-binding capacity usually decreased; storage iron (Prussian blue stain of bone marrow or serum ferritin concentration) usually increased.
- Iron deficiency anemia—serum iron concentration, percentage saturation of transferrin, and storage iron usually decreased; total iron-binding capacity usually increased.
- Serologic testing for EIA.

ANEMIA

IMAGING

• As indicated to diagnose underlying disease processes.
• Ultrasonography or radiography may assist in detecting thoracic or abdominal hemorrhage.

DIAGNOSTIC PROCEDURES

• Bone marrow aspiration or core biopsy—increased erythropoiesis in bone marrow with regenerative anemia, and possibly increased reticulocytes in bone marrow and decreased myeloid:erythroid ratio; decreased erythropoiesis in bone marrow with nonregenerative anemia, and possibly infiltration of abnormal cell types (e.g., myelodysplasia or myeloproliferative disorders)
• Abdominocentesis or thoracocentesis to detect internal hemorrhage
• Fecal occult blood to detect GI hemorrhage; however, this test may have many false-positive and -negative results.
• Endoscopy may assist in detecting respiratory or GI hemorrhage.

TREATMENT

APPROPRIATE HEALTH CARE

• Inpatient treatment may be necessary depending on severity of the anemia and of the underlying disease condition.
• Cross-matched whole blood or packed RBC transfusions if the anemia is severe and signs of tissue hypoxia are present.

NURSING CARE

Isotonic or hypertonic fluid therapy if patient is hypovolemic

ACTIVITY

• Decrease activity.
• Rest.

DIET

Oral iron supplementation with iron deficiency anemia

SURGICAL CONSIDERATIONS

May be indicated with significant uncontrolled internal hemorrhage.

MEDICATIONS

DRUGS AND FLUIDS

• Systemic corticosteroids if immune-mediated or oxidative hemolysis is suspected—dexamethasone (0.04–0.2 mg/kg IV or IM once or twice daily)
• Therapy indicated for the primary underlying disease process

CONTRAINDICATIONS

N/A

PRECAUTIONS

• Use caution in the administration of whole blood or blood products.
• Use caution in the administration of corticosteroids if a chronic infectious condition is suspected.

POSSIBLE INTERACTIONS

N/A

ALTERNATIVE DRUGS

N/A

FOLLOW-UP

PATIENT MONITORING

- Monitor PCV to assess marrow regenerative responses—PCV should begin to increase by an average of 0.5–1% per day within 3–5 days of an acute hemorrhagic or hemolytic episode.
- Additional monitoring as indicated by the underlying disease process.

POSSIBLE COMPLICATIONS

N/A

MISCELLANEOUS

ASSOCIATED CONDITIONS

N/A

AGE-RELATED FACTORS

N/A

ZOONOTIC POTENTIAL

N/A

PREGNANCY

N/A

SYNONYMS

N/A

SEE ALSO

- Anemia, aplastic (pure red cell aplasia)
- Anemia, Heinz body
- Anemia, immune-mediated
- Anemia, iron deficiency
- Coagulation defects, acquired
- Coagulation defects, inherited
- DIC
- EIA
- Hemorrhage, acute
- Hemorrhage, chronic
- Myeloproliferative diseases
- Pancytopenia
- Transfusion reactions

ABBREVIATIONS

- DIC = disseminated intravascular coagulation
- DMSO = dimethyl sulfoxide
- EIA = equine infectious anemia
- EIPH = exercise-induced pulmonary hemorrhage
- GI = gastrointestinal
- MCH = mean cell hemoglobin
- MCHC = mean cell hemoglobin concentration
- MCV = mean cell volume
- PCV = packed cell volume

Suggested Reading

Sellon DC. Diseases of the hematopoietic system. In: Kobluk CN, Ames TR, Geor RJ, eds. The horse. Diseases and clinical management. Philadelphia: WB Saunders, 1995:1073–1110.

Author Debra C. Sellon
Consulting Editor Debra C. Sellon

ANEMIA, APLASTIC (PURE RED CELL APLASIA)

BASICS

OVERVIEW

- Hematologic abnormality of racehorses that have been administered repeated doses of rhEPO
- Reduced or absent bone marrow RBC production despite adequate WBC and platelet production
- Occurs in the absence of other systemic disease.

SIGNALMENT

Most common in racing Standardbreds, Thoroughbreds, and possibly other breeds of performance horse

SIGNS

- Typically occurs in racehorses after administration of several doses of rhEPO.
- Various signs of anemia depending on the severity and duration of disease; poor performance, weight loss, depression, pale mucous membranes, and tachycardia may be seen.
- Prolonged or severe anemia may cause tissue hypoxia and heart failure; death may occur.

CAUSES AND RISK FACTORS

- Repeated administration of rhEPO to horses is believed to cause an immune response to the recombinant hormone. Anti-rhEPO antibodies may bind endogenous horse erythropoietin, preventing the hormone from stimulating terminal RBC differentiation and multiplication in bone marrow.
- Increased frequency of exposure likely leads to an exaggerated immune response and more severe clinical signs.

DIAGNOSIS

DIFFERENTIAL DIAGNOSIS

- Consider other causes of nonregenerative anemia, including folate deficiency after treatment of EPM with antifolate drugs, iron deficiency, and anemia of chronic disease or chronic renal failure. Anemia of chronic disease and renal failure is usually less severe; the former is associated with elevated plasma fibrinogen concentrations or WBC changes and the latter with azotemia.
- Chronic EIA may also cause significant bone marrow suppression. These horses are seropositive for EIAV.
- Regenerative anemia caused by external or internal hemorrhage and infectious, immune-mediated, or toxic hemolysis may be ruled out by the absence of icterus, normal bilirubin levels, normal urinalysis, and increased M:E ratio in the bone marrow.
- Primary myelophthisic disease may cause anemia in the presence of leukopenia or thrombocytopenia. The long survival of equine RBCs compared to WBCs or platelets means that other signs likely are present with anemia (e.g., infection, tendency to bleed).

CBC/BIOCHEMISTRY/URINALYSIS

- Anemia with normal WBC and platelet numbers
- Normal or only slightly elevated bilirubin
- Normal plasma fibrinogen
- Normal urinalysis

OTHER LABORATORY TESTS

- May be associated with increased serum iron and serum ferritin concentrations.
- Negative Coggins test for EIA and negative Coombs' test for immune-mediated hemolytic anemia.
- Rule out infectious causes with specific testing.
- Determine serum folate concentration if antifolate medication has been administered.

IMAGING

N/A

OTHER DIAGNOSTIC PROCEDURES

Bone marrow biopsy demonstrates an increased M:E ratio and erythroid hypoplasia, t confirming the nonregenerative anemia.

ANEMIA, APLASTIC (PURE RED CELL APLASIA)

TREATMENT

- Avoid further rhEPO administration.
- Blood transfusion from a cross-matched donor if anemia is severe and life-threatening

MEDICATION

DRUGS

Dexamethasone (0.05 mg/kg once daily) may be tried, but the efficacy is questionable. Monitor response to treatment, and adjust the dose accordingly.

CONTRAINDICATIONS/POSSIBLE INTERACTIONS

Avoid iron supplementation, because the iron binding-capacity of the serum may be exceeded, leading to hepatic necrosis.

FOLLOW-UP

Monitor the hematocrit over several weeks to months. Some horses appear to be nonresponsive and die despite multiple transfusions and steroid administration, whereas others recover completely.

MISCELLANEOUS

ASSOCIATED CONDITIONS

N/A

AGE-RELATED FACTORS

N/A

ZOONOTIC POTENTIAL

N/A

PREGNANCY

N/A

SEE ALSO

Anemia

ABBREVIATIONS

- EIA = equine infectious anemia
- EIAV = equine infectious anemia virus
- EPM = equine protozoal myeloencephalitis
- M:E = myeloid:erythroid
- rhEPO = recombinant human erythropoietin

Suggested Reading

Piercy RJ, Swardson CJ, Hinchcliff KW. Erythroid hypoplasia and anemia following administration of recombinant human erythropoietin to two horses. J Am Vet Med Assoc 1998;212:244–247.

Author Richard J. Piercy

Consulting Editor Debra C. Sellon

ANEMIA, HEINZ BODY

BASICS

DEFINITION

Acute or chronic RBC destruction caused by oxidative denaturation of hemoglobin with subsequent formation of Heinz bodies within the RBC, which produces a cell that is readily removed from the circulation by intravascular hemolysis or via macrophages as part of the reticuloendothelial system.

PATHOPHYSIOLOGY

- Known toxins, drugs, and chemicals associated with Heinz body production function as electron acceptors and act as an artificial link between cell components and the direct, oxidative action of molecular oxygen in the RBC.
- Denatured hemoglobin formed by this reaction precipitates during the formation of Heinz bodies and attaches to the RBC membrane, causing loss of critical ionic composition with resultant intravascular hemolysis or deformability changes with subsequent, premature RBC removal by the spleen.
- Many of these toxins also cause methemoglobin formation as ferrous iron in the hemoglobin molecule is oxidized to the ferric form.
- Methemoglobin cannot carry oxygen, resulting in tissue hypoxia and ischemia.

SYSTEMS AFFECTED

- Hemic/lymphatic/immune—generalized regenerative anemia
- Renal/urologic—possible pigment nephropathy and acute renal failure

INCIDENCE/PREVALENCE

Uncommon in adults

SIGNALMENT

Any age, breed, or sex

SIGNS

Historical Findings

- Access to wilted red-maple leaves or other oxidative toxins (e.g., phenothiazine, wild onions); dried red-maple leaves may remain toxic for as long as 30 days.
- Acute-onset lethargy and depression are common.
- May be a cause of sudden, unexplained death.

Physical Examination Findings

- Signs of anemia—exercise intolerance, weakness, pale or icteric mucous membranes, tachypnea, tachycardia, or holosystolic heart murmur
- Brown color to mucous membranes or blood with significant methemoglobin formation
- Fever
- Abdominal pain—ischemia
- Hemoglobinuria
- Rectal examination—enlarged spleen
- Severe cases—debilitation and death

CAUSES

- Phenothiazine toxicity
- Ingestion of wilted red-maple leaves
- Ingestion of wild onions

RISK FACTORS

Exposure to toxins (e.g., wilted red-maple leaves)

DIAGNOSIS

DIFFERENTIAL DIAGNOSIS

- Hemorrhage—usually evident from history; physical examination findings may suggest thoracic or abdominal disease.
- EIA—positive Coggins or C-ELISA test
- Babesiosis (i.e., piroplasmosis)—intracellular organisms on stained blood smear; seropositive or seroconversion on convalescent titer
- Granulocytic ehrlichiosis—intracellular organisms on stained blood smear; seropositive or seroconversion on convalescent titer
- Lymphosarcoma—usually a more chronic history, often including weight loss or organ-specific clinical signs
- Purpura hemorrhagica—usually a history of exposure to antigens of *Streptococcus equi* or other respiratory pathogens
- Familial methemoglobinemia—hereditary disorder described in some Standardbreds

CBC/BIOCHEMISTRY/URINALYSIS

- PCV—often <20%
- Heinz bodies on direct blood smear
- May be neutrophilic leukocytosis
- Increased MCH suggests intravascular hemolysis.
- Increased total bilirubin—indirect >> direct
- Increased BUN and creatinine concentrations with hemoglobinuric nephrosis
- Increased serum hepatic enzyme activity reflects hepatic ischemia
- Bilirubinuria and hemoglobinuria (no microscopic hematuria)

OTHER LABORATORY TESTS

- Negative direct antiglobulin test—Coombs
- Increased osmotic fragility
- Bone marrow aspiration—diffuse regenerative erythron (M:E ratio <0.5)
- Heinz bodies are best visualized with new methylene blue staining of a wet-mount preparation of blood; they appear as bluish-green, oval-to-serrated, refractile granules located near RBC margin or protruding from the cell.
- Blood methemoglobin concentration if mucous membranes or urine are brown-tinged—a normal value is <2% of total hemoglobin; affected horses may have >40% total hemoglobin.

IMAGING

- Splenic/hepatic ultrasonography—splenic/hepatic enlargement may appear hyperechoic or hypoechoic; some loss of architecture due to increased fluid component.
- Radiography—thorax usually within normal limits

DIAGNOSTIC PROCEDURES

Thorough diagnostic workup to rule out other causes of hemolytic anemia

PATHOLOGIC FINDINGS

- Enlarged liver and spleen; pale or icteric tissues
- Severe, diffuse congestion of the kidneys
- If chronic, possibly signs of congestive heart failure—pulmonary embolism, pulmonary edema, cardiomegaly, or hepatic congestion
- Histopathologic lesions might include renal tubular nephrosis with hemoglobin casts, centrilobular hepatic degeneration and necrosis, and phagocytized RBCs and hemosiderin in the spleen and liver.

ANEMIA, HEINZ BODY

TREATMENT

APPROPRIATE HEALTH CARE
- Identify and remove source of the oxidant.
- Cross-matched blood transfusion if clinically indicated—evidence of tissue hypoxia (usually PCV <8–12%).
- Monitor PCV closely for development of life-threatening anemia.
- IV fluid therapy to prevent pigment nephropathy
- Oxygen therapy may be useful but often is ineffective if hemoglobin oxygen-carrying capacity is too low.

NURSING CARE
As with other critical care cases (e.g., catheter asepsis, etc.)

ACTIVITY
- Minimize activity, but allow the animal access to fresh air and sunshine if possible.
- No forced exercise.

DIET
- Keep the horse eating a balanced diet, with good-quality hay and grain.
- Fresh water should be available ad libitum.

CLIENT EDUCATION
Explain the hazards of exposure to wilted red-maple leaves, and advise to remove branches blown down in storms or cut down where horse may have access to them.

SURGICAL CONSIDERATIONS
N/A

MEDICATIONS

DRUGS OF CHOICE
- No specific medicinal treatment for Heinz body anemia; treatment is mainly supportive.
- Treatment to prevent pigment nephropathy is critical and usually includes administration of isotonic IV fluids; furosemide or dopamine may be indicated in cases with oliguria or anuria.
- Dexamethasone may help to stabilize cellular membranes and decrease phagocytosis of damaged RBCs.

CONTRAINDICATIONS
Use of methylene blue or other reductive therapy may be detrimental, because these may enhance Heinz body formation.

PRECAUTIONS
N/A

POSSIBLE INTERACTIONS
N/A

ALTERNATIVE DRUGS
Vitamin C (30 mg/kg twice daily, diluted in IV fluids) may be useful as antioxidant therapy in cases involving methemoglobin-associated conditions.

FOLLOW-UP

PATIENT MONITORING
Close monitoring of PCV; as long as the PCV is stable or slowly increasing, the interval between tests may be increased.

PREVENTION/AVOIDANCE
Limiting access to excess phenothiazine, onions, or wilted red-maple leaves.

POSSIBLE COMPLICATIONS
- Laminitis
- Nephrosis
- General debilitation
- Abortion

EXPECTED COURSE AND PROGNOSIS
- If the inciting cause can be removed and methemoglobinemia is minimal, prognosis for recovery is fair to good.
- Several weeks may be required for full recovery.

MISCELLANEOUS

ASSOCIATED CONDITIONS
- Methemoglobinemia
- Pigment nephrosis

AGE-RELATED FACTORS
N/A

ZOONOTIC POTENTIAL
N/A

PREGNANCY
Severe cases with general debilitation may have abortion or weak foal at birth.

SYNONYMS
- Methemoglobinemia
- Oxidative hemoglobinemia

SEE ALSO
- Anemia
- Anemia, immune-mediated
- EIA

ABBREVIATIONS
- C-ELISA = competitive enzyme-linked immunoadsorbent assay
- EIA = equine infectious anemia
- MCH = mean corpuscular hemoglobin
- M:E = myeloid:erythroid
- PCV = packed cell volume

Suggested Reading

Divers TJ, George LW, George JW. Hemolytic anemia in horse after the ingestion of red maple leaves. J Am Vet Med Assoc 1982;180:300–302.

Pierce KR, Joyce JR, England RB, Jones LP. Acute hemolytic anemia caused by wild onion poisoning in horses. J Am Vet Med Assoc 1972;160:323–327.

Schmidt H, Christian TT, Smotherman WM. Is phenothiazine poisonous to horses? J Am Vet Med Assoc 1941:99:225–228.

Warner AE. Methemoglobinemia and hemolytic anemia in a horse with acute renal failure. Compend Contin Educ Pract Vet 1984;6:S465–S468.

Author Rebecca S. McConnico
Consulting Editor Debra C. Sellon

ANEMIA, IMMUNE-MEDIATED

BASICS

DEFINITION

Acute or chronic RBC destruction due to antierythrocyte antibody coating of RBCs and subsequent intravascular lysis or phagocytosis by macrophages of the reticuloendothelial system.

PATHOPHYSIOLOGY

- Antierythrocyte antibodies or circulating immune complexes bind to RBC membranes via direct antibody–antigen reaction or nonspecific immune complex binding. Antibody-coated RBCs are removed from the circulation by intravascular or extravascular hemolysis.
- Occasionally, the immune system produces true autoantibodies to normal erythrocyte antigens (primary or autoimmune hemolytic anemia).
- More commonly, antierythrocyte antibodies or immune complexes form secondary to sensitization by an exogenously administered drug or antigens from pathogenic microorganisms. Antibodies cross-react with drug or microorganism antigens and erythrocyte antigens.
- Neoplasia can result in production of antibodies that cross-react with both tumor antigen and normal RBC surface antigens; alternatively, neoplastic cells may produce abnormal antibodies.

SYSTEMS AFFECTED

- Hemic/lymphatic/immune—intravascular or extravascular hemolysis secondary to antibody or complement coating of circulating RBCs
- Renal/urologic—possible pigment nephropathy if significant intravascular hemolysis, especially with concurrent dehydration

INCIDENCE/PREVALENCE

- Neonatal isoerythrolysis—a form of IMHA; common in foals
- Uncommon in adults

SIGNALMENT

Any age, breed, or sex

SIGNS

General Comments

Often reflect a primary, underlying disease process—infection or neoplasia

Historical Findings

- History may reflect an underlying disease process—chronic weight loss with some neoplastic diseases; fever and inappetence with some infectious diseases
- History of exercise intolerance, weakness, or lethargy

Physical Examination Findings

- Signs referable to anemia—exercise intolerance, weakness, pale or icteric mucous membranes, fever, tachypnea, tachycardia, holosystolic heart murmur, abdominal pain (ischemia), and hemoglobinuria
- Rectal examination—enlarged spleen
- Severe debilitation and death may occur in severe, untreated cases.

CAUSES

Primary Immune-Mediated

- Neonatal isoerythrolysis
- Autoimmune hemolytic anemia
- Incompatible blood transfusion

Secondary Immune-Mediated

- Toxicosis—phenothiazine, wilted red-maple leaves, and wild onions
- Infectious—EIA, acute viral infections, bacterial infections, and septicemia
- Neoplastic—lymphosarcoma and others
- Drug-associated—penicillins, cephalosporins, and sulfas
- Microangiopathic—disseminated intravascular coagulation

RISK FACTORS

N/A

DIAGNOSIS

DIFFERENTIAL DIAGNOSIS

- Hemorrhage—often a history of external blood loss or signs referable to thoracic or abdominal disease
- Heinz-body anemia (red-maple leaf toxicosis, onion toxicosis, phenothiazine toxicosis)—history of exposure to oxidative toxins; Heinz bodies or methemoglobinemia evident on routine blood work
- Neonatal isoerythrolysis—usually in foals born to multiparous mares; acute-onset intravascular hemolysis, weakness, and icterus during the first few days of life
- EIA—seropositive for virus (Coggins or C-ELISA test)
- Equine babesiosis (piroplasmosis)—intravascular hemolysis; organisms often observed in stained blood smears; seropositive; rarely seen in the United States, except occasionally in Florida or Texas
- Equine granulocytic ehrlichiosis—organisms observed in neutrophils of stained blood smears; seropositive or seroconversion with acute and convalescent samples; neurologic signs (ataxia) often observed
- Lymphosarcoma—clinical signs can be extremely variable; often accompanied by chronic weight loss
- Purpura hemorrhagica—often a history of exposure to *Streptococcus equi var. equi* or other respiratory tract pathogens; edema of the legs, abdomen, and face is common; petechial hemorrhages of mucous membranes

CBC/BIOCHEMISTRY/URINALYSIS

- Anemia—PCV often <20%
- Often neutrophilic
- Autoagglutination of erythrocytes may be observed.
- Increased MCH suggests intravascular hemolysis.
- Increased serum total bilirubin (indirect much greater than direct)
- Bilirubinuria and hemoglobinuria (no microscopic hematuria)

OTHER LABORATORY TESTS

- Positive direct antiglobulin (Coombs') test
- In-saline autoagglutination—differentiated from rouleaux formation by diluting EDTA-anticoagulated blood (1:4) with physiologic saline solution; true autoagglutination does not disperse with saline dilution.
- Increased osmotic fragility
- Bone marrow aspiration reveals a diffuse, regenerative erythron (M:E ratio, <0.5)
- Positive serologic titer for infectious causes
- Evidence of hematologic parasites on direct blood smears

IMAGING

- Splenic/hepatic ultrasound—splenic/hepatic enlargement; may appear hyperechoic or hypoechoic; some loss of architecture due to increased fluid component
- Radiography—thorax usually within normal limits unless a primary neoplasia

DIAGNOSTIC PROCEDURES

Thorough diagnostic work-up to rule out neoplasia and infectious causes of secondary immune-mediated response

PATHOLOGIC FINDINGS

- Necropsy—enlarged liver and spleen; pale or icteric tissues
- If chronic in nature, possible signs of congestive heart failure—pulmonary embolism, pulmonary edema, cardiomegaly, and hepatic congestion

ANEMIA, IMMUNE-MEDIATED

TREATMENT

APPROPRIATE HEALTH CARE

- Most cases are treated as inpatients, especially if severe.
- Occasionally, emergency medical therapy with cross-matched blood transfusion is indicated for acute, severe cases.

NURSING CARE

- Cross-matched blood transfusion if clinically indicated by evidence of tissue hypoxia (PCV, <8–12%).
- IV fluid therapy if indicated and the horse is not drinking.
- Discontinue current medication to rule out drug-associated IMHA.

ACTIVITY

- Minimize activity, but allow the animal access to fresh air and sunshine if possible.
- No forced exercise.

DIET

- Make efforts to keep the horse eating a balanced diet, with good-quality hay and grain.
- Fresh water should be available ad libitum.

CLIENT EDUCATION

N/A

SURGICAL CONSIDERATIONS

Consider splenectomy if the primary cause cannot be identified.

MEDICATIONS

DRUGS OF CHOICE

Corticosteroids—dexamethasone phosphate (0.04–0.2 mg/kg IV or IM every 12–24 hours), then a decreasing-dose program of prednisolone or prednisone (beginning at ≅2–3 mg/kg)

CONTRAINDICATIONS

Corticosteroids may exacerbate underlying infectious diseases.

PRECAUTIONS

- Cross-match before blood transfusion.
- Corticosteroid therapy may predispose horses to laminitis.

POSSIBLE INTERACTIONS

N/A

ALTERNATIVE DRUGS

Azathioprine (3 mg/kg PO once daily) as an immune-suppressive agent in horses that are nonresponsive to corticosteroids

FOLLOW-UP

PATIENT MONITORING

Carfully monitor PCV, and increase the frequency of dexamethasone administration to twice daily if the PCV does not stabilize within 24–48 hours.

PREVENTION/AVOIDANCE

Avoid drugs known to have caused secondary IMHA.

POSSIBLE COMPLICATIONS

- Pigment nephropathy with intravascular hemolysis
- Laminitis

EXPECTED COURSE AND PROGNOSIS

- If the primary cause can be identified and successfully treated, the prognosis for IMHA is good.
- RBCs replenish as the immune-mediated response resolves; this may take several weeks in some patients.
- Horses requiring constant corticosteroid treatment may have an incurable underlying disease; the prognosis for these horses is poor.

MISCELLANEOUS

ASSOCIATED CONDITIONS

Possible pigment nephropathy

AGE-RELATED FACTORS

N/A

PREGNANCY

Use corticosteroids cautiously in pregnant mares.

SYNONYMS

- Autoimmune hemolytic anemia
- Immune-mediated hemolytic disease

SEE ALSO

- Anemia
- Anemia, Heinz-body
- Babesiosis
- EIA
- Hemorrhage, acute

ABBREVIATIONS

- C-ELISA = competitive enzyme-linked immunoadsorbent assay
- EIA = equine infectious anemia
- IMHA = immune-mediated hemolytic anemia
- MCH = mean corpuscular hemoglobin
- M:E = myeloid:erythroid ratio
- PCV = packed cell volume

Suggested Reading

Mair TS, Taylor FGR, Hillyer MH. Autoimmune haemolytic anaemia in eight horses. Vet Rec 1990;126:51.

McConnico RS, Roberts MC, Tompkins M. Penicillin-induced immune-mediated hemolytic anemia in a horse. J Am Vet Med Assoc 1992;201:1402–1403.

Morris DD. Immune-mediated hematologic disorders in horses. In: Proceedings of the Fourth Annual Forum of the American College of Veterinary Internal Medicine, Washington, DC, 1986:7–9.

Author Rebecca S. McConnico

Consulting Editor Debra C. Sellon

ANEMIA, IRON DEFICIENCY

BASICS

OVERVIEW

- Iron deficiency induces a reversible, nonregenerative anemia that is uncommon in horses; deficiency rarely is associated with insufficient iron intake in adult horses and usually results from chronic blood loss (i.e., two-thirds of total iron reserves are in circulating erythrocytes).
- Iron deficiency, and consequent diminished hemoglobin synthesis, cause a maturation arrest of erythrocytes during the late rubricyte stage in the bone marrow. Reduced numbers of small, hemoglobin-deficient erythrocytes are produced; anemia and reduced blood hemoglobin concentration lead to compromised oxygen delivery to tissues.
- When iron is deficient, depletion of other important, non-heme iron–containing enzymes (e.g., mitochondrial cytochromes essential for oxidative production of cellular energy) also may occur, and cell-mediated immunity and neutrophil killing of ingested bacteria may be impaired.
- Reduced gastric acid secretion, apathy, and irritability have been described in other species.

SIGNALMENT

- No breed or sex predilections
- Suckling foals not consuming forage or grain, especially with only limited access to pasture (i.e., dirt is iron-rich) are more susceptible, because mare's milk has a low iron concentration (0.88 μg/g of raw milk by 2 weeks and 0.6 μg/g by 8 weeks postpartum). Rapid growth is associated with high tissue demands for iron.
- Transient iron deficiency anemia not associated with clinical signs may occur in foals <4 months of age.

SIGNS

- Disease progression—first, second, and third stages
- First and second stages—clinical signs may be absent or mild/moderate; physiologic compensation for gradual reduction in oxygenation is efficient (e.g., improved tissue extraction of oxygen from hemoglobin offsets decreased tissue oxygen delivery).
- Lethargy, fatigue and exercise intolerance may be the first clinical signs noted.
- When PCV reaches ≅12%, tissue anoxia is associated with tachycardia, tachypnea, pale mucous membranes, systolic heart murmur, and lethargy.

CAUSES AND RISK FACTORS

- Chronic, low grade hemorrhage due to bleeding GI lesions (ulcers, NSAID toxicosis, neoplasia—especially gastric squamous cell carcinoma), internal parasitism (*Strongylus vulgaris*, small strongyli), external parasitism (heavy infestation of sucking lice—*Haematopinus asini*), and hemostatic defects
- Inadequate iron intake is uncommon in adult horses, because sufficient iron is available in pasture and feeds.
- Suckling foals denied access to forage, hay, and/or pasture dirt are more susceptible.

DIAGNOSIS

DIFFERENTIAL DIAGNOSES

Hemolysis

- Immune-mediated hemolysis
- Oxidant-induced hemolysis (phenothiazine drugs, onion ingestion, red maple leaf ingestion)
- Parasite-induced hemolysis (babesiosis)
- Hemolytic anemias are characterized by hemoglobinemia, hemoglobinuria, and a normal serum protein concentration; SI concentrations may be increased.

Decreased Erythrocyte Production

- Anemia of inflammatory disease—increased serum ferritin concentrations are typical in anemia of chronic disease.
- Aplastic anemia—bone marrow morphology is diagnostic for aplastic anemia.

CBC/BIOCHEMISTRY/URINALYSIS

- First and second stages—a normochromic, normocytic anemia is observed.
- Third stage (advanced disease)—microcytic hypochromic anemia may be present.
- Decreased TP and albumin concentrations.

OTHER LABORATORY TESTS

First Stage

- Decreased stainable iron (Prussian Blue stain) in bone marrow
- Decreased serum ferritin concentrations—reference range, 85–155 ng/mL; in phlebotomized horses, ≅50 ng/mL has been reported.

Second Stage

- Decreased SI concentration—reference range, 120–150 μg/dL
- Normal or increased TIBC (i.e., concentration of the iron-transporting protein transferrin)—reference range, 300–400 μg/dL
- Decreased percentage transferrin saturation ($100 \times SI/TIBC$)—reference range, 30–50% (Arabian horses, 68%); values <16% suggest that insufficient iron is available for erythropoiesis.
- Fecal occult blood test may be useful when chronic GI bleeding is suspected.

IMAGING

N/A

OTHER DIAGNOSTIC PROCEDURES

Bone marrow aspirate cytology shows erythrocyte maturation arrest at the late rubricyte stage; this test is useful in the diagnosis of early (first-stage) disease.

ANEMIA, IRON DEFICIENCY

TREATMENT

- Affected horses should be hospitalized to determine the underlying cause of anemia; this may require an extensive medical work-up, focusing on possible routes of chronic blood loss.
- Horses with lethargy, intolerance to mild exercise, or a PCV < 15% should be restricted to stall rest.

MEDICATIONS

DRUGS

- Appropriate treatment of the underlying disease process is essential to resolve chronic blood loss.
- Transfusion with compatible whole blood may be required if the anemia is life-threatening.
- Oral ferrous sulfate (1.0 g per 450 kg body wt)—ferrous sulfate is approximately 37% iron.
- Iron requirements for a 450-kg horse are ≅800 mg/day for maintenance and work and ≅1100–1300 mg/day during pregnancy and lactation.
- When IV administration of iron is essential, use only iron cacodylate (1 g/adult horse), and give the preparation slowly.

CONTRAINDICATIONS/POSSIBLE INTERACTIONS

- Do not administer iron dextrans because of likely idiosyncratic reactions, including anaphylaxis and sudden death.
- Iatrogenic iron overload has been reported in adult horses given unnecessary oral and/or parenteral iron supplementation.
- Do not give foals iron-containing products during the first 2 days of life because of the high SI and percentage transferrin saturation at this time and the efficiency with which the gut absorbs iron. Fatal toxic hepatopathy has been induced by administration of oral iron-containing products to newborn foals.

FOLLOW-UP

PATIENT MONITORING

- Monitor response to therapy of underlying disease; assure termination of chronic blood loss.
- Monitor response to treatment with evaluation of PCV/TP at daily to weekly intervals, depending on the severity of anemia.
- Monitor SI, TIBC, and percentage saturation at 2-week intervals.
- Discontinue iron supplementation when PCV, SI, TIBC, and percentage saturation return to reference ranges.

PREVENTION/AVOIDANCE

Ensure that suckling foals have access to pasture and, when of an appropriate age, forage and grain.

POSSIBLE COMPLICATIONS

May result in death if untreated.

EXPECTED COURSE AND PROGNOSIS

- If the underlying disease is successfully treated, iron deficiency anemia is reversible.
- Weeks of iron supplementation may be required, depending on the severity of anemia and the degree of iron store depletion.

MISCELLANEOUS

SEE ALSO

- Anemia
- Anemia, aplastic (pure red cell aplasia)
- Anemia, Heinz body
- Anemia, immune-mediated
- Hemorrhage, chronic
- Pancytopenia

ABBREVIATIONS

- GI = gastrointestinal
- PCV = packed cell volume
- SI = serum iron
- TIBC = total iron-binding capacity
- TP = total protein

Suggested Reading

Sellon DC. Diseases of the hematopoietic system. In: Kobluk CN, Ames TR, Geor RJ, eds. The horse. Diseases and clinical management. Philadelphia: WB Saunders, 1995:1073–1110.

Author Catherine W. Kohn
Consulting Editor Debra C. Sellon

ANESTRUS

BASICS

DEFINITION

Anestrus is the period of reproductive inactivity. The ovaries are small and inactive (no follicular activity). It is characterized by the mare's behavioral indifference in the presence of the stallion.

PATHOPHYSIOLOGY

The mare is seasonally polyestrus, with estrous cycles in the spring and summer months. Cyclicity is primarily regulated by photoperiod, which begins a cascade of events:

- Increasing day length decreases secretion of melatonin from the pineal gland.
- Decreasing melatonin allows increased production and release of GnRH.
- Increased GnRH stimulates gonadotropin release (FSH, LH).
- FSH promotes folliculogenesis and ultimately the onset of estrus behavior.
- When sufficient LH is present, ovulation occurs (end of vernal transition, onset of ovulatory period).
- Length of the average estrous cycle is 21 days (range: 19–22 days) and is defined as the period of time between ovulations that coincides with progesterone levels of <1 ng/mL.
- Estrus and estrous cycle lengths are quite repeatable by individual mare from cycle to cycle.

Key hormonal events/sequence of the equine estrous cycle:

- FSH (pituitary-origin) causes ovarian follicular growth.
- Estradiol (follicular origin) stimulates increased GnRH pulse frequency, resulting in secretion of LH (pituitary-origin).
- LH surge causes ovulation, after which estradiol returns to basal levels.
- Progesterone (CL origin) rises from basal levels (<1 ng/mL) at ovulation to >4 ng/mL by 4–7 days post-ovulation.
- Natural prostaglandin ($PGF_2\alpha$), of endometrial origin, is released 14–15 days post-ovulation, causes luteolysis, and a concurrent decline in progesterone levels.
- Interference with these normal hormonal events can result in anestrus.

SYSTEMS AFFECTED

- Reproductive
- Behavioral
- Hormonal

SIGNALMENT

Mares of any age and any breed may be affected.

SIGNS

General Comments

- Complete teasing records are essential to investigate suspected estrus abnormalities.
- Understand seasonal influences on reproduction. Individual variation in the onset/duration of cyclicity has bearing on presumed cases of anestrus.
- Individual reproductive history: estrous cycle length, response to teasing, foaling data, and injuries or infections of the genital tract may relate to current clinical abnormalities.
- Current and past history of drugs administered.

Historical Findings

The mare's failure to accept the stallion is the usual complaint. Rarely, stallion-like behavior is reported.

Physical Examination Findings

- Mares in poor body condition are more likely to exhibit anestrus.
- A vaginal examination can identify inflammation, adhesions, urine pooling, and conformational abnormalities. Speculum exam is one method of identifying the stage of the estrous cycle by assessing relaxation of the external cervical os.
- Clitoral enlargement, with the exception of intersex conditions, is most commonly observed following chronic anabolic steroid administration.
- Transrectal palpation by an experienced individual is essential to evaluate a problem mare. Features of uterine size and tone; ovarian size, shape, and location; and cervical relaxation must be noted in a complete examination. Serial examinations over the course of several weeks may be required to define the patient's status.
- Transrectal ultrasonography is an important adjunct to define abnormalities noted during palpation.

CAUSES

Normal Physiologic Variation

- Winter anestrus—Approximately 20% of mares continue to cycle during the winter months (November–January in the northern hemisphere), whereas the majority enter a period of ovarian quiescence. This is the time of year when failure to cycle is considered normal. Two transitional phases occur for the mare each year. Autumnal (fall), as the mare moves from cycling through autumnal transition into anestrus, and the vernal (spring), which progresses from anestrus through transition to resume cyclicity. Behavioral patterns vary during these transition periods. Individual variation in the onset and length of these phases is normal.

ANESTRUS

• Behavioral anestrus—These mares have normal estrous cycles as determined by serial transrectal palpations, but do not demonstrate estrus (see Abnormal Estrus Intervals).
• Pregnancy—With recognition of pregnancy, CL function and progesterone production continue. The majority of pregnant mare behavior is that of an anestrus mare.
• Pseudopregnancy—Embryonic death after maternal recognition of pregnancy or the formation of endometrial cups results in persistent luteal activity and behavioral anestrus.
• Postpartum anestrus—Most mares (>95%) re-establish cyclic activity within 20 days of parturition. Some fail to continue to cycle after the first postpartum ovulation (foal heat), due either to prolonged luteal function or ovarian inactivity.
• Age-related conditions—Puberty generally occurs between 12 and 24 months of age. Individual variations occur in response to age, weight, nutrition, and season. Aged mares tend to have protracted seasonal anestrus, and mares >25 years of age may stop cycling completely.

Congenital Abnormalities

• Gonadal dysgenesis—The absence of functional ovarian tissue can result in anestrus, erratic estrus, or persistent estrus. Behavioral estrus has been attributed to adrenal-origin steroid production in these mares in the absence of progesterone. Mares typically have a flaccid, often infantile uterus and hypoplastic endometrium in addition to small, non-functional ovaries. The most common chromosomal abnormality in these cases is XO monosomy (Turner's syndrome).
• Intersex conditions—XY sex reversal chromosomal abnormalities.
• Hormonal imbalances—Cushing's disease (hyperadrenocorticism), an adenomatous hyperplasia of the intermediate pituitary gland, can lead to destruction of FSH- and LH-secreting cells and/or the overproduction of glucocorticoids. This may be accompanied by increased levels of adrenal-origin androgens causing suppression of the normal hypothalamic-pituitary-ovarian axis. Primary hypothalamic-pituitary-ovarian axis interference has been proposed as a cause of anestrus in mares.

Ovarian Abnormalities

• Ovarian hematoma—See large ovary syndrome.
• Ovarian neoplasia—GCT/GTCT, cystadenoma, germ cell tumors. Affected mare behavior may be reflected as anestrus, stallion-like (increased aggression) behavior, or continuous estrus.

Uterine Abnormalities

Pyometra—Severe uterine infections can destroy the endometrium and prevent the formation and release of $PGF_2\alpha$ essential to regression of a CL. Clinically, this appears as prolonged diestrus.

Pharmacologic/Iatrogenic

• Anabolic steroids—Affected mares may behave as if in anestrus or having silent estrus, or become more aggressive (stallion-like).
• Progesterone/progestin administration—Continued administration effectively inhibits the expression of estrus.
• NSAIDs—These compounds suppress prostaglandin formation. There is no evidence that chronic administration at recommended therapeutic dosages inhibits the spontaneous formation and release of $PGF_2\alpha$ from the endometrium.

RISK FACTORS

Postpartum anestrus tends to occur more often in mares that foal early in the year and those that are in poor body condition at the time of parturition.

DIAGNOSIS

DIFFERENTIAL DIAGNOSIS

Differentiating Causes

• Critically review teasing records.
• Review general and reproductive history for infections, injuries, and medications that may affect current reproductive health.
• Every-other-day transrectal examinations over the course of 2–3 weeks' time should be sufficient to differentiate transitional anestrus, behavioral anestrus, and pregnancy from hypoplastic ovaries, large ovary syndrome/ovarian neoplasia, and pyometra.
• Gonadal dysgenesis and intersex conditions should be suspected based on history (anestrus, irregular estrus), palpation and ultrasound findings (small ovaries, flaccid uterus and cervix), repeated low serum progesterone concentrations (<1 ng/mL, q7 days for 5 weeks), and karyotype analysis.
• The diagnosis of hyperadrenocorticism is discussed elsewhere.

ANESTRUS

CBC/BIOCHEMISTRY/URINALYSIS
N/A

OTHER LABORATORY TESTS
- Serum progesterone concentrations. Basal levels of <1 ng/mL indicate no ovarian luteal tissue. Active CL function is associated with levels of >4 ng/mL.
- Serum testosterone and inhibin concentrations. Mares typically have testosterone values <50–60 pg/mL; values of >50–100 pg/mL have been observed in mares with GCT.
- Serum inhibin concentrations >0.7 ng/mL are usually produced by GTCT.
- Serum equine chorionic gonadotropin (eCG) levels, to rule-out embryonic death as the cause of anestrus. eCG is produced by the endometrial cups between 35- and 150 days of pregnancy.
- GnRH stimulation test to identify primary hypothalamic or pituitary dysfunction.
- Karyotype analysis, evaluating peripheral blood lymphocytes, is indicated for suspected gonadal dysgenesis or intersex conditions.

IMAGING
Transrectal ultrasonography is routinely used to evaluate the equine reproductive tract. The reader is referred to other texts for a comprehensive discussion on this technique.

DIAGNOSTIC PROCEDURES
Uterine cytology, culture, and biopsy techniques useful in the diagnosis and treatment of pyometra and endometritis. See also uterine disease, endometritis.

TREATMENT
- A case of behavioral anestrus may be solved simply by altering management techniques, e.g., varying teasing methods to elicit a response from a mare and basing the timing of AI on serial transrectal palpation and ultrasound findings.
- Artificial lighting can hasten the onset of vernal transition through manipulation of photoperiod. The actual duration of transition remains the same. Mares are kept in lighted conditions for 14.5–16 hr/day, or alternatively, by adding 1–2 hr of light 10 hr after dusk (*flash* lighting) for 60 days. Sixty days of supplemental lighting are required for the progression from anestrus to ovulatory period. Recommendation is to begin light supplementation by December 1 in the northern hemisphere.
- Mares due to foal early in the year may be placed under artificial lighting beginning 2 months prior to parturition to improve postpartum cyclicity and avoid the potential for lactational anestrus.
- Progesterone alone is not a recommended treatment for mares in deep anestrus. Coupling artificial lighting, as described above, for 60 days, followed by progesterone therapy for 12 days is an effective means to achieve the onset of early, regular estrous cycles.
- Ovarian tumors/ovariectomy—Removal of a GCT/GTCT allows the opposite ovary to recover from the effects of inhibin suppression by the tumor. Dependent on the season (available light) when the tumor is removed, there could be a longer latent period for activity to return (e.g., ovariectomy in autumn, the mare is exposed to normal increase in day length beginning at the end of winter).
- Pyometra management is discussed elsewhere.

MEDICATIONS

DRUG(S) OF CHOICE
- $PGF_{2}\alpha$ (Lutylase, 10 mg, IM, Upjohn, Kalamazoo, MI) for prolonged luteal activity. Multiple injections may be needed to lyse functional luteal tissue in cases of pseudopregnancy.
- Deslorelin (Ovuplant, 2.1 mg SC implant, Ft. Dodge), a GnRH analog, is used to induce ovulation within 48 hr in mares with a follicle(s) >30 mm in diameter. This method is useful for AI by appointment.
- Progesterone (altrenogest, 0.044 mg/kg SID, P/O) is used to shorten the duration of late vernal transition, providing the mares have some follicular development >20 mm in diameter and are showing behavioral estrus. Its use in seasonally anestrus mares is not recommended.

CONTRAINDICATIONS
N/A

PRECAUTIONS
- $PGF_{2}\alpha$ can cause sweating and colic-like symptoms due to stimulation of smooth muscle cells. Monitor mares for 1–2 hr, if required, treat symptomatically. $PGF_{2}\alpha$ administration can cause abortion in pregnant mares.
- Progesterone supplementation has been associated with decreased uterine clearance. Its use may be contraindicated in mares with a history of uterine infection.
- $PGF_{2}\alpha$ should not be handled by pregnant women.
- Altrenogest can be absorbed across the skin. Wear latex gloves.

POSSIBLE INTERACTIONS
N/A

FOLLOW-UP

PATIENT MONITORING

• Serial evaluation (three times weekly) of the reproductive tract during the physiologic breeding season is necessary to establish a tentative diagnosis for the origin of anestrus behavior.
• Pseudopregnant mares return to normal cyclic activity when the endometrial cups regress and eCG levels decrease. Serum eCG can persist for up to 150 days. In cases where embryonic death can be confirmed, delaying intervention until that length of time has passed may be indicated.

POSSIBLE COMPLICATIONS

Infertility may result in cases of intractable persistent anestrus.

MISCELLANEOUS

ASSOCIATED CONDITIONS

N/A

AGE-RELATED FACTORS

Postpartum anestrus tends to occur more often in older mares.

ZOONOTIC POTENTIAL

N/A

PREGNANCY

$PGF_2\alpha$ can cause pregnant mares to abort.

SYNONYMS

• Postpartum anestrus, lactational anestrus
• Gonadal dysgenesis, gonadal hypoplasia

SEE ALSO

• Early embryonic death/EED
• Endometritis
• Estrus, abnormal intervals
• Karyotype
• Large ovary syndrome
• Ovarian hypoplasia
• Pyometra
• Uterine disease

ABBREVIATIONS

• CL = corpus luteum
• eCG = equine chorionic gonadotropin
• EED = early embryonic death
• FSH = follicle stimulating hormone
• GCT/GTCT = granulosa cell tumor/granulosa-theca cell tumor
• GnRH = gonadotropin releasing hormone
• LH = luteinizing hormone
• $PGF_2\alpha$ = natural prostaglandin

Suggested Reading

Arbeiter K, Barth U, Jöchle W. Observations on the use of progesterone intravaginally and of deslorelin STI in acyclic mares for induction of ovulation. J Equine Vet Sci 1994;14:21-25.

Bowling AT, Hughes JP. Cytogenetic abnormalities. In: McKinnon AO, Voss JL, eds. Equine reproduction. Philadelphia: Lea & Febiger 1993;258-265.

Daels PF, Hughes JP. The abnormal estrous cycle. In: Equine reproduction. McKinnon AO and Voss JL, ed. Philadelphia: Lea & Febiger, 1993;144-160.

Hinrichs K. Irregularities of the estrous cycle and ovulation in mares. In: Current therapy in large animal theriogenology. Youngquist RS, ed. Philadelphia: WB Saunders, 1997;166-171.

Sharp, D, Robinson G, Cleaver B, Porter M. Role of photoperiod in regulating reproduction in mares: Basic and practical aspects. In: Youngquist RS, ed. Current therapy in large animal theriogenology. Philadelphia: WB Saunders, 1997;71-78.

Author Carole C. Miller
Consulting Editor Carla L. Carleton

ANGULAR LIMB DEFORMITY (ALD)

BASICS

DEFINITION

• Deviation from the normal axis of a limb, usually in one or two planes.
• Can be described as the appearance of the limbs as observed from the front or rear.
• Valgus (i.e., lateral deviation of the limb distal to the location of the deformity) or varus (i.e., medial deviation of the limb distal to the location of the deformity).

PATHOPHYSIOLOGY

Perinatal Factors

• Most foals are born with some degree of ALD, usually between 5–10%, that corrects on its own.
• Often associated with periarticular laxity, muscle weakness, or incomplete ossification of the cuboidal bones—carpi and tarsi. These deformities can easily be straightened with manual pressure.
• Normal cartilage templates of the cuboidal bones begin to ossify late in gestation. At birth, these bones are 42–62% calcified. Premature foals (<315 days of gestation) may have only 20–40% ossification, as may term foals with hyperplastic goiter—hypothyroidism.
• Bones that are not fully ossified have a higher plastic deformation. If the joints load unevenly while the bones are not ossified, deformation of the articular and precursor cartilage of the cuboidal bones may result. Once ossification occurs, an ALD develops because of the resultant, abnormally shaped cuboidal bones. If the condition is not noted and treated early, the deformity worsens and, eventually, becomes untreatable.
• Flaccidity of periarticular structures (i.e., soft tissue [collateral ligaments, joint capsule]) also may contribute in foals because of an unstable joint and result in abnormal loading of the articular surfaces, sometimes causing severe ALD.
• Foals may be born with a disproportionate growth of the metaphyseal region of the radius, uneven growth of the physis, or misshapen epiphysis. These deformities cannot be manually straightened.

Developmental Factors

• Old foals also may develop ALD.
• Unbalanced nutrition (e.g., excessive grain intake by dominant foals) may result in disproportionate growth at the level of the physis, causing deformity.
• Excessive exercise and trauma can lead to microfractures and crushing of the growth plate, leading in turn to early closure (i.e., Salter-Harris type V fracture) and development of ALD.

SYSTEM AFFECTED

Musculoskeletal—both the fore and hind limbs of foals, involving the carpus, tarsus, and fetlocks; one or more joints, with the carpus being the most commonly affected joint and valgus being the most frequently seen deformity.

SIGNALMENT

• All breeds, but there appears to be a predominance in Thoroughbreds; one study found an incidence of 11% in Thoroughbred foals.
• May be present at birth or develop later, during the first year of life.
• No gender predisposition

SIGNS

General Comments

Severity relates to the underlying cause and the duration before treatment.

Historical Findings

• Because ALD frequently occurs in immature or dysmature foals, a history of twinning or maternal placentitis may be present.
• Heavy parasite infestation, crib feeding of grain, and evidence of trauma may contribute to establishing the diagnosis.

Physical Examination Findings

• Interruption of the normal axis of the limb, either medially or laterally, distal to the location of the deformity.
• Sometimes joint effusion and decreased range of motion for the affected joint.
• May be swelling at the level of the growth plate if the deformity is secondary to physitis.
• Abnormal wear of the lateral and medial hoof walls with varus and valgus conditions, respectively.
• Generally not associated with lameness, unless with arthritis or septic or nonseptic physitis.

CAUSES

Perinatal Factors

• Prematurity
• Dysmaturity
• Hypothyroidism
• Intrauterine malpositioning
• Twin pregnancy
• Body pregnancy

Developmental Factors

• Nutritional imbalance
• Trauma
• Non–weight-bearing lameness in the opposite limb

RISK FACTORS

N/A

DIAGNOSIS

DIFFERENTIAL DIAGNOSIS

Perinatal ligament laxity and delayed cuboidal bone development must be distinguished from disproportionate physeal growth.

CBC/BIOCHEMISTRY/URINALYSIS

N/A

OTHER LABORATORY TESTS

Thyroid levels have been used in the diagnosis of hypothyroidism in foals with musculoskeletal abnormalities; however, because these levels can be influenced by several factors, such tests generally are not helpful.

IMAGING

Radiography—radiographs, especially anteroposterior and lateromedial views, should be taken of any premature foal or foal showing ALD; the degree of deviation can be accurately measured using a goniometer and the type of lesions determined.

DIAGNOSTIC PROCEDURES

• Simple observation and physical examination provide a presumptive diagnosis.
• Manipulation of the limbs to attempt to correct the deformity helps to rule out ALD caused by periarticular ligament laxity.

ANGULAR LIMB DEFORMITY (ALD)

TREATMENT

NONSURGICAL

Stall Rest

• Foals with incomplete ossification of the cuboidal bones and straight limbs—maximum period of 2 months; repeat radiography every 10–14 days to assess ossification.
• Foals with disproportionate growth at the level of the physis or diaphyseal deformities—4–6 weeks.
• Foals with flaccidity of periarticular supporting structures can benefit from stall rest with daily handwalking (10–15 minutes) for 4–6 weeks.

Splints and Casts

• Foals with incomplete ossification of the cuboidal bones and deviation of the limbs.
• Should end at the level of, or just proximal to, the fetlock joint to minimize tendon/ligament laxity and osteopenia.
• Change casts every 10–14 days.
• Change bandages with splints every 3–4 days.

Corrective Shoeing

• Corrective hoof trimming and glue-on shoes with lateral or medial extensions can be used alone or in combination with other treatment modalities.
• Valgus deformities—trim the lateral hoof wall, and apply a medial extension to the foot.
• Varus deformities—treat the opposite of varus deformities.

SURGICAL

Growth Acceleration (Periosteal Striping)

• Periosteal hemicircumferential transection and elevation on the concave side of the affected limb—the procedure is relatively easy; its maximum effect is seen within 2 months; and overcorrection has not been reported.
• Keep the surgical site clean and bandaged for 10–14 days.
• Stall rest for 2–3 weeks after surgery.

Growth Retardation (Transphyseal Bridging)

• Performed on young foals (<3 months) with severe ALD or foals with significant ALD in a bone after its rapid growth rate has been completed (MCIII/MTIII $\cong$2 mo, tibia $\cong$4 mo, radius $\cong$6 mo) on the convex side of the affected limb.
• The goal is to create compression across the physis, retarding growth on that side of the limb. The physis at the concave side is not affected.
• Current techniques—3.5-mm cortical bone screws with 18-G cerclage wire placed in a figure-eight pattern; a small, 2-7 mm DCP; or orthopedic staples.
• Keep the area in a clean bandage for 10–14 days.
• Stall rest for 2–3 days after surgery.
• Radiography every 10–14 days to assess degree of correction.
• Remove implants as soon as the deformity has been corrected, because overcorrection is possible.

Corrective Osteotomy

• Performed in foals with significant ALD after the growth plate has closed.
• Current techniques—a closing wedge ostectomy, a step osteotomy in a sagittal plane, and a step osteotomy in a frontal plane.
• Corrective osteotomy has been recommended primarily for deformities involving MCIII/MTIII but has also been described in the proximal phalanx and radius.
• Keep the limb in a bandage with a splint or cast for several weeks.

MEDICATIONS

DRUGS OF CHOICE

Anti-inflammatory medications (e.g., flunixin meglumine [0.5 mg/kg]) and antibiotics (e.g., gentamicin [6.6 mg/kg IV once daily], potassium penicillin [22,000 IU/kg IV QID]) for surgical cases during the perioperative period on a case-by-case basis.

CONTRAINDICATIONS

N/A

PRECAUTIONS

Foals are more sensitive to the ulcerogenic effects of NSAIDs.

POSSIBLE INTERACTIONS

N/A

ALTERNATIVE DRUGS

N/A

FOLLOW-UP

PATIENT MONITORING

• Radiography of foals with incomplete ossification of the cuboidal bones to evaluate the amount of calcification taking place.
• Daily evaluation of foals with splints or casts for heat or swelling of the limb. These foals may have difficulty standing and nursing; assist the foal in rising every hour to ensure it receives adequate nutrition.
• Monitor foals with transphyseal bridging closely to avoid overcorrection of the deformity.
• Continual observation of the foal's conformation is important, because more than one correction may be needed.

POSSIBLE COMPLICATIONS

• Foals with severe ALD may not be able to stand at birth and, thus, nurse the dam without assistance. These foals are at risk for failure of transfer of maternal antibodies and sepsis.
• If splints and casts are improperly applied, pressure sores may develop.
• Permanent deformities may develop if tarsal or carpal bones are crushed.

MISCELLANEOUS

ASSOCIATED CONDITIONS

N/A

AGE-RELATED FACTORS

The most rapid rate of change occurs during the active growth phase of the associated bone.

ZOONOTIC POTENTIAL

N/A

PREGNANCY

N/A

SYNONYMS

N/A

SEE ALSO

Flexural limb deformities

ABBREVIATIONS

• DCP = dynamic compression plate
• MCIII =
• MTIII =

Suggested Reading

Auer JA. Angular limb deformities. Equine Surg 1992;87:940–956.
Auer JA. Appendicular deviations. Curr Pract Equine Surg 1990;96:482–500.
Fretz, et al. Surgical correction of angular limb deformities in foals: a retrospective study. J Am Vet Med Assoc 1983;183:529–532.
O'Donohue, et al. The incidence of abnormal limb development in the Irish Thoroughbred from birth to 18 months. Equine Vet J 1992;24:305–309.

Author Jose M. Garcia-Lopez
Consulting Editor Mary Rose Paradis

ANHIDROSIS

BASICS

DEFINITION

The inability to sweat effectively in response to appropriate stimuli.

PATHOPHYSIOLOGY

- The exact mechanism is not yet fully elucidated, but the most probable cause is altered sweat gland–receptor function. Overstimulation of sweat gland β_2-receptors causes diminished function or a period of unresponsiveness through desensitization or down-regulation of the receptors.
- Other theories include the role of thyroid hormones, electrolyte abnormalities, and hyperkeratinization of sweat gland ducts.

SYSTEMS AFFECTED

- Skin/exocrine—sweat glands no longer function adequately.
- Respiratory—tachypnea

GENETICS

N/A

INCIDENCE/PREVALENCE

As many as 20% of horses may be affected when exercising in a hot, humid climate.

SIGNALMENT

No coat-color, age, sex, or breed predilections

SIGNS

Historical Findings

- Predominant complaints may be tachypnea (especially extended tachypnea after exercise) combined with a noticeable lack or reduction of sweating.
- Some horses, especially those recently introduced into a hot and humid climate, may sweat excessively before showing signs of anhidrosis.

Physical Examination Findings

- With acute onset, horses may demonstrate partial or complete absence of sweating when exposed to appropriate stimuli; however, remember that the rate of sweating depends on the ambient temperature and the intensity and duration of exercise.
- Horses with long-standing anhidrosis may exhibit dry and flaky skin with alopecia, lethargy, and decreased water intake. Body areas that may retain the ability to sweat include under the mane, the saddle and halter regions, and the axillary, inguinal, and perineal regions.

CAUSES

- Physiologic control of the equine sweat gland differs from that of other species. Horses have both humoral control by adrenergic agonists secreted from the adrenal medulla and nervous control by autonomic adrenergic nerves.
- Horses that experience heat stress may have higher-than-normal levels of circulating catecholamines. Anhidrotic horses have significantly higher levels of epinephrine compared with normal horses at rest. These catecholamines act as β_2-agonists and may overstimulate the sweat gland receptors, which results in either desensitization of the receptor (i.e., the receptor is sequestered away from its normal site to another site within the cell) or down-regulation (i.e., decreased number of receptors). Down-regulation is a long-term mechanism that may involve altered synthesis or degradation of receptor proteins.

RISK FACTORS

Horses maintained in hot, humid climates are at risk, and exercise magnifies this risk.

DIAGNOSIS

DIFFERENTIAL DIAGNOSIS

Respiratory diseases that cause an increase in the respiratory rate (both obstructive and restrictive diseases).

CBC/BIOCHEMISTRY/URINALYSIS

- Dehydration, as evidenced by prerenal azotemia
- Possibly increased urinary specific gravity

OTHER LABORATORY TESTS

Intradermal skin testing to evaluate sweat response

IMAGING

N/A

DIAGNOSTIC PROCEDURES

Intradermal injections, in the neck area below the mane, of a specific β_2-agonist (e.g., terbutaline sulfate, salbutamol sulfate), serial dilutions (10^{-3} to 10^{-8} [w/v]), and a control injection of sterile saline; read the results at 30 minutes. Normal horses sweat in response to all dilutions, whereas anhidrotic horses show a diminished response to some or all.

PATHOLOGIC FINDINGS

- Thickened basal lamina, evidence of poor myoepithelial contraction, thickened connective tissues, and marked reduction of vesicles in the secretory cells
- Luminal microvilli often are absent, and the lumen of the duct is obstructed with cellular debris.

TREATMENT

APPROPRIATE HEALTH CARE

- Horses with acute anhidrosis are at risk of heat stress–related lesions. Take such animals immediately to a cooler environment, and attempt to reduce the body temperature.
- Management and environmental changes are the most successful strategies for resolution of long-standing, chronic anhidrosis.

NURSING CARE

Restrict to a stall with adequate air movement (i.e., a fan) during hot periods of the day.

ACTIVITY

- If exercise is necessary, do so during the cooler periods of the day.
- After exercise, make sure the horse is "cooled off" adequately by hosing it down with water.

DIET

- Affected horses commonly are mildly anorexic.
- Normal diet can be maintained, but concentrates should be fed in decreased amounts.
- Additional supplements may include oral electrolytes.

CLIENT EDUCATION

- Advise clients that sound environmental management is the only reliable treatment option at present.
- Inform clients that these horses will be prone to poor performance and will only improve once the capability to sweat effectively has returned.
- Notify clients this usually is a lifelong problem, but under some circumstances, it may not occur again in a horse's lifetime. When it does occur, however, attempts to provide a cool, dry environment must be made.

SURGICAL CONSIDERATIONS

N/A

MEDICATIONS

DRUGS OF CHOICE

- Supplemental electrolytes, especially potassium salts, can be added to the feed or water.
- Some anecdotal reports of success with iodinated casein (10–15 g/day for 4–8 days) and with 1000–3000 U PO of vitamin E (i.e., natural α-tocopherol) daily for 1 month. If added to the water, plain water should be provided as well.
- Amino acid supplements, especially those with tyrosine, are commercially available. (Tyrosine is necessary for the resensitization of sequestered β_2-receptors.)

CONTRAINDICATIONS

N/A

PRECAUTIONS

Anaphylaxis has been reported when using injectable vitamin E.

POSSIBLE INTERACTIONS

N/A

ALTERNATIVE DRUGS

Drugs that either reduce down-regulation or decrease sympathetic drive are still in the investigative stages.

FOLLOW-UP

PATIENT MONITORING

- Monitoring the patient shortly after exercise is one way to recognize resolution or to ensure the horse does not become heat stressed.
- Normal thermoregulatory abilities allow a horse to reduce its body temperature to within normal limits approximately 30 minutes after exercise.

PREVENTION/AVOIDANCE

- Do not expose anhidrotic horses, especially when exercising, to extreme ambient temperatures.
- Exercising during the cooler periods of the day, and stall the horse in a cooler environment (e.g., an air-conditioned stall) during the hotter periods of the day.
- Relocating the horse to a more temperate climate may lead to resolution of the clinical signs.

POSSIBLE COMPLICATIONS

- Poor performance is the most common problem and usually is noted in athletic patients.
- Heat stroke may occur if horses are exercised during the hotter periods of the day.

EXPECTED COURSE AND PROGNOSIS

- Most horses respond to a change in environment and begin to sweat normally after a few days or weeks; moderately affected horses take ≅6 weeks for their signs to be relieved.
- Horses that have suffered from the disease before will usually, but not necessarily, become anhidrotic if exposed to hot, humid conditions again.

MISCELLANEOUS

ASSOCIATED CONDITIONS

Skin lesions—dry, flaky skin and alopecia, especially around the eyes and over the points of the shoulders.

AGE RELATED FACTORS

N/A

ZOONOTIC POTENTIAL

N/A

PREGNANCY

N/A

SYNONYMS

- Dry coat disease.
- Nonsweaters

SEE ALSO

Skin diseases

Suggested Reading

Evans CL. Physiological mechanisms that underlie sweating in the horse. Br Vet J 1966;122:117–123.

Hubert J, Beadle RE. Equine anhidrosis. Compend Cont Educ Pract Vet 1998; 20:846–852.

Mayhew IG, Ferguson HO. Clinical, clinicopathologic, and epidemiologic features of anhidrosis in central Florida Thoroughbred horses. J Vet Med 1987; 1:136–141.

Author Jeremy D. Hubert and Ralph E. Beadle

Consulting Editor Michel Levy

ANOREXIA AND DECREASED FOOD INTAKE

BASICS

DEFINITION

Anorexia is the complete loss of appetite or lack of desire for food. Some conditions that cause anorexia may not lead to complete loss of appetite, but merely reduced food intake.

PATHOPHYSIOLOGY

Appetite Suppression

Anorexia in general appears to be the result of a modification of central regulation of feeding behavior in the hypothalamus. Many factors and substances appear to be involved in regulating feed intake. Anorexia associated with alterations of smell and taste has not been shown in the horse. Decreased food intake has been associated with parasitic infections, but the mechanism is unknown. Pain and depression appear to cause anorexia, as well as causing dehydration, electrolyte imbalances, acid–base disorders, micronutrient deficiencies, and changes in concentrations of neurotransmitters, hormones or mediators. Serotonin agonists decrease food intake, apparently via central histaminergic activity. The neurotransmitter neuropeptide Y and various cytokines may cause cancer-related anorexia/cachexia syndrome (CACS). Cytokines induce anorexia when administered peripherally or directly into the brain. Administration of specific cytokine antagonists mitigates cachexia in experimental animal models. Other primary disease conditions, such as infection, inflammation, injury, toxins, immunologic reactions, and necrosis may cause anorexia via cytokines as well. In addition, a proteoglycan has been identified on the cell membranes of animals and has been named *satiomem*. It reduces food intake and may be a satiety or anorexigenic substance. Reduced food intake can also be caused by various conditions affecting the lips, mouth, tongue, pharynx, esophagus, or stomach, and may include painful conditions, mechanical obstructions, or nervous or neuromuscular dysfunctions.

SIGNALMENT

Any signalment

SIGNS

May be a lack of interest in food or an interest only in certain types of food. May note difficulty or inability in prehension, chewing, or swallowing of food, and food may appear at the nostrils. Nasal discharge and cough can occur due to foreign material entering trachea, acquired aspiration pneumonia, or both.

Some of the signs of anorexia may include the following:

• Increased salivation (ptyalism) due to inability to swallow • Hypoesthesia of the face (CN-V) • Neurogenic atrophy of the masticatory muscles (CN-V, motor component) • Bilateral paralysis of facial muscles (CN VII) • May expel partially chewed food ("quidding")

CAUSES

Anorexia

Commonly due to gastrointestinal or abdominal disorders, including colic.

May be secondary to one of the following primary disease processes in any organ system:

• Inflammation • Injury • Toxins • Immunologic reactions • Malignancy • Necrosis • Dehydration • Electrolyte imbalances • Acid–base disorders • Severe respiratory distress • Neurologic disorders • Uremia • Side effects of medications • Pain

Food prehension problems may be due to:

• Pain in lips, tongue, or mouth (e.g., ulcers, lacerations, dental "points") • Mechanical obstructions (e.g., severe swelling of the lips) • Nervous dysfunction of the lips or tongue

Mastication problems may be due to:

• Pain (in teeth, mandibles, maxilla, sinuses, muscles, or in tempero-mandibular joint) • Neurologic dysfunction

Swallowing problems may be due to:

• Pain (in pharynx or esophagus) • Mechanical obstructions in pharynx or esophagus • Neurologic dysfunction (e.g., CN-IX) • Unpalatable food due to contamination or spoilage

RISK FACTORS

Choke, which is the layperson's term for feed impaction of the esophagus, occurs more commonly in animals that bolt their food or have defective teeth.

DIAGNOSIS

DIFFERENTIAL DIAGNOSIS

Anorexia

• Colic • Esophagitis • Gastrointestinal ileus • Gastric ulcers and pyloric stenosis • Peritonitis • Renal failure (uremia) • Severe respiratory distress • Depression of the nervous system—especially cerebral disorders • Secondary to a primary disease process in any organ system • Inflammation or endotoxemia • Injury • Toxins (e.g., Monensin, lead) • Immunologic reactions • Malignancy • Necrosis • Secondary to diseases leading to dehydration, electrolyte imbalances, or acid–base disorders • Side effect of metronidazole

Dysphagia

Food prehension problems may be due to:

• Mucosal disease—oral erosions or ulcers, swellings, growths, or crusts • Vesicular stomatitis • Contact with chemical irritants • Phenylbutazone toxicity • Mechanical trauma; yellow bristle-grass, foxtails • Mechanical obstructions—severe swelling of the lips • Snake bites • Bee stings • Nervous dysfunction of the lips • Bilateral CN-VII damage • Yellow star thistle (nigropallidal encephalomalacia) poisoning • Rabies • Equine protozoal myelitis • Verminous encephalitis

Mastication problems may be due to:

• Musculoskeletal problems • Pain (in teeth, mandibles, or maxilla (e.g., fractured mandible), sinuses (e.g., sinusitis), temporomandibular joint • Pain or other problems of masticatory muscles • Vitamin E/selenium deficiency causing masseteric myopathy • Botulism or tick paralysis causing paresis of masticatory muscles and tongue • Tetanus causing trismus • Mechanical obstructions • Premolar caps (deciduous teeth) • Foreign body • Neurolgic problems • CN-V bilaterally • CN-XII damage • Rabies • Lead toxicity • Equine protozoal myelitis • Verminous encephalitis

Swallowing problems may be due to:

• Pain in pharynx or esophagus • Esophagitis • Pharyngitis or pharyngeal trauma • Pharyngeal abscess • Neoplasia • Strangles • Hyoid bone injury • Mechanical obstructions or abnormalities in pharynx or esophagus • Esophageal intraluminal occlusion; choke or foreign body • Esophageal stricture, stenosis, or diverticulum • Megaesophagus or esophageal ectasia • Persistent right aortic arch • Esophageal intramural inclusion cysts • Rostral displacement of the palatopharyngeal arch • Dorsal displacement of the soft palate in foals • Pharyngeal foreign body • Cysts: epiglottic, dorsal pharyngeal, aryepiglottic, soft palate, guttural pouch, or larynx • Strangles or other retropharyngeal abscess causing external compression • Cleft palate • Neoplasia of the tongue • Nervous or neuromuscular problems • Severe cerebrum or brain stem (forebrain) disease; hydrocephalus, trauma, leukoencephalomalacia, equine protozoal myelitis, verminous encephalitis • Lead toxicity • CN-IX damage • Guttural pouch disease (CN-IX to CN-XI damage) • White muscle disease—nutritional muscular dystrophy • Tetanus • Botulism • Tick paralysis • Weak suckle reflex, poor pharyngeal tone • Due to prematurity/dysmaturity, neonatal maladjustment sydrome, bacterial meningitis, viral encephalitis, hypoglycemia, or depression in foals • Electrolyte disorders (hypokalemia and hypocalcemia)

ANOREXIA AND DECREASED FOOD INTAKE

• Postanesthetic myasthenia • Myotonia congenita • Rabies • Ruptured rectus capitus ventralis muscle • Grass sickness • Pharyngeal–cricopharyngeal incoordination

CBC/BIOCHEMISTRY/URINALYSIS

• Free (unconjugated or indirect) bilirubin elevations, unless cachexic, in which case bilirubin levels may be normal. • Laboratory findings (CBC, biochemistry, fibrinogen) consistent with the primary disease process (e.g., inflammation, internal organ damage) • Laboratory findings (CBC, biochemistry, fibrinogen) consistent with a secondary disease (e.g., aspiration pneumonia)

OTHER LABORATORY TESTS

Various tests depending on primary disease process.

IMAGING

• Radiography of guttural pouches for swallowing problems • Fluoroscopy or radiography of barium swallow for swallowing problems • Radiography of mandible, temporo-mandibular joint and teeth for painful mastication • Radiographs of thorax for aspiration pneumonia • Abdominal ultrasound for primary inflammatory or neoplastic problems

OTHER DIAGNOSTIC PROCEDURES

• Examination of the food supply for evidence of contamination or spoilage • Careful observation of individual when offered food • Oral examination for painful chewing • Passage of a nasogastric tube (for difficulty swallowing) to rule out "choke" • Neurologic examination for difficulty swallowing • Endoscopy of guttural pouches for nervous cause of swallowing problems • Endoscopy of pharynx, larynx, and esophagus for swallowing problems • Rectal examination for internal organ disease

TREATMENT

Depends on the primary problem.

DIET–ACTIVITY

Offer highly palatable and varied feed in cases of anorexia. Supply feed that is easy to chew and swallow in case of dysphagia. Force-feeding by nasogastric intubation or parenteral nutrition may be required. Activity should be limited to stall rest or hand-walking in most cases.

MEDICATIONS

DRUG(S) OF CHOICE

• Depends on primary disease process • Oral administration of 40 g of KCl once or twice daily in anorectic patients

CONTRAINDICATIONS

KCl administration may be contraindicated in patients with abnormal renal function or those suspected of having hyperkalemic periodic paralysis.

FOLLOW-UP

PATIENT MONITORING

The patient should be monitored for dehydration, electrolyte imbalance, acid–base abnormalities, and weight loss, and in cases of dysphagia, for aspiration pneumonia.

POSSIBLE COMPLICATIONS

• Dehydration • Hypokalemia • Hypocalcemia • Metabolic alkalosis with salivary loss • Weight loss • Aspiration pneumonia with dysphagia

EXPECTED COURSE AND PROGNOSIS

Depends on the underlying cause.

MISCELLANEOUS

ASSOCIATED CONDITIONS

• Other primary disease conditions, such as infection, inflammation, injury, toxins, immunologic reactions, and necrosis. • Cancer-related anorexia/cachexia syndrome (CACS), a syndrome of anorexia and weight loss that occurs secondary to malignancy. • Guttural pouch disease can cause neurologic damage to CN-IX–CN-XI and impair chewing and swallowing as well as causing mechanical obstruction to swallowing. • Tetanus • Neonatal maladjustment syndrome may interfere with swallowing or the suckle reflex. • Moderate jaundice may occur due to increased indirect bilirubin levels in the blood. This is an idiosyncratic finding in the horse that occurs with fasting or decreased intake of feed. • Dehydration, electrolyte imbalances (hypokalemia, hypocalcemia), or acid–base disorders as a result of lack of intake of fluid and electrolytes, which may exacerbate the anorexia. • Salivary loss of electrolytes leads to metabolic alkalosis and hypochloremia, primarily. • Secondary or conditional protein–calorie malnutrition (PCM) that involves weight loss with prolonged anorexia. • Aspiration pneumonia occurs secondary to dysphagia.

AGE-RELATED FACTORS

Cleft palate, hydrocephalus and nutritional muscular dystrophy (White muscle disease) are noted most commonly in the neonatal period.

ZOONOTIC POTENTIAL

Rabies can cause anorexia or dysphagia. Precautions should be taken while examining and treating the patient.

SYNONYMS

Decreased appetite

SEE ALSO

• Aspiration pneumonia • Botulism • Cerebral disorders of the central nervous system • Choke • Colic • Dental disease • Epiglottic cysts • Esophagitis • Fractured mandible • Gastric ulcers • Gastrointestinal ileus • Guttural pouch disease • Lead toxicity • Monensin toxicity • Organophosphate toxicity • Peritonitis • Pharyngeal abscess • Phenylbutazone toxicity • Rabies • Renal failure (uremia) • Ruptured rectus capitis ventralis muscle • Sinusitis • Snake-bites • Strangles • Tetanus • Tick paralysis • Yellow star thistle poisoning • Vesicular stomatitis • Vitamin E/selenium deficiency causing swollen masseter muscles

ABBREVIATIONS

• CN = cranial nerve • CACS = cancer-related anorexia/cachexia syndrome • PCM = protein–calorie malnutrition

Suggested Reading

Barton MH. Nasal regurgitation of milk in foals. Compendium on Continuing Education, 1993;15:1, 81-91.

Mayhew IG. Large animal neurology: A handbook for veterinary clinicians. Philadelphia, Lea & Febiger, 1989.

Wilson GL, Osweiler GD, Garner HE. Experimental induction and review of lead toxicity in a Shetland pony. J Med Surg 1979;3:386-390.

Step DL, Divers TJ, Cooper B, Kallfelz FA, Karcher LF, Rebhun WC. Severe masseter myonecrosis in a horse. J Am Vet Med Assoc. 1991;198:1, 117-119.

Hanson PD, Frisbie DD, Dubielzig RR, Markel MD. Rhabdomyosarcoma of the tongue in a horse. J Am Vet Med Assoc 1993;202:8, 1281-1284.

Author Gail Abells Sutton

Consulting Editor Henry Stämpfli

ANTHRAX

BASICS

OVERVIEW

Anthrax is a septicemic disease of animals and human beings caused by *Bacillus anthracis,* which occurs in localized regions worldwide. In the horse, infection usually results from ingestion of soil, forage, or water contaminated with *B. anthracis* spores. In the animal, the organism produces exotoxins that impair phagocytosis and vascular integrity resulting in hemorrhage, edema, renal failure, shock, and almost invariably death. When *B. anthracis* is exposed to the environment, long-lasting spores are formed that are a potential source of infection for other animals.

SIGNALMENT

- Gender, age, or breed disposition have not been reported.
- In cattle, anthrax is reported to occur in adult animals, with males more frequently affected, probably due to differences in grazing habits.

SIGNS

- Fever, depression, and death in less than 4 days is characteristic of the acute form.
- Severe colic, bloody discharge from body orifices, and painful subcutaneous swellings may be noted.
- A chronic form resulting in pharyngeal edema has been described.
- The peracute form, in which death occurs with few clinical signs, appears to be less common in horses than in ruminants.

CAUSES AND RISK FACTORS

- The source of infection is usually soil contaminated by exudates from infected animals. *Bacillus anthracis* forms spores that are very resistant to environmental conditions and most disinfectants, and these spores may persist in the soil for decades. Ingestion of contaminated soil, feed, or water is the most common route of infection, but the organisms may also be inhaled or inoculated by biting insects.
- Anthrax is most common in tropical and subtropical climates, but is seen sporadically in temperate regions, usually in the summer. Anthrax usually occurs in regions with alkaline soils and with climatic cycles of heavy rain and drought.
- Overgrazing increases the risk of disease by increasing the ingestion of soil. Coarse forages may contribute to infection by causing breaks in the oral mucosa.

DIAGNOSIS

DIFFERENTIAL DIAGNOSIS

- Lightning strike can be differentiated on the basis of history of storms and absence of post-mortem findings typical of anthrax.
- Colic and enteritis can be differentiated by finding evidence of gastrointestinal disease at post mortem.
- Purpura hemorrhagica has similar signs but is not rapidly fatal.
- Toxicity can be differentiated based on history and lack of postmortem findings typical of anthrax.
- Leptospirosis causes hemolysis, not hemorrhagic disease.
- Malignant edema may appear similar, but the crepitation of swellings is not found with anthrax.

CBC/BIOCHEMISTRY/URINALYSIS

Routine laboratory findings have not been reported.

OTHER LABORATORY TESTS

Bacterial culture of blood is useful, although may be negative early in disease or if antibiotics have been administered. Cultures should only be performed in a facility capable of containment to prevent infection of laboratory personnel.

IMAGING

N/A

OTHER DIAGNOSTIC PROCEDURES

- Organisms may be seen by microscopic examination of blood smear or edema fluid. Bacilli are gram-positive, have blunt ends, are encapsulated, and occur singly or in short chains.
- Fluorescent antibody of blood or tissue may be diagnostic.

ANTHRAX

PATHOLOGIC FINDINGS

• Due to human health risk and danger of environmental contamination, necropsy should not be performed if anthrax is strongly suspected. Diagnosis can be made without necropsy.
• Dark, non-clotting blood from orifices; absence of rigor mortis; splenomegaly; and lymphadenopathy are hallmarks of anthrax.
• Serosal and mucosal hemorrhage and edema of many organs is seen.

TREATMENT

• The high mortality and rapid course of disease usually limits opportunity for treatment. The prognosis is poor even with treatment.
• Isolate affected and in-contact animals.

MEDICATIONS

DRUG(S) OF CHOICE

• Penicillin G 20,000–40,000 IU/kg IV q6h. Oxytetracycline (5–11 mg/kg IV q12h) is also considered effective. Continue treatment for at least 5 days.
• Anthrax antiserum may be useful but is not available in the United States.

CONTRAINDICATIONS/POSSIBLE INTERACTIONS

N/A

FOLLOW-UP

• Regulatory officials should be notified when anthrax is suspected and the premises placed under quarantine.
• Carcasses should not be opened, and may be disposed of by burning or deep (>6 ft) burial with lime. The area can be disinfected with 5% aqueous lye or 10% formaldehyde.
• Susceptible animals should be vaccinated. An avirulent live spore vaccine is administered subcutaneously and provides immunity in 1 week. Some authors recommend a second vaccination in 2–4 weeks. Annual boosters are required to maintain immunity. Severe adverse reactions have been reported; therefore, the vaccine is indicated only in endemic regions. No antibiotics should be administered within 5 days before or after vaccination, or the vaccine organism may be inactivated.

MISCELLANEOUS

ZOONOTIC POTENTIAL

Anthrax is a zoonosis. Gloves and mask should be worn if it is necessary to contact infected material or animals. Cutaneous anthrax is the most common form in human beings, resulting from inoculation of an open wound with spores, but disease may also result from inhalation or ingestion of spores.

SYNONYMS

• Woolsorters disease
• Charbon
• Splenic fever

Suggested Reading

Radostits OM, Blood DC, Gay CC, et al. Veterinary medicine. Philadelphia:Balliere Tindall. 1994: 671-676.
Pipkin AB. Anthrax. In: Smith BP, ed. Large animal internal medicine. Philadelphia: Mosby. 1996:1246-1248.

Author Laura K. Reilly
Consulting Editor Corinne R. Sweeney

ANTICOAGULANT RODENTICIDE TOXICOSIS

BASICS

OVERVIEW

- Ingestion of anticoagulant rodenticides interferes with normal blood clotting in horses.
- Anticoagulant rodenticides are the most commonly used class of rodenticides.
- First-generation anticoagulants (i.e., warfarin, pindone, coumafuryl, coumachlor) are short-acting coumarin derivatives requiring multiple feedings to result in toxicosis.
- Intermediate anticoagulants (i.e., chlorophacinone, diphacinone) require fewer feedings than first-generation chemicals and, thus, are more toxic to nontarget species.
- Second-generation anticoagulants (i.e., brodifacoum, bromadialone, difethialone) are highly toxic to nontarget species after a single feeding.
- Most anticoagulant rodenticides commonly used today are long-acting, second-generation anticoagulants, with activity in the body of $\cong$1 month.
- Coagulopathy has been reported in horses after a dose of brodifacoum of 0.125 mg/kg (equal to ingestion by an average-size horse of 1 kg of bait containing 0.005% brodifacoum).
- Warfarin has been used therapeutically (30–75 mg per 450 kg) in horses with navicular disease, laminitis, venous arteritis, DIC, and thrombophlebitis.

SIGNALMENT

- May affect all animals.
- Poisoning can occur after accidental ingestion of bait packages or as a result malicious intent.
- Poisoning is rare in horses because of the amount of bait needing to be ingested to cause signs.
- Iatrogenic warfarin toxicosis may result from overdosing, dietary vitamin K deficiency, or concurrent use of protein-bound drugs that increase the concentration of active, unbound warfarin.

SIGNS

- Bleeding diathesis ranging from mild to severe
- Hemorrhage—internal or external
- Signs generally manifest within 3–5 days after ingesting bait.
- Signs are similar to those seen with dicumarol toxicosis.

CAUSES AND RISK FACTORS

The mechanism of anticoagulant rodenticide toxicosis is the same as that for dicumarol toxicosis.

DIAGNOSIS

DIFFERENTIAL DIAGNOSIS

- Moldy sweet-clover ingestion
- DIC
- Severe liver disease

CBC/BIOCHEMISTRY/URINALYSIS

N/A

OTHER LABORATORY TESTS

- Elevated PT and APTT
- Chemical analysis of whole blood or liver tissue for specific anticoagulant

IMAGING

N/A

DIAGNOSTIC PROCEDURES

N/A

PATHOLOGIC FINDINGS

Hemorrhages may occur in any part of the body.

TREATMENT

- Blood or plasma transfusions may help.
- Handle horses with care to avoid stress and further hemorrhage.
- Attempt correction of organ dysfunction resulting from accumulation of extravascular blood (e.g., thoracocentesis) only if the situation is life-threatening and after normal blood coagulation is restored.
- Adding alfalfa hay to the diet may help to provide a source of increased dietary vitamin K_1.

ANTICOAGULANT RODENTICIDE TOXICOSIS

MEDICATIONS

DRUGS

• Vitamin K_1 (phytonadione, 2.5 mg/kg q12h, SQ initially then PO after ≅3 days and continuing for 3–5 weeks) effectively reverses the clotting defect.
• AC and a saline cathartic are useful if ingestion of bait has occurred within the last 12 hours.

CONTRAINDICATIONS/POSSIBLE INTERACTIONS

• Do not use vitamin K_3 (menadione) in horses. Vitamin K_3 is ineffective against dicumarol toxicosis and is nephrotoxic.
• Medications that are highly plasma protein bound may exacerbate toxicosis.
• Drugs generally contraindicated—NSAIDs, phenothiazine tranquilizers, local anesthetics, antihistamines, sulfonamide antibiotics, anabolic steroids, and epinephrine.

FOLLOW-UP

PATIENT MONITORING

• Continue monitoring for blood loss.
• Check PT 2–3 days after the last dose of vitamin K_1 to determine if additional treatment is necessary.

PREVENTION/AVOIDANCE

Prevent access to bait packages.

POSSIBLE COMPLICATIONS

N/A

EXPECTED COURSE AND PROGNOSIS

Prognosis is based on the severity of blood loss and damage to organ systems affected by hemorrhage.

MISCELLANEOUS

ASSOCIATED CONDITIONS

N/A

AGE-RELATED FACTORS

N/A

ZOONOTIC POTENTIAL

N/A

PREGNANCY

• Lactating mares may excrete anticoagulant rodenticides in their milk.
• Monitor foals for any coagulopathies, and treat with vitamin K_1 if PT rises.

SEE ALSO

Dicumarol (moldy sweet clover) toxicosis

ABBREVIATIONS

• AC = activated charcoal
• APTT = activated partial thromboplastin time
• DIC = disseminated intravascular coagulation
• PT = prothrombin time

Suggested Reading

McConnico RS, Copedge K, Bischoff KL. Brodifacoum toxicosis in two horses. J Am Vet Med Assoc 1997;211:882–886.

Author Anita M. Kore
Consulting Editor Robert H. Poppenga

ANURIA/OLIGURIA

BASICS

DEFINITION

- Anuria—lack of urine production
- Oliguria—decreased urine production (<0.25 mL/kg per hour, or <125 mL/hour in a 500-kg horse).

PATHOPHYSIOLOGY

Anuria

- May result from intrinsic ARF with a lack of urine production or from postrenal failure with complete obstruction of flow.
- May develop during the terminal stage of CRF.
- May be observed clinically with lower urinary tract obstruction or trauma or with bilateral ureteral rupture or bladder rupture resulting in urine accumulation in the abdomen.

Oliguria

- Physiologic—a normal response to hyperosmolality or renal hypoperfusion from hypotension, hypovolemia, or diversion of cardiac output to other tissues (e.g., to the muscles during exercise); characterized by production of lesser amounts of concentrated urine (specific gravity >1.035) in response to increased antidiuretic hormone activity on the collecting ducts and/or a decrease in GFR.
- Pathologic—a result of decreased GFR due to intrinsic renal parenchymal damage; characterized by production of lesser amounts of dilute urine (specific gravity <1.020), because tubular function also is compromised with renal parenchymal disease; may accompany incomplete obstruction of the lower urinary tract.

SYSTEM AFFECTED

Renal/Urologic

SIGNALMENT

Breed Predilections

None documented

Mean Age and Range

Ureteral and bladder rupture—more common in neonates

Predominant Sex

- Bladder rupture—more likely in male neonates or postpartum mares.
- Postpartum mares—may develop obstruction due to bladder displacement (e.g., prolapse or extrusion through a vaginal tear).
- Urethroliths or penile trauma causing obstruction are more common in adult males.

SIGNS

N/A

CAUSES

- Physiologic oliguria—hyperosmolality; renal hypoperfusion
- Pathologic anuria/oliguria—intrinsic ARF; terminal CRF; lower urinary tract disruption, trauma, or obstruction (i.e., urolithiasis); bladder displacement (mares)

RISK FACTORS

- Physiologic oliguria—any disease process leading to renal hypoperfusion (e.g., dehydration, hypotension, low cardiac output).
- Pathologic anuria/oliguria—risk factors for intrinsic ARF (e.g., ischemia, exposure to nephrotoxins) or birth trauma (e.g., dystocia) would increase the risk of urinary tract disruption and uroperitoneum in neonates and their dams; penile trauma is more common in breeding stallions.

DIAGNOSIS

DIFFERENTIAL DIAGNOSIS

Physiologic Oliguria

- Broad list of disease processes that may lead to hemorrhagic, hypovolemic, or endotoxic shock and accompanying renal hypoperfusion.
- Severe rhabdomyolysis, vasculitis, hemolytic diseases, or disseminated intravascular coagulation may compromise renal blood flow.

Pathologic Anuria/Oliguria

- Intrinsic ARF, terminal CRF, lower urinary tract disruption resulting in uroperitoneum, and urinary tract obstruction consequent to urolithiasis
- Bladder displacement
- Progressive abdominal distension should increase suspicion of uroperitoneum.
- Repeated posturing to urinate, with little urine passed, supports urinary tract obstruction

CBC/BIOCHEMISTRY/URINALYSIS

- Normal to high PCV in most cases; mild to moderate anemia may be found in horses with terminal CRF; variable leukopenia to leukocytosis; lymphopenia.
- CBC changes more often reflect underlying primary disease process with physiologic oliguria.
- Moderate to severe increases in BUN (50–150 mg/dL) and Cr (2.0–20 mg/dL).
- Variable hyponatremia, hypochloremia, hyperkalemia, hypocalcemia, and hyperphosphatemia—hyperkalemia and hyperphosphatemia more common with intrinsic ARF; hyperkalemia most apparent with urinary tract disruption and development of uroperitoneum.
- Mild to moderate metabolic acidosis—severity varies with the underlying disease process.
- Mild to moderate hyperglycemia—attributed to stress.
- Urine specific gravity—high (>1.035) with physiologic oliguria, low (<1.020) with oliguria due to intrinsic ARF; specific gravity best assessed in urine collected during initial patient evaluation (before rehydration) or while the horse is not receiving fluids; with some causes of physiologic oliguria (i.e., prolonged exercise), urine may less concentrated (specific gravity = 1.025–1.035) than with pure dehydration (specific gravity >1.035), as with water deprivation; more likely a consequence of increased intrarenal production of vasodilatory prostaglandins rather than of actual renal parenchymal damage.
- Oliguria with intrinsic ARF may be accompanied by mild to moderate proteinuria, glucosuria, pigmenturia, and increased numbers of RBCs and casts on sediment examination.
- Urine pH—normal to acidic, especially with concurrent depletion of body potassium stores.

OTHER LABORATORY TESTS

Perform quantitative urine culture in all cases of obstructive urolithiasis, because urinary tract infection often is a concurrent problem.

IMAGING

Transabdominal Ultrasonography

- Kidneys may be enlarged, with loss of detail of corticomedullary junction, in intrinsic ARF.
- Kidneys typically are reduced in size, with increased parenchymal echogenicity, in CRF.
- Uroperitoneum is supported by large amounts of free, echolucent fluid in the ventral portion of the abdominal cavity.
- Variable dilation of renal pelves with obstructive disease.
- Recurrent, obstructive urethrolithiasis may occur with upper urinary tract infection (i.e., pyelonephritis) and is an indication for renal ultrasonography.
- Ureterolithiasis may be further detected by imaging ureters and left kidney via transrectal ultrasonography.

Abdominal Radiography

- Retrograde contrast cystograms can be performed in foals <75 kg to further document bladder rupture as a cause of uroperitoneum.
- IV pyelography is less useful in foals than in small-animal patients.

Urethroscopy/Cystoscopy

Useful in adult horses with suspected obstructive disease, urethral obstruction, or bladder rupture.

DIAGNOSTIC PROCEDURES

Abdominocentesis—a ratio of abdominal fluid Cr concentration to serum Cr concentration of >2:1 supports uroperitoneum.

TREATMENT

- Whether physiologic or pathologic, initially treat anuria/oliguria as a medical emergency.
- Persistent renal hypoperfusion may lead to ischemic ARF.
- If untreated, metabolic disturbances, most notably hyperkalemia, may lead to cardiac arrhythmias and death. Similarly, life-threatening hyperkalemia can be a complication of uroperitoneum, or urinary tract obstruction may become further complicated by disruption and development of uroperitoneum.
- Once the patient is stabilized (largely with supportive treatment in the form of IV fluid therapy), pursue further diagnostic evaluation to determine if surgical intervention (for correction of uroperitoneum or relief of obstruction) is needed.
- Proper recognition and treatment of all underlying primary disease processes, usually on an inpatient basis for continuous fluid therapy, is warranted.
- Reassess dosage schedule of, and possibly discontinue, potentially nephrotoxic medications.

MEDICATIONS

DRUGS OF CHOICE

- Fluid therapy to correct renal hypoperfusion—after initial measurement of body weight, correct estimated dehydration with normal (0.9%) saline or another potassium-poor electrolyte solution over 6–12 hours; monitor closely for SC and pulmonary edema (i.e., increased respiratory rate and effort); conjunctival edema may develop rapidly in horses with intrinsic oliguric to anuric ARF; use maintenance fluid therapy judiciously in animals that are not clinically dehydrated; if hemorrhage is contributing to hypovolemia and renal hypoperfusion, initial treatment with hypertonic saline and/or a blood transfusion may have value.
- Severe hyperkalemia (>7.0 mEq/L) or cardiac arrhythmias—treat with agents that decrease serum potassium concentration (e.g., sodium bicarbonate [1–2 mEq/kg IV over 5–15 minutes]), or counteract the effects of hyperkalemia on cardiac conduction (e.g., calcium gluconate [0.5 mL/kg of a 10% solution by slow IV injection]).
- Furosemide—this diuretic may be administered two times (1–2 mg/kg IV) at 1–2-hour intervals; if effective, urination should be observed within 1 hour after administration of the second dose; if ineffective, discontinue.
- Mannitol—for patients unresponsive to furosemide; hypertonic mannitol (10%–20% solution) can be administered (0.5–1.0 g/kg IV) over 30–60 minutes; if effective, the treatment can be repeated 4–6 hours later.
- Dopamine—in persistently oliguric/anuric patients, dopamine infusion (3–5 μg/kg per minute IV in a 5% dextrose solution) can be given for 3–6 hours; monitor heart rate and rhythm regularly during dopamine infusion; may be combined with furosemide for potential synergistic effects.
- Antiulcer drugs (e.g., omeprazole [2–4 mg/kg PO q2 h], cimetidine [5–10 mg/kg IV q8h] in anorexic horses) may be useful in decreasing the risk of gastric ulcer disease associated with intrinsic ARF.

CONTRAINDICATIONS

- Dopamine—use cautiously may induce cardiac arrhythmias.
- Avoid all nephrotoxic medications unless specifically indicated for the underlying disease process, and then modify dosage accordingly.

PRECAUTIONS

- Monitor response to fluid therapy closely—as little as 40 mL/kg of IV fluids (20 L to a 500-kg horse) may produce significant pulmonary edema.
- Reassess dosage schedule of drugs eliminated by urinary excretion; consider discontinuing all potentially nephrotoxic medications (especially gentamicin, tetracycline, and NSAIDs).

POSSIBLE INTERACTIONS

Use of multiple anti-inflammatory drugs (e.g., corticosteroids and one or more NSAIDs) will have additive negative effects on renal blood flow; avoid combined administration in azotemic patients.

ALTERNATIVE DRUGS

N/A

FOLLOW-UP

PATIENT MONITORING

- Assess clinical status (emphasizing hydration), urine output, and body weight at least twice daily during the initial 24 hours of treatment and at least daily thereafter.
- Assess magnitude of azotemia and electrolyte and acid–basis status at least daily for the initial 3 days of treatment.
- Consider placing a central venous line to maintain central venous pressure <8 cm H_2O in more critical patients and neonates.

POSSIBLE COMPLICATIONS

- Severe hyperkalemia accompanied by cardiac arrhythmias, cardiac arrest, and death
- Pulmonary and peripheral edema; conjunctival edema may be dramatic.
- Disruption of the urinary tract in patients with initial obstruction.
- Urinary tract infection concurrent with obstructive disease.

MISCELLANEOUS

ASSOCIATED CONDITIONS

- Colic; enterocolitis
- Pleuritis; peritonitis; septicemia
- Exhausted horse syndrome—multiple organ failure

AGE-RELATED FACTORS

Neonates afflicted with hypoxic-ischemic multiple-organ damage or septicemia may be at increased risk of anuric/oliguric ARF.

ZOONOTIC POTENTIAL

Leptospirosis has infectious and zoonotic potential; avoid direct contact with infective urine.

PREGNANCY

N/A

SYNONYMS

N/A

SEE ALSO

- ARF
- CRF
- Urinary tract obstruction
- Uroperitoneum

ABBREVIATIONS

- ARF = acute renal failure
- CRF = chronic renal failure
- GFR = glomerular filtration rate
- PCV = packed cell volume

Suggested Reading

Bayly WM. Acute renal failure. In: Reed SM, Bayly WM, eds. Equine internal medicine. Philadelphia: WB Saunders, 1998:848–856.

Geor RJ. Acute renal failure. In: Robinson NE, ed. Current therapy in equine medicine 4. Philadelphia: WB Saunders, 1997:472–476.

Schott HC. Chronic renal failure. In: Reed SM, Bayly WM, eds. Equine internal medicine. Philadelphia: WB Saunders, 1998:856–875.

Schott HC. Obstructive disease of the urinary tract. In: Reed SM, Bayly WM, eds. Equine internal medicine. Philadelphia: WB Saunders, 1998:880–890.

Author Harold C. Schott II

Consulting Editor Harold C. Schott II

AORTIC REGURGITATION

BASICS

DEFINITION

• Occurs when the aortic valve becomes insufficient, allowing blood to leak backward into the left ventricular outflow tract during diastole and creating a holodiastolic decrescendo murmur with its PMI in the aortic valve area.
• The murmur radiates toward the left cardiac apex and the right side.

PATHOPHYSIOLOGY

• The aortic leaflets do not form a complete seal between the aorta and left ventricle.
• During diastole, blood regurgitates into the left ventricular outflow tract, causing a left ventricular volume overload. As this volume overload becomes more severe, stretching of the mitral annulus occurs, and mitral regurgitation often develops. Mitral regurgitation compounds the severe left ventricular volume overload, and these horses often rapidly develop congestive heart failure.
• Severe regurgitation results in decreased coronary artery blood flow and decreased myocardial perfusion.
• Ventricular arrhythmias may develop secondary to decreased myocardial perfusion.

SYSTEM AFFECTED

Cardiovascular

GENETICS

N/A

INCIDENCE/PREVALENCE

N/A

SIGNALMENT

Higher incidence of regurgitation in old horses—usually >10 years

SIGNS

General Comments

Usually an incidental finding during routine auscultation

Historical Findings

• Poor performance
• Possibly congestive heart failure

Physical Examination Findings

• Grade 1–6/6, decrescendo or musical holodiastolic murmur with PMI in the aortic valve area radiating to the left apex and right side
• Other, less common findings—bounding arterial pulses, atrial fibrillation, ventricular premature depolarizations, accentuated third heart sounds, and congestive heart failure

CAUSES

• Degenerative changes of the aortic leaflets
• Fenestration of aortic leaflets
• Nonvegetative valvulitis
• Flail aortic leaflet
• Bacterial endocarditis
• Ventricular septal defect
• Congenital malformation
• Disease of the aortic root

RISK FACTORS

Old age

DIAGNOSIS

DIFFERENTIAL DIAGNOSIS

Pulmonic regurgitation—rare; murmurs usually are soft or not detectable and should have PMI in the pulmonic valve area; bounding arterial pulses are not present; differentiate echocardiographically.

CBC/BIOCHEMISTRY/URINALYSIS

May have neutrophilic leukocytosis and hyperfibrinogenemia with bacterial endocarditis.

OTHER LABORATORY TESTS

• Elevated cardiac isoenzymes may be present (e.g., cardiac troponin I, CK-MB, HBDH, LDH 1 and 2) with concurrent myocardial disease.
• Positive blood culture may be obtained from horses with bacterial endocarditis.

IMAGING

Electrocardiography

• Ventricular premature depolarizations may be present in horses with severe regurgitation and be caused by poor myocardial perfusion.
• Atrial fibrillation often develops in horses with marked left ventricular volume overload and subsequent left atrial enlargement.

Echocardiography

• Most affected horses have thickened aortic valve leaflets.
• An echogenic band parallel to and a nodular thickening of the left coronary leaflet free edge are the most common findings.
• Prolapse of an aortic leaflet (usually the noncoronary or right coronary leaflet) into the left ventricular outflow tract frequently is detected.
• Fenestration of the aortic leaflet, flail aortic leaflet, bacterial endocarditis, or aortic root abnormalities infrequently are detected.
• Left ventricle—enlarged and dilated, with a rounded apex.
• Thinning of the left ventricular free wall and interventricular septum.
• Increased septal-to-E point separation may be present.
• Pattern of left ventricular volume overload.
• Normal or decreased fractional shortening in a horse with left ventricular enlargement is consistent with myocardial dysfunction.
• Dilatation of the aortic root in horses with long-standing regurgitation.
• High-frequency vibrations on the mitral valve septal leaflet usually are detected with M-mode echocardiography and are created by turbulence in the left ventricular outflow tract.
• In some horses, high-frequency vibrations may be visualized on the interventricular septum instead of, or in addition to, vibrations on the mitral valve septal leaflet.
• High-frequency vibrations on the aortic leaflets usually are visualized in horses with musical holodiastolic murmurs.
• Premature mitral valve closure may indicate more severe aortic insufficiency.

• Pulsed-wave or color-flow Doppler reveals a jet or jets of regurgitation in the left ventricular outflow tract. Size of the jet at its origin is a good indicator of severity. Size and extent of the regurgitation jet is another means of semiquantitating its severity, as is strength of the regurgitation signal.
• Continuous-wave Doppler assessment of the spectral tracing of the regurgitation jet also provides an estimate for the severity of regurgitation—a steep slope and a short pressure half-time indicate more severe regurgitation.

Thoracic Radiography

• Left-sided cardiac enlargement may be detected in horses with moderate to severe regurgitation.
• Pulmonary edema may be present in affected horses with congestive heart failure.

DIAGNOSTIC PROCEDURES

Cardiac Catheterization

• Right sided catheterization may reveal elevated pulmonary capillary wedge pressures and pulmonary arterial pressures in horses with severe regurgitation and concurrent mitral regurgitation.
• Right ventricular and atrial pressures may be elevated in affected horses with congestive heart failure.
• Oxygen saturation of blood obtained from the right atrium, right ventricle, and pulmonary artery should be normal.

Continuous 24-Hour Holter Monitoring

Useful in the diagnosis of horses with suspected ventricular premature depolarizations.

PATHOLOGIC FINDINGS

• Focal or diffuse thickening or distortion of one or more aortic leaflets may be present.
• Nodules, bands, plaques, and fenestrations have been described on the aortic leaflets at postmortem examination.
• Flail aortic leaflets, bacterial endocarditis, or congenital malformations of the aortic valve infrequently are detected.
• Aortic root dilatation usually is present in horses with severe, long-standing regurgitation.
• Jet lesions usually are detected on the ventricular side of the mitral valve septal leaflet and, less frequently, on the interventricular septum.
• Left ventricular enlargement and thinning of the left ventricular free wall and interventricular septum in horses with significant regurgitation.
• Atrial myocardial thinning with atrial dilatation has been documented in horses with atrial fibrillation and enlargement.
• Inflammatory cell infiltrate has been detected in horses with myocarditis and aortic regurgitation; however, most affected horses do not have significant underlying myocardial disease.

TREATMENT

APPROPRIATE HEALTH CARE

• Most affected horses require no treatment and can be monitored on an outpatient basis.
• Horses with moderate to severe regurgitation may benefit from long-term vasodilator therapy, particularly with ACE inhibitors.
• Treat horses with severe regurgitation and congestive heart failure for the congestive heart failure with positive inotropic drugs, vasodilators, and diuretics on an inpatient basis, if possible, and monitor response to therapy.

NURSING CARE

N/A

ACTIVITY

• Affected horses are safe to continue in full athletic work until the regurgitation becomes severe or ventricular arrhythmias develop.
• Monitor horses with moderate to severe regurgitation by ECG during high-intensity exercise to ensure they are safe to compete. These horses can be used for lower-level athletic competition until they begin to develop congestive heart failure.
• Horses with significant ventricular arrhythmias or pulmonary artery dilatation are no longer safe to ride.

DIET

N/A

CLIENT EDUCATION

• Regularly palpate the arterial pulses to monitor the progression of left ventricular volume overload. Bounding arterial pulses indicate significant left ventricular volume overload. Moderate to severe regurgitation usually is present in these horses.
• Regularly monitor cardiac rhythm; any irregularities other than second-degree AV block should prompt ECG.
• Carefully monitor for exercise intolerance, respiratory distress, prolonged recovery after exercise, increased resting respiratory rate or heart rate, or cough; if detected, seek a cardiac re-examination.

SURGICAL CONSIDERATIONS

N/A

AORTIC REGURGITATION

MEDICATIONS

DRUGS OF CHOICE

• Severe regurgitation—enalapril (0.25–0.5 mg/kg PO SID or BID) or another ACE inhibitor.
• ACE inhibitors prolong the time to valve replacement in humans with moderate to severe regurgitation.
• Horses with moderate to severe regurgitation have experienced a decrease in left ventricular chamber size with ACE inhibitors.
• Treatment of affected horses in heart failure include digoxin, furosemide, and vasodilators.

CONTRAINDICATIONS

Do not use ACE inhibitors in horses actively competing in types of athletic work for which drug testing occurs; these drugs must be withdrawn before competition to comply with the medication rules of the various governing bodies of equine sports.

PRECAUTIONS

ACE inhibitors can cause hypotension; thus, do not give a large dose without time to accommodate to this treatment.

POSSIBLE INTERACTIONS

N/A

ALTERNATIVE DRUGS

Most other vasodilatory drugs should have some beneficial effect in horses with moderate to severe regurgitation, but they may be less effective than the ACE inhibitors.

FOLLOW-UP

PATIENT MONITORING

• Frequently monitor arterial pulses and cardiac rhythm.
• Re-examine horses with mild to moderate regurgitation by ECG every year.
• Re-examine horses with severe regurgitation by echocardiography every 6 months to monitor progression of valvular insufficiency and determine if the horse continues to be safe to ride or drive.

PREVENTION/AVOIDANCE

N/A

POSSIBLE COMPLICATIONS

Chronic regurgitation—ventricular arrhythmias; atrial fibrillation; mitral regurgitation; congestive heart failure

EXPECTED COURSE AND PROGNOSIS

• Most affected horses have a normal performance life and life expectancy.
• Progression of regurgitation associated with degenerative valve disease usually is slow. With the typical onset of regurgitation that occurs in old horses, other problems are more likely to end of horse's performance career or shorten life expectancy.
• Affected horses with congestive heart failure usually have severe underlying valvular heart disease and myocardial disease and a guarded to grave prognosis for life. Most affected horses being treated for congestive heart failure respond to the supportive therapy and improve. This improvement usually is short lived, however, and and most are euthanized within 2–6 months of initiating treatment.

MISCELLANEOUS

ASSOCIATED CONDITIONS

N/A

AGE-RELATED FACTORS

Old horses are more likely to be affected.

AORTIC REGURGITATION

ZOONOTIC POTENTIAL

N/A

PREGNANCY

- Affected mares should not experience any problems with pregnancy unless the regurgitation is severe.
- Treat pregnant affected mares with congestive heart failure for the underlying cardiac disease with positive inotropic drugs and diuretics; ACE inhibitors are contraindicated because of potential adverse effects on the fetus.

SYNONYMS

Aortic insufficiency

SEE ALSO

- Bacterial endocarditis
- Congestive heart failure—left sided
- Diastolic murmurs
- Ventricular septal defect

ABBREVIATIONS

- ACE = angiotensin-converting enzyme
- AV = atrioventricular
- CK-MB = MB isoenzyme of creatine kinase
- HBDH = α-hydroxybutyrate dehydrogenase
- LDH = lactate dehydrogenase
- PMI = point of maximal intensity

Suggested Reading

Blissitt KJ, Bonagura JD. Colour flow Doppler echocardiography in horses with cardiac murmurs. Equine Vet J 1995;19(Suppl):82–85.

Else RW, Holmes JR. Cardiac pathology in the horse. I. Gross pathology. Equine Vet J 1972;4:1–8.

Marr CM. Equine echocardiography—sound advice at the heart of the matter. Br Vet J 1994;150:527–545.

Reef VB. Cardiovascular ultrasonography. In: Reef VB, ed. Equine diagnostic ultrasound. Philadelphia: WB Saunders, 1998:215–272.

Reef VB. Heart murmurs in horses: determining their significance with echocardiography. Equine Vet J 1995;19(Suppl):71–80.

Reef VB, Spencer P. Echocardiographic evaluation of equine aortic insufficiency. Am J Vet Res 1987;48:904–909.

Author Virginia B. Reef
Consulting Editor N/A

AORTIC ROOT RUPTURE

BASICS

DEFINITION
A defect in the wall of the aorta at the aortic root, usually associated with the right sinus of Valsalva.

PATHOPHYSIOLOGY
- Aortic rupture results in the exsanguination into the thoracic cavity, cardiac tamponade from an acute hemopericardium, or creation of a shunt between the aorta and heart.
- With an aortic rupture confined to the right sinus of Valsalva, an aorticocardiac fistula is created. Blood from the aorta shunts into the right side of the heart, either at the atrial or ventricular level, depending on the site of the rupture.
- Subendocardial dissection of blood into the interventricular septum is common, with subsequent rupture into the right or left ventricle (more commonly, the rupture is into the right ventricle).
- Often associated with a unifocal ventricular tachycardia that probably develops shortly after the rupture occurs and that may be associated with dissection of blood in the interventricular septum.

SYSTEM AFFECTED
Cardiovascular

GENETICS
N/A

INCIDENCE/PREVALENCE
More frequently occurs in old horses, particularly males.

SIGNALMENT
Often occurs after breeding or other exercise.

SIGNS

General Comments
Often interpreted by owners as colic, because the horse appears distressed, may be looking at its flanks, and acting uncomfortable.

Historical Findings
- Acute onset of colic or distress
- Usually after exercise—racing; breeding
- Other, less common findings—exercise intolerance; syncope

Physical Examination Findings
- Tachycardia—rapid and regular heart rhythm
- Tachypnea
- Continuous machinery murmur—usually loudest on the right side
- Bounding arterial pulses
- Other, less common findings— jugular pulses and distention, ventricular tachycardia (unifocal), and congestive heart failure

CAUSES
- A congenital aneurysm in the wall of the aortic root, usually in the right sinus of Valsalva, predisposes to aortic root rupture.
- Necrosis and degeneration of the aortic media have been associated, especially in old breeding stallions.
- Aberrant parasite migration in the ascending aorta must be considered but is unlikely.

RISK FACTORS
- Aortic aneurysm
- Aortitis

DIAGNOSIS

DIFFERENTIAL DIAGNOSIS

Ventricular Septal Defect with Aortic Regurgitation
- Murmurs are systolic (band shaped and pansystolic) and diastolic (holodiastolic and decrescendo), not continuous.
- Arterial pulses usually are not bounding, unless the associated aortic regurgitation is severe.
- No history of acute colic or distress.
- No unifocal ventricular tachycardia.
- Differentiate echocardiographically.

Patent Ductus Arteriosus
- No history of acute colic or distress.
- No unifocal ventricular tachycardia.
- Differentiate echocardiographically.

CBC/BIOCHEMISTRY/URINALYSIS
Elevated creatinine and BUN may occur because of impaired renal perfusion, which is associated with sustained ventricular tachycardia and any blood loss present.

OTHER LABORATORY TESTS
Cardiac troponin I and cardiac isoenzymes of creatine phosphokinase and lactate dehydrogenase may be elevated with significant myocardial cell injury, either from subendocardial dissection of blood or associated with hypoperfusion caused by sustained ventricular tachycardia.

IMAGING

ECG
Uniform ventricular tachycardia with a heart rate of >100 bpm usually is present acutely after aortic rupture associated with subendocardial dissection of blood into the interventricular septum.

Echocardiography
- A defect is visualized in the aortic root, usually in the right sinus of Valsalva.
- The rupture may be a small, irregular defect in the aortic wall (usually associated with the right aortic leaflet) or be visualized flailing in the right atrium or ventricle.
- Anechoic to echoic fluid may be detected dissecting subendocardially into the interventricular septum, most frequently along the right ventricular side; however, dissection of blood subendocardially along the left side also occurs.
- Significant right atrial or ventricular enlargement if the aorta has ruptured into one of these chambers.

AORTIC ROOT RUPTURE

- Paradoxic septal motion in horses with severe right ventricular volume overload.
- Ruptured tricuspid chordae tendineae or ruptured or flail tricuspid valve leaflet may be detected, particularly with rupture of an aneurysm of the sinus of Valsalva.
- Subendocardial dissection of blood along the left side of the interventricular septum may result in rupture into the left ventricle and left ventricular volume overload.
- Hyperdynamic interventricular septum and left ventricular free wall are associated with left ventricular volume overload, producing increased fractional shortening, until the myocardium starts to fail.
- Rupture of a mitral valve chorda tendineae and a flail mitral valve leaflet may occur, producing acute onset of severe mitral regurgitation.
- Significant left ventricular volume overload can lead to dilatation of the mitral annulus and mitral regurgitation.
- Two-dimensional echocardiography is diagnostic for a defect in the aortic root at the sinus of Valsalva or for a sinus of Valsalva aneurysm.
- Use color-flow Doppler, pulsed-wave Doppler, or contrast echocardiography to localize the shunt associated with the aortic cardiac fistula.
- Continuous-wave Doppler can be used to determine peak velocity of the shunt flow.

Thoracic Radiography

- An enlarged cardiac silhouette should be present in horses with a large aorticocardiac shunt.
- Pulmonary overcirculation and edema may be detected.

DIAGNOSTIC PROCEDURES

Cardiac Catheterization

- Elevated right ventricular pressure, pulmonary arterial pressure, pulmonary capillary wedge pressure, and oxygen saturation of the blood are detected in horses with aorticocardiac fistula into the right ventricle.
- With a shunt into the right atrium, right atrial pressures and oxygen saturation also are elevated.

Arterial Blood Pressure

Demonstrates the wide difference between peak systolic pressure and end-diastolic pressure associated with continuous shunting of blood from the aorta into the heart.

PATHOLOGIC FINDINGS

- Postmortem examination confirms the site and extent of the rupture and the presence of aorticocardiac fistula.
- Path of the dissection can be traced and the rupture into the right atrium, tricuspid valve, right ventricle, or left ventricle confirmed.
- Dissecting tracts into the interventricular septum usually are lined with immature and mature fibrous tissue, and disruption of the conduction system has been detected.
- Degeneration and necrosis of the aortic media have been reported in some horses with aortic root rupture but not in other affected horses.
- An absence of media in the right sinus of Valsalva was reported in one horse with a sinus of Valsalva (i.e., aortic root) aneurysm.
- Fibrosis and scarring of the rupture site have been reported in old breeding stallions that died of unrelated causes.
- Biatrial and biventricular enlargement usually is detected, and hepatic congestion and pulmonary edema may be present.

TREATMENT

APPROPRIATE HEALTH CARE

- Closely monitor affected horses with ventricular tachycardia if the tachycardia is uniform, the heart rate is <120 bpm, no R-on-T complexes are detected, and no clinical signs of cardiovascular collapse are observed.
- If ventricular tachycardia is multiform, R-on-T complexes are detected, heart rate is >120 bpm, or with clinical signs of cardiovascular collapse, institute antiarrhythmic treatment on an inpatient basis.
- If congestive heart failure also is present, institute treatment for congestive heart failure as well. Consider humane destruction, however, because the horse is no longer safe to use for athletic work.

NURSING CARE

- Perform continuous ECG monitoring during the attempted conversion from ventricular tachycardia to sinus rhythm.
- Keep horses quiet and unmoving during antiarrhythmic treatment.

ACTIVITY

- Stall confinement until conversion to sinus rhythm has been successfully achieved.
- Restrict athletic activity as much as possible once ventricular tachycardia has been converted, because exercise is associated with increased systemic blood pressure.

DIET

N/A

AORTIC ROOT RUPTURE

CLIENT EDUCATION

• Affected horses are not safe to ride or use for any type of athletic work because of the risk of sudden death associated with further aortic rupture or development of fatal ventricular arrhythmia.
• If the horse is a breeding stallion and such continued use is desired, warn the stallion and mare handlers (and all other personnel involved) about the risk of sudden death.
• Develop an emergency plan in the event the stallion becomes unsteady or unsafe to handle.

SURGICAL CONSIDERATIONS

N/A

MEDICATIONS

DRUGS OF CHOICE

Antiarrhythmics

• Indicated with multiform ventricular tachycardia, R-on-T complexes, heart rate > 120 bpm, or clinical signs of cardiovascular collapse.
• Drug selection depends on severity of ventricular tachycardia and associated clinical signs.
• IV lidocaine is rapidly acting and has a very short duration of action. However, it also had CNS in horses and, thus, must be used carefully.
• IV procainamide and quinidine gluconate have been effective in converting sustained, uniform ventricular tachycardia but have a slower onset of action.
• IV magnesium sulfate has been successful in converting sustained ventricular tachycardia and is not arrhythmogenic.

ACE Inhibitors

• May be indicated in stallions to decrease resistance to forward flow once ventricular tachycardia has been converted.
• Enalapril (0.5 mg/kg PO BID) has no effect on the stallion's libido, breeding performance, or fertility.
• Other vasodilators or antihypertensive drugs can be considered, but their effect on breeding stallions is unknown.

CONTRAINDICATIONS

Other vasodilators or antihypertensive drugs have the potential to adversely affect the stallion's libido, breeding performance, or fertility.

PRECAUTIONS

Affected horses could experience sudden death at any time; thus, everyone working around these horses must be aware of the safety issues involved.

POSSIBLE INTERACTIONS

Any antiarrhythmic drug has the potential to cause development of a more adverse arrhythmia as well as to convert to sinus rhythm.

ALTERNATIVE DRUGS

Propranolol

• The IV form is less likely to be effective but should be considered in affected horses with refractory ventricular tachycardia.
• Lowers systolic blood pressure.

Propafenone

• Very effective in converting refractory ventricular tachycardia.
• The IV form is not available in the U.S. (but is available abroad); only an oral form is available in this country.
• May have a synergistic effect with procainamide in horses with refractory ventricular tachycardia.

FOLLOW-UP

PATIENT MONITORING

• Routine monitoring of heart rate and of respiratory rate and rhythm after conversion to sinus rhythm.
• Persistent tachypnea, tachycardia, or new arrhythmias indicate deterioration in clinical status.
• Return of venous distention and jugular pulsations or development of ventral edema or coughing indicate the onset of congestive heart failure and worsening of ventricular volume overload.

PREVENTION/AVOIDANCE

• With congenital aneurysms of the sinus of Valsalva, control of systemic blood pressure may prolong the time until rupture occurs.
• With degenerative changes in the aortic media, antihypertensive drugs theoretically should have some benefit. However, identification of horses at risk has not yet been accomplished.
• Routine echocardiography of old breeding stallions and high-performance horses potentially at risk may help to identify these horses before development of a tear in the aortic root.

POSSIBLE COMPLICATIONS

• Deterioration of uniform ventricular tachycardia into fatal ventricular arrhythmia
• Severe, acute congestive heart failure from massive right atrial or ventricular, left atrial, and left ventricular volume overload
• Tricuspid valve rupture, leading to massive tricuspid regurgitation and congestive heart failure
• Rupture of a chordae tendineae of the tricuspid or mitral valve, leading to massive tricuspid or mitral regurgitation, respectively, and acute, right- or left-sided congestive heart failure
• Sudden death

AORTIC ROOT RUPTURE

EXPECTED COURSE AND PROGNOSIS

- If the rupture is extracardiac, the horse will experience sudden death, usually from exsanguination.
- If the rupture is into the pericardial sac, acute cardiac tamponade will occur secondary to the hemopericardium.
- If the rupture is intracardiac, an aorticocardiac fistula will be created. A direct communication between the aorta and either the right atrium or ventricle will be created, or blood from the aorta will dissect subendocardially down the interventricular septum and may rupture into the right or left ventricle. Most horses appear painful and experience a period of rapid, unifocal ventricular tachycardia. The pain (i.e., colic) or distress probably is associated with the rupture and acute subendocardial dissection. The unifocal ventricular tachycardia probably is associated with the dissection of blood into the interventricular septum.
- Prognosis for life in affected horses is grave, with sudden death expected in those with extracardiac or intrapericardial rupture.
- Onset of congestive heart failure is likely after development of an intracardiac fistula, and the speed of its development depends on the location and size of the shunt.

MISCELLANEOUS

ASSOCIATED CONDITIONS

Aortic root aneurysm

AGE-RELATED FACTORS

Old horses are more likely to be affected, but horses as young as 4 years have been diagnosed.

ZOONOTIC POTENTIAL

N/A

PREGNANCY

- Rupture of a sinus of Valsalva aneurysm has been seen in one late-gestation pregnant mare. The volume expansion of late pregnancy may predispose pregnant mares to aortic rupture at this time.
- Aortic root rupture has been seen in one mare during early pregnancy. This mare experienced acute onset of ventricular tachycardia and subendocardial dissection of blood into the interventricular septum, but survived to have the foal.

SYNONYMS

- Aortic cardiac fistula
- Aorticocardiac fistula

SEE ALSO

- Congestive heart failure—left sided
- Congestive heart failure—right sided
- Ventricular tachycardia

ABBREVIATIONS

ACE = angiotensin-converting enzyme

Suggested Reading

Lester GD, Lombard CW, Ackerman N. Echocardiographic detection of a dissecting aortic root aneurysm in a Thoroughbred stallion. Vet Radiol Ultrasound 1992;33:202–205.

Marr CM, Reef VB, Brazil T, Thomas W, Maxson AD, Reimer JM. Clinical and echocardiographic findings in horses with aortic root rupture. Vet Radiol Ultrasound 1998;39:22–31.

Reef VB, Klump S, Maxson AD, et al. Echocardiographic detection of an intact aneurysm in a horse. J Am Vet Med Assoc 1990;197:752–755.

Roby KA, Reef VB, Shaw DP, Sweeney CR. Rupture of an aortic sinus aneurysm in a 15-year-old broodmare. J Am Vet Med Assoc 1986;189:305–308.

Rooney JR, Prickett ME, Crowe MW. Aortic ring rupture in stallions. Pathol Vet 1967;4:268–274.

Van der Linde-Sipman JS, Kroneman J, Meulenaar H, Vos JH. Necrosis and rupture of the aorta and pulmonary trunk in four horses. Vet Pathol 1985;22:51–53.

Author Virginia B. Reef

Consulting Editor N/A

ARSENIC TOXICOSIS

BASICS

OVERVIEW

- Results from excessive exposure to arsenic-containing pesticides, arsenic-contaminated soils, burn piles, and water or feed.
- Ashes from CCA-treated lumber are high in arsenic.
- Toxicity depends on the form of arsenic ingested.
- Trivalent inorganic forms (e.g., arsenic trioxide; sodium, potassium and calcium salts of arsenite) are 10-fold more toxic than inorganic pentavalent forms (e.g., sodium, potassium, and calcium salts of arsenate).
- Toxicity of organic pentavalent forms used as growth promoter in swine (e.g., arsanilic acid, roxarsone) has not been determined for horses.
- Trivalent inorganic arsenicals inhibit cellular respiration and damage capillaries.
- Pentavalent inorganic arsenicals uncouple oxidative phosphorylation, leading to deficits in cell energy.

SIGNALMENT

No breed or sex predilections

SIGNS

- Peracute or acute syndromes are most likely.
- Peracute—patient often found dead; death caused by cardiovascular collapse
- Acute—intense abdominal pain, hypersalivation, severe watery diarrhea, decreased abdominal sounds, muscle tremors, weak and rapid pulse with signs of circulatory shock, ataxia, depression, and recumbency; if the animal survives for several days, oliguria and proteinuria secondary to renal damage
- Chronic—not described in horses

CAUSES AND RISK FACTORS

Ingestion of arsenic-containing products or arsenic-contaminated soils, water, or feed

DIAGNOSIS

DIFFERENTIAL DIAGNOSIS

- Lead toxicosis—evidence of neurologic dysfunction is likely
- Mercury toxicosis
- NSAID toxicosis—history of previous use
- Cantharidin toxicosis—evidence of cystitis
- Salmonellosis
- Colitis X
- Acute cyathastomiasis
- Clostridial colitis

CBC/BIOCHEMISTRY/URINALYSIS

- Reflect circulatory shock and possible liver and kidney damage
- Hemoconcentration—elevated PCV and plasma total protein
- Leukopenia with degenerative changes in PMNs
- Azotemia
- Electrolytes—hypokalemia; hyponatremia; hypochloremia
- Hyperglycemia
- Hyperbilirubinemia
- Elevated LDH and CK

OTHER LABORATORY TESTS

- Antemortem—measurement of arsenic in urine or GI contents
- Postmortem—measurement of arsenic in liver or kidney
- Chronic exposures—arsenic can be measured in hair
- Arsenic is rapidly excreted after exposure ceases.

IMAGING

N/A

DIAGNOSTIC PROCEDURES

N/A

PATHOLOGIC FINDINGS

Gross Findings

- GI hemorrhage, mucosal congestion, edema, and erosion, either localized or throughout the GI tract, which may be filled with watery, dark-green, black, or hemorrhagic ingesta, with necrotic material from mucosal sloughing.
- Pulmonary edema and epicardial and serosal hemorrhage.

Histopathologic Findings

Necrotizing, hemorrhagic typhlocolitis, with necrotizing vasculitis, renal tubular necrosis, and hepatic fatty degeneration

TREATMENT

- Emergency treatment is necessary.
- Remove animal from known or potential source of exposure.
- GI decontamination.
- Treat circulatory shock and acidosis.
- Control abdominal pain.
- Hasten elimination of absorbed arsenic with chelators.
- Appropriate fluid therapy.

ARSENIC TOXICOSIS

MEDICATIONS

DRUGS

- Dimercaprol (British anti-lewisite) is the classic arsenic chelator (loading dose of 4–5 mg/kg given by deep muscular injection, followed by 2–3 mg/kg q4h for 24 hours and then 1 mg/kg q4h for 2 days); adverse reactions include tremors, convulsions. and coma.
- DMSA is a less toxic chelator (equine dose not established, but 10 mg/kg PO q8h is suggested).
- Flunixin meglumine (1.1 mg/kg IV q12–24h) or butorphanol tartrate (0.1 mg/kg IV q3–4h up to 48 hours)
- Xylazine hydrochloride (1.1 mg/kg IV) may be used in conjunction with butorphanol (0.01–0.02 mg/kg IV).
- Demulcents—mineral oil or kaolin-pectin

CONTRAINDICATIONS/POSSIBLE INTERACTIONS

Use NSAIDs cautiously because of possible adverse GI and renal effects.

FOLLOW-UP

- Monitor renal and hepatic function.
- Provide a bland diet, containing reduced amounts of high-quality protein.
- Identify source of exposure, and properly dispose of source.
- Expected course and prognosis depend on the severity of clinical signs.
- If the animal survives, recovery should be complete.

MISCELLANEOUS

ASSOCIATED CONDITIONS

N/A

AGE-RELATED FACTORS

N/A

ZOONOTIC POTENTIAL

N/A

PREGNANCY

N/A

SEE ALSO

N/A

ABBREVIATIONS

- CCA = chromated copper arsenate
- CK = creatine kinase
- DMSA = 2,3-dimercaptosuccinic acid, succimer
- GI = gastrointestinal
- LDH = lactate dehydrogenase
- PCV = packed cell volume
- PMN = polymorphonucleocytes

Suggested Reading

Pace LW, Turnquist SE, Casteel SW, Johnson PJ, Frankeny RL. Acute arsenic toxicosis in five horses. Vet Pathol 1997;34:160–164.

Author Robert H. Poppenga
Consulting Editor Robert H. Poppenga

ARTIFICIAL INSEMINATION (AI)

BASICS

DEFINITION

Extended fresh, cooled, or frozen semen containing a minimum of 500–1000 × 10^6 progressively motile sperm is introduced into the mare's uterus using aseptic technique.

PATHOPHYSIOLOGY

Advantages of AI compared with natural breeding are many:

- Artificial breeding programs allow more efficient use of stallion semen.
- Ejaculate can be divided into several insemination doses, thereby increasing the number of mares that may be impregnated during a breeding season as well as the stallion's book of mares (i.e., those contracted to be bred to the stallion within a breeding season, e.g., 120 by AI vs. 40–80 by live cover).
- Allows wider use of genetically superior stallions.
- Eliminates the cost and risk of transporting mares with foals at side.
- Prevents genital infections by the addition of antibiotics to semen extenders.
- Decreases breeding injuries to mares and stallions.
- Allows continued use of stallions with musculoskeletal and behavioral problems.
- Protects mares with genital tract impairments or recent surgical repair from further breeding related trauma—rectovaginal fistulas, impaired cervical relaxation, and so on.
- Allows evaluation of semen quality before insemination.

SYSTEM AFFECTED

Reproductive

SIGNALMENT

- Thoroughbred, Standard Jack and Jennet, allow only natural breeding—live cover.
- All other breed registries allow AI but may impose separate, specific restrictions on semen storage and transport.

SIGNS

Historical Findings

Knowledge of the mare's previous estrous cycles helps to predict days in heat and time of ovulation.

Physical Examination Findings

- Timing of ovulation is critical and can be predicted by the mare's history, her response to teasing, and results from transrectal palpation/ultrasonography of the genital tract.
- During estrus, transrectal palpation reveals the presence of a large ovarian follicle (35+ mm), an edematous uterus, and a relaxing cervix.
- Increasing uterine estrual edema caused by circulating estradiol is evident during ultrasonography.
- Estrual edema usually begins to decrease 24–48 hours before ovulation.

DIAGNOSIS

PROCEDURAL ISSUES

Timing and Frequency of Breeding

- Dependent on semen longevity, which is affected by stallion idiosyncrasy and method of semen preservation—fresh, cooled, or frozen.
- Affected by estimates of how close the mare is to ovulation.
- Influenced by the short viability of equine ova—only 6–10 hours after ovulation.

Teasing and Examinations

- During estrus, mares are teased daily. On the second day of heat, begin daily or every-other-day transrectal palpations and perform ultrasonography as needed to determine the optimal time to breed.
- When the preovulatory follicle reaches 35 mm, GnRH analog (Ovuplant) or hCG (2500–3000 IU IV) may be administered to induce ovulation within 36–48 hours.
- Inseminate as close to ovulation as possible.
- In a problem mare, evaluate by ultrasonography 4–6 hours after AI for the presence of postbreeding intrauterine fluid and for ovulation.
- In a fertile mare, evaluate at the next regular farm visit (24–48 hours after breeding) for ovulation.

Fresh Extended Semen

- Mares are routinely bred every other day beginning on day 2 or 3 of estrus until they tease out, or only when a large preovulatory follicle is detected by transrectal palpation and ultrasonography.
- Insemination with fresh semen within 48 hours before ovulation is recommended to achieve acceptable pregnancy rates.

Cooled Transported Semen

- Mare management must be more intense, because the fertility of cooled semen from some stallions is reduced after 24 hours.
- Semen is ordered and inseminated no more than 24–36 hours before ovulation to achieve acceptable conception rates.
- When the preovulatory follicle is 30–35 mm, order semen (overnight shipment) and administer GnRH analogue (Ovuplant) or hCG.
- Semen from stallions with poor post-cooling fertility should be sent "counter to counter" (i.e. airline transport), and Ovuplant or hCG should be administered 24–36 hours before the expected semen arrival to assure that ovulation occurs very close to the time of insemination.

ARTIFICIAL INSEMINATION (AI)

Frozen Thawed Semen
• Insemination must be precisely timed, because after thawing, sperm longevity usually is reduced to ≤12–24 hours.
• Mare management consists of serial, daily teasing as well as transrectal palpation and ultrasonography.
• Administer Ovuplant or hCG when the dominant follicle reaches 30–35 mm.
• Transrectal palpation and scanning TID to QID ensures that insemination occurs as close before ovulation as possible and, most importantly, no more than 6–8 hours after ovulation.

General Comments
• Schedule re-examination of a mare to confirm ovulation in relationship to the time of breeding, or 6–8, 24, or 48 hours after insemination with frozen, cooled, or fresh semen, respectively.
• If ovulation has not occurred within these recommended time windows, re-inseminate the mare.

DIFFERENTIAL DIAGNOSIS
N/A

CBC/BIOCHEMISTRY/URINALYSIS
N/A

OTHER LABORATORY TESTS
Progesterone level of >1ng/mL confirms ovulation.

IMAGING
Ultrasonography:
• Used to assess follicular size and growth during estrus.
• A pre-ovulatory follicle may become softer and adopt a "pear" shape 6–12 hours before ovulation.
• Estrual edema of the uterine walls is described as having a cartwheel appearance.
• CH and/or CL is evidence of ovulation.
• Used to check for intrauterine fluid 4–6 hours after insemination and for pregnancy 15–16 days after ovulation.

DIAGNOSTIC PROCEDURES
Analysis of Semen
• Volume, motility, concentration, and morphology.
• A small sample of cooled or frozen semen should be saved and warmed (at 37°C or in the operator's pocket for 5–15 min) to evaluate immediately after insemination.
• Essential that the slide, coverslip, and pipette used to prepare the slide all be prewarmed, because stallion semen is very susceptible to cold shock.
• The total number of sperm should be at least 500–1000 × 10^6 progressively motile sperm (concentration [in millions of sperm per mL] × volume of the insemination × % progressively motile sperm × % normal morphology).

Disease Status of Stallion
Status should be known—negative for EVA, CEM, and so on.

Prebreeding Uterine Culture and Cytology of Mare
• Often performed to avoid transmitting infections to the stallion.
• For early identification of possible mare problems.
• To maximize the likelihood of conception at the first cycle.
• Especially helpful in managing problem mares or when breeding live cover, although some shipped semen operations may require these tests.

TREATMENT

INSEMINATION TECHNIQUE
• Equipment should be sterile and disposable. Mares are restrained, and the perineal area is thoroughly cleansed with a mild detergent, antiseptic solution, or soap and then rinsed completely to leave no residue (minimum of three times).
• The operator places a sterile sleeve on his or her arm. Nonspermicidal lubricant is applied to the dorsum of the hand.
• A 50–56-cm (20–22-inch) insemination pipette is carried in the gloved hand; index finger is first passed through the length of the cervix, acting as a guide alongside which the pipet can readily be advanced to a point no further than 2.5 cm into the uterine body.
• A syringe with a nonspermicidal plastic plunger (Air-tite) containing the calculated insemination dose of extended semen is attached to the pipette, and the semen is slowly deposited into the uterus. The remainder of the semen in the pipette then is passed using a small bolus of air (1 cc).
• Alternatively, if the pipette is attached during filling of the syringe, a bolus of air will be in the syringe equivalent to the length of the pipette. As the syringe is evacuated, the bolus is the last portion evacuated from the syringe and delivers all the insemination dose, removing the need to detach the syringe at all during insemination.

FRESH EXTENDED SEMEN
• Perform AI immediately after collection.
• If mares are resident on the farm with the stallion, semen collected can be mixed with an appropriate extender for immediate insemination at a semen:extender ratio of 1:1.

ARTIFICIAL INSEMINATION (AI)

COOLED TRANSPORTED SEMEN

- Semen is collected, diluted in semen extender, and cooled to 5–6 °C for 24–48 hours without losing its fertilizing capacity.
- A semen:extender ratio of 1:2 to 1:4 is acceptable, but semen longevity is maximized by extending the ejaculate to a final concentration of 25–50 × 10^6 sperm/mL.

FROZEN THAWED SEMEN

- Frozen semen is packed in 0.5- or 5-mL straws and stored in liquid nitrogen.
- A 5-mL straw contains from 600–1000 × 10^6 sperm cells; therefore, depending on postfreeze viability of the spermatozoa, only one straw may be needed.
- Thawing protocols vary and are specifically designed to be coupled with a particular freezing method. That is, no one acceptable universal standard (i.e., time and temperature) exists for thawing frozen semen.
- If specific details are not provided with frozen semen received, learn the details before the day of insemination to ensure proper handling.
- After thawing and using excellent technique, semen should be in the mare within 5 minutes.
- Postinsemination uterine treatment is strongly recommended.The high concentration of sperm cells in a straw and absence of seminal plasma, which has a natural protective effect in the uterus,in thawed semen may induce an acute, postmating endometritis.

POSTBREEDING

- Management involves ultrasonography 4–6 hours after AI to determine if intrauterine fluid, indicating inflammation, is accumulating.
- If so, treatment consists of uterine lavages with sterile saline or lactated Ringer's solution, followed by oxytocin beginning 4 hours after AI and repeated every 12–24 hours until the endometritis resolves.

MEDICATIONS

DRUGS OF CHOICE

- Induction of ovulation—ovulation may be induced when a follicle is ≥35 mm.
- Within 36–44 hours with hCG (2500–3000 IU IV).
- Within 40–42 hours with GnRH analogue (Ovuplant SC implants).
- Ecbolic drugs may be used to treat PMIE—see *Endometritis.*

CONTRAINDICATIONS

See *Endometritis.*

PRECAUTIONS

See *Endometritis.*

POSSIBLE INTERACTIONS

N/A

ALTERNATIVE DRUGS

N/A

FOLLOW-UP

PATIENT MONITORING

- Check for intrauterine fluid, the mare's response to insemination, 4–6 hours after breeding.
- Begin teasing within 11 days after ovulation for early detection of endometritis, which is indicated by a shortened cycle resulting from endogenous prostaglandin release.
- Perform ultrasonography for pregnancy 15 days after ovulation, including a check for one or more vesicles—twins.
- Perform follow-up transrectal palpation and ultrasonography between 24–30 days to confirm heartbeat in the embryo.
- Serial evaluation of pregnancy by transrectal palpation at 45, 60, 90, and 120 days

POSSIBLE COMPLICATIONS

- Semen collection—AV handling and maintenance.
- Evaluation of semen at the point of collection and adequacy of AI dose shipped or supplied frozen in straws.
- Packing method—Equitainer, one of reusable box cooling containers, or liquid nitrogen tank.
- Shipping—the entire breeding program with cooled semen is at the mercy of airlines/couriers.
- Operator skills to manipulate and place semen through the cervix, within the uterine lumen, in a proper and timely manner.
- Misidentification of stallions/mares.
- Transmission of EVA or CEM in shipped or frozen semen.
- Postbreeding inflammation; DUC.

MISCELLANEOUS

ASSOCIATED CONDITIONS

N/A

AGE-RELATED FACTORS

N/A

ZOONOTIC POTENTIAL

N/A

ARTIFICIAL INSEMINATION (AI)

PREGNANCY

Cooled Semen

Pregnancy rates per cycle are equivalent to on-farm insemination with fresh semen (60%–75%) if the semen quality remains good after a cooling period of 24 hours at 5–6°C.

Frozen Semen

- Pregnancy rates are reduced for most stallions.
- Spermatozoa suffer many stresses, and an attrition rate of ≅50% is associated with freezing and thawing.
- First-cycle pregnancy rates average 30%–40% (range, 0%–70%).
- Selection of candidates for breeding with frozen semen is important, with young. maiden mares being the best and old, barren mares the worst.

SYNONYM

Artificial breeding

SEE ALSO

- Conception failure
- DUC
- Early embryonic death
- Endometritis
- Semen evaluation—abnormal
- Semen evaluation—normal
- Venereal diseases

ABBREVIATIONS

- AV = artificial vagina
- CEM = contagious equine metritis
- CH = corpus hemorrhagicum
- CL = corpus luteum
- DUC = delayed uterine clearance
- EVA = equine viral arteritis
- GnRH = gonadotrophin-releasing hormone
- hCG = human chorionic gonadotropin
- PMIE = persistent mating-induced endometritis

Suggested Reading

Blanchard TL, Varner D, Schumacher J. Semen collection and artificial insemination. In: Manual of equine reproduction. St. Louis: Mosby–Year Book, 1998:111–125.

Brinsko SP, Varner DD. Artificial insemination. In:. McKinnon AO, Voss JL, eds. Equine reproduction. Philadelphia: Lea & Febiger, 1993:790–797.

Author Maria E. Cadario

Consulting Editor Carla L. Carleton

ARYTENOID CHONDRITIS

BASICS

DEFINITION

• A septic inflammatory process of one or both arytenoid cartilages, resulting in deformation with enlargement.
• This decreases the ability of the affected arytenoid cartilage to fully abduct during forced inspiration or to resist collapsing airway pressure during inspiration.
• The physical size of the cartilage also may contribute to airway obstruction during both inspiration and expiration.

PATHOPHYSIOLOGY

• The disease has been reproduced by creating a mucosal defect over the arytenoid cartilage, which allowed bacterial invasion of the perichondrium.
• The disease process results in fibrous tissue invasion and loss of normal cartilage framework as the infected arytenoid cartilage becomes deformed and unevenly enlarged.
• In advanced cases, granulomatous tissue may protrude into the laryngeal lumen.
• The size of the arytenoid cartilage and, perhaps, the pain associated with the disease process lead to loss of abductory function and, in turn, to an inspiratory obstruction.
• If the arytenoid cartilage becomes sufficiently enlarged, however, it also obstructs airflow during expiration.
• Airway obstruction also can result from decreased ability of the affected arytenoid cartilage to resist the subatmospheric pressure in the upper airway during exercise.
• Airflow limitation decreases ventilation, resulting in hypoxemia, hypercarbia, and diminished athletic performance.
• Horses respond to respiratory obstruction with one or more modifications to their natural breathing strategies during exercise to restore minute volume—more negative inspiratory pressure (with inspiratory obstruction), more positive expiratory pressure (with expiratory obstruction), increased inspiratory and expiratory time, and increased tidal volume by decreased respiratory frequency.

SYSTEM AFFECTED

Respiratory—upper respiratory tract

GENETICS

Unknown

INCIDENCE/PREVALENCE

Worldwide

SIGNALMENT

• Male and Thoroughbred racehorses are more commonly affected.
• Incidence increases with age.

SIGNS

• Upper respiratory noise, exercise intolerance, or both.
• The disease usually worsens gradually, with progressive involvement of one or both arytenoid cartilages.
• The condition leads to ventilation interference proportional to the loss of abductory function and the mechanical size of the affected arytenoid cartilages. The longer the high-intensity exercise occurs, the more severe the hypoventilation, so the horse does not "finish" or close well.
• In show horses, loss of points during competition because of upper respiratory noise is the main concern; this upper airway noise resembles that of horses with laryngeal hemiplegia.

CAUSES

• Physical trauma to the mucosa of the arytenoid cartilage caused by air turbulence or aspiration of track surface particles during exercise or severe coughing or intubation (e.g., endotracheal, nasogastric) procedures.
• Upper airway infection leading to cartilage sepsis.
• An association has been reported with lymphocyte antigens, suggesting that septic inflammation of the cartilage may result from lowered immunity in affected horses.
• In many cases, the inciting cause is never found.

RISK FACTORS

Procedures causing trauma to the arytenoid cartilage

DIAGNOSIS

DIFFERENTIAL DIAGNOSIS

• Laryngeal hemiplegia
• Congenital malformation of the laryngeal cartilages

CBC/BIOCHEMISTRY/URINALYSIS

Of no value

OTHER LABORATORY TESTS

• Arterial blood gases during exercise.
• Hypoventilation can be evaluated using arterial blood gases—typically at maximal exercise $PaCO_2$ can be >55 torr; PaO_2 may be <65 torr in affected horses.

IMAGING

Lateral radiography of the larynx may reveal enlarged laryngeal cartilages, sometimes with associated osseous metaplasia.

OTHER DIAGNOSTIC PROCEDURES

• The diagnosis is established on the basis of videoendoscopic examination at rest.
• The body of the arytenoid is irregular and thickened.
• A mass of granulation tissue may protrude from the axial surface of the arytenoid cartilage into the airway.
• The corniculate process may be deformed.
• Contact (i.e., "kissing") lesions may be observed on the contralateral arytenoid cartilage.
• With unilateral disease, asymmetry of the arytenoid cartilage is observed.
• Eventually, the condition leads to decreased or total inability of the affected arytenoid cartilage to abduct during inspiration.

PATHOLOGICAL FINDINGS

Gross Findings

Gross enlargement of the body and corniculate process of the arytenoid cartilage, with irregularity and focal elevation of granulation tissue on the axial surface of these structures.

Histopathologic Findings

• Consistent with those of a chronic recurrent inflammatory process.
• Involved cartilage is markedly thickened and laminated with fibrous connective tissue.
• Granulating sinus tracts sometimes are observed.

TREATMENT

APPROPRIATE HEALTH CARE

Medical treatment is indicated only in acute cases with mucosal ulceration and swellings.

NURSING CARE

N/A

ACTIVITY

N/A

DIET

N/A

CLIENT EDUCATION

Horses with upper airway noise should be evaluated by videoendoscopy to identify the early phase of this disease, before unilateral lesions become severely large or cause contact lesions on the contralateral arytenoid cartilage and, eventually, lead to bilateral disease.

SURGICAL CONSIDERATIONS

• Consider laser-assisted excision of intralaryngeal granulations if the affected arytenoid cartilage retains abductory function.
• Excision of the body and corniculate process of affected arytenoid cartilages is the treatment of choice to restore exercise capacity and to reduce upper airway noise.
• Permanent tracheotomy can be used in countries where athletic competition is allowed with this procedure and to salvage the animal for breeding purposes.

ARYTENOID CHONDRITIS

MEDICATIONS

DRUGS OF CHOICE

- None, other than routine perioperative antimicrobial and anti-inflammatory agents.
- With mucosal ulceration and swellings, broad-spectrum antibiotics and NSAIDs.
- Use of nasopharyngeal spray, consisting of various anti-inflammatory and antimicrobial agents (e.g., 250 mL of 90% DMSO, 500 mL of nitrofurazone, and 50 mL of prednisolone [25 mg/mL] mixed with 250 mL of glycerin) can be applied (20 mL BID) using a soft rubber feeding tube.
- If the airway is significantly compromised, a temporary tracheotomy may be needed until the swelling resolves.

CONTRAINDICATIONS

N/A

PRECAUTIONS

N/A

POSSIBLE INTERACTIONS

N/A

ALTERNATIVE DRUGS

N/A

FOLLOW-UP

PATIENT MONITORING

- Videoendoscopy of the upper airway for 6 weeks after surgery to monitor patient response.
- Final response to treatment or continuation of monitoring of affected horses is made on the basis of evaluating exercise tolerance and upper respiratory noise.

PREVENTION/AVOIDANCE

N/A

POSSIBLE COMPLICATIONS

- Horses undergoing removal of the corniculate and body of the arytenoid cartilage have a slightly increased risk for tracheal aspiration of feed during deglutition. In addition, these procedures do not fully restore the airway diameter, so a mild degree of airway obstruction persists, which may interfere with performance or result in upper airway noise during exercise.
- Bilateral arytenoidectomy increases the risk for tracheal aspiration of feed during deglutition and for glottic stenosis because of webbing at the resection site.

EXPECTED COURSE AND PROGNOSIS

- Horses with acute swelling of the arytenoid cartilage may respond favorably to NSAIDs, topical anti-inflammatory agents, and antibiotics.
- Untreated horses exhibit a progressive increase in exercise intolerance and upper respiratory noise.
- Some horses with focal elevated granulations on the axial surface of the arytenoid cartilage that maintains abductory function may respond to simple "lumpectomy," but most experience disease progression to generalized involvement of the affected cartilage.
- Horses with generalized involvement of an arytenoid cartilage and without surgical treatment often develop contralateral contact or "kissing" lesions.
- Horses with unilateral lesions treated surgically have a fair prognosis (50%) for elimination or significant reduction of exercise intolerance; however, the prognosis is guarded (20%) in horses with bilateral lesions.

MISCELLANEOUS

ASSOCIATED CONDITIONS

N/A

AGE-RELATED FACTORS

N/A

ZOONOTIC POTENTIAL

N/A

PREGNANCY

N/A

SYNONYMS

N/A

SEE ALSO

- Dynamic collapse of the upper airways
- Left laryngeal hemiparesis/hemiplegia

ABBREVIATION

DMSO = dimethyl sulfoxide

Suggested Reading

Dean PW, Cohen ND. Arytenoidectomy for advanced unilateral chondropathy with accompanying lesions. Vet Surg 1990;19:364–370.

Hay WP, Tulleners E. Excision of intralaryngeal granulation tissue in 25 horses using a neodymium:YAG laser (1986 to 1991). Vet Surg 1993:22:129–134.

Haynes PF, Snider TG, McLure JR, et al. Chronic chondritis of the equine arytenoid cartilage. J Am Vet Med Assoc 1980:177:1135–1142.

Lumsden JM, Derksen FJ, Stick JA, et al. Evaluation of partial arytenoidectomy as a treatment for equine laryngeal hemiplegia. Equine Vet J 1994;26:92–93.

McClure JJ, Koch C, Powell M, McClure JR. Association of arytenoid chondritis with equine lymphocyte antigens but no association with laryngeal hemiplegia, umbilical hernia and cryptorchidism. Anim Genet 1988;19:427–433.

Tulleners EP, Harrison IW, Raker CW. Management of arytenoid chondropathy and failed laryngoplasty in horses: 75 cases (1979–1985). J Am Vet Med Assoc 1988;192:670–675.

Authors Norm G. Ducharme and Richard P. Hackett

Consulting Editor Jean Pierre Lavoie

ASCARID INFESTATION

BASICS

OVERVIEW

Patent *Parascaris equorum* infection of the small intestine involves a direct life cycle starting with eggs passed in the feces that develop an infective larvae within 10 days. On ingestion, the eggs hatch larvae and migrate through the wall of the small intestine. The larvae are transported to the liver via the portal vein, and migrate through the liver to the hepatic vein, then enter the caudal vena cava and pulmonary circulation. Molting of larvae occurs in the lung parenchyma, and larvae then ascend the trachea and are swallowed. Final molting and maturation occurs in the small intestine. Heavy burdens of ascarids result in moderate enteritis or subnormal growth due to interference with digestion and absorption of nutrients within the small intestine.

SIGNALMENT

Horses, ponies, and donkeys of all ages may be affected. Patent infections are seen primarily in foals and weanlings up to 9–12 months of age. Older horses rarely have patent ascarid infections unless severe debilitation and immunocompromise exist.

SIGNS

Ascarid infection is characterized by an impaired growth rate, dull hair coat, dry skin, weakness, and a "pot-bellied" appearance. Other signs include decreased appetite, colic due to obstruction, or acute deterioration due to peritonitis from perforation of the intestinal wall. "Summer colds" (coughing, mucoid nasal discharge) may be seen in affected foals as large numbers of larvae migrate through the lungs.

CAUSES AND RISK FACTORS

Grazing from infected pastures provides an immense potential for reinfection or for transmission between foal crops in subsequent years on contaminated property.

DIAGNOSIS

DIFFERENTIAL DIAGNOSIS

Differential diagnoses for ill-thrift include other gastrointestinal parasites as well as chronic infection, abscessation, or poor nutrition. Colic is a nonspecific clinical sign associated with multiple causes of intra or extra-abdominal pain. Peritonitis may also occur with bowel rupture due to gastrointestinal ulceration or intestinal accidents.

CBC/BIOCHEMISTRY/URINALYSIS

Eosinophilia may be seen 10–40 days after infection, during the period of larval migration through the liver and lung. Hypoproteinemia may be detected in severe cases.

OTHER LABORATORY TESTS

N/A

IMAGING

N/A

DIAGNOSTIC PROCEDURES

Fecal flotation reveals numerous thick-walled eggs following the prepatent period of 10–12 weeks. Treatment is indicated for fecal egg cell counts >100 eggs per gram.

PATHOLOGIC FINDINGS

Multifocal white tracts within the liver appear histologically as fibrosis and cellular infiltration by eosinophils and lymphocytes appear in areas of previous larval migration. Lymphocytic nodules may also develop in lung tissue over time as an immunologic response to multiple episodes of reinfection as the foal ages.

TREATMENT

Contaminated facilities should be disinfected with a 5% phenolic compound and sprayed with a high-pressure hose. Frequent removal of manure from stalls and pastures also reduces the transmission between foals.

MEDICATIONS

DRUG(S) OF CHOICE

Routine anthelmintic treatment should be initiated at 6–8 weeks of age. Current anthelmintics in use are effective against the adult worms but do not eliminate migrating larvae. Therefore, preventative therapy should be continued every 6–8 weeks until 1 year of age. Mares should also be treated at monthly intervals during the last trimester of pregnancy to reduce environmental contamination for the foals. Appropriate anthelmintics to treat ascarid infections include:

- Moxidectin 0.4 mg/kg PO
- Ivermectin 0.2 mg/kg PO
- Pyrantel pamoate 6.6 mg/kg PO
- Levamisole 8 mg/kg PO
- Fenbendazole 10 mg/kg PO given for 5 consecutive days (Note: benzimidazoles vary in effectiveness against ascarids)
- Daily prophylactic administration of pyrantel tartrate (2.64 mg/kg) in the feed also prevents penetration of the intestinal wall by ascarid larvae

CONTRAINDICATIONS/POSSIBLE INTERACTIONS

Heavy ascarid burdens should not be treated with anthelmintics that result in paralysis of the parasites (e.g., pyrantel pamoate, piperazine, organophosphates, ivermectin). Complete paralysis of ascarids may cause impaction or complete bowel obstruction. Less efficacious anthelmintics such as benzimidazoles are therefore recommended in the early stages of treatment for heavy ascarid burdens.

FOLLOW-UP

PATIENT MONITORING

Fecal examinations should be performed on at least 10% of foals on each farm 2–3 times annually. Adequate control is reflected by <10% of tested foals passing eggs in the feces. Positive fecal results may occur for up to 2 weeks following treatment with ivermectin.

PREVENTION/AVOIDANCE

Parascaris equorum eggs can remain viable in the environment for many years due to their thick protective shell. Frequent removal of feces from pastures and drylots is essential in order to reduce the incidence of reinfection following treatment.

POSSIBLE COMPLICATIONS

Deworming with anthelmintics that cause rapid neuromuscular blockade and paralysis of ascarids (piperazine, ivermectin, levamisole, trichlorfon) may result in impaction or complete bowel obstruction.

EXPECTED COURSE AND PROGNOSIS

Infection rate decreases starting at 6 months of age. Foals and yearlings gradually develop an active, protective immunity, and adults maintain a continuously high antibody titer. Large numbers of ascarids are rarely seen in mature horses unless immunocompromise is present.

MISCELLANEOUS

ASSOCIATED CONDITIONS

N/A

AGE-RELATED FACTORS

Age-related immunity to ascarid infection starts to develop at 6 months of age.

ZOONOTIC POTENTIAL

None

PREGNANCY

Transplacental infection with *P. equorum* is not known to occur. Unlike other ascarid infections (*Toxocara cati, Toxocara canis, Toxocara vitulorum*), transfer of ascarid larvae in colostrum has not been proved in *P. equorum* infections.

SEE ALSO

N/A

ABBREVIATIONS

N/A

Suggested Reading

Bowman DD. Georgi's parasitology for veterinarians, 6th ed. Philadelphia: WB Saunders, 1994;203-212.

Author Joanne Hewson

Consulting Editor Henry Stämpfli

ASPARTATE AMINOTRANSFERASE (AST)

BASICS

DEFINITION

- Catalyzes transamination of 2-oxoglutarate and L-aspartate to glutamate and oxaloacetate.
- Present in many tissues—liver, striated muscle, erythrocytes, and others.
- Because of high activity in the liver and striated muscle, serum/plasma AST elevations are an indicator of hepatocellular and striated muscle damage.
- Two isoforms, cytoplasmic and mitochondrial, with most activity being in the cytoplasm.
- Reported normal serum AST activity in adult equine patients varies from 152–412 IU/L.

PATHOPHYSIOLOGY

- AST is an "injury" enzyme, escaping to the circulation when the cell cytoplasmic membrane is injured.
- Magnitude of the elevation generally is proportional to the number of hepatocytes affected, not to the severity of a particular insult.
- With skeletal muscle damage, magnitude of AST elevation is not necessarily proportional to the extent of tissue injury.
- Increases above the reference range can be seen with injections and downer animals.
- AST is a sensitive indicator of hepatocellular and striated muscle damage; however, because it is present in many tissues, AST lacks specificity. Other biochemical tests need to be examined concurrently with AST to localize the source of the increase.
- Such biochemical tests include SDH/IDH (i.e., a liver-specific enzyme) and CK (i.e., a striated muscle–specific enzyme).
- After respective tissue injury, AST activity increases in the circulation more slowly and remains elevated much longer than SDH (liver) or CK (muscle).
- The plasma half-life of AST in horses is 7–10 days, compared with only a few hours for either SDH or CK.
- Differences in appearance rates and half-lives of AST and SDH allow clinicians to better understand the chronology of an insult and to determine if it is ongoing. Elevated SDH, with normal or increased AST, indicates acute or ongoing hepatocellular injury. If serial serum chemistry analyses reveal continuously or progressively elevated activities of both enzymes, ongoing hepatocellular damage is likely. During treatment of hepatic disease, the enzymes can be used to monitor cessation of the insult. If, after documenting recent hepatocellular injury, serial serum chemistry analyses reveal elevated AST and progressively decreasing or normal SDH activity, cessation of the original insult is likely. Because of its longer half-life, AST may increase even after cessation of the original insult, and the levels may remain elevated for weeks.
- A similar interpretative approach is used when determining if muscle damage is present. Muscle and hepatocellular injury can occur concurrently, and increases in AST, CK, and SDH may be seen together.

SYSTEMS AFFECTED

Hepatic or muscular—severe necrosis of any tissue (e.g., kidney) may present with elevated AST values.

SIGNALMENT

- Given the breadth of most reference intervals, clear differences generally have not been evident.
- One draft breed (i.e., English Shire) appears to have values clustered at the lower reference interval (172 ± 28 IU/L).
- Fillies may have relatively higher activity compared to that in colts of the same age.
- Parturient mares receiving tetanus antitoxin appear to have an increased incidence of serum hepatitis, but this may simply reflect the higher incidence of antitoxin administration in this population.

SIGNS

Historical Findings

- Modest (generally <2-fold), transient increases in AST (and CK) may occur during strenuous exercise.
- Baseline and exercise-associated AST levels are higher early during training seasons and tend to decrease with better conditioning.
- Persistent, large elevations in AST may signal muscle injury associated with overtraining.

Physical Examination Findings

- Vary according to the primary cause.
- Typically, horses with muscle disorders exhibit a variety of signs—reluctance or inability to move, stiffness, and recumbency.
- Horses with liver disorders may exhibit jaundice, neurologic deficits, and many other nonspecific signs—anorexia, abdominal pain, weight loss, and fever.
- Horses may be presented with no significant clinical signs.
- Clinical signs of hepatic failure generally do not appear until 75% of the hepatic functional mass is lost.

CAUSES

- Degenerative conditions—cirrhosis, rhabdomyolysis, and choleliths
- Anomaly, congenital diseases—polysaccharide storage myopathy; biliary atresia
- Metabolic diseases—shock, hypovolemia, hypoxia caused by severe anemia or during anesthesia, and severe GI disease
- Neoplastic or nutritional diseases—primary neoplasia, metastatic neoplasia, leukemias, hepatic lipidosis, and vitamin E/selenium deficiency
- Infectious and immune-mediated diseases—hepatitis of various causes (e.g., viral, bacterial, protozoal, fungal, parasitic), serum sickness, amyloidosis, endotoxemia, and chronic active hepatitis

• Toxic or trauma—pyrrolizidine alkaloid–containing plants, cottonseed, castor bean, oaks, and alsike clover; fungal toxins, such as aflatoxins, cyclopiazonic acid, fumonisin, phalloidin (i.e., mushrooms), rubratoxins; blue-green algae; and chemical compounds/elements, such as ethanol, chlorinated hydrocarbons, carbon tetrachloride, monensin, copper, iron, and petroleum and its products.

RISK FACTORS

• Familial disease, exposure to infected animals, overweight and miniature ponies, poor nutrition, or exposure to toxic compound or plants.
• Risk factors vary according to the specific disease.
• The anesthetic halothane is metabolized by the liver. Prolonged anesthesia has been associated with transiently increased AST activity, and hypoxia during halothane anesthesia results in significantly greater evidence for hepatocellular injury than does similar hypoxia during isoflurane anesthesia.

DIAGNOSIS

DIFFERENTIAL DIAGNOSIS

• Once the origin of the increased AST has been localized to the liver or muscle by other clinical chemistry tests (e.g., SDH, CK), an appropriate differential list can be formulated.
• See *Causes.*
• A complete history, physical examination, diagnostic imaging findings, laboratory data, and microscopic examination of tissue help to narrow the list to the most likely causes.

LABORATORY FINDINGS

Drugs That May Alter Lab Results

A multitude of compounds may produce hepatocellular or muscular damage and lead to increased AST; however, most do not directly interfere with laboratory measurement.

Disorders That May Alter Laboratory Results

• Because of high AST activity in erythrocytes, hemolysis falsely elevates serum/plasma AST activity.
• Prolonged in vitro exposure of serum or plasma to erythrocytes falsely increases AST activity even before visible signs of hemolysis are present. To avoid this confounding factor, prompt separation of plasma/serum from the cellular components of blood is strongly recommended.
• If laboratory analysis will not occur within 1–2 days, freeze the plasma/serum.

Valid If Run in Human Lab?

Yes

CBC/BIOCHEMISTRY/URINALYSIS

CBC

• Erythrocytes—liver disease may cause nonregenerative anemia and morphologic changes (e.g., acanthocytes, target cells, nonspecific poikilocytosis, normochromic microcytosis in portosystemic vascular shunts); severe anemia of any cause may produce cellular damage from tissue hypoxia.
• Leukocytes—leukocytosis or leukopenia may be seen with inflammatory diseases and leukemias; morphologic changes of the leukocytes (e.g., neutrophil toxicity in inflammation; neoplastic cells) also may be seen.
• Platelets—quantitative decreases and increases may be seen with a variety of systemic diseases that may affect the liver or striated muscle.

Serum/Plasma Biochemistry Profile

• Glucose—increased in diabetes mellitus, glucocorticoid influence (e.g., exogenous, endogenous); decreased in end-stage liver disease, sepsis/endotoxemia
• BUN—increased in severe rhabdomyolysis from secondary renal damage; decreased in liver insufficiency and end-stage liver disease from decreased conversion of ammonia to urea
• Albumin—decreased in end-stage liver disease from decreased production; minimally to mildly decreased in inflammation
• Globulins—generally increased in end-stage liver disease
• SDH—increased with acute and ongoing hepatocellular injury
• ALP—increased with concurrent cholestatic disease
• GGT—increased with cholestatic disease or hepatocellular injury
• CK—increased with acute or ongoing muscle damage
• Conjugated bilirubin—increased in cholestatic disease
• Unconjugated bilirubin—increased with anorexia and prehepatic cholestasis (i.e., massive in vivo hemolysis)
• Cholesterol—may be increased with cholestasis and decreased in hepatic insufficiency; generally, cholesterol is within the reference interval in liver disease
• Triglycerides—increases may be associated with hepatic lipidosis

Urinalysis

Bilirubinuria—conjugated bilirubin, detected by the commonly used dipstick and diazo tablet methods, indicates cholestatic disease and should not be elevated if only hepatocellular injury is present.

ASPARTATE AMINOTRANSFERASE (AST)

OTHER LABORATORY TESTS

SBAs

- Fairly specific test for hepatobiliary disease, but not very specific for the type of disease
- May be elevated with cell injury, cholestasis, or hepatic insufficiency/decreased functional mass; specificity for the latter condition is greatly increased when SBAs are elevated in cases with normal or minimally elevated markers for hepatocellular injury (e.g., SDH, AST, GGT) and cholestasis (e.g., ALP, GGT, conjugated bilirubin).
- Main advantage over plasma ammonia, a more specific test for hepatic insufficiency/ decreased functional mass, is that immediate sample analysis is not necessary.

Plasma Ammonia

- Hepatic insufficiency/decreased functional mass is indicated if fasting or challenge ammonia levels are increased.
- A sensitive and specific test, because it is not affected by other factors (e.g., cholestasis). However, ammonia measurement requires special handling, which limits its general availability.
- Consult reference laboratory for specific requirements.

Sulfobromophthalein- and Indocyanine Green Dye–Clearance Tests

- Decreases in clearance of these dyes indicate hepatic insufficiency.
- These tests have largely been replaced by plasma ammonia and SBAs.

Coagulation Tests and Fibrinogen

- The liver manufactures many of the coagulation factors; significant decreases in liver function may lead to deficiencies in these factors and to coagulation abnormalities.
- Commonly used tests—APTT and PT.
- Decreased APTT and PT are seen when $<30\%$ of the activity of the factors is present.

Serologic Tests

Helpful in detecting infectious causes.

Toxicology

- Analysis of tissue biopsy material, feed, ingesta, serum/plasma, or other body fluids may indicate presence of a toxin.
- Contact reference laboratory regarding sample selection and submission recommendations.

Bacterial, Fungal, or Viral Culture

- May establish a definitive diagnosis regarding the infectious agent involved and help to guide treatment.
- Request bacterial antibiotic sensitivity to determine appropriate antibiotic therapy.
- Contact reference laboratory regarding sample selection and submission recommendations.

IMAGING

Ultrasonography

- Limited by position and size of the liver.
- Evaluate size, echogenicity, shape, and position.
- Useful for guidance when obtaining biopsy material for cytology, histopathology, and microbiology.
- Helpful in the evaluation of muscle and tendon injuries.

Radionucleotide Imaging

- Reveals information regarding liver architecture and function.
- Expensive and available only in selected institutions.

DIAGNOSTIC PROCEDURES

- Aspiration cytology and histopathology of formalin-fixed tissue.
- Cytology has the advantages of simplicity, quicker turnaround, better individual cellular detail, and better recognition of individual infectious organisms.
- Histopathology has the advantage of allowing examination of the architecture and lesion distribution.
- Success of these procedures depends on the quality of the sample, area sampled, and the disease process itself; some hepatic diseases do not have significant microscopic alterations.

TREATMENT

- Depends on the primary disease process and any secondary complications present.
- Choice of fluids depends on the primary cause of the disease and any metabolic imbalances (e.g., acid–base disturbances) present.

ASPARTATE AMINOTRANSFERASE (AST)

MEDICATIONS

DRUGS OF CHOICE
Choice of drugs depends on the primary cause and any complicating factors present.

CONTRAINDICATIONS
N/A

PRECAUTIONS
With suspected hepatic insufficiency, assess the relative safety/risk of invasive procedures (e.g., fine-needle aspiration, tissue biopsy, laparoscopy, surgery) in light of coagulation panel results.

POSSIBLE INTERACTIONS
N/A

ALTERNATIVE DRUGS
N/A

FOLLOW UP

PATIENT MONITORING
- Serial serum biochemical analyses to monitor progression or improvement of the disease process
- See *Pathophysiology*.

POSSIBLE COMPLICATIONS
If the primary disease is of infectious origin, take precautions not to contaminate the facilities and infect other horses by establishing appropriate quarantine/isolation and disinfection procedures.

MISCELLANEOUS

ASSOCIATED CONDITIONS
N/A

AGE-RELATED FACTORS
See *Signalment.*

ZOONOTIC POTENTIAL
Salmonellosis

PREGNANCY
See *Signalment.*

SYNONYMS
Previously known as glutamate oxaloacetate transaminase.

SEE ALSO
See *Causes.*

ABBREVIATIONS
- ALP = alkaline phosphatase
- APTT = Activated partial thromboplastin time
- CK = creatine kinase
- GGT = γ-glutamyltransferase
- GI = gastrointestinal
- IDH = idithiol dehydrogenase
- SBA = serum bile acid
- SDH = sorbitol dehydrogenase
- PT = prothrombin time

Suggested Reading

Cardinett GH. In: Kaneko JJ, Harvey JW, Bruss ML, eds. Clinical biochemistry of domestic animals. 5th ed. San Diego: Academic Press, 1997.

Harris PA. In: Reed SM, Bayly WM, eds. Equine internal medicine. Philadelphia: WB Saunders, 1998.

Barton HM, Deem MD. In: Reed SM, Bayly WM, eds. Equine internal medicine. Philadelphia: WB Saunders, 1998.

Kramer JW, Hoffmann WE. In: Kaneko JJ, Harvey JW, Bruss ML, eds. Clinical biochemistry of domestic animals. 5th ed. San Diego: Academic Press, 1997.

Authors Armando R. Irizarry-Rovira and John A. Christian

Consulting Editor Claire B. Andreasen

ASPIRATION PNEUMONIA (AP)

BASICS

OVERVIEW

• May develop after inhalation of foreign material and bacteria into the lower respiratory tract.
• Causes include dysphagia, obstructive esophageal disorders, GI reflux, and accidental inhalation of foreign material (e.g., accidental passage of a nasogastric tube into the trachea and the subsequent administration of medication into the lung).
• Characterized by cranioventral consolidation of the lungs.
• Other organ systems may be involved depending on the primary cause.

SIGNALMENT

• No sex or breed predisposition has been observed.
• Foals appear more prone to GI reflux and subsequent AP.

SIGNS

Historical findings

• Difficulty swallowing, ptyalism, or discharge of food or water from the nostrils may have been observed before the onset of respiratory signs.
• Recent history of drenching or nasogastric intubation should be investigated.

Physical Examination Findings

• Clinical signs—depression, anorexia, weight loss, fever, tachypnea, dyspnea, nasal discharge, and coughing.
• Foul-smelling breath or nasal discharge suggests anaerobic infection.
• Abnormal lung sounds often are heard on auscultation.
• Inhalation of large quantities of liquid may result in sudden death.

CAUSES AND RISK FACTORS

Dysphagia, esophageal disorders, GI reflux, or accidental inhalation of foreign material may cause AP.

Dysphagia

• Neurologic diseases affecting cranial nerves IX and X—guttural pouch diseases, botulism, lead toxicity, and viral encephalitis
• Primary myopathies of pharyngeal and laryngeal musculature—white muscle disease and hyperkalemic periodic paralysis
• Diseases causing pharyngeal obstruction—strangles, pharyngeal abscess, neoplasia, foreign body, follicular pharyngitis, dorsal displacement of the soft palate, rostral displacement of the palatopharyngeal arch, and pharyngeal and laryngeal cysts
• Congenital abnormalities—cleft palate and hypoplasia of the soft palate
• Iatrogenic causes—pharyngeal and laryngeal surgery

Esophageal Disorders

• Esophageal obstruction—foreign body, feed impaction, stricture, atresia, compression, and neoplasia
• Megaesophagus
• Esophagitis
• Esophageal diverticulum
• Esophageal fistula

GI Reflux

Gastric outflow obstruction is secondary to ulcer disease in foals.

Accidental Inhalation of a Foreign Body

After administration of fluids by drenching or nasogastric tube.

DIAGNOSIS

DIFFERENTIAL DIAGNOSIS

• Acute bronchopneumonia—often follows viral infection or stressful events (e.g., anesthesia, transportation, strenuous exercise, severe weather).
• Pleuropneumonia—possible complication of AP, bronchopneumonia, pulmonary abscess, or secondary to thoracic trauma or esophageal rupture; auscultation, percussion, ultrasonography, radiography, or thoracocentesis may confirm pleural effusion.
• Interstitial pneumonia—thoracic radiography most commonly reveals severe, diffuse increase in interstitial pulmonary opacity.
• Respiratory distress syndrome—severe respiratory distress noted 24–48 hours after birth caused by surfactant deficiency; thoracic radiography typically shows diffuse, ground-glass appearance of the lungs with air bronchograms.

CBC/BIOCHEMISTRY/URINALYSIS

• Elevated WBC count with absolute neutrophilia is common.
• Band neutrophils may be present.
• Hyperfibrinogenemia, hyperglobulinemia, and anemia are common findings with chronic pneumonia.

OTHER LABORATORY TESTS

• Various tests may help to diagnose the primary cause.
• Increased blood and tissue concentration of lead and erythrocyte concentration of δ-aminolevulinic acid are diagnostic for lead toxicity.
• Decreased whole-blood selenium concentration and glutathione peroxidase activity with increased serum creatinine kinase (CK) and Aspartate Amino Transferase (AST) are consistent with white muscle disease.
• Hyperkalemic periodic paralysis may be diagnosed by genetic testing and measurement of serum hyperkalemia during clinical episodes.

IMAGING

• Thoracic radiography commonly reveals cranioventral opacity and often results in loss of radiolucent space ventral to the cauda vena cava, caudal to the heart, and cranial to the diaphragm.
• Contrast radiography may help to diagnose causes of esophageal dysfunction.
• Thoracic ultrasonography is a sensitive means of detecting fluid accumulation in the pleural space.

ASPIRATION PNEUMONIA (AP)

DIAGNOSTIC PROCEDURES

- Obtain a fluid sample from a tracheobronchial aspiration for cytology, Gram stain, and culture (both aerobic and anaerobic); with pleural effusion, also obtain a fluid sample by thoracocentesis for cytology and culture.
- Endoscopy of the respiratory and upper GI tracts may help to identify the primary cause.

PATHOLOGIC FINDINGS

- Consolidation of the cranioventral region of the lungs.
- Acute cases—severely affected areas are hemorrhagic and edematous.
- Chronic cases—affected lung may be necrotic and filled with purulent material.
- Pleural space involvement—a fibrinous exudate and adhesion formation between visceral and parietal pleura.

TREATMENT

- Treat severe dyspnea according to the cause—restore airway patency, drain pleural effusion, etc.
- Horses with severe hypoxemia ($PaO_2 < 60$ torr) benefit from oxygen therapy.
- Positive-pressure ventilation may be used to correct hypoventilation ($PaCO_2 > 50$ torr).
- Treatment requires intensive medical care that can be provided only on an inpatient basis.
- The primary disease must be treated.
- Stall rest is imperative.
- Dysphagic horses may be fed via an indwelling nasogastric tube.
- With pleural effusion, thoracocentesis or placement of indwelling chest tubes can achieve drainage; a one-way valve attached to the tube prevents pneumothorax formation.
- Administer fluid therapy as needed.

MEDICATIONS

DRUGS

- Promptly initiate systemic administration of broad-spectrum antimicrobials while waiting for culture results.
- Preferred combinations include sodium or potassium penicillin (22,000–40,000 IU/kg IV q6h), aminoglycoside (gentamicin [6.6–8.8 mg/kg IV q24h] or amikacin [15–20 mg/kg IV or IM q24h] for foals), and metronidazole (15–25 mg/kg IV or PO q6h).
- Other antimicrobial choices include procaine penicillin G (22,000 IU/kg IM q12h), trimethoprim-sulfamethoxazole (30 mg/kg PO q12h), ceftiofur (1–5 mg/kg IV or IM q12h), or chloramphenicol (20–50 mg/kg PO q6–8h for adults and foals >1 week).
- Administer antimicrobial drugs systemically until the horse's condition is stable and improving; treatment may then be switched to long-term oral antimicrobials.
- NSAIDs are indicated for endotoxemia and inflammation—flunixin meglumine (0.25 mg/kg IV q8h to 1.1 mg/kg IV q12h).

CONTRAINDICATIONS/POSSIBLE INTERACTIONS

Use aminoglycosides and NSAIDs with caution in horses having compromised renal function or dehydration.

FOLLOW-UP

PATIENT MONITORING

- Monitor clinical signs, especially respiratory rate and efforts, and rectal temperature.
- Follow progress of pulmonary lesions by radiography.
- Ultrasonography helps to monitor pleural effusion.

PREVENTION/AVOIDANCE

- Prevent or avoid exposure to primary causes.
- Vitamin E and selenium supplementation for white muscle disease.

POSSIBLE COMPLICATIONS

- Lung abscessation
- Pleuritis
- Disseminated intravascular coagulation
- Laminitis
- Thrombophlebitis
- Septicemia

EXPECTED COURSE AND PROGNOSIS

- Expect a long and protracted course of treatment.
- Prognosis is guarded.

MISCELLANEOUS

ASSOCIATED CONDITIONS

N/A

AGE-RELATED FACTORS

N/A

ZOONOTIC POTENTIAL

N/A

PREGNANCY

N/A

SEE ALSO

- Hemorrhagic nasal discharge
- Pleuropneumonia
- Respiratory distress syndrome

ABBREVIATION

GI = gastrointestinal

Suggested Reading

Warner AE. Bacterial pneumonia in adult horses. In: Smith BP, ed. Large animal internal medicine. 2nd ed. St Louis: Mosby, 1996:566–572.

Author Laurent Couëtil
Consulting Editor Jean-Pierre Lavoie

ATHEROMA

BASICS

OVERVIEW

- An epidermal inclusion cyst of the false nostril (i.e., nasal diverticulum).
- Congenitally aberrant epithelial tissue between the skin and mucous membrane of the false nostril.
- Becomes apparent with age as the cyst enlarges.

SIGNALMENT

- Young horses
- No known sex or breed predilections

SIGNS

- Soft to firm, round swellings covered by normal skin in the caudal dorsal aspect of the false nostril.
- Typically unilateral, but can be bilateral.
- Not painful on palpation.
- Usually becomes apparent after weaning to 3 years of age, and can reach a size of up to 5 cm.
- Usually not associated with respiratory compromise unless very large.

CAUSES AND RISK FACTORS

N/A

DIAGNOSIS

DIFFERENTIAL DIAGNOSIS

- None
- Diagnosis is established on the characteristic location and physical features of the swellings.

CBC/BIOCHEMISTRY/URINALYSIS

N/A

OTHER LABORATORY TESTS

Aspirated cyst contents reveal a white to gray, creamy fluid that, under microscopy with rapid trichrome staining, reveals keratinized and nonkeratinized squamous epithelial cells and keratinous debris.

IMAGING

N/A

DIAGNOSTIC PROCEDURES

N/A

TREATMENT

- Usually not removed unless for cosmetic reasons or for airway noise or impairment from large swelling size.
- If removed surgically, it is imperative to remove the entire cyst lining to prevent recurrence.
- Total surgical removal can be done under general anesthesia or standing with sedation and local anesthesia of the infraorbital nerve.
- The cyst can be approached surgically through the skin over the dorsum of the swelling. The cyst then is dissected in its entirety, and the wound is closed.
- Another option is to open the cyst ventrally into the false nostril, drain the contents, and remove the lining using a burr instrument. In this technique, the wound is left open to heal by second intention.
- Usual precautions for tetanus prophylaxis and asepsis of the surgical site.

MEDICATIONS

DRUGS

Draining and cauterizing or sclerosing the cyst has been done using tincture of iodine, silver nitrate, or both followed by packing; this requires daily treatment and carries a high risk of recurrence.

CONTRAINDICATIONS/POSSIBLE INTERACTIONS

N/A

ATHEROMA

FOLLOW-UP

POSSIBLE COMPLICATIONS

- Transient swelling after surgery
- Recurrence
- Infection
- Scar formation
- White hair at surgery site

EXPECTED COURSE AND PROGNOSIS

Favorable prognosis for both leaving the atheroma untouched and for surgical removal if needed.

MISCELLANEOUS

ASSOCIATED CONDITIONS

N/A

AGE-RELATED FACTORS

N/A

ZOONOTIC POTENTIAL

N/A

PREGNANCY

N/A

SEE ALSO

N/A

Suggested Reading

Gaughan EM. Surgery of the upper respiratory tract. In: Kobluk CN, Ames TR, Geor RJ, eds. The horse. Philadelphia: WB Saunders, 1995:244.

Nickels FA, Tulleners EP. Nasal passages. In: Auer JA, ed. Equine surgery. Philadelphia: WB Saunders, 1992:435.

Schumacher J, Moll HD, Schumacher J, et al. A simple method to remove an epidermal inclusion cyst from the false nostril of horses. Equine Pract 1997;19:11–13.

Author Wendy Duckett

Consulting Editor Jean-Pierre Lavoie

ATRIAL FIBRILLATION

BASICS

DEFINITION

- An irregularly irregular cardiac rhythm, with variable-intensity heart sounds and variable-intensity pulses
- No consistent diastolic interval, with beats occurring sooner than expected and pauses in the rhythm
- A critical atrial mass must be present for the condition to occur.
- Predisposing factors—large atrial mass, high vagal tone, shortened effective refractory period, potassium depletion, atrial premature depolarizations, rapid atrial pacing, atrial enlargement, and atrial inhomogeneity

PATHOPHYSIOLOGY

- Produces no change in cardiac output in horses at rest without significant other underlying cardiac disease.
- During high-intensity exercise, however, the condition produces a marked increase in the heart rate response to exercise, with the average horse experiencing a 40–60 bpm increase for each level of exercise.
- Cardiac output falls during high-intensity exercise, and the horse no longer can perform up to expectations.
- Present in most horses with congestive heart failure but is not the cause of the congestive heart failure.

SYSTEM AFFECTED

Cardiovascular

GENETICS

N/A

INCIDENCE/PREVALENCE

N/A

SIGNALMENT

Higher incidence in Standardbred race horses, draft, and Warmblood horses.

SIGNS

General Comments

Most commonly associated with poor performance, but may be an incidental finding.

Historical Findings

- Exercise intolerance
- Exercise-induced pulmonary hemorrhage—often profuse
- Respiratory distress
- Congestive heart failure
- Ataxia
- Collapse
- Myositis

Physical Examination Findings

- Irregularly irregular heart rhythm
- Variable-intensity heart sounds
- Variable-intensity arterial pulses
- Absent fourth heart sound—S4
- Regurgitant murmurs may be present.

CAUSES

- Atrial enlargement
- Underlying atrial myocardial disease

RISK FACTORS

- Furosemide administration
- Bicarbonate milkshakes
- Mitral insufficiency
- Tricuspid insufficiency
- Congestive heart failure

DIAGNOSIS

DIFFERENTIAL DIAGNOSIS

- Second-degree AV block—regular rhythm is interrupted by pauses containing fourth heart sound.
- Atrial tachycardia with second-degree AV block—rhythm usually is regularly irregular; fourth heart sounds are present.
- Sinus rhythm with multifocal ventricular premature depolarizations—usually need ECG to differentiate, unless fourth heart sound is detected.

CBC/BIOCHEMISTRY/URINALYSIS

Low plasma potassium or urinary fractional excretion of potassium may be present.

OTHER LABORATORY TESTS

- Elevated cardiac isoenzymes (e.g., CK-MB, HBDH, LDH-1 and -2, cardiac troponin I) may be present.
- RBC potassium concentrations may be decreased.

IMAGING

ECG

- No P waves, which are replaced by baseline "f" (i.e., fibrillation) waves
- The "f" waves may be coarse or fine and may occur 300–500 times per minute.
- Irregular R-R interval
- Some variation in the amplitude of QRS and T complexes usually is present, but these complexes are normal in appearance.
- Unifocal ventricular extrasystoles in ≅ 10% of horses.

Echocardiography

- Most affected horses have little or no discernible underlying cardiac disease; therefore, the echocardiogram is normal.
- Affected horses often have a low-normal to low shortening fraction (24%–32%), related in part to loss of the atrial contraction that normally contributes to ventricular filling—decreased preload
- The shortening fraction should return to normal within several days of conversion to normal sinus rhythm.
- May reveal mild left atrial enlargement in horses with sustained atrial fibrillation.
- Insufficiency of the AV valves may be present along with atrial enlargement in horses with underlying myocardial or valvular heart disease.

DIAGNOSTIC PROCEDURES

Continuous 24-Hour Holter Monitoring

Useful in horses with suspected paroxysmal atrial fibrillation to be looking for increased frequency of atrial premature depolarizations.

Exercising ECG

- A stress test during high-speed exercise is useful to detect exercise-induced arrhythmias and to determine exercise limitations if the atrial fibrillation is not or cannot be converted.
- The high-speed treadmill provides a controlled environment in which cardiac rhythm can be evaluated during high-intensity exercise.

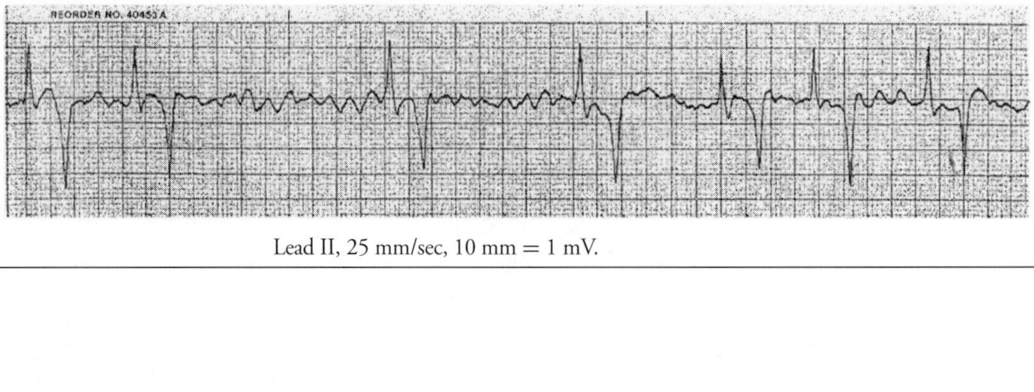

Lead II, 25 mm/sec, 10 mm = 1 mV.

PATHOLOGIC FINDINGS

- Normal heart, both grossly and histopathologically, in affected horses with no underlying cardiac disease.
- Focal or diffuse atrial fibrosis may be present in horses with long-standing atrial fibrillation.
- Inflammatory cell infiltrate has been documented in affected horses with myocarditis and atrial fibrillation.
- Myocardial necrosis has been detected in affected horses with toxic myocardial injury.
- Fatty infiltration has been reported.
- Thinning of the atrial myocardium with atrial dilatation has been documented in affected horses with atrial enlargement; however, most horses do not have significant underlying myocardial disease.
- Both atrial and ventricular enlargement in horses with significant AV valvular heart disease, along with valvular pathology.

TREATMENT

APPROPRIATE HEALTH CARE

- Monitor horses with acute-onset atrial fibrillation for 24–48 hours to determine if the condition will resolve without treatment (i.e., paroxysmal), unless congestive heart failure also is present.
- Once the atrial fibrillation is sustained, institute treatment on an inpatient basis if conversion to sinus rhythm is desired.
- In affected horses with congestive heart failure, institute treatment for congestive heart failure, ideally on an inpatient basis.

NURSING CARE

- Perform continuous ECG throughout attempted conversion to sinus rhythm.
- Keep horses quiet and unmoving during the quinidine treatment.

ACTIVITY

- Affected horses should not perform high-intensity exercise while in atrial fibrillation.
- Affected horses usually can perform successfully as pleasure horses, in lower-level athletic competition, as broodmares, and as breeding stallions.
- Once converted to sinus rhythm, affected horses without evidence of other underlying cardiac disease usually can resume normal work.

DIET

- Oral potassium supplementation may be indicated with low plasma potassium, low RED potassium, or low urinary fractional excretion of potassium or with excessive sweating.
- Potassium chloride salt can be added to the feed (1 tbsp BID, gradually increasing to 1 oz BID).

CLIENT EDUCATION

- Discuss treatment-associated risks with owners—see *Complications*.
- Discuss predisposing factors with owners to minimize the likelihood of future episodes.

SURGICAL CONSIDERATIONS

- Successful transvenous electrical conversion of horses with recent-onset atrial fibrillation has been described.
- Treated horses were converted with transvenous electrical pacing under general anesthesia.

MEDICATIONS

DRUGS OF CHOICE

The drug of choice for conversion is quinidine—sulfate or gluconate.

Quinidine Gluconate

- Indicated with recent-onset atrial fibrillation.
- Most successful when administered to horses with no other underlying cardiac disease and a duration of atrial fibrillation of ≤2 weeks.
- Administered in small boluses of 0.5–1 mg/kg every 5–10 minutes to a total dose of 10 mg/kg.

Quinidine Sulfate

- Indicated in horses with sustained atrial fibrillation.
- Administered via nasogastric intubation at 22 mg/kg q2h to a total of four to six treatments q2h or until the horse is toxic or has converted to sinus rhythm.
- Prolong treatment intervals to q6h if the horse has not converted after four to six treatments q2h and has not shown signs of quinidine toxicity.

CONTRAINDICATIONS

- Do not administer quinidine sulfate or gluconate to affected horses with congestive heart failure.
- Affected horses with a resting heart rate of >60 bpm are likely to be in congestive heart failure, unless there is another cause for their tachycardia.
- Horses with a grade 3/6 or louder systolic murmur are more likely to have congestive heart failure.

PRECAUTIONS

- Digoxin is recommended in conjunction with quinidine in horses with significant myocardial dysfunction (i.e., fractional shortening <24%), high resting heart rate that is very responsive to external stimuli, or rapid heart-rate response to quinidine treatment (i.e., persistent elevation of heart rate >100 bpm).
- If a heart rate >100 bpm develops with quinidine, treat the horse with digoxin—0.011 mg/kg PO or 0.0022 mg/kg IV.
- If a heart rate >150 bpm develops with quinidine, treat the horse with digoxin (0.0022 mg/kg IV) and sodium bicarbonate (1 mEq/kg IV).
- If the heart rate remains high, administer propranolol—0.03 mg/kg IV.
- If the blood pressure remains poor, administer phenylephrine—0.1–0.2 μg/kg per minute IV to effect).

ATRIAL FIBRILLATION

• If administering digoxin before or at the onset of quinidine treatment to control heart rate or in horses with significant myocardial dysfunction, administer orally BID for the first day.
• If a horse receiving quinidine only on day 1 does not convert, add digoxin orally on day 2.
• Base subsequent digoxin administration during quinidine treatment on serum digoxin concentration and need to control heart rate or to improve myocardial contractility.

POSSIBLE INTERACTIONS

Quinidine competes with digoxin for binding to plasma protein, causing elevated serum digoxin concentrations and potential digoxin toxicity.

ALTERNATIVE DRUGS

• Most other drugs with efficacy against atrial arrhythmias have been ineffective in converting affected horses with atrial fibrillation.
• Digoxin (0.011mg/kg PO BID) has converted one horse on two occasions.
• Procainamide (25–35 mg/kg PO TID) has converted one horse.
• Propafenone (0.5–1 mg/kg in 5% dextrose given slowly IV to effect over 5–8 minutes) has converted one horse.

FOLLOW-UP

PATIENT MONITORING

• Perform continuous ECG in all affected horses receiving treatment, because the antiarrhythmic drugs administered also are arrhythmogenic.
• Measure QRS duration before each quinidine treatment; a prolonged QRS duration >25% of the pretreatment duration should prompt discontinuation of treatment.
• Rapid supraventricular tachycardia with atrial fibrillation or a ventricular arrhythmia should prompt discontinuation of quinidine treatment.
• Colic, ataxia, convulsions, or bizarre behavior indicates quinidine toxicity and should prompt discontinuation of treatment.
• Urticaria, wheals, upper respiratory tract obstruction, or laminitis are infrequent adverse reactions to quinidine treatment and should prompt discontinuation.
• Severe diarrhea should prompt discontinuation of quinidine treatment.
• Following conversion, perform 24-hour Holter monitoring. If atrial ectopy is found, rest and corticosteroid therapy may be indicated.
• Owners and trainers should regularly monitor cardiac rhythm before high-intensity exercise; any irregularities, poor performance, or exercise-induced pulmonary hemorrhage should prompt cardiac re-examination.

PREVENTION AVOIDANCE

• Discontinue administration of furosemide (Lasix), if possible, or use the lowest possible dosage before a race to control exercise-induced pulmonary hemorrhage.
• Discontinue bicarbonate milkshakes.
• Administer potassium or other electrolyte supplementation on a daily basis, if indicated.
• Sudden discontinuation of electrolyte supplementation can result in transient potassium depletion.
• Horses with recent-onset atrial premature depolarizations should be rested and treated with corticosteroids or antiarrhythmics, if indicated, to reduce the frequency of atrial ectopy.

POSSIBLE COMPLICATIONS

• With sustained atrial fibrillation, continued detection of clinical signs the horse was presented for is expected.
• Exercise intolerance may develop in horses asked to perform higher-intensity exercise while in atrial fibrillation.

Cardiovascular

• Prolonged QRS duration—indicates quinidine toxicity.
• Rapid supraventricular tachycardia—treat aggressively with digoxin (see *Precautions*) to slow heart rate.
• Ventricular arrhythmias—treat with the appropriate antiarrhythmic drug unless ventricular rhythm is slow (<100 bpm), uniform, and no R-on-T is detected.
• Hypotension—monitor and treated, if severe, with phenylephrine (0.1–0.2 μg/kg per minute IV to effect).
• Congestive heart failure—treat with digoxin (0.0022 mg/kg IV) and furosemide (1–2 mg/kg IV), if needed.
• Sudden death—try to prevent with continuous ECG and treatment of any arrhythmias that occur.

Respiratory

Upper respiratory tract obstruction—treat with passage of a nasotracheal tube to relieve the upper airway obstruction; administer corticosteroids and antihistamines; emergency tracheotomy, if necessary.

Dermatologic

Urticaria and wheals—treat with corticosteroids and antihistamines.

Reproductive

Paraphimosis—resolves on return of plasma quinidine concentration to negligible levels.

Musculoskeletal

Laminitis—if the horse is uncomfortable, administer analgesics.

Neurologic

• Indicates quinidine toxicity.
• Ataxia—resolves on return of plasma quinidine concentration to negligible levels.
• Convulsions—administer anticonvulsants.
• Bizarre behavior—resolves on return of plasma quinidine concentration to negligible levels.

ATRIAL FIBRILLATION

GI

- Flatulence—resolves on return of quinidine plasma concentrations to negligible levels.
- Oral ulcerations—prevent by not administering drugs PO.
- Diarrhea—resolves on return of quinidine plasma concentrations to negligible levels.
- Colic—indicates quinidine toxicity; treat with analgesics as needed.

EXPECTED COURSE AND PROGNOSIS

- Most horses (90%) with little or no underlying cardiac disease convert to sinus rhythm with quinidine therapy.
- Recurrences occur in $\cong$25% of horses with a suspected duration of atrial fibrillation of $\leq$4 months.
- Recurrences occur in 60% of horses with a duration atrial fibrillation of >4 months.
- Recurrence is mostly likely during the first year after conversion but can occur at any time.
- Prognosis for return to the previous level of athletic performance is excellent in converted horses without significant underlying cardiovascular disease.
- Horses with sustained atrial fibrillation that did not convert to sinus rhythm with treatment or that are not candidates for conversion usually have a normal life expectancy and can be safely used for lower-level athletic performance.
- If an excessively high heart-rate response to exercise limits performance, digoxin (0.011 mg/kg PO BID) can be administered to slow heart rate.
- With significant valvular insufficiency, severity of the valvular heart disease and its progression determine the horse's useful performance life and life expectancy.
- Affected horses with congestive heart failure usually have severe underlying valvular heart or myocardial disease and have a guarded to grave prognosis for life.
- Most affected horses treated for congestive heart failure respond to the supportive therapy and improve for a short time but are euthanized within 2–6 months of initiating treatment.

MISCELLANEOUS

ASSOCIATED CONDITIONS

Any cardiac disease resulting in atrial enlargement predisposes to atrial fibrillation.

AGE-RELATED FACTORS

- Old horses are more likely to have significant underlying cardiac disease with valvular insufficiency and atrial enlargement.
- These horses usually are not candidates for conversion because of significant underlying cardiac disease.

ZOONOTIC POTENTIAL

N/A

PREGNANCY

- Affected pregnant mares without underlying cardiac disease and congestive heart failure should not experience any problems.
- Affected pregnant mares with congestive heart failure can be treated for the underlying cardiac disease with positive inotropic drugs (e.g., digoxin) and diuretics (e.g., furosemide).

SYNONYMS

A fib

SEE ALSO

- Congestive heart failure
- Mitral regurgitation
- Tricuspid regurgitation

ABBREVIATIONS

- AV = atrioventricular
- CK-MB = MB isoenzyme of creatine kinase
- GI = gastrointestinal
- HBDH = α-hydroxybutyrate dehydrogenase
- LDH = lactate dehydrogenase

Suggested Reading

Marr C, Reef VB, Reimer JM, et al. An echocardiographic study of atrial fibrillation in horses: before and after conversion to sinus rhythm. J Vet Intern Med 1995;9:57–67.

McGuirk SM, Muir WW, Sams RA. Pharmacokinetic analysis of intravenously and orally administered quinidine in horses. Am J Vet Res 1981;42:938–942.

Muir WW, Reed SM, McGuirk SM. Treatment of atrial fibrillation in horses by intravenous administration of quinidine. J Am Vet Med Assoc 1990;197:1607–1610.

Parraga ME, Kittleson MD, Drake CM. Quinidine administration increases steady state serum digoxin concentration in horses. Equine Vet J Suppl 1995;19:114–119.

Reef VB, Levitan CW, Spencer PA. Factors affecting prognosis and conversion in equine atrial fibrillation. J Vet Intern Med 1988;2:1–6.

Reef VB, Reimer JM, Spencer PA. Treatment of equine atrial fibrillation: new perspectives. J Vet Intern Med 1995;9:57–67.

Author Virginia B. Reef

Consulting Editor N/A

ATRIAL SEPTAL DEFECT (ASD)

BASICS

DEFINITION

- A congenital defect (i.e., hole) in the interatrial septum that creates a communication between the right and left atria.
- Can be located in the atrial septum immediately adjacent to the ventricular septum (i.e., atrium primum defect), in the area of the foramen ovale (i.e., atrium secundum defect), or in the most basilar portion of the interatrial septum (i.e., sinus venosus–type defect).
- The atrial septum forms in the fetus from the septum primum and the septum secundum. The slit-like communication between these septa (i.e., the foramen ovale) allows passage of blood from right to the left atrium in the fetus.
- The foramen ovale is functionally closed in neonates within 24–48 hours of birth, but anatomic closure may not be complete until 9 weeks.

PATHOPHYSIOLOGY

- A patent foramen ovale occurs when the foramen ovale fails to close.
- Failed formation of one of the two septa results in the other forms of ASD.
- Blood shunts from the higher-pressure left atrium to the lower-pressure right atrium in foals with ASD, creating a left atrial, right atrial, and right ventricular volume overload.
- Size of the ASD determines severity of the volume overload. In horses with a large ASD, the right and left atrial and right ventricular volume overload is severe.
- Over time, stretching of the tricuspid annulus occurs, and tricuspid regurgitation develops. As the tricuspid regurgitation becomes more severe, increases in right atrial pressure result in increased hepatic venous pressure and development of clinical signs of right-sided congestive heart failure.

SYSTEM AFFECTED

Cardiovascular

GENETICS

- Not yet determined in horses.
- Although heritable in other species, it is rare in horses.

INCIDENCE/PREVALENCE

These defects are uncommon as isolated congenital defects and more frequently occur in conjunction with complex congenital heart disease, particularly tricuspid and pulmonic atresia.

SIGNALMENT

Most frequently diagnosed in neonates, foals, and young horses, but may be diagnosed at any age.

SIGNS

General Comments

May be detected as an incidental finding, but usually is part of a more complex, congenital cardiac disorder.

Historical Findings

- Exercise intolerance—medium to large ASDs
- Congestive heart failure—large ASDs

Physical Examination Findings

- No murmur may be present, or a coarse, band- or ejection-shaped, holosystolic murmur with PMI in pulmonic valve area may be detected.
- Premature beats or an irregularly irregular heart rhythm of atrial fibrillation may be present with larger ASDs.

CAUSES

- Failed closure of the foramen ovale
- Congenital malformation of the interatrial septum

RISK FACTORS

- Premature foal
- Neonatal pulmonary hypertension
- Neonatal respiratory distress syndrome

DIAGNOSIS

DIFFERENTIAL DIAGNOSIS

- Physiologic flow murmur—differentiate echocardiographically.
- Pulmonic stenosis (rare)—murmur usually louder; differentiate echocardiographically.
- Aortic stenosis (rare)—murmur usually louder; weak arterial pulses; differentiate echocardiographically.
- Tricuspid atresia—murmur usually louder; foal is unthrifty, tachycardic, and hypoxemic; differentiate echocardiographically.
- Pulmonic atresia—murmur usually louder; may have a continuous machinery murmur; foal is unthrifty, tachycardic, and hypoxemic; differentiate echocardiographically.

CBC/BIOCHEMISTRY/URINALYSIS

N/A

OTHER LABORATORY TESTS

N/A

IMAGING

Electrocardiography

- Atrial premature depolarizations or atrial fibrillation may be present in horses with right and left atrial enlargement.
- Persistent atrial fibrillation has been reported in affected foals and horses.

Echocardiography

- Can determine location of the ASD.
- Atrial septal drop-out is detected at the ASD location and should be visualized in two mutually perpendicular planes.
- The left and right atria and right ventricle are enlarged, dilated, and have a rounded appearance.
- Paradoxic septal motion is detected with a severe right ventricular volume overload.
- Pulmonary artery dilatation is seen in horses with a large shunt.
- Interrogate the entire atrial septum with pulsed-wave or color-flow Doppler with suspected ASD.
- Contrast or color-flow Doppler reveals the shunt from the left to the right atrium through the ASD.
- A small amount of positive contrast may be seen in the left atrium in horses with normal pulmonary arterial pressures or with the Valsalva maneuver at contrast echocardiography.
- A jet of tricuspid regurgitation may be present in horses with a large ASD and marked right atrial and ventricular volume overload.

Thoracic Radiography

Increased pulmonary vascularity and cardiac enlargement may be detected in horses with large shunts.

DIAGNOSTIC PROCEDURES

Cardiac Catheterization

- Right-sided catheterization can be performed to directly measure right atrial, right ventricular, and pulmonary arterial pressures and to sample blood for oxygen content.
- Elevated right atrial, right ventricular, and pulmonary arterial pressures and increased oxygen saturation of right ventricular and pulmonary arterial blood in horses with larger ASDs.

24-Hour Holter Monitoring

Useful in establishing the diagnosis in horses with suspected atrial premature depolarizations.

PATHOLOGIC FINDINGS

- Jet lesions along the defect margins and on the adjacent right atrial endocardium.
- Left atrial, right atrial, and right ventricular enlargement and thinning of the left atrial, right atrial, and right ventricular free wall in horses with a significant shunt.
- Pulmonary artery dilatation in horses with a large shunt or that have developed pulmonary hypertension.
- With congestive heart failure, ventral and peripheral edema, pleural effusion, pericardial effusion, chronic hepatic congestion, and occasionally, ascites may be detected.

ATRIAL SEPTAL DEFECT (ASD)

TREATMENT

APPROPRIATE HEALTH CARE

- Most affected horses require no treatment and can be monitored on an outpatient basis.
- Monitor horses with large shunts on an annual basis.
- Affected horses with congestive heart failure can be treated for congestive heart failure with positive inotropic drugs, vasodilators, and diuretics. Consider humane destruction if congestive heart failure develops, however, because only short-term, symptomatic improvement can be expected.

NURSING CARE

N/A

ACTIVITY

- Affected horses are safe to continue in full athletic work until significant tricuspid regurgitation or atrial fibrillation develops.
- Horses with small defects can be in unrestricted activity and may be able to compete reasonably successfully in upper-level athletic competition.
- Monitor horses with hemodynamically significant defects echocardiographically on an annual basis to ensure they are safe to ride and compete. These horses can be used for lower-level athletic competition but are unlikely to compete at the upper levels of athletic performance.
- Affected horses that develop atrial fibrillation need a complete cardiovascular examination to determine if they are safe to use for lower-level athletic performance.
- Horses with significant pulmonary artery dilatation no longer are safe to ride.

DIET

N/A

CLIENT EDUCATION

- Regularly monitor cardiac rhythm; any irregularities of the rhythm, other than second-degree AV block, should prompt ECG.
- Carefully monitor for exercise intolerance, respiratory distress, prolonged recovery after exercise, increased resting respiratory or heart rate, cough, generalized venous distention, jugular pulses, or ventral edema; if detected, obtain a cardiac re-examination.

SURGICAL CONSIDERATIONS

- Closure of the ASD would be possible with a transvenous umbrella catheter if the diameter of the umbrella was large enough to close the defect.
- Surgical closure is not financially feasible or practical for obtaining equine athletes at this time.

MEDICATIONS

DRUGS OF CHOICE

N/A

CONTRAINDICATIONS

N/A

PRECAUTIONS

N/A

POSSIBLE INTERACTIONS

N/A

ALTERNATIVE DRUGS

N/A

FOLLOW-UP

PATIENT MONITORING

Frequently monitor cardiac rate, rhythm, and respiratory rate and effort.

PREVENTION/AVOIDANCE

N/A

POSSIBLE COMPLICATIONS

Large ASD—atrial fibrillation; congestive heart failure

EXPECTED COURSE AND PROGNOSIS

- Horses with small defects should have a normal performance life and life expectancy.
- Horses with moderate defects also have a normal life expectancy. These horses usually perform successfully only at lower levels of athletic competition, and they may develop atrial fibrillation.
- Horses with large defects have a guarded prognosis, because they may have a shortened life expectancy and performance life, even at the lower levels of athletic competition.
- Affected horses with congestive heart failure usually have a guarded to grave prognosis for life. Most such horses being treated for congestive heart failure should respond to the supportive therapy and transiently improve; however, once congestive heart failure develops, euthanasia is recommended.

MISCELLANEOUS

ASSOCIATED CONDITIONS

- Complex congenital cardiac disease, particularly tricuspid and pulmonic atresia, is likely.
- Tricuspid regurgitation can develop in horses with significant left atrial, right atrial, and right ventricular volume overload secondary to stretching of the tricuspid annulus.
- Pulmonic regurgitation can develop in horses with isolated defects.
- Pulmonic valve leaflets may no longer coapt with stretching of the pulmonary artery from the volume overload.

AGE-RELATED FACTORS

Young horses are more likely to be diagnosed.

ZOONOTIC POTENTIAL

N/A

PREGNANCY

Breeding affected horses is discouraged. The condition is rare, however, and the heritable nature of this defect in horses is not known.

SYNONYMS

N/A

SEE ALSO

- Congestive heart failure—right sided
- Systolic murmurs

ABBREVIATIONS

- AV = atrioventricular
- PMI = point of maximal intensity

Suggested Reading

Reef VB. Cardiovascular disease in the equine neonate. Vet Clin North Am Equine Pract 1985;1:117–129.

Reef VB. Cardiovascular ultrasonography. In: Reef VB, ed. Equine diagnostic ultrasound. Philadelphia: WB Saunders, 1998:215–272.

Reef VB. Echocardiographic findings in horses with congenital cardiac disease. Compend Contin Educ Pract Vet 1991;13:109–117.

Taylor FG, Wooton PR, Hillyer MH, Barr FJ, Luce VM. Atrial septal defect and atrial fibrillation in a foal. Vet Rec 1991; 128:80–81.

Wilson AP. Persistent foramen ovale in a foal. Vet Med 1943;38:491–492.

Author Virginia B. Reef

Consulting Editors N/A

AZOTEMIA AND UREMIA: CREATININE (CR) AND BUN

BASICS

DEFINITION

• Azotemia—the accumulation of nitrogenous waste (e.g., urea, Cr, other nitrogenous substance) in blood, plasma, or serum.
• Uremia—the clinical manifestation of azotemia; a multisystem disorder resulting from the effects of uremic toxins on cellular metabolism and function.
• Cr and BUN typically are measured in serum and used as indices of azotemia.

PATHOPHYSIOLOGY

• Azotemia can result from increased levels of dietary protein, or when urea is supplemented in the diet; fasting; decreased GFR; or resorption of formed urine into the circulatory system.
• In horses, fasting leads to enhanced protein catabolism to meet energy demands and increased BUN; however, in ponies, fasting leads to decreased BUN.
• Accelerated catabolism of endogenous proteins leads to elevated BUN.
• Decreased GFR may result from decreased renal perfusion (i.e., prerenal azotemia); primary renal disease, either insufficiency or failure (i.e., renal azotemia); or urinary obstruction (i.e., postrenal azotemia).
• Azotemia may result from resorption of urine when urinary tract rupture (i.e., postrenal azotemia) occurs.
• In equine azotemia, magnitude of the elevated BUN may be decreased proportional to the increased Cr because of hind-gut fermentation that includes urea-splitting bacteria.

SYSTEMS AFFECTED

• Generalized or systemic effects—depression, weakness, weight loss, edema, and dehydration
• GI—anorexia, diarrhea, uremic stomatitis, uriniferous breath, excessive dental tartar, gingivitis, oral ulceration, mild protein-losing enteropathy, and melena
• Neuromuscular—dullness, lethargy, gait imbalance, tremors, behavioral changes, seizures, and stupor
• Endocrine/metabolic—renal secondary hyperparathyroidism, inadequate production of erythropoietin and 1,25-dihydrocholecalciferol, decreased hormone clearance that prolongs plasma half-life (e.g., parathormone, gastrin), decreased tissue sensitivity (e.g., insulin, parathormone), decreased hormone production (i.e., testosterone), and hypersecretion to re-establish homeostasis (i.e., parathormone)
• Cardiovascular—elevated blood pressure, heart murmur, and cardiac dysrhythmia
• Respiratory—dyspnea
• Hemic/lymphatic/immune—depression anemia and immunodeficiency
• Ocular—scleral and conjunctival injection
• Skin/exocrine—pallor, bruising, dandruff, and dull hair coat

SIGNALMENT

All ages, breeds, and sexes

SIGNS

General Comments

• Azotemia does not always equate to clinical signs of disease described here.
• Unless the animal is uremic, clinical findings are limited to the process causing azotemia—dehydration, urinary outflow tract obstruction, or rupture

Historical Findings

• Weight loss
• Anorexia
• Abnormal urination
• Depression
• Lethargy
• Dental tartar
• Uriniferous breath
• Poor performance
• Lumbar pain
• Colic
• Abdominal distension
• Poor hair coat
• Prolonged posturing to urinate
• PU/PD

Physical Examination Findings

• Fever
• Anorexia
• Depression
• Oral pallor
• Poor body condition
• Ventral edema
• Oral ulceration
• Excessive dental tartar
• Scleral injection
• Colic
• Distended abdomen
• Urine scalding
• Dysuria
• Hematuria
• Halitosis

CAUSES

Prerenal Azotemia

• Renal hypoperfusion caused by decreased circulating volume or decreased blood pressure
• Protein catabolism associated with fever, infection, trauma, myositis, thermal injury, and corticosteroid therapy
• General anesthesia
• Prolonged exercise

Renal Azotemia

Acute or chronic renal failure—primary renal dysfunction affecting glomeruli, renal tubules, renal interstitium, or renal vasculature and impairing 75% of renal function

Postrenal Azotemia

• Obstruction of the urinary tract
• Rupture of the urinary outflow tract

RISK FACTORS

Medical Conditions

• Renal disease
• Diarrhea
• Endotoxemia
• Acute blood loss
• Septic shock
• Prolonged exercise
• Urolithiasis
• Exposure to nephrotoxic chemicals or plants
• Dehydration
• Acidosis
• Hepatic disease
• Neoplasia

Drugs

• Aminoglycosides
• NSAIDs
• Diuretics

Azotemia and Uremia: Creatinine (Cr) and BUN

DIAGNOSIS

DIFFERENTIAL DIAGNOSIS

• With dehydration, hypovolemia, acute blood loss, acute enteritis, some forms of colic, and exhaustive disease syndrome, rule out prerenal azotemia.
• With acute onset of altered urine output (increased or decreased), clinical signs indicating uremia, exposure to nephrotoxic drugs or chemicals, vasomotor nephropathy, and abnormal kidney size, rule out acute renal failure
• With progressive weight loss, PU/PD, pitting edema, dental tartar, oral ulcers, pallor, and signs of uremia that have occurred over several weeks or months, rule out chronic renal failure.
• With abrupt decrease in urine output and acute onset of signs of uremia, stranguria, abdominal distension, enlarged urinary bladder, and signs of colic, rule out postrenal azotemia.

LABORATORY FINDINGS

Drugs That May Alter Lab Results
N/A

Disorders That May Alter Lab Results
N/A

Valid If Run in Human Lab?
Yes

CBC/BIOCHEMISTRY/URINALYSIS

CBC
Nonregenerative anemia may be seen in chronic renal failure caused by decreased erythropoietin production.

Biochemistry
• Interpret BUN and Cr in light of hydration status, presenting complaint, and physical examination findings.
• In horses, the BUN:Cr ratio has been used to differentiate acute from chronic renal failure; however, this ratio can be very unreliable because of differences in diet (i.e., protein intake) and GI bacterial destruction of resorbed urea.
• With chronic renal failure, the BUN:Cr ratio often exceeds 10:1.
• Correcting dehydration deficits and restoring renal perfusion dramatically reduces BUN and Cr in patients with prerenal azotemia.
• Relieving outflow obstruction or correcting the rent in the excretory pathway rapidly decreases the degree of azotemia in patients with postrenal azotemia.
• Hyponatremia and hypochloremia are common in horses with renal disease and can occur with third-compartment spacing of fluid in the uroperitoneum.
• Hyperkalemia is a common finding in urinary tract disruption and uroperitoneum.
• Calcium and phosphorus levels vary in renal disease.
• Hypercalcemia and hypophosphatemia often are seen with chronic renal failure; hypocalcemia and hyperphosphatemia are noted with acute renal failure.
• Hypercalcemia in renal failure depends on dietary content and intake of calcium.

Urinalysis
• Urine specific gravity of >1.020 and urine osmolality of >500 mOsm/kg are consistent with prerenal azotemia.
• Fluid therapy and some medications (e.g., furosemide, α_2-receptor agonists, steroids) may render the urine specific gravity value uninterpretable.
• With dehydration, urine concentrating ability usually is lost in primary renal failure, and urine specific gravity and osmolality are <1.020 and <500 mOsm/kg, respectively.
• Urine specific gravity is not valuable in differentiating postrenal from prerenal or primary renal azotemia.

IMAGING

Radiography
Rarely is used to evaluate the urinary tract in adult horses but is useful in foals and miniature horses.

Ultrasonography
• The urinary tract can be examined transrectally or transabdominally.
• Bladder ultrasonography is best performed transrectally using a 5-MHz probe.
• Transcutaneous ultrasonography of the right or left kidney is best performed with a 2.5- or 3-MHz probe.
• Assess the size and shape of both kidneys and the architecture and echogenicity of the parenchyma.
• The renal medulla is more echolucent than the renal cortex, except for the renal pelvis, which varies in echogenicity.
• With acute renal failure, kidneys may be normal or enlarged, and parenchymal abnormalities often are not detected.
• With chronic renal failure, kidneys are smaller and more echogenic than normal.
• Cystic or mineralized areas more often are associated with chronic renal disease or congenital anomalies.
• Acoustic shadowing represents calculi formation.

Renal Scintigraphy
May be used to document renal function but commonly is not performed.

DIAGNOSTIC PROCEDURES

Urine GGT:Cr Ratio
• Reflects GGT leakage from damaged renal tubular epithelium containing GGT compared to the constant excretion of Cr.
• Calculated as (Urine GGT/Urine Cr) × 100.
• A ratio of >25 suggests proximal tubular damage; this elevation may occur before azotemia develops.
• Finding an elevated ratio depends on having enough remaining tubules that can leak GGT—severe renal fibrosis may yield values in the normal range.

AZOTEMIA AND UREMIA: CREATININE (CR) AND BUN

Fractional Excretion of Electrolytes
• Measurement of electrolytes in serum and urine can be compared to assess renal damage.
• Sodium is the most reliable indicator of choice for renal disease compared with potassium, chloride, and phosphorus.
• Fractional excretion assumes that clearance is relatively consistent, but these parameters can be affected by diet, drug treatment, and lactation.
• Calculated as (Urine [electrolyte] × Serum Cr)/(Serum [electrolyte] × Urine Cr).
• Reported reference intervals for sodium fractional excretion range from 0.01–0.70 in healthy horses.

Rectal Examination
• Bladder—determine size, wall thickness, and presence of calculi or mural mass.
• Left kidney (caudal pole)—determine size and texture.
• Ureter—usually not detectable; enlarged in association with pyelonephritis or ureterolithiasis.

Ultrasound-Guided Renal Biopsy
Can be used to confirm the diagnosis of primary renal failure, to differentiate acute from chronic renal disease, and to identify a specific cause.

Urinary Tract Endoscopy
• Extremely useful diagnostic aid when evaluating abnormal urination.
• In adult horses, a flexible endoscope with an outside diameter of <12 mm and a length of ≥ 1 m is adequate to evaluate the urethra and urinary bladder.
• Normal urethral mucosa is pale pink, with longitudinal folds.
• If the urethra is dilated with air (e.g., to aid passage of the endoscope), the mucosa may appear reddened, and a prominent vascular pattern may appear.
• The ischial arch and colliculus seminalis are the most common sites of posturination or postbreeding hemorrhage in geldings and stallions.
• In the dorsal aspect of the trigone, the ureteral openings can be visualized to determine the source of hematuria or pyuria.
• Biopsy of a bladder mass or collection of a sterile urine sample can also be obtained.

Renal Scintigraphy
May be used to document renal function but commonly is not performed.

TREATMENT

PRERENAL AZOTEMIA
• Based on correcting the underlying cause of renal hypoperfusion or correcting the dehydration deficit.
• Fluid replacement is primary therapy.
• More aggressive treatment in conditions that may lead to primary renal damage or failure.

PRIMARY RENAL AZOTEMIA
• Measures to stop or reverse the immediate cause.
• Supportive care to alleviate clinical signs of uremia; to correct fluid, electrolyte, and acid–base abnormalities; and to resolve the problems associated with decreased renal hormones.

POSTRENAL AZOTEMIA
• Based on eliminating urinary obstruction or correcting the cause of urine leakage.
• Surgical intervention often is required, but correction of any metabolic derangements is paramount.
• Solute diuresis can follow correction of postrenal azotemia; thus, additional fluid therapy may be required to prevent dehydration.

FLUIDS
• IV fluid therapy is indicated for most azotemic patients.
• Commonly used fluids—0.9% saline, Ringer, and lactated Ringer solution.
• Base the amount of fluid administered on the dehydration or volume deficit.
• Correction of the fluid deficit can occur during the first 6 hours without untoward effects, except in patients with hypoproteinemia/hypoalbuminemia and with signs of cardiac disease.

MEDICATIONS

DRUGS OF CHOICE
Treat any patient exhibiting signs of shock appropriately.

CONTRAINDICATIONS
Use nephrotoxic drugs (e.g., aminoglycosides, NSAIDs) with caution in patients with azotemia.

PRECAUTIONS
• Use caution when administering fluids to horses with chronic renal failure, because they can develop significant peripheral and pulmonary edema.
• Use IV fluids cautiously in oliguric or anuric patients to minimize overhydration.
• Use NSAIDs and corticosteroids cautiously. Although they can limit intrarenal inflammation, they also nonselectively block vasodilatory mediators of renal blood flow under conditions of renal hypoperfusion and are not recommended for chronic renal failure.
• Use caution with drugs requiring renal excretion. Horses should be well hydrated when using aminoglycosides and NSAIDs.
• Be aware of adverse reactions and toxic effects that may require altering dosage schedules.

AZOTEMIA AND UREMIA: CREATININE (CR) AND BUN

POSSIBLE INTERACTIONS
N/A

ALTERNATIVE DRUGS
N/A

FOLLOW-UP

PATIENT MONITORING
- Serum urea nitrogen, Cr, and electrolyte concentrations 24 hours after initiating fluid therapy; hydration status; and urine outflow.
- In neonates, monitoring body weight may be helpful.
- With severe acid–base derangements, more frequent monitoring may be required.

POSSIBLE COMPLICATIONS
- Failure to promptly correct prerenal azotemia caused by renal hypoperfusion may result in ischemic renal failure.
- Failure to correct renal azotemia may result in uremia.
- Failure to correct postrenal azotemia (e.g., urinary tract obstruction, uroperitoneum) may result in renal damage or death caused by hyperkalemia and uremia.

MISCELLANEOUS

ASSOCIATED CONDITIONS
N/A

AGE-RELATED FACTORS
- Primary renal failure may occur at any age, but old horses may be at higher risk for azotemia regardless of the cause.
- Postrenal azotemia caused by ruptured bladder is more common in neonatal foals.

ZOONOTIC POTENTIAL
Leptospirosis—rare cause in the horse

PREGNANCY
The ability of a mare to maintain a viable pregnancy decreases as renal function decreases.

SYNONYMS
N/A

SEE ALSO
- Renal failure, acute
- Renal failure, chronic
- Urinary tract obstruction

ABBREVIATIONS
- GFR = glomerular filtration rate
- GGT = γ-glutamyltransferase
- GI = gastrointestinal
- PU/PD = polyuria/polydipsia

Suggested Reading

Finco DR. Kidney function. In: Kaneko JJ, Harvey JW, Bruss ML, eds. Clinical biochemistry of domestic animals. 5th ed. San Diego: Academic Press, 1997:441–481.

Matthews HK, Andrews FM, Daniel GB, Jacobs WR. Measuring renal function in horses. Vet Med 1993;April:349–356.

Schott HC. The urinary system. In: Reed SM, Bayly WM, eds. Equine internal medicine. 1st ed. Philadelphia: WB Saunders, 1998:807–895.

Author Terry C. Gerros

Consulting Editor Claire Andreasen

BABESIOSIS

BASICS

DEFINITION

A tick-borne, noncontagious disease caused by infection of erythrocytes by either of two distinct protozoan parasites, *Babesia caballi* and *B. equi.*

PATHOPHYSIOLOGY

- Infection with *B. caballi* or *B. equi* results in clinical signs referable to infection and lysis of erythrocytes; dual infections are common.
- The erythrocytic stage of *B. equi* can lyse erythrocytes in the absence of specific immune responses; however, the precise role of immune responses to parasite antigens of *B. equi* and *B. caballi* in anemia is not known.
- Occlusion of capillaries within the pulmonary, hepatic, and central nervous system is common during acute infection with *B. caballi.*
- Those surviving acute infection are persistently infected and represent a problem for the international movement of horses, because several countries, including the United States, restrict the entry of horses based on their serologic status to *B. equi* and *B. caballi.*
- Intrauterine transmission appears to be frequent with *B. equi* but rare with *B. caballi* infections; abortions due to fetal infections have been reported for both parasites.

SYSTEMS AFFECTED

- Hemic/lymphatic/immune—lysis of infected erythrocytes leads to anemia and icterus.
- Nervous, hepatobiliary, respiratory—occlusion of capillaries by *B. caballi* can lead to dysfunction within these organ systems.

GENETICS

N/A

INCIDENCE/PREVALENCE

- Infection and clinical disease occur when susceptible horses move into endemic areas or persistently infected horses move into a nonendemic area with tick vectors capable of transmission. Compounding concerns about movement of persistently infected horses is the lack of knowledge about the ability of tick species in nonendemic areas to transmit *B. equi* and *B. caballi.*
- Disease and persistent infection have been reported in southern Florida, the U.S. Virgin Islands, part of Asia, Russia, India, the Middle East, Europe, Africa, Australia, South America, Central America, Mexico, the Philippines, and numerous Caribbean islands.
- Tick vectors include species of *Dermacentor, Hyalomma,* and *Rhipicephalus.*

SIGNALMENT

- Horses, donkeys, their cross-breeds, and zebras are susceptible to babesiosis.
- No known breed, age, or sex predilections.

SIGNS

General Comments

- Clinical signs depend on the immune status of the horse.
- Horses that survive acute infection are immune to clinical disease on reinfection; however, an exception may be those infected with *B. caballi* and cleared of infection by chemotherapy.
- In endemic areas, clinical babesiosis seldom is seen, except when nonimmune (i.e., uninfected) horses are introduced.

Historical Findings

- Acute disease—lethargy, anorexia, fever, anemia, petechial hemorrhages of mucous membranes, and icterus.
- Hemoglobinuria and subcutaneous edema can be observed during progression of *B. equi* infection.
- Exercise intolerance (related to the level of anemia) is common.

Physical Examination Findings

- Signs are common only during the acute phase of infection.
- During acute *B. caballi* infection, high fever, lethargy, hyperemia of mucous membranes with petechial hemorrhages, ventral edema, constipation, colic, dehydration, and icterus are seen.
- Acute *B. equi* infection is similar, with hemoglobinuria and a more pronounced icterus.

CAUSES

- Caused by infection of erythrocytes with the hemoprotozoan parasites *B. caballi* or *B. equi.*
- Anemia—result of hemolysis caused by replication of the erythrocyte-stage parasites.
- *B. caballi* sequesters in the capillaries of organ systems, including the CNS, leading to occlusion of blood flow.

RISK FACTORS

The primary risk factor is movement of uninfected (i.e., nonimmune) horses into endemic areas.

DIAGNOSIS

DIFFERENTIAL DIAGNOSIS

- EIAV—infected horses are seropositive.
- Purpura hemorrhagica—petechial hemorrhages and ventral edema are common; often a history of previous exposure to *Streptococcus equi* or other respiratory pathogens; hemolysis is uncommon.
- Equine viral arteritis virus—hemolysis is uncommon; diagnosis can be confirmed serologically or by viral isolation.
- Equine ehrlichiosis—hemolysis is uncommon.
- Trypanosomiasis
- Leptospirosis
- Red maple-leaf poisoning—Heinz bodies and methemoglobinemia common.

CBC/BIOCHEMISTRY/URINALYSIS

- Anemia
- Leukocytosis
- Hyperbilirubinemia
- Hemoglobinuria (*B. equi*)

OTHER LABORATORY TESTS

- Persistently infected horses have no indication of infection but for specific antiparasite antibody and, occasionally, a level of parasites in the peripheral blood detectable by light microscopy. Definitive diagnosis currently depends on identification of *Babesia* organisms in Giemsa-stained blood smears or by transfusion of blood into a susceptible animal.
- Direct parasitologic verification of chronic *B. caballi* infection is almost impossible but occasionally is successful with *B. equi* infection. The USDA in 1969 adopted CF as the official serologic test for equine babesiosis; this test measures antibodies against *B. equi* or *B. caballi.*
- Horses that test positive on CF assay are restricted from entry into the United States. Serum submitted to state diagnostic laboratories is forwarded to the National Veterinary Services Laboratory (Ames, IA) for testing.

• The CF test has several problems, including false-negative results. Sera with anticomplement activity are not testable.
• Competitive inhibition ELISAs have been developed for serologic detection of antibody against *B. equi* and *B. caballi.* These assays utilize monoclonal antibodies directed against immunodominant epitopes of the erythrocyte-stage parasites and are currently undergoing validation.
• Progress also has been made in routine culturing of *B. caballi* and *B. equi.*

IMAGING
N/A

DIAGNOSTIC PROCEDURES
N/A

PATHOLOGIC FINDINGS
• Horses that die of acute infection may demonstrate subcutaneous edema, serous exudates in the body cavities and pericardium, pronounced icterus, hepatomegaly, splenomegaly, glomerulonephropathy, and petechial hemorrhages of mucosal membranes.
• Histologically, the spleen contains macrophages with intracellular erythrocytes (erythrophagocytosis), the renal tubular epithelium often is degenerated, and hemoglobin is deposited in renal tubules.

TREATMENT

APPROPRIATE HEALTH CARE
Inpatient or outpatient, depending on the severity of clinical signs.

NURSING CARE
Routine care; intensive care usually not needed.

ACTIVITY
Restrict activity.

DIET
Normal diet.

CLIENT EDUCATION
Inform clients of the reportable nature of this infection and its significance regarding the international movement of horses.

SURGICAL CONSIDERATIONS
N/A

MEDICATIONS

DRUG OF CHOICE
• Imidocarb is the most effective and safest chemotherapy to date and eliminates *B. caballi* infections; however, effective therapy for elimination of *B. equi* infection has not been found. Recommended doses are, for *B. equi,* 4 mg/kg every third day for a total of four treatments and, for *B. caballi,* 2 mg/kg for 2 consecutive days for a total of two treatments. Each dose is given IM and divided among at least four injection sites.
• Colic, transient salivation, and purgation are common after imidocarb treatment.
• Do not initiate retreatment after use of imidocarb for *B. equi* infection 30 days after the first treatment.

CONTRAINDICATIONS
• In endemic regions, antibabesial therapy may lead to susceptibility on reinfection. This is especially true for *B. caballi* infections, in which chemotherapy clears persistent infections.
• Donkeys appear very susceptible to the toxic side effects of imidocarb and should not be treated with this drug.

PRECAUTIONS
N/A

POSSIBLE INTERACTIONS
N/A

ALTERNATIVE DRUGS
• Several chemotherapies with antibabesial activity have been tested; these therapies include phenamidine, benenil, and diampron.
• For *B. equi,* parvaquone and buparvaquone have been tested.
• Imidocarb is the most effective and safest of all therapies tested to date.

FOLLOW-UP

PATIENT MONITORING
Monitor hydration status and percentage parasitemia in the peripheral blood.

PREVENTION/AVOIDANCE
Control in endemic areas is most effectively directed at tick vectors.

POSSIBLE COMPLICATIONS
N/A

EXPECTED COURSE AND PROGNOSIS
• Horses that survive acute infection usually, with appropriate supportive care, can return to normal activity. Owners should be advised that such animals are persistently infected and remain a potential source of parasite transmission to susceptible horses.
• Although chemotherapy eliminates *B. caballi* infection in most cases, a chemotherapy has not been identified that eliminates *B. equi* infection.

MISCELLANEOUS

ASSOCIATED CONDITIONS
N/A

AGE-RELATED FACTORS
N/A

ZOONOTIC POTENTIAL
N/A

PREGNANCY
Abortion (especially with *B. equi* infection) is a possible outcome.

SYNONYMS
Piroplasmosis

SEE ALSO
N/A

ABBREVIATIONS
• CF = complement fixation
• EIAV = equine infectious anemia virus
• ELISA = enzyme-linked immunoadsorbent assay
• USDA = U.S. Department of Agriculture

Suggested Reading
Friedhoff KT. The piroplasms of Equidae—significance for international commerce. Berl Munch Tierarztl Wochenschr 1982;95:368–374.
Holman PJ, Chieves L, Frerichs WM, Olson D, Wagner GG. Culture confirmation of the carrier status of *Babesia caballi*–infected horses. J Clin Microbiol 1993;31:698–701.
Knowles DP. Control of *Babesia equi* parasitemia. Parasitol Today 1996;12:195–198.
Knowles RC. Equine babesiosis: epidemiology, control and chemotherapy. Equine Vet Sci 1988;8:61–64.

Author Don Knowles
Consulting Editor Debra C. Sellon

BACTEREMIA/SEPTICEMIA

BASICS

DEFINITION

• *Bacteremia* refers to the presence of viable bacteria in the circulating blood.
• *Septicemia* is defined as systemic disease caused by circulating microorganisms, including viral and fungal microorganisms, and their products.
• *Endotoxemia* specifically refers to the presence of endotoxin within the circulating blood and implies the presence of clinical signs associated with the circulating endotoxin.

PATHOPHYSIOLOGY

In cases of bacteremia, bacteria must gain access to the circulation, necessitating a breach of normal protective mechanisms. This occurs most commonly in the neonate, although adults may be affected, particularly if they are immunocompromised. Portals of entry commonly include the respiratory tract, gastrointestinal tract, placenta, umbilicus, and surgical and traumatic wounds. In a generally healthy animal, normal defense mechanisms rapidly clear circulating bacteria from the bloodstream.

In cases of septicemia, normal defense mechanisms are overwhelmed, allowing the establishment of localized or generalized infection. Passive acquisition of immunoglobulins from maternal colostrum provides for neutralizing and opsonizing activity in the neonate. The phagocytic and killing functions of polymorphonuclear neutrophils are crucial to the initial defense against invading pathogens. These functions, although present, appear to be impaired in the neonate. Other aspects of innate immunity appear to be less effective in the neonate than in the adult, increasing the risk of septicemia in the neonate. The large majority of pathogensassociated with neonatal septicemia are gram-negative bacteria, predominantly *Escherichia coli,* although gram-positive bacteria are gaining recognition in some geographic areas as a major cause of neonatal septicemia. Viral, fungal, and protozoal pathogens are also recognized causes of septicemia. In adults, septicemia can be associated with enterocolitis (e.g., *Salmonellosis*) because loss of the mucosal gastrointestinal barrier provides a route for entry of bacteria and fungi.

Endotoxemia results from the elucidation of lipopolysaccharide (LPS) from the bacteria cell wall of gram-negative pathogens. Endotoxemia is recognized as a sequellum to sepsis in the neonate. Endotoxemia in adults is frequently associated with enterocolitis and pleuropneumonia. Circulating LPS interacts with immune cells, macrophages, and lymphocytes to initiate production of a cascade of soluble immune mediators to produce a wide variety of systemic effects. Imbalance in the production of immune mediators (interleukins, prostaglandins, leukotrienes) can result in septic shock.

SYSTEMS AFFECTED

All body systems can be affected.
• Cardiovascular—Hyperdynamic responses in early septic shock, systemic hypoperfusion, and cardiac depression in later stages.
• Gastrointestinal
• Respiratory
• Renal/urogenital
• Neurologic
• Musculoskeletal
• Endocrine

GENETICS

N/A

SIGNALMENT

• Foals generally within the first 3 days of age, although may occur at almost any age.
• Adult horses of any age, sex or breed.

SIGNS

General Comments

A large variety of clinical signs are associated with infection, and specific signs depend on the stage of the disease process and the organ systems involved.

Historical Findings

• Foals with septicemia may have a history of perinatal problems, dystocia, premature/dysmature/postmature birth, previous abnormal siblings, etc. Failure of passive transfer is commonly reported. Poor management and poor environmental conditions may be present.
• Affected adults may have concurrent immunosuppression or other disease processes.

Physical Examination Findings

• Early signs: non-specific, vague, or non-existent. Easily attributable to other disease processes. Signs include lethargy, scleral injection, petechiation, mucous membrane injection, loss of suck reflex in foals, increased lethargy, or sleepiness.
• Fever is present inconsistently.
• Diarrhea may be the earliest localizing sign in septic foals.
• Other signs: seizures, colic, respiratory distress, uveitis, subcutaneous abscesses, lameness, gait abnormality, joint distention, and periarticular edema.
• Early septic shock: normal blood pressures and blood pressure gradient, variable fever, injected mucous membranes, normal to brisk capillary refill time, tachycardia, agitation, and depression.
• Late stage septic shock is characterized by hypoperfusion and cool distal limbs and extremities, depression, unresponsiveness, hypotension, hypothermia, and gray mucous membranes with delayed capillary refill time.

BACTEREMIA/SEPTICEMIA

DIAGNOSIS

DIFFERENTIAL DIAGNOSIS

Foals

Hypoxic ischemic asphyxial insult, prematurity, and viral sepsis.

Adults

Early sepsis can be confused with almost any disease process. Late stage septic shock is difficult to misdiagnose. Major differentials at that point are hypovolemic (e.g. blood loss) and cardiogenic shock.

CBC/BIOCHEMISTRY/URINALYSIS

CBC

Leukocytosis or leukopenia may be present. Increased numbers of band neutrophils in some cases. Neutropenia is common. Platelet counts may be decreased with associated disseminated intravascular coagulopathy (DIC). Fibrinogen may be normal, increased, or decreased (DIC), depending on stage of disease.

Biochemistry

Hypoglycemia is common in foals and some adult horses. There is metabolic acidosis with advancing hypoperfusion as well as increased lactate. Creatinine and serum urea nitrogen are increased, with dehydration and acute renal failure secondary to renal hypoperfusion in late stages. End stage sepsis is associated with multisystemic organ failure.

Urinalysis

With acute renal failure there is increased protein and cells, as well as altered fractional excretion of sodium and potassium. The animal shows a loss of the ability to concentrate. Urinary parameters may not be valid in animals on intravenous fluid therapy and may not reflect underlying pathology accurately.

OTHER LABORATORY TESTS

Arterial Blood Gas Analysis

Hypoxemia, hypercapnia, and/or acidosis (mixed respiratory and metabolic), particularly in animals with acute respiratory distress syndrome (ARDS) and/or pulmonary edema (PE).

DIAGNOSTIC PROCEDURES

- Blood culture required for definitive diagnosis.
- Culture from localized infection.
- Serial fecal cultures in cases of suspected salmonellosis, clostridiosis.
- Clostridial toxin determination from feces for suspected clostridiosis.

PATHOLOGIC FINDINGS

- Pathology is associated with affected organ systems.
- Pneumonia, focal abscess, pleuritis, peritonitis, enterocolitis, joint and/or physeal infection, menigitis, etc.
- Findings associated with DIC include jugular thrombosis, pulmonary thromboembolism, general or localized petechia and ecchymoses, sponateous hemorrhage, hemorrhage associated with venipuncture, and laminitis.
- Septic shock and end stage multiple organ failure finding may include pulmonary edema, tubular and interstitial nephritis, hepatic lipidosis, hepatic necrosis, myocardial necrosis, and/or gastrointestinal mucosal abnormalities.

IMAGING

- Radiographic abnormalities associated with organ systems involved.
- Thoracic radiography may demonstrate pneumonia or PE. Radiographs of affected joints may be normal at early stages, or may demonstrate radiolucency or other changes associated with the physis with advanced disease.
- Ultrasonsographic abnormalities associated with organ systems involved.
- Thoracic ultrasound may demonstrate pleural fluid or areas of pleural/parenchymal consolidation.
- Abdominal ultrasound may demonstrate thickened areas of small and large intestine, abnormal gastrointestinal motility, and increased peritoneal fluid.
- Cardiac ultrasonography demonstrates early increases in fractional shortening and decreased end-systolic volume, whereas later stages show decreased cardiac contractility and ejection fractions.

BACTEREMIA/SEPTICEMIA

TREATMENT

APPROPRIATE HEALTH CARE

Septic neonates and adults without evidence of septic shock may be treated at home. Horses and foals with evidence of early or late septic shock will benefit from referral to a facility where advanced 24-hr care can be more readily provided.

NURSING CARE

Nursing care in cases of septic shock may be intensive. Continuous intravenous fluid therapy is generally necessary, and intranasal oxygen supplementation should be considered. Affected foals will be recumbent and require frequent turning to prevent decubital sores and lung atelectasis. Hypothermia is common and may require heat lamps and warming blankets.

ACTIVITY

Activity should be restricted.

DIET

Septic foals and adults are frequently anorexic. In addition, gastrointestinal function may be compromised and gastrointestinal rest may be required. Parenteral nutrition should be considered for all foals and in adults in cases in which finances are not a primary concern. Foals with evidence of gastrointestinal discomfort and/or bloat should not be fed until signs resolve. Foals and adults with hypothermia should not be fed enterally, even if they demonstrate an appetite, until they are normothermic.

CLIENT EDUCATION

Foals and adults that do not have serious additional disease beyond localized or mild sepsis frequently respond to treatment and survive. Survival decreases with the onset of early septic shock, although rapid and aggressive intervention at this stage improves survival. Foals and adults with hypotensive septic shock have a guarded to grave prognosis, even with intensive care.

SURGICAL CONSIDERATIONS

- Localized abscesses that are readily accessible may be drained surgically.
- Infected umbilical remnants in foals may be removed surgically if the condition of the patient is stable enough to warrant general anesthesia.
- Lavage of infected joints may be indicated.

MEDICATIONS

DRUG(S) AND FLUIDS

- Broad-spectrum antimicrobial therapy in cases where culture is pending or culture results are negative. Antimicrobial therapy should then be based on culture and sensitivity results.
- Equine plasma should be administered to foals with failure of passive transfer of maternal antibody. Plasma should be given until serum IgG is >800 mg/dL. Plasma therapy may need to be repeated, and IgG may be consumed or lost due to disease processes.
- Plasma and/or whole blood are ideal volume expander fluids, but may not be readily and rapidly available for resuscitation.
- Hyperimmune anti-endotoxin plasma (J-5) therapy may benefit affected foals and adults.
- Adults and foals with dehydration and either early or late septic shock require the administration of intravenous fluids.
- Crystalloids may initially be administered rapidly in shock boluses of 20 mL/kg over 20 min. The patient should then be reassessed and additional boluses given as necessary.
- Colloidal fluids (Hetastarch) given at a dose of 10 mg/kg may aid in resuscitation of early or late septic shock.
- Cases with hypotensive septic shock may require pressor agents. Dopamine and dobutamine are commonly used and require adminstration at a constant rate of infusion. Use of these drugs requires that blood pressure and cardiac rate and rhythm be monitored constantly.
- Non-steroidal anti-inflammatory agents may aid in combating endotoxemia. Flunixine meglumine at 0.25 mg/kg is commonly administered TID IM or IV.
- Intravenous DMSO, although controversial, can be administered at 0.25–1.0 g/kg SID or BID as an anti-inflammatory agent and for diuresis.
- Short-acting corticosteroid therapy (dexamethasone 0.01–0.1 mg/kg IV SID) may be used with septic shock.

BACTEREMIA/SEPTICEMIA

CONTRAINDICATIONS/ PRECAUTIONS/POSSIBLE INTERACTIONS/ALTERNATIVE DRUGS

- Animals with sepsis and septic shock are in delicate physiologic balance. All interventions should be monitored carefully for any change in the patient's condition.
- Aminoglycoside antimicrobials are nephro- and ototoxic given at high dosages and dosage frequencies. Therapeutic drug monitoring should be performed.
- Corticosteroids have been associated with laminitis in the horse.
- Pressor agents may cause cardiac dysrhythmias or result in decreased renal perfusion at certain dosages.
- Non-steroidal anti-inflammatory agents have been associated with gastrointestinal ulceration and renal disease at high dosages and dose frequencies.

FOLLOW-UP

PATIENT MONITORING

- Patients with sepsis or septic shock must be monitored closely.
- Electrolyte and creatinine values should be obtained daily if animals are on intravenous fluids; otherwise, they should be obtained every other day. Urinary output should be monitored. Any decrease is suggestive of poor renal perfusion and possible renal failure.
- Blood glucose should be monitored twice daily if possible, particularly in septic shock patients.
- Frequent arterial blood gas determinations are desirable in cases of septic shock.
- Therapeutic drug monitoring is desirable.
- Arterial blood pressure should be monitored, along with heart rate and rhythm.
- Serial white blood cell counts and fibrinogen determinations aid in monitoring response to therapy. Antimicrobial treatment should continue until clinical signs are resolved and white blood count and fibrinogen are within normal range.

CLIENT EDUCATION

Sepsis and septic shock are best treated by prevention. Clients should be educated as to the importance of early ingestion of good-quality colostrum by neonates and good management practices.

MISCELLANEOUS

Suggested Reading

Freestone JF, Hietala S, Moulton J, Vivrette S. Acquired immunodeficiency in a seven-year-old horse. J Am Vet Med Assoc, 190:689-691, 1987.

Keusis B, Speir SJ. Endotoxemia. In: Equine Internal Medicine. Eds. SM Reed and WM Bayley. WB Saunders, Philadelphia, 1998, pp. 639-451.

Koterba AM, House JK. Neonatal Infection. In: Large Animal Internal Medicine. Ed. BP Smith, Mosby, Philadelphia, 1996, pp. 344-353.

Mackay RJ. Endotoxemia. In: Large Animal Internal Medicine. Ed. BP Smith, Mosby, Philadelphia, 1996, pp. 733-742.

Author Pamela A. Wilkins

Consulting Editor Corinne R. Sweeney

BASISPHENOID/BASIOCCIPITAL BONE FRACTURE

BASICS

OVERVIEW

- A neurologic disease resulting from a fracture of the floor of the calvaria and affecting the medulla oblongata and inner ear areas of the brain.
- Caused by trauma to the poll (i.e., nuchal crest).

SIGNALMENT

- No breed or sex predilection.
- Tends to occur in young, untrained horses.
- Also occurs in old horses under restrictive training methods.

SIGNS

- Many horses are unable to rise.
- Signs of depression, with an obtunded to comatose mentation due to damage to the reticular activating system.
- Affected horses may have nosebleed, bleeding from the ears, and air movement through the ears.
- Sluggish to absent pupillary light reflex and anisocoria.
- Signs associated with cerebral edema, hematoma, and/or parenchymal laceration.
- With brainstem or cerebellar involvement, extensor rigidity and abnormal breathing patterns may be seen.
- Involvement of the pons, medulla oblongata, and vestibular systems are indicated by head tilt and nystagmus.
- Ophthalmic examination may show alterations of retinal vasculature patterns, blurring of the optic disc, and papilledema due to increased intracranial pressure.

CAUSES AND RISK FACTORS

- Sharp trauma to the poll (i.e., nuchal crest) due to flipping over.
- Most commonly associated with training of young horses.
- Can be seen in old horses under restrictive training methods—sidelines; tying a rein around to the saddle to achieve bending.

DIAGNOSIS

DIFFERENTIAL DIAGNOSIS

- Other forms of trauma to the brain—history; physical examination; skull radiography.
- Rabies—postmortem IFA of the brain.
- Meningitis—CSF analysis.
- Encephalitis—CSF analysis.
- Cranial cervical spinal trauma—neurologic examination; radiographic examination.

CBC/BIOCHEMISTRY/URINALYSIS

Usually within normal limits.

OTHER LABORATORY TESTS

- CSF analysis.
- Fluid obtained from the atlanto-occipital space is contraindicated if signs of increased intracranial pressure are seen because of possible herniation of the cerebrum under the tentorium cerebella or through the foramen magnum.
- If fluid is obtained, it will likely have gross evidence of hemorrhage, including increased RBC numbers, increased total protein content, and increased albumin. Platelets, increased immunoglobulins, WBCs, erythrophagocytosis, and xanthochromia also may be seen.
- If the sample is obtained from the lumbosacral space acutely, it may well be within normal limits. If obtained in the subacute period, the sample will show similar changes as those seen with an atlanto-occipital sample.

IMAGING

- Skull radiography is essential but often unrewarding.
- Diagnostic views are difficult to obtain. In full-size horses, they require a focused grid, high-energy x-ray machine, and/or a fast-film screen combination.
- Oblique views, if the horse will allow its head to be moved, may help to highlight a fracture line.
- A fracture line in the basisphenoid or basioccipital bone, or separation of the suture line between these, is diagnostic. A nonossified suture may appear in the normal position. Look for fracture lines through occipital bones adjacent to the condyles.
- A few select referral centers can use CT or magnetic resonance imaging.

DIAGNOSTIC PROCEDURES

N/A

TREATMENT

- Keep the horse in quiet, dark stall, and minimize stimulation.
- Monitor for breathing difficulties, and provide support as necessary.
- Treat any lacerations or abrasions.
- Check for corneal abrasions and lacerations, and treat appropriately.
- Turn the horse frequently to minimize decubital ulcers.
- Use IV fluids cautiously to avoid increasing the intracranial pressure.

MEDICATIONS

DRUGS

NSAIDs

- Flunixin meglumine (1.1 mg/kg IV q12–24h).
- Phenylbutazone (2.2–4.4 mg/kg IV q12–24h).

Steroidal Anti-Inflammatory Agents

- Dexamethasone sodium phosphate (0.1–0.25 mg/kg IV q24h).
- Solu-delta Cortef (500 mg IV).

BASISPHENOID/BASIOCCIPITAL BONE FRACTURE

Diuretics
• DMSO (20–1000 mg/kg IV q12–24 h for 3 days in a 5%–10% solution).
• Mannitol (0.25–2 mg/kg IV)—contraindicated in cases with intracranial hemorrhage.
• Glycerol (0.5–2 mg/kg IV).
• Furosemide (1–3 mg/kg IV q12–24h)—monitor serum electrolytes.

Anticonvulsive Agents
• Diazepam (100–200 mg/kg IV as needed).
• Thiopental sodium (8–12 mg/kg IV to effect to control seizures).
• Glycerol guaiacolate (110 mg/kg IV).
• Chloral hydrate (40–100 mg/kg PO).

CONTRAINDICATIONS/POSSIBLE INTERACTIONS
• Phenothiazine tranquilizers—potentiate seizures.
• α2-Adrenergic agonist—increase intracranial pressure.
• Mannitol—increase edema in cases with intracranial hemorrhage.

FOLLOW-UP

PATIENT MONITORING
Serial neurologic examination to assess deterioration of condition.

PREVENTION/AOVIDANCE
Care, diligence, and patience during training.

EXPECTED COURSE AND PROGNOSIS
• If the horse can regain its feet in 4 hours or less, it will probably live. If not, the horse will either die or be euthanized.
• If the horse recovers, it will probably have residual neurologic and proprioceptive deficits.

MISCELLANEOUS

ASSOCIATED CONDITIONS
N/A

AGE-RELATED FACTORS
N/A

ZOONOTIC POTENTIAL
N/A

PREGNANCY
N/A

ABBREVIATIONS
• CSF = cerebrospinal fluid.
• DMSO = dimethyl sulfoxide.
• IFA = immunofluorescent antibody.

Suggested Reading

DeBowes RM, Gift L. Trauma of the brain and spinal cord. In: Robinson NE, ed. Current therapy in equine practice. 3rd ed. Philadelphia: WB Saunders, 1992:535–539.

Ragle CA. Head trauma. In: Honnas CM, Bertone AL, eds. Vet Clin N Am Equine Pract 1993;9:171–183.

Reed SM. Intracranial trauma. In: Robinson NE, ed. Current therapy in equine practice. 2nd ed. Philadelphia: WB Saunders, 1987:377–380.

Author R. Jay Bickers
Consulting Editor Joseph J. Bertone

BILE ACIDS

BASICS

DEFINITION

Total serum bile acid concentrations above the reference interval indicate hepatocellular mass dysfunction, e.g., $> 15\ \mu M/L$.
Horses do not have a diurnal variation or post-prandial change in bile acid concentration.

Pathophysiology

Bile acids are synthesized by the liver from cholesterol. The primary bile acids are conjugated with glycine or taurine and excreted in the bile. The conjugated bile acids form micelles, with fat for its solubilization and absorption. Most of the bile acids are reabsorbed by an active process in the ileum and carried by the portal circulation back to the liver for reuptake by hepatocytes and reexcretion. In the horse, 95% of the bile acids are reabsorbed and circulated back through the liver. It has been estimated that in ponies, bile acids can be circulated up to 38 times a day. More than 90% of the bile acids are removed by the liver on first passage, but a small amount gets past the liver into the systemic circulation. Higher than normal concentrations of bile acids appear in the serum for three reasons.
1. Hepatocellular damage prevents sufficient numbers of hepatocytes from removing adequate amounts from the portal circulation.
2. Cholestasis prevents the excretion of bile acids along with other products in the bile.
3. Portal–systemic shunts allow the portal blood containing high concentrations of reabsorbed bile acids to by-pass the liver.

Systems Affected

- Hepatobiliary—this is not only an indicator of hepatic damage, but retained bile acids can also be toxic to hepatocytes.
- Gastrointestinal—bile acids can damage the mucosal barrier and cause ulcerations, or in the colon induce excess secretion, causing diarrhea.
- Skin/exocrine—it is thought that bile acids deposited in the skin induce pruritus.

SIGNALMENT

Portal–caval shunts have been reported in foals. Horses of any age can have hepatic dysfunction.

SIGNS

Signs associated with hepatic disfunction include icterus, behavioral changes, weight loss, dermatitis of white areas, pruritus, diarrhea, coagulation disorders, and stridorous breathing. High concentrations of bile acid itself can cause ulceration with colic, bruxism, and gastric reflux, or hypersecretion and diarrhea, or pruritus.

CAUSES

The causes of increased bile acid concentration are hepatocellular damage, bile blockage, or portal–systemic shunts. Hepatocellular damage can occur from pyrrolidizine alkaloid toxicity; acute hepatitis (Theiler's disease, serum hepatitis); chronic active hepatitis; other hepatotoxins including plants, chemicals, and drugs; hyperlipemia; and in foals, iron toxicity and Tyzzer's disease. Some of these can also cause intrahepatic cholestasis. Extrahepatic cholestasis is uncommon, but may result from cholangitis, cholangiohepatitis, cholelithiasis, or parasites or tumors obstructing the bile duct. Portal–caval shunts have been reported in only a few foals.

RISK FACTORS

Exposure to pasture or hay containing hepatotoxic plants increases the risk. Giving products such as tetanus antitoxin or pregnant mare's serum to adult horses increases the risk of Theiler's disease.

DIAGNOSIS

DIFFERENTIAL DIAGNOSIS

Primary hepatobiliary disease may be suspected if there is a history of exposure to hepatotoxic plants or chemicals, or if equine serum products have been administered. Icterus and behavioral changes noted on physical examination also point to hepatocellular damage; however, many horses with liver disease are not icteric. Laboratory tests or liver biopsy are needed to differentiate between primary hepatocellular disease and bile obstruction, or between the different causes of hepatocellular disease.

LABORATORY FINDINGS

Drugs That May Alter Lab Results

N/A

Disorders That May Alter Lab Results

Ileal disease impairs reabsorption of bile acids.

Valid If Run in Human Lab?

Yes

CBC/BIOCHEMISTRY/URINALYSIS

High serum activity of gamma glutamyl transferase (GGT) would indicate cholestasis or hepatocellular disease. High serum activity of sorbitol dehydrogenase (SDH) or glutamate dehydrogenase (GDH) would indicate hepatocellular disease. High serum activity of alkaline phosphatase (ALP) would indicate cholestasis. High concentrations of direct reacting (conjugated) bilirubin would indicate cholestasis. High concentrations of either total or indirect reacting (unconjugated) bilirubin would indicate hepatocyte damage or hemolysis. Note that indirect bilirubin increases with anorexia in the horse. A direct to total ratio of bilirubin of >0.3 would indicate cholestasis in the horse. Absence of urobilinogen in fresh horse urine might indicate bile blockage. Increase of bilirubin in urine would indicate cholestasis. Very high concentrations of bile acids with minimal increases in bilirubin or liver derived enzymes would warrant the investigation of a possible portal–caval shunt. Blood (serum) urea nitrogen, glucose, clotting factors and albumin may be reduced in liver disease, but these are non-specific changes, and often do not occur until late in the disease process.

OTHER LABORATORY TESTS

Blood ammonia may be elevated in liver disease, and may be elevated and a causative factor in hepatic encephalopathy. Rapid analysis, including placing the plasma sample on ice, is required for ammonia concentration assays. Prolonged PT or PTT may indicate lack of clotting factors because of hepatocellular disease.

BILE ACIDS

IMAGING

Ultrasonographic Findings

Hyperechogenicity of the parenchyma occurs with cirrhosis or fatty change.

Hypoechogenicity occurs with passive congestion and suppuration. Abscesses may be identified. Bile duct obstruction may produce enlarged common and intrahepatic bile ducts and thickening. Choleliths can sometimes be identified. Ultrasound also is useful in guiding a liver biopsy instrument.

DIAGNOSTIC PROCEDURES

Liver biopsy is useful in differentiating the causes of liver disease or cholestasis. A blind percutaneous liver biopsy can be performed relatively safely on most horses. The biopsy specimen should be submitted for histopathologic evaluation and bacterial culture. The location within the liver lobule of the hepatocyte damage, the presence of inflammation, and the condition of the bile ducts may help rule out certain diseases.

TREATMENT

Treatment varies with the cause of the underlying disease. Diet changes may be necessary to support the liver with hepatic disease. A low-protein, high-quality protein diet containing higher amounts of branch-chain amino acids should be provided. Available energy should be increased by frequent feeding of energy-dense carbohydrates. Surgery may be needed for bile duct obstruction or shunts.

MEDICATIONS

DRUGS AND FLUIDS OF CHOICE

Vary depending on the underlying disease. Nothing specific is needed in most cases to reduce bile acid concentration, although in humans, cholestyramine has been used to bind bile acids in the gut and reduce the amount of its reabsorption.

CONTRAINDICATIONS

Vary depending on the underlying disease and medication used.

PRECAUTIONS

Vary depending on the underlying disease and medication used.

POSSIBLE INTERACTIONS

Vary depending on the underlying disease and medication used.

ALTERNATE DRUGS

Vary depending on the underlying disease.

FOLLOW-UP

PATIENT MONITORING

Recheck the bile acids and liver-derived enzymes, depending on underlying disease and progression of the clinical signs in the patient.

POSSIBLE COMPLICATIONS

Many causes of elevated bile acids are life-threatening, and some are not treatable. Bile acids themselves may induce gastric ulcers, secretory diarrhea, and pruritus.

MISCELLANEOUS

ASSOCIATED CONDITIONS

N/A

AGE-RELATED FACTORS

Oral iron toxicity and Tyzzer's disease are conditions of foals.

ZOONOTIC POTENTIAL

N/A

PREGNANCY

N/A

SYNONYMS

N/A

SEE ALSO

Liver enzymes, bilirubin, liver disease.

ABBREVIATIONS

- ALP = alkaline phosphatase
- GDH = glutamate dehydrogenase
- GGT = gamma glutamyl transferase
- PT = prothrombin time
- PTT = partial thromboplastin time
- SDH = sorbitol dehydrogenase

Suggested Reading

West HJ. Evaluation of total plasma bile acid concentrations for the diagnosis of hepatobiliary disease in horses. Res Vet Sci 1989;46:264-270.

Pearson EG. Diagnosis of liver disease. In: Smith BP, ed. Large animal internal medicine.2nd ed. St Louis: Mosby, 1996;913-920.

Anwer MS, Gronwall RR, Engelking LR, et al. Bile acid kinetics and bile secretion in the pony. Am J Physiol 1975;229:592.

Author Erwin G. Pearson

Consulting Editor Claire B. Andreasen

BILIRUBIN, HIGH

BASICS

DEFINITION

Serum or plasma concentrations exceeding the reference interval.

PATHOPHYSIOLOGY

• Most bilirubin in the blood of normal horses originates from the breakdown of hemoglobin by macrophages in the mononuclear phagocyte system that have phagocytized senescent or damaged erythrocytes.
• Macrophages release water-insoluble, unconjugated (i.e., indirect) bilirubin into the blood, where it then binds to albumin. This form of bilirubin does not normally pass through renal glomeruli into urine. Unconjugated bilirubin is removed by hepatocytes in a carrier-mediated process. Some unconjugated bilirubin is refluxed back into the blood; however, most is conjugated to a water-soluble form, which is secreted into the biliary system.
• In normal horses, very little conjugated (i.e., direct) bilirubin is regurgitated back into systemic circulation.
• Once in the intestines, conjugated bilirubin is metabolized by microflora into urobilinogen. A small amount of urobilinogen is absorbed into the portal circulation and excreted into urine.
• Conjugated bilirubin is filtered by the kidney, and increased blood concentrations are associated with bilirubinuria.
• Compared to many other species, normal horses have higher blood concentrations of bilirubin (primarily unconjugated).
• Hyperbilirubinemia occurs secondary to hemolytic anemia, hepatocellular disease, and biliary obstruction.

SYSTEM AFFECTED

Skin/Exocrine

• Yellow discoloration of the skin, sclera, or mucous membranes can be detected when plasma bilirubin concentrations exceed 2–3 mg/dL.
• Among normal horses, ≅10%–15% have a slight yellow discoloration of their sclera or mucous membranes.

Renal/Urologic

• Dark-colored urine caused by increased conjugated bilirubin.
• Hyperbilirubinuria often precedes detectable hyperbilirubinemia.

SIGNALMENT

• All ages and breeds.
• Newborns are at risk for neonatal isoerythrolysis.
• Young foals are predisposed to infectious hepatitis—*Bacillus piliformis*; herpes virus.
• Hyperlipidemia and hepatic lipidosis commonly occur in ponies and miniature horses.

SIGNS

Historical Findings

• Anorexia
• Depression
• Lethargy
• Weakness
• Icterus

Physical Examination Findings

• Hemolytic anemia—pale mucous membranes, tachycardia, tachypnea, and fever.
• Hepatocellular disease or posthepatic biliary obstruction—weight loss, behavioral/neurologic changes (i.e., hepatic encephalopathy), abdominal pain, fever, diarrhea, ascites, edema, hemorrhagic diathesis, photodermatitis, and pruritus.

CAUSES

Prehepatic Icterus

• Hemolytic disorders cause elevated total and unconjugated bilirubin when increased production overwhelms the ability of hepatocytes to uptake and metabolize bilirubin.
• Conjugated bilirubin may increase mildly because of increased hepatic production and associated regurgitation.
• Causes for hemolytic disorders—immune-mediated processes (e.g., neonatal isoerythrolysis, primary immune-mediated disease, immune-mediated disease secondary to drug therapy, infectious agents, neoplasia), infectious diseases (e.g., babesiosis, equine infectious anemia), oxidant-induced damage (e.g., red-maple leaf toxicity, onion toxicity), fragmentation (e.g., DIC), and severe hepatic failure.

Fasting Icterus

• The most common cause of hyperbilirubinemia.
• Occurs secondary to intestinal disorders and many systemic diseases.
• Anorexia or decreased food intake is associated with elevated unconjugated bilirubin levels in the blood within 12 hours of onset that plateau after 2–3 days.
• Hyperbilirubinemia rarely exceeds 6–8 mg/dL and is independent of hemolysis, hepatocellular disease, or biliary obstruction.
• The mechanism likely involves impaired bilirubin uptake by hepatocytes.
• Values normalize once sufficient food intake resumes.

Hepatic Icterus

• Hepatocellular disorders cause increased unconjugated and conjugated bilirubin because of impaired bilirubin uptake, conjugation, or secretion.
• Unconjugated bilirubin predominates.
• Suspect hepatic disease whenever conjugated bilirubin comprises 25%–30% of total bilirubin values.
• Acute hepatocellular diseases more commonly are associated with hyperbilirubinemia than with chronic diseases.
• Hepatocellular disorders associated with hyperbilirubinemia—Theiler's disease, infectious diseases (e.g., bacteria, herpes virus), toxic hepatopathies, chronic active hepatitis, neoplasia, and hepatic lipidosis.

Posthepatic Icterus

• Biliary tract obstruction causes decreased bilirubin excretion and subsequent elevated blood concentrations of unconjugated and conjugated bilirubin.
• Conjugated bilirubin levels rarely exceed 30%–40% of total bilirubin values.
• Causes of biliary obstruction—cholangitis, cholelithiasis, hepatitis, neoplasia, fibrosis, and biliary hyperplasia.

RISK FACTORS

• Hyperbilirubinemia frequently occurs secondary to fasting or anorexia.
• Mild hyperbilirubinemia may occur for several days after prolonged exercise in healthy horses.
• Anabolic steroids cause mild icterus because of cholestasis, which resolves after cessation of drug therapy.
• Hyperbilirubinemia may occur secondary to hemolytic disease.

BILIRUBIN, HIGH

DIAGNOSIS

DIFFERENTIAL DIAGNOSIS

Prehepatic icterus

- Acute history of depression, weakness, or lethargy.
- Physical examination reveals pale mucous membranes, mild icterus, and often, fever.
- With severe anemia, heart murmurs may be auscultated, and heart and respiratory rates increase.

Fasting Icterus

- History of anorexia of varying length.
- Physical examination reveals mild to moderate icterus.
- Clinical signs referable to the primary underlying disorder.

Hepatic or Posthepatic Icterus

- Acute to chronic history of anorexia, depression, weight loss, or polydipsia.
- Physical examination may reveal moderate to severe icterus, abdominal pain, behavioral changes, ascites, edema, fever, diarrhea, steatorrhea, hemorrhagic diathesis, photodermatitis, or pruritus.

LABORATORY FINDINGS

Drugs That May Alter Lab Results

- A number of drugs are reported to cause artifactual changes in total or conjugated bilirubin measurements, depending on the methodology used.
- Check with the laboratory performing the assay for possible interference.

Disorders That May Alter Lab Results

- Total and conjugated bilirubin usually are measured in serum or heparinized plasma using spectrophotometric or dry-reagent methods.
- Exposure to direct sunlight or fluorescent lighting may decrease total bilirubin concentration.
- Centrifuge whole blood within 4 hours of collection.
- Samples are stable up to 4 hours at room temperature, 7 days at 4°C, and 6 months at −20°C or lower.
- Hemolysis has variable effects on bilirubin concentrations measured using spectrophotometry and dry reagents.
- Lipemia falsely increases bilirubin measurements using spectrophotometric methods.

Valid if Run in Human Lab?

Yes

CBC/BIOCHEMISTRY/URINALYSIS

Prehepatic Icterus

- Severe decreases in RBC count, PCV, and hemoglobin concentration.
- If hemolysis is intravascular, hemoglobinemia and hemoglobinuria are expected.
- Total protein and albumin concentrations are normal.
- Microscopy of a blood smear may reveal agglutination, spherocytes, Heinz bodies, eccentrocytes, schistocytes, or erythroparasites.
- Neutrophilia with a left shift may be present.
- Liver enzymes (e.g., AST, SDH, LDH) are normal to slightly elevated secondary to hypoxia.

Fasting Icterus

- RBC count, PCV, and hemoglobin concentration are normal to slightly decreased.
- Liver enzymes are normal to minimally elevated.
- Bile acids may increase up to threefold in horses fasted for >3 days.

Hepatic Icterus

- RBC count, PCV, and hemoglobin concentration are normal to slightly decreased.
- Albumin concentrations usually are normal in acute and decreased in chronic hepatocellular disease.
- Globulin concentrations are normal to increased.
- Liver enzymes (e.g., AST, SDH, LDH, ALP, GGT) are significantly increased.
- Degree of elevation of some liver enzymes lessens with chronicity.
- With significant impairment of hepatic function, BUN, glucose, and cholesterol may decrease.
- Concentrations of bile acids and ammonia increase.
- Elevated triglycerides in horses or ponies with hyperlipemia and hepatic lipidosis.
- Urine contains increased bilirubin and detectable urobilinogen.

Posthepatic Icterus

- RBC count, PCV, and hemoglobin concentration are normal to slightly decreased.
- Total protein and albumin concentrations usually are normal.
- Enzymes indicative of hepatocellular damage (e.g., AST, SDH, LDH) are mildly increased; those indicative of biliary obstruction (e.g., ALP, GGT) are moderately to markedly increased.
- BUN, glucose, and cholesterol usually are normal.
- Bile acids are elevated.
- Urine contains increased bilirubin, and urobilinogen may be absent.

OTHER LABORATORY TESTS

- Prehepatic icterus—consider Coggins test, direct Coombs' test, antinuclear antibody test, osmotic fragility, or serology for babesiosis to determine cause of the anemia.
- Hepatic icterus—measurement of clotting times (i.e., PT, APTT) and FDP are recommended in horses with hemorrhagic diathesis or before surgery to assess risk of hemorrhage.

IMAGING

- Ultrasonography is useful to evaluate liver size, changes in hepatic parenchyma, and biliary patency.
- Radionucleotide imaging may detect altered blood flow or parenchymal changes.

BILIRUBIN, HIGH

DIAGNOSTIC PROCEDURES

Hepatic biopsy for histopathology and bacterial culture may elucidate the cause of hepatic or posthepatic icterus.

TREATMENT

PREHEPATIC ICTERUS

- Hospitalize patients for initial treatment, and restrict activity.
- Limitation of further erythrocyte destruction requires elimination of the inciting cause.
- IV fluid therapy to maintain cardiovascular function and renal perfusion.
- Compatible whole-blood or packed RBC transfusions are required to restore erythrocyte mass in severely anemic horses.

FASTING ICTERUS

- Identification and treatment of the underlying disorder are vital.
- No specific therapy for hyperbilirubinemia is required.
- Offer a high-quality diet; the icterus will resolve when food intake resumes.

HEPATIC OR POSTHEPATIC ICTERUS

- Treatment is supportive to maintain the horse until liver regeneration can occur.
- Hospitalize for initial treatment.
- Restrict activity, and protect horse from sunlight if photodermatitis is present.
- IV fluid therapy to maintain hydration and correct electrolyte imbalances.
- Provide a balanced, high-quality diet (e.g., high carbohydrates, low protein)—a mixture of one-part cracked corn and two-parts beet pulp in molasses (2.5 kg of feed per 100 kg of body weight per day) can be divided into six feedings; oat or grass hay is recommended.
- Administer vitamin B_1, K_1, and folic acid weekly.
- Surgery may be required in some cases of biliary obstruction.

MEDICATIONS

DRUGS OF CHOICE

Prehepatic Icterus

- Discontinue any current drug therapy to rule out drug-induced IMHA.
- Treatment of IMHA includes immunosuppressive doses of corticosteroids—dexamethasone (0.05–0.2 mg/kg IM or IV SID, decreasing gradually once PCV stabilizes).

Hepatic or Posthepatic Icterus

- No specific drug therapy.
- Bacterial hepatitis or cholangitis are best treated with antibiotics as determined by culture and sensitivity results.
- Chronic active hepatitis with a suspected immune-mediated origin may respond temporarily to corticosteroid therapy—dexamethasone (0.05–0.1 mg/kg IM or IV SID for 4–7 days, then gradually decreasing over several weeks).
- Hepatic encephalopathy—neomycin (10–100 mg/kg PO q6h for 1 day); lactulose (0.3 mL/kg via nasogastric tube q6h).
- Xylazine (0.5–1.0 mg/kg) may reduce agitation associated with hepatic encephalopathy.

CONTRAINDICATIONS

Hepatic or posthepatic icterus:

- Avoid drugs known to be hepatotoxic.
- Drugs that consistently cause hepatocellular disease in horses include phenothiazine and erythromycin.
- Drugs associated with idiosyncratic hepatotoxicity include aspirin, diazepam, erythromycin, halothane, isoniazid, nitrofurantoin, phenobarbital, phenytoin, rifampin, and sulfonamides.

PRECAUTIONS

Hepatic or posthepatic icterus:

- Use drugs cautiously in general, because many require biotransformation in the liver.
- Dosages of some drugs may need to be altered.
- Avoid analgesics, anesthetics, and barbiturates whenever possible.
- Avoid drugs that rely heavily on liver metabolism and excretion—chloramphenicol, erythromycin, and corticosteroids.

POSSIBLE INTERACTIONS

N/A

ALTERNATIVE DRUGS

N/A

BILIRUBIN, HIGH

FOLLOW-UP

PATIENT MONITORING

- Prehepatic icterus—serial CBCs as required by the underlying disease process.
- Hepatic or posthepatic icterus—regular measurement of liver enzymes, albumin, and bilirubin as required by the underlying disease process.

POSSIBLE COMPLICATIONS

N/A

MISCELLANEOUS

ASSOCIATED CONDITIONS

N/A

AGE-RELATED FACTORS

Bilirubin often is elevated in foals because of decreased hepatic uptake and conjugation and increased turnover of fetal hemoglobin with RBC destruction; values decrease to adult levels by 1 month of age.

ZOONOTIC POTENTIAL

N/A

PREGNANCY

N/A

SYNONYMS

- Hyperbilirubinemia
- Icterus
- Jaundice

SEE ALSO

- Hemolytic anemia
- Topics regarding liver disease

ABBREVIATIONS

- ALP = alkaline phosphatase
- APTT = activated partial thromboplastin time
- AST = aspartate aminotransferase
- DIC = disseminated intravascular coagulation
- FDP = fibrin degradation product
- GGT = γ-glutamyltransferase
- IMHA = immune-mediated hemolytic anemia.
- LDH = lactate dehydrogenase
- PCV = packed cell volume
- PT = prothrombin time
- SDH = sorbitol dehydrogenase

Suggested Reading

Barton MH, Morris DD. Diseases of the liver. In: Reed SM, Bayly WM, eds. Equine internal medicine. Philadelphia: WB Saunders, 1998.

Duncan JR, Prasse KW, Mahaffey EA. Veterinary laboratory medicine. 3rd ed. Ames, IA: Iowa State University Press, 1994:130–151.

Lofstedt J. Hepatobiliary diseases. In: Ogilivie TH, ed. Large animal internal medicine. Baltimore: Williams & Wilkins, 1998.

Morris DD. Diseases of the hemolymphatic system. In: Reed SM, Bayly WM, eds. Equine internal medicine. Philadelphia: WB Saunders, 1998.

Tennant BC. Hepatic function. In: Kaneko JJ, Harvey JW, Bruss ML, eds. Clinical biochemistry of domestic animals. 5th ed. San Diego: Academic Press, 1997.

Author Jennifer S. Thomas
Consulting Editor Claire B. Andreasen

BLADDER PARALYSIS AND INCONTINENCE

BASICS

DEFINITION

• Bladder paralysis results from partial or complete loss of detrusor function and most often manifests by urinary incontinence and scalding of the perineal area (mares) and inner aspect of the hind limbs (both sexes).
• Incontinence develops when intravesicular pressure exceeds resting urethral sphincter pressure, and, thus, also may occur with loss of urethral sphincter function despite normal detrusor function.
• In theory, a distinction between these two should be important clinically; however, most cases of bladder paralysis/incontinence are long-standing and complicated by UTI before clinical evaluation occurs.
• Response to treatment often is poor, unless the problem is a transient clinical sign of equine herpes myelitis or equine protozoal myeloencephalitis.
• In occasional mares with incontinence from decreased urethral sphincter tone, hypoestrogenism has been speculated as a cause, because successful long term management with estradiol has been reported.
• Incontinence in young horses most often results from ectopic ureter, for which surgical correction is indicated.

PATHOPHYSIOLOGY

• Bladder paralysis can be caused by a variety of disease processes and is pathogenetically separated into three types—reflex or UMN bladder (also known as spastic or autonomic bladder), paralytic or LMN bladder, and myogenic or noneurogenic bladder.
• Initially, UMN bladder is characterized by increased urethral resistance, leading to increased intravesicular pressure before voiding can occur. Voiding may occur as short bursts of urine passage, with incomplete bladder emptying, and rectal examination reveals a turgid bladder that is small to increased in size.
• LMN and myogenic bladder paresis result in chronic bladder distension from decreased or absent detrusor activity. Rectal palpation reveals a large, flaccid bladder, and urine usually can be expressed by placing pressure on the bladder.
• Initially, the signs of UMN bladder differ from those of the other two; this type of problem usually is not recognized in horses until more significant incontinence develops in association with progressive loss of detrusor function.
• LMN disease limited to the external urethral sphincter could result in incontinence with normal detrusor function; such a clinical syndrome has not been well documented in horses but may relate to hypoestrogenism in occasional mares. In fact, by the time incontinence develops into a clinically important problem, the pathogenetic mechanism usually cannot be specifically determined.
• Trauma during natural breeding or parturition is an additional mechanism by which direct injury to the urethral sphincter can occur and lead to a syndrome of urinary incontinence (and infertility).
• In both sexes, but perhaps more important in males, lower back pain has been a suggested cause for development of bladder paresis/paralysis. Lumbar pain could make it difficult for horses to posture to urinate and completely empty the bladder. Incomplete bladder emptying would lead to accumulation of crystalline sludge in the ventral aspect of the bladder (i.e., sabulous urolithiasis), progressive bladder distension, loss of detrusor function, and paralysis (i.e., myogenic bladder).
• In young horses, incontinence from ectopic ureter results from a developmental anomaly; affected horses also posture and urinate normally when ectopic ureter is a unilateral problem.

SYSTEM AFFECTED

• Renal/urologic
• Neurologic
• Musculoskeletal
• Reproductive

SIGNALMENT

Breed Predilections

None documented

Mean Age and Range

Ectopic ureter is a developmental anomaly and results in incontinence from birth.

Predominant Sex

• Bladder paralysis, accompanied by sabulous urolithiasis, appears more common in males due to the longer urethra.
• Postpartum mares may be at greater risk for incontinence from trauma sustained during parturition.
• Occasional mares may develop incontinence from hypoestrogenism.

SIGNS

• Urinary incontinence and scalding of the perineal area (mares) and inner aspect of the hind limbs (both sexes).
• Affected horses may appear painful while posturing to urinate or may not assume a normal voiding posture.
• Additional signs of neurologic disease—weakness, ataxia, etc., with bladder paralysis/incontinence from an underlying neurologic disease.
• Signs of systemic disease (e.g., fever, partial anorexia, weight loss) may be observed if complicated by upper UTI (e.g., pyelonephritis).

CAUSES

• Neurologic disease—equine herpes myelitis, equine protozoal myeloencephalitis, spinal cord trauma, cauda equine neuritis.
• Intoxication—grazing *Sorghum* sp. hybrids (e.g., Sudan grass, Johnson grass) containing hydrocyanic acid.
• Trauma—postbreeding or postpartum in mares.
• Hypoestrogenism—suspected cause of incontinence in occasional mares.
• Ectopic ureter—young horses.
• Idiopathic—possibly from lumbar pain/orthopedic disease, resulting in posturing difficulty and incomplete bladder emptying.

RISK FACTORS

• Trauma—to spinal cord or associated with breeding or parturition.
• Other neurologic diseases.
• Exposure to cyanogenic plants.
• Musculoskeletal problems affecting posturing to urinate.

BLADDER PARALYSIS AND INCONTINENCE

DIAGNOSIS

DIFFERENTIAL DIAGNOSIS

- Normal estrus behavior in mares can cause perineal staining with crystalloid material and be confused with incontinence.
- Accompanying neurologic disease—equine herpes myelitis, equine protozoal myeloencephalitis, spinal cord trauma, and cauda equine neuritis.

CBC/BIOCHEMISTRY/URINALYSIS

- CBC—usually normal unless UTI extends to upper urinary tract, leading to variable leukocytosis.
- BUN and Cr—normal unless complicated by moderate to severe bilateral pyelonephritis.
- Urinalysis—urine specific gravity usually is normal (1.020–1.035), but increased numbers of WBCs and bacteria may be seen on sediment examination if complicated by UTI.

OTHER LABORATORY TESTS

Perform quantitative urine culture in all cases.

IMAGING

- Transabdominal ultrasonography—renal parenchymal architecture may be abnormal (e.g., loss of detail of corticomedullary junction, cavitary lesions with abscess formation, nephrolithiasis) if complicated by pyelonephritis.
- Transrectal ultrasonography—confirms bladder size and may demonstrate accumulation of sabulous material in ventral aspect of the bladder.
- Abdominal radiography—IV pyelography (less useful in foals than in small-animal patients) may confirm ectopic ureter in foals with incontinence.
- Urethroscopy/cystoscopy—to assess bladder mucosa inflammation, accumulation of sabulous material, and integrity of ureteral orifices, which may be wide open with chronic bladder paralysis (supporting vesiculoureteral reflux and probable ascending pyelonephritis).

DIAGNOSTIC PROCEDURES

- Bulbocavernosus reflex (males)—when normal, contraction of the urethral sphincter can be palpated per rectum when the glans penis is gently squeezed by an assistant.
- Cystometry—continuous recording of intravesicular pressure during saline infusion to assess detrusor muscle function; threshold for onset of detrusor contraction in normal horses is 90 ± 20 cm H_2O.
- Urethral pressure profile—after passage of a balloon-tipped catheter into the bladder, pressure in the balloon is continuously recorded as the catheter is withdrawn through the urethral sphincter to assess external sphincter muscle function; in normal horses, pressure typically is >100 cm H_2O and waves of contractions can be appreciated on the tracing.
- Neurologic examination—to document additional neurologic deficits.
- CSF—cytology and Western blot analysis for equine protozoal myeloencephalitis.
- Electromyography—to assess perineal and tail muscles for evidence of denervation (i.e., LMN disease).
- Nuclear scintigraphy—may be useful to evaluate possible thoracolumbar musculoskeletal disease.

TREATMENT

- Proper recognition and treatment of all underlying primary neurologic disease processes.
- Removal from exposure to cyanogenic grasses.
- Medications to improve detrusor function (e.g., bethanecol) or enhance urethral sphincter tone (e.g., phenoxybenzamine or estradiol cypionate).
- Nursing care—daily cleaning of perineum and hind limbs to minimize skin irritation from incontinence; application of petrolatum to scalded areas.
- In cases of long-standing "idiopathic" bladder paralysis and associated incontinence, daily nursing care (i.e., cleaning of the perineum and hind limbs), prophylactic or therapeutic antimicrobial treatment, and possibly intermittent bladder lavage to remove sabulous material.
- Appropriate antimicrobial therapy for secondary UTIs.
- Surgical correction of ectopic ureter by unilateral nephrectomy or attachment of the distal ureter to the bladder neck.

MEDICATIONS

DRUGS OF CHOICE

Bethanecol

- 0.25–0.75 mg/kg SQ or PO q8h
- Parasympathomimetic agent with somewhat selective effect on smooth muscle of the GI tract and bladder.
- Stimulates postganglionic effector cells (i.e., detrusor myocytes) to improve detrusor muscle tone and strength of contraction.
- Response to treatment usually is poor because of long-standing detrusor paresis/paralysis before the problem is recognized clinically, except perhaps with acute herpes myelitis or equine protozoal myeloencephalitis.
- If no improvement within 3–5 days, discontinue therapy.

Phenoxybenzamine

- 0.7 mg/kg PO q6h
- α-Adrenergic blocker that can decrease urethral sphincter tone in UMN bladder; again, this condition has not been well documented in horses.

BLADDER PARALYSIS AND INCONTINENCE

Estradiol Cypionate

- 4 μg/kg IM every other day
- Estrogen appears to modulate the effect of norepinephrine on α-adrenergic–receptor activity in the urethral sphincter.
- Estrogen may improve urethral sphincter tone in mares with hypoestrogenism-associated incontinence.

Antimicrobials

- Sulfamethoxazole/trimethoprim or sulfadiazine/trimethoprim (preferable due to less hepatic metabolism of sulfadiazine than sulfamethoxazole) combinations (20 mg/kg PO q12–24 h) are the most practical long term treatment.
- These combinations can be used prophylactically or therapeutically for established UTI.
- Because they are concentrated nearly 100-fold in urine, they may achieve therapeutic minimum inhibitory concentrations against pathogens that are reported to be resistant.

NaCl

- 1–2 oz., twice daily, added to feed or mixed with water and administered as a PO slurry.
- Will increase flow of urine and decrease sedimentation of crystalloid material in ventral aspect of the bladder.

CONTRAINDICATIONS

N/A

PRECAUTIONS

Using bethanecol cautiously, because it may increase GI motility and lead to signs of colic.

POSSIBLE INTERACTIONS

N/A

ALTERNATIVE DRUGS

N/A

FOLLOW-UP

PATIENT MONITORING

- In cases of bladder paresis/paralysis and associated incontinence from neurological disease, regular repeat physical and neurologic examination; cystometry and urethral pressure profiles could be repeated at 2-4 week intervals if clinical improvement is uncertain.
- In cases of long-standing "idiopathic" bladder paralysis and associated incontinence, regular (weekly or monthly) assessment of overall condition—attitude, appetite, body weight, etc.

POSSIBLE COMPLICATIONS

- Moderate to severe dermatitis from urine scald.
- Sabulous urolithiasis
- UTI—cystitis, possibly complicated by ascending pyelonephritis.

EXPECTED COURSE AND PROGNOSIS

- The prognosis for recovery in cases of bladder paresis/paralysis and associated incontinence from neurological disease is guarded and depends on response to treatment of the underlying disease and duration of paresis/incontinence (generally more favorable if <2 weeks). Evidence of some detrusor function by cystometry and a normal urethral pressure profile improves the prognosis; such horses warrant aggressive treatment.
- The prognosis for recovery of cases of long standing "idiopathic" bladder paralysis and associated incontinence is poor; owner frustration often leads to a decision for euthanasia within a few months after the problem is first recognized.

BLADDER PARALYSIS AND INCONTINENCE

MISCELLANEOUS

ASSOCIATED CONDITIONS

- Equine herpes myelitis
- Equine protozoal myeloencephalitis
- Cauda equina neuritis
- Spinal cord trauma
- Thoracolumbar trauma/pain
- Hypoestrogenism
- Urine pooling and infertility—mares

AGE-RELATED FACTORS

- Hypoestrogenism is more likely in old mares.
- Ectopic ureter is more likely in young horses.

ZOONOTIC POTENTIAL

N/A

PREGNANCY

Increased risk of breeding and foaling trauma–induced incontinence.

SYNONYMS

Enzootic ataxia and cystitis—herd outbreaks associated with intoxication.

SEE ALSO

- UTI

ABBREVIATIONS

- CSF = cerebrospinal
- GI = gastrointestinal
- LMN = lower motor neuron
- UMN = upper motor neuron
- UTI = urinary tract infection

Suggested Reading

Bayly WM. Urinary incontinence and bladder dysfunction. In: Reed SM, Bayly WM, eds. Equine internal medicine. Philadelphia: WB Saunders, 1998:907–911.

Clark ES, Semrad SD, Bichsel P, Oliver JE. Cystometrography and urethral pressure profiles in healthy horse and pony mares. Am J Vet Res 1987;48:552–555.

Ronen N. Measurements of urethral pressure profiles in the male horse. Equine Vet J 1994;26:55–58.

Author Harold C. Schott II

Consulting Editor Harold C. Schott II

BLINDNESS ASSOCIATED WITH TRAUMA

DEFINITION
Head injuries associated with optic nerve or optic nuclei damage that have minimal other signs.

PATHOPHYSIOLOGY
Injuries to the back of the head can be associated with blindness. When blindness occurs, it is often associated with unilateral or bilateral rupture of the optic nerve. However, on occasion, horses with caudal head trauma that are blind can recover sight within a few days. In these cases, blindness may have been due to occipital cortical (optic cortex) edema or other pathology that resolves. There is a possibility that the optic nerves can be traumatized, but not completely ruptured.

SYSTEMS AFFECTED
Central nervous system and other traumatized tissues.

SIGNALMENT
No specific signalment.

SIGNS

Historical
A recent history of trauma, especially when the horse rolled backwards or received pol trauma.

Physical Examination
Lack of or sluggish pupillary light reflexes and menace response is indicative. Degrees of other central nervous system signs will depend on the extent of damage. Often the pupils are widely dilated in bilateral optic nerve rupture. Within the next 2 to 6 weeks, there is generalized retinal degeneration and optic nerve atrophy in the affected eye(s).

CAUSES
Trauma most often to the back of the head.

RISK FACTORS
N/A

DIAGNOSIS
Physical examination findings consistent with blindness and a recent history of trauma to most commonly the back of the head.

DIFFERENTIAL DIAGNOSIS
N/A

CBC/BIOCHEMISTRY/URINALYSIS
No specific abnormalities.

OTHER LABORATORY TESTS
N/A

IMAGING
Skull radiography may indicate trauma, but if blindness is the only abnormality, it is likely that there will be no changes evident.

OTHER DIAGNOSTIC PROCEDURES
N/A

PATHOLOGIC FINDINGS
Rupture of the optic nerves.

TREATMENT
No specific treatment is indicated unless the injury extends to other central nervous system tissues.

DRUGS
N/A

CONTRAINDICATIONS
N/A

PRECAUTIONS
N/A

POSSIBLE INTERACTIONS
N/A

ALTERNATIVE DRUGS
N/A

BLINDNESS ASSOCIATED WITH TRAUMA

FOLLOW-UP

N/A

PATIENT MONITORING

N/A

Observe the animal over the course of several days. This is to allow for cortical edema to resolve under the circumstances that this is the only abnormality.

POSSIBLE COMPLICATIONS

N/A

PROGNOSIS

No recovery if the nerves are ruptured.

MISCELLANEOUS

N/A

ASSOCIATED CONDITIONS

N/A

AGE-RELATED FACTORS

N/A

ZOONOTIC POTENTIAL

N/A

PREGNANCY

N/A

SYNONYMS

N/A

SEE ALSO

N/A

ABBREVIATIONS

N/A

Suggested Reading

Martin L, et al: Four cases of traumatic optic nerve blindness in the horse. *Equine Vet J* 18:133–137, 1986.

Author Joseph J Bertone, DVM, MS, Diplomate ACVIM

Consulting Editor Joseph J Bertone, DVM, MS, Diplomate ACVIM

BLOOD CULTURE

BASICS

DEFINITION

• A diagnostic procedure used to identify pathogenic microorganisms.
• A positive blood culture is one in which pathogens have been propagated and identified.
• Performing a blood culture involves aseptic collection of two or three 10–30-mL blood samples. These are collected during a rise in body temperature or at different times (minimum of 30–60 minutes apart) and before instituting antibiotic therapy. The blood samples are inoculated into broth culture media for propagation in both aerobic and anaerobic environments. Although not ideal, it is common for only a single blood sample to be cultured in foals with suspected neonatal septicemia.

PATHOPHYSIOLOGY

A positive culture occurs when microorganisms are present in the circulation because of systemic infection or local infection not contained at its primary site.

SYSTEM AFFECTED

• Hemic/lymph/immune—microorganisms, usually bacteremia, must be present in the circulation for a blood culture to be positive; therefore, the hemic system is always affected.
• Primary infections leading to positive cultures can affect any system—respiratory, cardiovascular, GI, nervous, hepatobiliary, renal/urologic, musculoskeletal, reproductive, and skin.

SIGNALMENT

• Any age, breed, or sex.
• Positive cultures are most common in neonatal foals with septicemia.
• Adult horses with infections not contained in the primary site can have positive cultures.

SIGNS

Historical Findings

• Inappetence, depression, and lethargy.
• Vary depending on location of the primary infection.

Physical Examination Findings

• Fever, anorexia, depression, tachycardia, tachypnea, and mucous membrane hyperemia.
• Signs referable to individual body systems where the primary infection is localized.
• Dehydration and shock in some animals.

CAUSES

Infectious Agents

Any condition that results in circulating microbial organisms, usually bacteria.

Neonatal Septicemia

• The most common disease associated with a positive blood culture.
• Many different bacteria can cause neonatal septicemia; most commonly, these are Gram-negative—*Escherichia coli, Actinobacillus equuli, Salmonella* sp., *Streptococcus* sp., *Klebsiella* sp., *Enterobacter* sp., *Staphylococcus* sp., *Clostridium* sp., and *Pasturella* sp.
• Mixed infections occur in approximately half of foals with septicemia.

Septicemia

• In adult horses, septicemia is not common, but positive blood cultures can occur when local infection is not contained at the primary site.
• Such conditions include endocarditis, abdominal abscess, pleuritis, pneumonia, renal abscess, retroperitoneal abscess, and pyometra.
• Blood cultures are not needed and, therefore, not performed when the primary site of infection can be identified and material from that area cultured.

RISK FACTORS

• Failure of passive transfer of immunoglobulins and heavy exposure to pathogens in the environment or uterus are associated with neonatal septicemia and, therefore, positive blood cultures.
• Failure of passive transfer is associated with premature lactation, colostrum with low antibody content, and insufficient intestinal absorption of immunoglobulins.
• Failure of passive transfer occurs more frequently in premature, weak, or orphaned foals.
• Other immunodeficiencies, such as combined immunodeficiency.
• Repeated doses of corticosteroids depress the immune response to infectious agents, increasing the likelihood of worsening infection and positive culture.
• Local infection or abscess.

DIAGNOSIS

DIFFERENTIAL DIAGNOSIS

Differentiate from a false-positive culture caused by contamination, which can result from errors in the collection, transfer, or incubation of samples.

LABORATORY FINDINGS

Drugs That May Alter Lab Results

• Antimicrobial agents can inhibit growth of microorganisms in culture.
• Blood culture should be performed before starting antibiotic therapy.

Disorders That May Alter Lab Results

N/A

Valid If Run in Human Lab?

• Yes; however, a veterinary laboratory may provide more useful results.
• Knowledge of the likely organisms can influence culture techniques, and the antibiotics used to determine microbial sensitivity in human labs often are not appropriate for treatment of horses.

CBC/BIOCHEMISTRY/URINALYSIS

CBC

• Leukopenia or leukocytosis, left shift, and increased fibrinogen.
• Hypoproteinemia with failure of passive transfer in foals.
• Elevated PCV and TP with dehydration or shock.

Biochemistry

• Abnormalities vary depending on the organ system involved.
• Hypoalbuminemia and hyperglobulinemia in animals with abscesses at primary sites of infection.
• Hypoglycemia is common in foals with neonatal septicemia.

OTHER LABORATORY TESTS

• If a specific septic focus is identified, culture a sample collected from that area; the likelihood of positive culture from the primary site is greater than that for blood culture.
• Serum IgG levels are low in neonatal foals with failure of passive transfer of immunoglobulins.
• Metabolic acidosis and hypoxemia are common blood-gas abnormalities in foals with neonatal septicemia.
• Abnormalities in the clotting profile (e.g., increased prothrombin time, partial thromboplastin, fibrin degradation products, thrombocytopenia) indicative of disseminated intravascular coagulation may occur in severely affected foals.
• Abnormalities can be present in abdominal, pleural, or cerebrospinal fluid if these are sites of primary infection—increased nucleated cell count, increased protein, degenerative changes in cell morphology, and intracellular bacteria.

IMAGING

Radiography, ultrasonography, and occasionally, nuclear scintigraphy can be useful in identifying the primary site of infection responsible for positive blood cultures.

DIAGNOSTIC PROCEDURES

- Depending on the focus of infection, abdominocentesis, thoracocentesis, cerebrospinal fluid tap, liver biopsy, renal biopsy, endoscopy, tracheal wash, and laparoscopy may be useful in diagnosing the primary reason for a positive blood culture.
- Samples collected from normally sterile sites should be cultured as well as evaluated microscopically.

TREATMENT

NEONATAL FOALS

- Neonatal foals with positive blood cultures require intensive care and generally should be treated on an inpatient basis.
- Medical management, in addition to appropriate antibiotic therapy, includes IV fluid therapy and supplying immunoglobulins, usually by administration of plasma.
- It also may involve total or partial parenteral nutrition, mechanical ventilation or nasal insufflation with oxygen, antiendotoxic medication (e.g., low-dose flunixin meglumine), and antiulcer medication (e.g., cimetidine, ranitidine, omeprazole).
- Consider surgical excision with acquired patent urachus or umbilical remnant infection.
- With septic arthritis, joint lavage should be performed.

ADULT HORSES

- Specific treatment depends on the focus of infection; hospitalization may be required.
- Medical management, in addition to appropriate antibiotic therapy, depends on the system involved.
- Surgical drainage of infected foci is indicated. This may require a surgical procedure, such as celiotomy to locate and excise, drain, or marsupialize an abdominal abscess.

NURSING CARE

- Keep horses and foals with positive cultures in a clean, dry stall.
- Do not ride adult horses with positive cultures.
- Anorexia occurs in many horses and foals with positive cultures. Therefore, monitor food intake, and supplement (e.g., total or partial parenteral nutrition, tube feeding) if indicated.

CLIENT EDUCATION

- Abdominal and other abscesses as well as endocarditis and pleuropneumonia can be difficult to treat successfully; treatment often is prolonged and expensive.
- Surgical drainage or excision of infected foci is not always possible but usually shortens the duration of treatment.

MEDICATIONS

DRUGS OF CHOICE

Antibiotics

- An essential part in treatment of bacterial infections.
- Choice is based on blood culture results.
- Broad-spectrum antibiotics can be initiated after collection of samples for culture.
- Commonly used broad-spectrum antibiotic combinations include sodium penicillin (22,000 IU/kg IV QID) and gentamicin (6.6 mg/kg IV SID) in adults and penicillin (22,000 IU/kg IV QID) and amikacin (4–8 mg/kg IV BID–TID) in foals.
- Monitor serum amikacin concentrations in critically ill and premature foals, because the dose per kilogram and the dose interval may need to be increased to maintain therapeutic levels without exceeding toxic trough values.

NSAIDs/Antiendotoxic Drugs

- Flunixen meglumine (0.25 mg/kg IV TID) with endotoxemia.
- Higher doses (1 mg/kg IV BID) for treatment of inflammation and fever reduction.

CONTRAINDICATIONS

Glucocorticoids:

- May temporarily alleviate clinical signs in animals with positive blood cultures, but repeated doses lead to immunosuppression and subsequent worsening of infection.
- Do not use as an antipyretic or anti-inflammatory drug in horses and foals with positive blood cultures.

PRECAUTIONS

N/A

ALTERNATIVE DRUGS

N/A

FOLLOW-UP

PATIENT MONITORING

- Foals with positive blood cultures associated with failure of passive transfer should have clinical parameters monitored frequently throughout each day.
- Blood gas analysis q6–12h in severely affected foals.
- CBC often is repeated daily during early stages of treatment.
- Other diagnostic tests are repeated depending on the system involved—radiographs of the chest or joints; depending on response to therapy.

POSSIBLE COMPLICATIONS

Depend on the underlying cause.

MISCELLANEOUS

ASSOCIATED CONDITIONS

N/A

AGE-RELATED FACTORS

- Blood cultures commonly are performed in neonatal foals to diagnose neonatal septicemia.
- Septicemia is much less common in adult horses.

ZOONOTIC POTENTIAL

Various bacteria identified on blood culture can infect humans, but this is not common and can be avoided by proper handling of samples.

PREGNANCY

Infections associated with positive blood cultures in pregnant mares also can affect the fetus, causing fetal death and abortion or neonatal septicemia.

SYNONYMS

N/A

SEE ALSO

- Abdominal abscesses
- Endocarditis
- Fever
- Neonatal septicemia
- Other diseases that result in bacteremia

ABBREVIATIONS

- GI = gastrointestinal
- PCV = packed cell volume
- TP = total protein

Suggested Reading

Forbes BA, Granato PA. Processing specimens for bacteria: blood. In: Murray PR, Baron EJ, Pfaller MA, Tenover FC, Yoken RH, eds. Manual of clinical microbiology. 6th ed. Washington, DC: ASM Press, 1995:267–271.

Paradis MR. Update on neonatal septicemia. Vet Clin North Am Equine Pract 1994;10:109–135.

Weinstein MP. Current blood culture methods and systems: clinical concepts, technology, and interpretation of results. Clin Infect Dis 1996;23:40–46.

Author Jill E. Parker

Consulting Editor Claire B. Andreasen

BLOOD TRANSFUSION REACTIONS

BASICS

OVERVIEW

• Acute, delayed, immune- or nonimmune-mediated reactions subsequent to blood transfusions.
• Acute hemolytic reactions are the most feared and caused by antibodies interacting with antigen on the surface of RBCs; antigen–antibody complexes and resultant complement activation lead to lysis of RBCs, release of vasoactive substances leading to hemodynamic alterations, and activation of the hemostatic system.
• Organ systems—hemic/lymphatic/immune, respiratory, skin/exocrine, gastrointestinal, and neuromuscular.
• Differences in inherited blood types, WBC and platelet antigens, and protein polymorphisms contribute to incidence.

SIGNALMENT

Horses and mules

SIGNS

Historical Findings

• Previous transfusion of blood or blood products.
• For NI, usually a multiparous mare.
• Transfusion of old, damaged, or hemolyzed blood.

Immune-Mediated Reactions

• Acute hemolytic reaction—hemoglobinuria, hemoglobinemia, fever, and hypotension.
• Delayed hemolytic reaction—poor response to RBC transfusion and mild to no icterus.
• Nonhemolytic febrile reaction—fever and chills.
• Systemic anaphylaxis—serious reaction characterized by respiratory distress and hypotension.
• Urticaria—development of small wheals over body, most often noticeable around the head.

Nonimmune-Mediated Reactions

• Sepsis—fever, tachycardia, tachypnea, leukopenia, and hypotension.
• Circulatory overload—hypertension and pulmonary edema.
• Citrate toxicity—muscle fasciculations and decrease in ionized calcium.
• Hemolysis—hemoglobinemia and hemoglobinuria.
• Infectious disease—signs pertain to the transmitted disease agent.

CAUSES AND RISK FACTORS

Immune-Mediated Reactions

• Acute hemolytic reaction—caused by recipient antibody against infused donor RBC antigen. Mare antibody against Aa or Qa can cause NI; mare antibody against a donkey RBC antigen can cause NI in mules.
• Delayed hemolytic reaction—minor reaction caused by recipient antibody against infused donor RBC antigen; hemolysis occurs after 3–14 days.
• Nonhemolytic febrile reaction—immune reaction to donor leukocyte, platelet, major histocompatibility antigens, or plasma protein antigens.
• Systemic anaphylaxis—caused by a reaction to soluble proteins in donor plasma.
• Urticaria—caused by a reaction to soluble proteins in donor plasma.

Nonimmune-Mediated Reactions

• Sepsis—contaminated blood from poor collection or storage techniques.
• Circulatory overload—more likely in neonates quickly receiving large volumes of blood.
• Citrate toxicity—caused by rapid infusion of large volumes of citrated blood or plasma.
• Hemolysis—transfusion of damaged and hemolyzed RBCs after excessive heating, freezing, or mechanical damage.
• Infectious disease—agents (e.g., EIAV) can be transmitted via blood transfusion.

Risk Factors

• Previous transfusion of blood or blood products.
• For NI, history of previous foals from that mare.
• Improper or aseptic handling and storage of blood or transfusion supplies and equipment.

DIAGNOSIS

DIFFERENTIAL DIAGNOSIS

• Hemolysis—rule out ongoing hemolytic disease.
• Fever, respiratory distress, hypotension—rule out underlying infectious or inflammatory disease.

CBC/BIOCHEMISTRY/URINALYSIS

Hemoglobinemia, hemoglobinuria, bilirubinemia, bilirubinuria, and leukopenia.

OTHER LABORATORY TESTS

• Repeat cross-match to confirm incompatibility.
• Coombs' test on foal with suspected NI or to determine presence of anti-RBC antibody in mare serum.

IMAGING

N/A

DIAGNOSTIC PROCEDURES

Culture of transfused blood or blood culture from patient with suspected sepsis.

BLOOD TRANSFUSION REACTIONS

TREATMENT

• Emergency inpatient intensive care.
• Stop transfusion; maintain IV access with appropriate crystalloid or colloid solution.
• Monitor heart and respiratory rates; determine blood pressure.
• Hypotension—initiate infusion of fluids.
• NI—remove foal from mare; if foal is severely anemic, transfuse with Aa- or Qa-negative blood.

MEDICATIONS

DRUGS

• Severe anaphylaxis—epinephrine (0.01 mg/kg of 1:1000 dilution [1.0 mg/ml] IM or 0.01 mg/kg of 1:10,000 dilution [0.1 mg/ml] IV).
• Dexamethasone (0.05–0.2 mg/kg IV) or prednisolone sodium succinate (0.25–2.0 mg/kg IV) may also be given.
• Less severe allergic reactions—dexamethasone (0.05–0.1 mg/kg IM or IV) or flunixin meglumine (0.25 mg/kg IV or IM).
• Septicemia—IV antibiotics and fluid therapy.
• Volume overload with pulmonary edema—diuretics (furosemide, 1 mg/kg IV) and intranasal oxygen (15 L/min).
• Hypocalcemia—calcium gluconate (4 mg/kg or 0.1–0.2 mEq/kg IV slowly) while monitoring the cardiac rate and rhythm.

CONTRAINDICATIONS/POSSIBLE INTERACTIONS

N/A

FOLLOW-UP

PATIENT MONITORING

Check vital signs, PCV/TS, and plasma color immediately before, during, and after transfusion.

PREVENTION/AVOIDANCE

• Use healthy donors; type or cross-match blood before transfusion.
• Collect, store, and administer blood appropriately.
• Blood type mares before breeding to identify those at risk for NI (i.e., negative for Aa or Qa); at-risk mares may be bred to Aa/Qa-negative stallions.
• Screen mare serum for antibody against RBC antigens 2-4 weeks before foaling.

POSSIBLE COMPLICATIONS

• Hemolysis can lead to renal failure and disseminated intravascular coagulation.
• Volume overload can lead to cardiac failure.

EXPECTED COURSE AND PROGNOSIS

• Most reactions follow an acute course.
• Prognosis—good in stable animals but guarded in severely ill animals or when not recognized.

MISCELLANEOUS

ASSOCIATED CONDITIONS

N/A

AGE-RELATED FACTORS

Neonatal foals exposed to anti-RBC colostral antibody can develop NI.

ZOONOTIC POTENTIAL

N/A

PREGNANCY

An acute, severe reaction with resultant hypotension and organ ischemia in a pregnant mare may result in death or abortion of the foal.

SEE ALSO

• Anemia
• Anemia, aplastic
• Anemia, Heinz body
• Anemia, immune-mediated
• Hemorrhage, acute
• Hemorrhage, chronic
• NI
• Thrombocytopenia

ABBREVIATIONS

• EIAV = equine infectious anemia virus
• NI = neonatal isoerythrolysis
• PCV = packed cell volume
• TS =

Suggested Reading

Divers TJ. General comments on blood transfusions. In: Orsini JA, Divers TJ, eds. Manual of equine emergencies. Philadelphia: WB Saunders, 1998:294–296.

Author K. Jane Wardrop
Consulting Editor Debra C. Sellon

BLUE-GREEN ALGAE TOXICOSIS

BASICS

OVERVIEW

- Acute intoxication caused by hepatotoxins or neurotoxins produced under certain environmental conditions by several genera of blue-green algae (cyanobacteria).
- Such algae are found in bodies of water such as reservoirs, lakes, and farm ponds.
- Toxigenic blue-green algae include *Microcystis, Anabaena,* and *Aphanizomenon* spp.
- *Microcystis* spp. produce the hepatotoxin microcystin; *Anabaena* spp. produce the neurotoxins anatoxin-a and anatoxin-a_s; and *Aphanizomenon* spp. produce anatoxin-a.
- Other potentially toxigenic blue-green algae include *Nodularia spumigena* and *Oscillatoria aghardii.*
- Documented equine cases of intoxication do not appear in the literature, but blue-green algae toxins are toxic to a wide variety of livestock species.
- Toxins are produced during environmental conditions favorable to rapid algal growth—"algal bloom".
- Microcystin causes acute and massive hepatic necrosis, intrahepatic hemorrhage, and hypovolemic shock.
- Anatoxin-a is a postsynaptic cholinergic agonist causing initial nicotinic-receptor stimulation and subsequent depolarizing neuromuscular blockade.
- Anatoxin-a_s is a cholinesterase inhibitor causing muscarinic- and nicotinic-receptor stimulation.

SIGNALMENT

N/A

SIGNS

Microcystin

- Weakness, reduced responsiveness, reluctance to move, anorexia, pallor of mucous membranes, poor capillary refill time, mental derangement, and bloody diarrhea.
- Death generally occurs within hours of the onset of clinical signs but may be delayed for several days.

Anatoxin-a

- Muscle fasciculations, collapse, exaggerated abdominal breathing, cyanosis, convulsions, and death.
- Affected animals often are found dead.

Anatoxin-a_s

- Signs attributable to muscarinic-receptor stimulation—colic, diarrhea, salivation, lacrimation, increased urination, and dyspnea.
- Muscle fasciculations caused by nicotinic stimulation.
- Cyanosis and seizures preceding death.

CAUSES AND RISK FACTORS

- Warm, sunny weather with high nutrient content in a body of water is conducive to algal blooms and toxin production.
- Steady winds that propel toxic blooms to shore allow for ingestion by drinking animals.

DIAGNOSIS

DIFFERENTIAL DIAGNOSIS

- Microcystin toxicosis—other causes of acute hepatic damage such as aflatoxicosis, iron and alsike clover disease, idiopathic drug sensitivity, Theiler's disease, and Tyzzer's disease (i.e., detection of toxicant, history)
- Anatoxin-a—acute intoxications such as cyanide, OP, and carbamate insecticides and yew (i.e., detection of toxicant)
- Anatoxin-a_s—OP and carbamate insecticides (i.e., detection of insecticide); slaframine

CBC/BIOCHEMISTRY/URINALYSIS

- Microcystin toxicosis—increases in serum bile acids, ALP, GGT, and AST
- Anatoxin-a toxicosis—no significant findings
- Anatoxin-a_s toxicosis—no significant findings

OTHER LABORATORY TESTS

- Anatoxin-a_s toxicosis—depressed cholinesterase activity in whole blood and diaphragm

IMAGING

N/A

DIAGNOSTIC PROCEDURES

- Microscopic examination of bloom material and stomach contents can identify characteristic algal structure.
- IP injection of a bloom extract into mice that results in characteristic clinical signs and postmortem findings can assist in confirming intoxication.
- Detection of specific toxins in bloom material is possible, but tests are not widely available.

BLUE-GREEN ALGAE TOXICOSIS

PATHOLOGIC FINDINGS

• Microcystin toxicosis—detection of algal clumps in GI tract, grossly evident hepatomegaly, histologic lesions including massive hepatocellular necrosis beginning centrilobularly and extending to periportal areas, and severe hepatic hemorrhage.
• Anatoxin-a toxicosis—detection of algal clumps in GI tract; no significant lesions.
• Anatoxin-a_s toxicosis—detection of algal clumps in GI tract; evidence of diarrhea and pulmonary congestion; often no significant lesions.

TREATMENT

• Often unsuccessful because of the rapid onset of clinical signs and death.
• If early after bloom ingestion, GI decontamination.
• Microcystin toxicosis—fluids for hypovolemia, glucose for hypoglycemia, and whole blood for blood loss; correct hyperkalemia and acid—base imbalances.
• Anatoxin-a_s toxicosis—atropine may reverse muscarinic signs.

MEDICATIONS

DRUGS

• AC (2–5 g/kg in water slurry [1 g of AC in 5 mL of water] PO)
• Anatoxin-a_s toxicosis—atropine to effect

CONTRAINDICATIONS/POSSIBLE INTERACTIONS

N/A

FOLLOW-UP

PATIENT MONITORING

Microcystin toxicosis—monitor liver function and coagulation status.

PREVENTION/AVOIDANCE

Chemical control of algal growth in water with copper sulfate or other algicides.

POSSIBLE COMPLICATIONS

Microcystin toxicosis—hepatic encephalopathy; secondary photosensitization.

EXPECTED COURSE AND PROGNOSIS

• Often rapid onset of clinical signs and death.
• Guarded prognosis

MISCELLANEOUS

ASSOCIATED CONDITIONS

N/A

AGE-RELATED FACTORS

N/A

ZOONOTIC POTENTIAL

N/A

PREGNANCY

N/A

SEE ALSO

N/A

ABBREVIATIONS

• AC = activated charcoal
• ALP = alkaline phosphatase
• AST = aspartate aminotransferase
• GGT = γ-glutamyltransferase
• GI = gastrointestinal
• OP = organophosphate insecticide

Suggested Reading

Beasley VR, Cook WO, Dahlem AM, Hooser SB, Lovell RA, Valentine WM. Algae intoxication in livestock and waterfowl. Vet Clin North Am Food Anim Pract 1988;5:345–361.

Author Robert H. Poppenga
Consulting Editor Robert H. Poppenga

BORDETELLA BRONCHISEPTICA

BASICS

OVERVIEW

Bordetella bronchiseptica is a respiratory pathogen in other species but its role in equine respiratory disease is unclear. It has been isolated as a primary pathogen and fairly frequently with other respiratory pathogens from horses with lower respiratory tract disease. In one report, it was associated with infertility in a mare.

SIGNALMENT

No breed, sex, or age predisposition.

SIGNS

Respiratory

Coughing, fever with associated inappetance, mucopurulent nasal discharge. Thoracic auscultation may reveal infrequent crackles and wheezes.

Reproductive

- Infertility
- Thickened uterine wall
- Hyperemic vaginal wall
- Uterine fluid

CAUSES AND RISK FACTORS

Bordetella is a small, aerobic, gram-negative rod. The frequency of isolation from transtracheal aspirates varies with geographic location. Factors associated with *B. bronchiseptica* as a pathogen in equine respiratory disease are not known. In other animal species, *B. bronchiseptica* can adhere to respiratory cilia and resist action of macrophages via filamentous hemagglutinin pertactin and fimbriae. It also produces a tracheal cytotoxin and adenylcyclase toxin, which inhibits phagocytic cells and causes damage to respiratory epithelium. This results in an acute inflammation, altered mucociliary clearance, and increased mucus secretion.

Factors compromising the normal airway defense mechanisms, such as transportation, confined close proximity, anesthesia, surgery, and antibiotics or recent viral infections, predispose horses to pneumonia in which *B. bronchiseptica* may be one of the pathogens.

DIAGNOSIS

DIFFERENTIAL DIAGNOSIS

Other infectious causes of lower respiratory tract disease can be differentiated with culture and cytology of transtracheal aspirates. Equine influenza, equine herpes-viruses 1 and 2, and equine viral arteritis can be differentiated by viral isolation from acute-phase collection of nasopharyngeal secretions and a four-fold increase in antibody titers from serum samples collected 2 weeks apart.

Noninfectious causes of coughing, such as allergic airway disease and upper airway disease, can be differentiated by lack of supportive laboratory data, endoscopic findings, transtracheal aspirate cytology, and lack of systemic illness. Other infectious causes of infertility can be differentiated with uterine culture and cytology.

CBC/BIOCHEMISTRY/URINALYSIS

Respiratory infection may be associated with elevated white cell count and fibrinogen.

OTHER LABORATORY TESTS

- Transtracheal aspirate (TTA)—cytology and culture. Cytologic examination reveals small gram-negative rods with a neutrophilic inflammation. This, however, does not differentiate *B. bronchiseptica* from other gram-negative infections. *Bordetella bronchiseptica* take up to 48 hr to grow on culture and grow easily on 5% sheep blood agar or MacConkey's agar plates.
- Uterine swab and lavage for culture and cytology.

IMAGING

- Thoracic radiography and ultrasonography are useful in evaluating the lower respiratory tract disease.
- Transrectal ultrasonography is useful in evaluation of the uterus.

DIAGNOSTIC PROCEDURES

Endoscopy

Assists in the evaluation of the upper respiratory tract and trachea and determining the origin of the nasal discharge and coughing.

Uterine Biopsy

Assists in the evaluation of uterine disease.

BORDETELLA BRONCHISEPTICA

TREATMENT

Horses reported with primary *B. bronchiseptica* respiratory disease could be managed as outpatients. Horses with other pathogens involved in the respiratory disease may require intensive management and monitoring, depending on the extent of lung and pleural involvement. The horse should be rested until several weeks after clinical signs have resolved.

MEDICATIONS

DRUG(S) OF CHOICE

Antimicrobial therapy should be based on susceptibility tests due to the variability of *B. bronchiseptica* susceptibility patterns. Most reported isolates are sensitive to gentamicin (6.6–8.8 mg q24h IV), oxytetracycline (6.6–11 mg/kg q12h IV), trimethoprim–sulpha combination (30 mg/kg q12h PO), and erythromycin (25 mg/kg q12h PO). Therapy should continue until clinical signs resolve. Antimicrobial therapy should cover any other pathogenic bacteria that are isolated. Intrauterine infusions for 5–7 days with antibiotics should be based on susceptibility tests.

FOLLOW-UP

PATIENT MONITORING

• Thoracic auscultation, temperature, white cell count, fibrinogen, thoracic, and ultrasonographic findings should be used to monitor response to therapy. • Uterine culture, cytology, and biopsy can be used to monitor response to therapy.

PREVENTION/AVOIDANCE

N/A

POSSIBLE COMPLICATIONS

When other pathogens are involved with *B. bronchiseptica,* complications with chronic pneumonia, such as abscess formation, pleuritis, and adhesions, may occur.

EXPECTED COURSE AND PROGNOSIS

Resolution of clinical signs usually occurs within 14 days with a primary *B. bronchiseptica* respiratory infection. Relapses have been reported to occur; however, further treatment with the same antibiotic regimen resulted in recovery. In small animals, the unresponsiveness to antibiotics is related to the presence of *B. bronchiseptica* within the lumen of the respiratory tree ratherthan the lung parenchyma. Thus, medication is often accompanied with nebulization of an aminoglycoside. This has not been reported in therapy for the affected horses. When other pathogens are involved with *B. bronchiseptica,* the treatment is for a longer period and complications associated with chronic pneumonia may occur. The reported *B. bronchiseptica* uterine infection resolved after 5 days of appropriate antibiotics.

MISCELLANEOUS

SEE ALSO

- Lower respiratory tract infection
- Pneumonia

Suggested Reading

Bayly WM, Reed SM, Foreman JH, Traub JL, McMurphy RM. Equine bronchopneumonia due to *Bordetella bronchiseptica.* Eq Pract 1982;4:25-32.

Author Jane E. Axon

Consulting Editor Corinne R. Sweeney

BORNA DISEASE

BASICS

OVERVIEW

Encephalitis that is caused by a flavivirus is also referred to as *Near Eastern equine encephalitis,* a significant disease in Europe and the Middle East. The clinical disease is not documented in the United States. Histologically, there is a diffuse, non-suppurative encephalitis. The characteristic microscopic lesion is the Joest–Degen inclusion body in the neuronal nucleus, found in the nerve cells of the hippocampus and olfactory lobes of the cerebral cortex.

SIGNALMENT

Infection is sporadic, with no known predilection—males and females are equally affected.

SIGNS

The incubation period is long (4 weeks to 6 months) due to time necessary for the virus to travel from the site of infection to the hippocampus. Typical signs for encephalitis include abnormal mentation; depression; head pressing or head tremors; circling; maniacal or compulsive behavior, such as chewing, biting the air, exhibiting a marching gait; and hyperesthesia, often progressing to coma or convulsions. Note: Not all signs are seen in every animal, and any combination of signs may occur.

CAUSES AND RISK FACTORS

Infections in horses occur in spring and early summer. Borna disease virus-specific antibodies have been detected in healthy horses in Europe, Asia, Africa, and the United States. The etiology of the development of the clinical disease is unknown.

DIAGNOSIS

DIFFERENTIAL DIAGNOSIS

Other viral encephalitides, such as Eastern equine encephalomyelitis, Western equine encephalomyelitis, and Venezuelan equine encephalomyelitis, present with identical signs, and differentiation is possible only by serologic testing for the presence of antibodies specific for Borna virus in the cerebrospinal fluid (CSF) and the serum.

Hepatic encephalopathy has similar signs and course and can be differentiated by laboratory tests for the evaluation of the liver, such as serum GGT, AST, blood ammonia, and bile acids.

Cerebral trauma, which may be indicated by abrasions or wounds located on the head, and skull fractures, which can be indicated by palpable crepitus of the skull, can not be definitively ruled out ante-mortem in the horse.

Equine protozoal myelitis often presents with signs of spinal disease but can also cause a diffuse encephalitis. This disease can be differentiated by detection of antibodies to *Sarcocystis neurona* in the CSF. This diagnosis can be complicated by compromise of the blood–CSF barrier that allows leakage of serum antibodies into the CSF.

Leukoencephalomalacia as seen with fumonisin poisoning can present with similar signs, although often more than one horse in a barn is affected. This disease can be differentiated antemortem only by history of exposure to moldy corn.

Bacterial meningitis can cause similar signs and can be differentiated by a history demonstrating recent fevers, leukocytosis, and cytologic examination of the CSF.

Rabies is a differential diagnosis in any animal with signs of cortical disease, depending on the occurrence of the disease within the region. No definitive antemortem diagnosis is possible.

CBC/BIOCHEMISTRY/URINALYSIS

Laboratory data is usually non-remarkable.

IMAGING

N/A

OTHER DIAGNOSTIC PROCEDURES

Collection of CSF, most commonly from the lumbosacral space. Cytologic examination of the CSF fluid may reveal increased numbers of nucleated cells, or may be normal. Due to the long incubation period of the organism, antibodies to the virus can be detected in both the serum and CSF of animals showing signs of acute neurologic disease.

PATHOLOGIC FINDINGS

N/A

TREATMENT

Mortality is high, and prognosis is grave. Patient requires hospitalization. Treatment is aimed at symptomatic care, and includes intravenous fluids at 50mL/kg/day and parenteral or nasogastric nutrition if animal is dysphagic. Frequent turning and treatment of decubital sores are necessary if the patient is recumbent. Confinement to a padded stall is recommended if compulsive activity or convulsions are present. A dark quiet environment is necessary if hyperesthesia is present. Evacuation of the bladder and rectum may be necessary.

MEDICATIONS

Treatment is aimed at decreasing cerebral inflammation and swelling, not at specifically eliminating the virus from the central nervous system. Dimethyl sulfoxide IV 1–4g/kg q24h as a 10% solution to decrease cerebral edema for 3–5 days. Dexamethasone IV at 0.02–0.15mg/lb q24h for 3–5 days, then gradually decrease dosage over the next 7 days. Flunixin meglumine 1.1mg/kg IV or PO BID for up to 7 days for anti-inflammatory effects. If hyperesthesia or convulsions are present, diazepam at 20–40mg/horse IV to effect or phenobarbital at 8–15mg/kg loading dose to effect, followed by 2–10 mg/kg IV or PO maintenance q24h.

FOLLOW-UP

EXPECTED COURSE AND PROGNOSIS

Prognosis is grave, with mortality approximately 80%. If the horse survives acute encephalitis, which usually lasts 1–3 weeks, residual miscellaneous neurologic deficits, such as dysphagia, ataxia, tremors, and convulsions, may be present.

PREVENTION/AVOIDANCE

A vaccine is available, but not used routinely due to the small incidence of disease.

COMPLICATIONS

Horses may develop laminitis secondary to steroid use. There may be self-inflicted trauma due to maniacal behavior or decubital ulcers due to recumbency. Repeated seizure activity can lead to permanent brain damage secondary to prolonged hypoxic events.

MISCELLANEOUS

ZOONOTIC POTENTIAL

Documented cases exist in sheep, cattle, goats, rabbits, cats, horses, and humans.

SEE ALSO

- Eastern equine encephalitis
- Western equine encephalitis
- Equine protozoal myelitis

Suggested Reading

Richt JA, et al. Borna disease virus infection in animals and humans. Emerg Infect Dis 1997;3(3):343-352.

Author Brett Dolente
Editor Corinne R. Sweeney

BORNA DISEASE

BASICS

DEFINITION
• A rare but severe neurologic disease of horses, cattle, sheep, and ostriches.
• Named after the city of Borna in Saxony.
• Near-Eastern equine encephalitis may be a similar or identical disease; ticks have been implicated in its transmission.

PATHOPHYSIOLOGY
• BDV is a single-stranded RNA virus.
• The virus has not been fully characterized, because cell-free virus has not been isolated.
• The clinical syndrome has been associated with virus-associated, cell-mediated, immunopathologic reactions.
• Prolonged incubation periods and persistent infections have been reported.

SYSTEMS AFFECTED
• CNS
• Secondary lower urinary tract

SIGNALMENT
Nonspecific

SIGNS
Historical Findings
• BDV seroconversion is widespread.
• Specific antibody has been identified in clinically normal horses in Germany, where clinical disease has been described.
• No clinical disease but seroconversion has been identified in other European countries, Israel, Japan, and the United States.

Physical Examination Findings
• Early disease is characterized by depression dysuria and hyperesthesia over large parts of the body.
• Abdominal discomfort also may occur, often in association with rectal impaction.
• Later, CNS signs become more pronounced; quadraparesis, ataxia, head-pressing, head tilt, compulsive/propulsive movements, muscular fasciculations, and death also are common.

CAUSES
BDV

RISK FACTORS
None identified

DIAGNOSIS
• Established by identifying Borna-disease specific antibodies in CSF with ELISA.
• A BDV polymerase chain reaction is available for premortem diagnosis.

DIFFERENTIAL DIAGNOSIS
Other regionally associated viral encephalitides.

CBC/BIOCHEMISTRY/URINALYSIS
No consistent abnormalities other than stress- and trauma-related changes.

OTHER LABORATORY TESTS
No consistent abnormalities.

IMAGING
N/A

DIAGNOSTIC PROCEDURES
N/A

PATHOLOGIC FINDINGS
• Gross findings—often no changes.
• Histopathologic findings—typical changes associated with viral encephalitides, including nonpurulent encephalomyelitis and patchy, discontinuous inflammatory lesions most prominent in the gray matter of the brain stem.

TREATMENT
Supportive care, with no specific treatment.

MEDICATIONS

DRUGS OF CHOICE
N/A

CONTRAINDICATIONS
N/A

PRECAUTIONS
N/A

POSSIBLE INTERACTIONS
N/A

ALTERNATIVE DRUGS
N/A

BORNA DISEASE

FOLLOW-UP

PATIENT MONITORING
N/A

POSSIBLE COMPLICATIONS
Affected animals usually are euthanized, because the mortality rate is very high and the virus can cause latent and persistent infection.

MISCELLANEOUS

ASSOCIATED CONDITIONS
N/A

AGE-RELATED FACTORS
Nonspecific

ZOONOTIC POTENTIAL
• Some lab animals are susceptible to disease from exposure to homogenates of infected brain.
• BDV has been implicated in the pathogenesis of some neuropsychiatric diseases in humans.

PREGNANCY
N/A

SYNONYMS
N/A

SEE ALSO
N/A

ABBREVIATIONS
• BDV = Borna disease virus
• CSF = cerebrospinal fluid
• ELISA = enzyme-linked immunoadsorbent assay

Suggested Reading

Briese T, et al. Borna disease virus, a negative-strand RNA virus, transcribes in the nucleus of infected cells. Proc Natl Acad Sci U S A 1992;89:11486–11489.

Author Joseph J. Bertone
Consulting Editor Joseph J. Bertone

BOTULISM

BASICS

DEFINITION

Gradually progressive, symmetric muscular weakness in horses characterized by dysphagia and eventual recumbency.

PATHOPHYSIOLOGY

• Caused by systemic absorption of a potent neurotoxin elaborated by *Clostridium botulinum* that impairs transmission of electrical impulse from the nerve fiber to the adjacent muscle.
• After absorption from the digestive tract or a wound previously infected with botulinum spores, botulinum toxin circulates in the bloodstream and, subsequently, is taken up by specific endopeptidase receptors on motor end plates. Once attached to the receptor, the toxin is translocated within the cell and bound to acetylcholine vesicles, preventing electrical signals from reaching the myoneural junctions.
• The process of initial attachment, translocation, and final binding depends on the dose and requires several hours. Thus, with relatively small doses of toxin, clinical signs may not become apparent for ≥ 10 days after ingestion. With massive doses (10^8 mouse lethal dose units), however, horses may become recumbent and die within 8 hours.
• Botulism spores are relatively ubiquitous in the environment. Ingestion rarely leads to clinical botulism, however, because the spores do not elaborate toxin unless present in an anaerobic environment with appropriate nutrients.
• Botulism spores are pH sensitive and do not form toxin at a pH < 4.5. If forages are harvested too dry and fermentation is inadequate, however, toxin may be elaborated.
• Three forms of the disease are recognized in horses. The most common in adult horses is ingestion of the preformed toxin. Horses also may contract toxicoinfectious botulism through ingestion of spores and subsequent sporulation. Toxin elaboration can occur in wounds as well; castrations and deep penetrating wounds, including deep IM injections, have been associated with wound botulism.

SYSTEMS AFFECTED

Neuromuscular

• Progressive muscular weakness during a period of several hours to days that frequently manifests as trembling of the larger muscle groups—triceps and large muscles of the rear limbs.
• As clinical signs progress, affected horses lie down more frequently than normal and, eventually, become so myasthenic they cannot stand.
• Affected foals attempt to suckle the mare, but milk drools from the foal's mouth.

GI

• Some affected adults exhibit colic or abdominal pain as the primary sign.
• In addition to the systemic muscular weakness, most horses develop variable degrees of intestinal ileus, which may result in abdominal pain.

Musculoskeletal

• Progressive, symmetric muscle weakness.
• Tetraparesis, not paraparesis.

Respiratory

• Respiratory distress is evident only during the terminal phases.
• Horses with type C botulism often have an unusual type of respiratory effort, characterized by decreased respiratory rate (often 6–12 per minute) and exaggerated abdominal lift during inspiration.

Ophthalmic

• Moderate mydriasis
• Intact pupillary light reflex

Renal/Urologic

Horses that remain standing can void the bladder, which helps to differentiate botulism from herpes.

GENETICS

N/A

INCIDENCE/PREVALENCE

Type B

• Almost always occurs preformed in forage and is unrelated to that contracted from ingested spores that thrive in decomposing animal carcasses.
• Most frequently occurs in the mid-Atlantic region of the eastern U.S., with a predominance in central Kentucky, Virginia, Maryland, Delaware, and southeastern Pennsylvania.
• In most cases, occurs on an individual basis.
• In unusual circumstances, several cases may occur over several days, where a point source of toxin may be present—feeding of silage to a group of horses or horses eating hay contaminated with botulinum toxin.

Type A

• Typically occurs in the western U.S.
• Can occur when carcass contaminates feed materials.

BOTULISM

SIGNALMENT

Breed Predilection

N/A

Mean Age and Range

- Foals—peak occurrence between 6 days and 6 weeks of age
- Adults—any age

Predominant Sex

N/A

SIGNS

Historical Findings

- Generalized muscle weakness (i.e., myasthenia) or dysphagia typically are the first clinical signs detected.
- Astute individuals also may detect mild depression, decreased exercise tolerance, and reluctance to eat hay or grain.

Physical Examination Findings

- Moderately affected horses walk with a shuffling gait, occasionally dragging their toes, and show evidence of muscle weakness.
- Decreased tail tone along with other signs of muscle weakness are early clinical signs.
- As the disease progresses, dysphagia becomes more obvious, and myasthenia leads to muscle tremors, difficulty in rising, and finally, recumbency.
- Clinical signs are always symmetric, progressive, and often result in recumbency followed by death caused by respiratory paralysis or euthanasia (for humane considerations).
- Reduced tongue tone and slow tongue retraction also are characteristic early signs.
- In advanced disease, before recumbency, affected horses retract the tongue very slowly, if at all. As the ability to retract the tongue diminishes, affected horses eat grain more slowly, and grain is mixed with more saliva than normal. The admixture of saliva and grain, with some grain falling out of the horse's lips during eating, is very characteristic and one of the earliest signs.
- Most normal horses consume an 8-oz cup of grain in <2 minutes. Accurate assessment of the time needed to consume a standard amount of grain (8 oz) and close observation of the horse eating the grain are essential in discerning early dysphagia. A delayed time to consume grain (>2 minutes) is one of the most sensitive indications of disease. The second most sensitive index is delayed tongue retraction into the mouth. Both of these signs must be evaluated first in normal horses to appreciate the variation from horse to horse.
- Horses with early dysphagia may attempt to eat hay but have difficulty swallowing. Inability to swallow water usually occurs after inability to swallow hay. Horses seem to respond differently to the inability to drink water—many refuse even to attempt to drink; others immerse their muzzles underwater.
- Recumbent horses are very difficult to assess with regard to swallowing ability, because the struggle to stand takes priority over eating and drinking.
- Vital signs, including capillary refill, are normal during the early stages of disease. Once the horse is recumbent, however, both the heart and respiratory rate increase in proportion to the intensity of the struggle to rise.
- Borborygmal sounds gradually reduce as affected horses eat less.

CAUSES

- The cause in most cases of individual equine botulism usually is not determined but most likely is ingestion of a small amount of preformed toxin in roughage (typically hay). It is nearly impossible to subsequently identify toxin in other roughage samples, because the offending material has been consumed.
- In herd outbreaks, the offending material usually is a point source, again most often roughage.
- Rarely has commercial grain been associated with equine botulism.
- Roughage contaminated with a carcass results in type C botulism.
- Microscopic examination of feed may reveal evidence of the offending material.
- Wound botulism results from infected castration sites, clamped umbilical hernias, and deep IM injections with counterirritants—iodine preparations.

RISK FACTORS

Never feed silage or fermented forages, because these may contain minute amounts of toxin.

BOTULISM

DIAGNOSIS

DIFFERENTIAL DIAGNOSIS
- Herpes myeloencephalopathy
- Ionophore toxicosis
- Equine protozoal myelitis may result in similar signs but often is asymmetric, as is guttural pouch mycosis.

CBC/BIOCHEMISTRY/URINALYSIS
Until affected horses are recumbent, CBC and biochemistry profiles are within normal limits.

OTHER LABORATORY TESTS
Other routinely available diagnostic tests, including electrodiagnostic testing or nerve conduction studies, have little value.

IMAGING
N/A

DIAGNOSTIC PROCEDURES
- Identification of toxin or spores in feed materials or GI contents has value only after the case is resolved, because these tests may take as long as 2 weeks to complete.
- Normal horses rarely, if ever, have detectable spores in their feces or GI contents.
- Laboratory identification of spores, together with compatible clinical signs, helps to confirm the diagnosis but is not definitive evidence.
- Detection of preformed toxin in serum or GI contents may be definitive but rarely is possible because of the exquisite sensitivity of horses to the toxin and the difficulty of identifying it.

TREATMENT

APPROPRIATE HEALTH CARE
Confine affected horses to a boxstall with no additional physical activity.

NURSING CARE
- Oral fluid therapy may be required in horses with complete dysphagia.
- Recumbent horses require an immense amount of nursing care to minimize decubital sores and other complications.
- Recumbent horses, especially males, also may need to have their bladder catheterized periodically to avoid necrosis of the bladder wall.

ACTIVITY
- Restrict the muscular activity of affected horses.
- Attempts to sling affected horses usually hasten their demise.
- Assistance to rise from recumbency should be less $<$3–4 times per 24 hours.

DIET
N/A

CLIENT EDUCATION
- Once botulism has occurred on a farm, annual vaccination of all horses is strongly recommended.
- After the occurrence of one case, owners should be very diligent for signs in other horses.

SURGICAL CONSIDERATIONS
N/A

MEDICATIONS

DRUGS OF CHOICE
- Multivalent botulinum antitoxin ($>$100,000 IU) administered as quickly as possible after the onset of clinical signs is the most important aspect of therapy. Only one IV dose is needed, because the half-life for equine origin antitoxin is $\cong$12 days in horses.
- Antitoxin will not reverse clinical signs, but it should stop progression of the disease and allow patients to improve by growing more motor end plates at the myoneural junctions.

CONTRAINDICATIONS

• Aminoglycosides, which slow myoneural transmission and reduce survival in humans.
• Metronidazole, which is ineffective and may predispose to toxicoinfectious botulism.
• Neostigmine and aminopyridines, which may provide transitory improvement but most often further deplete acetylcholine stores and exacerbate clinical signs.

PRECAUTIONS

N/A

POSSIBLE INTERACTIONS

N/A

ALTERNATIVE DRUGS

N/A

FOLLOW-UP

PATIENT MONITORING

• Monitor hydration status, and provide PO and parenteral fluid therapy as indicated.
• An initial dose of mineral oil (4 L) helps to minimize any impaction and to maintain intestinal function.
• During dysphagia, horses may be maintained with warm water (10–12 L) containing powdered alfalfa meal (2–3 kg) administered twice daily via nasogastric tube.
• A marine bilge pump works much better than a traditional stomach pump.

PREVENTION/AVOIDANCE

• Three doses of monovalent type B botulinum toxoid $\cong$4 weeks apart are recommended to provide the most complete protection.
• Annual revaccination with a single dose of toxoid is adequate to maintain effective protection.
• Adequately vaccinated mares provide passive protection to newborn foals for several weeks if colostral ingestion is adequate.
• Foals are immunocompetent for botulism at birth, and the initial dose of toxoid should be given within the first 2–3 weeks of life.

POSSIBLE COMPLICATIONS

• Inhalation pneumonia secondary to dysphagia is a major concern.
• Massive decubital sores may result from recumbency in adults with botulism.

EXPECTED COURSE AND PROGNOSIS

• The more rapid the onset of clinical signs, the poorer the prognosis for survival.
• In recumbent adults, the prognosis for survival is greatly reduced—usually <25%.
• Once given the antitoxin, horses remain stable for 2–4 days, then gradually improve during the next 5–10 days as they regain their ability to swallow both water and roughage. Muscle strength gradually returns during the next 30 days or so. Weak tongues may persist for several weeks, but affected horses seem to eat and swallow normally.

MISCELLANEOUS

ASSOCIATED CONDITIONS

N/A

AGE-RELATED FACTORS

N/A

ZOONOTIC POTENTIAL

N/A

PREGNANCY

N/A

SYNONYMS

Forage poisoning in adults.

SEE ALSO

N/A

ABBREVIATION

• GI = gastrointestinal

Suggested Reading

Kinde H, Betty RL, Ardans A, et al. *Clostridium botulinum* type-C intoxication associated with consumption of processed hay cubes in horses. J Am Vet Med Assoc 1991;199:742–746.

Whitlock RH, Buckley CA. Botulism. Vet Clin North Am Equine Pract 1997; April:107–128.

Author Robert H. Whitlock

Consulting Editor Robert H. Poppenga

BROAD LIGAMENT HEMATOMA

BASICS

DEFINITION

• A rupture of the utero-ovarian, middle uterine, or external iliac arteries near the time of parturition.
• Hemorrhage from the arteries can accumulate in the abdomen, in which case death is likely, or into the broad ligament, forming a hematoma.
• Mares with a hematoma may appear as if in shock, with pale mucous membranes, but death rarely occurs if the broad ligament remains intact and contains further hemorrhage.

PATHOPHYSIOLOGY

• With aging, the utero-ovarian and middle uterine artery walls undergo degenerative processes believed to result in loss of elasticity.
• Secondary to the increased size or stretching, the arteries are more prone to rupture.
• Pre-existing damage to the intima and underlying media of the external iliac arteries (e.g., parasites) may result in necrosis and accumulation of material, predisposing to thrombosis and rupture.

SYSTEMS AFFECTED

• Reproductive
• Cardiovascular

GENETICS

Whether an inherited weakness in the vessels causes loss of elasticity is unknown.

INCIDENCE/PREVALENCE

Can occur at any age, but most commonly reported in mares of >12 years.

SIGNALMENT

• Most common in horses >12 years.
• All breeds; any of breeding age.

SIGNS

General Comments

• Broad ligament hematoma (i.e., hemorrhage contained between separated layers of the broad ligament) usually is not fatal.
• Intraperitoneal hemorrhage (i.e., free blood into the abdomen) is fatal.

Historical Findings

• No cardinal, characteristic signs before artery rupture.
• Pale mucous membranes.
• After rupture and with accumulation of hemorrhage, mares may colic from pain associated with stretching of the mesometrium—portion of the broad ligament attached to the uterus.

Physical Examination Findings

• Transrectal palpation may reveal an enlarged broad ligament—unilateral is most common, but bilateral may occur.
• Mucous membranes may become pale from blood loss into the mesometrium.

CAUSES

• Degeneration of arterial vessel walls related to age.
• With increased weight of the uterus and greater fetal movement, vessels break rather than stretch.

RISK FACTORS

• Pregnancy
• Aging

DIAGNOSIS

DIFFERENTIAL DIAGNOSIS

• Colic—transrectal palpation of the broad ligaments and surroundings structures is the best means of distinguishing colic from hematoma.
• Old ilial fractures and pelvic abscesses may be present, but neither is associated with acute hemorrhage or pale mucous membranes.

CBC/BIOCHEMISTRY/URINALYSIS

N/A

OTHER LABORATORY TESTS

N/A

IMAGING

Ultrasonography to differentiate hemorrhage from purulent material.

DIAGNOSTIC PROCEDURES

Transrectal palpation is the preferred diagnostic method to confirm the condition.

PATHOLOGIC FINDINGS

Acute hemorrhagic enlargement in the mesometrium during the peripartal period.

TREATMENT

APPROPRIATE HEALTH CARE

• Avoid moving the mare.
• Prevent the mare from rolling, running, or becoming excited in any manner that might result in further bleeding from the weakened vessel or terminal rupture of the mesometrium, permitting blood to escape into the abdomen.

NURSING CARE

• Restrict movement.
• Maintain a quiet environment.

ACTIVITY

Restrict activity as much as possible, including hand walking, if necessary.

DIET

N/A

CLIENT EDUCATION

• Possibility of occurrence increases with age.
• Consider the possibility of arterial rupture before breeding an old mare.

SURGICAL CONSIDERATIONS

Attempts to ligate the damaged vessel may lead to further hemorrhage.

MEDICATIONS

DRUGS OF CHOICE

N/A

BROAD LIGAMENT HEMATOMA

CONTRAINDICATIONS

- Agents to enhance clotting have little or no value, because the primary mechanism to stem hemorrhage is not clot formation but the increased pressure within the broad ligament that prevents further accumulation of blood.
- Oxytocin is ill-advised—the bleeding is occurring in the broad ligament, and stimulation of uterine contractions may cause additional hemorrhage.

PRECAUTIONS

- Minimize movement of the mare.
- If broad ligament hemorrhage began prepartum, be careful when extracting a fetus if the mare is in dystocia.
- Transport to a veterinary hospital may be sufficient stimulus to rupture the damaged broad ligament, leaving the mare to bleed to death internally.

POSSIBLE INTERACTIONS

N/A

ALTERNATIVE DRUGS

N/A

FOLLOW-UP

PATIENT MONITORING

- Monitor PCV, packed solids, CRT, and color of mucous membranes if broad ligament hematoma has been diagnosed.
- Once a hematoma has been confirmed, subsequent serial transrectal palpations should be either avoided or brief and gentle to avoid iatrogenic rupture of a broad ligament that is stretched or under great pressure.

PREVENTION/AVOIDANCE

Avoid movement of the mare.

POSSIBLE COMPLICATIONS

- Death
- Abscessation after clotting and hematogenous contamination of the hematoma with bacteria.

EXPECTED COURSE AND PROGNOSIS

- Best outcome—slow regression of a hematoma; decreases in size; unlikely to return entirely to its prehematoma size and shape.
- Once affected, mares are at increased risk of future rupture.

MISCELLANEOUS

ASSOCIATED CONDITIONS

- Abscess formation within the affected broad ligament—mesometrium.
- Death
- Dystocia

AGE-RELATED FACTORS

All ages can be affected, but mares of > 12 years have a distinctly increased incidence.

ZOONOTIC POTENTIAL

N/A

PREGNANCY

Occurs either at or near term during an otherwise normal pregnancy.

SYNONYM

Mesometrial hematoma

SEE ALSO

- Dystocia
- Utero-ovarian, middle uterine, and iliac artery rupture.

ABBREVIATIONS

- CRT = capillary refill time
- PCV = packed cell volume

Suggested Reading

Asbury AC. Care of the mare after foaling. In: McKinnon AO, Voss JL, eds. Equine reproduction. Philadelphia: Lea & Febiger, 1993:979.

Pascoe RR. Rupture of the utero-ovarian or middle uterine artery in the mare at or near parturition. Vet Rec 1979:104:77–82.

Rooney JR. Internal hemorrhage related to gestation. In: Catcott EJ, Smithcors JF, eds. Progress in equine practice. Wheaton, IL: American Veterinary Publications, 1966:360–361.

Author Walter R. Threlfall

Consulting Editor Carla L. Carleton

BRUCELLOSIS

BASICS

OVERVIEW

Infection with *Brucella abortus,* a gram-negative coccobacillus, produces several outcomes in horses, the most common of which is supraspinous bursitis (fistulous withers), which results from the apparent predilection of the organism for synovial structures. Brucellosis, which is usually acquired from infected cattle, is difficult to treat and is a zoonosis. *Brucella suis,* transmitted from infected pigs, is a rare cause of bursitis or abortion in horses.

SIGNALMENT

No age, breed, or sex predilection has been reported.

SIGNS

- Most seropositive horses are asymptomatic. Supraspinous bursitis (fistulous withers) is the most common disease manifestation of *B. abortus* infection. This is marked by a painful swelling over the withers, which may open and drain purulent material.
- Fever, lameness, stiffness, and lethargy may be noted.
- Supraatlantal bursitis (poll evil) may also be caused by *B. abortus* infection.
- Osteomyelitis and osteoarthritis have been reported.
- Generalized illness marked by fever, stiffness, and lethargy may be seen.
- *B. abortus* infection is a rare cause of abortion in mares and infertility in the stallion.
- Uveitis has been associated with *B. abortus* infection, but evidence for this is weak.

CAUSES AND RISK FACTORS

Most infections result from contact with *Brucella*-positive cattle, especially placental tissue and newborn calves. The organism can survive in the environment for weeks, so horses grazing pasture recently vacated by infected cattle are at risk. In *Brucella*-free areas, the prevalence of *Brucella* infections in horses is low. In areas where *B. suis* exists, contact with infected pigs would also pose a risk to horses. The route of infection is usually ingestion. *Brucella abortus* then travels to the lymphatics and enters phagocytic cells, leading to formation of granulomas.

DIAGNOSIS

DIFFERENTIAL DIAGNOSIS

Fistulous withers may also result from infection of the supraspinous bursa by other agents, usually secondary to trauma or penetration of a foreign body. Failure to identify *Brucella* does not rule out infection because of the difficulty of isolating the organism and the common presence of secondary infection in cases that have developed fistulae. Radiographs or ultrasound may identify a foreign body or fracture of the spinous process.

Abortion in mares is usually a result of a noninfectious cause or an infection other than *Brucella.* History, culture, and histopathology of placental and fetal tissue may help identify the cause of abortion.

CBC/BIOCHEMISTRY/URINALYSIS

No consistent changes in CBC have been reported, but an elevated fibrinogen and neutrophilia may be detected.

OTHER LABORATORY TESTS

A rise in titer in paired serum samples 2 weeks apart is considered diagnostic. An elevated titer (>1:50 on the plate agglutination test) indicates exposure to the organism. However, a high titer in conjunction with a history of exposure to infected cattle and typical clinical signs is usually sufficient for diagnosis of brucellosis in horses. Acute cases should be retested in 2 weeks before *Brucella* infection is ruled out.

IMAGING

- Radiographs of the dorsal spinous processes may help rule out fractures secondary to trauma. Also, infectious causes of fistulous withers frequently have radiographic evidence of osteomyelitis.
- Contrast radiography of the fistulae may be used to determine the extent of the infection.
- Ultrasonography is useful for determining location of fluid pockets and fistulous tracts. Irregularities in the surface of the bone are suggestive of osteomyelitis.

OTHER DIAGNOSTIC PROCEDURES

- Aspirate and culture affected bursa or joint. *Brucella* is difficult to isolate and cultures should be performed in appropriate laboratories. If the withers has fistulated, secondary pathogens are usually isolated. If surgical excision is performed, a sample of material should be sent for culture.
- Intradermal testing is not considered reliable.
- In cases of abortion, the organism may be cultured from placenta, fetal stomach, and vaginal discharge.

PATHOLOGIC FINDINGS

- Affected bursae have a thickened capsule and clear fluid unless fistulated, in which case the exudate is usually purulent.
- Osteomyelitis of the dorsal spinous processes may be present.

TREATMENT

- State regulatory authorities should be notified when brucellosis is suspected. In some states, treatment of *Brucella*-positive animals is prohibited. In all cases, animals should be isolated from other animals and precautions should be taken to prevent infection of people involved in the patient's care.
- Lavage fistulous tracts with an antiseptic solution, such as 0.1% povidone iodine. Some recommend lavage with 10–50% DMSO solution.
- Hydrotherapy of the swollen withers may be useful.
- Horses with fistulous withers should not be ridden.
- Surgical curettage of the affected soft tissue and bone under general anesthesia is indicated in cases that do not respond to antibiotic treatment. Patients may require more than one surgery to resolve the symptoms.

MEDICATIONS

DRUGS

- Recommended antibiotics include trimethoprim–sulfamethoxazole (15–30 mg/kg PO q12h), chloramphenicol, and oxytetracycline. Many cases do not respond even after several weeks of therapy.
- Nonsteroidal anti-inflammatory drugs to reduce fever and inflammation, such as flunixin meglumine (1 mg/kg q12h) or phenylbutazone (2–4 mg/kg PO or IV q12 h).
- Vaccination with strain 19 vaccine has been described. Three subcutaneous doses (5 mL) 10 days apart, or a single dose (25 mL) IV are the most commonly cited regimens. Although some authors report success with this treatment, serious adverse affects, including death, may result. This is an extra-label use of the vaccine, and the efficacy has not been determined.

CONTRAINDICATIONS/POSSIBLE INTERACTIONS

- Informed consent should be obtained before treatment with strain 19 vaccine.
- Accidental injection of strain 19 vaccine may result in disease in humans.
- Before administration of the *Brucella* vaccine, animals should be treated with dexamethasone (0.25 mg/kg IV) and aspirin (35 mg/kg PO) or flunixin meglumine (1.1 mg/kg).

FOLLOW-UP

- The prevalence of this disease is declining in areas where brucellosis has been eradicated.
- Cases of transmission from horses to cattle have been reported.

MISCELLANEOUS

ZOONOTIC POTENTIAL

Humans can contract the disease via contact with skin or mucous membranes, ingestion, inhalation, or inoculation with live vaccine. Gloves, mask, and protective eyewear should be worn when working with affected animals.

SYNONYMS

- Bangs disease
- Undulant fever

Suggested Reading

Cohen ND, McMullan WC, Carter GK. Fistulous withers: the diagnosis and treatment of open and closed lesions. Vet Med 1991;86:416-426.

Author Laura K. Reilly

Consulting Editor Corinne R. Sweeney

BRUXISM

BASICS

DEFINITION
Bruxism is a behavior characterized by rhythmic or spasmodic grinding of the teeth and is accompanied by a distinctive loud grinding sound. Bruxism may occur intermittently or, in more severe cases, may become incessant.

PATHOPHYSIOLOGY
• Foals—Bruxism is most commonly associated with gastroduodenal ulceration. This is especially true when gastric outflow is inhibited by stricture of the pylorus or duodenum and subsequent gastroesophageal reflux results in corrosive esophagitis. Intermittent bruxism may also occur with any painful condition.
• Adults—Bruxism in adults is often associated with pharyngeal pain or pain at the distal esophagus in the area of the palatopharyngeal arch. This area can be irritated by nasogastric intubation and indwelling nasogastric tubes. However, bruxism may occur in response to almost any painful condition. It is also observed with esophagitis and certain neurologic conditions such as Borna disease. Bruxism may infrequently be observed with gastric ulceration in adults.

SYSTEM AFFECTED
N/A

SIGNALMENT
No age, breed, or sex predisposition.

SIGNS
Bruxism is a sign of pain, and can therefore be present with a variety of clinical signs associated with the primary disease.

Historical Findings
Historical findings generally associated with primary disease.

Physical Examination Findings
When associated with pharyngeal pain, mild dysphagia is often present and is frequently characterized by salivation or by holding saliva in the mouth for prolonged periods. With gastric ulceration, foals may exhibit poor appetite, intermittent nursing (may nurse for short period and then act mildly uncomfortable), episodes of mild colic, diarrhea, pot-bellied appearance, bruxism, salivation, or dorsal recumbency. Salivation and bruxism are usually indicative of severe glandular or duodenal ulcers with concurrent gastroesophageal reflux and delayed gastric emptying. Adults with gastric ulceration may exhibit poor appetite, lethargy, poor body condition, rough hair coat, and low-grade colic.

CAUSES
Trauma from nasogastric intubation, irritation from indwelling nasogastric tubes*, gastroduodenal ulceration*, reflux esophagitis, neurologic diseases such as Borna disease, any painful condition*.

RISK FACTORS
Passage of nasogastric tube, indwelling nasogastric tube, any painful illness.

DIAGNOSIS

DIFFERENTIAL DIAGNOSIS
The objective in the differential diagnosis is to determine the primary disease causing the horse to respond with bruxism. A history of recent nasogastric intubation or indwelling nasogastric tube would indicate traumatic pharyngitis/esophagitis as a likely cause. Foals exhibiting poor appetite, intermittent nursing (may nurse for short period and then act mildly uncomfortable), episodes of mild colic, diarrhea, pot-bellied appearance, or dorsal recumbency and adults exhibiting poor appetite, lethargy, poor body condition, rough hair coat, and low-grade colic should be suspected of having gastroduodenal ulceration. Neurologic disease would typically be accompanied by ataxia, proprioceptive defects, and possibly cranial nerve signs.

CBC/BIOCHEMISTRY/URINALYSIS
These parameters are unlikely to assist in differentiating the cause of bruxism.

OTHER LABORATORY TESTS
N/A

DIAGNOSTIC PROCEDURES

Endoscopic Examination
Endoscopy is of value in determining if bruxism is a response to traumatic pharyngitis or esophagitis, reflux esophagitis, and/or gastroduodenal ulceration. Pharyngitis might be obvious; however, in some cases the lesion is in or behind the palatopharyngeal arch and difficult to visualize.

TREATMENT
Many cases exhibiting bruxism have serious medical conditions that require inpatient monitoring and care. If the patient is not drinking or is losing fluids through salivation, appropriate intravenous fluid therapy should be administered. Nasogastric intubation should be avoided in cases of traumatic pharyngitis/esophagitis. Exercise should be limited to hand-walking or paddock turnout. Horses with traumatic pharyngitis/esophagitis might benefit by eating a wet gruel rather than dry feed. Esophageal perforation may require extensive treatment, intensive care, and could have a poor prognosis.

MEDICATIONS

DRUG(S) OF CHOICE
Patients with painful conditions may benefit from administration of NSAIDs for pain control. In general, flunixin meglumine and ketoprofen are preferred for pain originating in the gastrointestinal tract and phenylbutazone is preferred for musculoskeletal pain. Flunixin is administered at 1.1 mg/kg, ketoprofen at 2.2 mg/kg, and phenylbutazone at 4.4 mg/kg. However, NSAIDs may worsen gastroduodenal ulceration and can result in toxicosis if administered in excessive doses or if normal hydration is not maintained. Of the three, phenylbutazone has the greatest potential for toxicity. When frequent dosing is necessary, ketoprofen has been shown to have less potential for toxicosis than flunixin or phenylbutazone.
Gastric ulceration is treated with omeprazole or histamine H_2 receptor antagonists. Omeprazole is administered at 1–4 mg/kg PO once daily. Omeprazole has a time- and dose-related effect on healing of gastric ulcers. Therefore, higher doses result in more rapid and complete healing. However, lower doses are frequently effective in relieving clinical signs and promoting healing. Omeprazole requires 3–5 days treatment for maximum antisecretory effect to occur. Cimetidine is administered at 20–25 mg/kg PO or at 4-6 mg/kg IV bwt q6–8hr. Ranitidine is administered at 6–8 mg/kg PO or 1.5–2.0 mg/kg IV q6–8hr.

BRUXISM

CONTRAINDICATIONS
N/A

PRECAUTIONS
NSAIDs may worsen gastroduodenal ulceration and can result in toxicosis if administered in excessive doses or if normal hydration is not maintained. The first sign of toxicosis is poor appetite, followed by loose feces and, in some patients, oral ulceration. Serum total protein and especially albumin concentrations also decline.

POSSIBLE INTERACTIONS
Cimetidine and to a lesser extent omeprazole are hepatic cytochrome P450 inhibitors and might slow the metabolism of concurrently administered compounds that require this enzyme for metabolism and elimination. Drugs whose metabolism might be inhibited include phenylbutazone, diazepam, phenytoin, theophylline, and others.

ALTERNATIVE DRUGS
Butorphanol, xylazine, and detomodine may also be used for short-term relief of pain. For gastric ulceration, antacid compounds buffer gastric acid. They are impractical to use in most instances, and must be administered 4–6 times daily at approximately 250 mL/450 kg horse. Sucralfate is likely to be ineffective in the treatment of gastric stratified squamous lesions but could possibly be effective in glandular lesions. Sucralfate is administered as crushed tablets in syrup at 1 g/100 lbs (1g/45 kg) PO q6–8hr.

FOLLOW-UP

PATIENT MONITORING
Many patients exhibiting bruxism have serious medical problems and should be hospitalized for intensive monitoring. Foals exhibiting bruxism should be monitored carefully for development of gastroesophageal reflux and diminished gastric emptying.

POSSIBLE COMPLICATIONS
There are not significant complications associated with the bruxism itself. However, many complications may be associated with the primary disease process causing the patient to exhibit bruxism.

MISCELLANEOUS

ASSOCIATED CONDITIONS
Usually associated with primary disease.

AGE-RELATED FACTORS
N/A

ZOONOTIC POTENTIAL
In endemic areas, rabies should be considered in patients showing neurologic signs of undetermined etiology.

PREGNANCY
N/A

SYNONYMS
- Odontoprisis
- Teeth grinding

SEE ALSO
Gastric Erosions and Ulcers

ABBREVIATIONS
N/A

Suggested Reading

Hardy J, Stewart RH, Beard WL, et al. Complications of nasogastric intubation in horses: nine cases (1987–1989). J Am Vet Med Assoc 1992;201:483-486.

MacAllister CG. Medical therapy for equine gastric ulcers. Vet Med 1995;XX:1068-1076.

Murray MJ. Gastroduodenal ulceration. In: Reed SM, Bayly WM, eds. Equine internal medicine. Philadelphia: WB Saunders, 1998.

Author Charles G. MacAllister
Consulting Editor Henry Stämpfli

BURDOCK PAPPUS BRISTLE KERATOPATHY

BASICS

OVERVIEW

Burdock pappus (*Arctium* spp.) bristles are common conjunctival foreign bodies in the northeastern United States that can lead to chronic nonhealing lesions of the cornea.

System Affected

Ophthalmic

SIGNALMENT

All ages and breeds affected.

SIGNS

History of unilateral ocular signs, including photophobia, blepharospasm, lacrimation, ocular discharge characterized as either serous or mucopurulent, and a positive fluorescein dye uptake on the cornea. The corneal erosions or ulcerations persist despite topical antibiotic medication.

CAUSES AND RISK FACTORS

Burdock pappus bristles are a common source of small conjunctival foreign bodies.

DIAGNOSIS

DIFFERENTIAL DIAGNOSIS

Lid abnormalities such as distichiasis, trichiasis, and entropion; neuroparalytic and neurotrophic keratitis; keratoconjunctivitis sicca; corneal dystrophies; and corneal foreign bodies. Inappropriate topical corticosteroid therapy causing delayed corneal healing. Chronic epithelial erosion (indolent ulceration).

CBC/BIOCHEMISTRY/URINALYSIS

N/A

OTHER LABORATORY TESTS

Find the bristle. Rule out infectious causes (bacterial or fungal) with corneal scrapings for cytology and culture.

IMAGING

N/A

DIAGNOSTIC PROCEDURES

N/A

PATHOLOGIC FINDINGS

N/A

TREATMENT

Conjunctivalectomy of the bristle foreign body and surrounding tissue under sedation and auriculopalpebral nerve block.

BURDOCK PAPPUS BRISTLE KERATOPATHY

MEDICATIONS

DRUGS

After conjunctivalectomy: follow-up therapy with topical antibiotics 3 to 6 times daily (e.g., bacitracin–neomycin–polymyxin, chloramphenicol), topical 1% atropine SID to TID, and 1 to 2 gm phenylbutazone BID PO.

CONTRAINDICATIONS/POSSIBLE INTERACTIONS

N/A

FOLLOW-UP

EXPECTED COURSE AND PROGNOSIS

After removal of the bristle, healing of the corneal defect occurs within 3 to 14 days.

MISCELLANEOUS

ASSOCIATED CONDITIONS

Secondary bacterial infection.

SEE ALSO

- Equine corneal ulceration
- Equine corneal laceration
- Equine keratomycosis
- Equine corneal stromal abscessation
- Equine recurrent uveitis
- Equine glaucoma
- Equine nonulcerative keratouveitis
- Equine eosinophil keratitis
- Equine herpes keratitis
- Equine calcific band keratopathy
- Equine limbal keratopathy
- Equine superficial corneal erosions with anterior stromal sequestration

Suggested Reading

Brooks DE. Equine ophthalmology. In: Gelatt KN, ed. Veterinary ophthalmology. 3rd ed. Philadelphia: Lippincott Williams & Wilkins, 1999; chapter 30.

Author Andras M. Komaromy
Consulting Editor Dennis E. Brooks

CALCIFIC BAND KERATOPATHY

BASICS

OVERVIEW
Calcific band keratopathy consists of depositions of calcium (hydroxyapatite) in the corneal epithelium and stroma, and is a possible complication of uveitis.

System Affected

Ophthalmic

SIGNALMENT
All ages and breeds affected.

SIGNS
In addition to signs of chronic uveitis (e.g., synechiae, miosis, aqueous flare), dense, white, dystrophic bands are noted in the interpalpebral region of the central cornea, with scattered areas of fluorescein retention. Calcium deposited at the level of corneal epithelial basement membrane may accumulate and disrupt the epithelium, resulting in painful ulcers and uveitis.

CAUSES AND RISK FACTORS
The exact pathogenesis of calcium band keratopathy is unknown. It is an occasional complication of uveitis. The minimum time between onset of uveitis and onset of corneal lesions is 2 months, but in most cases is at least 1 year.

DIAGNOSIS

DIFFERENTIAL DIAGNOSIS
Lid abnormalities such as distichiasis, trichiasis, and entropion; neuroparalytic and neurotrophic keratitis; keratoconjunctivitis sicca; corneal dystrophies; and corneal foreign bodies. Inappropriate topical corticosteroid therapy causing delayed corneal healing. Chronic epithelial erosion (indolent ulceration).

CBC/BIOCHEMISTRY/URINALYSIS
N/A

OTHER LABORATORY TESTS
Rule out infectious causes (bacterial or fungal) with corneal scrapings for cytology and culture. Scraping procedure causes audible and tactile evidence of mineralization. Biopsy can be taken to support the diagnosis of calcific band keratopathy histologically.

IMAGING
N/A

DIAGNOSTIC PROCEDURES
N/A

PATHOLOGIC FINDINGS
Special stain (e.g., Kossa's method) confirms presence of calcium deposits at the level of the lamina propria of the epithelium and the underlying superficial stroma. Vascularization is noted.

CALCIFIC BAND KERATOPATHY

TREATMENT

Superficial keratectomy. If calcific deposits are not removed, affected eyes remain painful despite medical treatment because of persistent ulceration.

MEDICATIONS

DRUGS

Topically administered calcium chelating drugs (dipotassium ethylene diamine tetraacetate 13.8%, Sequester-Sol). Topical antibiotic (e.g., chloramphenicol, bacitracin–neomycin–polymyxin), atropine (1%), and systemic non-steroidal anti-inflammatory drugs (e.g., flunixin meglumine 0.25 to 1 mg/kg BID PO, IM, IV) until keratectomy site heals.

CONTRAINDICATIONS/POSSIBLE INTERACTIONS

Risk of opportunistic infections due to topical corticosteroids for treatment of uveitis.

FOLLOW-UP

EXPECTED COURSE AND PROGNOSIS

Healing of keratectomy sites can occur with severe scarring. Recurrence of calcium band keratopathy is possible with continued episodes of uveitis. The prognosis for vision is guarded because of subsequent corneal scarring and further uveitis episodes.

MISCELLANEOUS

ASSOCIATED CONDITIONS

Complication of uveitis.

SEE ALSO

- Equine corneal ulceration
- Equine corneal laceration
- Equine keratomycosis
- Equine corneal stromal abscessation
- Equine recurrent uveitis
- Equine glaucoma
- Equine nonulcerative keratouveitis
- Equine eosinophilic keratitis
- Equine herpes keratitis
- Equine burdock pappus bristle keratopathy
- Equine limbal keratopathy
- Equine superficial corneal erosions with anterior stromal sequestration

Suggested Reading

Brooks DE. Equine ophthalmology. In: Gelatt KN, ed. Veterinary ophthalmology. 3rd ed. Philadelphia: Lippincott Williams & Wilkins, 1999; chapter 30.

Author Andras M. Komaromy
Consulting Editor Dennis E. Brooks

CALCIUM, HYPERCALCEMIA

BASICS

DEFINITION

Serum total calcium greater than the reference interval, or >13.5 mg/dL.

PATHOPHYSIOLOGY

- PTH, calcitonin, and vitamin D act in conjunction with the intestine, bone, kidneys, and parathyroid glands to maintain calcium homeostasis.
- Equine serum calcium is closely dependent on dietary intake.
- The equine kidney is important in calcium regulation; horses excrete a larger proportion of absorbed calcium in the urine than other mammals do.
- Disturbances in calcium homeostasis leading to hypercalcemia occur with organ dysfunction or abnormalities in hormonal balance and control.
- Hypercalcemia of malignancy is associated with certain types of neoplasia. Tumor cells produce and secrete parathyroid-related or parathyroid-like hormone products, causing increased osteoclastic bone resorption and renal resorption of calcium.
- Hypercalcemic states can lead to widespread soft-tissue mineralization.

SYSTEMS AFFECTED

Cardiovascular

- ECG changes associated with increased serum calcium progress from bradycardia to tachycardia (with or without extrasystoles/ ectopic beats) to ventricular fibrillation.
- Hypervitaminosis D with secondary hypercalcemia and hyperphosphatemia can result in soft-tissue mineralization; lung, large vessels, endocardium are prone.

Endocrine/Metabolic

Hypercalcemia stimulates calcitonin release as a compensatory mechanism to decrease plasma calcium.

GI

Possible decreased contractility of GI smooth muscle.

Neuromuscular

Decreased neuromuscular irritability can result from hypercalcemia and contribute to decreased performance.

Renal

Soft-tissue mineralization may occur with concurrent hypercalcemia and hyperphosphatemia.

SIGNALMENT

Renal Failure

- Horses with chronic renal failure usually are adult to old.
- Suspect congenital abnormalities in young horses with renal failure.

Hypercalcemia of Malignancy

- Squamous cell carcinoma (e.g., cutaneous, GI, metastatic) generally occurs in adult and old animals.
- Cutaneous squamous cell carcinoma more commonly occurs in animals with an area of white skin; common sites are nonpigmented, sparsely haired areas near mucocutaneous junctions.
- Horses with lymphoma more often are young to middle-aged (2–9 years) but can be old as well.

SIGNS

General Comments

- Clinical signs in horses with hypercalcemia, regardless of cause, often are nonspecific.
- Weight loss, inappetence/anorexia, poor performance, and depression are most common.
- Clinical signs of hypervitaminosis D or hyperparathyroidism generally reflect the increased vitamin D or PTH activity causing increased renal and intestinal calcium reabsorption.

Historical Findings

- With renal disease/failure, poor performance may be the presenting complaint. Less frequently, mild colic signs or abnormal frequency or volume of urination are noted. Confirmation of exposure to potential nephrotoxins requires an excellent history and investigation.
- Depending on location of the alimentary tract squamous cell carcinoma, horses may exhibit signs of esophageal obstruction (e.g., dysphagia, ptyalism, choke), show a reluctance to eat or drink (despite interest in food and water), or have a prolonged history of anorexia and weight loss.
- Horses with hypervitaminosis D may exhibit limb stiffness, with painful flexor tendons and suspensory ligaments.
- In the documented case of primary hyperparathyroidism in an old pony, intermittent weakness was the presenting complaint.

Physical Examination Findings

Renal Failure:

- Ventral edema—frequently seen with glomerulonephritis
- Oral ulcerations
- Hematuria or PU/PD

Neoplasia:

- Proliferative or erosive masses or nonhealing wounds in the periorbital region, genitalia, lips, nose, or anus suggest cutaneous squamous cell carcinoma.
- During the late stages, metastasis to lymph nodes, lung, or bone can occur.
- Palpating abdominal masses or adhesions by rectal examination suggests GI tumors.
- Clinical findings in horses with lymphoma are nonspecific and relate to location of the tumor—cutaneous, alimentary, mediastinal, or multicentric.

CALCIUM, HYPERCALCEMIA

CAUSES

Chronic Renal Disease/Failure

• Hypercalcemia secondary to decreased excretion of calcium carbonate occurs with chronic renal disease.
• Hyper-, hypo-, or normocalcemia occurs with acute renal disease.
• Hypercalcemia in acute or chronic renal failure is more apt to develop in horses fed high-calcium rations.
• Cause is difficult to determine, because many conditions or diseases may predispose to chronic progressive renal disease/failure—glomerulonephritis from immune complex deposition (e.g., streptococcal infection, equine infectious anemia), nephrotoxins (e.g., aminoglycoside antibiotics, NSAIDs, vitamin K_3, heavy metals [especially mercury], hemoglobin, myoglobin), chronic urinary tract obstruction, interstitial nephritis, amyloidosis, pyelonephritis, nephrolithiasis and ureterolithiasis, and congenital abnormalities (e.g., renal hypoplasia, or polycystic kidneys).

Neoplasia

• The most common paraneoplastic finding in horses is hypercalcemia.
• Tumors associated with hypercalcemia—lymphoma (common), squamous cell carcinoma (common), adrenocortical carcinoma (uncommon), malignant mesenchymoma of the ovary (uncommon), and ameloblastoma (uncommon).

Hypervitaminosis D

Hypercalcemia from increased GI absorption and bone resorption is associated with ingestion of plants (e.g., *Cestrum diurnum* [wild jasmine] and certain *Solanum* sp., Hawaii) containing a vitamin D–like substance or excessive dietary supplementation with vitamin D–containing products.

Exercise

Calcium increases with exercise; however, because this ion is present in sweat, plasma concentrations may be reduced with large volumes of sweat loss.

Primary Hyperparathyroidism

• Potential causes—parathyroid adenoma, parathyroid hyperplasia, and carcinoma
• This condition is rare in horses but should be considered after ruling out all other causes of hypercalcemia.

RISK FACTORS

• Do not feed hypercalcemic horses legume hays (e.g., alfalfa, clover) or high-calcium rations.
• Fluid therapy for hypercalcemic horses should be devoid of calcium.

DIAGNOSIS

DIFFERENTIAL DIAGNOSIS

• Renal failure—azotemia, isosthenuria, and exposure to nephrotoxins.
• Squamous cell carcinoma, lymphoma, and other neoplasia—clinical signs related to neoplasia, identification of tumor by cytology, and histopathology.
• Hypervitaminosis D—hypercalcemia with concurrent hyperphosphatemia occurs with overzealous supplementation; hyperphosphatemia may be absent with plant intoxication.
• Primary hyperparathyroidism—hypercalcemia, hypophosphatemia, increased serum PTH concentration, increased fractional excretion of phosphorus, and low to normal vitamin D_3 concentration.

LABORATORY FINDINGS

Drugs That May Alter Lab Results

Anticoagulants containing EDTA, citrate, oxalate, or fluoride chelate calcium and falsely decrease calcium measurements.

Disorders That May Alter Lab Results

• Of total calcium, ≅50% is bound to protein, predominantly albumin.
• Abnormalities in serum albumin or protein concentration directly affect total serum calcium concentration, but the correlation is not as strong in horses as in dogs. Correction formulas as determined for dogs have not been validated in horses.
• Total serum calcium may be falsely increased with hyperproteinemia if hyperalbuminemia is present; hypoalbuminemia or hypoproteinemia may obscure hypercalcemia.
• Acid–base status affects the amount of ionized and protein-bound calcium. Acidosis increases the ionized calcium fraction by decreasing the fraction bound to protein; alkalosis decreases ionized calcium by increasing the fraction bound to protein. Total calcium, however, usually remains within the reference interval.
• Lipemia and hemolysis may falsely elevate total calcium.

Valid If Run in Human Lab?

Yes

CALCIUM, HYPERCALCEMIA

CBC/BIOCHEMISTRY/URINALYSIS

- Azotemia (increased serum creatinine and urea nitrogen) and isosthenuria (urine specific gravity, 1.008–1.015) support the diagnosis of renal failure, but other causes of azotemia with concurrent PU/PD must be ruled out.
- Hypophosphatemia, mild hyponatremia and hypochloridemia, and normo- or hyperkalemia can be present.
- Moderate to marked proteinuria is common with glomerulonephritis.
- Suspect urinary tract infection with moderate to many leukocytes in urine sediment.
- Hypercalcemia without concurrent azotemia or isosthenuria implies causes other than renal; suspect neoplasia.
- Consider vitaminosis D intoxication with concurrent hypercalcemia and hyperphosphatemia. Hyperphosphatemia is the earliest abnormality and may be more reliable for indicating hypervitaminosis D in oversupplementation than hypercalcemia. Hyperphosphatemia may be absent in plant intoxication. Urine specific gravity may be low.

OTHER LABORATORY TESTS

- Total serum calcium is reported during routine biochemical analysis.
- Measurement of ionized calcium concentration by ion-selective electrodes requires special sample handling and generally is not readily available.
- With suspected primary hyperparathyroidism after ruling out all other diseases, measurement of PTH is indicated.

IMAGING

Ultrasonography of kidneys during chronic renal failure may reveal increased echogenicity (i.e., fibrosis) and is useful in assessing abnormalities (e.g., polycystic kidneys).

DIAGNOSTIC PROCEDURES

- Fine-needle aspiration or tissue biopsy of masses (endoscopic or ultrasound-guided) are indicated for establishing the diagnosis of neoplasia.
- Abdominal or thoracic fluid cytology may reveal neoplastic cells.
- Renal biopsy sometimes is useful in determining the morphological disorder and cause.

TREATMENT

- Unless cutaneous or localized, neoplasia carries a guarded to poor prognosis. Surgical excision, radiotherapy, cryosurgery, or hypertherapy are options with some localized tumors.
- Treatment of chronic renal disease/failure seldom is curative. Supportive treatment options include fluids to correct dehydration and acid–base disorders and antibiotics for concurrent infection or sepsis. Salt restriction is indicated if ventral edema develops, and a diet of high-quality carbohydrates (e.g., corn, oats), roughage (e.g., grass hay), and free access to fresh water is recommended. Avoid feeds high in protein or calcium.
- Removal of vitamin D sources and time may result in recovery, but with soft-tissue mineralization in the heart or kidney, the prognosis is poor.

MEDICATIONS

DRUGS OF CHOICE

Chronic Renal Failure

- Good nutritional support and free access to fresh water, fluids and electrolytes, salt blocks if edema is absent (restrict if hypertension or edema develops), and vitamin B complex.
- Anabolic steroids may help to prevent muscle wasting.
- Supportive therapy may prolong life substantially in polyuric (urine output, >18 mL urine/kg per day), stabilized patients.

Hypervitaminosis D

- Removal of the source of vitamin D, fluid diuresis, corticosteroid administration, and low-calcium and -phosphorus feeds.
- In severe cases, treatment generally is unrewarding because of extensive soft-tissue mineralization.

CONTRAINDICATIONS

- Do not feed hypercalcemic horses legume hays (e.g., alfalfa, clover) or high-calcium rations.
- Fluid therapy for hypercalcemic horses should be devoid of calcium.
- Avoid aminoglycoside antibiotics and NSAIDs, or use with extreme caution because of potential nephrotoxic effects.

CALCIUM, HYPERCALCEMIA

PRECAUTIONS
N/A

POSSIBLE INTERACTIONS
N/A

ALTERNATIVE DRUGS
N/A

FOLLOW-UP

PATIENT MONITORING
Chronic renal failure—frequent blood samples to monitor sodium, potassium, calcium, and bicarbonate status.

POSSIBLE COMPLICATIONS
- Soft-tissue mineralization.
- See *Contraindications.*

MISCELLANEOUS

ASSOCIATED CONDITIONS
N/A

AGE-RELATED FACTORS
N/A

ZOONOTIC POTENTIAL
N/A

PREGNANCY
- Increased calcium concentration in mammary secretions is a good indicator of impending parturition.
- Serum calcium remains within reference intervals unless an underlying disease process is present.

SYNONYMS
Hypercalcemia of malignancy—humoral hypercalcemia of malignancy; pseudohyperparathyroidism.

SEE ALSO
- Hyperphosphatemia
- Hypocalcemia

ABBREVIATIONS
- GI = gastrointestinal
- PTH = parathyroid hormone
- PU/PD = Polyuria/polydipsia

Suggested Reading

Brewer BD. Disorders of equine calcium metabolism. Compend Contin Educ Pract Vet 1987;4:S244–S252.

Frank N, Hawkins JF, Couëtil LL, Raymond JT. Primary hyperparathyroidism with osteodystrophia fibrosa of the facial bones in a pony. J Am Vet Med Assoc 1998;212:84–86.

Peauroi JR, Fisher DJ, Mohr FC, Vivrette SL. Primary hyperparathyroidism caused by a functional parathyroid adenoma in a horse. J Am Vet Med Assoc 1998;212:1915–1918.

Pringle J, Ortenburger A. Diseases of the kidneys and ureters. In: Kobluk CN, Ames TR, Geor RJ, eds. The horse: diseases and clinical management. Philadelphia: WB Saunders, 1995:583–596.

Turrel JM. Oncology. In: Kobluk CN, Ames TR, Geor RJ, eds. The horse: diseases and clinical management. Philadelphia: WB Saunders, 1995:1111–1136.

Author Karen E. Russell

Consulting Editor Claire B. Andreasen

CALCIUM, HYPOCALCEMIA

BASICS

DEFINITION

Total serum calcium less than the reference interval, or <10.0 mg/dL.

PATHOPHYSIOLOGY

• Calcium, a major component of bone, also is necessary for blood coagulation, muscle contraction and neuromuscular excitability, hormone secretion, and enzyme activation.
• Fractions of total serum calcium occur as protein-bound (50%), ionized (40%), or complexed with other anions (10%).
• Ionized calcium is the physiologically active fraction.
• Of the protein-bound fraction, ≅50% is complexed with albumin.
• Serum albumin has a direct affect on total serum calcium concentration, but the correlation is not as strong in horses as in dogs. Ionized calcium usually is not affected by albumin concentrations. Acidosis increases the ionized calcium fraction by decreasing protein binding; alkalosis has the opposite effect. Total calcium usually remains within the reference interval.
• Hypocalcemia can be seen with dietary deficiency or imbalance, GI disease, hypocalcemic tetany (e.g., lactation, transport, idiopathic, eclampsia), hypoalbuminemia or hypoproteinemia, cantharidin (i.e., blister beetle) toxicosis, excessive sweating, renal disease, or pancreatic disease.

SYSTEMS AFFECTED

Skeletal

• In response to hypocalcemia, calcium is mobilized from bone to maintain other metabolic functions.
• Consequences include too little or abnormal bone formation, bone demineralization, and a skeleton more prone to injury.

Neuromuscular

Most acute cases manifest by tetany rather than paresis.

GI

Decreased contractility may lead to hypomotility and ileus, especially with decreased ionized calcium.

Cardiovascular

• SDF (i.e., contraction of one or both flanks coincident with heart beat) is thought to result from altered membrane potential of the phrenic nerve and its discharge in response to electrical impulses generated during myocardial depolarization.
• S_4–S_1 heart sounds may be obscured by thumping caused by contracture of the diaphragm.
• Hypocalcemia is the most consistent electrolyte abnormality in this condition.

SIGNALMENT

• Depends on underlying disease or condition.
• Lactation tetany most frequently occurs in mares ≅10 days postfoaling or 1–2 days postweaning.
• Draft breeds are more susceptible.

SIGNS

Historical Findings

• History varies with the underlying cause.
• Owners may describe fatigue or exhaustion; abdominal pain, anorexia, or depression after ingestion of alfalfa; lameness, swollen painful joints, or poor growth; or diets of high-grain content and low quality roughage or bran supplement added to grain (especially wheat or rice bran, which are high in phosphorus).

Physical Examination Findings

General Clinical Signs:
• Tetany, increased muscle tone, stiffness, muscle fasciculation, SDF, tachypnea, trismus, normal to high body temperature, and sweating.
• In very severe cases, inco-ordination, recumbency, convulsions, and death.

Dietary Calcium Deficiency or Imbalance:
• Clinical signs manifest in the skeletal system.
• Early signs include intermittent shifting-leg lameness, generalized joint tenderness, or stilted gait.
• As the disease progresses, abnormal bone formation and enlarged facial bones (e.g., NHP, bighead) occurs.

Cantharidin Toxicosis:
• Abdominal pain
• GI or urinary tract irritation
• Elevated respiratory and heart rates
• Watery feces
• Fever
• Sweating
• Shock

Pancreatic Disease:
• Weight loss
• Diarrhea
• Abdominal pain
• Gastric distention
• Shock

CAUSES

Hypoalbuminemia or Hypoproteinemia

• The protein-bound fraction of calcium is directly affected by serum protein concentration; low serum protein concentrations may mask hypercalcemia.
• Correction formulas determined for dogs have not been validated in horses.

CALCIUM, HYPOCALCEMIA

Dietary Calcium Deficiency or Imbalance

- Occurs from lack of dietary calcium or factors limiting calcium utilization—excess phosphorus (in the form of inorganic phosphorus, phylate phosphate); oxalic acid.
- Calcium deficiency may go undetected for many weeks or months; adults have large calcium reserves.
- In young animals, skeletal mass does not keep up with increasing body size; the skeleton is more prone to injury.
- NHP occurs from low calcium and excess phosphorus intake.
- PTH secretion increases a compensatory mechanism to correct disturbance in mineral homeostasis induced by nutritional imbalance.
- Rickets occurs from combined calcium and vitamin D deficiency.
- Young, growing animals with vitamin D deficiency may be hypocalcemic, hypophosphatemic, and have elevated ALP. The vitamin D deficiency causes defective mineralization of new bone, resulting in painful swelling of the physis and metaphysis of long bones and costochondral junctions, bowed limbs, and stiff gait.
- Natural cases of rickets in foals are not well documented and probably are quite rare.

Cantharidin Toxicosis

Ingestion of alfalfa hay or alfalfa-containing products contaminated with blister beetles (*Epicauta* sp.).

Hypocalcemic Tetany (Lactation, Transport)

- Lactation tetany generally occurs ≅10 days postfoaling or 2 days postweaning.
- Draft mares, mares that produce large amounts of milk, and mares on pasture only or a marginal plane of nutrition are at greatest risk.
- Prolonged transportation or strenuous activity can predispose to hypocalcemia and tetany.
- Concurrent hypomagnesemia is common in hypocalcemic tetany.

Excessive Sweating

- Horses lose calcium, chloride, and potassium in sweat.
- Endurance horses are especially prone to electrolyte imbalances and acid–base disturbances (e.g., alkalosis) after prolonged activity, and may develop SDF.

Renal Disease

Horses with acute renal failure may be hypo-, hyper-, or normocalcemic.

Pancreatic Disease

- Acute pancreatitis is difficult to diagnose antemortem.
- Horses in which pancreatic atrophy was the only abnormality at necropsy presented with SDF, tetany, generalized muscle tremors, and hypocalcemia.

GI Disease

- Plasma calcium concentrations may decline during the postoperative period after abdominal surgery and while receiving IV fluid therapy.
- Tendency to hypocalcemia may contribute to reduced GI smooth muscle activity, with gastric fluid accumulation and delayed fecal passage.

RISK FACTORS

See *Causes*.

DIAGNOSIS

DIFFERENTIAL DIAGNOSIS

- Diet, reproductive, and exercise history aid in differentiating many of the causes of hypocalcemia.
- Tetanus—normal serum calcium, history of wound, do not exhibit SDF, do not respond to treatment with calcium, hyperresponsive to sound, and show prolapse of the third eyelid.
- Strychnine—normal serum calcium.
- Exertional rhabdomyolysis, myositis—marked increases in CK and AST; myoglobinuria.
- Colic—abdominal pain; other signs of GI disease.
- Laminitis—extremely painful feet, bounding digital pulses, and characteristic stance.

CALCIUM, HYPOCALCEMIA

LABORATORY FINDINGS

Drugs That May Alter Lab Results

EDTA, citrate, or oxalate-containing anticoagulants chelate calcium, causing a false decrease in calcium measurements.

Disorders That May Alter Lab Results

- Of total calcium, ≅50% is bound to protein, predominantly albumin.
- Abnormalities in serum albumin or protein concentration directly affect total serum calcium concentration, but the correlation is not as strong in horses as in dogs. Correction formulas determined for dogs have not been validated in horses.
- Total serum calcium may be falsely decreased in the face of hypoproteinemia; hyperalbuminemia or hyperproteinemia may obscure hypocalcemia.
- Acid–base status affects the amount of ionized and protein-bound calcium. Acidosis increases the ionized calcium fraction by decreasing the fraction bound to protein; alkalosis decreases ionized calcium by increasing the fraction bound to protein. Total calcium usually remains within the reference range.
- Lipemia and hemolysis may falsely elevate total calcium.

Valid If Run in Human Lab?

Yes

CBC/BIOCHEMIATRY/URINALYSIS

- General—concurrent hypomagnesemia commonly is seen during many conditions associated with hypocalcemia.
- Cantharidin toxicosis—hypomagnesemia, hematuria, and normal to isosthenuric urine specific gravity.
- Excessive exercise, endurance events, SDF—hypocalcemia, hypokalemia, hypochloremia, and alkalosis.
- NHP—normal renal function; depending on stage of disease, hypocalcemia, hyperphosphatemia, and elevated ALP.
- Pancreatic disease—increased amylase, lipase, GGT, and peritoneal amylase.

OTHER LABORATORY TESTS

- Total serum calcium is reported with routine biochemical analysis.
- Measurement of ionized calcium concentration by ion-selective electrodes requires special sample handling and generally is not readily available.
- Dietary deficiency or imbalance—review of dietary history, inspection of feed, and chemical analysis for calcium and phosphorus.
- NHP—increased urinary phosphorus and decreased urinary calcium concentrations.
- Cantharidin toxicosis—presence of blister beetles in hay, determination of cantharidin in urine or stomach contents is definitive; loss of activity of toxic principle in urine occurs ≅5 days after consumption; urine collected early is most diagnostic.

IMAGING

Conventional radiology has little benefit in detecting loss of skeletal mineralization until losses exceed 30%.

DIAGNOSTIC PROCEDURES

N/A

TREATMENT

- General—often symptomatic to control pain with analgesics; maintain hydration with fluids; broad-spectrum antibiotics with suspected bacterial infections; supplementation with high-calcium feeds (e.g., alfalfa, legume hays).
- NHP—correct dietary deficiency or imbalance by supplying the deficient nutrient.
- Cantharidin toxicosis—no antidote available; remove contaminated feed; supportive therapy (e.g., vacuate GI tract, maintain hydration, control pain, diuretics).
- Sources of calcium include alfalfa or legume hay, molasses, limestone, bonemeal, or dicalcium phosphate.
- Dietary calcium:phosphorus ratio should not exceed 1.5–2:1.

MEDICATIONS

DRUGS OF CHOICE

IV calcium solutions—20% calcium borogluconate diluted with saline, dextrose, or lactated Ringer solution.

CONTRAINDICATIONS

N/A

PRECAUTIONS

- Calcium is cardiotoxic.
- Administer solutions containing calcium slowly, with constant monitoring of heart rate and rhythm.
- Stop treatment at once if dysrhythmia or bradycardia develops.

POSSIBLE INTERACTIONS

N/A

ALTERNATIVE DRUGS

N/A

FOLLOW UP

PATIENT MONITORING

With hypocalcemic tetany, recovery may take several days, and relapses can occur.

POSSIBLE COMPLICATIONS

N/A

MISCELLANEOUS

ASSOCIATED CONDITIONS

SDF has been associated with many diseases and conditions—PO administration of large quantities of sodium bicarbonate to hypochloremic and volume-depleted horses, salmonellosis, severe diarrhea, laminitis, abdominal disorders, postoperative rhabdomyolysis, myositis, uterine torsion, lactation tetany, overexertion, cantharidin toxicosis, thoracic hematoma, and trauma.

AGE-RELATED FACTORS

Young animals may be more prone to skeletal abnormalities resulting from dietary deficiency or imbalance.

ZOONOTIC POTENTIAL

N/A

PREGNANCY

See *Causes*—hypocalcemic tetany; lactation tetany

SYNONYMS

- NHP—bighead disease, bran disease, osteodystrophia fibrosa, and Miller's disease
- SDF—thumps

SEE ALSO

Hyperphosphatemia—NHP

ABBREVIATIONS

- ALP = alkaline phosphatase
- AST = aspartate aminotransferase
- CK = creatine kinase
- GGT = γ-glutamyltransferase
- GI = gastrointestinal
- NHP = nutritional secondary hyperparathyroidism
- PTH = parathyroid hormone
- SDF = synchronous diaphragmatic flutter

Suggested Reading

Brewer BD. Disorders of equine calcium metabolism. Compend Contin Educ Pract Vet 1987;4:S244–S252.

Capen CC. Nutritional secondary hyperparathyroidism. In: Robinson NE, ed. Current therapy in equine medicine. Philadelphia: WB Saunders, 1983:160–163.

Dart AJ, Snyder JR, Spier SJ, Sullivan KE. Ionized calcium concentration in horses with surgically managed gastrointestinal disease: 147 cases (1988–1990). J Am Vet Med Assoc 1992;1244–1248.

Helman RG, Edwards WC. Clinical features of blister beetle poisoning in equids: 70 cases (1983–1996). J Am Vet Med Assoc 1997;211:1018–1021.

Freestone JF, Melrose PA. Endocrine diseases. In: Kobluk CN, Amers TR, Geor RJ, eds. The horse: diseases and clinical management. Philadelphia: WB Saunders, 1995:1137–1164.

Author Karen E. Russell

Consulting Editor Claire B. Andreasen

CANTHARIDIN TOXICOSIS

BASICS

DEFINITION

• Cantharidin is a bicyclic, terpenoid vesicant in the hemolymph of blister beetles (*Epicauta* spp.).
• Toxicosis results from ingestion of baled alfalfa hay containing dead beetles.
• Horses poisoned by cantharidin display clinical signs of colic with lesions of ulceration or erosion throughout the digestive tract. Lesions also are reported in the urinary bladder and cardiac musculature.
• Cantharidin toxicosis can result in hypocalcemia, hypomagnesemia, renal failure, and cardiac abnormalities.
• The prognosis in affected horses is guarded.
• Poisoned horses should be treated aggressively.

PATHOPHYSIOLOGY

• Large swarms of blister beetles concentrate in alfalfa fields from the southwestern U.S. to the East Coast.
• Beetles consumed by horses result in cantharidin being rapidly absorbed from the GI tract and excreted in the urine.
• Because of the vesicant properties of cantharidin, irritation characterized by vesicle formation, ulceration, or erosions can occur where cantharidin contacts mucosal surfaces.
• Cantharidin inhibits phosphatase-2A, which controls cell proliferation, modulates phosphatases and protein kinases, and plays a role in the activity of cellular membrane channels and receptors.
• The pathophysiology of hypocalcemia, although not fully understood, is thought to be responsible for synchronous diaphragmatic flutter.

SYSTEMS AFFECTED

• GI—colic caused by the vesicant and irritating properties of cantharidin.
• Renal/urologic—mucosal hemorrhage in the urinary bladder, with resultant. hematuria.
• Cardiovascular—cardiac muscle necrosis; synchronous diaphragmatic flutter.
• Nervous—aggressive behavior and violent, seizure-like muscular activity can occur secondary to colic; muscle fasciculations and seizures before death.

GENETICS

N/A

INCIDENCE/PREVALENCE

• Associated primarily with feeding of alfalfa hay or alfalfa-containing products.
• Occasionally associated with blister beetles having been collected and fed in a malicious manner.

SIGNALMENT

Species

N/A

Breed Predilections

N/A

Mean Age and Range

N/A

Predominant Sex

N/A

SIGNS

General Comments

• Clinical signs and their severity depend on the amount of cantharidin ingested.
• In high doses, cantharidin can result in sudden death within several hours, with little or no evidence of struggle or severe shock and death.

Historical Findings

• Restlessness with sweating, pawing the ground, irritability, or other signs of abdominal pain or colic are most frequently reported.
• Violent, seizure-like activity and aggressive behavior have been reported secondary to severe colic.
• Some horses have diarrhea or play in water with their muzzles without drinking.
• Stranguria is common.

Physical Examination Findings

• Colic, fever, tachycardia, tachypnea, congested mucous membranes, and increased capillary refill times.
• Sweating, synchronous diaphragmatic flutter, muscle fasciculations, and evidence of blood in the urine occasionally are reported.

RISK FACTORS

Feeding of baled alfalfa or related alfalfa products increases risk.

DIAGNOSIS

DIFFERENTIAL DIAGNOSIS

• Consider any other cause of equine colic—intestinal displacement, impaction, intestinal torsion or volvulus, thromboembolism, gas-distended intestine, ulcers in the stomach or bowel, peritonitis, uterine torsion, mesenteric abscess, ovarian tumor, and abscess.
• Consider monensin toxicosis, endotoxic shock, or any other causes of peracute to acute abdominal crisis or shock.
• If observed, neurologic signs can be confused with rabies, other viral or bacterial encephalitides, hepatoencephalopathy, leukoencephalomalacia, thiamine deficiency, organochlorine or organophosphorus insecticide toxicosis, and trauma.
• Important findings that aid in differentiating cantharidiasis—history of feeding alfalfa or alfalfa-containing products, hypocalcemia with or without concurrent hypomagnesemia, discovery of beetles in hay or GI contents, and compatible lesions at postmortem examination.

CBC/BIOCHEMISTRY/URINALYSIS

• Consistent findings include hypocalcemia, hypomagnesemia, hyposthenuria despite hemoconcentration, mild azotemia, and increased serum creatine kinase concentrations.
• In experimental toxicosis, hypocalcemia and hypomagnesemia were the most persistent findings, even after all other values returned to baseline.
• Hematuria and renal epithelial cells can be observed at urinalysis; hemoconcentration and hypoproteinemia also can be detected.

OTHER LABORATORY TESTS

N/A

IMAGING

N/A

DIAGNOSTIC PROCEDURES

• Detection of cantharidin in urine or intestinal contents (500 mL each) at any level is considered clinically significant.
• Retrieve samples and send for analysis as early as possible because of the rapid renal clearance (3–4 days) of cantharidin.
• Liver, kidney, and serum samples can be used for analysis but are not the specimens of choice.

PATHOLOGIC FINDINGS

• Large doses can result in sudden death without gross lesions.
• Gross lesions are most common in the terminal esophagus and stomach, less frequent in the intestines, and consist of areas of ulceration or erosion that may (or may not) be hemorrhagic.
• Reddening of the mucosal lining of the GI tract and urinary bladder has been noted.
• Streaks of myocardial necrosis occasionally occur.

TREATMENT

APPROPRIATE HEALTH CARE

• Focus treatment on enhancing fecal and urinary elimination of cantharidin, correcting dehydration, managing serum calcium and magnesium abnormalities, and controlling pain.
• Intensive supportive treatment may be required for 3–10 days, depending on the severity of illness.

CANTHARIDIN TOXICOSIS

NURSING CARE

- Initiate fluid therapy to adequately rehydrate the horse, decrease serum cantharidin levels, and aid in toxin excretion via the kidneys.
- Monitor serum calcium frequently during treatment, and supplement fluids with calcium if indicated.
- Adult horses may receive 500 mL of a commercial calcium-containing fluid (not exceeding 23 g of calcium compound per 100 mL) if administered slowly. Dilute commercial calcium preparations in isotonic fluids to decrease the chance of adverse cardiac responses (e.g., heart block, severe bradyaprhythmia) and to allow more rapid administration. Dilute calcium in a ratio of 1:4 with saline or dextrose if frequent administration is required to control synchronous diaphragmatic flutter or muscle fasciculations.
- Decreased pulse rate and increased intensity of heartbeat on auscultation are noted when administering calcium.
- Do not include calcium in fluids containing sodium bicarbonate because of possible precipitation of calcium.
- Hypomagnesemia may require addition of magnesium as well as calcium to the isotonic fluids; oral supplementation with calcium lactate and magnesium oxide may be warranted.

ACTIVITY

Stall rest and limited activity for 5–10 days.

DIET

Remove all sources of contaminated alfalfa hay.

CLIENT EDUCATION

N/A

SURGICAL CONSIDERATIONS

N/A

MEDICATIONS

DRUGS OF CHOICE

- Prednisolone sodium succinate (50–100 mg as an initial dose) may be administered IV over 1 minute for severe shock.
- Administer AC (2–5 g/kg as a slurry) via nasogastric tube, then mineral oil (2–4 L 2–3 hours later) to prevent occupation of adsorptive sites on the AC.
- Some clinicians recommend repeated doses of mineral oil to aid in possible cantharidin binding and decreased GI transit time.
- Consider sucralfate (1 g per 45 kg PO q6–8h) in horses exhibiting clinical signs of gastritis—water playing). Ulcerative lesions in the lower digestive tract also benefit from sucralfate.
- Commonly prescribed analgesics (e.g., flunixin meglumine) may not provide adequate pain relief. Therefore, administer α_2-adrenergic agonists (e.g., detomidine [20–40 μg/kg IV], butorphanol tartrate [0.02–0.1 mg/kg IV q3–4h, not to exceed 48 hours]). Detomidine at 40 μg/kg should provide analgesia for 45–75 minutes.
- Broad-spectrum antibiotic therapy if septic complications from the ulceration or erosions present in the GI mucosa are likely.

CONTRAINDICATIONS

- Diuretics—furosemide
- Acepromazine maleate—may potentiate shock.
- Aminoglycosides—potential nephrotoxic effects.
- Use caution with corticosteroids—reported to cause laminitis.

PRECAUTIONS

N/A

POSSIBLE INTERACTIONS

Do not administer detomidine concurrently with potentiated sulfonamides (e.g., trimethoprim/sulfa), because fatal dysrythmias may result.

ALTERNATIVE DRUGS

Xylazine (1.1 mg/kg IV) also is an α_2-adrenergic agonist and may be substituted for detomidine for analgesia.

FOLLOW-UP

PATIENT MONITORING

Monitor hydration status, electrolytes (particularly serum calcium and magnesium), and response to analgesics.

PREVENTION/AVOIDANCE

- Because blister beetles prefer alfalfa field margins, avoid harvesting from these areas to decrease the risk of dead beetles being incorporated into hay bales.
- Spraying insecticides to control blister beetles has had some success.
- Owners should inspect individual flakes of hay for beetles when feeding. Shaking and shredding the flake by hand when placing in the feeding bunk allows detection of beetles caught in the hay during harvest.

POSSIBLE COMPLICATIONS

Complications are unusual, but laminitis has been reported.

EXPECTED COURSE AND PROGNOSIS

- Prognosis ranges from poor to excellent and depends on amount of cantharidin ingested, early recognition of intoxication, and aggressiveness of therapy.
- A more favorable prognosis may be given if the animal survives for 2–3 days after toxin exposure.
- In experimental cantharidiasis, persistent tachycardia and tachypnea as well as increased serum creatine kinase concentrations were associated with a poorer prognosis.

MISCELLANEOUS

ASSOCIATED CONDITIONS

N/A

AGE-RELATED FACTORS

N/A

ZOONOTIC POTENTIAL

N/A

PREGNANCY

Use corticosteroids with caution in pregnant mares, particularly during the later stages of gestation.

SYNONYMS

- Blister beetle poisoning
- Equine cantharidiasis

SEE ALSO

N/A

ABBREVIATIONS

- AC = activated charcoal
- GI = gastrointestinal

Suggested Reading

Helman RG, Edwards WC. Clinical features of blister beetle poisoning in equids: 70 cases (1983–1996). J Am Vet Med Assoc 1997;211:1018–1021.

Guglick MA, MacAllister CG, Panciera R. Equine cantharidiasis. Compend Contin Educ Pract Vet 1996;18:77–83.

Ray AC, Kyle ALG, Murphy MJ, et al. Etiologic agents, incidence, and improved diagnostic methods of cantharidin toxicosis in horses. Am J Vet Res 1989;50:187–191.

Schoeb TR, Panciera RJ. Blister beetle poisoning in horses. J Am Vet Med Assoc 1978;173:75–77.

Shawley RV, Rolf LL. Experimental cantharidiasis in the horse. Am J Vet Res 1984;45:2261–2266.

Author Eric L. Stair

Consulting Editor Robert H. Poppenga

CASTRATION

BASICS

DEFINITION
Surgical removal of testes.

Pathophysiology
The testes are removed from the stallion to prevent reproduction, curb objectionable male sexual behavior, eliminate neoplasia, remove an irreparably damaged testis, for hydrocoele and/or hematocoele, or as an adjunct during inguinal/scrotal hernia repair. One or both testes are removed, dependent on the circumstances.

System Affected
- Reproductive

SIGNALMENT
Intact male horses of any age.

SIGNS

Historical Findings
- Objectionable expression of stallion-like behavior.
- Recent history of breeding or semen collection.
- Gross changes in the size of the testis.
- Reduced fertility.
- Pain (generally colic-like symptoms).
- Reluctance to breed, jump, or walk.

Physical Examination Findings
- Scrotal testes of normal size, orientation, and/or texture.
- Increased or decreased scrotal size.
- Increased or decreased testicular size.
- Abnormal testicular texture (too soft or firm).
- Abnormal testicular position.
- Abnormal scrotal temperature (too warm or cold).
- Edema/engorgement of scrotum and/or contents.
- Derangements in systemic parameters (elevated HR, RR, inappetence, CBC abnormalities).

CAUSES AND RISK FACTORS
- Sexual maturation*
- Trauma*
- Cryptorchidism *
- Torsion of the spermatic cord*
- Testicular hematoma/rupture*
- Neoplasia*
- Testicular degeneration
- Testicular hypoplasia
- Orchitis/epididymitis
- Breeding activity (traumatic injury, herniation)
- Temperature extremes (scrotal hydrocoele, frostbite)

DIAGNOSIS

DIFFERENTIAL DIAGNOSIS

Differentiating Similar Signs
N/A

Differentiating Causes
See Scrotal Enlargement, Abnormal Testicular Size for pathologic conditions leading to castration.

CBC/BIOCHEMISTRY/URINALYSIS
Laboratory parameters should be normal prior to performing routine castration.

OTHER LABORATORY TESTS
N/A

IMAGING
N/A

DIAGNOSTIC PROCEDURES
N/A

TREATMENT

APPROPRIATE HEALTH CARE
Routine castration is generally managed as an outpatient procedure.

NURSING CARE
- Stall confinement for 24 hours after castration.
- Hydrotherapy: cold hose to affected area at least 15 minutes, SID, for 7 days.

ACTIVITY
Forced exercise (trotting on a longe line) for a minimum of 15 minutes, BID, for 2 weeks.

DIET
N/A

CLIENT EDUCATION
See Complications.

SURGICAL CONSIDERATIONS
- The reader is referred to an appropriate equine surgical textbook for a complete explanation of surgical technique. Factors to consider prior to performing castration are: position of the testes (2 scrotal testes present), position of the animal (recumbent vs standing), and technique (open vs closed castration).
- Castration of the recumbent horse requires general injectable anesthesia. Advantages of recumbent castration include safety to the surgeon (with a well-restrained and anesthetized animal), excellent surgical exposure, good analgesia, and muscle relaxation. Disadvantages include recovery from a recumbent position, anesthetic risks, and expense. Standing castration is advantageous due to decreased risk of injury to the animal during anesthetic recovery, shorter recovery time, and decreased expense. Disadvantages of standing castration include increased risk of injury to the surgeon and decreased exposure to the surgical site.

CASTRATION

• Open castration involves excision of the parietal (common) vaginal tunic and complete exposure of the testis, epididymis, and spermatic cord. The spermatic cord is transected close to the superficial inguinal ring. Using this technique, the vascular and the musculofibrous portions of the spermatic cord can be transected individually. With closed castration, the parietal vaginal tunic is dissected from the subcutaneous tissue, and the tunic is not incised. Emasculation of the entire cord occurs in one step.

MEDICATIONS

DRUG(S) OF CHOICE

• Anti-inflammatory therapy (phenylbutazone, 2-4 mg/kg, P/O or IV) is useful for 2- 3 days post-operatively to help control swelling.
• Antimicrobial therapy should not be necessary in an uncomplicated castration. Antimicrobial therapy should be considered in cases of orchitis/epididymitis and testicular trauma.
• Tetanus toxoid should be administered prior to surgery.

CONTRAINDICATIONS

N/A

PRECAUTIONS

N/A

POSSIBLE INTERACTIONS

N/A

ALTERNATIVE DRUGS

N/A

FOLLOW-UP

PATIENT MONITORING

The horse should be confined and monitored closely in the first 24 hours after the procedure for signs of excessive hemorrhage. The surgical site should be monitored once daily for 2 weeks post-operatively for signs of excessive swelling, infection, or evisceration.

POSSIBLE COMPLICATIONS

• Excessive hemorrhage
  • Improper emasculation frequently is the cause of excessive hemorrhage.
  • Minor hemorrhage may persist for hours, but significant hemorrhage should not persist for more than 30 minutes after castration.
  • Treatment is identification and ligation of the offending vessel. The horse may require general anesthesia to locate the vessel.
• Preputial/scrotal swelling occurs in moderate amounts after surgery.
  • Excessive swelling usually results from poor drainage at the surgical site.
  • Vigorous, forced exercise and patency of the incision site will help prevent excessive post-operative swelling.
  • Excessive swelling may also occur if the surgical area is infected. Antimicrobial therapy, anti-inflammatory therapy, and drainage are warranted if an infection is diagnosed.
• Infection of the spermatic cord (funiculitis, "schirrus cord") may occur as a result of improper drainage of the surgical site. Antimicrobial agents, drainage, hydrotherapy, and removal of the infected cord are the treatments of choice.
• Evisceration of the abdominal contents is an uncommon but possibly fatal complication of castration. If intestinal contents are noted in the incision, the horse should be anesthetized immediately to prevent further evisceration and trauma to the bowel. The intestinal contents and incision site should be cleaned meticulously and viable intestine should be replaced. Non-viable intestine must be resected. The superficial inguinal ring is sutured closed, or the inguinal canal is packed with sterile gauze and left open if the superficial ring is grossly contaminated and cannot be sutured. Gauze packing is left in place for 48-72 hours by suturing the scrotal incision closed. Care should be taken prior to removal of gauze to be certain the gauze has not adhered to intestinal contents.
• Persistent masculine behavior is a common post-castration complication. The behavior is often inappropriately attributed to epididymal remnants post-castration. The testes and adrenal cortices are the sole sources of androgens, i.e. not epididymides and spermatic cords. If both testes were completely removed at surgery, persistent stallion-like behavior in geldings results from learned behaviors, not hormonal influence.

MISCELLANEOUS

ASSOCIATED CONDITIONS

N/A

AGE-RELATED FACTORS

Older animals may have larger vessels within the spermatic cord. Crimping at emasculation site and/or ligation of the vessels may be necessary to prevent excessive hemorrhage.

ZOONOTIC POTENTIAL

N/A

PREGNANCY

N/A

SYNONYMS

Gelding

SEE ALSO

• Cryptorchidism
• Abnormal scrotal enlargement
• Abnormal testicular size

ABBREVIATIONS

N/A

Suggested Reading

Turner AS, McIlwraith CW. Techniques in large animal surgery, 2nd ed. Philadelphia: Lea & Febiger, 1989:177-184.
Varner DD, Schumacher J, Blanchard T, Johnson L. Diseases and management of breeding stallions. Goleta: American Veterinary Publications 1991.

Author Margo L. Macpherson
Consulting Editor Carla L. Carleton

CENTAUREA SPP. TOXICOSIS

BASICS

OVERVIEW
- *Centaurea solstitialis* (yellow star thistle) is an annual weed commonly found in the northwestern U.S. The plant is ≅1 m in height, and the flower is yellow, with a composite head and sharp thorns around the flowerhead.
- *C. repens* (Russian knapweed) is a perennial weed found mainly in the western U.S. but also in the eastern U.S. as well. The plant is ≅1 m in height and has a cone-shaped flowering head that is pinkish-purple in color as well as spreading rhizomes, which make control difficult. In general, it is not readily grazed.
- Ingestion of either plant can result in ENE or "chewing disease," which is characterized by the abrupt appearance of difficulties in eating and drinking.
- Typically, affected animals lose condition and die.

SIGNALMENT
No breed, age, or sex predilections.

SIGNS
- Drowsiness
- Difficulty eating and drinking
- Aimless walking, with the head low
- Hypertonicity of facial and lip muscles
- Tongue lolling
- Loss of body condition
- Dehydration
- Death

CAUSES AND RISK FACTORS
- Toxic principle not conclusively identified but suspected to be a sesquiterpene lactone.
- Lethal dose of fresh plant material has been reported as 2.3–2.6 kg per 100 kg for *C. solstitialis* and 1.8–2.5 kg per 100 kg for *C. repens.*

DIAGNOSIS

DIFFERENTIAL DIAGNOSIS
- Teeth or mouth abnormalities.
- Neurological conditions, particularly those affecting the cranial nerves—equine protozoal myeloencephalitis; guttural pouch mycosis.

CBC/BIOCHEMISTRY/URINALYSIS
N/A

OTHER LABORATORY TESTS
N/A

IMAGING
N/A

DIAGNOSTIC PROCEDURES
- Positive identification of plants.
- Evidence for consumption of *C. solstitialis* or *C. repens.*

PATHOLOGIC FINDINGS
ENE—foci of necrotic tissue in the brain, specifically in the globus pallidus and substantia nigra.

CENTAUREA SPP. TOXICOSIS

TREATMENT

- Removal from pasture or source of plants.
- Supportive care.

MEDICATIONS

DRUGS

N/A

CONTRAINDICATIONS/POSSIBLE INTERACTIONS

N/A

FOLLOW-UP

Remove any nonaffected animals from the suspected source.

MISCELLANEOUS

ASSOCIATED CONDITIONS

N/A

AGE-RELATED FACTORS

N/A

ZOONOTIC POTENTIAL

N/A

PREGNANCY

N/A

SEE ALSO

N/A

ABBREVIATION

ENE = equine nigropallidal encephalomalacia

Suggested Reading

Cordy DR. Centaurea species and equine nigropallidal encephalomalacia. In: Keeler RF, ed. Effects of poisonous plants on livestock. New York: Academic Press, 1978.

Author Larry J. Thompson
Consulting Editor Robert H. Poppenga

CERVICAL LESIONS

BASICS

DEFINITION

• Most common problems encountered—inflammation, lacerations and adhesions, and inability to dilate during estrus.
• Congenital abnormalities and neoplasia of the cervix—rare.

PATHOPHYSIOLOGY

May impair normal cervical function and competency, leading to infertility, repeated uterine infections, and possible pregnancy loss.

SYSTEM AFFECTED

Reproductive

GENETICS

N/A

INCIDENCE/PREVALANCE

More common in old mares.

SIGNALMENT

• Old (mean age, 12–13 years), pluriparous mares (mean parity before surgery, 6.2) after either normal parturition or dystocia.
• Old, pluriparous mares are more predisposed to cervicitis caused by pneumovagina, urovagina, or DUC.
• Young or old, nervous, maiden mares.

SIGNS

Historical Findings

• Infertility
• Recurrent uterine infections
• Pyometra
• Pregnancy loss

Physical Examination Findings

• Vaginal examination—pneumovagina or urovagina; vaginal discharge; purulent material coming through the cervix; cervical and vaginal mucosal irritation; cervical lacerations or mucosal roughness; adhesions between the cervix and vaginal fornix or in the cervical lumen; intrauterine fluid accumulation, with or without cervical adhesions.
• Intrauterine fluid accumulation after breeding.

CAUSES

Infectious

• Associated with anatomic abnormalities (e.g., pneumovagina), vaginitis, and endometritis.
• See also *Endometritis* and *Ascending Placentitis.*

Noninfectious

Cervical Trauma:
• Frequently occurs, resulting in full- or partial-thickness lacerations, during unassisted, prolonged parturition or dystocia—assisted, difficult foaling.
• Prolonged manipulation and traction and use of a fetotome aggravate the outcome.
• Lacerations most frequently occur in the vaginal portion of the cervix but may extend toward the uterus, affecting the internal os.
Adhesions:
• May be sequelae of cervical trauma during parturition or originate from use of irritating solutions for uterine therapy, pyometra, and rarely, chronic endometritis.
• May obliterate the cervical lumen and keep it from opening and closing properly.
Cervicitis:
• May be iatrogenic (e.g., chemical substances) or secondary to trauma (e.g., parturition, dystocia, obstetric manipulation) or infection (e.g., vaginitis, endometritis).
• Individual sensitivity exists to use of diluted iodine, chlorhexidine, or acetic acid. These products may produce mucosal irritation, ulceration, and necrosis, even at low dilutions.
• May occur with use of nonbuffered aminoglycosides, antibiotics, or antimycotics for endometritis.
• Pneumo- and urovagina result in vaginal, cervical, and uterine irritation.
Idiopathic:
• Some maiden mares (young or old) show impaired cervical relaxation during estrus.
• No associated fibrosis or adhesions.
• Affects ability to conceive by natural breeding, and causes DUC.
• Once affected mares conceive, the cervix dilates normally at parturition.
Neoplasia:
• Very rare
• Uterocervical leiomyoma has been reported.
Developmental Abnormalities
• Rare
• Cervical aplasia, hypoplasia, and double cervix.

RISK FACTORS

• Prolonged natural or assisted parturition.
• $>$2–3 cuts with the fetotome.
• Young or old maiden mares.
• Aggressive uterine therapy.
• Concurrent acute and chronic endometritis.
• Pyometra.

DIAGNOSIS

DIFFERENTIAL DIAGNOSIS

Other causes of vaginal discharge—endometritis; pyometra.

CBC/BIOCHEMISTRY/URINALYSIS

N/A

OTHER LABORATORY TESTS

N/A

IMAGING

Ultrasonography—fluid accumulation within the uterus caused by a tight cervix (e.g., while still in estrus, after breeding) or adhesions.

DIAGNOSTIC PROCEDURES

Cervical Examination

• The cervix is examined by transrectal palpation, direct visualization with a speculum, and direct vaginal/digital palpation.
• Transrectal palpation—determines the size, tone, and degree of relaxation.
• Vaginoscopy—provides information regarding cervical and vaginal color (e.g., hyperemia), presence of edema, secretions (e.g., pus, urine), or adhesions between the cervical os and vagina.
• Digital palpation of the cervix is essential to evaluate lacerations or intraluminal adhesions. It is performed by placing the index finger into the cervical lumen and the thumb on the vaginal side of the cervix, then carefully feeling for defects around its full perimeter.
• To assess its ability to relax and to detect intraluminal adhesions, perform cervical evaluation during estrus.
• To evaluate cervical closure and tone and for the presence and extent of lacerations, assessment is best conducted during diestrus.
• During the noncycling phase of the year, mares can be placed on exogenous progesterone for 7 days to evaluate cervical tone and its ability to close.

Timing of Repair in Postpartum Mares

• Postpartum mares may be evaluated for surgical readiness $\geq$30 days after foaling (i.e., after the 30-day heat) to allow for normal cervical involution.
• Alternatively, if a mare has foaled normally apart from its recurrent tear, breeding earlier can readily be accomplished: skip foal heat, short-cycle, and A.I. on the next estrus, with daily or every-other-day serial palpations to determine the day of ovulation. Surgical repair is ideally accomplished within 24–48 hours after ovulation. It must occur $\leq$72 hours after ovulation, such that inflammation induced by the surgical procedure will have abated before entry of the embryo into the uterus by 5.5–6 days. There is no need, nor should one attempt, to evaluate the repair before the mare's 16-day early pregnancy check. If normal cervical tone and competency have been restored and the mare is found to be pregnant, further cervical examination is unnecessary at that time.

PATHOLOGIC FINDINGS

N/A

CERVICAL LESIONS

TREATMENT

APPROPRIATE HEALTH CARE

• Mucosal and submucosal lacerations are treated daily with antimicrobial/steroidal anti-inflammatory ointment to avoid cervical adhesions.
• Recently formed adhesions are manually debrided daily, and ointment is applied BID.
• Mature cervical adhesions may be bypassed by AI or reduced surgically, with guarded prognosis for fertility.
• Treat postpartum mares with cervical lacerations immediately to prevent adhesions and infection.
• Infection—see *Endometritis* and *Ascending Placentitis*.
• Idiopathic—AI and treatment for DUC.

NURSING CARE

Treatment-induced inflammation—when using antiseptics or nonbuffered antibiotics, check for signs of acute mucosal irritation before administering subsequent treatments; stop and change to systemic treatment if inflammation is present.

ACTIVITY

N/A

DIET

N/A

CLIENT EDUCATION

N/A

SURGICAL CONSIDERATIONS

• Surgical repair may not be required when <50% of the vaginal portion of the cervix is affected (i.e., partial-thickness lacerations, competent cervical os). Progesterone supplementation may provide sufficient benefit by increasing cervical tone such that surgery is not required to overcome minor anatomic/functional damage.
• Longitudinal, full-thickness lacerations within the cervical muscle involving the internal cervical os and, therefore, ability of the cervix to close require surgical repair; however, the outcome usually is poor.
• Perform endometrial biopsy before surgery to evaluate ability of the uterus to carry a foal to term. Unnecessary repair and expense can be avoided if it is found that surgery cannot improve the eventual outcome.
• Anatomic defects resulting in cervicitis—pneumovagina and urovagina can be surgically corrected.

MEDICATIONS

DRUGS OF CHOICE

See *Endometritis*.

CONTRAINDICATIONS

See *Endometritis*.

PRECAUTIONS

• Be careful with use of antiseptics or nonbuffered antibiotics to treat infections of the vagina, cervix, or uterus.
• Minimize forced extraction during dystocia, use ample lubrication, and consider cesarean section in cases with poor dilation of the cervix or birth canal.

POSSIBLE INTERACTIONS

N/A

ALTERNATIVE DRUGS

N/A

FOLLOW-UP

PATIENT MONITORING

• Do not examine the cervix for competency or patency until ≥2 weeks after surgical repair.
• Thirty days of sexual rest are recommended before natural breeding.

PREVENTION/AVOIDANCE

N/A

POSSIBLE COMPLICATIONS

• The scar/site of repair lacks the elasticity of normal cervical tissue. A high percentage will tear again at the next foaling and require annual surgical repair after foaling.
• The decision to perform subsequent surgeries is based on the degree of cervical damage after the most recent foaling and assessment of surgical cost and breeding/treatment expenses versus the potential value of an additional foal.

EXPECTED COURSE AND PROGNOSIS

N/A

MISCELLANEOUS

ASSOCIATED CONDITIONS

N/A

AGE-RELATED FACTORS

Most common in old, pluriparous mares and young or old maiden mares.

ZOONOTIC POTENTIAL

N/A

PREGNANCY

Guarded prognosis for maintenance of pregnancy after repair of cervical lacerations.

SYNONYMS

N/A

SEE ALSO

• AI
• Dystocia
• Endometritis and DUC
• Pyometra

ABBREVIATIONS

• AI = artificial insemination
• DUC = delayed uterine clearance

Suggested Reading

Blanchard TL, Varner D, Schumacher J. Surgery of the mare reproductive tract. In: Manual of equine reproduction. St. Louis: Mosby–Year Book, 1998:165–167.

Sertich PL. Cervical problems in the mare. In: McKinnon AO, Voss JL, eds. Equine reproduction. Philadelphia: Lea & Febiger, 1993:404–407.

Author Maria E. Cadario
Consulting Editor Carla L. Carleton

CERVICAL VERTEBRAL MALFORMATION

BASICS

OVERVIEW

- A nervous system disease that occurs in two forms, in all breeds and in both sexes, but most commonly is seen in young male Thoroughbreds.
- The first form, CVI, occurs in horses 2 months to 2 years of age and consists of a dynamic subluxation of the C3 to C4 and/or C4 to C5 articulations, causing impingement of the spinal cord by the cranial epiphysis of the caudal vertebral body. This form is worsened by flexion of the neck.
- The second form, CSSM, is seen primarily in horses 5–10 years of age and consists of a constant narrowing of the C5 to C6 and/or C6 to C7 spinal canal. Hypertrophy of the supporting ligaments, joint capsule, and other surrounding soft tissues as well as degenerative joint disease of the dorsal articular facets encroach on the space of the spinal canal. This form is not worsened by flexion of the neck but is exacerbated by extreme extension of the neck.
- Both forms can present as an insidious, slowly progressive ataxia and weakness of the hind limbs or both the fore and hind limbs, with the hind limbs being more affected.

SIGNALMENT

- Primarily a disease of Thoroughbred colts.
- CVI occurs in horses 2 months to 2 years of age.
- CSSM occurs in horses 5–10 years of age.
- Both forms occur predominately in males—male:female prevalence, 3:1.
- Affected horses are large-frame, fast-growing horses that usually are described as being large for their age.
- The genetic basis of this disease remains under debate, but at least a predisposition for the disease is thought to exist. Breeding trails involving both affected males and females have been unable to produce affected offspring, but due to the strong breed prevalence, no clear answer has yet been found.

SIGNS

- Progressive weakness and ataxia—early in the disease, only the hind limbs are involved; as the disease progresses, the fore and hind limbs will be involved, with the hind limbs affected more severely.
- The neurological signs are those of L/UMN disease. Weakness and ataxia are characterized by knuckling of the fetlocks, toe dragging, a wide base stance, swaying of the body when moving, dysmetria, circumduction of the outside hind limb when tightly circled, the horse stepping on its own feet, abnormal placing responses, and a weak sway response. These signs usually are bilaterally symmetric and are exacerbated with backing. In addition, backing can reveal an inability or unwillingness to bend or flex the fore limbs, resulting in a stiff, awkward, dragging gait.
- Onset of signs may be acute or worsen acutely with trauma—flipping over, running into another horse or object, or hard playing and running.

CAUSES AND RISK FACTORS

- Osteochondrosis—commonly associated disease in affected horses; can occur in multiple joints, vertebrae, and articular facets.
- Fast/excessive growth—most commonly in big, "growthy" horses.
- Overnutrition/nutritional imbalances—excessive energy and carbohydrates; low levels of zinc and copper.
- Calcium:phosphorus ratio outside of 1.5:1.
- Excessive exercise and "rough housing" in predisposed horses.

DIAGNOSIS

DIFFERENTIAL DIAGNOSIS

- Cervical fractures—history and/or evidence of trauma; cervical radiography.
- EPM—CSF antibodies
- EDM
- EVH-1—matched CSF titers
- Intervertebral disc protrusion—rare in horses, but confirmed at myelography.
- Space-occupying masses—plasma cell tumor; hemangiosarcoma; reported but rare findings; myelography and necropsy will localize and confirm the lesion; usually old horses.
- Iliac artery thrombosis—weak and ataxic in appearance, but no other neurologic deficits.

CBC/BIOCHEMISTRY/URINALYSIS

Within normal limits.

IMAGING

Standing, Plain-Film, Lateral Cervical Radiography

- Must be absolutely lateral.
- Sagittal ratios of C1 through C7—measure width of the cranial vertebral orifice and of the widest portion of the epiphysis of the cranial vertebral body; divide width of the orifice by width of the body, which eliminates effects of magnification; ratios for unaffected horses for C2 through C6 are >0.56; ratios in affected horses are less; C7 ratios are >0.58 for unaffected and less for affected horses.

Myelography

- Requires general anesthesia, a focused grid, and a high-energy x-ray machine.
- An atlanto-occipital CSF tap is performed and CSF fluid removed; this fluid can be sent for titers and analysis, if needed.
- A radio-opaque contrast agent (e.g., metrizamide, iopamidole, iohexol, diatrizoate) is injected into the subarachnoid space.
- The head is elevated for 5 minutes, and then films of the entire cervical spine are obtained.
- This procedure is used to isolate the specific vertebral junctions that are involved as well as multiple junctions if surgery is contemplated.
- Obtain films with the horse in the neutral, flexed, and extended positions.

DIAGNOSTIC PROCEDURES

Electromyography:

- Prolonged insertion potentials (>5 seconds), positive sharp waves, and fibrillation potentials in the muscle groups of the neck that are supplied by the affected segments.
- Muscles of the fore and hind limbs have normal examinations.

CERVICAL VERTEBRAL MALFORMATION

TREATMENT

CONSERVATIVE THERAPY

- Stall confinement, with very limited turn out or hand walking.
- Diet balanced for trace minerals with 2× the NRC recommended level of zinc and 3.5 the recommended level of copper. The Ca:P ratio should be 1.5:1.
- TDN should start at 60%–65% of the NRC recommended levels and increase slowly to 75% as repeat examinations and radiography show improvement.
- Keep body condition score at 2 on a scale of 5.

SURGERY

Ventral Cervical Vertebral Stabilization:

- Uses a stainless-steel, Bagby basket filled with cancellous bone graft to fuse the vertebrae.
- Successful for both forms of the disease.
- Has replaced dorsal decompressive laminectomies.

MEDICATIONS

DRUGS

N/A

CONTRAINDICATIONS/POSSIBLE INTERACTIONS

N/A

FOLLOW-UP

PATIENT MONITORING

- Serial neurologic exams at 2–4-month intervals to monitor resolution or progression of clinical signs.
- Lateral cervical radiography at 2–4-month intervals to assess bony changes and, if surgery was performed, to monitor bony fusion.

EXPECTED COURSE AND PROGNOSIS

Conservative Therapy

- If mildly to moderately affected and <1 year of age, good prognosis for recovery to a functional athlete.
- If >1 year of age, not enough bone growth left to effect a cure.

Surgery

- Horses can take as long as a full year to completely recover from neurologic deficits, and some never fully recover but still become athletes.
- Signs of improvement should be noticed during the first 2–3 months.
- Owners should be aware this is a huge long-term commitment and that still liability issues remain if the horse is put into training.

MISCELLANEOUS

ASSOCIATED CONDITIONS

Very high incidence of osteochondrosis of the axial and appendicular skeleton in affected horses.

AGE-RELATED FACTORS

Ventral cervical stabilization is more effective than dorsal decompressive laminectomy in old horses with CSSM.

ZOONOTIC POTENTIAL

N/A

PREGNANCY

N/A

ABBREVIATIONS

- CSF = cerebrospinal fluid
- CSSM = cervical static stenotic malformation
- CVI = cervical vertebral instability
- EDM =
- EPM =
- EVH =
- L/UMN =
- NRC =
- TDN =

Suggested Reading

Donawick WJ, Mayhew IG, Galligan DT, Green SL, Stanley EK, Osborne J. Results of a low protein, low energy diet and confinement on young horses with wobbles. Proc AAEP 1993;39:125–127.

Mayhew IG, Whilock RH, de Lahunta A. Electromyographic and radiographic studies. Cornell Vet 1978;68(Suppl 6–7):44–68.

Moore BR, Reed SM, Biller DS, Kohn CW, Weisbrode SE. Assessment of vertebral canal diameter and bony malformations of the cervical part of the spine in horses with cervical stenotic myelopathy. Am J Vet Res 1994;55:5–13.

Nixon AJ, Stashak TS. Surgical management of Cervical Vertebral Malformation in the Horse. Proc AAEP, 1982;28:267–276.

Reed SM, Knight DA, Weisbrode SE, Stewart RH. The relationship of cervical vertebral malformation to developmental orthopedic disease. Proc AAEP, 1987;33:139–141.

Author R. Jay Bickers

Consulting Editor Joseph J. Bertone

CESTRUM DIURNUM (DAY-BLOOMING JESSAMINE) TOXICOSIS

BASICS

OVERVIEW

- *Cestrum diurnum* L. (day-blooming jessamine) is a large shrub with alternate, simple leaves having smooth margins and lanceolate or elliptic in shape.
- The fragrant and showy blooms are ≅2.5 cm in length and are five-parted flowers that appear in axillary clusters. The flowers are white and sweet-scented in the day.
- The fruit is a small berry that is spheric and black when mature.
- The plant, introduced into the U.S. from the West Indies, prefers the warmer areas and is used as an ornamental in the South. It also may be found wild in the Florida Keys and in south Texas.
- The plant is a member of the Solanaceae family and contains several toxins. The unripe berry contains solanine, a GI irritant, and a cholinesterase-inhibiting glycoalkaloid. The ripe berry contains tropane alkaloids. Traces of saponins and nicotine are found as well.
- The agent of greatest concern is 1,25-dihydroxy vitamin D-glucoside, which is found at high concentrations in the leaves; 1,25-dihydroxy vitamin D is the active metabolite of vitamin D.
- Ingestion of the plant results in hypercalcemia secondary to excessive calcium absorption and metastatic tissue calcification.

SIGNALMENT

N/A

SIGNS

- Progressive weight loss and lameness, increasing in severity during a 2–6-month period.
- Affected horses become stiff, are reluctant to move, and develop a short, choppy gait.
- Reluctance to move is especially evident when turning.
- Flexor and suspensory ligaments sensitive to palpation.
- Slight to moderate kyphosis.
- Elevated pulse and respiratory rates.

CAUSES AND RISK FACTORS

N/A

DIAGNOSIS

DIFFERENTIAL DIAGNOSIS

- Evidence of plant ingestion and compatible clinical signs.
- Vitamin D intoxication from other sources.

CBC/BIOCHEMISTRY/URINALYSIS

- Hypercalcemia
- Serum phosphorus remains within normal limits.

OTHER LABORATORY TESTS

N/A

IMAGING

Evidence of tissue calcification.

DIAGNOSTIC PROCEDURES

N/A

PATHOLOGIC FINDINGS

Gross Findings

- Hypervitaminosis D results in widespread soft-tissue mineralization (i.e., calcification), especially in arteries, ligaments, and tendons.
- Forelimb flexor tendons are more severely affected than those of the pelvic limb; however, all suspensory ligaments are calcified.
- Calcification occurs in the kidneys and lungs but is not a consistent finding.
- Cardiac calcification can occur, with the most severely calcified portion of the heart being the left atrium.
- Generalized osteoporosis and emaciation.

Histopathologic Findings

Hyperplasia of the parathyroid chief cells (i.e., C-cells).

TREATMENT

- No documented treatment.
- Treat hypercalcemia.

CESTRUM DIURNUM (DAY-BLOOMING JESSAMINE) TOXICOSIS

MEDICATIONS

DRUGS

- Promote diuresis and calciuresis with normal saline and furosemide.
- Corticosteroids (e.g., prednisone) decrease bone release and intestinal absorption of calcium and promote calciuresis.
- Salmon calcitonin promotes bone deposition of calcium.

CONTRAINDICATIONS/POSSIBLE INTERACTIONS

N/A

FOLLOW-UP

PATIENT MONITORING

Monitor serum calcium concentrations.

PREVENTION/AVOIDANCE

- Prevent access to the plant.
- When preventing access is impossible, remove the plant itself, because the dead leaves remain toxic.

POSSIBLE COMPLICATIONS

N/A

EXPECTED COURSE AND PROGNOSIS

N/A

MISCELLANEOUS

ASSOCIATED CONDITIONS

N/A

AGE-RELATED FACTORS

N/A

ZOONOTIC POTENTIAL

N/A

PREGNANCY

N/A

SEE ALSO

N/A

ABBREVIATION

GI = gastrointestinal

Suggested Reading

Krook L, Wasserman RH, Shively JN, Tashjian AH Jr, Brokken TD, Morton JF. Hypercalcemia and calcinosis in Florida horses: implication of the shrub, *Cestrum diurnum*, as the causative agent. Cornell Vet 1975;65:26–56.

Author Tam Garland

Consulting Editor Robert H. Poppenga

CHLORIDE, HYPERCHLOREMIA

BASICS

DEFINITIONS

Serum chloride concentration > the reference range—generally >111 mEq/L.

PATHOPHYSIOLOGY

- Chloride is the major anion in the ECF.
- Serum chloride concentrations often increase and decrease in proportion to changes in serum sodium concentrations; these proportional increases and decreases relate to changes in body water and sodium balance.
- Changes in serum chloride concentrations not proportional to those in serum sodium concentrations usually relate to acid–base abnormalities.
- Serum chloride concentrations tend to vary inversely with serum bicarbonate concentrations.
- Metabolic acidosis with a normal or low anion gap may be accompanied by hyperchloremia; in metabolic acidosis with a high anion gap, the serum chloride concentration is normal or low.
- Hyperchloremia also may occur when the serum bicarbonate concentration decreases in compensation for respiratory alkalosis.

SYSTEMS AFFECTED

- Depends on the underlying cause.
- Neuromuscular—severe hypernatremia and hyperchloremia, resulting in marked hyperosmolality, may cause neurologic abnormalities because of water loss from neurons.

SIGNALMENT

No breed, sex, or age predilections.

SIGNS

- May relate to either dehydration or acid–base abnormality.
- Severe hyperchloremia and hypernatremia may result in neurologic abnormalities—lethargy, weakness, seizures, coma, and death.
- In cases related to an acid–base abnormality, the respiratory rate may be increased or decreased.
- Other signs depend on the underlying abnormality.

CAUSES

Chloride Increased Proportionately to Sodium

- High total body chloride—excessive NaCl intake (i.e., salt poisoning) with water restriction (rare).
- Normal total body chloride with excessive free water loss—inadequate water intake; early stages of diarrhea; central or nephrogenic diabetes insipidus; prolonged hyperventilation.

Chloride Increased Disproportionately to Sodium

- Suggests an acid–base abnormality.
- Metabolic acidosis with a low or normal anion gap—renal tubular acidosis, an uncommon disorder in horses, results in striking hyperchloremia and metabolic acidosis.
- Compensated respiratory alkalosis—decreased bicarbonate as a compensatory response results in increased chloride.
- Acetazolamide treatment for hyperkalemic periodic paralysis.

RISK FACTORS

Inadequate water intake.

DIAGNOSIS

DIFFERENTIAL DIAGNOSIS

- History or physical examination to detect decreased water intake or excessive water loss resulting in dehydration.
- Diseases resulting in metabolic acidosis with a normal or low anion gap—renal tubular acidosis (uncommon) or renal failure.

LABORATORY FINDINGS

Drugs that May Alter Lab Results

N/A

Disorders that May Alter Lab Results

- Hemoglobin has a variable effect on serum chloride concentration; it may increase the concentrations with some methods.
- Bilirubin may falsely increase serum chloride concentrations.

Valid If Run In Human Lab?

Yes

CBC/BIOCHEMISTRY/URINALYSIS

Hyposthenuria in combination with hypochloremia and hyponatremia—consider diabetes insipidus (uncommon).

OTHER LABORATORY TESTS

- Blood gas analysis if the increase of chloride is disproportionate to that of sodium.
- Evaluate for primary metabolic acidosis or compensated respiratory alkalosis.
- Determine serum potassium and bicarbonate to calculate anion gap.

IMAGING

N/A

DIAGNOSTIC PROCEDURES

N/A

CHLORIDE, HYPERCHLOREMIA

TREATMENT

Treat the underlying cause.

MEDICATIONS

DRUGS OF CHOICE

- Treat the primary cause.
- If sodium and chloride increases are proportional, assure adequate water availability.
- If hypernatremia and hyperchloremia are long-standing, correction should be gradual to avoid neurologic damage.
- If chloride is increased disproportionately to sodium, evaluate and treat the acid–base imbalance.

CONTRAINDICATIONS

N/A

PRECAUTIONS

Rapid replacement of fluid deficit with water in markedly hyperosmotic animals may result in cerebral edema and neurologic abnormalities.

POSSIBLE INTERACTIONS

N/A

ALTERNATIVE DRUGS

N/A

FOLLOW-UP

PATIENT MONITORING

Serum electrolyte concentrations and acid–base status to monitor response to fluid therapy.

POSSIBLE COMPLICATIONS

- Depends on the underlying disorder.
- Hypernatremia—seizures, convulsions, and permanent neurologic damage are possible in severe cases.

MISCELLANEOUS

ASSOCIATED CONDITIONS

N/A

AGE-RELATED FACTORS

N/A

ZOONOTIC POTENTIAL

N/A

PREGNANCY

N/A

SYNONYMS

N/A

SEE ALSO

Hypernatremia

ABBREVIATION

ECF = extracellular fluid

Suggested Reading

Carlson GP. Clinical chemistry tests. In: Smith BP, ed. Large animal internal medicine. 2nd ed. St. Louis: Mosby, 1996.

Carlson GP. Fluid, electrolyte, and acid-base balance. In: Kaneko JJ, Harvey JW, Bruss ML, eds. Clinical biochemistry of domestic animals. 5th ed. New York, Academic Press, 1997.

Foreman JH. The exhausted horse syndrome. Vet Clin North Am Equine Pract 1998;14:205–219.

Hyyppä S, Pösö AR. Fluid, electrolyte, and acid-base responses to exercise in racehorses. Vet Clin North Am Equine Pract 1998;14:121–136.

Schmall LM. Fluid and electrolyte therapy. In: Robinson NE, ed. Current therapy in equine medicine 4. Philadelphia: WB Saunders, 1997.

Author E. Duane Lassen

Consulting Editor Claire B. Andreasen

CHLORIDE, HYPOCHLOREMIA

BASICS

DEFINITIONS

Serum chloride concentration < the reference range—generally <99 mEq/L.

PATHOPHYSIOLOGY

- Chloride is the major anion in the ECF.
- Serum chloride concentrations often increase and decrease in proportion to changes in serum sodium concentrations; these proportional increases and decreases relate to changes in body water and sodium balance.
- Changes in serum chloride concentrations not proportional to changes in serum sodium concentrations usually relate to acid–base abnormalities.
- Serum chloride concentrations tend to vary inversely with serum bicarbonate concentrations.
- Metabolic alkalosis usually is accompanied by, and may result from, hypochloremia, which also may occur when serum bicarbonate concentrations increase in compensation for respiratory acidosis.
- Metabolic acidosis with a high anion gap may result in serum chloride concentrations that are either normal or low.

SYSTEMS AFFECTED

- Depends on the underlying cause.
- If accompanied by markedly decreased sodium, see *Hyponatremia.*

SIGNALMENT

No breed, sex, or age predilections.

SIGNS

- If accompanied by severe and acute hyponatremia, lethargy, central blindness, seizures, tremors, and abnormal gait are possible.
- If related to acid–base abnormality, respiratory rate may be increased or decreased.
- Other signs depend on the underlying abnormality.

CAUSES

Proportionate Decreases in Serum Chloride and Sodium

Increased Total Body Water Compared with Sodium and Chloride

- Third spacing—occurs when abnormal fluid volumes accumulate in body spaces (e.g., abdominal and thoracic cavities, GI tract; specific abnormalities resulting in equine third spacing include ruptured urinary bladder in foals, abdominal effusions associated with colic, and peritonitis from a variety of causes.
- Iatrogenic—PO hypotonic fluids or excessive IV administration of 5% dextrose solution.
- Inappropriate water retention (rare) caused by congestive heart failure, hepatic fibrosis, severe hypoproteinemia, or inappropriate ADH secretion.

Disproportionate Loss of Sodium and Chloride Compared with Loss of Total Body Water

- Renal disease
- Some forms of diarrhea (e.g., secretory diarrhea) and other diseases causing fluid sequestration in the GI tract.
- Prolonged diuresis secondary to hyperglycemia and glucosuria may result in medullary washout and subsequent hyponatremia and hypochloremia.
- Adrenal insufficiency (i.e., iatrogenic) or adrenal exhaustion.
- Iatrogenic loss caused by GI fluid drainage via nasogastric intubation.
- Hemorrhage

Disproportionate Decrease in Serum Chloride Compared with Serum Sodium

- Primary metabolic alkalosis—serum chloride decreases in compensation for increased serum bicarbonate. Metabolic alkalosis may result from excessive sweating in horses. Because equine sweat contains a proportionally higher concentration of chloride than of sodium, excessive sweating can cause hypochloremia and metabolic alkalosis as a result of renal bicarbonate reabsorption in compensation for chloride loss.
- Compensatory response to a respiratory acidosis—serum bicarbonate concentration increases in compensation for the respiratory acidosis, and serum chloride concentration decreases to maintain electroneutrality.
- Metabolic acidosis with an increased anion gap (i.e., increased concentrations of anions other than chloride or bicarbonate)—frequently associated with colic. Serum bicarbonate decreases but serum chloride does not increase in compensation, because increased concentrations of other anions (e.g., lactate) provide the negative charges needed to maintain electroneutrality.
- Furosemide therapy—results in loss of chloride in the thick, ascending loop of the Henle.
- Sodium bicarbonate therapy—may lower serum chloride concentration in compensation for increased serum bicarbonate concentration.

RISK FACTORS

- Heavy sweating
- Colic and other GI disorders
- Furosemide treatment

DIAGNOSIS

DIFFERENTIAL DIAGNOSIS

Proportional Decreases in Serum Chloride and Sodium Concentrations

- Ascites suggests third spacing. In foals, consider ruptured urinary bladder, and check BUN/creatinine in serum and fluid. In adults consider peritonitis, congestive heart failure, and other causes of ascites. Perform abdominal fluid analysis.
- Thoracic effusion suggests third spacing. Consider pleuritis, neoplasia, and other causes of thoracic effusions, and perform thoracic fluid analysis.
- Diarrhea suggests GI loss.
- Polyuria/polydipsia indicates need to evaluate renal function.

Disproportionate Decrease in Chloride Compared with Sodium

- Normal or low anion gap—consider excessive sweating as a cause of metabolic alkalosis; evaluate respiratory system for possible cause of respiratory acidosis.
- Increased anion gap—consider possible colic and other causes of increased lactate, phosphate, sulfate, ketone, or protein concentrations.

LABORATORY FINDINGS

Drugs that May Alter Lab Results

N/A

Disorders that May Alter Lab Results

- Lipemia and hyperproteinemia may falsely lower chloride concentrations unless an ion-specific electrode used.
- Marked hyperglycemia causes dilution of serum chloride via osmotic water movement.
- Hemoglobin has a variable effect on serum chloride concentrations.

CHLORIDE, HYPOCHLOREMIA

Valid If Run in Human Lab?
Yes

CBC/BIOCHEMISTRY/URINALYSIS

- Depends on the underlying disorder.
- Concurrent hyponatremia indicates need to consider diseases altering water balance or resulting in loss of sodium and chloride.
- Decreased serum potassium is more typical of GI fluid loss.
- Increased potassium is more typical of renal disease or uroperitoneum.
- Increased bicarbonate indicates metabolic alkalosis or compensation for respiratory acidosis.
- Decreased bicarbonate and increased anion gap indicate increased concentrations of ions other than bicarbonate or chloride.
- Increased BUN/creatinine may indicate renal failure (with inadequate urine concentration) or uroperitoneum.

OTHER LABORATORY TESTS

- Urinary fractional excretion ($[Na_u^+/Na_s^+]/[Cr_u/Cr_s]$)—increased fractional excretion accompanying hypochloremia suggests renal disease or furosemide treatment.
- Blood gas analysis if the decrease of chloride is disproportionate to that of sodium. Evaluate for primary metabolic alkalosis or compensated respiratory acidosis.
- Serum potassium and bicarbonate to calculate anion gap.
- Abdominal or thoracic fluid examination if these fluids are present in abnormal volumes. In foals, abdominal fluid urea nitrogen or creatinine concentrations are indicated if rupture of the urinary bladder is suspected.

IMAGING

N/A

DIAGNOSTIC PROCEDURES

N/A

TREATMENT

Treat the underlying abnormality.

MEDICATIONS

DRUGS OF CHOICE

- Treat the primary cause.
- If sodium and chloride decreases are proportional, see the discussion of treatment in *Hyponatremia.*
- If chloride is decreased disproportionately compared with sodium, evaluate and treat the acid–base imbalance.

CONTRAINDICATIONS

N/A

PRECAUTIONS

N/A

POSSIBLE INTERACTIONS

N/A

ALTERNATIVE DRUGS

N/A

FOLLOW-UP

PATIENT MONITORING

Serum electrolyte concentrations and acid–base status to monitor response to fluid therapy.

POSSIBLE COMPLICATIONS

Depend on the underlying disorder.

MISCELLANEOUS

ASSOCIATED CONDITIONS

Other acid–base and electrolyte abnormalities.

AGE-RELATED FACTORS

N/A

ZOONOTIC POTENTIAL

N/A

PREGNANCY

N/A

SYNONYMS

N/A

SEE ALSO

Hyponatremia

ABBREVIATIONS

- ADH = antidiuretic hormone
- ECF = extracellular fluid
- GI = gastrointestinal tract

Suggested Reading

Carlson GP. Clinical chemistry tests. In: Smith BP, ed. Large animal internal medicine. 2nd ed. St. Louis: Mosby, 1996.

Carlson GP. Fluid, electrolyte, and acid-base balance. In: Kaneko JJ, Harvey JW, Bruss ML, eds. Clinical biochemistry of domestic animals. 5th ed. New York: Academic Press, 1997.

Foreman JH. The exhausted horse syndrome. Vet Clin North Am Equine Pract 1998;14:205–219.

Hyyppä S, Pösö AR. Fluid, electrolyte, and acid-base responses to exercise in racehorses. Vet Clin North Am Equine Pract 1998;14:121–136.

Schmall LM. Fluid and electrolyte therapy. In: Robinson NE, ed. Current therapy in equine medicine 4. Philadelphia: WB Saunders, 1997.

Author E. Duane Lassen

Consulting Editor Claire B. Andreasen

CHOLELITHIASIS

BASICS

OVERVIEW

• Refers to calculi in the biliary tree.
• Relatively uncommon
• The pathogenesis is not fully understood but possible involves conversion in the bile of conjugated bilirubin to unconjugated bilirubin by β-glucuronidase. The enzyme is present in the bile duct epithelium and in some bacteria.
• Many equine cases are associated with septic cholangitis, which suggests that bacterial enzymes may play a role.
• Unconjugated bilirubin combines with calcium in the bile to form calcium bilirubinate, which then precipitates to form the calculi, though many other compounds also are present—cholesterol, bile pigments, and sodium taurodeoxycholate.

SIGNALMENT

• Most affected horses are 5–15 years old.
• No breed or sex predilections.
• No reported geographic distribution.

SIGNS

• Intermittent abdominal pain
• Icterus
• Fever
• Depression
• Weight loss
• Hepatic encephalopathy
• Photosensitization

CAUSES AND RISK FACTORS

• The condition is sporadic.
• No clearly established risk factors have been identified.

DIAGNOSIS

DIFFERENTIAL DIAGNOSIS

• Other causes of chronic liver disease (e.g., chronic active hepatitis, toxic hepatitis) can be differentiated with ultrasonography and liver biopsy.
• Mild, recurrent abdominal pain more commonly may be caused by GI problems—parasitism, abdominal abscesses and neoplasms, sand accumulation, and enteroliths; however, most of these conditions are not accompanied by changes in serum liver enzymes or icterus.
• Fever is common in many equine infectious conditions, but the chronic, recurrent causes include pleuropneumonia, abdominal abscesses, endocarditis, and EIA. Clinical pathology and physical examination will assist in differentiation.
• Weight loss is a feature in many of the chronic conditions listed above but also includes malnutrition, dental disease, chronic laminitis, chronic severe arthritis, and malabsorption. Again, clinical signs and laboratory data assist in differentiation.

CBC/BIOCHEMISTRY/URINALYSIS

• Liver enzymes may be elevated from time to time—AST, GGT, ALP, and SDH (IDH).
• Total Bilirubin—both conjugated and unconjugated levels may be elevated.
• CBC—neutrophilia
• Fibrinogen and globulin—elevated

OTHER LABORATORY TESTS

N/A

IMAGING

• Ultrasonography of affected livers usually reveals dilation of the bile ducts, which are thickened; normally, equine bile ducts are not readily visualized.
• The liver usually is enlarged and more echogenic than normal.
• Choleliths—most readily seen on the right side of the liver at the sixth or seventh intercostal space; may be hyperechoic and cast an acoustic shadow, though some may be sonolucent.

DIAGNOSTIC PROCEDURES

Liver biopsy may be useful to define the nature of the pathology; a sample may be submitted for culture if septic cholangitis is suspected.

PATHOLOGIC FINDINGS

• In acute cases, the liver may be enlarged; in chronic cases; it may be smaller than normal.
• The liver surface may appear mottled, and the tissue is firm.
• Possible icterus
• Bile ducts often are dilated and contain one or more calculi, which usually are a greenish-brown in color.

CHOLELITHIASIS

TREATMENT

• Both choledocholithotomy and choledocholithotripsy have been described as treatment of cholelithiasis in three horses; thus, these treatments have not been fully evaluated.
• Basic principles focus on the relief of obstruction, treatment of underlying hepatic disease, and therapy for infection.

MEDICATIONS

DRUGS

• With suspected septic cholangitis, long-term antibiotic therapy is indicated.
• Gram-negative bacteria are the most frequently isolated; appropriate drugs include trimethoprim–sulfa combinations, chloramphenicol, ampicillin, and penicillin–gentamicin combinations.

CONTRAINDICATIONS/POSSIBLE INTERACTIONS

N/A

FOLLOW-UP

PATIENT MONITORING

N/A

PREVENTION/AVOIDANCE

N/A

POSSIBLE COMPLICATIONS

N/A

EXPECTED COURSE AND PROGNOSIS

• Prognosis depends on severity of the problem.
• Surgical intervention is not very feasible in many cases and gives only limited access to the biliary tree.
• With antimicrobial therapy, sequential ultrasonography may assist with in monitoring whether progress is being made.

MISCELLANEOUS

ASSOCIATED CONDITIONS

N/A

AGE-RELATED FACTORS

N/A

ZOONOTIC POTENTIAL

N/A

PREGNANCY

N/A

SEE ALSO

N/A

ABBREVIATIONS

• ALP = alkaline phosphatase
• AST = aspartate aminotransferase
• EIA = equine infection anemia
• GGT = γ-glutamyltransferase
• GI = gastrointestinal
• IDH = iditol dehydrogenase (SDH)
• SDH = sorbitol dehydrogenase (IDH)

Suggested Reading

Johnson JK, Divers TJ, Reef VB, et al. Cholelithiasis in horses: ten Cases (1982–1986). J Am Vet Med Assoc 1989;194:405–409.

Author Christopher M. Brown
Consulting Editor Michel Levy

CHORIORETINITIS

BASICS

OVERVIEW

Chorioretinitis is inflammation of the choroid and retina.

System Affected

Ophthalmic

SIGNALMENT

N/A

SIGNS

Chorioretinitis is manifest in equine eyes as "bullet-hole" retinal lesions, diffuse chorioretinal lesions, horizontal band lesions of the nontapetal retina, and peripapillary chorioretinitis.

- Bullet-hole lesions are focal or multifocal circular scars of the peripapillary and nontapetal regions. They develop over 2–4 weeks and consist of a depigmented periphery and a hyperpigmented central area. Acute lesions, which are uncommon, appear as white or gray exudative lesions. Vision is not impaired unless there are more than 10 to 20 bullet-hole lesions. Equine herpesvirus 1 (EHV-1) is associated with this type of lesion in horses.
- Diffuse chorioretinal lesions are vermiform, circular, or band-shaped lesions that are hyperreflective in the tapetal retina and depigmented in the nontapetal retina, with areas of hyperpigmentation. These lesions are uncommon. They represent widespread prior inflammatory disease or infarctive lesions with subsequent retinal degeneration and scarring. Optic nerve atrophy may accompany these lesions. Vision is markedly reduced.
- Horizontal band lesions of the nontapetal zone are multifocal chorioretinal lesions appearing one to two disc diameters ventral to the optic disc. They radiate in a horizontal fashion around the posterior pole.
- Peripapillary chorioretinitis is commonly associated with anterior uveitis. Fluffy, raised exudates adjacent to the optic disc are found in the active stage. Vasculitis can be observed in some cases with white or pale exudates surrounding affected retinal vessels. In the chronic stage, scar tissue develops, often but not necessarily in a butterfly shape around the papilla.

CAUSES AND RISK FACTORS

Lesions can be caused by infectious agents (e.g., leptospirosis, EHV-1, *Onchocerca cervicalis* microfilaria), immune-mediated uveitis of unknown origin, trauma, or vascular disease.

DIAGNOSIS

DIFFERENTIAL DIAGNOSIS

Chorioretinitis usually does not recur unless it is part of the equine recurrent uveitis (ERU) syndrome, where it is also associated with anterior uveitis.

CBC/BIOCHEMISTRY/URINALYSIS

Possible signs of systemic disease, such as infection or immune-mediated disorder.

OTHER LABORATORY TESTS

Rule out infectious causes of chorioretinitis by serologic testing for infectious agents.

IMAGING

N/A

DIAGNOSTIC PROCEDURES

Electroretinography helps in the assessment of the functionality of the retina.

PATHOLOGIC FINDINGS

Type of cellular reaction depends on underlying cause.

CHORIORETINITIS

TREATMENT

Remove underlying cause if known. Observed changes cannot be reversed. The goal of treatment is to stop the progression of the disease process. Chronic, inactive lesions do not require treatment.

MEDICATIONS

DRUGS

Systemic medication should be used according to the underlying cause. In addition, nonsteroidal drugs, such as flunixin meglumine (0.25 to 1.0 mg/kg BID, PO), phenylbutazone (1 gm BID, IV or PO), or aspirin (25 mg/kg BID, PO), may be administered. The following topical medications are indicated only if anterior uveitis is also present: prednisolone acetate (1%) or dexamethasone (0.1%) at least 4 to 6 times a day; atropine (1%) SID to TID.

CONTRAINDICATIONS/POSSIBLE INTERACTIONS

N/A

FOLLOW-UP

EXPECTED COURSE AND PROGNOSIS

The goal of the treatment for chorioretinitis is to preserve the present status, i.e., to prevent progression of the disease.

MISCELLANEOUS

ASSOCIATED CONDITIONS

Possible signs of systemic infection.

AGE-RELATED FACTORS

N/A

PREGNANCY

Some infectious agents causing chorioretinitis can threaten pregnancy (e.g., *Leptospira*).

SEE ALSO

- Equine recurrent uveitis
- Equine stationary night blindness
- Equine progressive retinal atrophy
- Equine retinal detachment
- Equine optic neuropathy

ABREVIATIONS

- EHV-1 = equine herpesvirus 1
- ERU = equine recurrent uveitis

Suggested Reading

Brooks DE. Equine ophthalmology. In: Gelatt KN, ed. Veterinary ophthalmology. 3rd ed. Philadelphia: Lippincott Williams & Wilkins, 1999; chapter 30.

Author Andras M. Komaromy
Consulting Editor Dennis E. Brooks

CHRONIC ACTIVE HEPATITIS

BASICS

OVERVIEW

- A condition of unknown cause characterized by a chronic inflammatory process in the liver
- The diagnosis is established based primarily on histopathologic findings; in some cases, large numbers of mononuclear cells suggest an immune-mediated etiology.
- The liver is the primary organ affected, but cutaneous lesions also may occur.

SIGNALMENT

- No breed or sex predispositions.
- Most affected horses are mature.
- No geographic distribution
- The condition is sporadic.

SIGNS

- Depression
- Weight loss
- Lethargy
- Icterus
- Fever
- Occasional cases—necrotic lesions on the coronary bands.

CAUSES AND RISK FACTORS

- Unknown cause
- Autoimmune mechanisms, hepatitis B infection, non-A/non-B viral hepatitis, Wilson's disease, α-1-antitrypsin deficiency, and occasional drug reactions cause similar conditions in humans, but none has been proved to be the cause in horses.
- In some equine cases, the condition appears to be secondary to septic cholangiohepatitis.

DIAGNOSIS

DIFFERENTIAL DIAGNOSIS

- Toxic hepatopathy and cholelithiasis—differentiated based on ultrasonography and liver biopsy.
- Weight loss, dental disease, parasitism, pleuropneumonia, abdominal abscess, EIA, laminitis, malabsorption—differentiated based on physical findings and laboratory data.

CBC/BIOCHEMISTRY/URINALYSIS

- Elevated liver-derived enzymes—AST, ALP, and GGT
- Serum bile acids—elevated
- Bilirubin— elevated (particularly conjugated)
- Serum protein—increased
- May have neutrophilia
- Bilirubinuria

OTHER LABORATORY TESTS

BSP half-life—prolonged

IMAGING

Ultrasonography may help in assessing liver size and rule out the presence of calculi.

DIAGNOSTIC PROCEDURES

Liver biopsy

PATHOLOGIC FINDINGS

Gross Findings

The liver is pale brown to green in color and firm to the touch.

Histologic Findings

- The periportal areas are infiltrated with mononuclear cells and, in some cases, neutrophils.
- Hepatocellular necrosis, bile ductule hyperplasia, and fibrosis.
- With suspected bacterial infection, submit a sample for culture and sensitivity.

CHRONIC ACTIVE HEPATITIS

TREATMENT

• General supportive care, depending on the severity of clinical signs.
• Diet—low in protein and rich in carbohydrate (e.g., two parts beet pulp and one part cracked corn); the protein should be rich in BCAAs; oat or grass hay is preferred.

MEDICATIONS

DRUGS

• If many mononuclear cells are present, corticosteroids may be beneficial, at least initially—dexamethasone (0.05–0.1 mg/kg per day for 4–7 days, then gradually reducing over the next 2–3 weeks)
• If infection is suspected, antibiotics may be indicated, with the selection based on culture and sensitivity results; this treatment will be long term, at least 4 weeks and possible longer.

CONTRAINDICATIONS/POSSIBLE INTERACTIONS

N/A

FOLLOW-UP

PATIENT MONITORING

• Duration of therapy is influenced by response to therapy.
• Serial biochemical monitoring.

PREVENTION/AVOIDANCE

N/A

POSSIBLE COMPLICATIONS

N/A

EXPECTED COURSE AND PROGNOSIS

• With extensive fibrosis on histopathology and well-developed signs of liver failure, the prognosis is poor.
• If detected early and the pathology is primarily a monocytic infiltrate, some horses respond well to corticosteroid therapy; however, long-term survival in these cases often remains poor.

MISCELLANEOUS

ASSOCIATED CONDITIONS

N/A

AGE-RELATED FACTORS

N/A

ZOONOTIC POTENTIAL

N/A

PREGNANCY

N/A

SEE ALSO

N/A

ABBREVIATIONS

• ALP = alkaline phosphatase
• AST = aspartate aminotransferase
• BCAAs = branched-chain amino acids
• BSP = bromosulfophtalein
• EIA = equine infectious anemia
• GGT = gamma-glutamyl transferase

Suggested Reading

Pearson EG. Chronic active hepatitis. In: Smith BP, ed. Large animal internal medicine. St. Louis: Mosby, 1996:927–928.

Author Christopher M. Brown
Consulting Editor Michel Levy

CHRONIC/RECURRENT ADULT ABDOMINAL PAIN–CHRONIC COLIC

BASICS

DEFINITION

Chronic abdominal pain–discomfort (colic) originating usually, but not exclusively, from the gastrointestinal tract and that has been present constantly or intermittently for more than 3 days. It may also originate from other abdominal organs such as liver, spleen, kidney, uterus, and peritoneum.

PATHOPHYSIOLOGY

Pain from within the intestinal tract may result from intramural tension, tension on a mesentery, inflammation, spasm associated with hypermotility, or a combination of those. Most cases of chronic colic usually exclude strangulating obstructive events.

SYSTEMS AFFECTED

Gastrointestinal

The cardiovascular system may be affected due to progressive dehydration, toxemia, or shock secondary to gastrointestinal events.

Other Systems Affected

Other systems such as urinary, reproductive, or hepatic may be involved, and details should be consulted in those sections.

SIGNALMENT

Non-specific; for example, small intestinal intussusceptions are more commonly seen in young animals. Previous abdominal surgery results in a risk of adhesions leading to chronic colic.

SIGNS

General Comments

Signs of chronic/recurrent abdominal pain are usually mild to moderate in nature.

Historical Findings

There may be a recent history of change in diet or exercise regimen, lack of access to drinking water, deworming, weight loss, previous infection, or abdominal surgery. Furthermore, a change in attitude (depression), appetite, and fecal output may be noticed. *Chronic abdominal pain* refers to continuous or intermittent signs of abdominal pain of more than 3 days duration. *Recurrent abdominal pain* refers to several episodes of transient or prolonged abdominal pain separated by a period of a few days or weeks in which the horse is usually normal. The signs of abdominal pain are usually of mild to moderate intensity and may include extended neck and rolling of the upper lip (Flehmen-like response), teeth grinding, pawing at the ground, flank watching, kicking of the abdomen with the hind legs, ears pinned back, lying down more frequently, and attempting to roll.

Physical Examination Findings

Vital signs are usually normal to moderately elevated. The following signs might be observed:

- General findings—none to moderate abdominal distention.
- Cardiovascular findings—normal to mild changes in color of the mucous membrane, normal or mild increase in capillary refill time, normal to moderate increase in heart rate, and dehydration may occur with time. May have signs of endotoxemia such as hyperemic mucous membranes and increase in heart rate if the problem is related to a septic process or enteritis/colitis.
- Gastrointestinal findings—normal, decrease, or increase in gut motility; abnormal sounds may be heard in sand impactions; may have a gas-filled viscus on percussion; may have presence of gastric reflux on passage of the nasogastric tube. If gastric reflux is present, lesion most likely located at the level of the stomach or small intestine. The pH of the gastric reflux may also be helpful in identifying the origin of the reflux. Feces are normal, reduced, or absent, or there may be diarrhea.
- Abnormalities on rectal examination—distension of a viscus by gas, liquid, or food; displacement of a viscus; uterine or renal abnormalities. May have a painful response on palpation of a specific area.

CAUSES

The most common cause of chronic colic located at the gastrointestinal level is impaction of the large colon, but there are a variety of others causes, such as chronic peritonitis, enteritis/colitis, colonic displacement, ulceration (colonic and gastric), and intussusception. For recurrent abdominal pain, the most common cause is spasmodic colic but also includes inflammatory processes such as chronic ulceration, non-total disturbance of the intestinal lumen due to adhesions, intussusception, enteroliths, intra-abdominal masses such as abscesses and neoplasms, and sand impactions. Many of these conditions are related to altered motility, and intestinal parasitism probably has a significant role in the etiology of this.

Gastrointestinal

- Gastric—gastric ulcer, gastric neoplasia.
- Small intestine—duodenal ulcer, duodenojejunal enteritis, adhesions, stricture, intussusception, neoplasia, impaction, etc.
- Large intestine, cecum, and small colon—impaction, ulceration, spasmodic colic, enteroliths, sand impaction, neoplasia, displacement.

Reproductive

- Uterine torsion
- Late stage of pregnancy

Renal/Urologic

- Renal/ureteral/bladder/urethral calculi
- Pyelonephritis
- Cystitis
- Renal inflammatory process

Hepatobiliary

- Hepatitis
- Hepatobiliary calculi
- Abscesses

Other Systems Affected

- Peritonitis
- Mesenteric abscesses
- Abdominal neoplasia (e.g., lymphosarcoma)

RISK FACTORS

Previous surgery, diet (feeding coastal grass hay), environment, excessive use of NSAIDs, *Anoplocephala* infestation, no access to water, sudden change in exercise, history of deworming, pregnancy. Horses with severe dental disease may fail to masticate coarse herbage and be prone to impactions.

DIFFERENTIAL DIAGNOSIS

Other causes of pain that might resemble pain originating from the abdominal cavity include myositis, pleuropneumonia, neurologic, and musculoskeletal injury.

CBC/BIOCHEMISTRY/URINALYSIS

Increase in PCV and TP might be present due to dehydration. Hypoproteinemia secondary to intestinal loss is seen in conditions such as chronic ulceration, intussusception, neoplasia, and inflammatory bowel disease. Leukocytosis in chronic inflammatory process may be present. Anemia may result from chronic inflammatory processes or chronic bleeding (ulceration, neoplasia). Hypochloremia, hyponatremia, and low bicarbonate concentrations is seen in colitis. In cases of abdominal pain related to renal problems, an increase in leukocyte count, red blood cells, and pH may be observed in the urine. Presence of azotemia occurs in severely dehydrated horses or in cases of renal disease. Liver enzymes may also be increased if hepatic disease is present.

OTHER LABORATORY TESTS

- Abdominal paracentesis—Cytology of the abdominal fluid may be normal or may reveal presence of an inflammatory process. This is indicated by an elevation of the protein level and leukocyte count. The presence of abnormal or mitotic cells may suggest lymphosarcoma. Bacteriology of abdominal fluid in cases of peritonitis may be helpful in isolating an agent and appropriately choose the antibiotic therapy.

- Melena in feces—Ulcerative disease, intussusceptions of the small intestine.
- Fecal analysis for the presence of parasitic eggs and sand.
- Fecal bacteriology might help identifying the cause of inflammatory abdominal pain (*Salmonella* spp., *Clostridia* spp.). Culture and sensitivity of abdominal fluid if peritonitis is present.
- Urinanalysis—A change in specific gravity or an increase in leukocyte content, red blood cell, and pH may be noticed if renal disease is present.

IMAGING

- Radiographs—May be useful in identification of sand impaction or enteroliths.
- Ultrasonography—Evaluation of the amount, quality, and characteristics of abdominal fluids; evaluation of wall thickness and diameter of small intestine; evaluation of the nephrosplenic space; and abnormal findings such as intussusception, abscess, or adhesions. Also useful in evaluating the kidneys, liver, spleen, and uterus.
- Endoscopy/gastroscopy—Evaluation of the glandular and non glandular part of the stomach for ulcer or impaction. The duodenum may be also observed in small horses.
- Cystoscopy—Evaluation of the urethra, bladder, and opening of the ureters for inflammation urolithiasis.
- Laparoscopy—visualization of abdominal viscera.

DIAGNOSTIC PROCEDURES

- Biopsy—Liver or renal biopsy for histology.
- Histology—Biopsy of kidney or liver if these are suspected to be the origin of the problem; intestinal biopsy (requires an exploratory laparotomy or laparascopy).
- Exploratory laparotomy or laparascopy—To identify the origin of the problem if has not been determined by other tests.

TREATMENT

The treatment depends on the source of the problem. The treatment may be supportive or curative, medical or surgical. Moderate or severe cases of cecal impaction are an indication to perform exploratory laparotomy to prevent cecal rupture.

MEDICATIONS

DRUG(S) OF CHOICE

Analgesics

Analgesics control the abdominal pain, and include:

- Non-steroidal anti-inflammatory drugs—flunixin meglumine (0.5–1.1 mg/kg q8–12hr), (10 mg/kg).
- Alpha-2-blockers, such as xylazine (0.25–0.5 mg/kg IV or IM) or romifidine (0.02–0.05 mg/kg IV or IM), can also be given in more severe cases.
- Although usually not needed unless signs of pain are severe, the narcotic analgesics such as utorphanol or meperidine (pethidine) can be given alone or in conjunction to xylazine.

Spasmolytic

Hyoscine (20–30 mL IV)

Laxative

To soften ingesta; mainly used for impaction.

- Mineral oil–10 mL/kg via nasogastric tube.
- Osmotic laxative–diluted magnesium sulfate(0.5–1 g/kg) in 4L warm water via nasogastric tube.
- Dioctyl sodium succinate (DSS) (10–30 mg/kg of a 30% solution) intravenous fluid of balanced electrolytes solution (100–200 mL/kg/day).

Fluids

- Parenteral—In case of dehydration or moderate to severe impaction, intravenous fluidotherapy should be initiated with a balanced electrolyte solution (LRS). Unbalanced electrolytes should be corrected, especially hypokaliemia and hypocalcemia, which are important for intestinal motility.
- Orally—In cases of impaction where good gastrointestinal motility is present, -5 L of water every 2 hr can be given per nasogastric tube (check for gastric reflux prior to giving water).

Antibiotic Therapy

Antibiotic therapy should be started if peritonitis is suspected or surgery is performed. Usually, broad-spectrum antibiotics such as a combination of penicillin (20,000 UI/kg IV qid) and gentamicin (6.6 mg/kg IV sid) or trimetroprim–sulfa (30 mg/kg IV bid) are given. Surgical exploration may be necessary to determine the cause of chronic or recurrent signs of abdominal discomfort. Other treatments are specific according to diagnosis, such as sand impaction, enteroliths, and parasitism.

PRECAUTIONS

Repeated use of alpha-2-blockers and butorphanol causes prolonged ileus. Repeat doses of NSAIDs, especially in cases of dehydration, can result in gastric or large colon ulceration as well as renal damage.

POSSIBLE INTERACTIONS

N/A

ALTERNATIVE DRUGS

N/A

FOLLOW-UP

PATIENT MONITORING

The heart rate and cardiovascular status of the horse should be monitored closely to detect any deterioration.

POSSIBLE COMPLICATIONS

Chronic signs of pain non-responsive to medical treatment, intestinal rupture secondary to intestinal necrosis due to an enterolith, and severe impaction are indications for an exploratory laparotomy.

ZOONOTIC POTENTIAL

N/A

PREGNANCY

Late stage of pregnancy can result in intermittent mild signs of abdominal discomfort.

SYNONYM

Chronic/recurrent colic

Suggested Reading

Hillyer MH, Mair TS. Recurrent colic in the mature horse: A retrospective reviews of 58 cases. Eq Vet J 1997:29:421-424.

Hillyer MH, Mair TS. Chronic colic in the mature horse: A retrospective review of 106 cases. Eq Vet J 1997:29:415-420.

White NA. Epidemiology and etiology of colic. In: White NA (Ed.), The equine acute abdomen. Philadelphia: Lea & Febiger, 1990.

Schramme M. Investigation and management of recurrent colic in the horse. In Pract. 1995:17:303-314.

Author Nathalie Coté

Consulting Editor Henry Stämpfli

CHRONIC RENAL FAILURE (CRF)

BASICS

DEFINITION

Results from a substantial and permanent decrease in GFR.

PATHOPHYSIOLOGY

- Usually a consequence of GN or CIN.
- CIN is a catch-all term for non-GN causes of CRF—permanent loss of renal function after a bout of hemodynamic/ischemic or toxic ARF, analgesic (NSAID) nephropathy, or pyelonephritis.
- The hallmark of CIN is development of interstitial fibrosis.
- Less commonly, renal anomalies (e.g., hypoplasia, dysplasia) or polycystic kidney disease may cause CRF.
- Impaired urine concentrating ability (i.e., isosthenuria) occurs when more than of two-thirds of nephron function is lost.
- Azotemia develops after loss of more than three-fourths of nephron function.
- Disturbances in fluid, electrolyte, and acid–base homeostasis are less severe than with ARF, but the loss of renal function is irreversible.

SYSTEM AFFECTED

- Renal/urologic—failure
- Endocrine/metabolic—disturbances in electrolyte and acid–base homeostasis; decreased erythropoietin production.
- GI—inappetance, possible diarrhea, and increased risk of ulcers.
- Nervous/neuromuscular—occasional ataxia or dementia in severe CRF; tremors or muscle fasciculations may accompany metabolic disturbances.
- Hemic/lymphatic/immune—alterations in hemostasis (i.e., platelet dysfunction); increased susceptibility to infection.

GENETICS

N/A

INCIDENCE/PREVALENCE

Reported to be 0.12%, increasing to 0.51% for stallions >15 years.

SIGNALMENT

Breed Predilections

- May be more common in Clydesdales.
- A heritable form of polycystic kidney disease may occur in Paints.

Mean Age and Range

Old horses (>15 years) are at greater risk.

Predominant Sex

Old stallions may be at greater risk; however, this may reflect more extensive diagnostic investigation of valuable breeding animals.

SIGNS

Historical Findings

- Because CRF can be a long-term sequel to other underlying disease processes (e.g., colic, diarrhea, prolonged exercise, rhabdomyolysis, purpura hemorrhagica, or neonatal septicemia) that initially led to ischemic ARF or GN, historical questioning should broadly pursue all previous medical and surgical problems.
- May develop months to years after nephrotoxin-induced acute tubular necrosis or papillary necrosis associated with use of NSAIDs.
- Most affected horses are presented for evaluation of insidious-onset mild depression, partial anorexia, and weight loss.
- Some astute owners may complain of ventral edema and mild polyuria and polydipsia (with clear-appearing urine).
- If detected at an earlier stage, a decrease in performance may be the initial presenting complaint.

Physical Examination Findings

- Weight loss and rough hair coat with mild depression, lethargy, reduced appetite, edema, excessive dental tartar, or an uremic odor in the oral cavity may be found.
- Affected horses usually are not clinically dehydrated.
- Voided urine usually is clear yellow, unlike the cloudy urine of normal horses.
- Rectal examination may reveal a small, firm left kidney with an irregular surface and, rarely, bilateral ureteral distension due to obstruction with uroliths.
- With end-stage disease, anuria may develop with anorexia, and more marked depression may be accompanied by ataxia, hypermetria, and mental obtundation.

CAUSES

- Immune-mediated GN initiated by chronic infections (e.g., equine infectious anemia, streptococcal diseases) or autoimmune disease.
- May be a sequel to ischemic or nephrotoxic ARF, leading to CIN.
- Less commonly, ascending infections may lead to bilateral pyelonephritis and nephrolithiasis/ureterolithiasis.
- Long-term use of NSAIDs with papillary necrosis and nephrolithiasis.
- Amyloidosis and renal neoplasia—rare.
- In horses <5 years and with no history of medical problems, anomalies of development—renal hypoplasia or dysplasia; polycystic kidney disease.

RISK FACTORS

- Previous episodes of ARF or UTI likely are important risk factors.
- Long-term use of NSAIDs.

CHRONIC RENAL FAILURE (CRF)

DIAGNOSIS

DIFFERENTIAL DIAGNOSIS

- A broad list of disorders that may lead to depression, partial anorexia, and weight loss (i.e., syndrome of ill thrift).
- Physical examination findings with CRF are nonspecific, but detection of azotemia, especially when accompanied by hypercalcemia, makes CRF rise to the top of the list.
- Prerenal or intrinsic ARF—supported by another underlying disease process producing renal ischemia or recent/concurrent exposure to nephrotoxic agents.
- Postrenal ARF—supported by stranguria, anuria, or uroperitoneum.

CBC/BIOCHEMISTRY/URINALYSIS

- Normal to low PCV (attributed to decreased serum erythropoietin concentration and shortened RBC life span), leukocyte count usually within normal ranges, and platelets normal to decreased.
- Increased BUN (100–250 mg/dL) and Cr (2.0–20 mg/dL); BUN:Cr ratio usually >10; Cr usually >5.0 mg/dL with horses presented for chronic ill thrift.
- Variable hyponatremia, hypochloremia, and hyperkalemia—hypercalcemia and hypophosphatemia with CRF are somewhat unique to horses; the former appears to result from decreased renal calcium excretion in the face of ongoing intestinal absorption, because elevated plasma parathormone concentrations have not been found in horses with CRF and hypercalcemia.
- Mild to moderate hypoalbuminemia.
- Mild to moderate hypertriglyceridemia (i.e., hyperlipemia) and hypercholesterolemia.
- Mild to moderate metabolic acidosis may accompany end-stage disease.
- Urine specific gravity—isosthenuria (1.008–1.014) is a hallmark feature.
- Mild to moderate proteinuria in some—may increase urine specific gravity to 1.020.
- Urine sediment is relatively devoid of crystals, but otherwise may be unremarkable. Increased RBCs support lithiasis or neoplasia, and increased leukocytes support UTI.

OTHER LABORATORY TESTS

- Increased fractional clearances (i.e., excretions) of sodium and chloride with advanced disease.
- Increased urine protein:creatinine ratio (>2:1) supports proteinuria.
- Include quantitative urine culture in the diagnostic evaluation of all affected horses, because significant bacteriuria may occur without pyuria.

IMAGING

Transabdominal Ultrasonography

- Kidneys may be small (diameter, <6 cm; length, <12 cm), with irregular surfaces.
- Parenchymal echogenicity may be increased, with loss of detail of corticomedullary junction.
- Bilateral nephrolithiasis/ureterolithiasis and variable hydronephrosis may be depicted.
- Multiple cystic structures may be depicted with polycystic kidney disease or pyelonephritis.

TRANSPECTAL ULTRASONOGRAPHT

- Greater detail of changes in the left kidney may be depicted.

Urethroscopy/Cystoscopy

- Useful with suspected obstructive disease or pyelonephritis.
- Urine samples may be collected from each ureter during cystoscopy by passing tubing through the biopsy channel of the endoscope.

DIAGNOSTIC PROCEDURES

GFR

- Measuring changes in GFR over time may be the most accurate way to follow the accompanying, progressive decrease in renal function.
- A simple method to estimate decline in GFR is to plot the inverse of Cr over time; alternatively, plasma disappearance of sodium sulfanilate, exogenous Cr, or radionuclides can be used.
- Timed urine collections to measure endogenous Cr clearance or clearance of inulin or radionuclides provide the most accurate measures.

Biopsy

- Percutaneous renal biopsy with routine immunohistochemistry and electron microscopy of the sample may provide information regarding cause (i.e., GN vs. CIN) but rarely affects prognosis or supportive treatment.
- Pursue biopsy with caution, because life-threatening hemorrhage can be a complication.

PATHOLOGIC FINDINGS

Gross Findings

- Characterized by firm, shrunken kidneys, with irregular surfaces.
- Renal capsule often adhered to parenchyma
- On cut section, kidneys typically are pale, with narrowed cortices.
- Nephroliths may be present within the parenchyma or the pelves.
- Hydronephrosis may accompany nephrolithiasis and ureterolithiasis.
- Abscesses and nephroliths often accompany chronic pyelonephritis.
- Enlarged kidneys with multiple cysts are found with polycystic kidney disease.

Histopathologic Findings

- Variable glomerular, tubular, and interstitial changes.
- End-stage kidney disease may preclude histologic categorization of the initiating cause.

TREATMENT

APPROPRIATE HEALTH CARE

- Proper recognition and treatment of all underlying disease processes.
- Fluid therapy, usually on an inpatient basis, to rule out ARF or acute-on-chronic disease.
- Discontinue potentially nephrotoxic medications.

CHRONIC RENAL FAILURE (CRF)

NURSING CARE

Fluid Therapy

- After initial measurement of body weight, magnitude of azotemia, and urine specific gravity, patients can be diuresed with 5% dextrose or normal (0.9%) saline at 2–3-fold the maintenance rate for 12–24 hours.
- Monitor closely, because significant pulmonary edema may develop after administering as little as 40 mL/kg of IV fluids.
- Increased urine output and decreased azotemia should occur in patients with ARF of acute-on-chronic disease.
- Horses with CRF typically develop more severe edema, with little decrease in magnitude of azotemia.

Oral Electrolyte Supplementation

- Sodium chloride (30 g) can be administered in concentrate feed or as an oral slurry/paste twice daily to replace urinary losses.
- With serum bicarbonate <20 mEq/L, a similar dose of sodium bicarbonate may be administered daily.
- Both should be discontinued if sodium supplementation produces or exacerbates edema.

ACTIVITY

- When clinical signs are mild and the horse's attitude is good, light exercise (e.g., 30 minutes of walking) can be continued daily or a few days each week.
- Maintain on high-quality pasture with walk-in shelter or in a stall with frequent hand-walking for grazing grass if appetite is poor.

DIET

- Access to fresh water at all times.
- The ideal diet for affected horses provides adequate caloric intake without excessive protein intake.
- Offering a variety of concentrate feeds, bran mash, and access to good-quality pasture is the recommended diet. Grass hay is preferred to alfalfa due to the higher protein and calcium content of the latter; however, if appetite for grass hay is poor, feed alfalfa.
- Supplementation with fat (rice bran or up to 12–16 oz. of oil added to concentrate feed) effectively increases caloric intake.

CLIENT EDUCATION

Inform clients that prognosis is poor for long-term survival but fair to guarded for short-term survival, especially when Cr < 5.0 mg/dL.

SURGICAL CONSIDERATIONS

Surgery is only required for acute-on-chronic disease due to obstructive urolithiasis—ureteral, cystic, or urethral calculi.

MEDICATIONS

DRUG(S) OF CHOICE

- Judicious use of oral electrolytes—see above.
- Antioxidant supplements—see above.
- Antiulcer drugs (e.g., omeprazole [2–4 mg/kg PO q24h]) may be useful in combating decreased feed intake in affected horses with accompanying gastric ulcers.

CONTRAINDICATIONS

- Corticosteroids and NSAIDs may exacerbate renal hypoperfusion and decline in GFR.
- Avoid all nephrotoxic medications unless specifically indicated for a concurrent disease process, and then modify dosage accordingly.

PRECAUTIONS

- Monitor response to fluid therapy closely—as little as 40 mL/kg of IV fluids (20 L to a 500-kg horse) may produce significant pulmonary edema in oliguric/anuric patients.
- Discontinue oral electrolyte supplementation if sodium supplementation produces or exacerbates edema.

POSSIBLE INTERACTIONS

N/A

ALTERNATIVE DRUGS

N/A

FOLLOW-UP

PATIENT MONITORING

- Assess clinical status (emphasizing attitude and appetite), edema formation, body weight, and magnitude of azotemia at least monthly during the initial few months of supportive care and every 2–3 months thereafter.
- Assess electrolyte and acid–basis status whenever changes in clinical status are noted.

CHRONIC RENAL FAILURE (CRF)

PREVENTION/AVOIDANCE

- Anticipate compromised renal function in patients with other diseases or undergoing prolonged anesthesia and surgery; institute appropriate treatment to minimize dehydration and potential renal damage.
- Ensure adequate hydration status in patients receiving nephrotoxic medications.
- Avoid prolonged use of NSAIDs unless necessary.

POSSIBLE COMPLICATIONS

- Pulmonary and peripheral edema with fluid therapy.
- Oral and GI ulceration or GI bleeding.
- Signs of neurologic impairment—ataxia; mental obtundation.

EXPECTED COURSE AND PROGNOSIS

- Issue a poor prognosis and consider euthanasia for horses that are emaciated, anuric, or have a Cr > 10 mg/dL at initial evaluation.
- Issue a guarded prognosis for short-term survival for patients with a Cr of 5–10 mg/dL at initial evaluation.
- Issue a fair prognosis for short-term survival for patients with a Cr <5 mg/dL that are in good body condition at initial evaluation.

MISCELLANEOUS

ASSOCIATED CONDITIONS

- UTI
- Urolithiasis

AGE-RELATED FACTORS

- Renal function decreases with aging; old horses likely are at greater risk.
- In horses <5 years, likely due to a developmental anomaly—renal hypoplasia or dysplasia.

ZOONOTIC POTENTIAL

N/A

PREGNANCY

Although not well documented, pregnant mares may be at increased risk of UTI.

SYNONYMS

- Kidney failure
- Chronic renal disease

SEE ALSO

- ARF
- Urolithiasis
- Urinary tract infection

ABBREVIATIONS

- ARF = acute renal failure
- CRF = chronic renal failure
- CIN = chronic interstitial nephritis
- GFR = glomerular filtration rate
- GI = gastrointestinal
- GN = glomerulonephritis
- PCV = packed cell volume
- UTI = urinary tract infection

Suggested Reading

King AB, Schott HC. Chronic renal failure. In: Robinson NE, ed. Current therapy in equine medicine 4. Philadelphia: WB Saunders, 1997:478–482.

Schott HC. Chronic renal failure. In: Reed SM, Bayly WM, eds. Equine internal medicine. Philadelphia: WB Saunders, 1998:856–875.

Author Harold C. Schott II

Consulting Editor Harold C. Schott II

CHRONIC WEIGHT LOSS

BASICS

DEFINITION

Chronic weight loss is not a specific problem of the digestive system but it is a common clinical manifestation of gastrointestinal disease. It can be defined as loss of body weight over time (over 4–5 weeks) and may be due to decreased fat and muscle mass or loss of gastrointestinal content and total body water, or a combination of these factors.

PATHOPHYSIOLOGY

Weight loss can result from many different clinical conditions. Loss of weight in the horse can occur due to lack of adequate food and/or water, poor-quality food, inability to prehend or swallow, maldigestion or malabsorption of food, increased loss of nutrients once absorbed, and increased catabolism. Inadequate caloric intake is likely the most common cause of weight loss, with endoparasitism following suit, and may also be due to specific nutrient deficiencies, chronic liver disease, neoplasia, and malabsorption. The pathophysiologic events leading to weight loss are multifold and depend on underlying causes. For details, see specific problems.

SYSTEM AFFECTED

Gastrointestinal

- Dental diseases
- Oral ulcerations
- Tongue paralysis
- Pharyngeal paresis or paralysis
- Retropharyngeal masses
- Esophageal strictures
- Gastric ulceration
- Duodenal and jejunal malabsorption
- Maldigestion
- Intestinal infections and non-infectious infiltrative and neoplastic disorders
- Chronic diarrhea
- Intestinal motility disturbances
- Intra-abdominal abscesses
- Parasitism
- Chronic grass sickness

Endocrine/Metabolic

- Pituitary adenoma of the pars intermedia in the horse due to increased metabolic rate, including muscle wasting induced by hyperadrenocorticism.
- Diabetes mellitus due to endocrine pancreatic insufficiency.

Hemic/Lymphatic/Immune

- Lymphoma leading to cancer cachexia.
- Inflammatory bowel disease leading to malabsorption.
- EIA

Hepatobiliary

Chronic hepatic failure

Cardiovascular

- Congestive heart failure, leading to decreased liver and gastrointestinal function.
- Valvular endocarditis due to occult infections.

Renal/Urologic

Chronic renal failure

Neuromuscular

Equine motor neuron disease and associated muscle wasting.

Behavioral

- Cribbing
- Oral stereotypy

Respiratory

- Severe COPD
- Chronic pleuropneumonia

Skin/Exocrine

Pemphigus foliaceus

Musculoskeletal

Chronic painful lameness (e.g., severe laminitis)

Nervous

Neurologic conditions that impair prehension, chewing, and swallowing.

Ophthalmic

N/A

Reproductive

N/A

Chronic Weight Loss

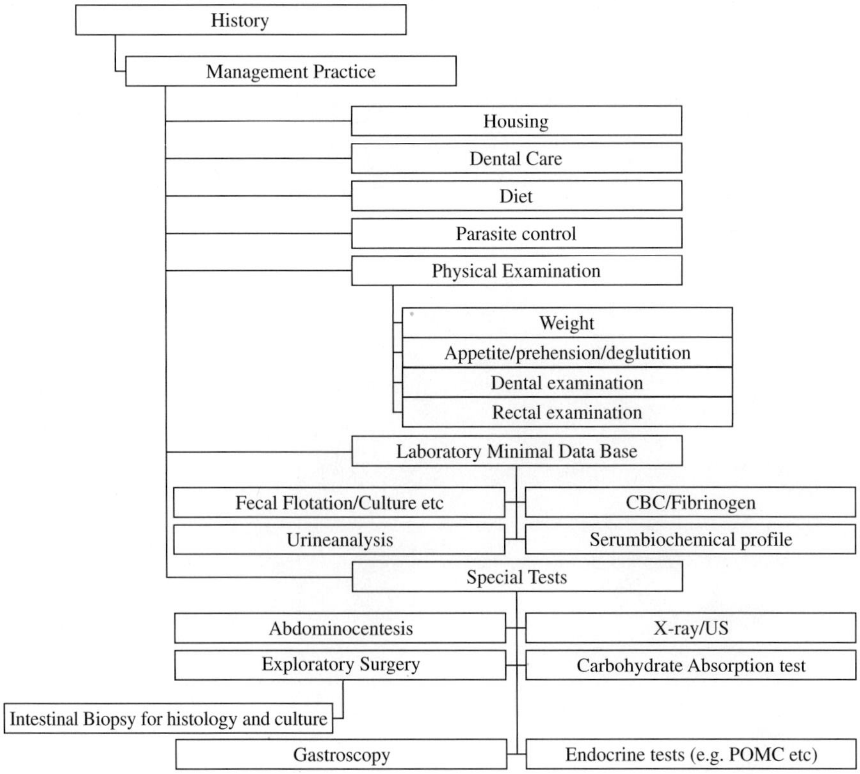

CHRONIC WEIGHT LOSS

SIGNALMENT
Age is important, especially in cases where parasitism is suspected (young horses), various bacterial diseases (*Rhodococcus equi, Lawsonia intracellularis*), or neoplasia, which is more commonly observed in older horses.

SIGNS
Signs vary according to the primary condition, but commonly, decrease in body condition and reduced appetite are observed.

CAUSES
A search of weight loss on Consultant® (Maurice White Cornell, 1999) listed 278 possible causes of weight loss in the horse. The causes include occult infections*, such as abdominal abscesses, pulmonary abscesses, pleuro-pneumonia, sinusitis, valvular endocarditis, and tooth problems; the whole group of malabsorption syndromes, including IBD and neoplasia; chronic renal failure; chronic hepatic failures; chronic parasitism; chronic viral infections (EIA); and endocrinopathies.

RISK FACTORS
Any condition leading to catabolic situations.

DIAGNOSIS

DIFFERENTIAL DIAGNOSIS
N/A

CBC/BIOCHEMISTRY/URINALYSIS
To work up a chronic weight loss case, a minimal database should include CBC, serum biochemical profile, and fibrinogen. CBC may be very non-specific, but total protein might be increased (e.g., due to hyperglobulinemia in occult infections) or decreased (e.g., due to protein-losing enteropathies). Anemia of chronic disease might be present with a hematocrit of <0.3 L/L ($<30\%$). There might be leukocytosis.
Biochemistry should help to differentiate between specific organ failure problems such as hepatic or renal diseases. Serum electrophoresis might assist in characterizing dysproteinemias and in separating conditions such as occult infections from neoplasia or parasitism.

OTHER LABORATORY TESTS
Hyperfibrinogenemia in inflammatory or neoplastic disease (>10 g/L or 1000 mg/dL).

IMAGING
N/A

DIAGNOSTIC PROCEDURES
- Abdominocentesis can be useful in identifying the abdomen to be the site of occult infections.
- Ultrasonography is used to detect abscesses (abdominal, pleural, etc).
- In individual cases, exploratory laparatomy might be required.
- Glucose and xylose absorption tests where small intestine malabsorption is suspected.
- When stomach ulcers are suspected, gastroscopy should be performed.

TREATMENT
See specific conditions.

MEDICATIONS

DRUG(S) OF CHOICE
See specific conditions.

CONTRAINDICATIONS
N/A

PRECAUTIONS
N/A

POSSIBLE INTERACTIONS
N/A

ALTERNATIVE DRUGS
N/A

FOLLOW-UP

PATIENT MONITORING
Monitoring feed intake and body weight of animal.

POSSIBLE COMPLICATIONS
Secondary infections due to debilitated immune system of the horse.

MISCELLANEOUS

ASSOCIATED CONDITIONS
N/A

AGE-RELATED FACTORS
Poor dentition might be a major factor in weight loss in older horses.

ZOONOTIC POTENTIAL
Chronic salmonellosis

PREGNANCY
N/A

SYNONYMS
N/A

SEE ALSO
N/A

ABBREVIATIONS
- IBD = inflammatory bowel disease
- EIA = equine infectious anemia

Suggested Reading

Brown CM. Chronic weight loss. In: Brown CM (Ed.): Chapter 2, Problems in equine medicine. Philadelphia: Lea & Febiger, 1989:6-21.
Roberts MC. Malabsorption syndromes in the horse. Compend Contin Educ. 1985:7:S637-S647.
McClure JJ. Chronic weight loss without diarrhea, pain, or icterus. In: Anderson NV: Chapter 27, Veterinary gastroenterology, 2nd ed. Philadelphia: Lea & Febiger, 1992.

Authors Olimpo Oliver and Henry Stämpfli
Consulting Editor Henry Stämpfli

CLEFT PALATE

BASICS

OVERVIEW

Cleft palate (palatoschisis) is a rare congenital abnormality of horses. Embryologically, the lateral palatine processes fuse at approximately day 47 of gestation in the horse. Failure of fusion of this process is manifest by cleft palate. Fusion occurs in a rostral to caudal direction, and therefore defects in the caudal soft palate occur more commonly than combined soft and hard palate clefts. Failure of palatine process fusion can be divided into two distinct conditions: a cleft in the primary palate, consisting of the lips and nares, or a cleft in the secondary palate, consisting of the hard and soft palates. These conditions are distinct, although they may occur together.

SIGNALMENT

Cleft palate is a congenital condition. Breed and sex predilections have not been reported.

SIGNS

The most common clinical signs include uni- or bilateral nasal discharge following nursing. However, other signs referable to aspiration pneumonia and malnourishment may be evident.

CAUSES AND RISK FACTORS

There is little information on the causes of cleft palate in the horse. In humans, however, it appears that the expression of cleft palates is a combination of teratogens and genetic factors with a potential modifying role of transforming growth factor alpha. Teratogens that have been identified in humans include ethanol, retinoids, and folate antagonists. In addition, epidemiologic studies have implicated maternal cigarette smoking. Moreover, animal models for this condition can be created by decreasing their PaO_2 during the time of palate closure. The role of conditions that decrease PaO_2 in horses might be speculated to cause cleft palate abnormalities.

DIFFERENTIAL DIAGNOSIS

Differential diagnoses for the clinical signs seen in neonates include causes of regurgitation, either physiologic (e.g., overfeeding) or pathologic (e.g., obstruction, achalasia, diverticul). In older animals, differentials for chronic pneumonia nasal discharge and ill thrift may be considered.

CBC/BIOCHEMISTRY/URINALYSIS

N/A

OTHER LABORATORY TESTS

N/A

IMAGING

Endoscopy is useful for confirming the diagnosis of cleft palate in the horse. Partial clefts of the caudal soft palate may be difficult to diagnose. Endoscopic findings consistent with cleft palates include a lack of palatal tissue contacting the epiglottis and an appearance that the epiglottis is ventrally displaced. Epiglotic entrapment, submucosal clefting, nasal septal deviation, and nasal mucosal inflammation may also be present.

DIAGNOSTIC PROCEDURES

Direct visualization of the cleft on oral examination is often difficult due to the long and narrow nature of the equine mouth and oropharynx.

TREATMENT

Curative treatment requires surgical intervention. The timing of surgical correction (palatoplasty) depends on the severity of the deformity as well as the concurrent associated medical problems, including sinusitis and regurgitation pneumonia. Early treatment of healthy individuals may prevent serious medical sequela and allows consumption of a liquid diet postoperatively. Delayed repair for animals sufficiently stable may allow development of the palatal tissues and avoids surgical scarring of developing tissues. The most common surgical approach is ventrally via a mandibular symphysiotomy, although a pharyngotomy has also been performed to achieve improved access to the caudal aspect of the soft palate when exposure via symphysiotomy is inadequate. One- and two-stage procedures have been proposed with these two techniques. Involvement of the hard palate requires more complex procedures, including mucoperiosteal sliding flaps for small caudal defects and mucoperiosteal reflected flaps for more severe defects. Reconstruction of palatine musculature has also been performed to improve postoperative function, and relief incisions as well as pterygoid bone osteotomies have been performed to decrease tension on the palate repair. The use of lidocaine containing epinephrine has been advocated to "tense tissues" and provide hemostasis. Despite these methods, postoperative complications remain very problematic.

CLEFT PALATE

MEDICATIONS

DRUG(S) OF CHOICE

Medical therapy is aimed at concurrent or associated conditions such as aspiration pneumonia.

CONTRAINDICATIONS/POSSIBLE INTERACTIONS

N/A

FOLLOW-UP

PATIENT MONITORING

Postoperatively, horses require antimicrobial therapy due to the contaminated surgical field and anti-inflammatory drugs to decrease postoperative swelling of the tongue and surrounding tissues. Broad-spectrum antibiotics should be prescribed, and if aspiration pneumonia is present, culture and sensitivity results of transtracheal aspiration may guide the appropriate choice of antimicrobial therapy. Foals should be encouraged to nurse postoperatively; however, morbidity may require alimentary support, including parenteral nutrition or stomach tubing. The oral cavity should be flushed daily to ensure removal of debris from the palate repair. Sutures in the palate are usually left in place, unless there is a specific indication for their removal.

PREVENTION/AVOIDANCE

Particular care must be taken to avoid exposure to teratogens, particularly at the time of closure of the lateral palatine processes (day 47 of gestation). Horses with cleft palates should not be bred due to the potential genetic etiology of this condition.

POSSIBLE COMPLICATIONS

Complications following surgical correction are frequent and serious. In one report, 100% of animals experienced postoperative complications. Complications include dehiscence of the suture line with formation of an oro-nasal fistula, osteomyelitis of the mandibular symphysis, dehiscence of the lower lip, failure to thrive, and chronic nasal discharge.

EXPECTED COURSE AND PROGNOSIS

The prognosis is dependent on the severity of the cleft and the involvement of the hard palate. Severe cleft palates with hard-palate involvement carry an extremely poor prognosis due to the retardation to alimentation, the development of more severe aspiration pneumonia, and the requirement for more complex surgical closure. Some foals with soft-palate clefts may survive without surgical intervention, but growth rates are commonly retarded. Complications following surgery approach 100%, and clinical signs may persist despite palate closure. Due to alterations to the function of the soft palate, horses with successfully repaired cleft palates may not be candidates for strenuous athletic pursuits.

MISCELLANEOUS

ASSOCIATED CONDITIONS

Associated conditions include inanition, malnutrition, failure of passive transfer, dysphagia, aspiration pneumonia and sinusitis.

AGE-RELATED FACTORS

Cleft palate is a congenital condition. There are case reports of older animals diagnosed and treated for cleft palates that were thereafter able to develop despite this condition.

Suggested Reading

Bowman KF. Cleft palate. In: Robinson, NE, ed. Current therapy in equine medicine, 2nd ed. Philadelphia: WB Saunders Co. 1987:1-3.

Author Simon G. Pearce

Consulting Editor Henry Stämpfli

CLITORAL ENLARGEMENT

BASICS

OVERVIEW

• The clitoris appears larger than normal and may appear to protrude through the vulvar lips at the ventral commissure.
• The clitoris develops from the embryonic genital tubercle in the absence of testicular testosterone production or its conversion to the active form, dihydrotestosterone. It is the female homologue of the penis.
• Corpus cavernosum clitoris—erectile tissue.
• Corpus clitoris (body of the clitoris)—5 cm in length.
• Crura—attached to the ischial arch.
• Glans clitoris—2.5 cm in diameter; situated in fossa at the ventral commissure of the vulva; well-developed median sinus and lateral sinuses may be present.

SIGNALMENT

• Females
• Congenital
• Iatrogenic drug administration—anabolic, progestational steroid
• Intersex conditions

SIGNS

• Historical findings—known drug administration; female offspring of treated mare.
• Enlargement of the glans clitoris beyond the expected norm.
• May be visible externally as swelling of the ventral vulval commissure.
• May protrude from the clitoral sinus between labia.
• May be associated with other genital anomalies—internal; external.

CAUSES AND RISK FACTORS

• Administration of anabolic steroids.
• Progestin (altrenogest) usage for estrus control, behavior modification, and pregnancy maintenance—female progeny have associated altered gonadotropin secretion and increased clitoral size to 21 months of age; no effect on reproductive function.
• Aberrant endogenous sex-steroid production—granulosa cell tumor in dam during. gestation.

DIAGNOSIS

DIFFERENTIAL DIAGNOSIS

Intersex Conditions

Pseudohermaphrodite—associated with clitoral enlargement.

Hypospadia Penis

• Hypoplastic penis with incomplete closure of embryonic urethral folds.
• Associated with prominent perineal median raphe, ventrally displaced vulva, and caudad direction of penis.
• Most common presentation—64,XX male.

CBC/BIOCHEMISTRY/URINALYSIS

N/A

OTHER LABORATORY TESTS

Hormonal Assay

• Testosterone/hCG challenge—baseline sample; administer 3000 IU of hCG, with additional samples at 3 and 24 hours; increased testosterone indicates testicular tissue is present (i.e., Leydig cell production).
• Estrone sulfate—produced by Sertoli cells in the testicle; couple with hCG challenge to improve diagnostic accuracy.

Immunology

• Test for presence of 5α-reductase or cytosolic receptor.
• Use labial skin only, because the receptors are site specific.

IMAGING

Ultrasonography—coupled with transrectal palpation of internal genitalia for ovarian pathology or internal genital anomaly.

DIAGNOSTIC PROCEDURES

N/A

PATHOLOGIC FINDINGS

N/A

TREATMENT

N/A

MEDICATIONS

DRUGS

N/A

CONTRAINDICATIONS/POSSIBLE INTERACTIONS

N/A

CLITORAL ENLARGEMENT

FOLLOW-UP

For control/prevention:

- Rational causative drug usage
- If genetic, elimination of parent stock from breeding pool

MISCELLANEOUS

ASSOCIATED CONDITIONS

Intersex conditions

AGE-RELATED FACTORS

Congenital

ZOONOTIC POTENTIAL

N/A

PREGNANCY

Associated abnormalities may preclude fertility.

SYNONYMS

N/A

SEE ALSO

Disorders of sexual development.

ABBREVIATION

hCG = human chorionic gonadotropin

Suggested Reading

Hughes JP. Developmental anomalies of the female reproductive tract. In: McKinnon AO, Voss JL, eds. Equine reproduction. Philadelphia: Lea & Febiger, 1993:409–410.

Noden J, Squires EL, Nett TM. Effect of maternal treatment with altrenogest on age at puberty, hormone concentrations, pituitary response to exogenous GnRH, oestrous cycle characteristics and fertility of fillies. J Reprod Fertil 1990;88:185–195.

Author Peter R. Morresey

Consulting Editor Carla L. Carleton

CLOSTRIDIAL MYOSITIS

BASICS

DEFINITION

Clostridial myositis is an infection of muscle by *Clostridium* spp. most frequently associated with intramuscular injection. The infection may remain localized and form a focal abscess or migrate along fascial planes, resulting in diffuse cellulitis.

PATHOPHYSIOLOGY

The frequent temporal association between intramuscular injections and clostridial myositis suggests entry of the organism at the time of injection. However, injection of irritating substances may produce local tissue necrosis and an anaerobic environment ideal for proliferation of spores already present in muscle. In cattle, *Clostridium* spp. are thought to be absorbed from the gastrointestinal tract and remain dormant in tissue until conditions exist for proliferation. Due to the ubiquitous nature of clostridial organisms, they may contaminate wounds and surgical sites. Clostridial organisms are also common in subsolar abscesses. Regardless of the origin, the release of potent clostridial exotoxins leads to local tissue necrosis, systemic toxemia, and organ dysfunction. In this most severe form, the term "*malignant edema*", is used to reflect the systemic involvement and high mortality.

SYSTEM AFFECTED

Musculoskeletal

This is the primary system affected. Necrotizing toxins released by the organism lead to local tissue necrosis.

Cardiovascular, Respiratory, Renal, and Hemic

Exotoxins absorbed from the site of infection cause damage to cell membranes, leading to hemolysis, increased capillary permeability, and multiple organ dysfunction.

GENETICS

N/A

INCIDENCE/PREVALENCE

Some geographic areas may have a greater incidence due to higher environmental contamination by clostridial organisms.

SIGNALMENT

Clostridial myositis occurs in horses of any breed or age. Horses on a high plane of nutrition may be predisposed due to proliferation of clostridial organisms in the alimentary tract.

SIGNS

Historical Findings

Intramuscular injection with a non-antibiotic medication is the most common cause of clostridial myositis, and thus owners should be questioned about recent medications, treatments, or illnesses. Depending on the site of infection, horses may be stiff and reluctant to walk, lame, or unwilling to raise or lower the head to eat. Pain and systemic toxemia may lead to anorexia and tachypnea. Vague signs of discomfort are easily mistaken for colic.

Physical Examination Findings

If myonecrosis is related to intramuscular injection, common sites of injection should be palpated for heat, pain, swelling, and crepitus. Small puncture wounds are occasionally only visible once the hair over the affected area is clipped. Swellings that are initially warm and painful later become cool, firm, and necrotic. Muscle pain may cause a lame or stiff gait, reluctance to walk, depression, anorexia, tachypnea, and tachycardia. Dehydration, depression, delayed capillary refill time, poor peripheral pulses, and cool extremities suggest systemic toxemia and inadequate peripheral perfusion and shock. Oral mucous membranes may be dark red to blue. Fever is common.

CAUSES

Clostridial myositis has been associated with *C. perfringens* (type A), *C. chauvoei*, *C. septicum*, and *C. novyi*.

RISK FACTORS

Although any intramuscular injection could potentially result in a clostridial infection, medications that are irritating and result in tissue necrosis are frequently associated with this syndrome.

DIAGNOSIS

DIFFERENTIAL DIAGNOSIS

When clostridial myositis is secondary to an injection, the diagnosis can be complicated by previous medical problems. Pain associated with myonecrosis may be confused with colic, exertional myopathy, laminitis, or abscesses from other causes. Severe pain, fever, toxemia, and shock rarely result from an abscess due to other less virulent organisms.

CBC/BIOCHEMISTRY

If clostridial infection is localized into an abscess, a CBC may reveal only a modest leukocytosis with left shift and neutrophilia. Hyperfibrinogenemia may be present if infection is present for more than a few days. When severe systemic toxemia develops, leukopenia and hemolysis can occur. Increases in muscle enzymes CPK and AST may be mild compared to the apparent severity of toxemia perhaps due to the focal nature of the disease, destruction of enzyme, or lack of enzyme absorption into systemic circulation. Dehydration and shock may result in azotemia and hemoconcentration.

OTHER LABORATORY TESTS

Clostridial toxins may result in disseminated intravascular coagulation and alterations in platelet count, PT, PTT, and antithrombin-III.

IMAGING

Ultrasonography may reveal an encapsulated abscess or diffuse tissue edema, necrosis, cellulitis, and echogenic foci of emphysema. Differentiation between focal abscesses and diffuse cellulitis aids in defining areas for treatment. Abscesses should be lanced and lavaged. Fasciotomy is appropriate if diffuse cellulitis and myonecrosis are present.

DIAGNOSTIC PROCEDURES

A tentative diagnosis can be made based on a history of intramuscular injection or wound and a rapid onset of severe heat, pain, and swelling of affected tissues. Diagnosis can be confirmed by aspiration of purulent or serosanguinous material for anaerobic culture, cytology, or fluorescent antibody identification. Care should be taken to properly prepare sites for aspiration to avoid contamination with surface organisms. Samples should be collected and placed in media designed for transportation of anaerobic specimens and submitted to a laboratory as soon as possible. Muscle biopsies frequently reveal characteristic gram-positive rods.

PATHOLOGIC FINDINGS

Systemic toxemia results in the degeneration of parenchymatous tissues. Malodorous serosanguinous fluid and emphysema are present in dark-colored necrotic muscle.

CLOSTRIDIAL MYOSITIS

TREATMENT

APPROPRIATE HEALTH CARE
Treatment options are dictated by the severity of the disease. Focal encapsulated abscesses may be managed in the field; however, referral should be considered for horses with signs of systemic toxemia (tachycardia, increased CRT, abnormal mucous membrane color, poor peripheral pulses, or cool extremities).

NURSING CARE
Oral fluids are indicated if dehydration is present and balanced polyionic fluids (lactated or acetated Ringer solution) should be administered if there are signs of shock. Hot-packing may aid in drainage of abscesses, whereas later in the course of the disease cold hydrotherapy may decrease activity of inflammatory mediators. Feed should be provided at head level for horses with neck pain associated with infection of cervical musculature.

ACTIVITY
Activity should be limited to decrease movement of bacteria along fascial planes.

DIET
N/A

CLIENT EDUCATION
Clients should be educated about proper intramuscular injection techniques.

SURGICAL CONSIDERATIONS
Focal abscesses may be drained by incision, lavage, and placement of a drain. Diffuse cellulitis and tissue edema are important to identify sonographically because medical management may be more appropriate for this type of infection. However, when severe toxemia occurs, fenestration of infected tissue with vertical incisions is helpful in reducing an anaerobic environment. Incisions are made through skin and necrotic muscle so as to aerate tissues and reduce pressure associated with severe edema. Minimal sedation and hemostasis are frequently necessary due to the necrotic nature of the tissue incised.

MEDICATIONS

DRUG(S) OF CHOICE
Horses with severe systemic signs are initially given potassium or sodium penicillin (44,000 IU/kg IV) every 2 to 4 hr until stabilized and then four times daily. Focal abscesses can be managed with drainage and penicillin (22,000 IU/kg IM q12h). Metronidazole (15–25 mg/kg PO q6h) is also effective against *Clostridium* spp. and can be given orally. Analgesics and anti-inflammatory medications (flunixin meglumine 1 mg/kg IV q12h) are indicated.

CONTRAINDICATIONS
N/A

PRECAUTIONS
Hydration and renal function should be monitored when using nonsteroidal anti-inflammatory medications in horses with severe systemic disease.

POSSIBLE INTERACTIONS
N/A

ALTERNATIVE DRUGS
Chloramphenicol (50 mg/kg PO q6h) also has activity against anaerobic bacteria; however, due to the potential for irreversible aplastic anemia in people, its use should be avoided if possible. Trimethoprim-potentiated sulfonamides are efficacious *in-vitro* but have questionable *in-vivo* efficacy. Rifampin is effective against most *Clostridium* spp.; however, it is generally used in combination with other antimicrobials due to the development of resistance.

FOLLOW-UP

PATIENT MONITORING
N/A

PREVENTION/AVOIDANCE
Clostridial myonecrosis may result from intramuscular injections even when proper technique is followed. Avoiding intramuscular injection of irritating substances may reduce the incidence of this disease.

POSSIBLE COMPLICATIONS
Severe toxemia may lead to shock, renal insufficiency, laminitis, intravascular hemolysis, disseminated intravascular coagulation, or death.

EXPECTED COURSE AND PROGNOSIS
Focal abscesses respond well to drainage and systemic antimicrobials. Horses with diffuse myositis, toxemia, and shock have a guarded to poor prognosis in spite of aggressive therapy. *Clostridium septicum* and *C. chauvoei* infections are usually fatal; however, *C. perfringens* infections have a better prognosis.

MISCELLANEOUS

ASSOCIATED CONDITIONS
N/A

AGE-RELATED FACTORS
N/A

ZOONOTIC POTENTIAL
Clostridium perfringens is the most common cause of malignant edema in people.

PREGNANCY
N/A

SYNONYMS
- Malignant edema
- Clostridial myonecrosis

SEE ALSO
- Botulism
- Tetanus
- Tyzzer's disease
- Enteric clostridiosis

ABBREVIATIONS
N/A

Suggested Reading

Rebhun WC, Shin SJ, King JM, et al. Malignant edema in horses. J Am Vet Med Assoc. 1985,187:732-736.

Author Mark T. Donaldson
Consulting Editor Corinne R. Sweeney

CLOSTRIDIUM DIFFICILE ENTEROCOLITIS

BASICS

DEFINITION

Clostridium difficile enterocolitis is an inflammation of the colon due to overgrowth of toxigenic strains of *C. difficile*, most commonly causing diarrhea and varying degrees of toxemia.

PATHOPHYSIOLOGY

Clostridium difficile may be acquired through oral inoculation or may be present in low numbers in the gastrointestinal tract. In many cases, it is not known why proliferation of this organism occurs, but it is assumed to be due to a disruption of the normal, protective gastrointestinal microflora and in some cases follows the use of antibiotics. This organism produces two toxins, a cytotoxin and an enterotoxin, that work synergistically. These toxins cause clinical signs both by their direct toxic effects on the colon and through proinflammatory effects on neutrophils. The net result is varying degrees of fluid secretion, mucosal damage, and intestinal inflammation.

SYSTEMS AFFECTED

Gastrointestinal

Overgrowth of *C. difficile* can cause a diarrhea ranging in severity from mild, cow-pie consistency feces to profuse and watery feces. Borborygmi may be increased or decreased in intensity, but typically have a fluid sound. Mild to severe colic may be present.

Cardiovascular

Dehydration and cardiovascular shock can ensue. Venous thrombosis of injection or catheter sites can occur.

Musculoskeletal

Peripheral edema is common because hypoproteinemia is frequent. Laminitis is a common sequel.

INCIDENCE/PREVALENCE

This is a sporadic condition. It is more commonly reported in certain geographic areas, but this is likely because the techniques to diagnose this condition are not being used in all regions.

SIGNALMENT

There are no reported breed, age, or sex predilections.

SIGNS

Historical Findings

There is occasionally a history of depression, anorexia, and pyrexia. Diarrhea is not always an initial complaint. When present, diarrhea can range from cow-pie consistency to profuse and watery. There may be a history of recent antibiotic use.

Physical Examination Findings

Diarrhea is present in most cases. Dehydration may be present, suggested by decreased skin turgor, tacky oral mucous membranes, and increased capillary refill time. Rectal temperature may be subnormal, normal, or increased. Tachycardia is often present. Hypermotile or hypomotile but fluid-sounding gastrointestinal sounds may be present. Signs of endotoxemia may be present. Colic may result from fluid distension of the intestinal tract. Peripheral edema may be present if the animal is hypoproteinemic.

CAUSES

Infectious

Intestinal proliferation and exotoxin production by toxigenic strains of the anaerobic gram-positive bacterium *C. difficile.*

RISK FACTORS

Risk factors for *C. difficile* enterocolitis have not been explored in the horse. It is presumed that any condition altering the normal intestinal microflora could allow proliferation of toxigenic *C. difficile.* Antibiotic use is a well-documented risk factor in cases in which humans developed *C. difficile* colitis. Antibiotic disruption of the intestinal microflora is presumed to be a significant risk factor in the horse. *Clostridium difficile* colitis has also been reported in mares whose foals were being treated with erythromycin succinate, presumably through low-dose antibiotic exposure. This syndrome has recently been reproduced experimentally. This pathogen is also a major nosocomial pathogen in human medicine, so hospitalization may be a risk factor as well. Other stressors, such as surgery and transportation, may play a role.

DIAGNOSIS

DIFFERENTIAL DIAGNOSIS

- Salmonellosis
- Potomac horse fever
- *Clostridium perfringens* enterocolitis
- Cyathostomiasis
- NSAID-induced colitis
- Cantharidin toxicosis
- Chronic sand impaction
- Idiopathic colitis

CBC/BIOCHEMISTRY/URINALYSIS

CBC

The packed cell volume is often elevated, depending on the degree of dehydration. Total protein levels are variable and may be increased due to hemoconcentration or decreased due to protein loss into the intestinal tract. It is important to interpret the total protein level relative to the hydration status. Leukopenia with neutropenia is often present, frequently with a left shift. Neutrophils may be degenerate. A leukocytosis develops at later stages of the disease.

Biochemistry

Hyponatremia and hypochloremia are characteristic. Hypokalemia is sometimes present, but hyperkalemia in response to a metabolic acidosis is common. Hypocalcemia and hypoalbuminemia are also common. A prerenal azotemia is common in dehydrated animals.

OTHER LABORATORY TESTS

Culture of this organism is difficult, time-consuming, and requires specialized equipment for anaerobic culture. Selective culture media are required because this organism is readily overgrown by other intestinal organisms. Because approximately 25% of *C. difficile* strains are non-toxigenic, definitive diagnosis requires identification of toxins in the feces. Toxin presence can be detected with the use of an ELISA for either or both toxins. Bacterial culture for *Salmonella* spp. should also be performed because it is a major differential diagnosis.

IMAGING

Abdominal ultrasonography may be performed, and the large colon may appear hypoechoic with increased motility.

DIAGNOSTIC PROCEDURES

Palpation per rectum should always be performed in cases of colitis to ensure that signs of colic, depression, and toxemia are not related to another gastrointestinal lesion.

PATHOLOGIC FINDINGS

The pathologic lesions in *C. difficile* colitis are not well described in horses. The large intestine, including the cecum, is the main site affected in adult horses. The only gross abnormality may be fluid intestinal contents. More severe cases may have marked intestinal edema and hemorrhage, with petechia and ecchymoses throughout. Histologically, there is mild to severe inflammation, and hemorrhagic necrotizing enterocolitis may be present.

TREATMENT

APPROPRIATE HEALTH CARE

This condition is best managed with intensive inpatient care due to the frequent need for aggressive fluid therapy and the incidence of secondary problems. If the diarrhea is not very severe and adequate hydration can be maintained, treatment on the farm could be attempted.

NURSING CARE

Intravenous fluid therapy is the most important treatment of this condition. A balanced polyionic electrolyte solution should be administered via an intravenous catheter. Two catheters may be required in severe cases. The rate of fluid administration depends on the degree of dehydration and the amount and fluid content of the diarrhea. Mild to moderate cases of metabolic acidosis typically resolve with fluid therapy. Sodium bicarbonate may be required in certain cases to correct a severe metabolic acidosis. In severely hypokalemic horses, 20–40 mEq/L of potassium chloride can be added to the intravenous fluids. Intravenous administration of KCl should not exceed 0.5 mEq/kg/hr.

An oral electrolyte solution containing 35 g KCl and 70 g of NaCl in 10 L of water should be provided, along with clean, fresh drinking water. Intravenous administration of hypertonic saline (4–6 mL/kg of 5–7.5% NaCl) may be indicated in severely dehydrated animals. This provides rapid volume expansion and also appears to increase myocardial contractility, vasodilation, and peripheral perfusion. It is essential that isotonic fluid therapy follow the use of hypertonic saline.

Due to the high incidence of venous thrombosis in colitis, the catheter site should be monitored frequently. If distal limb edema develops due to hypoproteinemia, then leg wraps should be applied and changed daily. Deep bedding should be provided if there are any signs of laminitis.

CLOSTRIDIUM DIFFICILE ENTEROCOLITIS

ACTIVITY

Activity is commonly restricted due to the need for intravenous fluid therapy and the potential for disease transmission. Horses that display signs of colic may benefit from short walks to stimulate progressive motility and help pass diarrhea. Because diarrheic horses should be considered infectious, an isolated area should be used and it should be disinfected appropriately.

DIET

Affected horses should be provided with free choice hay. This may help stabilize the disrupted gastrointestinal flora, provide electrolytes such as potassium and calcium, and decrease weight loss, as affected animals can become very catabolic. It is recommended to feed hay in a hay net because hypoproteinemic horses eating off the ground may develop severe facial edema. Higher energy feeds can also be provided. Large amounts of grain should be avoided due to the risk of further gastrointestinal flora disruption.

Due to the severe catabolic state that occurs in many cases of colitis, forced enteral feeding or partial or total parenteral nutrition may be required. The cost of parenteral nutrition is often prohibitive.

CLIENT EDUCATION

Clients should be made aware of the potential for mortality and the serious risk of secondary problems such as laminitis and jugular vein thrombosis. They should also be warned that the horse should be considered infectious, and appropriate sanitation of contaminated areas should be recommended.

SURGICAL CONSIDERATION

N/A

MEDICATIONS

DRUG(S) OF CHOICE

- Metronidazole—15–25 mg/kg q6–8-hr.
- Flunixin meglumine: 0.25 mg/kg q8-hr can be used for its purported anti-endotoxic effects,1.1 mg/kg can be used for analgesia.
- Fresh-frozen plasma is beneficial in severely hypoproteinemic animals (<40 g/L) (4.0g/dL) Although not proved to be of added benefit in cases of colitis, some clinicians believe that the use of serum from horses hyperimmunized to *Escherichia coli* J5 strain helps moderate the effects of endotoxemia.
- Potassium chloride—25–50 g PO q12–24h. If the horse is eating but remains hypokalemic, oral administration of KCl once or twice a day is an easy and cost-effective route of supplementation.
- Lamitinis treatment—See the appropriate chapter in this text.

CONTRAINDICATIONS

Metronidazole may be teratogenic and is therefore contraindicated in pregnant mares.

PRECAUTIONS

The 1.1mg/kg dose of flunixin meglumine may be nephrotoxic in dehydrated animals. It can also mask severe pain that might indicate a surgical lesion, and should be used judiciously in cases where the diagnosis is still in question.

POSSIBLE INTERACTIONS

Cimetidine should not be used concurrently with metronidazole because there is interaction through hepatic inhibition.

ALTERNATIVE DRUGS

N/A

FOLLOW-UP

PATIENT MONITORING

Affected animals should be monitored frequently to evaluate hydration status, character and volume of diarrhea, presence of edema, and to observe for signs of colic. Packed cell volume and total protein levels should be evaluated at least daily during the initial course of disease to monitor hydration and protein status. If increases in urea and creatinine were present on presentation, this should be re-evaluated after the animal is rehydrated to ensure it was due to pre-renal azotemia and not to renal failure. Serum or plasma electrolyte levels should be monitored to determine whether electrolyte supplementation, especially potassium and calcium, is required. The intravenous catheter site should be monitored frequently. The feet should be checked frequently for increased digital pulses or hoof wall temperature, indicative of laminitis.

PREVENTION/AVOIDANCE

Antibiotics should be used judiciously to decrease the risk of disruption of the gastrointesinal microflora.

POSSIBLE COMPLICATIONS

- Endotoxemia
- Laminitis
- Jugular vein thrombosis
- Renal failure

CLOSTRIDIUM DIFFICILE ENTEROCOLITIS

EXPECTED COURSE AND PROGNOSIS

Overall mortality rates for colitis in animals presented to a referral center ranged from 10% to 40%. Death can occur from the primary gastrointestinal disease; however, euthanasia is often opted for due to expense of treatment, poor response to initial treatment, or development of severe laminitis. Mortality rates for *C. difficile* enterocolitis have not been studied extensively. The prognosis is good in cases where the diarrhea resolves shortly after presentation and no signs of laminitis occur.

MISCELLANEOUS

ASSOCIATED CONDITIONS

- Laminitis
- Venous thrombosis

AGE-RELATED FACTORS

N/A

ZOONOTIC POTENTIAL

As the causative organism is an important cause of colitis in humans, it may be advisable to treat all affected horses as zoonotic risks.

PREGNANCY

Metronidazole should not be administered to pregnant mares. An increased risk of abortion may be present due to endotoxemia and hypovolemic shock.

SYNONYMS

N/A

SEE ALSO

Laminitis

ABBREVIATIONS

N/A

Suggested Reading

Baverud V, Gustafsson A, Franklin A, Lindholm A, Gunnersson A. *Clostridium difficile* associated with acute colitis in mature horses treated with antibiotics. Eq Vet J 1997;29:279-284.

Jones RL, Shideler RK, Cockerell GL. Association of *Clostridium difficile* with foal diarrhea. In: Equine infectious diseases V. Lexington: University of Kentucky Press. 1988;5:236-240.

Knoop FC, Owens M, Crocker IC. *Clostridium difficile:* Clinical disease and diagnosis. Clin Microbiol Rev. 1993;6:251-265.

Weese JS, Parsons DA, Stämpfli HR. Association of *Clostridium difficile* with enterocolitis and lactose intolerance in a foal. J Am Vet Med Assoc. 1999;214:229-232.

Author J. Scott Weese
Consulting Editor Henry Stämpfli

CLOTTING FACTOR DEFICIENCIES

BASICS

DEFINITION

Bleeding disorder characterized by decreased concentration or functional activity of one or more factors in the coagulation system.

PATHOPHYSIOLOGY

The formation and remodeling of a thrombus involves interactions between the blood vessel wall, platelets, the coagulation system and its inhibitors (e.g., antithrombin III [ATIII]), and the fibrinolytic system. Proper functioning of the coagulation system requires sequential activation of a series of coagulation factors. Exposure of a negatively charged surface (e.g., platelet plug, subendothelium) and release of tissue factor initiate activation of the intrinsic and extrinsic coagulation pathways, respectively. These pathways converge at the activation of factor X, which cleaves prothrombin to thrombin in the common pathway. Thrombin converts fibrinogen into fibrin, which stabilizes the platelet plug at the site of vessel injury. A defect in one or more coagulation factors may result in defective thrombus formation.

SYSTEM AFFECTED

Clotting factor deficiencies are associated with hemorrhage into any tissue or organ system. Prolonged or excessive bleeding may result from trauma or surgery. Common sites for hemorrhage include subcutaneous tissues, joint cavities, body cavities, or muscles. Bleeding into the laryngeal region or the pleural cavity causes respiratory distress. Bleeding into the central nervous system may be life-threatening because tissue expansion is limited by the bones in the skull.

SIGNALMENT

Hereditary Defects

Hereditary deficiency of factor VIII or IX is a sex-linked disorder that may cause severe spontaneous bleeding. These disorders affect primarily males and are first recognized at a young age; females are usually asymptomatic carriers. Factor VIII deficiency is most common and has been reported in quarter-horses, thoroughbreds, and standardbreds. A combined factor IX and XI deficiency has been reported in an Arabian. Deficiency of prekallikrein, a factor involved in contact activation of the intrinsic coagulation system, occurs in Belgians and miniature horses. Prekallikrein deficiency may go undetected until a horse is hemostatically challenged (e.g., surgery, trauma).

Acquired Defects

All ages and breeds are affected.

SIGNS

Historical Findings

Spontaneous hemorrhage or excessive bleeding following trauma or surgery.

Physical Findings

Subcutaneous hematoma formation, lameness associated with hemarthrosis or muscle hemorrhage, ecchymoses, and pale mucous membranes. Bleeding into body cavities may cause depression, dyspnea, or abdominal pain. Melena, hematuria, and epistaxis are commonly associated with platelet defects or DIC, but may occur with some coagulation factor defects.

CAUSES

Coagulation defects result from decreased production of a coagulation factor, production of dysfunctional coagulation factors, or the presence of circulating inhibitors of coagulation. Inherited clotting factor defects occur much less frequently than acquired defects. Common causes for acquired defects include: (1) DIC; (2) hepatic disease; (3) vitamin K antagonism (e.g., exposure to coumarin or coumarin derivatives in rodenticide anticoagulants or moldy sweet clover hay) or deficiency (e.g., biliary obstruction); or (4) administration of drugs that inhibit coagulation (e.g., heparin). DIC is most common, and occurs secondary to an underlying disorder (e.g., gastrointestinal disorders, bacterial sepsis, endotoxemia, neoplasia) that causes overwhelming activation of the hemostatic pathways. Initially, microthrombi form, and may be followed by hemorrhagic diathesis due to fibrinolysis and consumption of coagulation factors, inhibitors, and platelets. Vitamin K antagonism or deficiency causes the production of non-functional factors II, VII, IX, and X. Hepatic disease is associated with laboratory evidence of a coagulation defect because the liver is the production site for most coagulation factors and inhibitors.

RISK FACTORS

Exposure to vitamin K antagonists should be investigated in adult horses with acute onset of unexplained bleeding. Therapeutic administration of coumarin derivatives for thrombotic disease must be carefully monitored to prevent toxicity. Administration of drugs that bind extensively to plasma proteins (e.g., phenylbutazone) may displace protein-bound coumarin and cause toxicity. Diets low in vitamin K may potentiate toxicosis.

DIAGNOSIS

DIFFERENTIAL DIAGNOSIS

- Local disease processes (e.g., trauma, neoplasia) are the most common cause for hemorrhage. History, physical findings, and normal coagulation test results are necessary to rule out an underlying coagulation defect.
- Inherited deficiencies of factor VIII or IX should be suspected in foals with unexplained hemorrhage, hematoma formation, or hemarthrosis. Bleeding often occurs repeatedly through the animal's life. Family histories should be obtained to determine if relatives are affected. Deficiencies of prekallikrein or factor XI are either asymptomatic and detected with laboratory testing, or associated with mild bleeding following surgery or trauma.
- Acquired coagulation defects occur in horses with no prior history of bleeding problems. Horses with DIC present with signs referable to the underlying disease process as well as evidence of organ failure associated with microthrombi formation. Horses may have evidence of hemorrhagic diathesis. Horses with hepatic disease present with anorexia, weight loss, abdominal pain, fever, icterus, or neurologic signs due to hepatic encephalopathy. Horses with vitamin K antagonism have acute subcutaneous hematoma formation, and hemorrhage into body cavities, causing abdominal pain or dyspnea, melena, or epistaxis.
- Patients with quantitative or qualitative platelet defects usually have petechial hemorrhages on mucosal surfaces or non-haired skin, epistaxis, hematuria, melena, or spontaneous hemorrhage from other mucosal surfaces. Hematoma formation and bleeding into body cavities are not common. Horses with platelet defects have normal PT and APTT. Deficiency of von Willebrand factor (vWF) is rarely recognized in horses; clinical signs and history are similar to a platelet defect. Affected horses have normal platelet number, normal clotting times, and decreased concentrations of plasma vWF.

LABORATORY FINDINGS

Drugs That May Alter Lab Results

Heparin may cause prolonged clotting times.

Disorders That May Alter Lab Results

Care must be taken when collecting blood for coagulation testing. Excessive tissue trauma during venipuncture activates the coagulation system and alters clotting times. Proper dilution of blood with anticoagulant is critical (9 parts blood plus 1 part 3.8% trisodium citrate). Underfilling of collection tubes may prolong clotting times. Collection directly into a syringe containing anticoagulant is preferred. Blood should be immediately centrifuged to separate plasma. If laboratory testing is not performed within 2–3 hr of collection, the plasma should be frozen in small aliquots (<1 mL/tube) because some coagulation factors are labile at room temperature. Repeated thawing and freezing of samples should be avoided. If sent to a laboratory, samples should be mailed overnight on dry ice or ice packs to ensure that they remain frozen. Plasma from a normal horse should be sent with the patient sample to detect any alterations associated with transport. Lipemia or hemolysis may affect clotting times measured with some analyzers.

CLOTTING FACTOR DEFICIENCIES

Valid If Run in Human Lab

The sensitivity of coagulation assays varies with methodology and reagents. Assays measured in human laboratories are valid if normal equine plasma is used as a control.

CBC/BIOCHEMISTRY/URINALYSIS

Anemia and hypoproteinemia (decreased albumin and globulin concentrations) are expected in horses with severe hemorrhage due to hereditary or acquired clotting factor defects. Platelet counts should be performed in all horses with a bleeding disorder. Horses with inherited coagulation defects or with vitamin K antagonism/deficiency have normal platelet counts unless hemorrhage is severe enough to cause a mild, transient thrombocytopenia. Thrombocytopenia is expected in horses with DIC. Elevated liver enzymes, decreased albumin concentrations, hyperbilirubinemia, or elevated bile acids occur in horses with hepatic disease.

OTHER LABORATORY TESTING

Clotting Times

The PT and APTT evaluate the extrinsic and intrinsic coagulation pathways, respectively. The ACT and WBCT are less sensitive assays that can substitute for the APTT. Prolonged PT with normal APTT occurs with a hereditary deficiency of factor VII (not reported in horses), early vitamin K antagonism (generally before clinical signs of hemorrhage are present), or hepatic disease. Prolonged APTT with normal PT suggests a deficiency of one or more factors in the intrinsic pathway (VIII, IX, XI, XII, prekallikrein, high molecular weight kininogen) due to a hereditary deficiency or hepatic disease. Prolonged PT and APTT suggest either a hereditary single factor defect in the common pathway (X, V, II, fibrinogen) or multiple factor deficiencies due to vitamin K antagonism/deficiency, DIC, or hepatic disease. If a hereditary deficiency is suspected, correction factor assays can be performed to determine the specific factors involved.

Other Hemostatic Assays

FDPs increase and ATIII activity decrease in many patients with DIC or hepatic disease. Blood must be collected into a special tube for measurement of FDP.

DIAGNOSTIC PROCEDURES

Bleeding time: A small incision is made in a mucous membrane (e.g., inside of the lip) or non-haired skin (e.g., shaved area of the neck), being careful to avoid puncturing any visible vessels. Spring-loaded devices (e.g., Surgicutt, ITC, Edison, NJ) are available to make the incision. The time until bleeding stops is measured. The reported reference range for horses is 2–6 min. Bleeding time is prolonged in patients with qualitative or quantitative platelet defects (including DIC) or von Willebrand's disease. Properly performed bleeding times are within the reference intervals in patients with uncomplicated clotting factor deficiencies.

TREATMENT

Horses should be hospitalized and activity restricted until hemorrhage is controlled. Administration of compatible whole blood (for patients with severe anemia) or fresh or fresh-frozen plasma (4–30 mL/kg) is recommended for patients with life-threatening hemorrhage. Repeated transfusions may be necessary if bleeding continues. Intravenous fluid therapy is vital to maintain tissue perfusion and to correct acid–base and electrolyte abnormalities in patients with DIC or hepatic disease.

MEDICATIONS

DRUG(S) OF CHOICE

Vitamin K_1 (0.5–1 mg/kg SC every 6 hr) is recommended for horses with suspected vitamin K antagonism. Because some coumarin derivatives have a long half-life, treatment may need to continue for several weeks. DIC therapy is multifaceted; it is vital that the underlying disease be treated. Antibiotic therapy is appropriate for horses with sepsis. Flunixin meglumine (0.25 mg/kg IV q8hr) is useful in horses with endotoxemia. The use of heparin in horses with DIC is controversial.

CLOTTING FACTOR DEFICIENCIES

CONTRAINDICATIONS

Administration of drugs that inhibit platelet function (e.g., aspirin or other NSAIDs) may potentiate bleeding. Do not use vitamin K_3 because it has limited therapeutic efficacy and is nephrotoxic. Drugs that normally bind to plasma proteins (e.g., phenylbutazone, chloral hydrate) may potentiate coumarin toxicity. Heparin should not be used in horses with low ATIII activity unless a source of ATIII is provided.

PRECAUTIONS

Intramuscular injections should be avoided. Intravenous administration of vitamin K_1 may induce anaphylaxis.

FOLLOW-UP

PATIENT MONITORING

Cessation of clinical bleeding in conjunction with serial clotting times should be monitored to assess effectiveness of therapy. PT is the preferred assay for patients with vitamin K antagonism. Administration of vitamin K_1 should cause shortening of the PT within 24 hr. If the PT does not stay within the reference range on 2 consecutive days following cessation of vitamin K_1 therapy, then therapy should be resumed.

POSSIBLE COMPLICATIONS

There is no cure for horses with inherited clotting factor deficiencies.

MISCELLANEOUS

AGE-RELATED FACTORS

PT and APTT are prolonged at birth, but normalize in foals 4–7 days of age.

SYNONYMS

- Coagulopathies
- Coagulation defects

SEE ALSO

- Thrombocytopenia
- DIC
- Vasculitis

ABBREVIATIONS

- ACT = activated clotting time
- APTT = activated partial thromboplastin time
- ATIII = antithrombin III
- FDP = fibrin degradation product
- PT = prothrombin time
- WBCT = whole blood clotting time

Suggested Reading

Collatos C. Hemostatic dysfunction. In: Robinson NE, ed. Current therapy in equine medicine 4. Philadelphia: WB Saunders Company, 1997.

Dodds WJ. Hemostasis. In: Kaneko JJ, Harvey JW, Bruss ML, eds. Clinical biochemistry of domestic animals. Fifth ed. San Diego: Academic Press, 1997.

Lassen ED, Swardson CJ. Hematology and hemostasis in the horse: Normal functions and common abnormalities. Vet Clin N Amer [Eq Pract] 1995;11:352-389.

Morris DD. Diseases associated with blood loss or hemostatic dysfunction. In: Smith BP. Large animal internal medicine. St. Louis: Mosby, 1996.

Morris DD. Diseases of the hemolymphatic system. In: Reed SM, Bayly WM, eds. Equine internal medicine. Philadelphia: WB Saunders Company, 1998.

Author Jennifer S. Thomas

Consulting Editor Claire B. Andreasen

COAGULATION DEFECTS, ACQUIRED

BASICS

DEFINITION

Acquired disorders characterized by the inability to form a stable fibrin clot, resulting in loss of blood from the vasculature.

PATHOPHYSIOLOGY

- Vasculitis—immune-mediated/ hypersensitivity vasculitis results from the immune response to an antigenic stimulus; usually induced by a microbe, drug, toxin, or protein. Deposition of immune complexes in vessel walls results in complement activation and chemoattractant production.
- Platelet defects—function defects may occur with DIC, end-stage hepatic disease, or renal failure; decreased platelet numbers occur with immune-mediated thrombocytopenia, bone marrow infiltrative disorders, and DIC. (Thrombocytopenia is discussed in detail elsewhere.)
- Coagulation defects—may occur with DIC, anticoagulant toxicosis, and hepatic failure. (DIC and hepatic failure are discussed in detail elsewhere.)
- Anticoagulant toxicosis—warfarin, brodifacoum, bromodiolone, diphacinone, and moldy sweet clover (dicoumarin). First- and second-generation anti-coagulant rodenticides act on the enzyme vitamin K epoxide reductase, which is required for production of vitamin K–dependent clotting factors (primarily II, VII, IX, and X). Vitamin K epoxide reductase is necessary for recycling vitamin K; when inhibited, body stores of vitamin K diminish, synthesis of vitamin K–dependent clotting factors ceases, and eventually, hemorrhagic crisis develops.
- DIC—a multifactorial disorder characterized by inappropriate activation of coagulative and fibrinolytic cascades. (DIC is discussed in detail elsewhere.)

SYSTEMS AFFECTED

- Hemic/lymphatic/immune—immune-mediated vasculitis with associated problems (plaques of pitting edema, fever, swollen limbs, or possible parenchymal [liver, kidney, pulmonary] infarcts) and myopathy. Anticoagulant rodenticide results in depletion of activated clotting factors and hemorrhage.
- Other systems—may be affected, depending on sites of hemorrhage.

SIGNALMENT

Any sex, breed, and age.

SIGNS

General Comments

History and physical examination findings depend on the type of coagulation problem and its cause.

Historical Findings

- Recent exposure to infectious diseases—strangles, EIA, EVA, or EE
- Inappropriate hemorrhage after relatively minor trauma or surgery
- Unexplained swellings
- Epistaxis, hematuria, hematochezia, or other unexplained hemorrhage

Physical Examination Findings

- Vasculitis—petechial and ecchymotic hemorrhages and hyperemia are common; demarcated areas of dermal or subcutaneous edema may develop, sometimes severe enough to cause skin, muscle, or organ infarction, necrosis, and exudation.
- Platelet disorders and vitamin K–dependent clotting dysfunction cause diffuse hemorrhage from small blood vessels, characterized by petechial hemorrhages on the mucosal membranes, third eyelid, or sclera.
- Epistaxis, occult melena, hyphema, and hematuria are not uncommon.
- Prolonged bleeding from wounds or injection sites is not unusual.
- Dyspnea and coughing may be observed with pulmonary involvement.

CAUSES

- Vasculitis—immune response secondary to infection with EIA, EVA, EE, influenza virus, or *Streptococcus* sp. infection.
- Ingestion of moldy sweet-clover hay or rodenticides containing first- or second-generation anticoagulants.
- Causes of DIC, platelet dysfunction, and hepatic failure are discussed in detail elsewhere.

RISK FACTORS

- Anticoagulant rodenticides—small, repeated doses are more serious, although a single ingestion may be lethal.
- May be more common during the spring and fall, when rodenticides are used more often.

DIAGNOSIS

DIFFERENTIAL DIAGNOSIS

- Vasculitis—EIA, EVA, EE, and purpura hemorrhagica.
- Anticoagulant rodenticide toxicosis—congenital coagulation disorders (e.g., hemophilia A or factor VIII deficiency), thrombocytopenia, and infectious viral disease (e.g., EVA, EIA).

CBC/BIOCHEMISTRY/URINALYSIS

- Vasculitis—neutrophilia, mild anemia, hyperglobulinemia, hyperfibrinogenemia, moderate to severe anemia, thrombocytopenia in many cases, elevated CPK and AST in cases with myopathy, elevated BUN or creatinine in cases of pigment or vasculitis-associated nephropathy.
- Anticoagulant rodenticide toxicosis—anemia (mild to marked).

OTHER LABORATORY TESTS

- Vasculitis—serology for EIV, EVA, EIA, and EE is indicated.
- Anticoagulant rodenticide toxicosis—monitor coagulation times (PT and PTT) daily for 2–4 days, then twice weekly after PT and PTT have normalized; ACT (a simplified variation of PTT) may be more useful for clinicians.

IMAGING

- Vasculitis—thoracic radiography may reveal pulmonary infiltrate suggestive of hemorrhage or infarcted lung; ultrasonography may reveal areas of hypoechogenicity in muscle or parenchymal tissues, indicating hemorrhage or edema.
- Anticoagulant rodenticide/moldy sweet-clover ingestion—thoracic radiography may show tissue hemorrhage (pulmonary infiltrate or hemothorax); ultrasonography may show areas of hypoechogenicity (e.g., kidney, liver, or spleen).

DIAGNOSTIC PROCEDURES

- Vasculitis—full-thickness, skin-punch biopsies (preserved in Michels media) show neutrophilic infiltration of venules in dermal and SC tissues. Leukocytoclasis and fibrinoid necrosis are also present; immunofluorescence may show immune complexes.
- Anticoagulant rodenticides—see *Other Laboratory Tests.*

PATHOLOGIC FINDINGS

Tissue hemorrhage and icteric tissues (if chronic in nature).

TREATMENT

APPROPRIATE HEALTH CARE

- Anticoagulant rodenticide toxicosis—most cases should be managed as inpatients to monitor closely for hemorrhage; emergency medical care with whole-blood transfusions may be needed in severe cases.
- Vasculitis—may be handled as inpatients or outpatients, depending on the severity of clinical signs; if an infectious cause is suspected (e.g., EIA, EVA, or *S. equi*), consider isolation from other horses.
- Minimize trauma and venipunctures.
- Whole-blood transfusions may be indicated in horses with severe hemorrhage.

NURSING CARE

Support wraps of distal limbs, controlled exercise (hand-walking), and cold hosing may be beneficial for limb edema associated with vasculitis.

ACTIVITY

Minimal exercise and trauma.

DIET

Good-quality alfalfa hay (i.e., vitamin K rich) is recommended.

MEDICATIONS

DRUGS OF CHOICE

- Anticoagulant rodenticide toxicosis—vitamin K_1 (2.5 mg/kg PO or SC q12h); continue for 1 week when treating first-generation anticoagulant exposure (i.e., warfarin) or 3–5 weeks when treating second-generation anticoagulant rodenticide toxicity (i.e., brodifacoum), with continued monitoring of PT and PTT after treatment is discontinued.
- Vasculitis—dexamethasone sodium phosphate (0.04–0.2 mg/kg IV or IM q12–24 h); when condition is stabilized, gradually decrease the daily dose or switch to prednisolone or prednisone (initial dose of 2–3 mg/kg PO daily).

CONTRAINDICATIONS

- Drugs that may interfere with vitamin K_1 binding—phenylbutazone, xyphenbutazone, heparin, phenytoin, salicylates, quinidine, potentiated sulfas, and steroid hormones.
- Menadione (i.e., vitamin K_3)—may cause renal failure.

PRECAUTIONS

Menadione (i.e., vitamin K_3)—may cause renal failure.

POSSIBLE INTERACTIONS

Some drugs may interfere with vitamin K_1 binding—phenylbutazone, oxyphenbutazone, heparin, phenytoin, salicylates, quinidine, potentiated sulfas, and steroid hormones.

ALTERNATIVE DRUGS

N/A

FOLLOW-UP

PATIENT MONITORING

- Continuous monitoring of clotting profile—PT, PTT, ACT, and platelet count.
- Some patients may be nonresponsive and die if not recognized and treated appropriately.

POSSIBLE COMPLICATIONS

- Anticoagulant rodenticide toxicosis—possible secondary infections (e.g., pneumonia) due to pulmonary or other tissue hemorrhage.
- Vasculitis—sloughing of skin, especially on distal limbs; laminitis.

EXPECTED COURSE AND PROGNOSIS

Good to fair if recognized and treated early—vasculitis and rodenticide anticoagulant toxicosis.

MISCELLANEOUS

ASSOCIATED CONDITIONS

N/A

AGE RELATED FACTORS

N/A

ZOONOTIC POTENTIAL

N/A

PREGNANCY

Rodenticides may pass through the placenta and cause coagulation defects in the fetus.

SYNONYMS

N/A

SEE ALSO

- Coagulation defects, inherited
- DIC
- Ehrlichiosis, equine granulocytic
- EIA
- EVA
- Hemorrhage, acute
- Hepatic disease
- Purpura hemorrhagica
- *S. equi* (strangles)
- Thrombocytopenia
- Vasculitis

ABBREVIATIONS

- ACT = activated clotting time
- AST = aspartate aminotransferase
- CPK = creatine phosphokinase
- DIC = disseminated intravascular coagulation
- EE = equine ehrlichiosis
- EIA = equine infectious anemia
- EIV =
- EVA = equine viral arteritis
- PT = prothrombin time
- PTT = partial thromboplastin time

Suggested Reading

Byars TD. Warfarin toxicosis. In: Robinson NE, ed. Current therapy in equine medicine 2. Philadelphia: WB Saunders, 1987:305–306.

Feldman BF, Carroll EJ, Jain NC: Coagulation and its disorders. In: Jain NC, ed. Schalm's veterinary hematology. 4th ed. Philadelphia: Lea & Febiger, 1986:388–430.

McConnico RS, Copedge K, Bischoff KL. Brodifacoum toxicosis in two horses. J Am Vet Med Assoc. 1997;211:882–886.

Author Rebecca S. McConnico

Consulting Editor Debra C. Sellon

COAGULATION DEFECTS, INHERITED

BASICS

DEFINITION

Abnormal hemostasis associated with hereditary defects in the quantity or function of soluble coagulation factors.

PATHOPHYSIOLOGY

- Inherited coagulation disorders that involve defects in secondary hemostasis (i.e. the interaction of soluble coagulation factors produce a stable fibrin mesh that reinforces the platelet plug formed during the primary phase of hemostasis).
- Clinical significance—depends on the underlying defect in coagulation function. Disorders involving initiation of the contact phase (i.e., interaction of factor XII, high-molecular-weight kininogen, and prekallikrein that activates factor XI) do not result in spontaneous hemorrhage, but bleeding tendency may be increased after trauma or surgery. In contrast, deficiency of any other coagulation factor results in profound hemorrhagic tendencies.
- Factor VIII deficiency (i.e., hemophilia A)—the most commonly reported inherited defect of equine hemostasis. Synthesis and secretion of factor VIII:C is decreased in patients with hemophilia A; deficiency of factor VIII:C compromises the intrinsic coagulation pathway. Severity of clinical signs varies inversely with factor VIII:C activity in plasma. Severe hemophilic bleeding occurs with factor VIII:C activity <1% of normal, whereas a mild syndrome accompanies coagulant activity between 5–20%.

SYSTEMS AFFECTED

- Hemic/lymphatic/immune—hemorrhagic diathesis is the major clinical manifestation.
- Musculoskeletal—with hemophilia A, SC or IM hematomas and joint swellings due to hemarthroses are the prominent clinical signs.
- Respiratory—dyspnea associated with bleeding in the thoracic cavity (hemophilia A).
- GI—abdominal pain associated with hemoperitoneum (hemophilia A).
- Cardiovascular—severe hemorrhage in horses with hemophilia A may result in hypovolemic shock.

GENETICS

- Factor VIII deficiency—transmitted as an X-linked recessive trait; only hemizygous males are clinically affected.
- The mode of inheritance for other hereditary coagulation disorders in horses has not been determined.

INCIDENCE/PREVALENCE

N/A

SIGNALMENT

- Factor VIII deficiency (hemophilia A) has been diagnosed in Thoroughbred, Standardbred, Quarter Horse, and Arabian colts; hemophilia A occurs exclusively in males and usually manifests within the first few weeks of life.
- Prekallikrein deficiency has been described in a family of miniature horses and of Belgian horses.
- Single cases of von Willebrand disease (Quarter Horse filly) and protein C deficiency (2-year-old Thoroughbred colt) have been reported.

SIGNS

General Comments

Hemophilia A (factor VIII deficiency)—the most common inherited coagulopathy.

Historical Findings

Inherited coagulation disorders should be suspected in young horses with evidence of inappropriate bleeding but no history of underlying disease or in horses of any age that bleed excessively after minor trauma or surgery.

Physical Examination Findings

- Prominent clinical signs in hemophilia A—SC or IM hematomas and joint swellings associated with hemarthroses; affected colts may demonstrate a shifting-leg lameness; joints are not painful when palpated.
- Trauma may result in hemothorax or hemoperitoneum, with signs of labored respiration and mild abdominal discomfort, respectively.
- Episodes of oral bleeding, conjunctival hemorrhage, and prolonged bleeding at injection sites were reported in the single case of von Willebrand disease.
- Prekallikrein deficiency is not associated with spontaneous bleeding tendency; however, affected animals may bleed excessively after trauma or surgery, particularly procedures such as castration when vessels are not ligated.

CAUSES

- Factor VIII deficiency (hemophilia A)
- Von Willebrand disease
- Defects in the contact phase of coagulation—prekallikrein deficiency
- Protein C deficiency

RISK FACTORS

N/A

DIAGNOSIS

DIFFERENTIAL DIAGNOSIS

- Differentiate hereditary coagulation disorders from acquired disorders of hemostatic function (e.g., DIC, vitamin K deficiency, warfarin toxicity, and thrombocytopenia) based on clinical presentation and coagulation function testing.
- Acquired hemostatic disorders, particularly DIC, often are accompanied by a severe, underlying systemic disorder and multiple coagulation parameter abnormalities.

CBC/BIOCHEMISTRY/URINALYSIS

- Little or no changes in hemogram, leukogram, platelet count, serum biochemistry, and urinalysis.
- Hematocrit may be low in hemophiliacs because of severe hemorrhage.
- Large hematomas may result in increased serum bilirubin concentration.

OTHER LABORATORY TESTS

- Differentiation of inherited from acquired hemostatic disorders requires assessment of coagulation function—PT, APTT, platelet count, and plasma fibrinogen and FDP concentrations should be measured; particularly when a human laboratory will be used, also collect blood samples from a clinically healthy, control horse.
- With hemophilia A and plasma prekallikrein deficiency, defects in the intrinsic coagulation pathway result in prolonged APTT but normal PT. Platelet counts, plasma fibrinogen, and FDPs are within normal limits, but DIC often results in abnormalities of all these measures.
- Coagulation function (i.e., APTT, PT, and FDPs) and platelet count are normal in von Willebrand disease, allowing differentiation from acquired thrombocytopenia.
- Definitive diagnosis requires specialized tests not routinely available in most laboratories.
- Hemophilia A— factor VIII:C activity <20% of normal.
- Prekallikrein deficiency—low prekallikrein activity, with normal activity of other contact-phase coagulation factors.
- Von Willebrand disease—specialized tests for assessment of vWF quantity and activity may be available.

IMAGING
Thoracic radiography as well as thoracic and abdominal ultrasonography may be indicated if hemothorax or hemoperitoneum is suspected.

DIAGNOSTIC PROCEDURES
Thoracic or abdominal centesis to confirm internal hemorrhage.

PATHOLOGIC FINDINGS
Hemophiliacs may have widely distributed hematomas.

TREATMENT

APPROPRIATE HEALTH CARE
On the farm or in the hospital.

NURSING CARE
- Patients with hemorrhagic diathesis should be rested in a safe enclosure to minimize trauma.
- Severe hemorrhage after surgery or in hemophiliacs may require whole-blood transfusion.
- The only effective treatment for hemophilia is repeated transfusion with fresh plasma (15–20 mL/kg IV); because the half-life of transfused factor VIII:C is only 8–12 hours, daily transfusions are necessary.

ACTIVITY
Keep the patient as quiet as possible.

DIET
N/A

CLIENT EDUCATION
- Inherited disorders of coagulation are incurable.
- Do not use affected animals and carrier parents for breeding.
- Recommend humane destruction for hemophiliacs with severe, recurrent hemorrhagic episodes.

SURGICAL CONSIDERATIONS
N/A

MEDICATIONS

CONTRAINDICATIONS
N/A

PRECAUTIONS
N/A

POSSIBLE INTERACTIONS
N/A

ALTERNATIVE DRUGS
N/A

FOLLOW-UP

PATIENT MONITORING
Hemophiliacs require close monitoring because of recurrent hemorrhagic episodes.

PREVENTION/AVOIDANCE
- Affected animals and their parents are unsuitable as breeding stock.
- Surgery of horses with inherited coagulopathies carries the risk of severe postsurgical bleeding; identify a suitable donor and collect blood before elective surgery.
- Castration procedures should include placement of ligatures around vascular stumps.

EXPECTED COURSE AND PROGNOSIS
- Prognosis with hemophilia A is grave; most affected animals die or are destroyed within the first year of life.
- Contact-phase coagulation disorders are not life threatening but require precautions during surgery.

MISCELLANEOUS

ASSOCIATED CONDITIONS
N/A

AGE-RELATED FACTORS
N/A

ZOONOTIC POTENTIAL
N/A

PREGNANCY
Do not breed affected horses.

SYNONYMS
- Clotting factor deficiencies
- Coagulopathies

SEE ALSO
- Anemia
- Coagulopathies, acquired/induced
- Hemorrhage, acute
- Hemorrhage, chronic

ABBREVIATIONS
- APTT = activated partial thromboplastin time
- DIC = disseminated intravascular coagulation
- FDP = fibrin degradation product
- GI = gastrointestinal
- PT = prothrombin time
- vWF = von Willebrand factor

Suggested Reading

Brooks M, Leith GS, Allen AK, et al. Bleeding disorder (von Willebrand disease) in a Quarter Horse. J Am Vet Med Assoc 1991;198:114–116.

Geor RJ, Jackson ML, Lewis KD, Fretz PB. Prekallikrein deficiency in a family of Belgian horses. J Am Vet Med Assoc 1990;197:741–745.

Littlewood JD, Bevan A. Haemophilia A (classic haemophilia, factor VIII deficiency) in a Thoroughbred colt. Equine Vet J 1991;23:70–72.

Author Raymond J. Geor
Consulting Editor Debra C. Sellon

COCCIDIOIDOMYCOSIS

BASICS

OVERVIEW

Coccidioidomycosis is a systemic fungal infection of animals and humans caused by the dimorphic fungus, *Coccidioides immitis,* which grows in soil of arid or semi-arid regions of the southwestern United States and South America. Disease results from inhalation of arthrospores, although rarely disease may result from ingestion or cutaneous inoculation of the organism. Infection most commonly produces granulomatous lesions in the respiratory system and associated lymph nodes. Osteomyelitis, abortion, and nasal granuloma have also been reported. The incubation period is not known.

SIGNALMENT

The influence of age, gender, and pregnancy status has not been determined. Arabian horses may be over-represented in the case population.

SIGNS

Weight loss and respiratory symptoms (cough, nasal discharge, tachypnea) are the most common findings. Thoracic auscultation frequently reveals wheezes and/or areas of dullness corresponding with a pleural effusion or a pulmonary mass. Other signs include:

- Fever
- Lameness
- Intermittent colic
- Vaginal discharge, abortion
- Cutaneous abscesses
- Ventral edema

CAUSES AND RISK FACTORS

Coccidioides immitis is endemic in localized areas of California, Arizona, New Mexico, Texas, Nevada, and Utah.

DIAGNOSIS

DIFFERENTIAL DIAGNOSIS

- Bacterial pneumonia may appear similar, but bacteria are usually identified by culture or cytology of tracheal aspirate.
- Chronic obstructive pulmonary disease (COPD) patients usually are not febrile and have normal hematology and fibrinogen concentrations.
- Neoplasia, such as lymphosarcoma, could appear similar but often has abnormal cells and a negative culture of tracheal aspirate or pleural effusion.
- Infectious and noninfectious causes of abortion may be diagnosed by history, culture, and histopathology of placental and fetal tissues.

CBC/BIOCHEMISTRY/URINALYSIS

- Hyperfibrinogenemia
- Hyperproteinemia
- Leukocytosis
- Neutrophilia
- Anemia

OTHER LABORATORY TESTS

Serologic testing (complement fixation, agar gel immunodiffusion) is indicated when coccidioidomycosis is suspected. A positive titer is considered diagnostic of infection.

IMAGING

- Thoracic radiography may show increased interstitial pattern in the lung and evidence of enlarged mediastinal lymph nodes. Pleural effusion may also be detected. Osteomyelitis of vertebrae has been reported. These findings are not specific for coccidioidomycosis.
- Thoracic ultrasonography may reveal pleural effusion or abscess, although these findings are not pathognomonic for coccidioidomycosis.

DIAGNOSTIC PROCEDURES

- Culture of pleural fluid, peritoneal fluid, or transtracheal aspirate may yield *C. immitis.*
- Pleural and peritoneal fluids may be tested for *C. immitis* antibodies.
- Pleural and peritoneal fluids may have an elevated protein and white blood cell count, but these changes not diagnostic for coccidioidomycosis.
- Intradermal testing with coccidiodin is nonspecific.
- In cases of abortion, the organism may be cultured from vaginal discharge or placental or fetal tissue.

COCCIDIOIDOMYCOSIS

PATHOLOGIC FINDINGS

Histopathology reveals granulomas or pyogranulomas in pulmonary parenchyma, thoracic lymph nodes, and often other sites, such as liver, bone, and peritoneum. The organism may be observed microscopically.

TREATMENT

• Treatment of coccidioidomycosis is difficult and costly. Most reported cases have not responded to treatment.
• If treatment is elected, many patients may be managed as outpatients. Others, however, require intensive support, including intravenous fluids and nutritional supplementation, and may be best managed in a hospital.
• If infection is limited to the nasal cavity, surgical excision may be beneficial, although recurrence is possible.

MEDICATIONS

DRUG(S) OF CHOICE

Treatment with ketoconazole or amphotericin B has been attempted with no reported success. Itraconazole (2.6 mg/kg PO q12h) was successful in one case after several months of treatment.

FOLLOW-UP

• Clinical signs and hematology should improve if treatment is effective.
• There is no vaccine for this disease and the organism cannot be eliminated from the soil. If possible, control dust in endemic areas.
• Prognosis is grave. Most reported cases died or were euthanized. Treatment of generalized cases is likely to be expensive and ineffective, although itraconazole may prove useful. In other species, some cases resolve without treatment. It is not known if this is the case in horses.

MISCELLANEOUS

ZOONOTIC POTENTIAL

This disease is not considered contagious, but care should be taken to avoid aerosolization of infected fluids or tissue.

Suggested Reading

Zeimer EL, Pappagianis D, Madigan JE, et al. Coccidioidomycosis in horses: 15 cases 1975–1984. J Am Vet Med Assoc 1992;201:910-916.

Foley JP, Legendre AM. Treatment of coccidioidomycosis osteomyelitis with itraconazole in a horse. A brief report. J Vet Int Med 1992;6:333-334.

Author Laura K. Reilly

Consulting Editor Corinne R. Sweeney

COCCIDIOSIS

BASICS

OVERVIEW

Equine coccidiosis is a protozoal infection of the intestinal tract of equids. It is difficult to talk of pathophysiologic changes in the equine coccidiosis because it has not been clearly demonstrated that the causative organism has any pathogenic capacity. Oocysts of *Eimeria leukarti* have been identified in the feces of normal horses and horses with diarrhea. The prepatent period is normally between 16 and 36 days. The meronts (schizonts) develop in the jejunum and ileum, mainly in the lacteal of these intestinal sections. This infestation has a world-wide distribution and has been reported in the five continents. International reports indicated a prevalence of 0.6–2.6% in horses but mainly in foals.

SIGNALMENT

Detection of the causative organism is more prevalent in foals but it also occurs in adult horses. The organism is also a parasite of donkeys.

SIGNS

Because there are so many doubts of the pathogenic properties of the etiologic agent of equine coccidiosis, its presence is recorded as an incidental finding. Signs associated with this infestation are profuse diarrhea, massive intestinal hemorrhage, chronic diarrhea, catarrhal inflammation of the jejunum, and cecocolic intussusception.

CAUSES AND RISK FACTORS

The causative organism of equine coccidiosis is *Eimeria leuckarti.*

COCCIDIOSIS

DIAGNOSIS

DIFFERENTIAL DIAGNOSIS

The finding of oocysts in the feces of any horse with diarrhea should not be taken as evidence of cause and effect. A thorough investigation for other causes (e.g., salmonellosis, potomac horse fever, cyathastomiasis) should be undertaken.

CBC/BIOCHEMISTRY/URINALYSIS

N/A

OTHER LABORATORY TESTS

Fecal flotation is the main diagnostic method. Saturated sodium nitrate gives better concentration of oocysts of *E. leuckarti.*

TREATMENT

There is no therapeutic regimen reported for equine cocccidial infestation.

Suggested Reading

Lyons, ET, Drudge, JH, Tolliver, SC. Natural infection with *Eimeria leuckarti*: prevalence of oocysts in feces of horse foals on several farms in Kentucky during 1986. Am J Vet Res. 1988;49:96-98.

Author Oliver E. Olimpo

Consulting Editor Henry Stämpfli

CONCEPTION FAILURE

BASICS

DEFINITION
Maternal structural or functional defects that prevent:
• The fertilized ovum from normal embryonic development.
• Transport of the embryo into the uterus on day 6 after ovulation.
• Embryonic survival until pregnancy is diagnosed by transrectal ultrasound at ≥14 days after ovulation.

PATHOPHYSIOLOGY
• Defective embryo
• Unsuitable oviductal or uterine environment
• Early CL regression
• Failure of "maternal recognition of pregnancy"
• Luteal insufficiency—anecdotal
• Oviductal blockage or impaired function

SYSTEM AFFECTED
Reproductive

GENETICS
N/A

INCIDENCE/PREVALENCE
The "normal" rate of conception failure is ≅30% but approaches 50%–70% in old, subfertile mares.

SIGNALMENT
• Old (>15 years) mares
• Certain heterospecific matings—stallion × jenny

SIGNS
Historical Findings
• Diagnosis of failure of pregnancy by transrectal ultrasound at ≥14 days after ovulation following appropriately timed breeding with semen of normal fertility.
• Diagnosis of failure of pregnancy by transrectal palpation at ≥25 days after ovulation following appropriately timed breeding with semen of normal fertility.
• Return (possibly early) to estrus after appropriately timed breeding with semen of normal fertility.

Physical Examination Findings
• Nonpregnant uterus, possibly with edema of endometrial folds or accumulation of intrauterine fluid.
• Absence of CL
• Mucoid or mucopurulent vulvar discharge

CAUSES
Defective Embryos
• Old mares
• Seasonal effects

Endometritis
• Early CL regression
• Unsuitable/hostile uterine environment

Unsuitable Uterine Environment
• Endometritis
• Endometrial lymphatic cysts of sufficient size to impede embryonic mobility, resulting in failure of "maternal recognition of pregnancy".
• Inadequate secretion of histotrophs.

Xenobiotics
• Equine fescue toxicosis
• Phytoestrogens—anecdotal

Oviductal Disease
• Unsuitable/hostile environment for embryonic development
• Oviductal blockage

Endocrine Disorders
• Hypothyroidism—anecdotal
• Luteal insufficiency—anecdotal

Maternal Disease
• Fever
• Pain—anecdotal

RISK FACTORS
• Age of >15 years
• Anatomic defects predisposing the genital tract to endometritis
• Seasonal effects
• Foal heat breeding—anecdotal
• Inadequate nutrition
• Exposure to xenobiotics—fescue toxicosis
• Some heterospecific matings—stallion × jenny

DIAGNOSIS

DIFFERENTIAL DIAGNOSIS
Mistiming of Insemination or Breeding
• Monitor follicular development and ovulation by transrectal palpation or ultrasonography.
• Appropriate timing of insemination or breeding.
• Ovulation induction to complement timing of insemination or breeding.

EED
Transrectal ultrasonography to detect pregnancy at ≥14 days but that is absent on subsequent examination at <40 days of gestation.

Pregnancy Undetected by Transrectal Ultrasonography
• Careful, systematic visualization of the entire uterus—horns, body, and region near cervix.
• A slow sweep, twice per examination, over the entire tract will reduce "misses."

Ovulation Failure
• Transrectal palpation or ultrasonography (preferred) to confirm ovulation and formation of a CL.
• Serum progesterone level 6–7 days after ovulation or at end of estrus.

Poor Semen Quality
Monitoring/examination of ejaculate for adequate number of spermatozoa and evaluation of progressive motility and normal morphology.

Ejaculation Failure
• Observation of "flagging" of stallion's tail.
• Palpation of ventral penile surface during live cover or collection of semen in an AV to confirm ejaculation was complete—6–10 pulses of the urethra.
• Examination of dismount semen sample for motile spermatozoa.

Mishandling of Semen

Systematic review of all procedures and examination of semen collection equipment, extenders, incubator temperature, and any containers coming into contact with semen that may be causing death of spermatozoa.

Impaired Spermatozoal Transport

- Transrectal ultrasonography to ensure absence of intrauterine fluid at insemination or breeding.
- Vaginal speculum and digital cervical examination to assess cervical patency and to rule out urovagina.

CBC/BIOCHEMISTRY/URINALYSIS

Not indicated, unless signs of concurrent systemic disease are present.

OTHER LABORATORY TESTS

Maternal Progesterone

- May be indicated at >6 days after ovulation to evaluate CL function.
- ELISA or RIA for progesterone—acceptable levels vary from >1 to >4 ng/mL, depending on the reference lab.

Maternal T_3/T_4 Levels

- Anecdotal reports of lower levels in mares with history of conception failure, EED, or abortion.
- Significance of low T_4 levels is not clear at present.

Cytogenetic Studies

May be indicated with suspected maternal chromosomal abnormalities.

Feed Analysis

May be indicated for specific xenobiotics (e.g., ergopeptine alkaloids, phytoestrogens, heavy metals) or endophyte (*Neotyphodium coenophialum*).

IMAGING

Transrectal ultrasonography—essential to confirm ovulation and early pregnancy and to detect intrauterine fluid and endometrial cysts.

DIAGNOSTIC PROCEDURES

Thorough Reproductive Evaluation

- Indicated for individuals predisposed to conception failure (e.g., barren, old mares, history of conception failure) prebreeding.
- Transrectal ultrasonography, vaginal speculum, endometrial cytology/culture, and endometrial biopsy to detect anatomic defects, endometritis, or fibrosis.

Transrectal Ultrasonography

If performed earlier than normal, at 10 days, to determine presence of embryo, confusion with endometrial cysts often results.

Embryo Recovery

- Same procedure as for embryo transfer
- Performed to detect embryonic transport—into uterus (6–8 days after ovulation) or oviduct (2–4 days after ovulation)
- Flush may be therapeutic as well

Hysteroscopy

Endoscopy of uterine lumen and uterotubal junction.

Oviductal Patency

- Starch granules or microspheres are deposited on the ovarian surface.
- Uterine lavage is then performed.
- Recovery of starch granules/microspheres in the lavage fluid is evaluated.

Laparoscopy

To evaluate normal structure and function of ovarian-uterine tubal interaction.

PATHOLOGIC FINDINGS

Endometrial biopsy—presence of moderate to severe, chronic endometritis or fibrosis.

TREATMENT

APPROPRIATE HEALTH CARE

- Treat pre-existing endometritis before insemination or breeding of mares during physiologic breeding season when they have adequate body condition.
- Inseminate or breed foal heat mares if ovulation occurs ≥10 days postpartum and no intrauterine fluid is present.
- Progestin supplementation.
- Anecdotal reports of oviductal flushing to resolve oviductal occlusion.
- Various forms of advanced reproductive technologies (e.g., embryo, zygote) to retrieve embryos from the uterus (days 6–8 after ovulation) or oviduct (≅days 2–4 after ovulation); successful in vitro fertilization is in the early stages of development.
- Primary, age-related (most are from aged mares) embryonic defects are refractory to treatment.
- Most cases of conception failure can be handled in an ambulatory situation.
- Increased frequency of ultrasonographic monitoring of follicular development and ovulation, or to permit insemination closer to ovulation, as well as more technical diagnostic procedures, may need to be performed in a hospital setting.
- Adequate restraint and optimal lighting (usually the problem is an excess of light) may not be available in the field to permit quality ultrasonography.

NURSING CARE

- Generally requires none.
- Minimal nursing care after more invasive diagnostic and therapeutic procedures.

CONCEPTION FAILURE

ACTIVITY

• Generally no restriction of broodmare activity, unless contraindicated by concurrent maternal disease or diagnostic or therapeutic procedures.
• Preference may be to restrict activity of mares in competition because of the impact of stress on cyclicity and ovulation.

DIET

Generally no restriction, unless indicated by concurrent maternal disease.

CLIENT EDUCATION

• Emphasize the effects of aged mares on conception failure and their refractoriness to treatment.
• Inform regarding the cause, diagnosis, and treatment of endometritis.
• Inform regarding the seasonal aspects and nutritional requirements of conception.
• Inform regarding the role that endophyte-infected fescue and certain heterospecific breedings might play in conception failure.

SURGICAL CONSIDERATIONS

• Indicated for repair of anatomic defects predisposing mares to endometritis.
• Certain diagnostic and therapeutic procedures.

MEDICATIONS

DRUGS OF CHOICE

• See specific sections for drug recommendations.
• Mares with a history of conception failure or moderate to severe endometritis (i.e., no active, infectious component) or fibrosis—altrenogest (Regu-mate, Hoechst-Roussel Agri-Vet; 0.044–0.088 mg/kg PO SID; begin 2–3 days after ovulation or at diagnosis of pregnancy and continue until at least day 100 of gestation; taper daily dose over a 14-day period at the end of treatment).
• Altrenogest administration may be started later during gestation, continued longer, or used for only short periods of time, depending on serum progesterone levels during the first 80 days of gestation (>1 to >4 ng/mL, depending on the reference lab), clinical circumstances, risk factors, and clinician preference.
• If used near term, altrenogest frequently is discontinued 7–14 days before the expected foaling date, depending on the case, unless otherwise indicated by assessment of fetal maturity/viability or by questions regarding the accuracy of gestational length.

CONTRAINDICATIONS

Use altrenogest only to prevent conception failure of noninfectious endometritis.

PRECAUTIONS

• Use transrectal ultrasonography to diagnose pregnancy at ≥14–16 days after ovulation to identify intrauterine fluid or pyometra early in the disease course for appropriate treatment.
• If pregnancy is diagnosed, frequent monitoring (weekly initially) may be indicated to detect EED.
• Altrenogest is absorbed through the skin, so persons handling this preparation should wear gloves and wash their hands.
• Although supplemental progestins are used widely to treat cases of conception failure, any reported success is purely anecdotal. Primary, age-related embryonic defects do not respond to supplemental progestins.

POSSIBLE INTERACTIONS

N/A

ALTERNATIVE DRUGS

• Injectable progesterone (150–500 mg/day, oil base) can be administered IM SID instead of the oral formulation. Variations, contraindications, and precautions are similar to those associated with altrenogest.
• Other injectable and implantable progestin preparations are available commercially for use in other species. Any use in horses of these products is off-label, and no scientific data are available regarding their efficacy.
• Thyroxine supplementation has been successful (anecdotally) for treating mares with histories of subfertility. Its use remains controversial, however, and is considered deleterious by some clinicians.

FOLLOW-UP

PATIENT MONITORING

• Accurate teasing records.
• Re-examination of mares treated for endometritis before breeding.
• Early examination for pregnancy by transrectal ultrasonography.
• Monitor embryonic and fetal development with transrectal or transabdominal ultrasonography.

PREVENTION/AVOIDANCE

• Recognition of at-risk mares.
• Management of endometritis before breeding.
• Removal of mares from fescue pasture after breeding and during early gestation.
• Prudent use of medications in bred mares.
• Avoiding exposure to known toxicants.

POSSIBLE COMPLICATIONS

• Later EED
• High-risk pregnancy
• Abortion

EXPECTED COURSE AND PROGNOSIS

• Young mares with resolved cases of endometritis may have a fair to good prognosis for conception and completion of pregnancy.
• Old mares (>15 years) with a history of conception failure or chronic, moderate to severe endometritis or fibrosis have a guarded to poor prognosis for conception and completion of pregnancy.

CONCEPTION FAILURE

MISCELLANEOUS

ASSOCIATED CONDITIONS
- Abortion
- Conception failure—stallions
- EED
- Embryo transfer
- Endometritis
- Metritis

AGE-RELATED FACTORS
- Development of chronic endometritis and endometrial fibrosis
- Age-related embryonic defects

ZOONOTIC POTENTIAL
N/A

PREGNANCY
- Condition is pregnancy-associated by definition
- Increased risk of EED or abortion

SYNONYMS
N/A

SEE ALSO
- Abortion
- Conception failure—stallions
- EED
- Ejaculation failure
- Embryo transfer
- Endometrial biopsy
- Endometritis
- Metritis
- Ovulation failure
- Pregnancy diagnosis
- Semen abnormalities

ABBREVIATIONS
- AV = artificial vagina
- CL = corpus luteum
- EED = early embryonic death
- ELISA = enzyme-linked immunoadsorbent assay
- RIA = radioimmunoassay
- T_3 = triiodothyronine
- T_4 = thyroxine

Suggested Reading

Ball BA, Daels PF. Early pregnancy loss in mares: application for progestin therapy. In: Robinson NE, ed. Current therapy in equine medicine 4. Philadelphia: WB Saunders, 1997:531–533.

Brendemuehl JP. Reproductive aspects of fescue toxicosis. In: Robinson NE, ed. Current therapy in equine medicine 4. Philadelphia: WB Saunders, 1997:571–573.

LeBlanc MM. Diseases of the embryo. In: Colahan PT, Mayhew IG, Merritt AM, Moore JM, eds. Equine medicine and surgery, 5th ed. St. Louis: Mosby, 1999;2:1199–1202.

LeBlanc MM. Diseases of the oviduct. In: Colahan PT, Mayhew IG, Merritt AM, Moore JM, eds. Equine medicine and surgery, 5th ed. St. Louis: Mosby, 1999;2:1164.

Ley WB, Bowen JM, Purswell BJ, et al. Modified technique to evaluate uterine tubal patency in the mare. Proc Am Assoc Equine Pract 1998;56–59.

Author Tim J. Evans

Consulting Editor Carla L. Carleton

CONGENITAL CEREBELLAR DISEASES

BASICS

DEFINITION
Disease associated with cerebellar dysfunction identified either at birth or early in life.

PATHOPHYSIOLOGY
- Cerebellar disorders in neonates are rare, and the causes are unknown.
- Cerebellar hypoplasia, abiotrophy, transient cerebellar dysfunction, and occipital atlantoaxial malformation have been described.

Cerebellar Hypoplasia
A hypoplastic cerebellum is evident at necropsy.

Cerebellar Abiotrophy
- Cerebellar abiotrophy seems to be associated with an inherited metabolic defect of cortical cerebellar neurons.
- The result is formation and then premature death of these neurons during late fetal or early postnatal life.

Transient Cerebellar Dysfunction
The pathology of this disease is not well described, because given time, foals recover.

Occipital Atlantoaxial Malformation
Malformation of the occipital calvarium and cervical vertebrae 1 and 2 occurs.

SYSTEM AFFECTED
CNS

SIGNALMENT

Cerebellar Hypoplasia and Abiotrophy
- Foals may be affected at birth, but disease often is not evident until a few months of age.
- Arabian foals seem to be affected, but cases have been identified in several breeds.

Occipital Atlantoaxial Malformation
- Foals may be affected at birth, but disease often is not evident until a few months of age.
- Arabian foals seem to be affected, but cases have been identified in several breeds.

Transient Cerebellar Dysfunction
- Foals develop the disease most commonly at a few months of age.
- Foals afflicted at birth have recovered after a few months of age.
- Thoroughbreds seem to be affected, but cases have been identified in several breeds.

SIGNS

Historical Findings
- No specific historical features are evident.
- Foals are can be affected at birth but are more commonly identified at a few months of age with cerebellar hypoplasia, abiotrophy, and atlantoaxial malformation.
- Transient cerebellar dysfunction usually occurs later in life, but foals may be affected at birth and recover after a few months.

Physical Examination Findings
- The cerebellum processes peripheral proprioceptive sensory input from afferent pathways. The cerebellum then dictates the quality of motor activity through its efferent pathways. Hence, cerebellar disorders are expressed as inappropriate rate, range, and force of body movement, resulting in hypermetria, spasticity, and intention tremors.
- The feature isolating cerebellar defects from white-matter spinal cord disease is the lack of paresis in the former. In addition, the menace response may be poor or absent because of interference with the pathway from the occipital cortex to the facial nucleus.
- With transient cerebellar disease, the menace response may be normal to slow or missing, but intention tremors often are not present. This could place the lesion in the spinocerebellar tracts rather than the cerebellum, but this remains to be elucidated.
- With occipital atlantoaxial malformation, the wings of the atlas often are palpably malformed. Foals may be born dead because of severe parturient compression of the medulla oblongata and spinal cord by the unstable craniovertebral bones, or foals may be tetraparetic or tetraplegic. The atlas is palpably abnormal, and the atlas wings often are small. These horses often posture with the head and neck extended. In some cases, horses present with progressive ataxia and tetraparesis, usually caused by spinal cord compression resulting from accumulation of fibrous tissue associated with the unstable atlantoaxial joint.

CAUSES
The causes of these diseases are unknown, but there is a hereditary implication.

RISK FACTORS
Unknown

DIAGNOSIS

DIFFERENTIAL DIAGNOSIS
- Cerebellar hypoplasia
- Cerebellar abiotrophy
- Occipital atlantoaxial malformation
- Transient cerebellar dysfunction

CBC/BIOCHEMISTRY/URINALYSIS
No specific abnormalities

OTHER LABORATORY TESTS
N/A

CONGENITAL CEREBELLAR DISEASES

IMAGING

The various malformations evident with occipital atlantoaxial malformation often can be depicted.

OTHER DIAGNOSTIC PROCEDURES

- Signalment and clinical signs
- Necropsy is definitive for abiotrophy and hypoplasia.

PATHOLOGIC FINDINGS

Cerebellar Hypoplasia

- Reduced cerebellar mass is evident grossly.
- Diffuse cerebellar cortical tissue scarcity is evident histopathologically.

Cerebellar Abiotrophy

- Gross necropsy findings may not be evident.
- The cerebellum may weight less than normal.
- Histopatholgoic changes include reduced numbers as well as degeneration and disorientation of Purkinje cells.
- In the Arabian syndrome, thinning and depletion of the granular and molecular layers of the cerebellar cortex, with mineralized neuronal cell bodies, are common.

Occipital Atlantoaxial Malformation

- Destructive malformation of the caudal calvarium and proximal spinal column.
- Brainstem malformations can vary and seem to be associated with the degree of bony malformation.
- Malformations include fusion of the atlas to the occiput as well as atlas and dens hypoplasia.
- Scoliosis may occur in association with extra bone formations.

Transient Cerebellar Dysfunction

The lesions have not been well characterized, because affected animals recover.

TREATMENT

N/A

MEDICATIONS

DRUGS

N/A

CONTRAINDICATIONS

N/A

PRECAUTIONS

N/A

POSSIBLE INTERACTIONS

N/A

ALTERNATIVE DRUGS

N/A

FOLLOW-UP

PATIENT MONITORING

N/A

POSSIBLE COMPLICATIONS

N/A

EXPECTED COURSE AND PROGNOSIS

- In transient cerebellar dysfunction, the prognosis is excellent.
- The prognosis is guarded in other disorders.

MISCELLANEOUS

ASSOCIATED CONDITIONS

N/A

AGE-RELATED FACTORS

N/A

ZOONOTIC POTENTIAL

N/A

PREGNANCY

N/A

SYNONYMS

N/A

SEE ALSO

N/A

Suggested Reading

Beatty MT, et al. Cerebellar disease in Arabian horses. Proc Annu Conv AAEP 1985;31:241–245.

De Bowes RM, et al. Cerebellar abiotrophy. Vet Clin North Am 1987;3:345–352.

De Lahunta A. Comparative cerebellar disease in domestic animals. Compend Contin Educ Pract Vet 1980;11:8–19.

Mayhew IG, Schneiders DH. An unusual familial neurological syndrome in newborn Thoroughbred foals. Vet Rec 1993;133:447–448.

Sponseller ML: Equine cerebellar hypoplasia and degeneration. Proc Annu Conv AAEP 1967;13:123–126.

Author Joseph J. Bertone

Consulting Editor Joseph J. Bertone

CONIUM MACULATUM (POISON HEMLOCK) TOXICOSIS

BASICS

OVERVIEW

- A potent toxic plant causing neurotoxicity and rapid death in horses.
- *Conium maculatum* (poison hemlock) also is known as spotted hemlock, European hemlock, and Nebraska or California fern.
- The plant is a biennial herb with a fern-like appearance and growing up to 10 feet in height, with a smooth, hollow, purple-spotted stem and a stout, white to pale yellow taproot.
- The lacy, triangular leaves resemble those of a carrot and have a musky odor, like that of a parsnip, when crushed.
- Small, white flowers cluster in flat-topped umbels 4–6 cm across.
- Grayish, round, tiny fruit with flattened ridges are produced during the second year.
- The plant commonly grows in disturbed soil along roadsides, field edges, railroad tracks, and stream banks throughout the U.S.
- The whole green plant is toxic at doses of $\cong$1% of body weight; 4–5 pounds of fresh leaves are lethal for horses.
- The plant contains numerous piperidine alkaloids, with the most toxic being *N*-methyl coniine and γ-coniceine; coniine acts similarly to nicotine, first causing stimulation and then depression of the CNS.

SIGNALMENT

- All animals
- Horses readily eat the plant even if other forage is present.

SIGNS

- The clinical course is rapid, and horses may be found dead or die within a few hours.
- Initial signs include mydriasis, salivation, hypotension, colic, and diarrhea.
- Neurologic signs develop rapidly and include apprehension, muscle tremors, muscular weakness, inco-ordination, recumbency, paralysis, and coma.
- Death results from respiratory failure.

CAUSES AND RISK FACTORS

- The plant appears during the early spring, and most toxicoses occur at this time, when the plant is most palatable.
- The level of *N*-methyl coniine increases as the plant matures; the root becomes toxic only later in the year.
- The highest alkaloid concentration is in the seeds.
- Drying seems to reduce, but not eliminate, the toxicity.

DIAGNOSIS

DIFFERENTIAL DIAGNOSIS

Other causes of sudden death in horses

CBC/BIOCHEMISTRY/URINALYSIS

N/A

OTHER LABORATORY TESTS

- Evidence of plant consumption
- Chemical analysis for coniine in the stomach contents and urine is available.

IMAGING

N/A

DIAGNOSTIC PROCEDURES

N/A

PATHOLOGIC FINDINGS

- No diagnostic postmortem findings, but the toxin is eliminated via the kidneys and lungs, giving the urine and exhaled air a characteristic mousy odor.
- Nonspecific necropsy findings include diffuse congestion of the lungs, liver, and myocardium.

CONIUM MACULATUM (POISON HEMLOCK) TOXICOSIS

TREATMENT

- No specific treatment
- Early GI decontamination may be useful.
- Respiratory support by mechanical ventilation may be helpful.
- Adequate nursing care of recumbent animals.

MEDICATIONS

DRUGS

- AC (2–5 g/kg PO in water slurry [1 g of AC in 5 mL of water]).
- One dose of a cathartic PO with AC if no diarrhea or ileus—70% sorbitol (3 mL/kg) or sodium or magnesium sulfate (250–500 mg/kg).
- Maintain body fluid and electrolyte balance.

CONTRAINDICATIONS/POSSIBLE INTERACTIONS

N/A

FOLLOW-UP

PATIENT MONITORING

N/A

PREVENTION/AVOIDANCE

- Remove poison hemlock from all areas accessible by horses. Treatment with herbicides may be attempted. Ensure all plants are dead before reintroducing horses, however, because herbicide-treated plants may be more palatable.
- Feed little or no hay that contains poison hemlock. Seeds may contaminate grains, making these feeds unsafe for consumption.

POSSIBLE COMPLICATIONS

N/A

EXPECTED COURSE AND PROGNOSIS

- Very guarded early prognosis.
- Clinical course may last several hours to a day or two.
- Onset of signs occurs within ≅2 hours of ingestion.
- In severe cases, death occurs within 5–10 hours of the onset of signs.
- Because both the quantity of alkaloid in the plant and the quantity of plant consumed vary, not all horses that eat poison hemlock die.

MISCELLANEOUS

ASSOCIATED CONDITIONS

N/A

AGE-RELATED FACTORS

N/A

ZOONOTIC POTENTIAL

N/A

PREGNANCY

Poison hemlock has teratogenic effects in cattle and pigs; however, teratogenicity has not been reported in horses.

SEE ALSO

N/A

ABBREVIATIONS

- AC = activated charcoal
- GI = gastrointestinal

Suggested Reading

Galey FD, Holstege DM, Fisher EG. Toxicosis in dairy cattle exposed to poison hemlock (*Conium maculatum*) in hay: isolation of conium alkaloids in plants, hay, and urine. J Vet Diagn Invest 1992;4:60–64.

Knight AP. Poison hemlock. Compend Contin Educ Pract Vet 1987;9:F256–F257.

Author Anita M. Kore

Consulting Editor Robert H. Poppenga

CONJUNCTIVAL DISEASES

BASICS

DEFINITION

Conjunctivitis is inflammation of the mucous membrane that covers the posterior aspects of the eyelids and nictitating membrane (palpebral conjunctiva) and the sclera (bulbar conjunctiva). Dermoids (choristoma) are reported to occur on the conjunctiva of foals. Squamous cell carcinoma is the most common neoplasm affecting the equine conjunctiva. Habronemiasis is a parasitic disease resulting in conjunctival and ocular granulomas. Onchocerciasis is a parasitic disease that can cause inflammation of the conjunctiva, cornea, and anterior uvea. *Thelazia lacrymalis,* a commensal parasite of the conjunctival fornices and nasolacrimal ducts of horses, can incite a parasitic conjunctivitis. Horses with *Thelazia* are usually asymptomatic, but may develop conjunctivitis, superficial keratitis, dacryocystitis, and mild eyelid swelling.

Pathophysiology

Conjunctivitis is a nonspecific finding that indicates ocular inflammation, and may also be seen in systemic disease. Infectious and noninfectious diseases of the lids, cornea, sclera, anterior uvea, nasolacrimal system, and orbit can result in conjunctivitis. The conjunctiva is a mucous membrane that can reflect systemic dysfunction through color changes, as in anemia and jaundice. Neoplasia may involve the conjunctiva. Environmental allergies may cause conjunctivitis. Habronemiasis is a parasitic conjunctivitis caused by aberrant migration of *Habronema megastoma, H. muscae,* and *Draschia megastoma* larvae in ocular adnexa. The vectors are stable and house flies that deposit the larvae in moist body areas and wounds. Habronemiasis may occur concurrently with squamous cell carcinoma. Onchocerciasis can cause conjunctivitis, keratitis, and keratouveitis. The causative agent is *Onchocerca cervicalis,* and the vector is female *Culicoides* spp. Adult *Onchocerca* organisms live in the nuchal ligament, and migrating larvae may invade the conjunctiva, cornea, and anterior uvea, resulting in inflammation.

Systems Affected

Ophthalmic

SIGNALMENT

Breed Predilections

There are no breed predilections for conjunctivitis. Squamous cell carcinoma has a high prevalance in draft horses, Appaloosas, and Paints.

Mean Age and Range

Neonates—Conjunctivitis associated with neonatal maladjustment syndrome, septicemia, immune-mediated hemolytic anemia, environmental irritants, dermoids, subconjunctival or episcleral hemorrhages secondary to birth trauma, and neonatal maladjustment syndrome. Conjunctivitis secondary to pneumonia is seen most commonly in 1- to 6-month-old foals. Prevalence of ocular squamous cell carcinoma increases with age.

Genetics

No proven genetic basis for conjunctivitis, but breed predilection for ocular squamous cell carcinoma suggests genetic influence.

Predominant Sex

No proven sex predilection.

SIGNS

- Conjunctivitis—Conjunctival hyperemia (redness) and chemosis (edema of the conjunctiva); ocular discharge varies with type of disease: serous (viral, allergic), mucopurulent to purulent (bacterial); lymphoid follicle formation.
- Onchocerciasis—Limbal conjunctival thickening and depigmentation, corneal edema, vascularization, and stromal cellular infiltrate.
- Squamous cell carcinoma has two characteristic appearances: proliferative mass, which may be ulcerated; or diffuse thickening and ulceration of tissue. May be complicated secondarily with habronemiasis.
- Habronemiasis—Appearance ranges from granulomas or nodules to small, raised, caseated plaques on the conjunctiva. May be nonhealing and ulcerated.
- Dermoid—Pigmented mass; may have hair follicle development.

CAUSES

Causes of Infectious Conjunctivitis

- Parasitic—*Habronema megastoma**, *H. muscae**, *Draschia megastoma, Onchocerca cervicalis,* and *Thelazia lacrimalis.*
- Viral—Adenovirus, equine herpesvirus type 4, equine infectious anemia, equine viral arteritis, and influenza type A2.
- Bacterial—*Moraxella equi, Streptococcus equi* subspecies *equi, Rhodococcus, Actinobacillus* spp., and leptospirosis.
- Mycotic
- Protozoal—Equine protozoal myeloencephalitis.

Causes of Neoplastic Conjunctivitis

- Squamous cell carcinoma*
- Lymphoma
- Papilloma
- Hemangioma
- Hemangiosarcoma
- Multiple myeloma

Secondary to Other Ocular/Adnexal Disease

- Ulcerative keratitis*
- Corneal stromal abscess*
- Anterior uveitis*
- Equine recurrent uveitis*
- Keratomycosis*
- Obstructed nasolacrimal duct
- Imperforate punctum
- Entropion
- Keratoconjunctivitis sicca
- Distichiasis
- Ectopic cilia

Secondary to Environmental Causes

- Foreign bodies and debris*
- Trauma*
- Allergic reactions to dust and environmental pollutants
- Chemical sprays

Secondary to Systemic Disease

- Polyneuritis equi
- Vestibular disease syndrome
- African Horse Sickness
- Epizootic lymphangitis
- Neonatal maladjustment syndrome
- Septicemia
- Immune-mediated hemolytic anemia

RISK FACTORS

Recumbent foals are at risk for conjunctivitis secondary to environmental irritants. White, gray-white, and palomino hair color predisposes to ocular squamous cell carcinoma. Warm weather and climates with a heavy fly population are a risk factor for habronemiasis.

DIAGNOSIS

Differential Diagnosis

Conjunctivitis is a nonspecific sign, reflecting the eye's limited response mechanisms to injury. It is critical to differentiate primary conjunctivitis from conjunctivitis associated with ocular or systemic disease. Conjunctival hyperemia must be differentiated from episcleral injection, as episcleral injection indicates serious ocular disease. Conjunctival vasculature has extensive branching, is freely moveable, and blanches when a sympathomimetic drug is applied topically. Episcleral vasculature has a radial pattern from the limbus, is not freely moveable, and does not blanch when a sympathomimetic drug is applied topically. Nodular/mass lesions of conjunctiva include:

- Habronemiasis
- Squamous cell carcinoma
- Mastocytoma
- Hemangioma
- Hemangiosarcoma
- Papilloma
- Fungal granulomas
- Nodular necrobiosis
- Dermoid
- Foreign body reaction

CBC/BIOCHEMISTRY/URINALYSIS

Results are usually normal unless conjunctival disease is associated with systemic disease.

OTHER LABORATORY TESTS

- Cytology to identify mycotic, bacterial causes of conjunctivitis.
- Culture and sensitivity of mucopurulent discharge may be considered if primary bacterial cause suspected.
- Habronemiasis—Conjunctival scraping reveals eosinophils, mast cells, neutrophils, plasma cells, rarely larvae.
- Biopsy and histopathology for mass lesions.
- Other specific tests as indicated when systemic disease suspected.

IMAGING

N/A

DIAGNOSTIC PROCEDURES

Complete ophthalmic examination is indicated to identify adnexal and ocular causes of conjunctivitis. Thorough adnexal exam, fluorescein stain, examination for signs of anterior uveitis (aqueous flare, miosis, hypotony), and schirmer tear test. Compare pupil size: will not vary between eyes if primary conjunctivitis; anisocoria may be seen if ocular disease present. Examination behind nictitans may reveal foreign body or debris. Consider cannulation and flushing of nasolacrimal duct to rule out nasolacrimal disease. If conjunctival laceration with hypotony and/or hyphema are present, rule out scleral laceration.

PATHOLOGIC FINDINGS

Conjunctival Biopsy

- Onchocerciasis—Microfilaria, eosinophils, lymphocytes.
- Habronemiasis—Eosinophils, mast cells, neutrophils, plasma cells, larvae (rare).
- Squamous cell carcinoma—Epithelial cells with neoplastic characteristics.
- Lymphoma—Large population monomorphic lymphocytes with neoplastic characteristics.
- Multiple myeloma—Large population neoplastic plasma cells.
- Other histopathologic findings possible depending on type of neoplasia present.

TREATMENT

APPROPRIATE HEALTH CARE

Most horses with conjunctivitis associated with parasitic, bacterial, viral, and environmental causes can be treated on an outpatient basis. Treatment of some systemic (septicemia, neonatal maladjustment syndrome, equine protozoal myelitis) and ocular (severe ulcerative keratitis, corneal stromal abscess, keratomycosis, squamous cell carcinoma) diseases associated with conjunctivitis may require hospitalization.

CONJUNCTIVAL DISEASES

ACTIVITY
Restriction of activity may be required in cases where conjunctival disease is associated with systemic illness. If environmental irritation is suspected, then exposure to the inciting substance should be restricted or eliminated. Animals with ocular involvement/disease should not be ridden if visual status is compromised.

DIET
No change in diet is necessary. Hay should be fed at ground level rather than elevated hayracks or bags to avoid further irritation of the conjunctiva by dust and debris.

CLIENT EDUCATION
If there is evidence of self-trauma, a protective hood covering the affected eye should be placed on the horse. The client should be instructed to contact the veterinarian if the condition worsens in any way. The problem may not be responding appropriately to treatment, may be progressing, or the patient may be having an adverse response to the medication.

SURGICAL CONSIDERATIONS
Treatment of corneal stromal abscessation and keratomycosis may require conjunctival flap procedures, lamellar keratectomy, or penetrating keratoplasty. Treatment of conjunctival neoplasia may involve local resection, with adjunctive beta-irradiation, brachytherapy, cryotherapy, radiofrequency hyperthermia, or intralesional chemotherapy. Enucleation or exenteration may be necessary, depending on the type of neoplasia and extent of invasion. Management of obstructed nasolacrimal duct may require surgical intervention. Small lacerations of the conjunctiva will heal without primary closure. Large lacerations should be sutured with fine absorbable suture. Conjunctival foreign bodies and debris can usually be removed with topical anesthesia and liberal flushing of conjunctival fornices.

MEDICATIONS

DRUGS OF CHOICE

Parasitic Conjunctivitis
- Habronemiasis—Topical 0.03% Echothiophate iodide (phospholine iodide) and ophthalmic neomycin/polymixin B with dexamethasone (Maxitrol) q12h.
- Multifocal lesions—Oral ivermectin (200 μg/kg). Intralesional triamcinolone may reduce size of granulomas.
- Onchocerciasis—Systemic ivermectin with topical anti-inflammatories.
- Thelazia—Topical phospholine iodide, flush conjunctival fornix.

Mycotic Conjunctivitis
Topical Natamycin q6–12h depending on severity of disease.

Bacterial Conjunctivitis
Topical broad-spectrum antibiotic initially (triple antibiotic usually appropriate), may change after results of bacterial culture and sensitivity. Treat q6–12h, depending on severity of disease.

Conjunctival Lacerations
Treat with topical prophylactic broad-spectrum antibiotic.

Allergic Conjunctivitis
- Topical corticosteroid; reduce/eliminate exposure to inciting cause if possible.

Squamous Cell Carcinoma
See Ocular Squamous Cell Carcinoma section.

Ocular Diseases Inciting Conjunctivitis
See appropriate section. Other systemic medication as indicated by concurrent systemic disease.

CONTRAINDICATIONS
N/A

PRECAUTIONS
Most antifungal drugs are slightly irritating. Miconazole is not available as an ophthalmic preparation. The intravenous and vaginal preparations can be used as topical ophthalmic medications. The dermatologic preparation of miconazole contains alcohol, which can be very irritating. Topical organophosphates, corticosteroids, dimethyl sulfoxide, antibiotics, and petroleum ointment have been suggested for treatment of habronemiasis. These may have corneal and/or conjunctival toxicity, and should be used with caution.

POSSIBLE INTERACTIONS
N/A

ALTERNATIVE DRUGS
Other antifungal medications include natamycin, nystatin, and pyrimidines.

FOLLOW-UP

PATIENT MONITORING

The patient should be rechecked soon after beginning therapy (3–4 days), with the specific time frame determined by the disease and its severity. Subsequent rechecks are dictated by severity of disease and response to treatment.

PREVENTION/AVOIDANCE

Fly control in barns and pastures, fly hoods, and frequent periocular administration of insect repellent can help prevent the development of habronemiasis. A preventative health program, including regular deworming with ivermectin, helps prevent habronemiasis and onchocerciasis. The incidence of allergic/environmental conjunctivitis can be reduced/prevented by avoidance of the inciting agent. Treat any underlying ocular or systemic disease that may be promoting the conjunctival disease.

POSSIBLE COMPLICATIONS

Potential complications of conjunctival neoplasia and its treatment vary with the specific type of tumor. Possible complications of treatment include depigmentation in region of treatment, recurrence of the neoplasia, and metastatic disease.

EXPECTED COURSE AND PROGNOSIS

Infectious conjunctivitis usually responds to appropriate treatment. Failure to respond or recurrence suggests an unidentified underlying cause (i.e., recurrent bacterial conjunctivitis associated with an unrecognized foreign body). Course and prognosis of conjunctival neoplasia depend on the specific type of neoplasia and the extent of invasion of surrounding tissues. Allergic conjunctivitis is often difficult to eliminate completely due to the nature of the horse's environment. Prognosis associated with conjunctivitis secondary to systemic or ocular disease varies with the specific disease.

MISCELLANEOUS

ASSOCIATED CONDITIONS

N/A

AGE-RELATED FACTORS

N/A

ZOONOTIC POTENTIAL

N/A

PREGNANCY

Systemic absorption of topically applied medication is possible. Benefits of treatment should be considered against any risks posed to the fetus.

SYNONYMS

N/A

SEE ALSO

- Ocular squamous cell carcinoma
- Ocular problems in the neonate
- Eyelid diseases
- Corneal ulceration
- Keratomycosis
- Corneal stromal abscessation

ABBREVIATIONS

N/A

Suggested Reading

Brooks DE: Equine Ophthalmology. In: Gelatt KN (ed). Veterinary Ophthalmology, Chapter 30. 1999. Philadelphia: Lippincott Williams & Wilkins.

Author Heidi M. Denis, DVM

Consulting Editor D. E. Brooks

CONTAGIOUS EQUINE METRITIS (CEM)

BASICS

DEFINITION

• Genital infection of stallions and mares caused by *Taylorella equigenitalis*.
• A reportable, highly contagious disease transmitted primarily by coitus.
• Transmission also may occur by contaminated equipment.
• Stallions are asymptomatic carriers, with the organism harbored in fossa glandis, urethral sinus, and smegma. It is also recoverable from the terminal urethra, preputial surface, and pre-ejaculatory fluid.
• Clinical signs only occur in mares and range from none to acute endometritis.
• The organism can persist in the clitoral sinuses and fossa, and mares may be mechanical carriers via smegma of the clitoral fossa.

PATHOPHYSIOLOGY

Stallions

The organism is harbored in various external regions of the genital tract and is transmitted primarily by coitus.

Mares

• Clinical signs range from none to acute endometritis.
• The organism initially is found in the endometrium and cervix.
• The organism less frequently is found in the vagina, vulva, clitoris, and oviducts.
• From 3 weeks to 4 months, the organism occasionally is recoverable from the ovarian surface, oviduct, uterus, cervix, and vagina.
• The organism is more reliably isolated from clitoral fossa and sinuses.
• Local IgA, IgM, and systemic IgG response.
• The organism also is recoverable from placentae of positive mares and genitalia of colts and fillies—acquired in utero or at parturition.

SYSTEM AFFECTED

Reproductive

GENETICS

N/A

INCIDENCE/PREVALENCE

Dependent on carrier stallion or contaminated equipment for transmission.

SIGNALMENT

Breeding-age mares and stallions from countries identified as CEM-affected.

SIGNS

Stallions

Inapparent infection

Mares

• Within 2–7 days of infection, mares develop varying amount of odorless, grayish, mucopurulent discharge.
• Severe diffuse endometritis and cervicitis—more severe and plasmacytic by 14 days, then declines and persists as mild, diffuse, and multifocal for as long as 2 weeks.
• Shortened diestrus period because of premature luteolysis.
• Temporary infertility.
• No systemic involvement.

CAUSES

• Two strains of *T. equigenitalis*—streptomycin resistant; streptomycin sensitive.
• Contaminated equipment (e.g., specula, artificial insemination) and handling personnel (e.g., gloves).

RISK FACTORS

• Carrier stallion
• Contaminated equipment
• No lifelong immunity
• Previous exposure does not afford absolute protection against subsequent challenge.

DIAGNOSIS

DIFFERENTIAL DIAGNOSIS

• Bacterial or fungal endometritis
• Pyometra
• Vaginitis
• Urinary tract infection
• Urine pooling
• Neoplasia of the uterus or vagina
• Persistent hymen

CBC/BIOCHEMISTRY/URINALYSIS

Unremarkable

OTHER LABORATORY TESTS

• Speculum examination
• Collection of cervical discharge
• Isolation of organism

IMAGING

Ultrasonography—intrauterine fluid suggestive of endometritis.

DIAGNOSTIC PROCEDURES

Serology

• Detectable antibody in acute cases—mares only.
• No value in stallions, because contamination is surface only.

Bacterial Cultures

• Stallions—urethral fossa and urethral sinus, distal urethra, penile skin, and preputial folds.
• Mares—clitoral sinus and fossa; endometrium, vaginal fluid, and cervix of estrous mare.
• Exacting culture requirements for *T. equigenitalis*—immediately place swabs in Amies charcoal medium, kept at 4°C for transport; plate samples within 24 hours of collection.
• Colonies usually form in 2–3 days; a recent streptomycin-sensitive strain may take as long as 6 days.
• Reportable disease that requires a federally approved laboratory for identification.

Cytology (Mares)

• Presence of PMNs, indicating endometritis.
• Presence of morphologically similar bacteria—free or phagocytized.

Test Breeding (Stallions)

Breed to known uninfected (i.e., virgin) mares.

PCR

Developed, but not yet sufficiently validated.

CONTAGIOUS EQUINE METRITIS (CEM)

TREATMENT

APPROPRIATE HEALTH CARE

Under federal supervision at approved quarantine station.

Mares

- Intrauterine antibiotics—crystalline penicillin (5–10 million U for 5–7 days).
- Cleansing of the clitoral fossa and sinuses with chlorhexidine scrub to remove all smegma.
- Pack with nitrofurazone ointment.

Stallions

- Completely extrude and wash penis in chlorhexidine scrub.
- Remove all smegma, especially from the urethral fossa and skin folds of prepuce.
- Nitrofurazone dressing for 5 days.

NURSING CARE

N/A

ACTIVITY

N/A

DIET

N/A

CLIENT EDUCATION

N/A

SURGICAL CONSIDERATIONS

Mares—clitoral sinusectomy or clitorectomy for intractable cases.

MEDICATIONS

DRUGS OF CHOICE

- Chlorhexidine (2%–4%)—higher concentrations can lead to penile irritation.
- Nitrofurazone (0.2% ointment).

CONTRAINDICATIONS

N/A

PRECAUTIONS

N/A

POSSIBLE INTERACTIONS

N/A

ALTERNATIVE DRUGS

N/A

FOLLOW-UP

PATIENT MONITORING

Culture (Timing)

- Swabs 7 days after the last day of treatment for three consecutive sets of negatives.
- Stallions—every 2 days for three sets.
- Mares—three consecutive estrus periods.

Culture (Locations)

- Mares—swab the clitoris and endometrium at estrus before breeding; swab during abnormal estrous intervals.
- Stallions— swabs from teaser and breeding stallions before season begins.

Culture (Equipment)

- Disposable gloves, sleeves, and speculum.
- Use AI when feasible or permitted by breed-society regulations.

PREVENTION/AVOIDANCE

- All horses older than 2 years entering the United States from CEM-affected countries must follow treatment and testing protocol.
- Mares—test three times in 7 days, then treat for 5 days; if three negative cultures are obtained, the mare is released.
- Stallions—require negative culture and negative test breeding to two mares; if positive, repeat cycle until three consecutive, negative culture results are obtained.

POSSIBLE COMPLICATIONS

N/A

EXPECTED COURSE AND PROGNOSIS

Recovery with treatment as described.

MISCELLANEOUS

ASSOCIATED CONDITIONS

N/A

AGE-RELATED FACTORS

N/A

ZOONOTIC POTENTIAL

N/A

PREGNANCY

N/A

SYNONYMS

Formerly *Haemophilus equigenitalis*

SEE ALSO

Venereal diseases

ABBREVIATIONS

- AI = artificial insemination
- PCR = polymerase chain reaction
- PMN = polymorphonuclear

Suggested Reading

Blanchard TL, Kenney RM, Timoney PJ. Venereal disease. Vet Clin North Am Equine Pract 1992;8:193–195.

Timoney PJ. Aspects of the occurrence, diagnosis and control of selected venereal diseases of the stallion. In: Proceedings of the Stallion Symposium, Sponsored by the ACT/SFT, Hastings, Nebraska, December 1998:76–78.

Watson ED. Swabbing protocols in screening for contagious equine metritis. Vet Rec 1997;140:268–271.

Author Peter R. Morresey
Consulting Editor Carla L. Carleton

CORNEAL/SCLERAL LACERATIONS

BASICS

OVERVIEW

• Ocular trauma results from a redistribution of kinetic energy, with no boundaries regarding the possible effects on any ocular structure; thus, ocular injury can have a variety of manifestations.
• Blunt injuries carry a worse prognosis than injury from sharp objects or missiles, because blunt forces are transmitted throughout the eye but sharp, penetrating forces are localized to the site of impact.

SIGNALMENT

Any age and breed.

SIGNS

• The eye may be cloudy, red, and painful.
• Blepharospasm and lacrimation are present with focal or generalized corneal edema.
• Slight droopiness of the upper lid eyelashes may be a subtle sign of corneal ulceration.
• Full-thickness corneal/scleral perforations usually are associated with iris prolapse, shallow anterior chamber, and hyphema.
• If the corneal lesion extends to the limbus, check the sclera carefully for perforation, because the scleral wound can be obscured by conjunctival chemosis and hemorrhage.

CAUSES AND RISK FACTORS

Trauma from whips, nails, buckets, light fixtures, vegetative material, and tree branches.

DIAGNOSIS

DIFFERENTIAL DIAGNOSIS

Ocular pain also may be found with corneal ulcers, uveitis, conjunctivitis, glaucoma, blepharitis, and dacryocystitis.

CBC/BIOCHEMISTRY/URINALYSIS

N/A

OTHER LABORATORY TESTS

N/A

IMAGING

N/A

DIAGNOSTIC PROCEDURES

Staining the cornea with fluorescein dye reveals the laceration; fluorescein dye may enter the anterior chamber.

TREATMENT

• For superficial, nonperforating lacerations, medical therapy should be sufficient. Deep or irregular corneal lacerations require surgical support of the cornea and more aggressive therapy for iridocyclitis. Direct corneal suturing and conjunctival flaps are indicated to restore corneal integrity more rapidly.
• Both small and large full-thickness corneal perforations should be repaired surgically. Complications include infection, iris prolapse, anterior synechiae, cataract formation, and persistent iridocyclitis. Left untreated, both small and large corneal or scleral full-thickness defects can result in phthisis bulbi.
• Traumatic corneal perforation that defies repair, extensive extrusion of intraocular contents, severe intraocular hemorrhage, or evidence of bacterial infection require enucleation.

MEDICATIONS

DRUGS

• Medical therapy alone should be sufficient for superficial, nonperforating lacerations.
• Topically applied antibiotics (chloramphenicol, bacitracin-neomycin-polymyxin B, gentamicin; QID), atropine (1%; QID), and serum (QID).
• Systemic NSAIDs (phenylbutazone [2 mg/kg PO BID] or flunixin meglumine [1 mg/kg PO, IM, or IV BID]) and broad-spectrum parenteral antibiotics are also indicated for full-thickness lesions.

CONTRAINDICATIONS/POSSIBLE INTERACTIONS

N/A

CORNEAL/SCLERAL LACERATIONS

FOLLOW-UP

PATIENT MONITORING

- Monitor horses with corneal lacerations for continued blepharospasm and colic.
- Protect the horse from self-trauma with hard or soft cup hoods.
- Horses with corneal lacerations and secondary uveitis should be stall rested until the condition heals; intraocular hemorrhage and increased severity of uveitis are sequela to overexertion.
- Diet should be consistent with the training level of the horse.

PREVENTION/AVOIDANCE

N/A

POSSIBLE COMPLICATIONS

- Failure to detect a scleral tear results in chronic hypotony and globe atrophy (i.e., phthisis bulbi).
- The equine eye does not tolerate much damage to its vasculature; severe intraocular hemorrhage usually results in phthisis bulbi.
- Injury to the lens, iris, and retina can accompany blunt or sharp corneal/scleral trauma.
- Septic intrusion into the globe results in painful endophthalmitis; such infection can spread to surrounding soft tissues and necessitates enucleation.

EXPECTED COURSE AND PROGNOSIS

- Small corneal lacerations can heal quickly with prompt surgical and medical therapy.
- Larger lesions are associated with more uveitis and heal more slowly.

MISCELLANEOUS

ASSOCIATED CONDITIONS

Corneal lacerations always are accompanied by varying degrees of iridocyclitis.

AGE-RELATED FACTORS

N/A

ZOONOTIC POTENTIAL

N/A

PREGNANCY

N/A

SEE ALSO

Iris prolapse

Suggested Reading

Brooks DE. Equine Ophthalmology. In Gelatt KN, ed. Veterinary ophthalmology. 3rd ed. Philadelphia, Lippincot, Williams & Wilkins, 1999.

Author Dennis E. Brooks
Consulting Editor Dennis E. Brooks

CORNEAL STROMAL ABSCESSES

BASICS

OVERVIEW

- A corneal abscess may develop after epithelial cells adjacent to a small epithelial puncture divide and migrate over the wound to seal infectious agents or foreign bodies in the stroma.
- The re-epithelialization forms a barrier that protects the bacteria or fungi from topically administered antimicrobial medications.

SIGNALMENT

All ages and breeds in all types of environments.

SIGNS

- The eye may be cloudy, red, and painful.
- Blepharospasm and tearing
- Slight droopiness of the upper eyelid lashes may be a subtle sign of corneal abscessation.
- Stromal abscessation—a focal, yellow-white, stromal infiltrate with associated corneal edema; single or multiple abscesses; mild to fulminating iridocyclitis secondary to what appears initially to be a relatively benign corneal disease, causing severe pain and possible blindness; variable corneal vascularization.
- Most cases initially have clinical signs suggestive of minor corneal trauma; fluorescein dye retention either is negative or is positive over a much smaller area than the corneal lesion diameter.

CAUSES AND RISK FACTORS

Corneal stromal abscesses can be sterile or infected with bacteria or fungi.

DIAGNOSIS

DIFFERENTIAL DIAGNOSIS

- Ocular pain may be associated with corneal ulcers, ERU, glaucoma, conjunctivitis, blepharitis, and dacryocystitis.
- Differentiating a chronic stromal abscess with secondary uveitis from the NKU keratopathy noticed in the southern United States may be difficult. History of previous trauma, evidence of corneal ulceration, yellow-white stromal infiltrate, and varying corneal position of the stromal abscesses help to make the distinction. NKU cases have a pink, fleshy, stromal lesion at the limbus, with very painful anterior uveitis.
- Although melting and infected equine ulcers also are associated with severe anterior uveitis, each is distinct in general appearance from a stromal abscess, with ulcers invariably retaining fluorescein stain over most of the lesion and stromal abscesses only over a small area of the lesion during the acute stages (if at all).

CBC/BIOCHEMISTRY/URINALYSIS

N/A

OTHER LABORATORY TESTS

N/A

IMAGING

N/A

DIAGNOSTIC PROCEDURES

- Many cytologic, microbiologic, and histologic specimens may fail to yield diagnostic results. It may be that bacteria and fungi are killed by the initial medical treatment regimen, and that the toxins subsequently released by the dying bacteria and fungi and the degenerating leukocytes continue the stimulus for this interstitial keratitis, prolonging the anterior uveitis.
- Keratectomy specimens may be the only way to obtain a definitive causative diagnosis for the institution of proper antimicrobial therapy.

TREATMENT

- Many superficial stromal abscesses initially respond positively (i.e., with less uveitis) to topical mydriatic/cycloplegics and topical and systemic antibiotic and NSAID therapy but then gradually worsen clinically, requiring surgical intervention.
- Scraping over the stromal abscess may aid drug penetration and abscess healing during the early stages.
- If significant improvement in signs associated with stromal abscess does not occur within the first 48–72 hours of intense and appropriate medical therapy, surgery can improve results and reduce the duration of medical therapy.
- Carefully adjust systemic NSAIDs if medical therapy is used alone to allow for control of the anterior uveitis without significantly inhibiting the corneal vascularization necessary to heal the corneal stromal abscesses.
- Deep corneal abscesses respond poorly to medical therapy.
- Most stromal abscesses involving Descemet's membrane are fungal infections.
- Deep lamellar and penetrating keratoplasties are used in eyes with abscesses near Descemet's membrane and in eyes with rupture of the abscess into the anterior chamber. This aggressive surgical therapy can be very successful in eliminating antigenic stimulation from the sequestered organisms and removing the necrotic debris, metabolites, and toxins from the degenerating leukocytes and microbes in the abscess.
- Horses that undergo surgery early during the course of disease tend to have a more rapid recovery than those in which surgery is delayed. If a positive response to medical therapy is not seen quickly, especially when stromal abscesses are deep or with severe uveitis, consider surgery.
- The decision to perform surgery is based on continued progression of anterior uveitis despite intense medical therapy, imminent or pre-existing rupture of the abscess into the anterior chamber, severe and unrelenting endophthalmitis, or anticipated poor visual outcome resulting from lack of vascularization of the stromal abscess.
- Penetrating keratoplasty or corneal transplantation for treatment of deep corneal stromal abscesses, with or without conjunctival pedicle grafts, is effective.

CORNEAL STROMAL ABSCESSES

MEDICATIONS

DRUGS

- Initially, doxycycline (3 mg/kg PO BID) or gentamicin (2 mg/kg IV or IM BID)/K penicillin (10,000 IU/kg IM or IV BID).
- Topically applied antibiotics (e.g., chloramphenicol, bacitracin-neomycin-polymyxin B, gentamicin; QID), atropine (1%; QID), and serum (QID) are recommended.
- Systemic NSAIDs—phenylbutazone (2 mg/kg PO BID) or flunixin meglumine (1 mg/kg PO, IM, or IV BID).
- Topical natamycin or other antifungals are strongly recommended for deeper abscesses.
- Intraocular injection of miconazole and fluconazole (0.1 mg/0.1 mL solution), which can be performed at the time of surgery, has been an effective adjunctive treatment of deep fungal stromal abscesses.

CONTRAINDICATIONS/POSSIBLE INTERACTIONS

N/A

FOLLOW-UP

PATIENT MONITORING

- Monitor ocular pain, which should diminish with resolution of the abscess.
- Protect the horse from self-trauma with hard or soft cup hoods.
- Topically administered atropine is associated with colic.
- Horses with stromal abscesses should be stall rested until the condition heals; intraocular hemorrhage and increased severity of uveitis are sequela to overexertion.
- Diet should be consistent with the training level of the horse.

PREVENTION/AVOIDANCE

N/A

POSSIBLE COMPLICATIONS

Stromal abscesses—endophthalmitis, persistent uveitis, iris prolapse, ERU, and corneal ulcers.

EXPECTED COURSE AND PROGNOSIS

- Stromal abscesses do not heal completely until they become vascularized, either directly from a conjunctival graft or indirectly from centripetal corneal vascular ingrowth.
- Deep and superficial corneal vascularization must occur in deep stromal abscesses for the lesion to resolve. Although some degree of corneal vascularization generally is present, it appears to grow much more slowly than the 1–2 mm/day described for the horse.
- Re-epithelialization after corneal scrapings of medically treated horses is rapid and dramatic.
- Scraping over the stromal abscess may aid in drug penetration and abscess healing during the early stages; less benefit may be attained with scraping during the chronic stages.
- Enucleation of painful blind eyes has been necessary in a few cases.

MISCELLANEOUS

ASSOCIATED CONDITIONS

N/A

AGE-RELATED FACTORS

N/A

ZOONOTIC POTENTIAL

N/A

PREGNANCY

N/A

SEE ALSO

NKU

ABBREVIATIONS

- ERU = equine recurrent uveitis
- NKU = nonulcerative keratouveitis

Suggested Reading

Brooks DE: Equine ophthalmology. In Gelatt KN, ed. Veterinary ophthalmology. 3rd ed. Philadelphia: Lippincott Williams & Wilkins, 1999.

Hendrix DVH, Brooks DE, Smith PJ, Gelatt KN, Miller TR, Whittaker C, Pellicane C, Chmielewski. Corneal stromal abscesses in the horse: a review of 24 cases. Equine Vet J 1995;27:440–447.

Author Dennis E. Brooks

Consulting Editor Dennis E. Brooks

CORNEAL ULCERATION (EXPANDED)

BASICS

DEFINITION

- A sight-threatening disease requiring early clinical diagnosis, laboratory confirmation, and appropriate medical and surgical therapy.
- Both bacterial and fungal keratitis may present with a mild, early clinical course but require prompt therapy to avoid serious ocular complications.
- Ulcers can range from simple, superficial breaks or abrasions in the corneal epithelium to full-thickness corneal perforations with iris prolapse.

PATHOPHYSIOLOGY

- Thickness of the equine cornea—1.0–1.5 mm.
- The normal equine corneal epithelium is 8–10 cell layers thick but increases to 10–15 cell layers with hypertrophy of the basal epithelial cells after corneal injury. The epithelial basement membrane is not completely formed 6 weeks after corneal injury in the horse, despite the epithelium completely covering the ulcer site. Healing time for a 7-mm diameter, midstromal-depth, corneal trephine wound is nearly 12 days in horses with noninfected wounds.
- The environment of the horse constantly exposes the conjunctiva and cornea to bacteria and fungi. The equine conjunctival microbial flora varies, depending on the season and geographic area. Many bacterial and fungal organisms normally found in equine conjunctival flora are potential ocular pathogens. *Staphylococcus, Streptococcus, Pseudomonas, Aspergillus,* and *Fusarium* sp. are common causes of equine corneal ulceration.
- The equine corneal epithelium is a formidable barrier to invasion by bacteria or fungi. A defect in the corneal epithelium, however, allows bacteria or fungi to adhere to the cornea and to initiate infection. Epithelial defects need not be full thickness; corneas with partial-thickness epithelial defects are more susceptible to adherence by *Pseudomonas* sp. than corneas with a fully intact epithelium.
- Tear-film neutrophils, and some bacteria and fungi, are associated with highly destructive protease and collagenase enzymes that can result in rapid corneal stromal thinning and perforation. Excessive protease activity is termed *melting* and results in a gelatinous appearance to the stroma. Total corneal ulceration ultimately requires the degradation of collagen, which forms the framework of the corneal stroma.
- Equine corneas demonstrate a strong fibrovascular healing response.

SYSTEM AFFECTED

Ophthalmic

GENETICS

No proven genetic predisposition to equine corneal ulceration, but the unique corneal healing properties of the horse regarding excessive corneal vascularization and fibrosis appear to be strongly species specific.

INCIDENCE/PREVALENCE

Corneal ulceration is a common course of equine ophthalmic disease and may be associated with bacterial and fungal infection.

SIGNALMENT

All ages and breeds in all types of environment are at risk.

SIGNS

- The eye may be cloudy, red, and painful.
- Blepharospasm and tearing
- Slight droopiness of the upper lid eyelashes may be a subtle sign of corneal ulceration.
- Corneal edema may surround the ulcer or involve the entire cornea.
- Signs of anterior uveitis are found with every equine corneal ulcer—miosis, fibrin, hyphema, or hypopyon.

CAUSES

- Trauma is the most common cause.
- Infection should be considered likely in every equine corneal ulcer.
- Infectious keratitis in horses develops in eyes with traumatic corneal abrasions and in those with epithelial defects caused by chronic edema, KCS, exposure keratitis, neurotropic keratitis, and neuroparalytic keratitis.
- Fungal involvement should be suspected if a history of corneal injury with vegetative material or if a corneal ulcer has received prolonged antibiotic and/or corticosteroid therapy with slight or no improvement.
- Foreign bodies, chemical burns, and immune mechanisms.
- Persistent superficial ulcers may become indolent because of hyaline membrane formation on the ulcer bed.

RISK FACTORS

The prominent eye of the horse may predispose to injury.

DIAGNOSIS

DIFFERENTIAL DIAGNOSIS

- Fluorescein dye retention is diagnostic.
- Painful eye—uveitis, blepharitis, conjunctivitis, glaucoma, and dacryocystitis.

CBC/BIOCHEMISTRY/URINALYSIS

N/A

OTHER LABORATORY TESTS

- Microbial culture and sensitivity for bacteria and fungi in horses with rapidly progressive and deep corneal ulcers. Corneal culture specimens should be obtained first, followed by corneal scrapings for cytology. Mixed bacterial and fungal infections can be present.
- Vigorous corneal scrapings, at the edge and base of the lesion to detect bacteria and deep hyphal elements, can be obtained with the handle end of a sterile scalpel and topical anesthesia.
- Superficial swabbing cannot be expected to yield the organisms in a high percentage of cases.
- Stain cytologic specimens with Gram, Giemsa, or Wright's.

IMAGING

N/A

DIAGNOSTIC PROCEDURES

- Fluorescein stain all corneal injuries to detect corneal ulcers; small corneal abrasions are detected with oblique transillumination and fluorescein dye retention.
- A "crater-like" defect that retains fluorescein dye at its periphery but is clear in the center is a descemetocele and indicates that the globe is at high risk of rupture.

PATHOLOGIC FINDINGS

- Many early cases of equine ulcerative keratitis initially present as minor corneal epithelial ulcers or infiltrates, with slight pain, blepharospasm, epiphora, and photophobia.
- At first, anterior uveitis and corneal vascularization may not be clinically pronounced.
- Superficial and deep corneal vascularization, and painful uveitis may occur. Extensive intrastromal lesions, vascularization, conjunctival injection, and corneal edema then may become evident.
- Corneal collagen breakdown or melting appears as a gelatinous, gray opacity at the margins and/or central regions of an ulcer.
- A descemetocele can be recognized as a clearing at the bottom of a deep ulcer. It does retain not fluorescein dye, whereas deep ulcers retain fluorescein.
- Deep penetration of the stroma to Descemet's membrane with perforation of the cornea is a possible sequela to all equine corneal ulcers.

TREATMENT

APPROPRIATE HEALTH CARE

- Always consider corneal ulceration an emergency. The equine cornea can rapidly deteriorate if ulcerated and is prone to infection.

- Employ subpalpebral or nasolacrimal lavage treatment systems for a fractious horse or one with a painful eye needing frequent therapy.

NURSING CARE

N/A

ACTIVITY

- Stall rest horses with corneal ulcers and secondary uveitis until the condition heals.
- Intraocular hemorrhage and increased severity of uveitis are sequelae to overexertion.

DIET

Should be consistent with the training level of the horse.

CLIENT EDUCATION

- A slowly progressive, indolent course often belies the seriousness of the ulcer.
- Corneal ulcers may rapidly progress to descemetoceles.
- Corneal ulcers often are very slow to heal.
- Anterior uveitis may be difficult to control.
- Corneal scarring and vascularization are common after ulceration.

SURGICAL CONSIDERATIONS

- Surgical placement of a conjunctival flap, corneoconjunctival transposition, or corneal transplantation may be indicated for rapidly progressive and deep corneal ulcers.
- Removing necrotic tissue by keratectomy speeds healing, minimizes scarring, and decreases the stimulus for iridocyclitis.
- Conjunctival grafts or flaps frequently are used for clinical management of deep, melting, and large corneal ulcers, descemetoceles, and perforated corneal ulcers both with and without iris prolapse.
- Nictitating membrane flaps are used for superficial corneal diseases, including corneal erosions, neuroparalytic and neurotropic keratitis, temporary exposure keratitis, and superficial corneal ulcers, and to reinforce bulbar conjunctival grafts.
- Panophthalmitis after perforation through a corneal stromal ulcer has a grave prognosis; to spare the affected horse this chronic discomfort, enucleation is the humane alternative.
- Persistent ulcers may need surgical debridement and grid keratotomy to remove the hyaline membrane that slows healing.

MEDICATIONS

DRUGS OF CHOICE

- Topically applied antibiotics (e.g., chloramphenicol, gentamicin, ciprofloxacin, or tobramycin ophthalmic solutions) may be used to treat bacterial ulcers. Amikacin (10 mg/ml) also may be used topically. Frequency of medication varies from q2–8h.
- Topically applied atropine (1–2%) is effective for stabilizing the blood–aqueous barrier, minimizing pain from ciliary muscle spasm, and causing pupillary dilatation. Atropine may used as often as q4h, with the frequency being reduced as soon as the pupil dilates.
- Topically administered autogenous serum is used in ulcers with evidence of collagenolysis, infection, or chronicity. The serum can be administered topically as often as possible and is replaced by new serum every 5 days. Acetylcysteine (10%) or sodium EDTA also can be administered until stromal liquefaction diminishes; in some horses, both acetylcysteine and serum may be needed to arrest melting.
- Systemic and topically administered NSAIDs (e.g., phenylbutazone [1 g PO BID] or flunixin meglumine [1 mg/kg IV, IM, or PO BID]) are effective in reducing uveal exudation and in relieving ocular discomfort from the anterior uveitis in horses with ulcers.

CONTRAINDICATIONS

Topical corticosteroids may encourage growth of bacterial and fungal opportunists by interfering with nonspecific inflammatory reactions and cellular immunity.

PRECAUTIONS

- Monitor horses receiving topically administered atropine for signs of colic.
- Intestinal hypomotility can be induced with topical atropine in a small percentage of horses.

POSSIBLE INTERACTIONS

N/A

ALTERNATIVE DRUGS

Autogenous serum administered topically can reduce tear film and corneal protease activity in equine corneal ulcers.

FOLLOW-UP

PATIENT MONITORING

- Monitor clarity of the cornea, depth and size of the ulcer, degree of corneal vascularization, amount of tearing, pupil size, and intensity of the anterior uveitis. Serial fluorescein staining of the ulcer is indicated to assess healing.
- As the cornea heals, the stimulus for the uveitis diminishes, and the pupil dilates with minimal atropine therapy.
- Reduce self-trauma by using hard or soft cup hoods.

PREVENTION/AVOIDANCE

Equine corneal ulcers, no matter how small or superficial, should be treated aggressively.

POSSIBLE COMPLICATIONS

Globe rupture, phthisis bulbi, and blindness are possible sequelae to equine corneal ulceration.

EXPECTED COURSE AND PROGNOSIS

- The typical equine corneal ulcer heals slowly and with scarring and has a strong tendency to vascularize.
- If replication and spread of bacteria are not halted by the host response or instillation of antibiotics, stromal degradation and melting ultimately lead to total loss of stromal tissue and to corneal perforation.
- Conjunctival flaps are necessary to save the globe and vision but are associated with scarring of the ulcer site. They generally are left in place 4–6 weeks.

MISCELLANEOUS

ASSOCIATED CONDITIONS

- Corneal infection and iridocyclitis are always major concerns, even with the slightest corneal ulcerations.
- Iridocyclitis or uveitis is present in all types of corneal ulcers and must be treated to preserve vision.

AGE-RELATED FACTORS

N/A

ZOONOTIC POTENTIAL

N/A

PREGNANCY

N/A

SYNONYMS

N/A

SEE ALSO

N/A

ABBREVIATION

- KCS = keratoconjunctivitis sicca

Suggested Reading

Brooks DE: Equine ophthalmology. In Gelatt KN, ed. Veterinary ophthalmology. 3rd ed. Philadelphia: Lippincott Williams & Wilkins, 1999.

Author Dennis E. Brooks

Consulting Editor Dennis E. Brooks

CORYNEBACTERIUM PSEUDOTUBERCULOSIS INFECTION

BASICS

DEFINITION

Several clinical manifestations of infection in the horse caused by the gram-positive bacterium *Corynebacterium pseudotuberculosis.* The three clinical presentations in the horse include cutaneous abscesses, most commonly of the pectoral and/or ventral regions; ulcerative lymphadenitis; and uncommonly, internal abscesses. The organism causes lymphadenitis and abscesses in sheep and goats.

PATHOPHYSIOLOGY

Corynebacterium pseudotuberculosis is a gram-positive facultative intracellular anaerobic rod that lives in the soil and survives well in the environment, especially in arid conditions. Mode of transmission is unknown, but thought to involve entry of the bacteria through wounds or abrasions in the skin, and then spreads in the body through the lymphatic system. Various insects have been investigated as possible vectors; however, none have been confirmed experimentally as the mode of transmission. Once in the body the bacteria is phagocytosed and is able to survive the host's defense mechanisms and replicate intracellularly. The incubation period is thought to be 3–4 weeks. Two factors are considered to contribute to the organism's ability to survive intracellularly: lipids in the organism's cell wall and a phospholipase D–protein exotoxin. The bacterial cell wall lipids are suspected to aid in survival in macrophages. The exotoxin helps fend off the host's defense systems by a variety of methods, including inhibiting neutrophil chemotaxis and reducing opsonization of the bacteria. Other effects of the exotoxin include increased vascular permeability and endothelium degradation, thereby increasing spread of infection both locally and along lymphatic tracts. This also results in localized edema. No theories have been postulated on why different forms of the disease exist.

Once the infection has resolved, there is a low rate of recurrence. It is believed that like sheep and goats, host resistance in horses includes both humoral and cell-mediated immune responses. Strains isolated from horses are distinct from strains that affect sheep and goats. Natural transmission between species does not seem to take place.

SYSTEM AFFECTED

Lymphatic and Associated Organs

Cutaneous abscesses generally occur in the pectoral region and/or along the ventral midline; however, abscesses can be found in a variety of other locations, such as the head, axillary, or inguinal regions and the mammary glands. Internal abscesses can arise anywhere in the body, including either or both the thoracic or abdominal cavities. These abscesses affect the organ system in which the infection is located—for example, the liver, pulmonary parenchyma, or the urogenital tract.

Ulcerative lymphangitis affects one or more limbs.

GENETICS

N/A

INCIDENCE/PREVALENCE

Geographic distribution of the cutaneous abscesses form of the disease is limited to the western United States and Brazil. Infection with *C. pseudotuberculosis* can occur at any time of the year, but in the western United States the highest incidence is during the fall (the dry time of the year). Although all ages of horses can be affected, the disease is most common in young horses between 6 months and 5 years of age.

Ulcerative lymphangitis has a sporadic worldwide distribution. This form can be endemic to a farm, and may affect several horses.

SIGNALMENT

Nonspecific

SIGNS

General Comments

Variable signs, depending on clinical form of the infection.

Historical Findings

Variable history, depending on the clinical form of infection. In cases of cutaneous abscesses and ulcerative lymphangitis, the origin of the problem is often more obvious than with internal abscesses. With these forms of infection, history of a non-healing wound is common. History with internal abscesses may be nonspecific, and include depression, weight loss, and/or fever of unknown origin.

CORYNEBACTERIUM PSEUDOTUBERCULOSIS INFECTION

Physical Examination Findings

Cutaneous abscesses:
- Focal swelling(s), typically in the pectoral region or along the ventral midline
- Fever
- Lameness, especially notable with deep abscesses in the axilla or inguinal regions
- Ventral midline dermatitis
- Weight loss
- Depression
- Anorexia
- Mastitis

Internal abscesses:
- Fever
- Weight loss
- Colic
- Depression
- Ventral edema
- Ventral midline dermatitis
- Anorexia
- Nasal discharge
- Rarely, hematuria, ataxia, or abortion

Ulcerative lymphangitis:
- Hot, painful, and swollen limb(s) with small ulcerative nodules and/or multiple small abscesses
- Fever
- Lameness
- Depression
- Anorexia

CAUSE

Infection with *C. pseudotuberculosis.*

RISK FACTORS

- Wounds
- Ventral midline dermatitis
- Poor hygiene
- Endemic regions

DIAGNOSIS

DIFFERENTIAL DIAGNOSIS

Other causes of pectoral swelling:
- Trauma-induced hematoma or seroma.
- Foreign body

Other etiologic agents causing cutaneous abscesses in the horse include *Streptococcus equi* var *S. zooepidemicus, Actinobacillus equuli,* and in particular with submandibular abscesses, *Streptococcus equi* var *equi* (strangles).

Other causes of weight loss, ventral edema, and fever include neoplasia and pleural pneumonia.

Other causes of cellulitis/lymphangitis with nodules in one or more limb include:
- Cutaneous glanders or farcy, a rare disease caused by *Pseudomonas mallei.*
- Epizootic lymphangitis caused by the fungus *Histoplasma farciminosus.*
- Sporotrichosis caused by the fungus *Sporothrix schenckii.*
- Pythiosis (swamp cancer) caused by the protozoal organism *Pythium insidiosum*

Most of these infectious causes of lymphangitis are not common and are restricted geographically. Other bacteria, such as *Pseudomonas aeruginosa* and staphylococcal and streptococcal species, have been implicated as etiologic agents in lymphangitis.

CBC/BIOCHEMISTRY/URINALYSIS

Inflammatory leukocyte response. Typically a leukocytosis with a neutrophilia, hyperfibrinogenemia, and hyperproteinemia. Anemia of chronic disease is common, especially with internal abscesses. Results of serum biochemistry panel and urinalysis are usually normal. However, abnormalities may be noted due to local effects of infection—for example, increased liver enzyme activity with abscesses localized to the hepatic region.

OTHER LABORATORY TESTS

- Gram's stain of exudate from abscess aspiration reveals gram-positive pleomorphic rods.
- Culture of exudate
- The exudate is characteristically tan in color and odorless. The organism yields growth of small, white, opaque colonies readily on blood agar in 24–48 hr.
- Synergistic hemolysis inhibition (SHI) test measures the host's antibody (IgG) titer to an exotoxin of *C. pseudotuberculosis.* Interpretation of results from this test can be confusing. A positive titer indicates exposure to the bacteria and not necessarily disease; however, a titer >256–512 is thought to be indicative of active infection. Also, false-negative results can occur, especially with cutaneous abscesses.

IMAGING

Ultrasonographic examination is helpful to aid in diagnosis and help localize deep cutaneous and some internal abscesses.

CORYNEBACTERIUM PSEUDOTUBERCULOSIS INFECTION

DIAGNOSTIC PROCEDURES

Rectal evaluation to aid diagnosis of internal abscesses, possibly with trans-rectal imaging. Also, consider analysis of peritoneal fluid. Other diagnostic methods sometimes helpful in diagnosing internal abscesses include culture of tracheal aspirate and blood culture. In some cases of internal abdominal abscesses, surgical exploration may be required to document the presence of an abscess. If an abscess is noted during surgical exploration, it is prudent to obtain an aspirate if possible for culture to aid in identifying an etiologic agent.

PATHOLOGIC FINDINGS

Thick-walled abscesses with tan odorless exudate in a wide variety of locations.

TREATMENT

APPROPRIATE HEALTH CARE

Isolation of an infected animal has not been shown to be necessary; however, removal of exudative material from drained abscesses, proper disposal of contaminated bedding, insect control, and good hygiene practices should all be recommended. The diagnostic work-up needed to demonstrate the presence of an internal abscess may entail hospitalization. Both internal abscesses and ulcerative lymphangitis cases require long-term antimicrobial therapy; therefore, reliable client compliance is needed.

NURSING CARE

Cutaneous Abscesses

Hot pack or apply a poultice agent to abscessed areas until they soften to allow drainage. Once the abscess is open, daily irrigation is recommended.

Ulcerative Lymphangitis

- Keep affected limbs clean and dry.
- Attempt to decrease swelling with hydrotherapy, massage, and bandaging.
- In all situations, good hygiene practices should be followed.

ACTIVITY

Ulcerative lymphangitis cases may benefit from enforced light exercise (hand walking) to help decrease limb edema.

DIET

Offer a variety of feeds if the animal is anorexic.

CLIENT EDUCATION

Stress good sanitation practices and insect control.

SURGICAL CONSIDERATIONS

Once a cutaneous abscess is mature, it is recommended to surgically lance, drain, and lavage. Some internal abscesses can be resolved with surgical drainage or rarely with marsupialization.

MEDICATIONS

DRUG(S) OF CHOICE

Antimicrobial Agents

In vitro sensitivities generally indicate the organism to be susceptible to most all commonly used antimicrobials. However, selection of an appropriate drug requires consideration of several factors, including location of the abscess, expected duration of treatment, and safety and ease of administration. Successful treatment has been seen with procaine penicillin (20,000 IU/kg IM BID) or potassium penicillin (20,000–40,000 IU/kg IV QID) used alone or in combination with a potentiated sulfa agent (15 mg/kg PO BID). Also, the use of erythromycin estolate (15 mg/kg BID to TID) has been recommended. Rifampin (2.5–5 mg/kg PO BID) used in combination with any one of the drugs listed above is a good choice for treatment of internal abscesses.

CONTRAINDICATIONS

The use of antimicrobials for cutaneous abscesses is controversial. Their use instead of external drainage of the abscess likely does not shorten the recovery period, and may even prolong it.

PRECAUTIONS

Rifampin is often an excellent antimicrobial choice, but should not be used alone because of the rapid development of resistance. When using any antimicrobial in the horse, the animal should be monitored for the development of diarrhea.

POSSIBLE INTERACTIONS

N/A

ALTERNATIVE DRUGS

Nonsteroidal agents such as phenylbutazone or flunixin meglumine at standard dosages may aid in reducing inflammation and pain.

FOLLOW-UP

PATIENT MONITORING

With internal abscesses, following abnormal parameters, such as fibrinogen concentration or ultrasonographic appearance of the abscess, is helpful to determine the duration of antimicrobial administration.

CORYNEBACTERIUM PSEUDOTUBERCULOSIS INFECTION

PREVENTION/AVOIDANCE

Because mode of transmission is poorly understood, definitive recommendations are difficult to make. Removing any drainage expressed, insect control, and good hygiene is recommended. Autologous vaccines have been use in a limited number of cases in the horse. No studies have been performed to test their effectiveness or safety.

POSSIBLE COMPLICATIONS

- Failure of antimicrobial treatment to affect a cure with internal abcesses.
- Laminitis, especially in the contra-lateral limb in horses affected with ulcerative lymphangitis.

EXPECTED COURSE AND PROGNOSIS

Prognosis for full recovery in cases of cutaneous abscesses is very good. Prognosis for internal abscess and ulcerative lymphangitis is more guarded, and typically requires long-term (several months minimum) treatment. Ulcerative lymphangitis cases have intermittent recurrence of lymphangitis due to permanent damage to lymphatic drainage.

MISCELLANEOUS

ASSOCIATED CONDITIONS

N/A

AGE-RELATED FACTORS

Low incidence of the disease in foals >6 months of age is consistent with possible protection via passive transfer of specific antibodies from previously exposed mares.

ZOONOTIC POTENTIAL

No reports of infection transmitted from a horse to a human were found in a limited search of the literature, but there are sporadic reports of people infected from outbreaks of caseous lymphadenitis in sheep. The risk of transmission was increased in immuno-suppressed individuals.

PREGNANCY

Report of abortion in a mare related to infection with *C. pseudotuberculosis.*

SYNONYMS

- Pigeon fever
- Pigeon breast
- Dryland distemper
- Colorado or Wyoming strangles

SEE ALSO

N/A

ABBREVIATIONS

- *C. pseudotuberculosis* = *Corynebacterium pseudotuberculosis*
- SHI = synergistic hemolysis inhibition

Suggested Reading

Aleman M, et al. *Corynebacterium pseudotuberculosis* infection in horses: 538 cases (1982–1993). J Am Vet Med Assoc 1996;209:804-809.

Davis EW. *Corynebacterium pseudotuberculosis* infection in animals. In: Smith BP, ed. Large animal internal medicine, 2nd ed. St. Louis: Mosby, 1996:1251-1257.

Doherr MG, et al. Evaluation of temporal and spatial clustering of horses with *Corynebacterium pseudotuberculosis* infection. Am J Vet Res 1999; 60:284-291.

Somerville B, et al. Subcutaneous abscesses caused by *Corynebacterium pseudotuberculosis.* In: Robinson NE, ed. Current therapy in equine medicine 4. Philadelphia: WB Saunders, 1997:393–395.

Author Peggy S. Marsh

Consulting Editor Corinne R. Sweeney

COUGH

BASICS

DEFINITION

A sudden, forceful, noisy expulsion of air through the glottis to clear mucus, particles, and other material from the tracheobronchial tree and glottis.

PATHOPHYSIOLOGY

- This reflex is a protective respiratory defense mechanism that, together with the mucociliary escalator, clears undesired material from the tracheobronchial tree proximal to the level of segmental bronchi.
- Initiated by stimulation of irritant receptors that ramify between epithelial cells from the level of the larynx down to the distal bronchioles and by receptors located in the lung parenchyma and pleura.
- Receptors are stimulated by mechanical deformation, chemically inert dusts, foreign bodies, pollutant gases, inflammatory conditions, and chemical mediators—histamine.
- Afferent and efferent components of the reflex are co-ordinated by centers in the medulla oblongata.
- Cough begins with a deep inspiration, which is followed (in sequence) by an inspiratory pause, closure of the glottis, relaxation of the diaphragm synchronous with contraction of intercostal and abdominal musculature against the closed glottis to increase intrathoracic pressure, and finally, rapid opening of the glottis to permit expulsion of air at high velocity.

SYSTEMS AFFECTED

- Respiratory
- Musculoskeletal
- Cardiovascular
- Nervous

SIGNALMENT

- All ages, breeds, and sexes.
- Particular causes have a specific or general age predilection.
- Aspiration pneumonia is more common in neonatal foals.
- Pneumonia caused by *Rhodococcus equi* and other bacteria is most common in foals aged from 4 weeks and 6 months.
- Viral infections are most common in weanlings, yearlings, and young adult performance horses.
- Heaves is most common in mature horses stabled in dusty environments.

SIGNS

Historical Findings

Season and Activity:

- Cough associated with heaves typically has a higher incidence from autumn through early spring, when horses are confined indoors.
- Summer pasture-associated obstructive airway disease and bacterial pneumonia in foals typically occur during late spring and summer.
- Influenza and other viral respiratory infections may have a seasonal pattern, reflecting circumstances in which horses from different sources congregate at shows, sales, and performance events.
- Lungworm infection occurs in horses cograzed with donkeys or mules, which typically happens during late spring and summer in temperate zones and during winter and early spring in arid climates with winter rainfall.
- Recent prolonged transportation, viral infection, strenuous exercise, or anesthesia are common historical features of horses with pleuropneumonia.

Housing and Feeding Practices:

- Cough associated with heaves occurs primarily in stabled horses fed hay and bedded on straw in poorly ventilated buildings.
- Silicosis typically occurs in horses fed on the ground or grazed in bare, dusty paddocks in areas such as the Monterey Peninsula of California, which have exposed crystobalite silica shale.

Speed of Onset, Contagiousness, Duration, and Characteristics:

- May suggest the underlying cause.
- Sudden onset and rapid spread are characteristics of viral infection, particularly influenza and EHV.
- Cough-associated aspiration of food or a foreign body into the tracheobronchial tree is sudden in onset but does not spread to affect other horses.
- Gradual onset and chronic course are typical for lower airway inflammatory disease, heaves, interstitial pneumonia, fungal pneumonia, and thoracic neoplasia.
- Cough associated with lungworm infection typically has a sudden onset and chronic course, may affect multiple horses, but does not have the rapid pattern of spread characteristic of highly contagious diseases.
- Onset in bacterial pneumonia and pleuropneumonia may be sudden or gradual, and more than one foal or horse may be affected.
- Harsh, persistent cough suggests involvement of the major airways or exudate in the large airways secondary to pulmonary disease or aspiration.
- Soft, infrequent cough often reflects early heaves, interstitial lung disease, or pulmonary edema secondary to cardiac failure.
- Guarded cough is a feature of inflammatory pleural disease (e.g., pleuropneumonia) and of painful pharyngeal or laryngeal disease (e.g., strangles, epiglottic ulceration, laryngeal foreign body).
- Productive cough frequently is reflected by swallowing movements afterward or by nasal discharge.

• Productive cough typically suggests fluid or mucus in large airways, whereas dry cough often indicates airway inflammation or foreign body without excess production of mucus or fluid.
• Exercise or activity frequently precipitates cough caused by many conditions, particularly those associated with airway irritation or fluid accumulation in airways. Cough associated only with exercise, however, often is a feature of EIPH or lower airway inflammatory disease, including early heaves.

Physical Examination Findings

• Fever—usually indicates a primary infectious cause or secondary infection superimposed on a noninfectious cause; a typical, but not invariable, feature of aspiration pneumonia, bacterial pneumonia, pulmonary abscess, viral respiratory tract infection, strangles, fungal pneumonia, pleuropneumonia (e.g., bacterial, viral, mycoplasmal), acute bronchointerstitial pneumonia, and thoracic neoplasia.
• No fever—typically found in heaves, abnormalities of the larynx or pharynx (other than retropharyngeal abscess), parasitic pneumonia, EIPH, tracheobronchial foreign body, tracheal collapse, and airway-oriented neoplasia (e.g., bronchial carcinoma).
• Food return via the nose—typically indicates esophageal obstruction (i.e., choke), aspiration of food secondary to anatomic or neurologic derangement in the upper airway, severe pharyngeal inflammation (e.g., in acute strangles), or cleft palate.
• Pleurodynia—typically occurs with pleuropneumonia and other less common pleural inflammatory diseases.
• Nasal discharge—reflects disease characterized by exudation or drainage of mucus or purulent exudate into the lower airways or, less commonly, aspiration of exudate draining into the pharynx or nasal passages secondary to guttural pouch or sinus disease.

CAUSES

Upper Respiratory Tract Diseases

• Nasopharyngeal—rhinitis; sinusitis; pharyngitis/pharyngeal lymphoid hyperplasia; nasopharyngeal foreign body, cyst, hematoma, or tumor; strangles; cleft palate; dorsal or rostral displacement of the soft palate; guttural pouch empyema, tympany, or mycosis.
• Laryngeal—hemiplegia, inflammation, epiglottic entrapment, epiglottic ulcer, foreign body, injuries, chondritis of the arytenoid cartilages, tumors, previous laryngeal or pharyngeal surgery (e.g., laryngeal prosthesis, staphylectomy).
• Tracheal—inflammation (e.g., inhalation of irritating substances, heat, smoke inhalation), infection (e.g., viral, bacterial), foreign body, collapse, and tumor.

Lower Respiratory Tract Diseases

• Bronchial—inflammation, infection (e.g., viral, bacterial, parasitic), allergy, foreign body, and tumor.
• Pulmonary—inflammation, infection (e.g., viral, bacterial, fungal, parasitic), allergic (e.g., heaves, summer pasture-associated obstructive pulmonary disease), aspiration pneumonia, pulmonary edema, tumor, acute bronchointerstitial pneumonia, pneumoconiosis (e.g., silica or other inorganic dusts), and granulomatous pneumonia.
• Pulmonary vascular—thrombosis/embolism, congestive cardiac failure, and pulmonary hypertension.
• Pleural—inflammation, infection (e.g., bacterial, fungal), hernia, and tumor.

Other Diseases

Esophageal—obstruction (e.g., choke caused by foreign body, stricture, diverticulum, motility disorder), ulceration, inflammation, and tumor.

RISK FACTORS

• Prolonged transportation predisposes to pleuropneumonia.
• Indoor housing in dusty environments, feeding of dusty hay, use of dusty bedding, and previous viral respiratory infection may predispose to heaves.
• Viral respiratory infection predisposes to bacterial pneumonia and pleuropneumonia.
• Hot, dry, dusty outdoor conditions predispose foals to *R. equi* pneumonia.
• Mixing with other horses at shows, sales, and events predisposes to viral infections and strangles.
• Cograzing with donkeys or mules predisposes to lungworm infection.
• High ambient temperature or transportation of foals during hot weather predisposes to acute bronchointerstitial pneumonia.
• Poor parasite-control regimens predispose to parasitic pneumonitis resulting from ascarid migration.
• Congenital or acquired pharyngeal, palatal, and esophageal disorders and corrective upper airway surgery (e.g., laryngeal prosthesis) predispose to aspiration pneumonia.

DIAGNOSIS

DIFFERENTIAL DIAGNOSIS

Differentiating Similar Signs

Because horses do not sneeze or vomit like humans or small animals, cough is not easily confused with other signs.

COUGH

Differentiating Causes

See the sections on historical findings, physical examination findings, and risk factors.

CBC/BIOCHEMISTRY/URINALYSIS

- CBC typically is normal in noninflammatory diseases, whereas neutrophilia, with or without a left shift, and hyperfibrinogenemia are common in inflammatory diseases, particularly those caused by infection.
- Eosinophilia is not typical of equine allergic airway disease (e.g., heaves) but is a common finding in lungworm infection and some horses with granulomatous interstitial lung disease.
- Serum globulin concentrations frequently are elevated in chronic inflammatory disease involving the lungs or pleura.

OTHER LABORATORY TESTS

- Serologic tests—for equine influenza, EHV-4, EHV-1, or equine viral arteritis.
- Arterial blood gases in patients with signs of respiratory distress or cyanosis.

IMAGING

- Thoracic ultrasonography in patients with suspected pulmonary consolidation, pulmonary abscesses or other masses, inflammatory pleural disease, pleural effusion, primary cardiac disease, and right heart disease secondary to a pulmonary condition.
- Thoracic radiography (i.e., lateral projections) for differentiating types of lower respiratory tract disorders, particularly those involving consolidation, mass lesions, infiltrative interstitial disease, and pleural effusion.
- Radiography of the nasal passages, pharynx, larynx, guttural pouches, retropharyngeal structures, proximal esophagus, and trachea also may provide useful information.

OTHER DIAGNOSTIC PROCEDURES

- Endoscopy of the upper airway, guttural pouches, trachea, and bronchi detects anatomic, physiologic, and pathologic lesions and the source of discharges.
- Bronchoalveolar lavage and collection of biopsy specimens of lesions or airway walls can be performed via the endoscope during bronchoscopy.
- Collection of nasal or nasopharyngeal swabs from horses with acute onset cough and fever help to establish the diagnosis of acute viral infection and strangles. Diagnostic tests such as antigen-capture ELISA for influenza and PCR for herpesviruses, supplemented by viral isolation and serology, facilitate rapid diagnosis of viral infection. Bacterial culture of nasal swabs does not yield useful information in horses with lower airway disease but is important for early diagnosis of strangles.
- Transtracheal aspiration with cytology and culture for evaluation of lower respiratory tract disorders, particularly those in which an infectious agent is suspected to be the cause.
- Bronchoalveolar lavage with cytology for evaluation of lower respiratory tract disorders, particularly those that are diffusely distributed and have a noninfectious cause—heaves, inflammatory lower airway disease, silicosis, and granulomatous lung disease.
- Thoracocentesis with cytology if pleural effusion is present. Culture and determination of pH, LDH, and glucose concentration in aspirated fluid help to differentiate septic from nonseptic exudates.
- Direct and flotation fecal tests (e.g., Baermann) to detect respiratory parasites and ova; however, lungworm infection rarely is patent. Testing of donkeys or mules cograzed with affected horses may document asymptomatic infestation and shedding of lungworm ova.
- Lung biopsy and histologic examination is indicated for horses with suspected or confirmed diffuse, nonseptic lung disease or discreet pulmonary masses resembling tumors.
- Echocardiography and electrocardiography in patients with evidence of cardiac disease.

TREATMENT

- Horses presented with cough usually can be evaluated and managed as outpatients, unless respiratory distress, profound hypoxemia, serious choke, pleural effusion, pulmonary infarction, or congestive cardiac failure also are features of the disease process.
- Housing in a dust-free environment and exercise restriction are best until a cause for the cough is established and corrected, especially when activity aggravates the cough.
- Horses with suspected viral respiratory disease and contacts in the same airspace should be isolated as a group, either in the location currently occupied by the sick horses or in a separate isolation facility. Do not allow other horses to enter the same airspace occupied by sick horses.
- Inform owners that a wide variety of conditions can be responsible for the cough, and that a fairly extensive workup may be required to define and treat the underlying cause.

COUGH

MEDICATIONS

DRUGS OF CHOICE

Treatment is directed at the suspected or confirmed underlying cause rather than at attempting symptomatic relief by using cough suppressants (see relevant sections on individual diseases).

CONTRAINDICATIONS

- Do not use corticosteroids, except in foals with acute respiratory distress syndrome (i.e., acute bronchointerstitial pneumonia), unless allergic disease, hyperreactive airway disease, or anaphylaxis is suspected or confirmed and evidence of infection, parasitic infestation, or cardiac disease is lacking.
- Do not use cough suppressants with any patient in which a respiratory infection or clinically significant heart disease is suspected.

PRECAUTIONS

- Cough suppressants—indiscriminate use may obscure warning signs of serious pulmonary or cardiac disorders and predispose to life-threatening complications.
- Bronchodilator therapy may exacerbate hypoxemia in patients with V/Q mismatch secondary to pulmonary consolidation or edema.

POSSIBLE INTERACTIONS

N/A

ALTERNATIVE DRUGS

N/A

FOLLOW-UP

PATIENT MONITORING

- Regularly communicate with owners regarding resolution of the disease process concerning cough.
- Cough may persist for several weeks after resolution of other signs in horses with infectious respiratory disease, because restoration of normal structure and function in the respiratory mucosa take several weeks.
- Continue exercise restriction until the cough disappears.

POSSIBLE COMPLICATIONS

Some diseases that cause cough also can induce prolonged or permanent respiratory dysfunction and even death.

MISCELLANEOUS

ASSOCIATED CONDITIONS

N/A

AGE-RELATED FACTORS

See discussion of historical findings.

ZOONOTIC POTENTIAL

N/A

PREGNANCY

N/A

SYNONYMS

N/A

SEE ALSO

- See the section on causes.
- Nasal discharge
- Respiratory distress
- Tachypnea

ABBREVIATIONS

- EHV = equine herpes virus
- EIPH = exercise-induced pulmonary hemorrhage
- ELISA = enzyme-linked immunoadsorbent assay
- LDH = lactate dehydrogenase
- PCR = polymerase chain reaction
- V/Q = ventilation-perfusion ratio

Suggested Reading

Kopos J, Tomori Z. Cough and other respiratory reflexes. Prog Resp Rec 1979;12:15–188.

Wilson WD, Lofstedt J. Cough. In: Smith BP, ed. Large animal internal medicine. 2nd ed. St. Louis: Mosby, 1996:46–53.

Author W. David Wilson

Consulting Editor Jean-Pierre Lavoie

CREATINE KINASE (CK)

BASICS

DEFINITION

Serum CK activity significantly greater than the upper limit of the reference interval provided by the laboratory.

PATHOPHYSIOLOGY

- Increased serum activity indicates increased leakage from muscle—cardiac or skeletal.
- The condition may or may not be reversible.
- Three CK isoenzymes are known.
- Isoenzymes are found in many tissues, but most serum CK originates from skeletal and cardiac muscle, making it essentially muscle specific.
- Analysis of individual isoenzymes, although useful in assessing human cardiac disease, has minimal benefit in differentiating equine myocardial disease from skeletal muscle disease.
- Plasma half-life of CK is <2 hours in horses.
- After injury, serum activity typically peaks within 12 hours and returns to normal in 2–3 days (or, sometimes, as long as 7 days), provided the damage is not active and persistent.

SYSTEMS AFFECTED

- Increased serum activity is a result of a pathologic condition, not a cause.
- Systems affected in a given patient depend on the cause of the increased CK, not on the increased CK per se.

SIGNALMENT

- Depends on the specific cause.
- With polysaccharide storage disease, onset occurs at an early age, and there may be a familial pattern in Quarter Horses and Belgian Draft Horses.
- Hyperkalemic periodic paralysis generally is seen in Quarter Horses.
- Otherwise, no convincing predilections for age, breed, or sex.

SIGNS

Historical Findings

- Trauma
- Recent injections (up to 1 week previously)
- Surgery or recumbency
- Vigorous exercise, particularly after periods of rest
- Discolored urine
- Incorrect or difficult venipuncture
- Seizures
- Exposure to feed containing monensin
- Halothane anesthesia
- Vitamin E/selenium–deficient feed

Physical Examination Findings

- Muscle pain, reluctance to move or gait abnormality, recumbency, and seizure activity—skeletal muscle origin.
- Exercise intolerance—cardiac or muscle origin.

CAUSES

Musculoskeletal

- Exertional rhabdomyolysis—azoturia, myositis, tying-up; chronic or acute
- Trauma
- Prolonged recumbency
- Recent injections
- Improper venipuncture
- Exercise/endurance event
- Clostridial myositis
- Equine influenza
- Streptococcal infection—purpura hemorrhagica
- Surgery
- Vitamin E/selenium deficiency—nutritional myodegeneration
- Hyperthermia
- Malignant hyperthermia secondary to halothane anesthesia
- Capture myopathy
- Electric shock
- Hyperkalemic periodic paralysis
- Polysaccharide storage disease
- Lower motor neuron disease

Cardiovascular

- Traumatic myocarditis
- Monensin-induced myocardial degeneration
- Bacterial endocarditis
- Cardiomyopathy

Nervous

- Disorders resulting in seizures, excessive muscular activity, or prolonged recumbency.
- **NOTE**: the serum CK is of muscular origin.

RISK FACTORS

- Improper conditioning
- Heavy training after prolonged rest
- Prolonged recumbency from any cause
- Monensin administration
- Trauma
- Medications administered by IM injection
- Seizures
- Poor nutrition

DIAGNOSIS

DIFFERENTIAL DIAGNOSIS

- History and physical examination (e.g., firm, swollen muscles; sweating; increased heart rate, body temperature, or respiratory rate) and degree of CK increase may suggest exertional rhabdomyolysis or capture myopathy and rule out other causes for gait abnormalities or discomfort.
- History and physical examination may indicate trauma, recent injections, or prolonged recumbency.
- Systemic signs and CBC, comprehensive chemistry profile, and urinalysis may suggest metabolic or infectious causes for recumbency, myositis, or endocarditis.
- A thorough history may elucidate recent IM injections, recent surgery, traumatic myocarditis, monensin toxicosis, cardiac causes (e.g., exercise intolerance), and seizures.
- Signalment is helpful in identifying polysaccharide storage disease.
- Signalment plus serum potassium determinations during an episode or induction of an episode by oral potassium challenge may suggest hyperkalemic periodic paralysis (**NOTE**: CK will be normal to moderately increased).
- If multiple farm animals are affected and feed quality is poor, suspect vitamin E/selenium deficiency.

LABORATORY FINDINGS

Drugs That May Alter Lab Results

N/A

Disorders That May Alter Lab Results

- Improper sample handling (consult with laboratory); gross hemolysis.
- Very high serum activity itself can alter reported values, because serum contains inhibitors of CK activity. Sample dilution may be necessary to bring extremely high values into the range of linearity for the instrument, but the resultant reduction in serum volume fraction reduces the inhibitor concentrations, resulting in higher CK values. This becomes important when CK values are monitored over time, because the actual value obtained from a diluted sample may not be accurate.

Valid if Run in Human Lab?

Yes

CBC/BIOCHEMISTRY/URINALYSIS

- Increased fibrinogen (with or without inflammatory leukogram) may be present with infectious causes, and physiologic leukocytosis may be present in horses that are excited, nervous, or in pain from myonecrosis.
- Increased AST often is seen with increased CK, depending on the time course.
- Initially, CK increases (peaks in 5–12 hours), and if muscle damage is not continuous, CK returns to baseline (usually by 2–3 days, but sometimes as long as 7 days).
- AST may take several days to peak, has a more modest increase, and takes longer to return to baseline (may take several weeks).
- Samples should be taken over time, because increases in CK and AST indicate recent/active muscle damage.
- If CK remains increased, myonecrosis is ongoing; if AST remains increased but CK is falling, myonecrosis is not likely to be progressing.

CREATINE KINASE (CK)

- The degree of increase in CK may be helpful.
- Modest increases (<1000 IU/L), usually in the absence of increased AST, occur in normal horses from training, transport, or exercise.
- Endurance events may increase CK to >1000 IU/L, but activities generally return to baseline within 24–48 hours.
- Improper venipuncture and IM injections result in relatively mild to moderate increases, but values in more extensive myonecrosis (e.g., vitamin E/Selenium deficiency, exertional rhabdomyolysis) generally are well into the thousands and may exceed 100,000 IU/L.
- In milder forms of chronic exertional rhabdomyolysis, CK may be <1500–10,000 IU/L.
- Hyperkalemic periodic paralysis results in normal to moderately increased serum activity, even during an episode.
- Acid–base status is variable, depending on the cause and progression of myopathy.
- Moderate to severe myonecrosis results in myoglobinuria, regardless of the cause, but the absence of myoglobinuria does not rule out mild forms of chronic exertional rhabdomyolysis.

OTHER LABORATORY TESTS

Vitamin E/selenium determinations when indicated.

IMAGING

Scintigraphy for localizing muscle pathology.

DIAGNOSTIC PROCEDURES

- Biopsy for histopathology or muscle function tests to identify subtle cases of chronic exertional rhabdomyolysis or polysaccharide storage disease. The laboratory must specialize in muscle evaluation and be consulted before sample collection.
- Electromyography to rule out neuromuscular disease; also helpful in hyperkalemic periodic paralysis.

TREATMENT

- Supportive care includes minimizing movement, diminishing pain and anxiety, and maintaining fluid and electrolyte balance.
- IV fluid therapy with balanced electrolytes is indicated with moderate to severe cases, especially if myoglobinuria or sweating is present.
- Continue IV fluids at least until hydration is restored and urine is clear.

MEDICATIONS

DRUGS OF CHOICE

- No drug therapy is needed to specifically reduce CK, because increased serum activity is not harmful per se.
- With acute, severe myonecrosis, medications that reduce pain and anxiety may be of benefit—flunixin meglumine (1 mg/kg IV), ketoprofen (0.5 mg/kg), or phenylbutazone.
- Acepromazine at low doses for vasodilation and anxiety relief.
- With extreme pain, IV butorphanol (0.01–0.020 mg/kg) combined with xylazine (0.3–0.6 mg/kg) or detomidine (0.005–0.020 mg/kg).
- Recumbent, violent horses may be treated with phenobarbital by slow IV infusion to effect.
- Dantrolene sodium (recommended dosage varies by author: 2 or 10 mg/kg as a loading dose; alternatively, 2.5 mg/kg q1h) diluted in normal saline and administered by stomach tube to reduce calcium release from sarcoplasmic reticulum.

CONTRAINDICATIONS

Diuretics in muscle necrosis.

PRECAUTIONS

- Avoid phenylbutazone in cases of myoglobinuria because of potential renal toxicity.
- Do not treat for acid–base abnormalities without blood gas data, because patients could be acidotic or alkalotic.
- Acepromazine at high doses is not recommended overall and is contraindicated at any dose in dehydration.
- If phenobarbital is used, titrate the dose to the patient.

FOLLOW-UP

PATIENT MONITORING

- CK and AST determinations over several days—during the initial episode, 24–48 hours later, and several days to a week after that. Reassessment if parameters have not normalized.
- BUN, creatinine, and electrolyte determinations at similar timepoints to monitor renal and electrolyte status and response to therapy in cases of moderate to severe myonecrosis.

POSSIBLE COMPLICATIONS

- None solely caused by increased serum activity.
- Myoglobin released from damaged muscles can cause irreversible renal failure without aggressive supportive care.

MISCELLANEOUS

AGE-RELATED FACTORS

None known

ZOONOTIC POTENTIAL

None known

PREGNANCY

N/A

SYNONYMS

Creatinine phosphokinase

SEE ALSO

- Myoglobin
- See *Causes.*

ABBREVATIONS

AST = aspartate aminotransferase

Suggested Reading

Beech J. Chronic exertional rhabdomyolysis. Vet Clin North Am Equine Pract 1997;13:145–168.

Cardinet GH. Skeletal muscle function. In: Kaneko JJ, Harvey JW, Bruss ML, eds. Clinical biochemistry of domestic animals. 5th ed. San Diego: Academic Press, 1997.

Duncan JR, Prasse KW, Mahaffey EA. Muscle. In: Veterinary laboratory medicine. 3rd ed. Ames: Iowa State University Press, 1994.

Spier SJ, Carlson GP, Holliday TA, Cardinet GH, Pickar DC. Hyperkalemic periodic paralysis in horses. J Am Vet Med Assoc 1990;197:1009–1017.

Valberg SJ, Hodgson DR. Diseases of muscle. In: Smith BP, ed. Large animal internal medicine. St. Louis: Mosby, 1996.

Author Ellen W. Evans

Consulting Editor Claire B. Andreasen

CRYPTOCOCCAL MENINGOENCEPHALOMYELITIS

BASICS

DEFINITION
Meningoencephalomyelitis associated with the encapsulated, yeast-like fungus *Cryptococcus neoformans.*

PATHOPHYSIOLOGY
Meningeal and cerebral localization occurs after hematogenous or direct spread from a benign or clinical focus in the respiratory tract.

SYSTEMS AFFECTED
- CNS—rarely involved
- Extraneural associated abnormalities are most common with myxomatous lesions of the lips, nasal cavity, paranasal sinuses, ocular orbits, intestinal tract, lungs, and skin.

SIGNALMENT
No associated signalment.

SIGNS
Physical Examination Findings:
- Signs may be acute or insidious in onset, but usually progress.
- Signs typical of diffuse meningitis, with dementia, blindness, dysphagia, hyperesthesia, and rigidity, are common.
- Signs progress to weakness, recumbency, convulsions, coma, and death.
- Unusual cases involve signs consistent with spinal cord gray matter, which can include muscle atrophy.
- Pelvic limb-gait abnormalities, atony, areflexia of the tail and anus, and perineal hypalgesia can occur.

CAUSES
- Meningoencephalomyelitis associated with the encapsulated, yeast-like fungus. *Cryptococcus neoformans*
- *C. neoformans* is a saprophyte commonly found in soil and feces, especially in feces of pigeons and chickens.

RISK FACTORS
Exposure to feces of pigeons and chickens.

DIAGNOSIS

DIFFERENTIAL DIAGNOSIS
Other diseases that may cause similar clinical signs, including viral and bacterial encephalitides.

CBC/BIOCHEMISTRY/URINALYSIS
No specific associated changes.

OTHER LABORATORY TESTS
N/A

IMAGING
N/A

DIAGNOSTIC PROCEDURES
- India ink preparation or routine laboratory stain of CSF samples can be examined cytopathologically antemortem.
- Clinical CNS signs and the findings of large, oval to round, encapsulated organisms are highly suggestive.
- A positive latex-agglutination test for cryptococcal antigen in the CSF has been developed.
- Clinical evidence of peripheral cryptococcal masses is highly suggestive.

PATHOLOGIC FINDINGS

Gross Findings

Myxomatous masses within the CNS and extraneural tissues.

Histopathologic Findings

- Characteristic budding, yeast-like organisms in the meninges, surrounding blood vessels in the brain parenchyma, or within lesions in the brain or spinal cord.
- Cellular reaction to cryptococcal organisms is predominantly mononuclear and characterized by lymphocytes and giant cells.

TREATMENT
None available

MEDICATIONS

DRUGS OF CHOICE
- Treatment does not seem to be effective.
- In humans, the disease is treated effectively by combined systemic and intrathecal administration of amphotericin B and flucytosine, alone or in combination, for a minimum of 6–10 weeks.
- A suggested, but unproven, regimen for a 450-kg horse is amphotericin B (100–150 mg) in 4 L of 5% dextrose administered on alternate days for at least 6 weeks.
- In addition, amphotericin B (5–15 mg) could be administered intrathecally, under anesthesia, once weekly for at least the first 4 weeks.

CRYPTOCOCCAL MENINGOENCEPHALOMYELITIS

CONTRAINDICATIONS
N/A

PRECAUTIONS
- Side effects of treatments with amphotericin B—systemic nephrotoxicity; topical neurotoxicity.
- Avoid contact with infected tissues and secretions.

POSSIBLE INTERACTIONS
N/A

ALTERNATIVE DRUGS
N/A

FOLLOW-UP

PATIENT MONITORING
Poor prognosis

POSSIBLE COMPLICATIONS
Trauma associated with dementia is likely.

MISCELLANEOUS

ASSOCIATED CONDITIONS
N/A

AGE-RELATED FACTORS
N/A

ZOONOTIC POTENTIAL
- Possible, but unlikely
- Use caution when handling infected tissues, and reduce exposure to infected secretions.

PREGNANCY
N/A

SYNONYMS
N/A

SEE ALSO
N/A

ABBREVIATIONS
CSF = cerebrospinal fluid

Suggested Reading

Barron CN. Cryptococcosis in animals. J Am Vet Med Assoc 1955;124:125–127.

Bennett JE, et al. A comparison of amphotericin B alone and combined with flucytosine in the treatment of cryptococcal meningitis. N Engl J Med 1979;301:126–131.

Steckel RR, et al. Antemortem diagnosis and treatment of cryptococcal meningitis in a horse. J Am Vet Med Assoc 1982;180:1085–1089.

Author Joseph J. Bertone

Consulting Editor Joseph J. Bertone

CRYPTORCHIDISM

BASICS

DEFINITION

• Failure of one or both testes to descend completely into its associated scrotal sac.
• Affected males are referred to as rigs, riglings, originals, or if the testis is located in the inguinal canal, high flankers.
• False rig—a true castrate that retains some degree of stallion-like behavior.
• Complete abdominal cryptorchid—when the testis and entire epididymis are contained within the abdomen.
• Incomplete abdominal cryptorchid—when the testis and most of the epididymis are intra-abdominal but the ductus deferens and epididymal cauda (i.e., tail) are located in the inguinal canal.
• Inguinal cryptorchid—when the testis is located in the inguinal canal.
• Ectopic cryptorchid—when testis is subcutaneous and cannot be displaced manually into the scrotum.

PATHOPHYSIOLOGY

• Embryologically, testes develop adjacent to the kidneys and are situated in the dorsal abdomen.
• Normal descent—both testes descend ventrally through the abdominal cavity and inguinal canals into the scrotum sometime during the last 30 days of gestation or first 10 days after birth.
• Abnormal descent—failure to descend may result from faults in development of the gubernaculum, vaginal process, vaginal ring, inguinal canal, or testis or from persistence of the testicular suspensory ligament.
• Cryptorchidism—unilateral is more common, but may be bilateral.
• Spermatogenesis of abdominal testes is thermally suppressed with development arrested at the spermatogonia stage.
• Unilateral cryptorchids have normal fertility.
• Bilateral cryptorchidism results in sterility.
• If testes are retained in the inguinal canal, development may proceed to the primary spermatocyte stage.
• Palpation of a retained testis—if inguinal, the testis often is palpable; if abdominal, the testis is difficult to locate by palpation (i.e., small and soft) but may be visualized at ultrasonography.

SYSTEM AFFECTED

Reproductive

GENETICS

There appears to be some genetic link/heritability, but this does not explain the entire population of individuals affected by cryptorchidism.

INCIDENCE/PREVALENCE

• Higher incidence/risk—Quarter Horse, Percheron, Saddlebred, and pony breeds.
• Lower incidence/risk—Thoroughbreds, Standardbreds, Morgans, and Tennessee Walking horses.
• Cryptorchidism is relatively common in horses, with a higher prevalence compared with that in dogs and cats.

SIGNALMENT

• All breeds.
• Absence of a palpable testis in the scrotal sac by one month of age is presumptive evidence of cryptorchidism. After 12 months, inguinal-retained testes rarely enter the scrotum but, reportedly, have entered in horses as old as 2–3 years of age.
• Unilateral is ≅10-fold more prevalent than bilateral.
• The left testis is retained slightly more often than the right in horses, which contrasts with dogs and cats, in which the right testis is twice as likely as the left to be retained.
• Left testes more often are intra-abdominal; right testes are equally likely to be inguinal or abdominal.

SIGNS

Historical Findings

• Stallion-like behavior in presumed geldings.
• Testes produce androgens regardless of location; even bilaterally affected individuals develop normal secondary sex characteristics and sexual behavior.
• Rarely associated with pain or other signs of disease.
• Isolated reports of torsion of the retained testis and of intestinal strangulation in association with a retained testis.

Physical Examination Findings

Undescended testes are smaller and softer than scrotal testes.

CAUSES AND RISK FACTORS

• Cause unknown.
• Genetic research suggests a complex mechanism of inheritance involving several genes. The decreasing incidence of cryptorchidism in certain lines of horses suggests that *selective breeding influences the incidence.*
• Both autosomal dominant and autosomal recessive modes of inheritance have been proposed.
• In addition to genetics, other factors implicated in abnormal testicular descent include inadequate gonadotropic stimulation, intrinsically defective testes, and mechanical impediment of descent, all of which may, in turn, have a genetic basis.
• Cryptorchidism has been associated with intersexuality and abnormal karyotypes.

DIAGNOSIS

• Complete history.
• Behavioral observation.
• Often diagnostic to conduct a thorough visual examination and to palpate the scrotum and external inguinal region.
• External deep inguinal palpation and transrectal palpation often require tranquilization or sedation.

DIFFERENTIAL DIAGNOSIS

• Bilateral cryptorchid stallion.
• Cryptorchid hemicastrate.
• Gelding.
• True anorchidism, in which neither testis develops, is extremely rare.
• Monorchid animals, having failed to develop a second testis, have been described in isolated reports.

CBC/BIOCHEMISTRY/URINALYSIS

N/A

OTHER LABORATORY TESTS

hCG Stimulation Test

• Administer hCG (10,000 U IV), and collect preadministration, 1-hour, and 2-hour samples.
• Stallions and cryptorchids show a 2–3-fold increase in serum testosterone levels.
• Geldings show no change in testosterone levels.

Serum Conjugated Estrogen Concentration

• Estrone sulfate.
• Stallions and cryptorchids, >400 pg/mL.
• Geldings, <50 pg/mL.
• Not reliable in horses of <3 years and in donkeys of any age—donkeys have no detectable conjugated estrogens.

CRYPTORCHIDISM

Fecal Conjugated Estrogen Concentration

- Noninvasive technique.
- Estrogens are stable in feces for at least 1 week.

Serum Testosterone Concentration

- Stallion and cryptorchids, >100 pg/mL.
- Geldings, <40 pg/mL.
- Unreliable in horses of <18 months of age
- Less reliable than hCG stimulation test and conjugated estrogen determination because of wide seasonal variation in basal concentrations.

Serum Inhibin Concentration

- Stallions, 1–3 ng/mL.
- Gelding, negligible.

IMAGING

- Parenchyma of a cryptorchid testis is less echogenic and smaller than that of a normal descended testis.
- Percutaneous ultrasonography may help to identify an inguinal testis.
- Transrectal ultrasonography may help to identify an abdominal testis.

DIAGNOSTIC PROCEDURES

- Laparoscopy to identify an abdominal testis
- Less invasive procedures usually are sufficient to diagnose the problem and often are used in conjunction with laparoscopic cryptorchidectomy.

PATHOLOGIC FINDINGS

- Thermally induced arrest of spermatogenesis in abdominal testis
- Spermatocytogenic development may reach the primary spermatocyte stage if the testis is inguinal.
- Seminiferous tubule development is impeded.
- Elevated body temperature may induce interstitial cell hyperplasia.

TREATMENT

APPROPRIATE HEALTH CARE

Surgical removal of the retained testis.

NURSING CARE

N/A

ACTIVITY

N/A

DIET

N/A

CLIENT CONSIDERATIONS

N/A

SURGICAL CONSIDERATIONS

- Cryptorchidectomy via standard or laparoscopic approaches.
- Standard approaches—inguinal, parainguinal, paramedian, suprapubic, and flank; choice is dictated by the location of the testis.
- Laparoscopy can be performed with the horse standing or in dorsal recumbency. Remove the retained testis before the descended testis.
- Another, less reliable technique involves laparoscopic cautery and transection of the spermatic cord to induce avascular necrosis of the testis. Revascularization can occur, with subsequent production of testosterone.
- Orchiopexy (i.e., surgical placement of a retained testis into the scrotum) is considered unethical.

MEDICATIONS

DRUGS OF CHOICE

N/A

CONTRAINDICATIONS

N/A

PRECAUTIONS

N/A

POSSIBLE INTERACTIONS

N/A

ALTERNATIVE DRUGS

N/A

FOLLOW-UP

PATIENT MONITORING

- Cessation of stallion-like behavior occurs concomitant with decreasing androgen levels and may require 6–8 weeks.
- Some stallions castrated at an older age or, after having bred mares, retain stallion-like behavior even after removal of all testicular tissue.

POSSIBLE COMPLICATIONS

- Complications are uncommon, usually those associated with cryptorchidectomy.
- Possible sequelae—infection, hemorrhage, adhesion formation, eventration, and incomplete castration.

MISCELLANEOUS

ASSOCIATED CONDITIONS

Testicular cysts and neoplasia (e.g., teratoma, interstitial cell tumor, seminoma, Sertoli cell tumor) have been reported.

AGE-RELATED FACTORS

Endocrine assay is not reliable as a diagnostic tool in prepubertal males.

ZOONOTIC POTENTIAL

N/A

PREGNANCY

N/A

SYNONYMS

Lay terms include rigs, riglings, originals, or if the retained testis is inguinal, high flanker.

SEE ALSO

- Scrotal evaluation
- Semen evaluation—abnormal
- Semen evaluation—normal
- Testicular enlargement
- Testicular tumors

ABBREVIATION

hCG = human chorionic gonadotropin

Suggested Reading

Mueller POE, Parks H. Cryptorchidism in horses. Equine Vet Educ 1999;11:77–86.

Rodgerson DH, Hanson RR. Cryptorchidism in horses. Part I. Anatomy, causes and diagnosis. Compend Contin Educ Pract Vet 1997;19:1280–1288.

Rodgerson DH, Hanson RR. Cryptorchidism in horses. Part II. Treatment. Compend Contin Educ Pract Vet 1997;19: 1372–1379.

Author Jane A. Barber

Consulting Editor Carla L. Carleton

CUSHING'S SYNDROME (CD)

BASICS

DEFINITION

A syndrome associated with functional adenomas or adenomatous hyperplasia of the pars intermedia of the pituitary gland, with excessive production and secretion of ACTH and other peptides.

PATHOPHYSIOLOGY

- The pars distalis and pars intermedia of the pituitary gland secrete the same precursor molecule, POMC, but they process it into different hormones.
- The corticotroph cells of the pars distalis cleave POMC into ACTH and β-endorphin–related peptides.
- The melanotroph cells of the pars intermedia cleave POMC mainly into MSH and β-endorphin–related peptides, with relatively small amounts of ACTH.
- In health, glucocorticoid levels are maintained by ACTH secretion from the corticotroph cells.
- Control of the pars intermedia appears to be via tonic inhibition of melanotrophs by dopamine secreted from hypothalamic neurons. Horses with ECD show loss of dopaminergic neurons of the hypothalamus and, consequently, decreased inhibition of the melanotrophs. This results in hyperplasia of the melanotrophs, significantly increasing POMC-related peptide synthesis and secretion (including ACTH).

SYSTEMS AFFECTED

Skin/Exocrine

Clinical signs most often include hirsutism, abnormal hair coat–shedding pattern, and hyperhidrosis.

Endocrine/Metabolic

- Polyuria/polydipsia may be multifactorial.
- Excess cortisol can increase the GFR and antagonize the effect of ADH on water reabsorption in the renal tubules.
- Hyperglycemia can lead to an osmotic diuresis, although polyuria/polydipsia also is observed in euglycemic horses.
- Compression or destruction of the pars nervosa by enlargement of the pars intermedia can decreased ADH secretion.

Musculoskeletal

Laminitis, particularly in ponies

Behavioral

The more docile behavior of some patients has been suggested to result from increased production of β-endorphin.

GENETICS

N/A

INCIDENCE/PREVALENCE

The reported prevalence varies from 0.1–0.5% of equine hospital caseloads but probably is an underestimation, because private practitioners treat a large number of cases.

SIGNALMENT

- All breeds, but prevalent appears to be greater in ponies.
- Old horses—range, 10–35 yeas; mean, 20 years.
- No sex predilection.

SIGNS

Historical Findings

Affected horses may have various complaints not necessarily directly related to a disease of the pituitary gland—weight loss, recurrent laminitis, infertility, or chronic infections.

Physical Examination Findings

- Hirsutism is the most common sign and is characterized by a long, wavy hair coat.
- In some, shedding of the winter coat is delayed; in others, hair grows earlier and faster during the fall months.
- Excessive sweating, primarily in horses with hirsutism.
- Polyuria and polydipsia in >50% of cases; however, this may not be noticed if the horse is on pasture for prolonged periods.
- Weight loss is common and may be associated with parasitism, poor dentition, or concurrent infection.
- Horses with ECD but without concurrent infections maintain normal body weight but may show decreased muscle mass, particularly over the back, and a pot-bellied appearance.
- Less frequent signs—chronic laminitis, tachycardia, sinusitis, gingivitis, pneumonia, skin infections, delayed wound healing, infertility, lethargy, blindness, seizures, and abnormal bulging of supraorbital fat pads

CAUSES

The pituitary lesion has been described as pituitary basophil or chromophobe adenomas or a diffuse hyperplasia of the melanotroph cells.

RISK FACTORS

None known

CUSHING'S SYNDROME (CD)

DIAGNOSIS

DIFFERENTIAL DIAGNOSIS

• Hirsutism is pathognomonic, except in breeds with a long hair coat—Missouri Foxtrotter or Bashkin.
• Chronic weight loss—poor management, parasitism, poor dentition, hypothyroidism, other chronic systemic diseases, or neoplasia.
• Polyuria/polydipsia can be a sign of chronic renal failure, diabetes insipidus, or diabetes mellitus, although the latter two diseases are rare in horses.
• Pheochromocytoma may cause episodes of hyperthermia, hyperhidrosis, tachypnea, and weight loss.

CBC/CHEMISTRY/URINALYSIS

• No consistent changes in laboratory values, although ≅60% show hyperglycemia.
• Hyperlipidemia is noted frequently in ponies.
• Serum liver enzyme activity may be elevated.
• CBC—may show a stress leukogram.

OTHER LABORATORY TESTS

Endocrinologic testing of the pituitary adrenal axis most often confirms the diagnosis.

Resting Plasma Cortisol Concentration

• Wide range of normal values—horses with pars intermedia dysfunction often are within the normal limits.
• Physiologic elevation of cortisol can occur secondary to exercise, hypoglycemia, or stress.
• Equine plasma cortisol levels have a diurnal rhythm, with morning values higher than evening values. Affected horses appear to lose the diurnal variation. However, this cannot be used for a definitive diagnosis, because the rhythm also may be absent in normal horses.
• If a horse does have a marked diurnal variation, it probably does not have ECD.

Dexamethasone Suppression Test

• The most commonly used test for pituitary adrenocortical function and, in the author's experience, the test of choice in most cases.
• Plasma cortisol concentration is measured in samples collected immediately before and 19 hours after administration of dexamethasone (40 μg/kg IM).
• Normal horses—administration in the late afternoon depresses cortisol production to >10 ng/mL (1 μg/dL) by the following morning.
• Affected horses—administration produces a small degree of suppression, but not to the extent of normal horses; affected horses also rebound more quickly.

ACTH Stimulation Test

• Measurement of plasma or serum cortisol levels before and 8 hours after administration of ACTH gel (1 IU/kg IM) or 2 hours after synthetic ACTH gel (100 IU IV).
• Normal horses—2- to 3-fold increase in plasma cortisol within 4–8 hours.
• Affected horses—exaggerated response, with cortisol levels sometimes rising at least 4-fold.
• Because of the variable responsiveness of affected horses and the overlap in values with those of normal horses, this test fails to consistently differentiate affected and nonaffected animals.

Resting Plasma ACTH Level

• Measurement of plasma endogenous ACTH concentration is valuable in establishing the diagnosis.
• Normal values may vary between laboratories.
• Sampling of plasma requires special handling—blood must be collected in cold disodium EDTA tubes, kept at 4° C, promptly centrifuged, and the plasma stored at −70° C until assayed.
• Values in stressed normal horses and those with early ECD can overlap.

TRH Response Test

• Affected horses with respond uniquely to administration of TRH. (1 mg IV)—in addition to the expected elevations in T_3 and T_4, plasma cortisol production increases significantly by 15–30 minutes and lasts for up to 90 minutes.
• Normal horses—cortisol level slightly decreases.
• This test has been used in horses with clinical signs of ECD and ambiguous dexamethasone suppression test results.
• Recommended for use when dexamethasone is contraindicated—laminitis.
• This test has been recently reviewed, and its specificity has been questioned.

Combined Dexamethasone/TRH Stimulation Test

• Collect a baseline blood sample, and administer dexamethasone (40 μg/kg IV).
• Collect a second blood sample 3 hours later, and then administer TRH (1.1 mg/kg IV).
• Collect a third blood sample 30 minutes after TRH administration.
• Normal horses—cortisol levels decrease, as expected after dexamethasone administration, and remain low after TRH administration.
• Affected horses—plasma cortisol concentration decrease somewhat after dexamethasone administration but return to normal after TRH administration.

Glucose Tolerance Test, Insulin Levels, and Insulin Tolerance Test

• Affected horses have a deranged glycoregulatory mechanism and often are insulin resistant.
• Normal horses challenged with glucose (0.5 g/kg IV) show an immediate rise in plasma glucose concentration and return to baseline level in 1.5 hours.

CUSHING'S SYNDROME (CD)

• Affected horses show a delayed return of plasma glucose concentration to baseline; basal insulin levels also are persistently increased, with or without hyperglycemia.
• When subjected to an exogenous insulin tolerance test (0.4 IU/kg IV), affected horses show no significant decline in blood glucose.

Urinary Corticoid:Creatinine Ratio

• The urinary corticoid:creatinine ratio was determined in eight horses with ECD and found to be significantly greater than that in control horses. Urine was collected in the morning, but values of affected and nonaffected horses overlapped.
• Do not use as the sole test to confirm the diagnosis.

IMAGING

• Computed tomography has been used to evaluate the pituitary gland.
• Ventrodorsal radiography with contrast venography has been described.

DIAGNOSTIC PROCEDURES

N/A

PATHOLOGIC FINDINGS

• Necropsy usually reveals an enlarged pituitary gland (three- to fourfold normal weight).
• Tumors are composed of large columnar or polyhedral cells with hyperchromatic nuclei.
• No metastases
• Enlargement of the adrenals and multiple sites of infections often are present.

TREATMENT

APPROPRIATE HEALTH CARE

Pay particular attention to regular deworming, dental care, and foot trimming.

NURSING CARE

Body clipping and appropriate blanketing are recommended for horses with heavy hair coat.

ACTIVITY

No need to decrease activity unless infections or laminitis are present.

DIET

Iincrease the energy content of the ration for horses showing signs of weight loss.

CLIENT EDUCATION

• Remind owners about the importance of husbandry.
• Owners need to be vigilant for intercurrent complications (e.g., sinusitis, gingivitis, laminitis, nonhealing wounds), to readily recognize signs of disease, and to seek veterinary help early.

SURGICAL CONSIDERATIONS

Bilateral adrenalectomy has not been successful in the long term.

MEDICATIONS

DRUGS OF CHOICE

• Dopamine agonists (e.g., bromocriptine, pergolide) or serotonin antagonists (e.g., cyproheptadine).
• Pergolide mesylate is an expensive, long-acting, type 2 dopaminergic agonist that provides dopamine replacement therapy. Treatment recommendations are based on information extrapolated from human literature and anecdotal clinical accounts. The recommended starting dose is 0.001 mg/kg (0.5 mg for an average-size horse) PO once a day. Some ponies can be successfully maintained on 0.25 mg/day. Clinical improvement should be noted within a few weeks. The dose can be increased by 0.25–0.5 mg/day, to a maximum of 0.011 mg/kg, if horses show no improvement at lower doses. If anorexia, colic, diarrhea, worsening of signs of laminitis, or other undesirable effects develop, decrease the dose.
• Bromocriptine can be given orally but apparently has poor bioavailability. It can be prepared in an injectable solution for intramuscular administration. Reported effective oral doses range from 0.03–0.09 mg/kg twice a day or 0.04 mg/kg PO in the morning and 0.02 mg/kg PO in the evening.

• Information regarding the basic pharmacokinetic behavior and metabolism of cyproheptadine in horses has not been collected. Reports of clinical efficacy vary from 35–75%. Initial recommended dose is 0.25 mg/kg PO once a day for 1 month. The dose can be increased to 0.3–0.5 mg/kg if no clinical response occurs.
• Cyproheptadine is less expensive than pergolide; cases in which cyproheptadine is unsuccessful often respond to pergolide treatment.
• A complete treatment plan also should include symptomatic therapy such as NSAIDs for laminitis and/or antibiotics for focal bacterial infections.

CONTRAINDICATIONS

N/A

PRECAUTIONS

N/A

POSSIBLE INTERACTIONS

Unknown

ALTERNATIVE DRUGS

There is one report of insulin used to treat the hyperglycemia associated with ECD; improvement was temporary because of the development of anti-insulin antibodies.

FOLLOW-UP

PATIENT MONITORING

• Clinical improvement manifests by decreased water consumption in polyuric/polydipsic horses, disappearance of pain associated with laminitis, increased weight, or shedding of the long hair (replaced by a shinier coat).
• Improvement also may be marked by a return to normal blood glucose levels in hyperglycemic horses.
• Objectively evaluate the efficacy of treatment by repeating a dexamethasone suppression test or re-evaluating endogenous ACTH levels.

PREVENTION/AVOIDANCE

N/A

POSSIBLE COMPLICATIONS

N/A

EXPECTED COURSE AND PROGNOSIS

Prognosis varies, depending on the severity of clinical signs.

MISCELLANEOUS

ASSOCIATED CONDITIONS

In the lay literature, ECD often is associated with hypothyroidism. In more than 30 affected horses tested, the response of the thyroid to TRH stimulation was normal.

AGE RELATED FACTORS

N/A

ZOONOTIC POTENTIAL

N/A

PREGNANCY

Abortion is a significant possibility in pregnant, affected mares.

SYNONYMS

• Hyperadrenocorticism
• Pituitary adenoma
• Pituitary-dependent hyperadrenocorticism
• Pituitary pars intermedia dysfunction

SEE ALSO

• Glucose-hyperglycemia
• TRH and TSH stimulation tests

ABBREVIATIONS

• ADH = antidiuretic hormone
• GFR = glomerular filtration rate
• MSH =
• POMC = pro-opiomelanocortin
• TRH = thyroid-releasing hormone

Suggested Readings

Couëtil L, Paradis MR, Knoll J. Plasma adrenocorticotropin concentration in healthy horses and in horses with clinical signs of hyperadrenocorticism. J Vet Intern Med 1996;10:1–6.
Dybdal NO. Endocrine disorders. In: Smith BP, ed. Large animal medicine. 2nd ed. St. Louis: Mosby, 1996.
Levy M, Sojka JE, Dybdal NO. Update on therapeutics: diagnosis and treatment of equine Cushing's disease. Compend Contin Educ Pract Vet 1999;21:766–769.
Van der Kolk H. Diseases of the pituitary gland including hyperadrenocorticism. In: Watson T, ed. Metabolic and endocrine problems of the horse. London: WB Saunders, 1998.

Author Michel Levy
Consulting Editor Michel Levy

CYANIDE TOXICOSIS

BASICS

OVERVIEW

- Ingestion of plants containing cyanogenic glycosides can result in cyanide toxicosis.
- Although 55 different cyanogenic glycosides are reported (e.g., amygdalin, prunasin, dhurrin) in >1000 different plant species, the most important sources for animals have been in the genera *Prunus, Sorghum, Triglochin, Pyrus, Suckleya*, and *Amelanchier*.
- Damage to the plant, including wilting and mastication, results in enzymatic degradation of the glycoside, with release of cyanide.
- The cyanide ion has great affinity for the iron in cytochrome oxidase and inhibits both electron transport and cellular respiration. Blood can carry oxygen, but it cannot be used by the cells, resulting in tissue anoxia.

SIGNALMENT

No breed, size, sex, or age predilections.

SIGNS

- Onset usually is rapid (20–120 minutes) after large ingestion
- Tachypnea
- Dyspnea
- Weakness
- Tachycardia
- Bright red mucous membranes
- Recumbency
- Terminal seizure-like activity
- Death

CAUSES AND RISK FACTORS

- Ingesting large amounts of (usually wilted) plant material containing high concentrations of cyanogenic glycosides.
- Typical scenario—ingestion of fresh but wilted cherry leaves from branches broken off during storms.
- Reports indicate 100 g of wild black cherry leaves can be fatal to a 100-lb animal.
- Cyanide is volatile, and dried cherry leaves or hay made from sorghum species generally are safe.

DIAGNOSIS

DIFFERENTIAL DIAGNOSIS

Carbon monoxide poisoning

CBC/BIOCHEMISTRY/URINALYSIS

N/A

OTHER LABORATORY TESTS

- Cyanide analysis of suspect material or stomach contents.
- Place samples in air-tight containers and freeze immediately.
- Identification of suspect plant material in ingesta.

IMAGING

N/A

DIAGNOSTIC PROCEDURES

N/A

PATHOLOGIC FINDINGS

- Blood is bright red in color.
- Tracheal or pulmonary congestion or hemorrhage.
- Other nonspecific agonal changes may be present.

TREATMENT

- Supportive care
- Supplemental oxygen administration

CYANIDE TOXICOSIS

MEDICATIONS

DRUGS

- Treatment must be administered soon after clinical signs are exhibited to be effective.
- Sodium nitrite (10–20 mg/kg as a 20% solution) is used to induce methemoglobinemia, causing cyanide to disassociate from cytochrome oxidase and to react with methemoglobin to form cyanmethemoglobin.
- Sodium thiosulfate (30–40 mg/kg as a 20% solution) converts cyanide (by the enzyme rhodanese) to thiocyanate, which is excreted.
- Sodium nitrite and sodium thiosulfate can be administered IV as a mixture of 1 mL of 20% sodium nitrite and 3 mL of 20% sodium thiosulfate at 4 mL per 45 kg.
- AC may help to bind cyanide remaining in the GI tract.
- Sodium thiosulfate ($\leq$20 g in solution PO) also may help to detoxify cyanide in the GI tract.

CONTRAINDICATIONS/POSSIBLE INTERACTIONS

N/A

FOLLOW-UP

PATIENT MONITORING

N/A

PREVENTION/AVOIDANCE

Avoid additional exposure to cyanide-containing plants.

POSSIBLE COMPLICATIONS

N/A

EXPECTED COURSE AND PROGNOSIS

Death or recovery occurs rapidly.

MISCELLANEOUS

ASSOCIATED CONDITIONS

- Sorghum cystitis ataxia syndrome has been reported after long-term grazing on exclusively sorghum pastures.
- Syndrome is characterized by hindlimb ataxia, urinary incontinence, and subsequent skin irritation or scalding and cystitis.
- The lumbar and sacral segments of the spinal cord may have focal axonal degeneration and demyelination.
- Probably caused by thiocyanates formed from high, sublethal cyanide ingestion.

AGE-RELATED FACTORS

N/A

ZOONOTIC POTENTIAL

N/A

PREGNANCY

N/A

SEE ALSO

N/A

ABBREVIATIONS

- AC = activated charcoal
- GI = gastrointestinal

Suggested Reading

Cheeke PR. Natural toxicants in feeds, forages, and poisonous plants. Danville, IL: Interstate Publishers, 1998.

Author Larry J. Thompson
Consulting Editor Robert H. Poppenga

CYATHOSTOMIASIS (SMALL STRONGYLE INFESTATION)

BASICS

OVERVIEW

Cyathostomiasis is currently recognized as the most significant intestinal parasitic infection in horses. Cyathostome eggs within the feces hatch and develop to the L_3 larval stage in 1–3 weeks. Ingested L_3 and L_4 larvae penetrate the intestinal mucosa of the cecum and large colon, with eventual encapsulation of the larvae within the submucosa. Larvae may remain encysted (hypobiosis) for varying periods of time before emerging to mature into adults in the intestinal lumen. The host inflammatory response to larvae includes a granulomatous reaction. A second inflammatory response occurs on rupturing of the cysts and release of encysted larvae. These inflammatory reactions result in widespread dysfunction of the intestine due to extensive edema; catarrhal, hemorrhagic, or fibrinous inflammation; and ulceration, causing loss of intestinal absorption, nutrients, and motility. Synchronous emergence of hypobiotic larvae in the late winter (spring rise) may result in seasonal episodes of clinical signs such as diarrhea and ill-thrift. Large numbers of adults within the intestinal lumen may also cause damage by digesting small plugs of mucosa, resulting in pinpoint or coalescing ulcer formation.

PATHOPHYSIOLOGY

Lesions include generalized inflammation, edema, and pinpoint ulcerations or regional areas of denuded mucosa within the cecum and large colon. There may be catarrhal, hemorrhagic, or fibrinous enteritis with multiple nodules on the mucosal surface from larval cysts or visible larvae beneath the mucosal wall. Adult parasites (6–20 mm) may be present in large numbers within the intestinal lumen.

SIGNALMENT

Equids of all ages can be infected, although young or naïve animals are at greatest risk.

SIGNS

Seasonal or continuous signs of acute or chronic severe enteritis with anorexia and dramatic weight loss have been recognized in association with cyathostomiasis in horses. Less specific signs, such as recurrent colic, transient fever of unknown origin, episodic diarrhea, ventral abdominal edema, anemia, and generalized slow debilitation may also occur.

CAUSES AND RISK FACTORS

High stocking density and overgrazing of paddocks and pastures leads to an extremely high level of contamination with larvae.

DIAGNOSIS

DIFFERENTIAL DIAGNOSIS

Differential diagnoses for acute or chronic diarrhea include salmonellosis, *Clostridium* spp., ehrlichiosis, and antibiotic- or NSAID-induced colitis. Possible causes of ill-thrift include other gastrointestinal parasites as well as chronic infection, abscessation, dental disease, or poor nutrition. Colic is a nonspecific clinical sign associated with multiple causes of intra- or extra-abdominal pain.

CBC/BIOCHEMISTRY/URINALYSIS

Mild neutrophilia has been recognized in several cases but transient systemic eosinophilia is rare. Hypoalbuminemia may be present as a result of extensive intestinal protein loss.

OTHER LABORATORY TESTS

N/A

IMAGING

N/A

DIAGNOSTIC PROCEDURES

As the prepatent period is highly variable (5 weeks–20 months), perhaps due to hypobiosis, routine fecal flotation is often negative for parasitic ova. Treatment is indicated for fecal egg cell counts >200 eggs per gram.

TREATMENT

Stocking density on pastures or turnout facilities should ideally provide 2–3 acres per horse. More intense stocking densities are frequently encountered and require special pasture management to control gastrointestinal parasitism. Removal of manure from turnout facilities twice a week is optimal in order to remove eggs before infective larvae develop. Pasture rotation or grazing horse pastures with cattle or small ruminants (which are resistant to strongyle infection) also assists in reducing herbage contamination with infective strongyle larvae. Horses with acute enteritis from larval cyathostomiasis often require hospitalization for intensive supportive therapy (intravenous colloids or crystalloids) in addition to repeated administration of appropriate anthelmintics.

MEDICATIONS

DRUG(S) OF CHOICE

- Ivermectin (0.2 mg/kg PO) is often effective against mature cyathostomes, but does not eliminate encysted larvae reliably.
- Oxfendazole (10 mg/kg PO), or fenbendazole (30–60 mg/kg PO once, or 7.5–10 mg/kg PO daily for 5 consecutive days) may be used against adult cyathostomes, although benzimidazole resistance has been identified in some cyathostome populations.

CYATHOSTOMIASIS (SMALL STRONGYLE INFESTATION)

- Pyrantel tartrate (2.2 mg/kg/day PO) kills ingested larvae, preventing subsequent infection.
- Moxidectin (0.4 mg/kg PO) is effective against encysted cyathostome larvae in addition to benzimidazole-resistant intraluminal forms of the parasite. This drug provides protection against cyathostomiasis for up to 3 months following treatment.

CONTRAINDICATIONS/POSSIBLE INTERACTIONS

N/A

FOLLOW-UP

PATIENT MONITORING

Fecal examinations should be performed weekly following anthelmintic treatment. Retreatment is indicated when 25–30% of horses tested have fecal strongyle-type egg counts >200 eggs per gram of feces.

PREVENTION/AVOIDANCE

Frequent removal of feces from pastures and drylots is essential in order to reduce the incidence of infection. Infective-stage larvae and cyathostome eggs can remain viable in the environment for extended periods of time, including overwintering. Hatching occurs when ambient temperatures are between 7.2° and 37.7°C. Dry, hot weather often destroys hatched larvae by desiccation and inhibition of larval migration on herbage. Pasture harrowing during dry, hot weather may facilitate reduction of pasture contamination.

POSSIBLE COMPLICATIONS

Acute colitis may result in severe dehydration and dramatic weight loss as a result of extensive destruction and inflammation of the intestinal wall.

EXPECTED COURSE AND PROGNOSIS

Adult equids are less susceptible to infection with high numbers of cyathostome larvae. Infection in these animals is often subclinical, although undetected reductions in feed conversion may occur. Younger horses may be less tolerant of cyathostome infection and may show clinical signs with lower infection rates. Approximately 40% of horses affected with acute diarrhea from larval cyathostomiasis survive if treated with appropriate anthelmintic and supportive therapy. Return to normal intestinal function may be slow.

MISCELLANEOUS

ASSOCIATED CONDITIONS

N/A

AGE-RELATED FACTORS

Adult horses tend to be less susceptible to infection with small strongyles.

ZOONOTIC POTENTIAL

N/A

PREGNANCY

N/A

SEE ALSO

N/A

ABBREVIATIONS

N/A

Suggested Reading

Collobert C, Bernard N, Clement F, Hubert J, Kerboeuf D, Flochlay A, Blond-Riou F. Efficacy of oral moxidectin gel against benzimidazole-resistant cyathostomes in horses both naturally and artificially infected with a field population. J Eq Vet Sci 1998;18:588-590.

DiPietro JA, Hutchens DE, Lock TF, Walker AJP, Shipley C, Rulli D. Clinical trial of moxidectin oral gel in horses. Vet Parasit 1997;72:167-177.

Love S. Parasite-associated equine diarrhea. Comp Contin Ed Prac Vet 1992;14(5):642-663.

Author Joanne Hewson

Consulting Editor Henry Stämpfli

CYTOLOGY OF BRONCHOALVEOLAR LAVAGE (BAL) FLUID

BASICS

DEFINITION

- Collection of material from the small airways and alveoli by flushing with sterile saline and suctioning back through an endoscope in a bronchus.
- Fluid is collected into EDTA for cytology and, for bacterial culture, into a sterile clot tube.
- Direct smears, sediment preparations, or cytocentrifuged slides of fluid may be made.
- Cytologic assessment and differential cell counts usually are made from smears stained with Wright's or Dif-Quick.
- Total nucleated cells may be counted on a hemocytometer. This is not routine, however, because standardizing the amount of saline recovered is difficult; Thus, the value of total cell counts is questionable.
- Total protein of a wash fluid is low, so protein content also is not routine.
- BAL fluid from normal horses predominantly contains macrophages, with small numbers of lymphocytes, columnar epithelial cells, and nondegenerate neutrophils. Rarely, mast cells and eosinophils are seen.
- Most samples contain a small amount of mucus, which appears as fibrillar strands of purple material.
- Presence of squamous epithelial cells, often with adherent bacteria, indicates contamination from the oropharynx.

PATHOPHYSIOLOGY

- Material present in fluid from bronchoalveolar flushes represents the region of lung being sampled.
- Detected abnormalities can include inflammatory cells; organisms, including bacteria, fungi, and rarely, lungworm larvae; evidence of hemorrhage; increased mucus and goblet cells; and material (e.g., pollens, particulates) that passes the mucociliary clearance apparatus.
- Chronic inflammation or irritation of any type causes increased mucus production by epithelial cells of the airways.
- Neoplastic cells from metastatic or primary lung tumors typically are not found in BAL samples.
- This technique may not be diagnostic for focal lung lesions, mild diffuse disease, or severe, chronic small airway disease that prevents lavage fluid from reaching affected alveoli.

SYSTEMS AFFECTED

- Respiratory
- Hemic/lymphatic/immune

SIGNALMENT

Any breed or sex

SIGNS

- Coughing
- Dyspnea
- Exercise intolerance
- Nasal discharge
- Fever

CAUSES

- Acute or chronic inflammation—bacterial, fungal, or viral
- COPD
- EIPH
- Parasitic inflammation
- Hypersensitivity
- Neoplasia

RISK FACTORS

N/A

DIAGNOSIS

DIFFERENTIAL DIAGNOSIS

Acute or Chronic Inflammation

- Acute pulmonary inflammation is associated with increased neutrophil numbers, which may appear degenerate if bacteria are present.
- Bacteria may be intra- or extracellular. If primarily extracellular, examine cytologic samples for oropharyngeal contamination, which may lead to a false diagnosis of sepsis.
- As inflammation becomes more chronic, the macrophage numbers typically increase, and neutrophils may seem relatively fewer but are, in fact, still present in increased numbers.
- Fungal elements may be observed, usually in association with increased macrophage and neutrophil numbers.
- Viral infection of the lungs does not produce a typical inflammatory pattern in equine BAL fluid.
- *Pneumocystis carinii* may be observed during pneumonias in immunosuppressed horses.

COPD

- Typical findings—increased numbers of nondegenerate neutrophils ($\geq 5\%$) and increased mucus production, as evidenced by amount of mucus, Curschmann's spirals (i.e., casts of inspissated mucus from small airways), or increased goblet cells (i.e., columnar epithelial cells with distinct, round, purple granules of mucus in the cytoplasm).
- Eosinophil and mast cell numbers may increase mildly in BAL fluid from horses with COPD.
- Severity of chronic small airway disease may not correlate well with cytologic findings in many cases.

EIPH

- Varied numbers of erythrocytes may be seen in BAL fluid from normal horses if mild trauma occurs during sampling.
- Phagocytized RBCs or macrophages containing breakdown products of hemoglobin (e.g., hemosiderin) is most typical of pulmonary hemorrhage before sampling.

Parasitic Inflammation

- Infection with the lungworm *Dictyocaulus arnfeldi* is associated with large numbers of eosinophils and macrophages in BAL fluid.
- Larvae typically are not seen.

Hypersensitivity

- Respiratory allergic reactions typically are associated with increased numbers of eosinophils.
- Increased numbers of mast cells, neutrophils, and lymphocytes also may be seen.

CYTOLOGY OF BRONCHOALVEOLAR LAVAGE (BAL) FLUID

Neoplasia

BAL is not usually considered a useful technique in the diagnosis of equine pulmonary neoplasia.

LABORATORY FINDINGS

Drugs That May Alter Lab Results

N/A

Disorders That May Alter Lab Results

N/A

Valid If Run in Human Lab?

Equine cytology requires specialized veterinary training.

CBC/BIOCHEMISTRY/URINALYSIS

Inflammatory respiratory disease may be associated with neutrophilia, left shift, and hyperfibrinogenemia; however, these changes are neither consistent nor specific for respiratory disease.

OTHER LABORATORY TESTS

- Bacterial or fungal culture of BAL fluid when indicated; contamination often occurs while obtaining a sample and must be considered when interpreting culture results.
- Blood gas analysis to evaluate gas exchange.
- Baermann funnel fecal examination to detect lungworms.

IMAGING

Radiology and ultrasonography may be useful in localizing and characterizing lung lesions.

DIAGNOSTIC PROCEDURES

- Bronchoscopy
- Lung biopsy

TREATMENT

Directed at the underlying cause.

MEDICATIONS

DRUGS OF CHOICE

N/A

CONTRAINDICATIONS

N/A

PRECAUTIONS

N/A

POSSIBLE INTERACTIONS

N/A

ALTERNATIVE DRUGS

N/A

FOLLOW UP

PATIENT MONITORING

Within 48 hours of BAL with sterile saline, a significant influx of neutrophils occurs into the lavaged region of the lung; recognize this effect if repeated BALs are performed.

POSSIBLE COMPLICATIONS

N/A

MISCELLANEOUS

ASSOCIATED CONDITIONS

N/A

AGE-RELATED FACTORS

N/A

ZOONOTIC POTENTIAL

N/A

PREGNANCY

N/A

SYNONYMS

N/A

SEE ALSO

N/A

ABBREVIATIONS

- COPD = chronic obstructive pulmonary disease
- EIPH = exercise-induced pulmonary hemorrhage

Suggested Reading

Derksen FJ, Brown CM, Sonea I, Darien BJ, Robinson NE. Comparison of transtracheal aspirate and bronchoalveolar lavage cytology in 50 horses with chronic lung disease. Equine Vet J 1989;21:23–26.

Mair TS, Stokes CR, Bourne FJ. Cellular content of secretions obtained by lavage from different levels of the equine respiratory tract. Equine Vet J 1987;19:458–462.

Sweeney, CR, Rossier Y, Ziemer EL, Lindborg SR. Effect of prior lavage on broncho-alveolar lavage fluid cell population of lavaged and unlavaged lung segments in horses. Am J Vet Res 1994;55:1501–1504.

Zinkl JG. The lower respiratory tract. In: Cowell RL, Tyler RD, eds. Cytology and hematology of the horse. Goleta, CA: American Veterinary Publications, 1992:77–87.

Author Susan J. Tornquist

Consulting Editor Claire B. Andreasen

CYTOLOGY OF TRANSTRACHEAL ASPIRATION (TTA) FLUID

BASICS

DEFINITION

- Aspiration of fluid from the tracheal lumen using a sterile, polyethylene catheter inserted between the tracheal rings.
- Sterile saline (20–60 mL) is instilled and recovered by applying suction with a syringe.
- Retrieved fluid that appears cloudy or flocculent indicates a good sample has been obtained.
- The sample is aliquoted into a sterile tube for culture and into a tube containing EDTA for cytology.
- Direct smears, sediment preparations, or cytocentrifuged slides may be made.
- Most commonly, air-dried slides are stained with Wright's or Dif-Quick.
- Cell counts rarely are performed, because the amount of fluid infused and recovered is variable.
- Protein content is also not commonly determined, because wash fluids usually are low in protein.
- In aspirates from normal horses, columnar epithelial cells, which may appear ciliated or nonciliated, are most common. Macrophages also are present in moderate numbers, along with small numbers of nondegenerate neutrophils and occasional eosinophils and lymphocytes. Multinucleated macrophages may be seen in low numbers; increased numbers may indicate disease.
- Mucus is present in most samples and appears as strands of purple fibrillar material.
- Squamous epithelial cells, organisms, and debris from the oropharynx or skin may be present and indicate contamination.

PATHOPHYSIOLOGY

- Samples from normal horses have a wide range of cell types and generally do not contain the same cell types as those obtained using BAL. This reflects differences in cell populations in the trachea and those lining alveolar spaces, and that TTA samples material in both small and large airways.
- Acute inflammation, especially bacterial, of the respiratory tract most often causes widespread migration of inflammatory cells to the trachea, facilitating a diagnosis based on findings in TTA samples.
- Other conditions (e.g., COPD) may not be diagnosed as readily by TTA compared with BAL.
- With suspected septic conditions, sterile collection of material by TTA is preferred over BAL; however, bacteria in the trachea without cytologic evidence of neutrophilic inflammation suggests nonpathogenic colonization of the trachea.
- Chronic inflammation or irritation of any type causes increased mucus production by epithelial cells of the airways.

SYSTEMS AFFECTED

- Respiratory
- Hemic/lymphatic/immune

SIGNALMENT

Any breed or sex

SIGNS

- Coughing
- Dyspnea
- Exercise intolerance
- Nasal discharge
- Fever

CAUSES

- Acute or chronic inflammation—bacterial, fungal, or viral
- COPD
- EIPH
- Parasitic inflammation
- Hypersensitivity
- Neoplasia

RISK FACTORS

N/A

DIAGNOSIS

DIFFERENTIAL DIAGNOSIS

Acute or Chronic Inflammation

- Acute pulmonary inflammation is characterized by increased neutrophil numbers.
- Bacterial infection often causes neutrophil degeneration.
- Bacteria may be present intra- or extracellularly. If primarily extracellular and increased numbers of degenerate neutrophils are not seen, examine cytologic samples for signs of oropharyngeal contamination, which may lead to a false diagnosis of sepsis.
- As inflammation becomes more chronic, macrophage numbers typically increase, and neutrophils may appear relatively fewer but, in fact, are still present in increased numbers.
- Fungal elements may be observed, usually in association with increased macrophage and neutrophil numbers.
- Viral infection of the lungs does not produce a typical inflammatory pattern.
- *Pneumocystis carinii* may be observed during pneumonias in immunosuppressed horses.

COPD

- In chronic small airway inflammation, increased numbers of nondegenerate neutrophils ($\geq$5%) and macrophages are seen, with no evidence of causative agents.
- Evidence of increased mucus production—increased mucus, Curschmann's spirals (i.e., casts of inspissated mucus from small airways), or increased goblet cells (i.e., columnar epithelial cells with distinct, round, purple granules of mucus in the cytoplasm).
- Numbers of eosinophils and mast cells may increase mildly in horses with COPD.
- Severity of chronic small airway disease may not correlate well with cytologic findings in many cases.

CYTOLOGY OF TRANSTRACHEAL ASPIRATION (TTA) FLUID

EIPH

• Few to moderate numbers of intact RBCs because of mild hemorrhage during TTA are common.

• Phagocytized RBCs or macrophages containing the breakdown products of hemoglobin (e.g., hemosiderin) are consistent with pulmonary hemorrhage before sampling.

Parasitic Inflammation

• Infection with the lungworm *Dictyocaulus arnfeldi* most often results in large numbers of eosinophils and macrophages in the sample.

• Larvae have been found in unfixed, unstained sediment of tracheal fluid.

Hypersensitivity

• Respiratory allergic reactions typically are associated with increased numbers of eosinophils.

• Mast cells, neutrophils, and lymphocytes also may be present.

Neoplasia

TTA is not usually considered a useful technique for the diagnosis of equine pulmonary neoplasia.

LABORATORY FINDINGS

Drugs That May Alter Lab Results

N/A

Disorders That May Alter Lab Results

N/A

Valid If Run in Human Lab?

Equine cytology requires specialized veterinary training.

CBC/BIOCHEMISTRY/URINALYSIS

Inflammatory respiratory disease may be associated with neutrophilia, left shift, and hyperfibrinogenemia; however, these findings are neither consistent nor specific for respiratory disease.

OTHER LABORATORY TESTS

• Bacterial or fungal culture of aspirated fluid.

• Baermann funnel technique to detect lungworm larvae in feces may be indicated with marked eosinophilic inflammation and appropriate history.

IMAGING

Radiology and ultrasonography may be useful in localizing and characterizing lung lesions.

DIAGNOSTIC PROCEDURES

• Bronchoscopy
• Lung biopsy

TREATMENT

Directed at the underlying cause.

MEDICATIONS

DRUGS OF CHOICE

N/A

CONTRAINDICATIONS

N/A

PRECAUTIONS

N/A

POSSIBLE INTERACTIONS

N/A

ALTERNATIVE DRUGS

N/A

FOLLOW UP

PATIENT MONITORING

N/A

POSSIBLE COMPLICATIONS

Uncommon complications—infection, hemorrhage, or emphysema at the site.

MISCELLANEOUS

ASSOCIATED CONDITIONS

N/A

AGE-RELATED FACTORS

Foals normally may have increased neutrophil numbers.

ZOONOTIC POTENTIAL

N/A

PREGNANCY

N/A

SYNONYMS

• Tracheobronchial aspirate
• Transtracheal wash

SEE ALSO

N/A

ABBREVIATIONS

• BAL = bronchoalveolar lavage
• COPD = chronic obstructive pulmonary disease
• EIPH = exercise-induced pulmonary hemorrhage

Suggested Reading

Bain F. Cytology of the respiratory tract. Vet Clin North Am Equine Pract 1997;13:477–486.

Derksen FJ, Brown CM, Sonea I, Darien BJ, Robinson NE. Comparison of transtracheal aspirate and bronchoalveolar lavage cytology in 50 horses with chronic lung disease. Equine Vet J 1989;21:23–26.

Zinkl JG. The lower respiratory tract. In: Cowell RL, Tyler RD, eds. Cytology and hematology of the horse. Goleta, CA: American Veterinary Publications, 1992:77–87.

Author Susan J. Tornquist
Consulting Editor Claire B. Andreasen

DACRYOCYSTITIS

BASICS

OVERVIEW

Definition

The nasolacrimal system has both secretory and drainage components. Drainage of ocular secretions occurs through the upper and lower eyelid puncta into the nasolacrimal canaliculi and subsequently the nasolacrimal sac. The nasolacrimal duct then extends from the lacrimal sac in the lacrimal bone into the maxilla, opening into the ventrolateral nasal cavity. Dacryocystitis is inflammation of the lacrimal sac and nasolacrimal duct. It is seen frequently in horses.

PATHOPHYSIOLOGY

Dacryocystitis may develop as a primary problem or secondary to duct obstruction. Eyelid puncta atresia, nasolacrimal duct agenesis, and nasal puncta atresia are congenital abnormalities that can result in severe dacryocystitis. There are many potential causes of acquired obstruction of the nasolacrimal system (fractures, foreign bodies, neoplasia, granulomas, sinusitis), although often an underlying cause cannot be determined.

SYSTEMS AFFECTED

Ophthalmic

GENETICS

No known genetic influence on development of dacryocystitis.

SIGNALMENT

Breed Predilections

There are no breed predilections for dacryocystitis.

Mean Age and Range

Dacryocystitis associated with a congenital abnormality of the nasolacrimal system is usually seen within the first 3 to 4 months of life, and occasionally not until 1 to 2 years of age.

Predominant Sex

No proven sex predilection.

SIGNS

Thick, mucopurulent discharge at medial canthus; reflux exudation on manipulation of the medial eyelid; mild conjunctival hyperemia. May be unilateral or bilateral when associated with congenital causes; acquired obstruction usually unilateral. Atresia of the nasal puncta is most commonly unilateral. Globe and conjunctiva are usually not involved, unless chronic dacryocystitis has resulted in blepharoconjunctivitis.

CAUSES

Congenital Obstruction

- Nasal puncta atresia*
- Nasolacrimal duct agenesis
- Eyelid puncta atresia

Acquired Obstruction

- Traumatic disruption*
- Foreign body*
- Neoplasia (squamous cell carcinoma)
- Granuloma (habronemiasis)
- Sinusitis, rhinitis
- Periodontitis
- Fibrosis secondary to chronic inflammation
- *Thelazia lacrymalis*

RISK FACTORS

White, gray-white, and palomino hair color predisposes to ocular squamous cell carcinoma. Warm weather and climates with heavy fly population are a risk factor for habronemiasis.

DIAGNOSIS

DIFFERENTIAL DIAGNOSIS

Must differentiate dacryocystitis from other causes of mucopurulent ocular discharge, including bacterial or parasitic conjunctivitis, neoplasia of eyelid or conjunctiva, secondary infection of ocular or eyelid injury, or ocular foreign body.

CBC/BIOCHEMISTRY/URINALYSIS

Results usually normal.

OTHER LABORATORY TESTS

- Aerobic and anaerobic bacterial culture and sensitivity of material flushed from puncta.
- Habronemiasis—Scraping of the granuloma reveals eosinophils, mast cells, neutrophils, plasma cells, rarely larvae. Biopsy and histopathology for mass lesions.

IMAGING

Skull radiographs if fracture suspected from history or physical exam. Contrast dacryocystorhinography assists in identifying cause of obstruction. It involves instillation of 4–6 mL of radiopaque solution into puncta. Rhinoscopy indicated if sinusitis/rhinitis suspected.

DIAGNOSTIC PROCEDURES

Complete ophthalmic examination is indicated to identify any primary ocular problem causing mucopurulent discharge or secondary ocular involvement. Patency of duct may be assessed initially by Jones dye test. Fluorescein dye is instilled into the eye, and the nasal puncta is observed for appearance of fluorescein within 5 min. An attempt should be made to flush the duct with saline or irrigating solution from patent puncta. Topical anesthetic should be applied to both nasal mucosa and conjunctiva. Cannulation of nasolacrimal duct is performed using 5 French urinary catheter or polyethylene tubing (size 160) inserted through nasal or eyelid puncta. The catheter may hit a blind end several centimeters from nasal puncta opening, and should be directed laterally. Dental and oral examination should be performed if dental disease is suspected as inciting cause of dacryocystitis.

HISTOPATHOLOGIC FINDINGS

- Habronemiasis—Eosinophils, mast cells, neutrophils, plasma cells, rarely larvae.
- Squamous cell carcinoma—Epithelial cells with neoplastic characteristics.
- Other histopathologic findings possible depending on type of neoplasia present.

DACRYOCYSTITIS

TREATMENT

APPROPRIATE HEALTH CARE

Patients that require surgical intervention to reestablish patency of duct would be hospitalized for a short-term basis. Those in which patency is reestablished with simple irrigation or cannulation can be treated on an outpatient basis.

ACTIVITY

Restriction of activity may be required for a short time following surgical procedures.

DIET

No change in diet is necessary. Hay should be fed at ground level rather than elevated hayracks or bags if ocular disease is present.

CLIENT EDUCATION

The client should be informed of potential for recurrence, especially in cases of acquired obstruction or unidentified cause.

SURGICAL CONSIDERATIONS

Nasolacrimal duct agenesis accompanied by nasal or eyelid puncta atresia necessitates surgical creation of a proximal or distal opening. If the duct is present, flushing of the nasolacrimal system results in dilation of tissue overlying the site of the atretic puncta. An incision through overlying tissue establishes patency, and a stent placed in the nasolacrimal duct allows epithelialization of new puncta. Severe hemorrhage may occur following incision over the atretic nasal puncta. Ends of the stent are sutured to the skin of the muzzle and near medial canthus, and the stent is left in place for 2 to 3 weeks. Acquired obstructions all treated by removal of the inciting cause when possible, irrigating the duct, and catheterization of the duct for 2 to 3 weeks. The indwelling stent is sutured to the skin as described for congenital lesions. Conjunctivorhinostomy involves creation of mucous membrane–lined fistula between the lacrimal lake and nasal cavity. This procedure is indicated for nasolacrimal duct obstruction that cannot be relieved with flushing or cannulation.

MEDICATIONS

DRUGS OF CHOICE

Topical triple antibiotic solution placed in the eye three times daily until stent removal. Systemic antibiotics based on culture and sensitivity results for 7 to 10 days. Appropriate antibiotic solution should be flushed through the indwelling stent on a daily or every other day basis.

CONTRAINDICATIONS

N/A

PRECAUTIONS

N/A

POSSIBLE INTERACTIONS

N/A

ALTERNATIVE DRUGS

N/A

FOLLOW-UP

PATIENT MONITORING

The patient should be rechecked soon after the initial procedure to establish patency (7–10 days), with the specific time frame determined by severity. Subsequent rechecks are dictated by severity of the disease and response to treatment.

PREVENTION/AVOIDANCE

Fly control in barns and pastures, fly hoods, frequent periocular administration of insect repellant, and regular deworming with ivermectin can help prevent the development of habronemiasis.

POSSIBLE COMPLICATIONS

Potential complications vary with the inciting cause. They include recurrence of the dacryocystitis and failure to maintain patency of the duct.

EXPECTED COURSE AND PROGNOSIS

Acquired obstructions resulting in dacryocystitis are more difficult to treat than congenital abnormalities. Foreign body and periodontal causes have the best response to therapy of acquired obstructions. Cannulation of the duct may be impossible in cases of neoplasia and maxillary fractures, and permanent correction of the obstruction and subsequent dacryocystitis may not be possible.

MISCELLANEOUS

ASSOCIATED CONDITIONS

N/A

AGE-RELATED FACTORS

N/A

ZOONOTIC POTENTIAL

N/A

PREGNANCY

Systemic absorption of topically applied medication is possible. Benefits of treatment should be considered against any risks posed to the fetus.

SYNONYMS

N/A

SEE ALSO

Ocular problems in the neonate; ocular squamous cell carcinoma.

ABBREVIATIONS

N/A

Suggested Reading

Moore CP. Eyelid and nasolacrimal disease. Vet Clin N Am 8(3); 1992.

Author Heidi Denis, DVM
Consulting Editor D. E. Brooks, DVM

DEGENERATIVE MYELOENCEPHALOPATHY (DM)

BASICS

DEFINITION

A neurologic disease of young, growing horses that affects all major equine breeds and results in a diffuse, degenerative disease in select areas of the brainstem and spinal cord.

PATHOPHYSIOLOGY

- The exact pathogenesis remains speculative.
- Histopathologic findings include degrees of neuroaxonal dystrophy affecting the spinal cord and brainstem nuclei, with neuronal fiber degeneration within ascending and descending spinal cord pathways.
- Exposure to toxins (e.g., organophosphates) and deficiencies of vitamins (e.g., vitamin E) or minerals (e.g., copper) have produced the pathologic change of neuroaxonal dystrophy.
- Risk factors—use of insecticides on foals, exposure of foals to wood preservatives, foals that frequently spend time on dirt lots, and use of feeds with very low vitamin E levels
- Foals with access to green pastures appear to have a protective effect against development of the condition.
- Evidence suggests that vitamin E concentrations less than control values of 1–4 mg/L have a causative role in this condition.
- Low to deficient serum or plasma α-tocopherol values have been reported in several studies.
- Prophylactic administration of vitamin E to foals from sires known to produce affected foals has resulted in a decreased incidence of the disease.
- Five affected horses treated with 6000 IU/day of α-tocopherol showed improved neurologic score.
- Vitamin E has been suggested to act as an intracellular oxidant that protects lipid membranes from free radicals generated by normal oxidative processes of metabolism and inflammation.
- Inadequate amounts of vitamin E result in lipid peroxidation of cellular membranes, especially in the CNS.
- Vitamin E deficiency has been suggested to occur from deficient feed levels, decreased GI absorption, deficient blood transport lipoproteins, lack of hepatic transfer proteins, decrease or absence of cellular receptors, and increased utilization or excretion.
- Current evidence supports the hypothesis that the condition is a vitamin E deficiency having a genetic predisposition along with the proposed familial tendency.

SYSTEMS AFFECTED

Neurologic:

- A diffuse, degenerative disease of the brain and spinal cord
- Gross pathologic lesions do not appear in the nervous system.
- Neuronal fiber degeneration may be particularly prominent in the thoracolumbar region of the spinal cord and lateral cuneate nuclei of the caudal portion of the medulla.

GENETICS

- A vitamin E–responsive disorder of horses and zebras, with possible familial predisposition
- Inheritance in a polygenic mode or as a dominant disorder with variable expression has been suggested.

INCIDENCE/PREVALENCE

- Reported in horses throughout the United States, but most commonly in the northeastern regions.
- Also documented in England and Germany.

SIGNALMENT

Species

- Domestic horses
- Wild horses and zebras

Breed Predilections

Most of the common breeds in the United States are affected—Appaloosas, Arabians, Quarter Horses, Thoroughbreds, Standardbreds, Paso Fino, and Morgans

Mean Age and Range

- Most affected animals exhibit clinical signs of ataxia during the first year of life.
- Onset of clinical signs has been reported as early as birth and as late as 12 years of age, but rarely after 2 years.
- Most frequently, signs are first seen in suckling and weanling foals.

Predominant Sex

N/A

SIGNS

General Comments

- More severely affected horses usually exhibit clinical signs before 6 months of age.
- Mildly affected horses may not exhibit clinical signs until 1–2 years of age.

Historical Findings

- Clinical signs may be very acute in onset.
- Many cases involve horses that tended to be clumsy during the first few months of life and progressed slowly to visible ataxia at 6 months to 2 years.
- Owners have reported lameness of one limb that progressed to ataxia and is often described as having an acute onset after a traumatic fall or injury. The fall may have been caused by a neurologic dysfunction that was unnoticed.

Physical Examination Findings

- Bilaterally symmetric ataxia, weakness, and hypermetria
- All limbs may be affected, but the rear limbs usually are one to three grades more severe than the fore limbs.
- Deficits in the fore limbs may be too subtle to notice.
- Characteristic signs—clumsiness, inability to do complicated movements (e.g., backing, tight turns), incorrect positioning of limbs at rest and during movement, and ataxia of the limbs
- Proprioceptive deficits—awkward placement of limbs and circumduction of the outside limb when turning in a tight circle
- Response to the slap test may be decreased or absent, and hyporeflexia or areflexia of the cutaneous trunci reflex is a major sign that can help to differentiate CSM from EDM.
- No evidence of cranial nerve deficits or muscle atrophy

CAUSES AND RISK FACTORS

- Exposure to toxins—insecticides on foals (organophosphates)
- Exposure of foals to wood preservatives
- Foals frequently spending time on dirt lots with no grass
- Deficiencies of vitamins—vitamin E (6 weeks to 10 months is apparently the most critical)
- Familial predisposition

DIAGNOSIS

DIFFERENTIAL DIAGNOSIS

Other Causes of Ataxia in Horses <2 Years:

- Trauma can be diagnosed at radiography if vertebral fractures occur. Trauma may only cause injury to the spinal cord without bone involvement, resulting in unobservable radiographic lesions.
- CSM usually is diagnosed at radiography, along with myelography, to identify sites of spinal cord compression. Horses with CSM do not have hyporeflexia of the cutaneous trunci reflex and usually improve after treatment with corticosteroids. Horses with EDM fail to show this improvement with corticosteroids.
- Occipital-atlanto-axial malformation and cerebellar abiotrophy usually are seen in Arabian horses. Signs occur within the first 6 months to 1 year of life, and radiography usually is helpful in diagnosing the malformation. Foals with cerebellar abiotrophy present with head tremors.

DEGENERATIVE MYELOENCEPHALOPATHY (DM)

• EPM can occur at any age, and the resulting lesions can be located in any area of the CNS, resulting in different clinical signs. EPM can be acute or have a slow, insidious onset. CSF analysis usually has increased protein content, with a normal nucleated cell count. Cerebrospinal fluid IgG indexes (increased) and albumin quotients (normal) should be run in conjunction with the CSF antibody titer. Antibody titers found in the CSF (by Western blot analysis) to *Sarcocystis neurona* is the diagnostic test used to identify this disease.
• EHV-1 usually is associated with outbreaks of respiratory disease or abortion. Onset usually is rapid, with affected horses showing signs of ataxia and lower motor neuron signs of incontinence, with a flaccid anal sphincter and decreased tail tone. Horses with EHV-1 usually experience the greatest deterioration during the first 24 hours and then begin to recover. A definitive diagnosis can be made based on a rising serum and/or CSF titer to EHV-1. A xanthochromic CSF tap and increased total protein content with a normal cell count is common. IgG indexes usually are normal, and albumin quotients are increased in horses.

CBC/BIOCHEMISTRY/URINALYSIS
N/A

OTHER LABORATORY TESTS
• Currently no definitive, antemortem diagnostic test
• The only abnormal CSF constituent in affected horses is creatine kinase (increased, and rarely) during the active phase of the disease. Increased creatine kinase is not specific for the disease, however, and only reflects myelin and neuronal damage.
• Low serum α-tocopherol values may indicate EDM or be a nutritional deficiency. Some normal horses may have low serum α-tocopherol values, making this test unreliable for diagnosis.

IMAGING
Radiography may help in differentiating other causes of neurologic disease.

DIAGNOSTIC PROCEDURES
CSF analysis in affected horses may show increased creatine kinase during the acute period of the disease.

PATHOLOGIC FINDINGS
N/A

TREATMENT

• Allow access to ample pasture and properly cured hay containing high amounts of vitamin E.
• Improper curing of hay results in low levels vitamin E; therefore, properly cured hay should be fed.

MEDICATIONS

DRUGS OF CHOICE
• No therapeutic agents are available to quickly return an affected horse to normal.
• Vitamin E has shown promise in prophylaxis on affected farms and as a treatment after signs appear.
• Prophylaxis—supplement at least 2000 IU/day of α-tocopherol.
• Therapeutic—6000 IU/day of α-tocopherol mixed in grain has improved neurologic scores of affected horses; improvement may be evident during the first 3–4 weeks, with slower improvements observed during the next year.
• The earlier any gait deficits are recognized and treatment is started, the better the response to therapy.

CONTRAINDICATIONS
Toxic levels of vitamin E in horses are unknown.

PRECAUTIONS
Refer to the manufacturer's label for specific recommendations.

POSSIBLE INTERACTIONS
Refer to the manufacturer's label for specific recommendations.

ALTERNATIVE DRUGS
N/A

FOLLOW-UP

PATIENT MONITORING
• Monitor horses receiving vitamin E therapy for α-tocopherol levels in plasma and serum to ensure adequate absorption. If levels have not increased in 30 days, run a vitamin E–absorption test to rule out malabsorption of the fat-soluble vitamin.
• Each affected horse should undergo follow-up neurologic examinations to enable continued assessment of its condition.

PREVENTION/AVOIDANCE
N/A

POSSIBLE COMPLICATIONS
N/A

EXPECTED COURSE AND PROGNOSIS
N/A

MISCELLANEOUS

ASSOCIATED CONDITIONS
N/A

AGE-RELATED FACTORS
Young horses with a familial tendency for the disease should be monitored closely and given adequate vitamin E supplementation as needed.

ZOONOTIC POTENTIAL
N/A

PREGNANCY
N/A

SYNONYMS
N/A

SEE ALSO
N/A

ABBREVIATIONS
• CSF = cerebrospinal fluid
• CSM = cervical stenotic myelopathy
• EPM = equine protozoal myelopathy
• EHV = equine herpes virus
• GI = gastrointestinal

Suggested Reading

Blythe LL, Craig AM. Equine degenerative myeloencephalopathy. Part 1. Clinical signs and pathogenesis. Compend Contin Educ Pract Vet 1992;14:1215–1221.
Blythe LL, Craig AM. Equine degenerative myeloencephalopathy. Part 2. Diagnosis and treatment. Compend Contin Educ Pract Vet 1992;14:1633–1636.
Dill SJ, Correa MT, Erb HN, et al. Factors associated with the development of equine degenerative myeloencephalopathy. Am J Vet Res 1990;51:1300–1305.
Mathew IG. II: The diseased spinal cord. Am Assoc Equine Pract Proc 1999;45:67–84.
Mayhew IG, Brown CM, Stowe HD, et al. Equine degenerative myeloencephalopathy: a vitamin E deficiency that may be familial. J Vet Intern Med 1987;1:45–50.
Mayhew IG, de Lahunta A, Whitlock RH, et al: Spinal cord disease in the horse. Cornell Vet 1978;68(Suppl 6):1–207.

Author Steven T. Grubbs
Consulting Editor Joseph J. Bertone

DELAYED UTERINE INVOLUTION

BASICS

DEFINITION

- Any delay in return of the uterus to its prepartum state
- Delays may be of size, tone, endometrial regeneration, or elimination of bacteria from the uterine lumen.
- In normal mares, endometrial involution is complete by 13–25 days, with the exception of normal size, which may require as long as 35 days.

PATHOPHYSIOLOGY

- DUC can be mechanical (e.g., decreased muscular contractions), inflammatory (e.g., PMN function), or immunologic (e.g., Ig) in origin.
- DUC may follow dystocia or retained fetal membranes and is characterized by compromised ability to eliminate postpartum debris and bacteria from the uterus.

SYSTEM AFFECTED

Reproductive

GENETICS

N/A

INCIDENCE/PREVALENCE

- Old mares
- Dystocia
- Increased contamination of the uterus at parturition.

SIGNALMENT

- All breeds
- Any mare of breeding age.
- More prevalent in old mares.

SIGNS

General Comments

Because foal heat and rebreeding can occur within 5–18 days postpartum, it is extremely important for the uterus to return to normal rapidly postpartum.

Historical Findings

A history of postpartum delayed involution may be suspected because of failure to conceive when bred during an early foal heat.

Physical Examination Findings

- Evaluate uterine size and tone, and record if fluid is present.
- Note any abnormal discharge from the vulva.
- Any of the above may indicate delayed uterine involution.

CAUSES

- Multiple; great variation within the total population.
- Predisposition to slower involution.
- Hormonal
- Immunologic
- Mechanical—myometrial contractions.
- Management—greater contamination at parturition may increase the time needed for involution.

RISK FACTORS

- Increasing age
- Dystocia
- Unsanitary foaling conditions.
- Decreased oxytocin release—endogenous.
- Failure of the uterus to respond to oxytocin—endogenous or exogenous.

DIAGNOSIS

DIFFERENTIAL DIAGNOSIS

- Important to distinguish metritis from delayed uterine involution.
- Delayed uterine involution may accompany infection or inflammation of the uterus, but these are not necessarily codependent.

CBC/BIOCHEMISTRY/URINALYSIS

N/A

OTHER LABORATORY TESTS

Endometrial cytology—determine characteristics of the uterine fluid.

IMAGING

Ultrasonography:

- Fluid within the postpartum uterine lumen.
- Presence or absence of other findings (e.g., decreased uterine tone, increased uterine size) that are linked with delayed involution.

DIAGNOSTIC PROCEDURES

Endometrial cytology—presence of PMNs.

PATHOLOGIC FINDINGS

Indicators of delayed uterine involution, between 12–15-days postpartum.

Uterus

- Intraluminal fluid
- Enlarged uterus
- Decreased tone
- Endometrial cytology—increased number of leukocytes.

Vulva/Vulvar

Discharge is abnormal at this time postpartum.

TREATMENT

APPROPRIATE HEALTH CARE

- DUC may accompany uterine infections or inflammation and should be differentiated from a combination of delayed involution with metritis.
- Delayed involution does not have an effect systemically, so systemic antibiotics are not needed.
- Local, intrauterine instillation of antibiotics may be contraindicated.
- Uterine flushes or use of hormonal stimulants (e.g., oxytocin, $PGF_2\alpha$) may be more appropriate therapy.

NURSING CARE

N/A

ACTIVITY

Normal activity

DIET

N/A

CLIENT EDUCATION

- Not all mares are breedable at foal heat.
- Transrectal palpations to determine the degree of uterine involution are advisable to select mares with the highest probability of conceiving if bred on a postpartum estrus.

SURGICAL CONSIDERATIONS

N/A

DELAYED UTERINE INVOLUTION

MEDICATIONS

DRUGS OF CHOICE

- Oxytocin and $PGF_2\alpha$ are the hormones of choice for aiding involution of the uterus.
- Uterine flushes (i.e., sterile saline or water), when indicated, may aid involution.
- Instillation of irritants or antiseptics (e.g. Lugol's solution) sometimes has value to further stimulate uterine involution.

CONTRAINDICATIONS

N/A

PRECAUTIONS

Do not overtreat delayed uterine involution with unnecessary antibiotics or other local or systemic medications. Such treatments may further retard return of the uterus to normal and cost the owner additional expense without providing any measurable benefit.

POSSIBLE INTERACTIONS

N/A

ALTERNATIVE DRUGS

N/A

FOLLOW-UP

PATIENT MONITORING

Examination of the uterus to determine return to normal is essential after therapy—transrectal palpation; ultrasonography.

PREVENTION/AVOIDANCE

- Light exercise during late gestation and postpartum can aid uterine involution.
- Barn hygiene—foal in stalls bedded with clean straw; keep stalls clean during the first several days postpartum; expense of bedding and labor is offset by improved reproductive health.

POSSIBLE COMPLICATIONS

- Failure to conceive.
- EED

EXPECTED COURSE AND PROGNOSIS

- Majority mares return to normal without treatment; the only difference is the increased time necessary for involution to be complete.
- In some cases, involution remains incomplete and may prevent conception or pregnancy maintenance.

MISCELLANEOUS

ASSOCIATED CONDITIONS

May be coupled with a uterine infection or occur in the absence of such infection.

AGE-RELATED FACTORS

Increase occurrence in old mares.

ZOONOTIC POTENTIAL

N/A

PREGNANCY

Postpartum

SYNONYMS

N/A

SEE ALSO

- Dystocia
- Postpartum problems
- Retained fetal membranes
- Uterine infection
- Vaginitis and vulvar discharge

ABBREVIATIONS

- DUC = delayed uterine clearance
- EED = early embryonic death
- PMN = polymorphonuclear

Suggested Reading

McKinnon AO, et al. Ultrasonographic studies on the reproductive tract of mares after parturition: effect of involution and uterine fluid on pregnancy rates in mares with normal and delayed first postpartum ovulatory cycles. J Am Vet Med Assoc 1988;192:350–353.

Roberts SJ. Veterinary obstetrics and genital diseases (theriogenology). 3rd ed. Woodstock, VT: published by the author, 1986:584. Stewart DR, et al. Concentrations of 15-keto-13,14-dihydro-prostaglandin $PGF_2\alpha$ in the mare during spontaneous and oxytocin induced foaling. Equine Vet J 1984;16:270–274.

Vandeplassche M, et al. Observations on involution and puerperal endometritis in mares. Ir Vet J 1983;37:126–132.

Author Walter R. Threlfall

Consulting Editor Carla L. Carleton

DIABETES MELLITUS (DM)

BASICS

OVERVIEW

- A group of metabolic diseases characterized by hyperglycemia resulting from defects in insulin secretion, insulin action, or both.
- In humans, DM represents an etiologically and clinically heterogeneous group of disorders sharing hyperglycemia in common.
- An international committee under the sponsorship of the American Diabetes Association recently proposed a classification based on cause rather than treatment modalities—type 1, type 2, and other specific types.
- Type 1 DM (previously classified as insulin-dependent DM and juvenile-onset DM)—primarily due to β-cell destruction, usually leading to insulin deficiency (immune mediated or idiopathic).
- Type 2 DM (previously classified as noninsulin-dependent DM)—may range from insulin resistance with relative insulin deficiency to a predominantly secretory defect with insulin resistance.
- Other specific types of DM—this group encompasses genetic defects in β-cell function, genetic defects in insulin action, diseases of the exocrine pancreas, endocrinopathies, drug or chemical induced, infections, and other genetic syndromes associated with DM and gestational DM.
- Equine DM most commonly is associated with insulin resistance secondary to a tumor or hyperplasia of the pars intermedia of the pituitary gland—ECD.
- Type 2 DM, or DM secondary to pancreatic damage, bilateral granulosa cell tumors (insulin resistance of unknown causes), and pheochromocytoma, also have been reported but are rare conditions.
- Organ systems involved in ECD are described elsewhere; the primary organ systems involved in DM resulting from causes other than pituitary gland dysfunction include endocrine, metabolic, and musculoskeletal.

SIGNALMENT

- ECD affects horses between 10–35 years.
- Reported cases of DM other than ECD usually have involved older horses.
- No breed or sex predilections

SIGNS

- Progressive weight loss, anorexia or polyphagia, polyuria/polydipsia, laminitis, rough hair coat, and irregular estrous cycle have been associated with DM from pancreatitis, granulosa cell tumor, and type 2 DM.
- These signs may be observed with DM from ECD as well.
- Anorexia, abdominal pain, sweating, tachycardia, and diarrhea are associated with pheochromocytoma.

CAUSES AND RISK FACTORS

- The most common cause of equine DM is a functional adenoma or hyperplasia of the pars intermedia of the pituitary gland.
- Other reported causes—granulosa cell tumor, pheochromocytoma, and chronic pancreatitis; the latter can result from migration of *Strongylus equinus* or *S. edentatus* larvae or be idiopathic.

DIAGNOSIS

DIFFERENTIAL DIAGNOSIS

- Causes of transient and persistent hyperglycemia
- Transient elevations of blood glucose result from physiologic causes (e.g., carbohydrate meal, stress, strenuous exercise), iatrogenic causes (α_2-agonists or glucocorticoid administration, glucose therapy), or pathologic states (e.g., endotoxemia); in these cases, a second sample shows normal glucose levels.
- Persistent hyperglycemia most commonly is associated with adenomas of the pars intermedia of the pituitary gland. Endocrinologic testing of the pituitary-adrenal axis (e.g., dexamethasone suppression test, resting plasma ACTH levels) most often confirms the diagnosis of ECD.
- Hyperglycemia also is reported in horses affected with pheochromocytoma. In these patients, clinical signs include colic, excessive sweating tachycardia, and renal failure; the diagnosis is confirmed by repeated elevation of blood or urine catecholamines.

CBC/BIOCHEMISTRY/URINALYSIS

- Hematologic parameters—usually normal
- Hyperglycemia, glucosuria, and ketonuria are the main abnormalities detected in routine laboratory tests.
- Azotemia and metabolic acidosis with hyperkalemia may be present with a pheochromocytoma.

OTHER LABORATORY TESTS

- IV glucose tolerance test with measurement of insulin levels is useful to confirm the diagnosis and to characterize the type of DM. In healthy animals, glucose infusion stimulates an immediate insulin response, and glucose returns to baseline in <3 hours. With DM from insulin deficiency, insulin levels do not rise significantly, and glucose remains elevated >3 hours.
- Elevated serum testosterone and/or inhibin confirm the diagnosis of granulosa cell tumors of the ovaries. Documenting an elevated catecholamine concentration to confirm the diagnosis of pheochromocytoma is technically difficult. Serum catecholamine levels vary rapidly with the status of the patient (e.g., stress, nervousness) and are very unstable. Urinary catecholamines are more useful. Laboratories that offer an assay and reference values for equine catecholamine may be difficult to find.

IMAGING

- Pancreatic ultrasonography has not been fully described in the horse. A large, heterogeneous mass medial to the right kidney and right lobe of the liver, however, was visualized in a horse that was later diagnosed with an enlarged pancreas caused by severe necrotizing pancreatitis.
- With granulosa cell tumors, transrectal ultrasonography of the enlarged ovary may reveal a structure composed of numerous anechoic cysts with different diameters. Granulosa cell tumors also may be uniloculated or, rarely, appear as hyperechoic, dense, and without cyst.

DIAGNOSTIC PROCEDURES

- With suspected pancreatic disease, exploratory laparotomy with biopsy of the pancreas may yield information on the nature of the disease.
- Surgical excision and histopathology of the ovaries provides the definitive diagnosis of granulosa cell tumor.

DIABETES MELLITUS (DM)

PATHOLOGIC FINDINGS

- Horses with DM other than that resulting from ECD may show lesions of chronic pancreatitis, with fibrosis and abscesses.
- Lesions in cases of bilateral granulosa cell tumor include enlarged ovaries containing multiple, thick-walled, fluid-filled cysts.
- Pheochromocytomas usually are unilateral and appear as unique or multiple, nodular masses of variable size within the adrenal gland.

TREATMENT

With DM secondary to granulosa cell tumor or pheochromocytoma, surgical ablation of the tumor should be curative.

MEDICATIONS

DRUGS

- Horses with insulin deficiency (either type 1 DM or secondary to pancreatitis) require administration of insulin. In one report of a 7-year-old pony with DM, regular insulin at dosage of as much as 8 U/kg IV failed to normalize blood glucose levels. Protamine zinc insulin at 0.5–1 U/kg IM effectively controlled the hyperglycemia. When treatment was discontinued, however, the clinical signs recurred. Determining the appropriate insulin dosage requires frequent monitoring of the patient's serum glucose.
- Treatment of DM, secondary to a functional pituitary adenoma, has been described elsewhere and involves pergolide mesylate (Permax) or cyproheptadine hydrochloride (Periactin). One report of a stallion with pituitary adenoma, treated using insulin showed improvement in the clinical signs for 6 weeks. The signs then worsened, suggesting refractoriness to treatment, probably caused by production of antibodies against insulin.
- Severe hypoglycemia is a risk associated with insulin administration in horses; thus, dextrose for injection should always be available. Signs of hypoglycemia include muscle trembling, ataxia, nystagmus, depression, convulsion, coma, and death.

CONTRAINDICATIONS/POSSIBLE INTERACTIONS

N/A

FOLLOW-UP

- In diabetic horses with ECD, clinical improvement and euglycemia indicate improvement. Repeating the dexamethasone suppression test allows an objective evaluation of treatment, but a strict correlation between clinical improvement and a normal test has not been established.
- A positive response to insulin therapy manifests by disappearance of clinical signs. Once glycemic control is established, periodic evaluation of insulin therapy can be implemented every 2–4 months by serial serum glucose measurements.

MISCELLANEOUS

ASSOCIATED CONDITIONS

N/A

AGE-RELATED FACTORS

N/A

ZOONOTIC POTENTIAL

N/A

PREGNANCY

N/A

SEE ALSO

- ECD
- Glucose-hyperglycemia
- Glucose tolerance test
- Pheochromocytoma

ABBREVIATION

- ECD = equine Cushing's disease

Suggested Reading

McCoy DJ. Diabetes mellitus associated with bilateral granulosa cell tumors in a mare. J Am Vet Med Assoc 1986;188:733–735.

Muylle E, Van den Hende C, Deprez P, Nuytten J, Oyaert W. Non-insulin dependent diabetes mellitus in a horse. Equine Vet J 1986;18:145–146.

Ruoff WW, Baker DC, Morgan SJ, Abbitt B. Type II diabetes mellitus in a horse. Equine Vet J 1986;18:143–144.

Author Michel Levy
Consulting Editor Michel Levy

DIAPHRAGMATIC HERNIA

BASIC

OVERVIEW

- Herniation of abdominal viscera into the thoracic cavity through a diaphragmatic defect
- Generally results in simple or strangulated obstruction of the herniated GI viscera, hemorrhage into the abdominal or thoracic cavity, and hypoventilation.

SIGNALMENT

- No sex or breed predilections, but most frequently observed in adults.
- History of trauma is common.

SIGNS

- Abdominal pain, which can vary from mild, intermittent episodes of colic to severe and intractable.
- Altered respiratory pattern of variable severity, depending on the volume of herniated tissue in the thoracic cavity; signs may vary from mild exercise intolerance to respiratory distress.
- Clinical signs suggestive of hypovolemic shock (e.g., blanched mucous membranes, tachycardia, collapse) may be observed with severe hemorrhage into the abdominal or thoracic cavity.

CAUSES AND RISK FACTORS

- Congenital or acquired
- Congenital defects result from incomplete fusion of the pleuroperitoneal folds, causing an enlarged esophageal hiatus.
- Acquired defects result from sudden increases in intrathoracic or intra-abdominal pressure and usually are observed after external trauma, strenuous exercise, GI distension, or pregnancy.

DIAGNOSIS

DIFFERENTIAL DIAGNOSIS

- All disorders causing acute abdominal pain in the horse should be included; therefore, intestinal conditions requiring surgical correction and severe medical conditions of the GI tract (e.g., salmonellosis, idiopathic colitis, Potomac horse fever) should be included. Making a definitive diagnosis depends on a complete physical examination and appropriate auxiliary testing.
- Pneumonia and pleuritis—horses with diaphragmatic hernias usually are not pyrexic and generally do not have an inflammatory leukogram.
- Horses with diaphragmatic hernia may be exercise intolerant; therefore, any disorder of the respiratory, circulatory, and musculoskeletal systems that results in exercise intolerance must be included.

CBC/BIOCHEMISTRY/URINALYSIS

Anemia and hypoproteinemia may be present with severe hemorrhage.

OTHER LABORATORY TESTS

Blood gas analysis usually reveals hypercapnia, resulting from hypoventilation caused by thoracic pain or compression of the lungs by herniated viscera.

IMAGING

- Thoracic radiography—standing lateral thoracic radiography to confirm the diagnosis; radiographic signs include gas-filled intestinal loops in the thoracic cavity, increased ventral thoracic density, and absence of the cardiac shadow and diaphragmatic silhouette.
- Thoracic ultrasonography—reveals pleural fluid and abdominal viscera in the thoracic cavity; viscera may not be visualized in the absence of fluid.

DIAGNOSTIC PROCEDURES

- Thoracic auscultation reveals areas of dullness or reduced cardiac sounds on the side with herniated abdominal contents. Referred GI sounds frequently are heard over the caudoventral thorax in normal horses and cannot be considered as supporting a definitive diagnosis.
- Abdominal palpation per rectum may reveal an empty caudal abdomen, but this is not a consistent finding.
- Abdominal paracentesis usually yields normal abdominal fluid, but with acute acquired diaphragmatic defects, abundant hemorrhagic fluid may be obtained.
- Electrocardiography may reveal decreased amplitude of the QRS complex, caused by the herniated abdominal viscera that surrounds the heart and impairs conduction of electrical impulses to the skin to form surface potentials.

DIAPHRAGMATIC HERNIA

TREATMENT

- Emergency exploratory celiotomy under general anesthesia with assisted, positive-pressure ventilation—surgical treatment consists of reducing herniated viscera, resecting devitalized intestines and intestinal anastomosis, and repairing diaphragmatic defect.
- Acute diaphragmatic defects secondary to trauma—surgery may be delayed if the animal is stable, allowing development of fibrosis of the defect's edges and easier surgical closure.
- Preoperative fluid volume replacement therapy—lactated Ringer solution (6—12 mL/kg per hour); this solution also is used for postoperative maintenance fluid therapy.

MEDICATIONS

DRUGS

Pre- and postoperative medication consists of systemic antibiotics (sodium penicillin G [20,000 IU/kg IV QID] and gentamicin sulfate [6.6 mg/kg IV SID]) and NSAIDs (flunixin meglumine [1 mg/kg IV BID]).

CONTRAINDICATIONS/POSSIBLE INTERACTIONS

Use α2-agonist agents (e.g., xylazine, detomidine) cautiously in horses with diaphragmatic hernia, because these drugs have depressant effects on cardiovascular and respiratory function.

FOLLOW-UP

- Postsurgical monitoring for pneumothorax, pleural effusion, or recurrence
- Restrict exercise for 90 days after surgical correction.
- Prognosis for survival is poor to guarded.

MISCELLANEOUS

ASSOCIATED CONDITIONS

Colic

AGE-RELATED FACTORS

N/A

ZOONOTIC POTENTIAL

N/A

PREGNANCY

N/A

SEE ALSO

- Expiratory dyspnea
- Inspiratory dyspnea
- Pleuropneumonia
- Thoracic trauma

ABBREVIATION

GI = gastrointestinal

Suggested Reading

Bristol DG. Diaphragmatic hernias in horses and cattle. Compend Cont Educ Pract Vet 1986;8:S407–S412.

Santschi EM, Juzwiak JS, Moll HD, et al. Diaphragmatic hernia repair in three young horses. Vet Surg 1997;26:242–245.

Author Ludovic Bouré

Consulting Editor Jean-Pierre Lavoie

DIARRHEA, NEONATAL

BASICS

DEFINITION

• Diarrhea—increased fecal water
• Neonatal foal—a foal <30 days of age

PATHOPHYSIOLOGY

• Complex and varies with the cause.
• Can result from active secretion, passive secretion, intraluminal osmotic effects, and altered GI transit time.
• Unlike adult horses, in which diarrhea principally involves colonic dysfunction, the small or large intestine may be affected in neonates.
• Loss of large volumes of electrolyte-rich fluid can result in electrolyte, fluid, and acid–base derangements and in multiple organ dysfunction associated with hypovolemic or septic shock.
• Bacterial infections (e.g., salmonellosis) can disseminate to other organs (e.g., joints).

SYSTEMS AFFECTED

• GI—increased fluid secretion into the GI tract results in increased fecal water; depending on the cause, inflammation, ischemia, and disruption of the mucosal barrier can occur.
• Cardiovascular—with severe fluid loss from the vascular space to the intestinal lumen, hypovolemic shock may occur.

GENETICS

N/A

INCIDENCE/PREVALENCE

N/A

SIGNALMENT

• By definition, any foal <30 days of age
• Signs generally are more severe in Arabian foals with SCID.

CLINICAL SIGNS

Historical Findings

• Often acute in onset
• More than one foal may be affected.
• Important to determine dietary history, deworming history, housing and other management practices, and medications administered.

Physical Examination Findings

• Consistency of diarrhea can vary from pasty to watery, and color of feces can vary from yellow to red, with the latter color resulting from hematochezia.
• Foals may show signs of colic (e.g., rolling up on their backs, pawing), abdominal distention, tenesmus, etc.
• Depression, dehydration, and fever are common.

CAUSES

Infectious Causes

• Bacterial—common: *Salmonella* sp., other Gram-negative sepsis/endotoxemia, *Clostridium* (*difficile, perfringens,* rarely others), *Rhodococcus equi* (usually >3 weeks of age); rare: *Escherichia coli, Campylobacter* sp., *Lawsonia intracellularis, Bacteroides* sp., and *Leptospira* sp.
• Viral—common: rotavirus; rare: adenovirus, coronavirus, and parvovirus
• Protozoal—common: *Cryptosporidium* sp.; rare: *Giardia* sp. and *Eimeria leukarti*
• Parasitic—uncommon: *Strongyloides westeri, Strongylus vulgaris,* and *Parascaris equorum*

Noninfectious Causes

• Foal heat diarrhea is a self-limiting diarrhea in foals during the first 2 weeks of life. Proposed causes include changes in milk composition, overfeeding, coprophagia, and enterocyte maturation.
• Antibiotic-induced (i.e., potentiated sulfonamides), flunixin meglumine, and other NSAIDs, although evidence is weak that these cause diarrhea.

RISK FACTORS

• SCID, high population density, poor hygiene, farm history of infectious diarrhea, and sepsis are risk factors.
• Failure of passive transfer does not appear to be a risk factor.

DIAGNOSIS

DIFFERENTIAL DIAGNOSIS

• Other causes of abdominal signs
• Mechanical obstruction—meconium impaction, ileal impaction, umbilical or inguinal hernia, etc.
• Ileus
• Gastric/duodenal ulceration
• Congenital causes of colic—atresias, aganglionosis, etc.
• Peritonitis
• Uroperitoneum

CBC/BIOCHEMISTRY/URINALYSIS

• Often leukopenic with neutropenia (± left shift; ± toxic changes in neutrophils); may show leukocytosis/neutrophilia or normal WBC.

- Often hypoproteinemic, depending on the cause; be careful to interpret protein in light of fluid loss—TP may be lower than it seems initially.
- Often acidemic (e.g., increased pH, lowered CO_2) hyponatremic, and hypochloremic, with varying potassium concentration—often low with diarrhea
- May be hypoglycemic from failure to nurse adequately.
- May be azotemic—pre-renal or renal origin
- Leukopenia with severe lymphopenia and SCID in Arabian foals

OTHER LABORATORY TESTS

Infectious Causes

- Frank blood or hematochezia in neonates is consistent with clostridial diarrhea.
- Culture feces or blood for *Salmonella* sp., *Clostridium* sp., and other bacteria.
- Gram stain feces—many Gram-positive rods indicate clostridial diarrhea.
- Test feces using immunoassays for clostridial toxins—*C. difficile* toxins A or B, and *C. perfringens* toxins.
- Test feces by acid-fast staining or IFA for *Cryptosporidium* sp. and *Giardia* sp.
- Test feces for rotavirus by immunoassay or electron microscopy.
- Test feces by fecal floatation for nematode parasites—rarely cause diarrhea in neonates.
- Look for other evidence of *R. equi,* including disease in other foals.
- RID for immunoglobulins and lymph node biopsy in Arabian foals with suspected SCID, or DNA testing.

Noninfectious Causes

Lactose absorption test (to detect lactase deficiency)—rarely necessary

IMAGING

Abdominal Radiography

- Helpful in detecting evidence of gas- or fluid-filled intestines, free fluid in abdomen, intra-abdominal masses, and erectile loops of small intestine that suggest mechanical obstruction.
- Contrast radiography with barium sulfate (administered by nasogastric tube at a dose of 5 mL/kg as a 30% [w/v] solution, or administered by Foley catheter per rectum at a dose of 5–20 mL/kg using gravity flow) helps to delineate any intestinal obstruction.

Ultrasonography

Can identify free fluid in abdomen (e.g., uroperitoneum, peritonitis), thickening and distention of small intestinal segments, thickening of the large intestine, contraction of small intestinal segments, intussusceptions, or other intra-abdominal masses.

DIAGNOSTIC PROCEDURES

- Measure abdominal circumference in a systematic fashion to monitor progression of distention.
- Abdominocentesis for evidence of peritonitis (normal WBC count in peritoneal fluid in foals is lower [<1500 cells/γL] than in adults) or creatinine concentration to compare with serum results.
- Pass nasogastric tube for evidence of reflux/ileus.
- Stomach endoscopy to detect ulceration

TREATMENT

APPROPRIATE HEALTH CARE

- Fluid therapy is needed to restore circulatory volume and to correct electrolyte and metabolic derangement.
- Depending on the degree of dehydration, fluid may be administered IV or PO.
- IV administration of lactated Ringer solution often is adequate.
- With severe acidosis, isotonic sodium bicarbonate (1.3%; 13 g of sodium bicarbonate per 1 L of distilled water) may be used.
- Dextrose solutions (2.5–5.0%) may promote intracellular movement of potassium, and they provide a small proportion of the foal's caloric needs.
- With hypoglycemia and an unknown electrolyte and acid–base status, a 2.5% dextrose and 0.45% saline solution has been recommended.
- With less severe derangement of fluid and electrolyte balance, oral solutions can be used. Oral electrolyte solutions containing glucose are preferred because of glucose-ionic cotransport; foals that do not consume these solutions voluntarily (not uncommon) can be fed through a nasogastric tube.
- Administration of plasma or *Salmonella typhimurium* antiserum to hypoproteinemic, endotoxemic foals helps to restore normal protein levels, can increase IgG levels, and may help to neutralize circulating endotoxin.

DIARRHEA, NEONATAL

NURSING CARE

- Important
- Vaseline or zinc oxide around the perineum and back of hind legs helps to prevent hair loss and scalding of the skin.
- Ophthalmic ointment may be useful in lubricating eyes if the foal is excessively recumbent.

ACTIVITY

N/A

DIET

N/A

CLIENT EDUCATION

N/A

SURGICAL CONSIDERATIONS

MEDICATIONS

DRUGS OF CHOICE

Broad-Spectrum Antimicrobial Therapy

- Penicillin (22,000 IU/kg q6h) or a first-generation cephalosporin and an aminoglycoside (e.g., amikacin [20–25 mg/kg SID]) may be indicated in foals with suspected primary or secondary bacterial enteritis, primary or secondary peritonitis, or primary or secondary bacteremia.
- Parenteral antimicrobials that do not undergo significant enterohepatic circulation generally are preferred to diminish the potential for exacerbation of diarrhea.
- With suspected clostridial enteritis, metronidazole (10–15 mg/kg PO or IV q8h) is recommended.

Antiulcer Medication

May be given for treatment or prophylaxis—cimetidine, ranitidine, omeprazole, sucralfate, etc.

Intestinal Protectants

- Agents such as bismuth subsalicylate (2–6 ounces PO q6–8h) may aid in decreasing intestinal inflammation.
- Psyllium (0.5–2 ounces PO q6–8h) adds bulk to stool.
- Constipation can result from (over)use of these products.
- Delay/cessation of fecal passage in toxemic animals may lead to increased time for absorption of toxins from the gut.

Loperamide

May benefit some foals (2–4 mg PO q8–12h)

General Comments

- Some foals improve with administration of probiotic preparations PO or by gavage.
- Discontinue intestinal protectants, loperamide, or probiotics if no improvement occurs within 72 hours.

CONTRAINDICATIONS

- Avoid oral antimicrobials, particularly those associated with inducing diarrhea (e.g., erythromycin).
- Avoid enteral nutrition in foals with clostridial colitis.

PRECAUTIONS

- Use of intestinal protectants and loperamide, particularly bismuth subsalicylate, may cause constipation and allow for increased absorption of toxins from the gut.
- Implement isolation measures to control/prevent the spread of possible infectious agents—protective clothing and footwear, footbaths, good hygiene, traffic management of people and horses in barn to minimize contact, appropriate disposal of manure, and careful cleaning and disinfecting

POSSIBLE INTERACTIONS

N/A

ALTERNATIVE DRUGS

N/A

FOLLOW-UP

PATIENT MONITORING

- Monitor attitude, appetite, fecal color and consistency, hydration status, abdominal distention, CBC, serum electrolytes and biochemistry, radiographic or ultrasonographic abnormalities, and response to treatment.
- Monitor other foals for signs of diarrhea or colic.
- Foals may deteriorate rapidly and require intensive care.
- It may be difficult initially to distinguish colic resulting from diarrhea from that resulting from other causes, some of which may require surgery.

POSSIBLE COMPLICATIONS

- Sepsis
- Hypovolemic shock
- Septic peritonitis
- Septic arthritis
- Peripheral arterial or venous thrombosis—distal limbs; jugular veins
- Cerebral edema
- Gastric ulceration

MISCELLANEOUS

ASSOCIATED CONDITIONS

- Septicemia
- SCID
- Peritonitis
- Gastric ulceration

AGE-RELATED FACTORS

- Foals commonly develop a non–life-threatening diarrhea (i.e., foal heat diarrhea) at 5–10 days of age.
- High index of suspicion for clostridial enterocolitis in foals with hemorrhagic diarrhea <1 week of age
- Cryptosporidiosis is most common in foals 2–4 weeks of age.
- *R. equi* is an uncommon cause

ZOONOTIC POTENTIAL

- *Salmonella* sp.
- *Cryptosporidium* sp.
- Enterohemorrhagic *E. coli*

PREGNANCY

Mares often are the source of *Salmonella* sp. in foals.

SYNONYMS

N/A

SEE ALSO

- Acute abdominal pain in foals
- Gastric ulcers
- Neonatal shock

ABBREVIATIONS

- GI = gastrointestinal
- IFA = immunofluorescence assay
- RID = radioimmunodetection
- SCID = Severe combined immunodeficiency disease
- TP = total protein

Suggested Reading

Bernard WV. Differentiating enteritis and conditions that require surgery in foals. Compend Contin Educ Pract Vet 1992;14:535–537.

Cohen ND, Chaffin MK. Colic in foals: infectious and noninfectious causes of diarrhea and enteritis in foals. Compend Contin Educ Pract Vet 1995;18:568–574.

Wilson JH, Cudd TA. Common gastrointestinal diseases. In: Koterba AM, Drummond WH, Kosch PC, eds. Equine clinical neonatology. Philadelphia: Lea & Febiger, 1990:331–341.

Author Noah D. Cohen

Consulting Editor Mary Rose Paradis

DICUMAROL (MOLDY SWEET CLOVER) TOXICOSIS

BASICS

OVERVIEW

- Sweet clover has erect stems and leaves divided into three segments and spikes of flowers, white or yellow, that give off a sweet odor when crushed.
- The white variety can grow as tall as 8 feet; the yellow variety grows to $\cong$6 feet.
- The plant grows in moist soils throughout the U.S. and Canada.
- In some areas, sweet clover is grown for hay and compares favorably with alfalfa in nutrient value; it also may become a weed invading pastures and growing along roadsides.
- Ingestion of moldy sweet clover hay interferes with normal blood clotting in horses.
- Sweet clovers (*Melilotus alba, M. officinalis*) and sweet vernal (*Anthoxanthum odoratum*) contain the nontoxic compound coumarin. When cut and baled for hay under high-moisture conditions, various molds metabolize coumarin to form dicumarol, which inhibits vitamin K epoxide reductase, in turn decreasing vitamin K_1 formation and leading to decreased prothrombin formation and bleeding.
- Dicumarol levels in hay >20 ppm suggest potential toxicity problems; most toxicoses in livestock are reported at levels >30 ppm.

SIGNALMENT

- All animals
- Poisoning occurs more commonly in cattle than in horses, because horses rarely eat moldy sweet clover hay.

SIGNS

- Bleeding diathesis, ranging from mild to severe
- Generally, horses show symptoms within 3–8 weeks after initial ingestion.
- Hemorrhage may be internal or external—epistaxis; fecal blood
- Swellings may appear over bony protuberances of the body because of bruising and hematoma formation.
- Lameness can result from hemorrhage into joint capsules, and soreness may result from muscle hematomas.
- Profuse hemorrhage can occur during minor surgical procedures.
- Symptoms include anemia, pale mucous membranes, weakness, abnormal heartbeat, and death.
- Sudden death often is marked by massive hemorrhage into the thorax or abdominal cavity or around the brain.

CAUSES AND RISK FACTORS

Dicumarol interferes with normal blood clotting because of reduction in the concentrations of the active forms of clotting factors II (i.e., prothrombin), VII, IX, and X. This results from competitive inhibition between vitamin K epoxide and dicumarol for the enzyme vitamin K epoxide reductase, which converts inactive vitamin K epoxide back to its active vitamin K form in the body. Thus, dicumarol causes vitamin K deficiency by inhibiting regeneration of the active form of vitamin K.

DIAGNOSIS

DIFFERENTIAL DIAGNOSIS

- DIC—reduced plasma concentrations of platelets and coagulant and anticoagulant proteins; increased concentrations of coagulant byproducts; petechial hemorrhages
- Severe liver disease—altered liver function tests
- Inherited deficiencies of coagulation factors—measurement of specific coagulation factors
- IMTP—thrombocytopenia; petechial hemorrhages

CBC/BIOCHEMISTRY/URINALYSIS

Blood loss anemia

OTHER LABORATORY TESTS

- Elevated PT and APTT
- Chemical analysis of suspect hay for dicumarol content
- Liver tissue also may be analyzed.

IMAGING

N/A

DIAGNOSTIC PROCEDURES

N/A

PATHOLOGIC FINDINGS

Hemorrhages may occur in any part of the body.

DICUMAROL (MOLDY SWEET CLOVER) TOXICOSIS

TREATMENT

• Massive blood or plasma transfusions may be helpful.
• Handle horses with care to avoid stress and further hemorrhaging.
• Attempt correction of organ dysfunction resulting from accumulation of extravascular blood (e.g., thoracocentesis) only if life-threatening and after normal blood coagulation has been restored.
• Adding alfalfa hay to the diet may help to provide a source of increased dietary vitamin K_1.

MEDICATIONS

DRUGS

• Vitamin K_1 (i.e., phytonadione; 1.5 mg/kg SC or IM BID for up to 3 days) effectively reverses the clotting defect.
• Improvement in PT after vitamin K_1 therapy usually is observed within 24 hours.

CONTRAINDICATIONS/POSSIBLE INTERACTIONS

Do not use vitamin K_3 (i.e., menadione), which is ineffective against dicumarol toxicosis and is nephrotoxic in horses.

FOLLOW-UP

PATIENT MONITORING

Monitor for blood loss.

PREVENTION/AVOIDANCE

• Remove all moldy sweet clover hay from diet.
• Grazing sweet clover in a pasture has not been associated with coagulopathy.

POSSIBLE COMPLICATIONS

N/A

EXPECTED COURSE AND PROGNOSIS

• The time required to exhibit observable clinical signs in healthy horses fed contaminated hay depends on the dicumarol concentrations in that hay; onset of toxicosis is more delayed with lower dicumarol concentrations in the hay.
• Prognosis is based on the severity of blood loss and damage to organ systems affected by hemorrhage.

MISCELLANEOUS

ASSOCIATED CONDITIONS

N/A

AGE-RELATED FACTORS

N/A

ZOONOTIC POTENTIAL

N/A

PREGNANCY

Late-term abortions have been reported in cattle after moldy sweet clover intoxication, but this effect has not been specifically reported in horses.

SEE ALSO

Anticoagulant rodenticides

ABBREVIATIONS

• DIC = disseminated intravascular coagulation
• IMTP = immune-mediated thrombocytopenia
• PT = one-stage prothrombin time
• PTT = activated partial thromboplastin time

Suggested Reading

Hintz HF. Molds, mycotoxins, and mycotoxicosis. Vet Clin North Am Equine Pract 1990;6:419–431.

Author Anita M. Kore
Consulting Editor Robert H. Poppenga

DIGOXIN TOXICOSIS

BASICS

OVERVIEW

Dose-related, cardiovascular failure caused by altered cardiac conduction

SIGNALMENT

No age, breed, or sex predispositions

SIGNS

- Depression, anorexia, and diarrhea
- ECG changes—marked sinus bradycardia, disturbances of atrioventricular conduction, supraventricular and ventricular arrhythmias, widened QRS intervals, and bundle-branch block

CAUSES AND RISK FACTORS

- Patients receiving digoxin—overdose, dose not calculated on basis of lean body mass, or rapid IV administration; hypokalemia increases myocardial sensitivity; hypoproteinemia or displacement from protein-binding sites increases portion of unbound digoxin.
- Renal failure reduces elimination.
- Concurrent quinidine or verapamil administration can reduce renal clearance.

DIAGNOSIS

DIFFERENTIAL DIAGNOSIS

- Clinical signs may be similar to those associated with the primary disease being treated and confused with therapeutic failure, leading to a fatal decision to increase the dose.
- Differentiation is based on sequential monitoring of ECG and sequential TDM of circulating digoxin concentrations.

CBC/BIOCHEMISTRY/URINALYSIS

- No pathognomonic changes
- Evaluate electrolytes, creatinine, and BUN for evidence of predisposing causes of intoxication.

OTHER LABORATORY TESTS

N/A

IMAGING

N/A

DIAGNOSTIC PROCEDURES

TDM—therapeutic concentrations range from 0.5–2.0 ng/mL of plasma; hypokalemia can cause lower concentrations to be toxic.

TREATMENT

- Discontinue digoxin administration.
- Restrict activity by stall confinement.
- Provide supportive care.

MEDICATIONS

DRUGS

- PO supplementation with potassium salts
- Antiarrhythmic medication as indicated by the arrhythmia present
- Antidigoxin antibodies
- Dialysis
- Administer polyionic fluids with caution to avoid worsening the cardiac workload.

CONTRAINDICATIONS/POSSIBLE INTERACTIONS

See *Causes and Risk Factors*.

DIGOXIN TOXICOSIS

FOLLOW-UP

PATIENT MONITORING

• Monitor circulating concentrations and time-course of digoxin, and adjust dosage regimen as indicated by results to maintain concentrations in the therapeutic range.
• Monitor circulating concentrations and fractional renal clearance of electrolytes.
• Supplement potassium as needed to maintain physiologic concentrations.

PREVENTION/AVOIDANCE

N/A

POSSIBLE COMPLICATIONS

N/A

EXPECTED COURSE AND PROGNOSIS

N/A

MISCELLANEOUS

ASSOCIATED CONDITIONS

N/A

AGE-RELATED FACTORS

N/A

ZOONOTIC POTENTIAL

N/A

PREGNANCY

N/A

ABBREVIATION

TDM = therapeutic drug monitoring

Suggested Reading

Brumbaugh GW. Toxicity of pharmacological agents. In: Robinson NE, ed. Current therapy in equine medicine. Philadelphia: WB Saunders, 1992:353–358.

Author Gordon W. Brumbaugh
Consulting Editor Robert H. Poppenga

DISEASES OF THE EQUINE NICTITANS

BASICS

DEFINITION

• The nictitating membrane consists of a T-shaped cartilage with a seromucoid gland located at its base; this gland secretes a significant portion of the aqueous tear film.
• The nictitans is covered on both the palpebral and bulbar surfaces with conjunctiva, and diseases affecting the conjunctiva also may involve the nictitans.
• Movement of the nictitans distributes the tear film and protects the cornea.
• Protrusion of the membrane is passive and occurs secondary to retraction of the globe into the orbit.
• Sympathetic innervation functions to retract the nictitans.
• Horner's syndrome—sympathetic denervation

PATHOPHYSIOLOGY

• Protrusion of the membrane usually is a nonspecific sign of pain. Ocular diseases often result in ocular pain and secondary nictitans protrusion, but systemic disease also can result in protrusion.
• Horner's syndrome can result from central, preganglionic, or postganglionic lesions of the sympathetic innervation of the eye; the subsequent oculosympathetic paralysis is reflected in the loss of sympathetically mediated functions.
• Tetanus may be a complication of elective surgery or accidental wounds. Contamination of wounds by *Clostridium tetani* and the subsequent production of a neurotoxin results in the classical "sawhorse stance."

SYSTEM AFFECTED

Ophthalmic

GENETICS

Breed predilection for ocular squamous cell carcinoma suggests a genetic influence.

SIGNALMENT

Breed Predilection

• No breed predilections for Horner's syndrome
• Hyperkalemic periodic paralysis can cause protrusion of the nictitans and most commonly occurs in Quarter Horses.
• Squamous cell carcinoma, the most common neoplasm affecting the equine nictitans, has a high prevalence in draft horses, Appaloosas, and Paints.

Mean Age and Range

• No detected age distribution for Horner's syndrome or protrusion
• Prevalence of ocular squamous cell carcinoma increases with age.

Predominant Sex

No proven sex predilection

SIGNS

• Protrusion of the membrane, conjunctival hyperemia, chemosis, follicle development, and ocular discharge
• Horner's syndrome—ptosis, nictitans protrusion, slight miosis, hyperemia of nasal and conjunctival mucosa, and increased temperature and sweating of the base of ear, side of the face, and neck of the affected side
• Squamous cell carcinoma may have different appearances (e.g., proliferative/ulcerated, thickening/ulceration of tissue) and may be complicated by habronemiasis.
• Habronemiasis—granulomas, nodules, and often a yellow, caseous exudate and necrotic, mineralized tissue; may be nonhealing and ulcerated.
• Tetanus causes bilateral protrusion, spasms of the masseter muscles, stiff gait, and increased sensitivity to external stimulation.

CAUSES

Protrusion

• Ocular pain
• Neoplasia—squamous cell carcinoma is most common.
• Secondary to environmental causes—foreign bodies and debris; trauma
• Horner's syndrome
• Tetanus
• Inflammation—bacterial, parasitic (i.e., habronemiasis), or trauma
• Enophthalmos
• Space-occupying orbital mass
• Loss of orbital mass—starvation or dehydration
• Decreased ocular mass—microphthalmos or phthisis bulbi
• Secondary to systemic disease—hyperkalemic periodic paralysis
• Congenital lack of pigmentation on the leading edge—optical illusion of protrusion

RISK FACTORS

• Ocular squamous cell carcinoma—white, gray-white, and palomino hair color
• Habronemiasis—warm weather and climates with a heavy fly population
• Tetanus—deficient vaccination programs

DIAGNOSIS

DIFFERENTIAL DIAGNOSIS

• Ocular pain—ulcerative keratitis, corneal stromal abscess, anterior uveitis, keratomycosis, corneal laceration, and conjunctivitis
• Horner's syndrome—jugular vein and carotid artery injections, cervical abscesses, guttural pouch infections, neoplasia of the neck and thoracic inlet, trauma to the neck and thorax, and mediastinal and thoracic masses
• Nodular/mass lesions of the nictitans—squamous cell carcinoma, habronemiasis, mastocytoma, hemangioma, hemangiosarcoma, papilloma, fungal granulomas, nodular necrobiosis, and foreign-body reaction
• Space-occupying orbital mass—neoplasia, abscess, hematoma, and arteriovenous fistula

CBC/BIOCHEMISTRY/URINALYSIS

Usually normal, unless nictitans disease is associated with systemic disease.

OTHER LABORATORY TESTS

• Habronemiasis—conjuctival scraping reveals eosinophils, mast cells, neutrophils, plasma cells, and rarely, larvae.
• Mass lesions—biopsy and histopathology
• Consider bacterial culture and sensitivity if bacterial inflammation is suspected.
• Other specific tests as indicated when systemic disease is suspected.

IMAGING

N/A

DIAGNOSTIC PROCEDURES

• Complete ophthalmic examination to identify ocular causes—fluorescein stain and examination for signs of anterior uveitis (e.g., aqueous flare, miosis, hypotony); examination behind the nictitans may reveal a foreign body or debris.
• Pharmacologic testing to differentiate central/preganglionic from postganglionic lesions in Horner's syndrome has not been evaluated in horses.
• Topical application of 1% phenylephrine or 0.1% epinephrine—rapid mydriasis within 20 minutes indicates postganglionic lesion; slow mydriasis within 30–40 minutes indicates preganglionic lesion.
• Topical application of 0.1% pilocarpine—rapid miosis within 20 minutes indicates postganglionic lesion; no miosis indicates preganglionic lesion.

PATHOLOGIC FINDINGS

• Habronemiasis—eosinophils, mast cells, neutrophils, plasma cells, and rarely, larvae
• Squamous cell carcinoma—epithelial cells with neoplastic characteristics
• Lymphoma—large population of monomorphic lymphocytes with neoplastic characteristics
• Multiple myeloma—large population of neoplastic plasma cells
• Other histopathologic findings are possible depending on the type of neoplasia.

DISEASES OF THE EQUINE NICTITANS

TREATMENT

APPROPRIATE HEALTH CARE

- Most horses with protrusion or Horner's syndrome can be treated on an outpatient basis.
- Treatment of some ocular (e.g., severe ulcerative keratitis, corneal stromal abscess, keratomycosis, squamous cell carcinoma) and systemic (e.g., tetanus, severe hyperkalemic periodic paralysis) diseases associated with secondary nictitans involvement may require hospitalization.

ACTIVITY

- Restriction may be required in cases of hyperkalemic periodic paralysis associated with nictitans protrusion.
- If environmental irritation is suspected, restrict or eliminate exposure to the inciting substance.
- Do not ride animals with ocular involvement/ disease if visual status is compromised.
- Keep animals with tetanus in a quiet, dark environment.

DIET

- No changes necessary
- Feed hay at ground level rather than in elevated hayracks or bags.

CLIENT EDUCATION

- With evidence of self trauma, place a protective hood over the affected eye.
- Instruct the client to contact the veterinarian if the condition worsens in any way—the problem may not be responding appropriately to treatment or may be progressing, or the patient may be having an adverse response to the medication.
- With hyperkalemic periodic paralysis, inform the client regarding the genetic basis of this disease, and advise against breeding the affected animal.

SURGICAL CONSIDERATIONS

- Squamous cell carcinoma—surgical resection of the nictitans, with adjunctive cryotherapy or chemotherapy; enucleation or exenteration may be necessary depending on the type of neoplasia and the extent of surrounding tissue invasion.
- Foreign bodies and debris—usually can be removed with topical anesthesia and liberal flushing of the conjunctival fornices.
- Surgical management of ocular diseases causing protrusion of the membrane is addressed in the appropriate chapters. Treatment of corneal stromal abscessation and keratomycosis may require conjunctival flap procedures, lamellar keratectomy, or penetrating keratoplasty.
- Tetanus—thorough wound lavage and debridement

MEDICATIONS

DRUGS OF CHOICE

- Habronemiasis—topical 0.03% echothiophate iodide (Phospholine) and ophthalmic neomycin/polymyxin B with dexamethasone (Maxitrol) q12h.
- Multifocal lesions—ivermectin (200 μg/kg PO); intralesional triamcinolone (10–40 mg/lesion) may reduce the size of granulomas.
- Bacterial inflammation—topical, broad-spectrum antibiotic initially (triple antibiotic usually appropriate); may change based on results of bacterial culture and sensitivity; treat q6–12h, depending on the severity of disease.
- Squamous cell carcinoma—see the *Ocular Squamous Cell Carcinoma section.*
- Ocular diseases inciting protrusion—see the appropriate section.
- Tetanus—tetanus antitoxin (IM or IV) to neutralize circulating exotoxin; tetanus toxoid (IM) to induce humeral immunity, penicillin, and muscle relaxants/tranquilizers as needed to control muscle spasms.
- Other systemic medication as indicated by any concurrent systemic disease.

CONTRAINDICATIONS

N/A

PRECAUTIONS

N/A

POSSIBLE INTERACTIONS

N/A

ALTERNATE DRUGS

N/A

FOLLOW-UP

PATIENT MONITORING

- Recheck the patient soon after beginning therapy (3–4 days), with the specific time frame determined by the disease and its severity.
- Subsequent rechecks as dictated by the severity of disease and response to treatment

PREVENTION/AVOIDANCE

- Fly control in barns and pastures, fly hoods, frequent periocular administration of insect repellant, and regular deworming with ivermectin can help to prevent habronemiasis.
- Treat any underlying ocular or systemic disease that may be inciting the nictitans disease.

POSSIBLE COMPLICATIONS

Potential complications from neoplasia of the nictitans and its treatment vary with the specific type of tumor; possibilities include recurrence of the neoplasia and metastatic disease.

EXPECTED COURSE AND PROGNOSIS

- Course and prognosis of nictitating membrane neoplasia depend on the specific type of neoplasia and the extent of surrounding tissue invasion.
- Horner's syndrome may be reversible, depending on the cause. Resolution of cervical abscesses and guttural pouch disease may resolve associated Horner's syndrome, but neoplastic and traumatic causes are less likely to be correctable.
- Prognosis of nictitans protrusion secondary to systemic or ocular disease varies with the specific disease.
- Tetanus is a life-threatening disease with a prolonged recovery phase requiring intense supportive care.

MISCELLANEOUS

ASSOCIATED CONDITIONS

N/A

AGE-RELATED FACTORS

N/A

ZOONOTIC POTENTIAL

N/A

PREGNANCY

Systemic absorption of topically applied medication is possible; weigh the benefits of treatment against any risks posed to the fetus.

SYNONYMS

N/A

SEE ALSO

- Conjunctivitis
- Corneal stromal abscessation
- Corneal ulceration
- Hyperkalemic periodic paralysis
- Keratomycosis
- Ocular squamous cell carcinoma
- Tetanus

Suggested Reading

Brooks DE. Equine ophthalmology. In: Gelatt KN, ed. Veterinary ophthalmology. Philadelphia: Lippincott Williams & Wilkins, 1999.

Author Heidi M. Dennis
Consulting Editor Dennis E. Brooks

DISORDERS OF SEXUAL DEVELOPMENT

BASICS

DEFINITION

- Sexual differentiation occurs sequentially at three levels—genetic, gonadal, and phenotypic.
- Errors at any level lead to varying degrees of genital ambiguity and aberrant reproductive function.
- Affected animals are known as intersexes or as particular classes of hermaphrodites—true hermaphrodites or pseudohermaphrodites, with the latter further divided into male and female.

PATHOPHYSIOLOGY

- Genetic sex is established at fertilization.
- Gonadal sex is controlled by genetic sex determination.
- Phenotypic sex is governed by gonadal function and target-organ sensitivity.

Disorders of Genetic Sex

- Sex chromosomes—abnormal number (aneuploidy); abnormal structure (deletion, duplication/insertion, reciprocal exchange, fusion, inversion).
- Chimeras—individual with coexisting, genetically distinct cell populations admixed in utero from different genetic sources.
- Mosaics—individual with coexisting, genetically distinct cell populations caused by errors in chromosomal segregation during division of a single genetic source.
- Normality of genetic sex development depends on normality of sex chromosomal pairings during gametogenesis and fertilization.
- Spontaneous errors affecting gonadal development may occur early during embryonic life.
- *Sry* gene initiates testicular development; if present, the animal develops testicular tissue regardless of the number of X chromosomes present.
- 63,XO (most common)—ovarian dysgenesis, small stature, phenotypic female; similar to Turner's syndrome.
- 65,XXY—hypoplastic testes, genitalia normal to hypoplastic, phenotypic male; similar to Klinefelter's syndrome.
- Numerous possible combinations (mixoploidies) are reported.

Disorders of Gonadal Sex

- Sex reversal syndromes—gonadal and genetic sex may disagree because of autosomal recessive genes or translocation of TDF to X chromosomes.
- XY with no testes—hypoplastic ovary/streak gonad; acyclic, sterile; female phenotype, but is XY female.
- XX with varying degrees of testicular development—extreme form is XX male; otherwise, a true hermaphrodite forms.
- True hermaphrodite with ovotestes—ambiguous genitalia; named by genetic makeup, either XX or XY.

Disorders of Phenotypic Sex

- Genetic and gonadal sex agree, but ambiguous external genitalia present.
- Phenotypic sex development involves differentiation of tubular genitalia (mesonephric and paramesonephric ducts) and external genitalia under direction of the gonad.
- Degree of masculinization of external genitalia relates to the proportion of testicular tissue on the intersex gonad.
- Male reproductive tract—gonad must produce testosterone (Leydig cells) and mullerian-inhibitory substance (Sertoli cells) at correct time.
- Target tissue (duct system) must have cytosolic receptors for testosterone and enzyme 5α-reductase to produce dihydrotestosterone, the androgen responsible for tubular and external genitalia differentiation.
- Hypospadia—urethra opens ventrally on penis.
- Epispadia—urethra opens dorsally on penis.
- Pseudohermaphrodite—named by the gonadal tissue present; male, testes; female, ovary.
- Testicular feminization—genetic/gonadal male but external genitalia female; target-organ insensitivity.

GENETICS

See *Pathophysiology.*

INCIDENCE/PREVALENCE

N/A

SIGNALMENT

- Congenital disorders, by definition, mean present at birth.
- Normal external genitalia may delay detection of problem until the affected individual enters a breeding program.

SIGNS

Historical Findings

- Failure to display appropriate reproductive behavior with opposite sex; attraction to same sex.
- Infertility; sterility.

Physical Examination Findings

External:

- Female—normal or hypoplastic vulva; enlarged clitoris; presence of os clitoris; purulent vulval discharge.
- Male—penis, prepuce normal, hypoplastic; testes, scrotal or cryptorchid; hypospadia, epispadia (abnormal position of urinary orifice, closure of urethra).

Internal:

- Abnormal gonadal position (cryptorchid), form (hypoplastic, fibrous) or type (ovotestis).
- Aberrant ductal derivatives—aplasia, hypoplasia, or cysts.

CAUSES

- Congenital—heritable or spontaneous.
- Genetic abnormalities—zygote fusion.
- Placental admixture not reported in equines.
- Exogenous—steroid hormone use during pregnancy.
- Progestins, androgens—masculinize females.
- Estrogens, antiandrogens—feminize males.

DIAGNOSIS

DIFFERENTIAL DIAGNOSIS

If phenotypically normal:

- Infectious infertility—female, endometritis (see also *Venereal Disease*); male, see *Venereal Disease.*
- Noninfectious infertility—female, endometrial degeneration; male, testicular hypoplasia or degeneration.

CBC/BIOCHEMISTRY/URINALYSIS

Unremarkable, unless cystitis or infection results from aberrant genital structure.

OTHER LABORATORY TESTS

Hormonal Assays

Testosterone:

- hCG challenge—baseline sample; administer 3000 IU hCG; blood samples at 3 and 24 hours.
- Increase in testosterone indicates testicular tissue is present—Leydig cell production.

Estrone Sulfate:

- Source in male is the testicles—Sertoli cells.
- Couple with testosterone (hCG challenge) to improve diagnostic accuracy.

DISORDERS OF SEXUAL DEVELOPMENT

Immunology

- Test for 5α-reductase or cytosolic receptor.
- Use labial skin only, because receptors are site specific.

IMAGING

Ultrasonography—coupled with transrectal palpation; discovery of mass (neoplastic) or cyst (segmental aplasia with fluid dilations).

PATHOLOGIC FINDINGS

- Disorders are characterized by histopathology of gonad, morphology of tubular genitalia (duct derivatives), accessory glands (male), and external genitalia (increased anogenital distance, vulval folds, blind ended vagina).
- Karyotyping—culture of peripheral blood leukocytes and examination of metaphase spreads; collect whole blood in heparin or ACD; send samples unrefrigerated by rapid courier; cultures require 48–72 hours.
- PCR
- Detection of *Sry*—whole blood in EDTA.

TREATMENT

APPROPRIATE HEALTH CARE

N/A, unless resulting pathology or physical/behavioral problems develop that require gonadectomy or hysterectomy to modify behavior.

NURSING CARE

N/A

ACTIVITY

N/A

DIET

N/A

CLIENT EDUCATION

N/A

SURGICAL CONSIDERATIONS

See *Appropriate Health Care.*

MEDICATIONS

DRUGS OF CHOICE

N/A

CONTRAINDICATIONS

N/A

PRECAUTIONS

N/A

POSSIBLE INTERACTIONS

N/A

ALTERNATIVE DRUGS

N/A

FOLLOW-UP

PATIENT MONITORING

Only if physical or behavioral complications develop.

PREVENTION/AVOIDANCE

Remove carrier animals from the breeding population—gonadectomy.

POSSIBLE COMPLICATIONS

N/A

EXPECTED COURSE AND PROGNOSIS

N/A

MISCELLANEOUS

ASSOCIATED CONDITIONS

If not detected early—pyometra; cystitis; hematuria; gonadal neoplasia (intra-abdominal testis).

AGE-RELATED FACTORS

Congenital

ZOONOTIC POTENTIAL

N/A

PREGNANCY

Fertility is rare in affected animals.

SYNONYMS

- Hermaphrodite
- Intersex
- Klinefelter's syndrome—trisomy
- Mesonephric—wolffian
- Paramesonephric—mullerian
- Pseudohermaphrodite
- Turner's syndrome—monosomy X

ABBREVIATIONS

- ACD = acid citrate dextrose
- hCG = human chorionic gonadotropin
- PCR = polymerase chain reaction
- *Sry* = sex-determining region of the Y chromosome
- TDF = testis-determining factor

Suggested Reading

Bowling AT, Hughes JP. Cytogenetic abnormalities. In: McKinnon AO, Voss JL, eds. Equine reproduction. Malvern: Lea & Febiger, 1993:258–265.

Halnan CR. Equine cytogenetics: role in equine veterinary practice. Equine Vet J 1985;17:173–177.

Meyers-Wallen VN. Normal sexual development and intersex conditions in domestic animals. In: Proceedings of the Reproductive Pathology Symposium. Sponsored by the ACT/SFT. Hastings, Nebraska, 1997:18–28.

Meyers-Wallen VN, Hurtgen J, Schlafer D, et al. *Sry*-negative XX true hermaphroditism in a Pasa Fino horse. Equine Vet J 1997; 29:404–408.

Milliken JE, Paccamonti DL, Shoemaker S, Green WH. XX male pseudohermaphroditism in a horse. J Am Vet Med Assoc 1995;207:77–79.

Author Peter R. Morresey

Consulting Editor Carla L. Carleton

DISSEMINATED INTRAVASCULAR COAGULATION (DIC)

BASICS

DEFINITION

Pathologic disruption of hemostasis, with early microvascular thrombosis leading to clotting factor consumption; consumptive coagulopathy and actions of fibrinolytic byproducts may lead to fatal hemorrhagic diathesis.

PATHOPHYSIOLOGY

- Any disease that activates the coagulation cascade or exposes subendothelial phospholipid to blood can cause DIC. The character, severity, and duration of the procoagulant stimulus determine the clinical manifestation.
- Chronic or localized forms exist, but usually is acute and systemic
- Endotoxemia is the most common underlying cause. Endotoxin initiates intrinsic coagulation through activation of factor XII, initiates extrinsic coagulation by stimulating expression of mononuclear cell–associated tissue factor, causes direct damage to vascular endothelium, and causes thromboxane-mediated platelet activation. Endotoxin also inhibits fibrinolysis; thus, producing concurrent accelerated clot formation and inhibited clot resolution.
- Initial thrombus formation in capillary beds causes localized tissue ischemia and necrosis; the associated inflammation further stimulates coagulation. Inhibited fibrinolysis and progressive consumption of the anticoagulants antithrombin III and protein C perpetuate coagulopathy.
- The mononuclear phagocyte system cannot cope with accumulated byproducts of coagulation and fibrinolysis. Intravascular accumulation of fibrin degradation products inhibits thrombin, causes platelet dysfunction, and decreases fibrin polymerization, all of which contribute to unregulated hemostasis.
- Terminally, clotting factors are depleted and thrombosis replaced by consumptive coagulopathy with associated hemorrhagic diathesis.

SYSTEMS AFFECTED

- Cardiovascular—early DIC may manifest as an enhanced tendency toward vessel thrombosis; later, hemorrhage predominates.
- Hemic/lymphatic/immune—tendency toward thrombosis (early) or hemorrhage (as clotting factors are depleted)
- Renal/urologic—microvascular thrombosis may result in renal ischemia, hematuria, and oliguria.
- Hepatobiliary—microvascular thrombosis may result in ischemic hepatic dysfunction.
- GI—colic due to microvascular thrombosis
- Respiratory—thrombosis of the pulmonary vessels

GENETICS

N/A

INCIDENCE/PREVALENCE

N/A

SIGNALMENT

N/A

SIGNS

General Comments

- Most early clinical signs are referable to the primary underlying disease process.
- May result in microthrombosis of almost any body system; a wide variety of clinical signs are described.

Historical Findings

Depend on the primary underlying disease process

Physical Examination Findings

- Organ system microthrombosis may cause colic, laminitis, oliguria, dyspnea, tachypnea, or abnormal mentation.
- Catheter- and venipuncture-site thrombosis is common.
- Ironically, signs of hemorrhage are unusual; however, petechial or ecchymotic hemorrhage or prolonged bleeding after venipuncture may be noticed. Epistaxis, hyphema, and melena are uncommon, and life-threatening hemorrhage is rare.

CAUSES

- Endotoxemia, secondary to ischemic or inflammatory GI diseases, and gram-negative bacterial sepsis are the most common causes in horses.
- Less commonly associated—metritis, pleuropneumonia, hemolytic anemia, viremia, vasculitis, burns, neoplasia, and renal or hepatic failure

RISK FACTORS

Any disease that activates coagulation or causes significant endothelial damage

DIAGNOSIS

DIFFERENTIAL DIAGNOSIS

- Early detection is a more significant diagnostic challenge than differentiation from other diseases.
- Severity of signs associated with the inciting disease may mask early evidence of DIC.
- Rarely, occurs secondary to a disease in which laboratory and clinical abnormalities associated with the primary disease may mirror those signifying the onset of DIC (e.g., thrombocytopenia accompanying hemolytic anemia or vasculitis).

CBC/BIOCHEMISTRY/URINALYSIS

- Laboratory findings—inconsistent
- Early diagnosis depends on astute clinical observation, recognition of a likely predisposing primary disease, and supportive laboratory evidence.
- Thrombocytopenia is the most common CBC abnormality.
- The primary disease process usually involves acute, severe inflammation; therefore, hypofibrinoginemia is rare.
- Biochemical indications of organ system ischemia secondary to microvascular thrombosis are nonspecific and commonly include azotemia and increased serum hepatic enzyme concentrations.

OTHER LABORATORY TESTS

- In addition to thrombocytopenia, increased serum fibrin degradation products ($>40\ \mu g/mL$) and decreased serum antithrombin III are the most common clinicopathologic abnormalities.
- PT, APTT, and TT are crude indicators in horses and vary with the stage of disease. A trend toward prolongation of PT, APTT, and TT with repeated measurement is consistent with the diagnosis but only occurs when the disease process is advanced.
- Laboratory test findings—best interpreted serially and in conjunction with careful and repeated clinical assessment
- Poor venipuncture technique and sample handling can result in erroneous laboratory findings, particularly when hemostatic testing is in question.

DISSEMINATED INTRAVASCULAR COAGULATION (DIC)

IMAGING
N/A

DIAGNOSTIC PROCEDURES
N/A

PATHOLOGIC FINDINGS
- Generally reflect the primary underlying disease process
- Thrombosis, petechiation, and ecchymoses may be evident grossly or histologically.

TREATMENT

APPROPRIATE HEALTH CARE
This life-threatening condition always warrants hospitalization and intensive care.

NURSING CARE
Venipuncture technique, catheter maintenance, and frequent clinical assessment are critical.

ACTIVITY
Strictly limited

DIET
Horses should be encouraged to eat a balanced diet, based on any restrictions appropriate to the primary disease.

CLIENT EDUCATION
Poor prognosis; clients should be prepared accordingly.

SURGICAL CONSIDERATIONS
If a surgical GI disease is also present, the prognosis is grave; consider euthanasia.

MEDICATIONS

DRUGS OF CHOICE
- Treatment is highly controversial.
- Address the underlying disease aggressively.
- Consider treatments aimed at limiting the deleterious affects of endotoxemia—low-dose flunixin meglumine (0.25 mg/kg IV BID) and antiendotoxin antiserum
- Support of tissue perfusion with IV fluids is mandatory.
- Fresh plasma transfusion (15–30 mL/kg) may be warranted by severe thrombocytopenia and uncontrolled bleeding, but cost and availability may make this impractical.
- Administration of heparin to reduce thrombosis is problematic. Detrimental as well as beneficial effects are possible, selection of a rational dosage regimen is difficult, and commercially available products vary widely in composition. The antithrombotic activity of heparin depends on adequate serum concentrations of antithrombin III. Heparin likely is most beneficial if administered early during the course of severe GI diseases (i.e., before onset of DIC). Administer sodium heparin for no more than 3 days, due to the likely development of erythrocyte agglutination, and at a dosage no greater than 40 IU/kg SC every 12 hours.

CONTRAINDICATIONS
Avoid potentially nephrotoxic drugs and those requiring hepatic metabolism.

POSSIBLE INTERACTIONS
N/A

ALTERNATIVE DRUGS
N/A

FOLLOW-UP

PATIENT MONITORING
- Physical examination every 2–4 hours, with particular attention to gait (laminitis) and evidence of bleeding or thrombosis
- Check platelet count, fibrin degradation products, PT and APTT, and serum creatinine and hepatic enzyme concentrations daily.
- Check PCV and plasma protein every 12 hours.

PREVENTION/AVOIDANCE
Early detection and aggressive treatment of predisposing diseases

POSSIBLE COMPLICATIONS
- Septic thrombophlebitis
- Laminitis
- Colic
- Acute renal failure
- Acute hepatic failure

EXPECTED COURSE AND PROGNOSIS
With early detection and aggressive treatment of the underlying disease, DIC occasionally can be arrested; more commonly, DIC is so advanced at its detection that the outcome is fatal.

MISCELLANEOUS

ASSOCIATED CONDITIONS
- Laminitis
- Jugular vein thrombosis

AGE-RELATED FACTORS
N/A

ZOONOTIC POTENTIAL
N/A

PREGNANCY
N/A

SYNONYMS
- Consumptive coagulopathy
- Defibrination syndrome
- Intravascular coagulation or fibrinolysis

SEE ALSO
- Coagulation defects, acquired/induced
- Hemorrhage, acute

ABBREVIATIONS
- APTT = activated partial thromboplastin time
- GI = gastrointestinal
- PCV = packed cell volume
- PT = prothrombin time
- TT = thrombin time

Suggested Reading

Morris DD. Diseases of the hemolymphatic system. In: Reed SM, Bayly WM, eds. Equine internal medicine. Philadelphia: WB Saunders, 1998:558–602.

Author Chrysann Collatos
Consulting Editor Debra C. Sellon

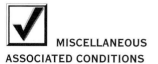

DORSAL DISPLACEMENT OF THE SOFT PALATE (DDSP)

BASICS

OVERVIEW

• A performance-limiting, upper airway condition identified in 1.3% of 479 racehorses examined endoscopically at rest. The true prevalence probably is higher, however, because palate displacement is a dynamic condition that most frequently occurs during intense exercise, making diagnosis at rest difficult.

• Horse are obligate nasal breathers, perhaps to allow maintenance of the olfactory senses during deglutition. The normal epiglottis is dorsal to the soft palate and contacts the caudal free margin, forming a tight seal around the base of the soft palate. The pillars of the soft palate converge dorsally, forming the palatopharyngeal arch. When the soft palate displaces dorsally, the epiglottis cannot be seen within the nasopharynx and is within the oropharynx, and the caudal free margin of the soft palate billows across the rima glottis during exhalation, creating airway obstruction.

• Organ system—respiratory

SIGNALMENT

Any horse participating in intense exercise is at risk.

SIGNS

• Intermittent DDSP occurs in athletic horses during intense exercise.

• Horses with intermittent DDSP generally have a history of exercise intolerance and may make a loud noise during exhalation; concurrent with these signs is open-mouth breathing.

• Frequently, affected horses have a history of respiratory tract infection.

CAUSES AND RISK FACTORS

• Despite DDSP first being reported in 1949, the cause remains unknown.

• The condition has been attributed to many anatomic and functional abnormalities—excessive caudal retraction of the larynx, overly long soft palate, epiglottic hypoplasia or malformation, caudal retraction of the tongue and opening the mouth, and neuromuscular dysfunction.

• A few affected horses have been diagnosed with equine protozoal myelitis; DDSP was the only sign of neuromuscular dysfunction.

DIAGNOSIS

DIFFERENTIAL DIAGNOSIS

• Any dynamic upper airway obstruction—laryngeal hemiplegia, epiglottic entrapment, and aryepiglottic fold collapse; endoscopy of the upper airway both at rest and while exercising on a treadmill may be required to differentiate these conditions from DDSP.

• Complete physical examination to rule out other causes of exercise intolerance—pulmonary disease, cardiac abnormalities, lameness, and neurologic disease

CBC/BIOCHEMISTRY/URINALYSIS

N/A

OTHER LABORATORY TESTS

N/A

IMAGING

N/A

DIAGNOSTIC PROCEDURES

• The diagnosis of intermittent DDSP is based on a history of poor performance associated with respiratory noise, observation of the horse competing or racing, physical examination findings, and endoscopy of the upper airway at rest and while exercising on a treadmill.

DORSAL DISPLACEMENT OF THE SOFT PALATE (DDSP)

• Endoscopy of the upper airway at rest usually is normal. A nasal occlusion test may be performed to mimic intense breathing efforts that occur during exercise, and this test may induce DDSP. When the soft palate displaces dorsally, the epiglottis cannot be seen within the nasopharynx.
• To date, the best diagnostic test is treadmill endoscopy, in which the horse completes an incremental exercise test with the endoscope placed in the nasopharynx.

TREATMENT

• Treatment initially is directed at modifying or eliminating factors associated with the occurrence of DDSP.
• Condition and re-evaluate unfit horses before considering surgery.
• If upper respiratory tract inflammation was diagnosed during the examination, treatment should include judicious use of systemic anti-inflammatory medication.
• Several surgical therapies and combination surgical therapies currently are performed as treatment—sternothyrohyoid myectomy, staphylectomy, epiglottic augmentation, and combinations of these techniques.

MEDICATIONS

DRUGS
N/A

CONTRAINDICATIONS/POSSIBLE INTERACTIONS
N/A

FOLLOW-UP

EXPECTED COURSE AND PROGNOSIS
• Continue medical treatment for 30–60 days, rest the horse for 30–60 days, and then re-evaluate before resuming training or considering surgery.
• Prognosis after surgery is approximately 60%.

MISCELLANOUS

ASSOCIATED CONDITIONS
N/A

AGE-RELATED FACTORS
N/A

ZOONOTIC POTENTIAL
N/A

PREGNANCY
N/A

SEE ALSO
Dynamic collapse of the upper airway

Suggested Reading

Robertson JT. Pharynx and larynx. In: Beech J, ed. Equine respiratory disorders. 1st ed. Philadelphia: Lea & Febiger, 1991:331–388.

Author Susan J. Holcombe
Consulting Editor Jean-Pierre Lavoie

DOURINE

BASICS

DEFINITION
• Disease of equidae
• Natural infections reported only in horses and donkeys.
• Causative agent—*Trypanosoma equiperdum.*
• Venereal-only transmission.
• Requires no vector host; transmissible by direct contact.
• Tropism for genital mucosa; cannot survive outside host.
• Mortality high; debilitation; predisposition to other diseases.

PATHOPHYSIOLOGY
• Limited to venereal transmission.
• The organism has a predilection for genital mucosa.
• Acute disease after incubation is characterized by pyrexia, debility, and multisystemic disease.

SYSTEMS AFFECTED
• GI—weight loss; emaciation.
• Cardiovascular—intense anemia, dependent edema, and urticaria.
• Lymphatic—peripheral lymphadenopathy.
• Nervous—meningoencephalitis, progressive weakness, paresis, and paralysis.
• Musculoskeletal—progressive weakness.
• Reproductive—abortion.
• Ophthalmic—keratoconjunctivitis.

GENETICS
N/A

INCIDENCE/PREVALENCE
• Enzootic; endemic in Africa, Asia, Central and South America.
• Low prevalence in parts of Europe.
• 50% mortality with acute disease.

SIGNALMENT
Breeding mares and stallions.

SIGNS
• Depend on strain and general health of the horse population.
• Incubation period—1 week to 3 months.
• $\cong$50% of affected animals die of acute disease in 6–8 weeks.
• Hindquarter weakness; ataxia.
• Hyperesthesia; hyperalgia.
• Anemia, wasting, and intermittent pyrexia.
• Course of disease—usually 1–2 months, but may last from 2–4 years.

Females
• severe, edematous vulval and perineal swelling.
• Mucopurulent vulval discharge.
• Frequent, painful attempts at urination because of vaginal mucosal irritation.
• Chronic cases develop urticarial subcutaneous plaques in vulva and surrounding tissues, which may regress within hours or days to areas of depigmentation.
• Abortion, if pregnant.

Males
• Edema of prepuce, urethral process, penis, testes, and scrotum.
• Paraphimosis may ensue.
• Inguinal lymph node enlargement.
• Plaques and depigmented lesions, as in females.

CAUSES
• Exposure to *T. equiperdum.*
• Infection occurs across intact genital mucosal barriers.

RISK FACTORS
• Presence of asymptomatic carriers.
• The organism periodically may be unrecoverable from the urethra or vagina.
• Transmission is not certain, even from matings with known-infected animals.
• Transport of horses from known-infected areas.
• Intact male discharges from urethra.
• Males may serve as noninfected mechanical carriers after breeding of infected females.

DIAGNOSIS

DIFFERENTIAL DIAGNOSIS
• Equine herpes virus 3
• Equine infectious anemia
• Equine viral arteritis
• Endometritis

CBC/BIOCHEMISTRY/URINALYSIS
• Acute infection—leukocytosis; other inflammatory changes.
• Chronic, debilitating infection results in anemia and extensive multisystemic disease.

OTHER LABORATORY TESTS

Cytology/Histopathology
• Causative organism in smears of body fluid or lymph node aspirates.
• Seminal fluid, mucus from prepuce, and vaginal discharges.

Serology
• CF test is the most widely used and reliable.
• Also available—AGID, IFA, and ELISA tests.

IMAGING
N/A

DIAGNOSTIC PROCEDURES
In the nervous form, the organism can be recovered from the lumbar and sacral spinal cord, sciatic and obturator nerves, and CSF.

PATHOLOGIC FINDINGS
Primarily emaciation with enlargement of lymph nodes, spleen, liver; periportal infiltrations in liver; and petechial hemorrhages in kidney.

DOURINE

TREATMENT

APPROPRIATE HEALTH CARE
- May be successful if treated early in the course of disease.
- Chronic cases in particular are unresponsive to treatment.

NURSING CARE
N/A

ACTIVITY
N/A

DIET
N/A

CLIENT EDUCATION
Recovered treated animals may become asymptomatic carriers.

SURGICAL CONSIDERATIONS
N/A

MEDICATIONS

DRUGS OF CHOICE
Quinapyramine sulfate—5mg/kg divided doses SC.

CONTRAINDICATIONS
N/A

PRECAUTIONS
N/A

POSSIBLE INTERACTIONS
N/A

ALTERNATIVE DRUGS
- Diminazene—7mg/kg as 5% solution injected SC; repeat at half-dose 24 hours later.
- Suramin—10mg/kg IV 2–3 times at weekly intervals.

FOLLOW-UP

PATIENT MONITORING
- Body weight and condition.
- CBC
- Neurologic examination.

PREVENTION/AVOIDANCE
- Prohibit movement of horses from infected areas.
- Control breeding practices.
- Eradication—serology with slaughter of infected animals.
- Consecutive negative tests at least 1 month apart indicate freedom from disease.

POSSIBLE COMPLICATIONS
Multisystemic nature of the disease predisposes to multiple system failure.

EXPECTED COURSE AND PROGNOSIS
- Incubation period—1 week to 3 months.
- ≅50% of affected animals die of acute disease in 6–8 weeks.
- Hindquarter weakness; ataxia.
- Hyperesthesia and hyperalgia.
- Anemia, wasting, and intermittent pyrexia.
- Course of disease—usually 1–2 months, but may last from 2–4 years.

MISCELLANEOUS

ASSOCIATED CONDITIONS
N/A

AGE-RELATED CONDITIONS
N/A

ZOONOTIC POTENTIAL
N/A

PREGNANCY
Abortion

SYNONYMS
N/A

SEE ALSO
Venereal diseases

ABBREVIATIONS
- AGID = agar gel immunodiffusion
- CF = complement fixation
- CSF = cerebrospinal fluid
- ELISA = enzyme-linked immunoadsorbent assay
- GI = gastrointestinal
- IFA = immunofluorescent assay

Suggested Reading

Barrowman PR. Observations on the transmission, immunology, clinical signs and chemotherapy of dourine (*Trypanosoma equiperdum* infection) in horses, with special reference to cerebrospinal fluid. Onderstepoort J Vet Res 1976;43:55–66.

Hagebock JM, Chieves L, Frerichs WM, Miller CD. Evaluation of agar gel immunodiffusion and indirect fluorescent antibody assays as supplemental tests for dourine in equids. Am J Vet Res 1993;54:1201–1208.

Radositis OM, Blood DC, Gay CC. Veterinary medicine. 8th ed. London: Balliere Tindall, 1994:1220–1222.

Author Peter R. Morresey

Consulting Editor Carla L. Carleton

DUODENITIS–PROXIMAL JEJUNITIS (ANTERIOR ENTERITIS, PROXIMAL ENTERITIS)

BASICS

DEFINITION

A condition in which inflammation of the proximal small intestine results in small intestinal distension and gastric reflux through excessive fluid and electrolyte secretion.

PATHOPHYSIOLOGY

- Idiopathic condition
- Lesions tend to be restricted to the duodenum and proximal jejunum.
- Whatever the inciting factor, fluid and electrolyte accumulation occurs in the small intestine proximal to the site of disease.
- As the intestine distends, signs of abdominal pain are displayed; with further distension, the intestine becomes compromised, resulting in increased secretion, decreased absorption, and poor perfusion.
- Ileus may result from distension, pain, toxemia or hypokalemia, and other electrolyte disturbances.
- Net fluid movement into the small intestine combined with lack of aboral movement eventually result in gastric distension, which can develop to the point of rupture if the stomach is not decompressed.

SYSTEMS AFFECTED

GI

- Increased fluid secretion, decreased fluid absorption, and lack of aboral movement cause small intestinal distension, mainly in the duodenum and proximal jejunum.
- Fluid accumulation in the small intestine progresses to gastric distension.
- Signs of abdominal pain result from intestinal and gastric distension.

Cardiovascular

As large volumes of fluid are sequestered in the proximal GI tract or removed through gastric decompression, dehydration can ensue.

Musculoskeletal

- Laminitis is a relatively common secondary problem.
- Marked muscle loss can result from the severe catabolic state and restricted food intake.

GENETICS

No known genetic basis

INCIDENCE/PREVALENCE

- Anecdotal reports indicate a greater prevalence in the southern United States; however, cases can occur in any region.
- More often seen during the summer months.

SIGNALMENT

- Horses >2 years are primarily affected, with a high proportion in those >9 years.
- No sex predisposition

SIGNS

Historical Findings

- Affected horses usually present with acute-onset colic, and signs can progress quickly.
- Sometimes, a history of recent introduction of a higher-energy diet or to lush pasture.

Physical Examination Findings

- Tachycardia, with the heart rate usually within 40–80 bpm, is typical.
- Dehydration, depending on the severity and duration of disease.
- Animals tend to be more depressed than painful, especially after gastric decompression.
- Initial volumes of gastric reflux may reach 20 L.
- Reflux fluid has a variable appearance, from green to brownish-red, and with or without a fetid odor.
- Many horses also are pyrexic.
- A distended small intestine is usually, but not always, palpable per rectum.
- Clinical signs are very similar to those of an obstructive small intestinal lesion. Differentiation is critical, because medical treatment of horses with obstructive lesions can result in a poorer prognosis because of a delay in surgical intervention. In general, horses with DPJ tend to be more depressed and to have a lower heart rate, significantly more reflux, a less palpable distended small intestine, more GI sounds, and lower peritoneal WBC counts (with elevated peritoneal protein levels) compared to horses with surgical small intestinal lesions. None of these signs alone are diagnostic, however, and a definitive diagnosis often is arrived at only during surgical exploration or necropsy.

CAUSES

- Unknown, but an infectious agent is suspected.
- *Salmonella* and *Clostridium* sp. have been recovered from clinical cases, but attempts to reproduce the disease with these isolates have been unsuccessful.
- Mycotoxins have been explored but not proven.
- A diet high in concentrate, or a recent dietary change, may be a predisposing factor, perhaps because of development of an intestinal dysbacteriosis.

RISK FACTORS

A recent dietary change, with introduction of a higher level or concentrates or into a lush pasture, may predispose patients to this condition.

DIAGNOSIS

DIFFERENTIAL DIAGNOSIS

- Any condition causing colic and gastric reflux.
- Strangulating or nonstrangulating obstructive small intestinal lesions
- Ileus
- Large colon impaction, causing small intestinal compression

CBC/BIOCHEMISTRY/URINALYSIS

A leukocytosis may be present but is not diagnostic.

OTHER LABORATORY TESTS

A metabolic alkalosis may be present from the loss of gastric HCl, but many animals are acidotic because of hypovolemia and decreased tissue perfusion.

IMAGING

Abdominal ultrasonography—small intestinal distension not palpable per rectum may be visualized, but DPJ cannot be differentiated at imaging from other conditions causing small intestinal distension.

DIAGNOSTIC PROCEDURES

- Surgery—a definitive diagnosis usually is arrived at only by exploratory laparotomy or necropsy.
- Abdominocentesis—a high peritoneal fluid protein level (>30 g/L, and possibly >45 g/L) with normal WBC numbers (<5–10×10^9 cells/L) is suggestive but is not diagnostic.

DUODENITIS–PROXIMAL JEJUNITIS (ANTERIOR ENTERITIS, PROXIMAL ENTERITIS)

PATHOLOGIC FINDINGS

Gross Findings

- Lesions are present invariably in the duodenum, often in the jejunum, and occasionally in the pyloric region of the stomach.
- The serosal surface typically contains petechial and ecchymotic hemorrhages.
- The intestinal wall may be thickened from edema and inflammation.
- The mucosa tends to be hyperemic.

Histopathologic Findings

- Lesions include fibrinopurulent exudation on the serosal surface, intramural hemorrhage, and hyperemia and edema of the mucosa and submucosa.
- Depending on severity, there may be villous epithelial degeneration, epithelial cell sloughing, and neutrophilic infiltration.
- In some cases, no gross or histologic lesions may be present.

TREATMENT

APPROPRIATE HEALTH CARE

- Because of the difficulty in differentiating this condition from that of a surgical lesion and the intensive treatment and monitoring that are required, affected horses should be managed on an emergency inpatient basis.
- Hyperimmune serum directed against the Gram-negative core antigens (i.e., "anti-endotoxin" serum) can be administered in horses with signs of toxemia.

NURSING CARE

- Frequent monitoring is essential, especially early in the course of treatment, when the presence of a surgical lesion remains unclear.
- Signs of colic and tachycardia indicate the need for gastric decompression.
- Deep bedding may be beneficial considering the risk for development of laminitis.

IV Fluid Therapy

- Invariably indicated, with a balanced electrolyte solution.
- Administer daily maintenance (65 mL/kg per day) plus correction of fluid deficits from dehydration and replacement of the fluid volume lost during refluxing. Initially, 50–100 L/day may be required.
- IV fluid therapy initially may increase the volume of reflux obtained because of reduced intravascular oncotic pressure and increased capillary perfusion pressure.
- Monitor serum electrolyte levels.
- Approach IV supplementation of potassium with caution—20–40 mEq/L of KCl can be added to lactated Ringer solution or saline in hypokalemic animals, but the rate of infusion should not exceed 0.5 mEq/kg per hour.
- Hypocalcemia also is frequently encountered and can be treated with slow IV infusion (500 mL of 23% calcium borogluconate).

Gastric Decompression

- A crucial component of treatment to relieve pain and prevent gastric rupture.
- Initially, refluxing may be needed every 1–2 hours. A siphon must be established each time, because passage of a nasogastric tube does not always result in reflux, even with a distended stomach.
- If <5 L of fluid are obtained, the interval between refluxing can be increased.
- If signs of colic or an elevated heart rate are observed, the stomach should be refluxed.
- Leave the tube in place until refluxing has either ceased or decreased to 1–2 L every 4 hours.

ACTIVITY

If no signs of laminitis are present, it may be beneficial to walk the horse frequently for short periods of time to stimulate GI motility.

DIET

- Nothing should be given orally until the nasogastric tube is removed, after which a slow reintroduction of feed can begin. No concentrates should be fed initially.
- Because there may be no food intake for a prolonged period in some cases, partial or total parenteral nutrition may be indicated.

CLIENT EDUCATION

- This condition can be frustrating and expensive to treat.
- Reported survival rates range from 25–94%.
- Owners should be aware that the affected horses may reflux for >1 week, and that expensive therapy (e.g., total or partial parenteral nutrition) may be indicated.
- Laminitis is a common secondary problem, especially in larger horses.
- Death most often occurs from complications (e.g., laminitis, adhesions), or horses are euthanized because of economic concerns.

SURGICAL CONSIDERATIONS

- Surgical intervention is common during the early stages of this condition, because differentiation from a surgical small intestinal lesion is very difficult.
- Surgery may be beneficial in the short term by confirming the diagnosis and decompressing the small intestine, but the possibility for secondary problems from the stress of anesthesia and risk of adhesion formation increases.

DUODENITIS–PROXIMAL JEJUNITIS (ANTERIOR ENTERITIS, PROXIMAL ENTERITIS)

MEDICATIONS

DRUGS OF CHOICE

• Intestinal clostridiosis has been suggested as a cause; thus, penicillin may be administered—sodium penicillin (20,000 IU/kg IV q6h).
• Broad-spectrum antibiotics are indicated with signs of toxemia or bacteremia. Options include a penicillin/aminoglycoside combination (sodium penicillin [20,000 IU/kg IV q6h]/gentamicin [6.6 mg/kg IV q24h]), trimethoprim-sulfamethoxazole (24 mg/kg IV q12h), or ceftiofur sodium (2 mg/kg IV q12h).
• Low-dose flunixin meglumine (0.25 mg/kg IV q8h) can be administered for its purported antiendotoxin effects.
• If the stomach is decompressed, there usually is little need for analgesics.
• Analgesics should be administered judiciously, because they may mask the progression of clinical signs that might indicate a surgical lesion. If analgesia is required, flunixin meglumine (1.1 mg/kg IV q12h) can be administered.
• H_2-receptor antagonists (e.g., cimetidine [20 mg/kg PO q6–8h]) may be indicated after refluxing has ceased because of gastric irritation from distension, the primary disease process, and prolonged nasogastric intubation.
• Dimethyl sulfoxide (20 mg/kg to 1g/kg as a 10% solution q8–12h) has been recommended by some authors for laminitis prophylaxis.
• Heparin (40–100 IU/kg SC q8–12h) has been suggested to reduce the incidence of intestinal adhesions and laminitis; monitor the PCV concurrently if this treatment is used.
• Various prokinetics have been tried by clinicians. Success has been sporadic, however, and no definitive results are available regarding the efficacy of these agents.

CONTRAINDICATIONS

Prokinetic agents are contraindicated if an obstructive small intestinal lesion may be present. Reserve their use for the later stages in medical treatment, once an obstructive lesion has been ruled out or when DPJ has been diagnosed via exploratory laparotomy.

PRECAUTIONS

• Aminoglycosides and NSAIDs are potentially nephrotoxic and should not be administered until the patient's hydration status is normal.
• Antibiotics have been implicated in the development of colitis.

POTENTIAL INTERACTIONS

N/A

ALTERNATIVE DRUGS

N/A

FOLLOW-UP

PATIENT MONITORING

During the recovery period, monitor for signs of recrudescence of disease.

PREVENTION/AVOIDANCE

Because an intestinal dysbacteriosis may be involved in pathogenesis, institute feeding changes gradually.

POSSIBLE COMPLICATIONS

• Laminitis is the most common complication.
• Intestinal adhesions are relatively uncommon, unless surgical exploration was undertaken.
• Other less common complications—peritonitis, aspiration pneumonia, and myocardial or renal infarcts

EXPECTED COURSE AND PROGNOSIS

• Duration of reflux may be as short as 24 hours but typically lasts for 3–7 days (and may be even longer).
• Reported survival rates range from 25–94%.
• Prognosis is relatively good for horses that stop refluxing within 72 hours.
• Death most often results from economic concerns or complications—laminitis or adhesions

Duodenitis-Proximal Jejunitis (Anterior Enteritis, Proximal Enteritis)

MISCELLANEOUS

ASSOCIATED CONDITIONS

- Aspiration pneumonia
- Intestinal adhesions
- Laminitis
- Peritonitis

AGE-RELATED FACTORS

N/A

ZOONOTIC POTENTIAL

N/A

PREGNANCY

Pregnant mares may be at greater risk for abortion because of endotoxemia, systemic compromise from dehydration, and severe loss of body condition.

SYNONYMS

- Anterior enteritis
- Proximal enteritis

SEE ALSO

- Intestinal adhesions
- Laminitis
- Peritonitis

ABBREVIATIONS

- DPJ = duodenitis–proximal jejunitis
- GI = gastrointestinal
- PCV = packed cell volume

Suggested Reading

Allen DA, Clark ES. Duodenitis-proximal jejunitis. In: Robinson NE, ed. Current therapy in equine medicine. 3rd ed. Toronto: WB Saunders, 1992.

White NA II, Tyler DE, Blackwell RB, Allen D. Hemorrhagic fibrinonecrotic duodenitis-proximal jejunitis in horses: 20 cases (1977–1984). J Am Vet Med Assoc 1987;190:311–315.

Author J. Scott Weese

Consulting Editor Henry R Stämpfli

DYNAMIC COLLAPSE OF THE UPPER AIRWAY

BASICS

DEFINITION

- Causes a transient obstruction to respiration within the pharynx, larynx, or both.
- Often cyclic and synchronous with inspiration.
- Results from fatigue of the musculature that normally maintains luminal patency of the pharynx and larynx.

PATHOPHYSIOLOGY

- The pathophysiologies for many of the abnormalities resulting in this condition have not yet been specifically characterized. All appear to be different forms of neuromuscular dysfunction or fatigue, however, and most occur during the inspiratory phase of respiration, under the pull of high negative inspiratory pressures.
- With increased respiratory effort and muscular fatigue, the condition worsens, the obstruction becomes more severe, and a vicious cycle ensues.
- Airway turbulence may result in abnormal respiratory noise but is not always present.

SYSTEMS AFFECTED

- Upper respiratory tract
- With severe, more chronic conditions, the cardiopulmonary system may undergo secondary changes from repeated, high negative intrathoracic pressures and hypoxia.

GENETICS

N/A

INCIDENCE/PREVALENCE

N/A

SIGNALMENT

- Any age or breed.
- More commonly diagnosed in racehorses because of the high negative inspiratory pressures created during strenuous exercise.
- Thoroughbreds (2–3 years) are the largest group affected.
- To date, axial deviation of the aryepiglottic folds has been identified only in racehorses.
- Quarterhorses with hyperkalemic periodic paralysis can have paroxysmal spasms of the pharynx and larynx during "paralytic episodes" that result in severe upper respiratory obstruction.

SIGNS

- Exercise intolerance or poor performance
- Abnormal upper respiratory noise during inspiration may occur depending on the degree and type of obstruction.
- Only dorsal displacement of the soft palate results in expiratory noise.
- Coughing
- Dysphagia

CAUSES

- Laryngeal hemiplegia most commonly affects the left arytenoid cartilage, results from idiopathic degeneration of the left recurrent laryngeal nerve, and cause a paresis of the primary abductor of the left arytenoid, or of the cricoarytenoideus dorsalis muscle.
- Infrequently, trauma to either the left or right recurrent laryngeal nerve associated with jugular thrombophlebitis can result in laryngeal hemiplegia.
- Epiglottic retroversion is presumed to be a dysfunction of the hypoepiglotticus muscle on the basis of experimental reproduction of the disorder after anesthetic blockade of the nerve (i.e., the hypoglossal) that supplies the hypoepiglotticus.
- Other forms of collapse are thought to represent either specific muscle dysfunction within the pharynx or disproportionate force between the muscle groups.

RISK FACTORS

- High-speed exercise
- Hyperkalemic periodic paralysis in Quarterhorses

DIAGNOSIS

DIFFERENTIAL DIAGNOSIS

- Laryngeal hemiplegia
- Vocal cord collapse
- Dorsal displacement of the soft palate
- Pharyngeal collapse
- Epiglottic retroversion
- Axial deviation of the aryepiglottic folds
- Combinations of any of the above-mentioned distinct disorders

CBC/BIOCHEMISTRY/URINALYSIS

N/A

OTHER LABORATORY TESTS

N/A

IMAGING

N/A

DIAGNOSTIC PROCEDURES

Resting Endoscopy

- Helps to evaluate any structural abnormalities predisposing to dynamic obstruction during exercise but rarely is definitive for a dynamic abnormality.
- More difficult to speculate on pharyngeal than on laryngeal forms of dynamic collapse.
- Assess laryngeal and pharyngeal function during normal breathing, nasal occlusion, and swallowing.
- Horses normally demonstrate some dorsal roof collapse of the pharynx and have air pass between the aryepiglottic folds and pharyngeal ostium during nasal occlusion. This is not an indication of a pharyngeal abnormality during exercise.
- With prolonged nasal occlusion, 60% of horses can be made to displace their palates, but they do not experience dynamic collapse during exercise.
- Horses that very readily displace their soft palate are more likely to displace during a race.
- Horses that leave their palates displaced for an extended period of time or have difficulty replacing their palates with a swallow are more likely to have a pharyngeal abnormality during high-speed exercise. This may be a crude indication of some pharyngeal weakness.
- A certain degree of laryngeal hemiplegia is very prevalent.
- Horses commonly demonstrate asymmetry and asynchrony to their arytenoid movement yet achieve full abduction of both arytenoids during nasal occlusion or after swallowing (grade 2 on a scale of 1–4). These horses do not experience dynamic collapse during exercise. Horses that cannot fully and symmetrically abduct both arytenoids after swallowing or nasal occlusion (grade 3) are considered to be impaired.
- The degree of dynamic collapse depends on the degree of paresis and on the intensity of exercise. Racehorses likely undergo significant respiratory compromise with grade 3 laryngeal hemiplegia; show horses are more likely be asymptomatic.

High-Speed Treadmill Endoscopy

• Often required to see the cause of upper respiratory collapse.
• Minimum requirements to ensure a valid test—Holter monitor to record heart rate during exercise, to determine heart rate relative to the horse's speed, and to guarantee the horse is maximally exerting itself by achieving a heart rate of ≅220 bpm or greater; videoendoscope linked to a video recorder to visualize the abnormality and play back the video in slow motion if the obstruction occurs too quickly to see in real time; and a physiologically fit horse exercised in tack (harness for Standardbreds) to minimize spurious results.
• Typical racehorse protocol—phase 1: warm up, 2 m/sec for 4 minutes, 4.5 m/sec for 1 minute, 7 m/sec for 2 minutes; phase 2: walk until heart rate <90 bpm, stop and insert endoscope; phase 3: gradually accelerate to 9 m/sec, incline treadmill to 3° (for Thoroughbreds); accelerate to 11 m/sec, continue for 400 meters; accelerate to 12 m/sec, continue for 400 meters; accelerate to 14 m/sec, continue for 1600 meters; then decelerate to 12 m/s, continue for 400 meters.
• Horses are unlikely to be capable of completing these steps as described; therefore, they are exercised as close to the desired speed as possible for the predetermined distances. Most horses require at least one schooling episode to become familiar enough with the treadmill to exercise at an adequate speed.
• Measurements of upper respiratory pressures and use of flow–volume loops during treadmill exercise can document respiratory obstruction but cannot discriminate between the many different abnormalities.

PATHOLOGIC FINDINGS
N/A

TREATMENT

APPROPRIATE HEALTH CARE
N/A

NURSING CARE
N/A

ACTIVITY
N/A

DIET
N/A

CLIENT EDUCATION
N/A

SURGICAL CONSIDERATIONS
• Laryngeal hemiplegia is treated with surgical laryngoplasty (i.e., tieback procedure). The affected arytenoid is held in a fixed, partially abducted position with a nonabsorbable suture simulating the contracted cricoarytenoideus muscle. An adjunctive procedure (i.e., ventriculocordectomy) also can be performed to minimize obstruction at the ventral aspect of the glottis after a tieback.
• Axial deviation of the aryepiglottic folds has been treated effectively both with rest and with laser resection of the offending soft tissue; however, surgery affords a quicker return to training.
• In addition to rest, several surgical procedures are available.
• Rest and oral anti-inflammatory treatment has been the only mode of therapy for other forms of dynamic collapse.

MEDICATIONS

DRUGS OF CHOICE
A 3–4-week course of an anti-inflammatory drug may be indicated during the period of rest to resolve any presumed inflammatory component causing the dysfunction.

CONTRAINDICATIONS
N/A

PRECAUTIONS
N/A

POSSIBLE INTERACTIONS
N/A

ALTERNATIVE DRUGS
N/A

FOLLOW-UP

PATIENT MONITORING
• Resting endoscopy is necessary several weeks after any surgical intervention, and though it will not be definitive for determining the success of the surgery, it will determine the capability of the horse to resume training.
• An increase in performance or diminution of noise often is the criterion used to determine a successful treatment.
• Repeat high-speed treadmill endoscopy is the best method to determine a successful outcome from any treatment, but only after the horse has regained fitness.

PREVENTION/AVOIDANCE
N/A

POSSIBLE COMPLICATIONS
N/A

EXPECTED COURSE AND PROGNOSIS
N/A

MISCELLANEOUS

ASSOCIATED CONDITIONS
N/A

AGE-RELATED FACTORS
N/A

ZOONOTIC POTENTIAL
N/A

PREGNANCY
N/A

SYNONYMS
N/A

SEE ALSO
• Arytenoid chrondritis
• Epiglottic entrapment
• Laryngeal hemiplegia
• Dorsal displacement of the soft palate

Suggested Reading

Parente EJ. Treadmill endoscopy. In: Traub-Dargatz JL, Brown CM, eds. Equine endoscopy. Philadelphia: Mosby, 1997.
Parente EJ, Martin BB. Correlation between standing endoscopic examinations and those made during high-speed exercise in horses: 150 cases. Proc Am Assoc Equine Pract 1995:170.

Author Eric J. Parente
Consulting Editor Jean-Pierre Lavoie

DYSMATURITY

BASICS

DEFINITION

A clinical term applied to foals born after ≥320 days of gestation that show clinical signs of immaturity.

PATHOPHYSIOLOGY

- Frequently associated with signs of placental pathology resulting in IUGR.
- Decreased placental size, maternal/fetal diffusion pathway abnormalities, and degenerative changes in the endometrium secondary to age and parity may contribute to hypoxemia and fetal starvation.
- Signs generally parallel those of premature foals, except for the pulmonary system, which usually is less affected by a lack of surfactant, and the skin, which is more likely to have a normal-length hair coat.
- Insufficient thyroid hormone production results in maturational delays of virtually all body systems.

SYSTEM AFFECTED

Musculoskeletal—dysmature foals usually are small for gestational age; often appear generally emaciated, with decreased muscle mass, which probably is secondary to decreased nutrition in utero; and may evidence incomplete ossification of the cuboidal bones.

SIGNALMENT

- Any breed of foal
- No gender predilection
- By definition, the foal is born after a normal-length or prolonged gestation.

SIGNS

Historical Findings

- Old mares are more likely to produce dysmature foals.
- Possible history of maternal illness.

Physical Examination Findings

- Placenta may be heavy or abnormally thickened if placental infection is present; conversely, areas of the chorionic surface may appear denuded or underdeveloped if corresponding uterine areas are abnormal—scarring or cysts.
- Foals can be weak at birth and may require delivery assistance.
- Normal or low birth weight
- Small for gestational age
- Increased flexor tendon laxity (**EXCEPTION:** hypothyroid foals often have flexural deformities with or without rupture of the common digital extensor tendon, characterized by fluid swelling dorsolateral to the radiocarpal joint).
- Floppy ears in some
- Normal or depressed mentation—may show signs of neonatal maladjustment syndrome (i.e., hypoxic ischemic encephalopathy).
- Normal or irregular breathing, dependent on lung maturity and mental status; if lungs are very immature, may progress to respiratory distress.
- Progressive, angular limb deformity of carpi or hocks secondary to crushing of poorly calcified cuboidal bones; onset depends on exercise and activity level of the foal.
- In hypothyroid foals, poor thermoregulation, mandibular brachygnathism, and poorly developed pectoral muscles may be seen.

CAUSES

Multiple causes have been recognized that delay equine fetal maturation, with or without evidence of disease in the broodmare.

Severe Maternal Illness

- May lead to poor nutritional intake by a sick broodmare in combination with the effects of hypoxia, endotoxemia, or drugs.
- Congestive heart failure or advanced chronic obstructive pulmonary disease may contribute to fetal hypoxia.
- Chronic laminitis with prolonged recumbency and high levels of NSAIDs (e.g., phenylbutazone) may produce a small-for-gestational-age foal.
- Equine protozoal myeloencephalitis treated with high doses of trimethoprim sulfa and pyrimethamine can result in abnormal fetal development.

Placental Insufficiency

Affects fetal growth when associated with conditions such as twinning, placentitis, body pregnancy, endometrial scarring, or partial separation from the endometrial surface.

Fescue Toxicosis

- Regional disease, restricted to temperate areas where fescue pastures are commonly employed for grazing broodmares.
- Some fescue grasses are infested with endophytes, which results in agalactia and prolonged gestations.

Congenital Hypothyroidism

- Most common in areas with iodine-deficient soils (e.g., the U.S. Great Lakes states, the plains provinces of western Canada), but can occur on any farm if inadequate iodine is provided or high nitrate exposure occurs.

RISK FACTORS

- Old broodmares
- Chronic drug administration during pregnancy
- Grazing endophyte-infested fescue pasture
- Insufficient dietary iodine

DIAGNOSIS

DIFFERENTIAL DIAGNOSIS

- Congenital defects of the heart or vasculature
- Prematurity rather than dysmaturity because of errors in estimating length of gestation
- Intrauterine equine herpes virus 1 infection

CBC/BIOCHEMISTRY/URINALYSIS

- No pathognomonic abnormalities
- Foals that are dysmature because of bacterial placentitis may have elevated neutrophil and serum fibrinogen concentrations.
- If sepsis develops in affected foals, leukopenia or leukocytosis, toxic changes of neutrophils, left shift, and elevated fibrinogen may be noted.
- Elevated liver enzymes, BUN, and creatinine may indicate reduced liver and kidney function.
- Electrolyte abnormalities can result from enteritis and renal or adrenal disease.

OTHER LABORATORY TESTS

- Measure serum IgG levels in foals between 12–24 hours after birth to check for FPT.
- With suspected congenital hypothyroidism, serum T_3 or T_4 may be lower than age-specific normal values.
- With suspected in utero sepsis or septicemia, collect blood aseptically for bacteriologic culture.

IMAGING

Carpal/Tarsal Radiography

- Used to assess maturity of the cuboidal bones.
- Immaturity is indicated by wider-than-normal spaces between the cuboidal bones and growth plates of the long bones as well as by rounded corners of the cuboidal bones.
- With angular deformities, collapse of the carpal or tarsal bones may be noted or, more rarely, crushing of the distal radial epiphysis.

Thoracic Radiography

May assist in assessing lung maturity or concurrent pneumonia.

Ultrasonography

- Common digital extensor tendon at the musculotendonous junction of hypothyroid foals—may reveal complete or partial rupture of the tendon, with accompanying hemorrhage.
- Lungs—may provide information on the degree of aeration versus consolidation.

DIAGNOSTIC PROCEDURES

N/A

PATHOLOGIC FINDINGS

- Placental pathology may be present.
- Increased weight or thickness of the placenta may be noted.
- Areas of scarring or cyst formation may decrease surface area of the placental exchange.

• Evidence of fungal or bacterial infection may be present.
• With congenital hypothyroidism, the thyroid glands may be slightly darker in appearance.
• Microscopically, thyroid hyperplasia is evident, with reduced colloid.

TREATMENT

• Early recognition is critical for successful outcome.
• With respiratory distress, maintain the foal in a sternal position, and if available, administer humidified oxygen.
• Assist with standing and nursing, ensure adequate colostral intake, and verify absorption.
• IV plasma administration in cases with serum IgG <800 mg/dL.
• Strongly consider prophylactic antibiotics because of the risk of septicemia; monitor closely for early evidence of sepsis.
• With marked tendon laxity, protect the fetlocks with a light bandage, or place extended heel shoes on the feet to prevent damage to the heels or caudal fetlock. Restrict exercise until normal limb angulation is achieved; ultrasound therapy for the lax flexor tendons may accelerate development of tone.
• If carpal or tarsal bones are not fully calcified, restrict the foal and mare to a stall. Splint to prevent uneven weight distribution on these bones if sufficient padding is provided and splints are reset at least daily. Intermittent splinting for periods when the foal is standing also is an option if sufficient personnel are available. Continue exercise restriction and splinting until the bones are completely ossified.
• Provide adequate hydration and nutritional intake if the foal cannot nurse effectively.
• If fescue toxicosis is the underlying cause, the dam may have poor udder development and little milk. Consider substitute nurse-mare, milk replacer, or treatment of the mare with domperidone.

MEDICATIONS

DRUGS
No specific medications for dysmaturity

CONTRAINDICATIONS
N/A

PRECAUTIONS
Avoid long-term use of drugs such as phenylbutazone or trimethoprim sulfa in pregnant mares.

POSSIBLE INTERACTIONS
N/A

ALTERNATIVE DRUGS
N/A

FOLLOW UP

PATIENT MONITORING
• Closely monitor affected foals to ascertain that adequate caloric and fluid intake occurs.
• With splints, scrutinize foals at least daily for pressure sores.
• With immature cuboidal bones, repeat radiography of the affected limbs to verify complete ossification of the cuboidal bones before splinting is discontinued, after which exercise may be gradually increased.

POSSIBLE COMPLICATIONS
• Foals that are small for gestational age at birth may be smaller than genetically expected as adults.
• Long-term effects of IUGR in foals are unknown.
• With carpal or tarsal bone collapse, arthritis is likely.

MISCELLANEOUS

ASSOCIATED CONDITIONS
N/A

AGE-RELATED FACTORS
N/A

ZOONOTIC POTENTIAL
N/A

PRENANCY
N/A

SYNONYMS
• IUGR
• Small for gestational age

SEE ALSO
• Angular limb deformity
• Flexural limb deformity
• Prematurity
• Seizures/coma
• Septicemia

ABBREVIATIONS
• FPT = failure of passive transfer
• IUGR = intrauterine growth retardation
• T3 = triiodothyronine
• T4 = thyroxine

Suggested Reading

Allen AL, Townsend HGG, Doige CE, et al. A case-control study of the congenital hypothyroidism and dysmaturity syndrome of foals. Can Vet J 1996;37:349–358.
Rossdale PD, Ousey JC. The Dorothy Russell Havemeyer Foundation Third International Workshop on equine perinatology: comparative aspects. Equine Vet J 1998;30:455–466.

Author Julia H. Wilson
Consulting Editor Mary Rose Paradis

DYSTOCIA

BASICS

DEFINITION

Any difficult delivery with or without assistance.

Standard System To Describe Obstetric Problems

- Presentation—relationship of the spinal axis of the fetus to the spinal axis of the dam (e.g., anterior, posterior, or transverse presentation).
- Position—relationship of the dorsum of the fetus to a quadrant of the maternal pelvis (e.g., dorsosacral, dorsoilial, dorsopubic; exceptions to this are the transverse and vertical positions of the head of the fetus in relation to the quadrants of the pelvis).
- Posture—relationship of the fetal extremities to the fetal trunk; unrelated to the dam's anatomy.
- In normal parturition, fetal presentation is anterior longitudinal, position is dorsosacral, and the fetal head, neck, and forelimbs are extended.

Stages of Labor

Stage I:

- Lasts from 1–4 hours.
- Signs—anorexia; defecates/urinates frequently in small amounts; $<$2 hours prepartum becomes more restless, signs of colic, paws, sweating begins front of shoulder to neck and side, milk may begin squirting from the teats; activity peaks coincident with uterine contractions (i.e., intermittent periods: 1–2 minutes to 20 minutes in length).
- Internally—uterine contractions beginning, fetus and fluid forced against the cervix, pressure causes cervical dilation; chorioallantoic membrane up against the cervix ruptures, and allantoic fluid escapes (amber colored, watery consistency), signaling end of the first stage.

Stage II:

- Average length is 20 minutes; maximum normal length is 1 hour.
- Fetus passes through the birth canal.
- Signs—mare usually lying down, may bite her flank or chew on hay or straw, may roll, amniotic membrane protrudes through the vulvar lips, fetus is within the amniotic sac; with active labor (i.e., abdominal contractions), membrane breaks when the fetus is less than midway through the birth canal.
- Internally—normal delivery is dorsosacral position, one forelimb extended $\cong$20 cm ahead of the other, soles of both feet directed ventrally; neck is straight, and the head rests on forelimbs in the area of the carpal joints; rear limbs are extended so that the rear hooves are the first part to be delivered.

Stage III:

- Begins after the foal is expelled.
- Includes the expulsion of the placenta ($\leq$3 hours).
- Some definitions include time required for involution ($\leq$1 month).

PATHOPHYSIOLOGY

Multifactorial

Hereditary Causes:

- Abnormality of the genital tract.
- Twinning
- Size of head
- Ankyloses of joints
- Hydrocephalus

Nutritional and Management Causes:

- Pelvic size—if dam has been nutritionally stunted.
- Fat in pelvic cavity.
- Failure to observe animals near term (and uterine inertia develops).
- Close confinement of mares during entire gestation.

Infectious Conditions of the Placenta or Fetus May Contribute To:

- Uterine inertia
- Incomplete cervical dilation.
- Postural abnormalities caused by fetal death.
- Loss of placental attachment sites.

Traumatic Causes:

- Damage to the abdominal wall inhibiting normal abdominal contractions.
- Uterine torsion
- Fractured pelvis

Miscellaneous Causes:

- Unexplainable fetal postural changes.
- Posterior presentation
- Transverse presentation

Causes of Uterine Inertia:

- Primary—uterine overstretching or overloading (i.e., hydrops, twins), increased incidence in older or debilitated animals; uterine infections may predispose to inertia; failure of oxytocin to be released or to have an effect on uterus.
- Secondary—as a result of dystocia, uterine muscle is exhausted; after failure of labor caused by pain to the dam; fatigue after prolonged dystocia and its strong circular contractions; uterus may rupture if forced extraction is attempted.

Immediate

- Those causes of dystocia that are relieved at delivery, divided into maternal and fetal origin.
- Most immediate causes of dystocia are fetal in origin.
- Maternal causes—birth canal stenosis, small pelvis, hypoplastic genital tract, genital tract lacerations and scars, pelvic tumors, persistent hymen, failure of cervical dilation, uterine inertia, abortions, or twinning.
- Fetal causes—abnormal presentation, position, and posture; excessive fetal size; fetal anasarca or ascites; fetal tumors; hydrocephalus, fetal monsters; posterior presentation; wry neck; or transverse or longitudinal presentation.

SYSTEMS AFFECTED

- Reproductive
- May become multisystemic as the condition progresses.

DYSTOCIA

GENETICS
See *Pathophysiology.*

INCIDENCE/PREVALENCE
Dystocia rate—1%.

SIGNALMENT
• All breeds
• All breeding ages.

SIGNS

General Comments
• Approach—this is an emergency.
• Take a complete history, and perform a routine physical examination.
• Include an examination of the reproductive tract and fetus before deciding how to handle a dystocia.

Historical Findings
• Obtain a complete history, including current due date, problems associated with previous gestations (e.g., dystocia, systemic disease, length of active labor [i.e., stages I and II], premature allantoic or amniotic membrane rupture, any assistance given), and if the mare is able to stand and walk.
• Mares in stage II labor of >70 minutes or that have a fetus with an abnormal presentation, position, and/or posture require assistance as soon as possible. This also may include those with premature separation (i.e., detachment) of the placenta with the fetus remaining within the uterus.

Physical Examination Findings
• Is the mare able to move normally? If the mare is down and unable to rise, determine cause.
• Evaluate hydration status, CRT, mucous membrane color, and likelihood of being in shock or going into shock before the procedure is complete.
• Is the mare stable enough to administer local anesthetics, epidurals, or general anesthesia or sedation if necessary?
• Transrectal examination of the mare—for fetal viability, for any lacerations of the uterus before attempting vaginal exam or delivery, and to determine the amount of uterine contracture around the fetus (i.e., contractions and loss of fluid from the uterus); increases risk of uterine tears.
• Proper preparation/washing of the vulvar region before conducting a genital examination is essential.
• Vaginal examination—use liberal amounts of lubrication; evaluate condition of the vulva, vagina, cervix and uterus, if possible, for lacerations before obstetrical manipulation; inform the owner before proceeding; assess amount of space between the fetus and maternal pelvis; determine degree of cervical relaxation.
• Determine fetal viability—press gently over eye (to stimulate a blink response); place fingers in mouth of fetus or more caudal on its tongue (to stimulate suck reflex); pull on or maximally flex fetal limb (resistance, pulling away from your effort); if only a foot is within reach, pinch on coronary band with a Kelly forceps (very painful, stimulates response); if the fetus is in a posterior presentation, place finger in anus (stimulates contraction); transabdominal ultrasonography for fetal heartbeat.
• If the fetus is dead, determine approximate TOD—if the corneas are gray or cloudy, 6–12 hours; if emphysematous or hair is sloughing, 24–48+ hours.
• Determine fetal presentation, position, and posture.

CAUSES
Fetal Causes of Dystocia Include:
• All posterior presentations
• Any deviation from dorsosacral (i.e., normal) position—dorsoilial; dorsopubic.
• Flexion of the extremities (i.e., limbs, head, and neck)—the most common fetal cause of dystocia is flexion of the extremities or of its head and neck.
• Ankyloses of the joints.
• Hydrocephalus
• Fetal anasarca

RISK FACTORS
• The major cause of dystocia involves fetal malpostures.
• Impossible to state precisely why the fetus moves from an anterior presentation, dorsosacral position, with extension of the head and neck and both forelimbs (i.e., normal posture); any variation from that is considered an abnormality.
• Old mares and mares with insufficient exercise experience increased incidence of dystocia for unknown reasons.

DIAGNOSIS

DIFFERENTIAL DIAGNOSIS
• Primary differential is prepartum colic. The signs can be very similar, especially during the early stages of dystocia.
• With colic, signs of abdominal distress worsen.
• With dystocia, it becomes obvious that the mare is experiencing more than abdominal pain and also is straining.
• With true breech deliveries (i.e., fetus in posterior presentation, both rear legs flexed), point pressure on the cervix is absent so straining may be absent, and thus the mare may fail to enter stage II labor.
• Palpation, including transrectal and vaginal examinations, is most helpful to differentiate these conditions.

CBC/BIOCHEMISTRY/URINALYSIS
CBCs and profiles are indicated if the animal is hospitalized and results are rapidly available.

OTHER LABORATORY TESTS
N/A

IMAGING
Transabominal ultrasonography of the mare at term for determining fetal viability and presence of a fetal heartbeat.

DIAGNOSTIC PROCEDURES
N/A

PATHOLOGIC FINDINGS
Dependent on the cause.

DYSTOCIA

TREATMENT

APPROPRIATE HEALTH CARE

- Best handled on the farm early during stage II labor.
- Vaginal delivery is preferred and is best accomplished shortly after dystocia is diagnosed, whether mutation, forced extraction, or fetotomy is necessary.
- Additional transport and time may preclude vaginal delivery.

NURSING CARE

- Thorough examination of the uterus, cervix, vagina, vestibule, and vulva after delivery.
- Intrauterine antibiotics to reduce contaminants invariably introduced during corrective procedures.
- Uterine stimulants (e.g., oxytocin) to hasten involution.
- Systemic antibiotics with signs of systemic infection.
- Uterine flushes or infusions as indicated to hasten involution.
- Additional postoperative care may be indicated for mares after cesarean sections.

ACTIVITY

- No restriction after vaginal delivery.
- Stall rest for mares undergoing cesarean section.

DIET

Normal

CLIENT EDUCATION

- Emphasize that prolonged labor reduces the likely survivability of the neonate.
- Train owners about normal stages of labor and to recognize early warning signs of dystocia including—abnormal orientation of the fetal limbs protruding from the vulva.

SURGICAL CONSIDERATIONS

- If a cesarean section is to be performed, timing is critical. Decide early if this is the best approach. Considerations include viability and value of the fetus, value of dam, costs, facilities, and support staff and services (e.g., anesthesia).
- If the fetus cannot be delivered alive, consider a fetotomy, especially if a resolution can be achieved with one or two cuts.

MEDICATIONS

DRUGS OF CHOICE

- Epidural anesthesia can assist in the delivery process by reducing contractions of the mare during assisted delivery—2% carbocaine (≅1 ml per 40 kg).
- Xylazine (0.5–1.0 mg/kg) can be used for sedation alone or combined with acepromazine (0.04 mg/ kg).
- After delivery—oxytocin (20 U per 500 kg IM) to enhance uterine contractions and involution of the postpartum uterus.

CONTRAINDICATIONS

Never administer oxytocin prepartum because of the potential to induce further uterine contracture and to further reduce the available space for fetal manipulation.

PRECAUTIONS

None

POSSIBLE INTERACTIONS

None

ALTERNATIVE DRUGS

Pain relief, sedation—butorphenol, dormosodan, or morphine (0.6 mg/kg).

FOLLOW-UP

PATIENT MONITORING

Postpartum Monitoring of the At-Risk Mare:

- At-risk mares—assisted delivery; history of postpartum infection.
- Transrectal palpation of the reproductive tract daily or every other day to assess uterine size and tone.
- Ultrasonography coupled with palpation for uterine fluid and its volume and character.

PREVENTION/AVOIDANCE

No method to prevent dystocia other than pre-emptive cesarean section.

DYSTOCIA

POSSIBLE COMPLICATIONS
- Lacerations of the cervix, vagina, vestibule, or vulva.
- Lacerations of the uterus also are possible.
- Uterine inflammation or infection.

EXPECTED COURSE AND PROGNOSIS
Obstetrical inexperience of the veterinarian or owner/manager, posterior presentation, dorsopubic position, lateral flexion of the head and neck, and prolonged duration of stage II lower the prognosis for the dam and/or fetus.

Duration of Stage II
- Mare survival—prognosis grave if >24 hours; related to increased contamination and subsequent infection of the uterus, possibility of peritonitis.
- Fetal survival—prognosis guarded if >70 minutes; related to strenuous nature of stage II in the mare, rapid detachment of placenta with active labor, long birth canal, and long fetal extremities (i.e., mutation more difficult than with a bovine fetus).

MISCELLANEOUS

ASSOCIATED CONDITIONS
N/A

AGE-RELATED FACTORS
Slight increase in the incidence of dystocia among old mares; possibly related to decreased uterine contractility.

ZOONOTIC POTENTIAL
N/A

PREGNANCY
Only affects pregnant mares.

SYNONYMS
N/A

SEE ALSO
- Broad ligament hematoma
- Delayed uterine involution
- Perineal lacerations/rectovaginal fistulas
- Premature placental separation
- Prepubic tendon rupture
- Retained fetal membranes
- Uterine inertia
- Uterine torsion

ABBREVIATIONS
- CRT = capillary refill time
- TOD = time of death

Suggested Reading

Asbury AC. Care of the mare after foaling. In: McKinnon AO, Voss JL, eds. Equine reproduction. Philadelphia: Lea & Febiger, 1993:578–587.

Roberts SJ. Veterinary obstetrics and genital diseases (theriogenology). 3rd ed. Woodstock, VT: Published by the author, 1986:326–351.

Author Walter R. Threlfall

Consulting Editor Carla L. Carleton

EARLY EMBRYONIC DEATH (EED)

BASICS

DEFINITION

Maternal structural or functional defects preventing normal embryonic development from early pregnancy diagnosis at 14–15 days to the beginning of the fetal stage at 40 days of gestation.

PATHOPHYSIOLOGY

- Defective embryo.
- Unsuitable uterine environment.
- Early regression of CL.
- Luteal insufficiency—anecdotal.

SYSTEM AFFECTED

Reproductive

GENETICS

N/A

INCIDENCE/PREVALENCE

- Normal rate is ≅5%–10%.
- Incidence may be much higher in old, subfertile mares.

SIGNALMENT

- Mares of >15 years
- Certain heterospecific matings—stallion × jenny.

SIGNS

Historical Findings

- At ≤40 days, failure to detect pregnancies previously diagnosed by transrectal ultrasonography at 14–15 days after ovulation.
- Return to estrus after previous diagnosis of pregnancy.

Physical Examination Findings

- At ≤40 days after ovulation, no evidence by transrectal ultrasonography of previously diagnosed pregnancy.
- At ≤40 days after ovulation, evidence by transrectal ultrasonography of previously diagnosed pregnancy undergoing EED (e.g., decreasing size, change in appearance of fluid, absence of heartbeat)—nonpregnant uterus (possibly with endometrial folds or intrauterine fluid); possible absence of CL; none or mucoid or mucopurulent vulvar discharge.

CAUSES

- Defective embryos—old mares; seasonal effects.
- Endometritis—early CL regression; unsuitable uterine environment.
- Unsuitable uterine environment—endometritis; occurrence of endometrial cysts large enough to impede embryonic mobility and failure of maternal recognition of pregnancy (more likely conception failure); endometrosis; inadequate secretion of histotrophs.
- Xenobiotics—fescue toxicosis; phytoestrogens (anecdotal).
- Endocrine disorders—hypothyroidism (anecdotal); luteal insufficiency (anecdotal).
- Maternal disease—fever; pain (anecdotal).

RISK FACTORS

- Age of >15 years.
- Anatomic defects predisposing to endometritis.
- Seasonal effects.
- Foal heat breedings—anecdotal.
- Inadequate nutrition.
- Exposure to xenobiotics—fescue toxicosis.
- Some heterospecific matings—stallion × jenny.

DIAGNOSIS

DIFFERENTIAL DIAGNOSIS

- Conception failure—failure to detect a 14-day pregnancy by transrectal ultrasonography.
- Previous misdiagnosis of pregnancy by transrectal ultrasonography—endometrial cysts, intrauterine fluid, paraovarian cystic structures, and small ovarian follicles are distinguished from pregnancies based on shape, size, location, and re-examination (pregnancies move at <16 days after ovulation, grow, and develop heartbeats).

CBC/BIOCHEMISTRY/URINALYSIS

Not indicated, unless signs of concurrent systemic disease are present.

OTHER LABORATORY TESTS

Maternal Progesterone

- May be indicated at initial pregnancy examination to check for functional CL.
- ELISA or RIA for progesterone—acceptable levels vary from >1 to >4 ng/mL, depending on the reference.

Maternal T_3/T_4 Levels

- Anecdotal reports of lower levels in mares with history of failure of conception, early embryonic loss, or abortion.
- Significance of low T_4 levels is not clear at present.

Cytogenetic Studies

May be indicated with suspected maternal chromosomal abnormalities.

Feed Analysis

May be indicated for specific xenobiotics (e.g., ergopeptine alkaloids, phytoestrogens, heavy metals) or endophyte (*Neotyphodium coenophialum*).

IMAGING

Transrectal ultrasonography is essential to confirm early pregnancy and to detect embryonic death, intrauterine fluid, and endometrial cysts.

DIAGNOSTIC PROCEDURES

Reproductive Evaluation of Mares

• In predisposed individuals (i.e., barren, old mares or mares with history of EED), evaluation before breeding is indicated.
• Transrectal ultrasonography, vaginal examination (speculum and manual digital), endometrial cytology/culture, and endometrial biopsy should detect anatomic defects and endometrial inflammation or fibrosis that may predispose a mare to conception failure (see *Endometritis* and *Endometrial Biopsy*).

Transrectal Ultrasonography

Performed at weekly intervals in mares with history of EED or biweekly in normal mares to detect EED, follow embryonic growth and development, and distinguish the conceptus from cysts.

PATHOLOGIC FINDINGS

Endometrial biopsy—presence of moderate to severe, chronic endometrial inflammation and/or fibrosis (see *Endometrial Biopsy*)

TREATMENT

APPROPRIATE HEALTH CARE

• Treatment of pre-existing endometritis
• Insemination or breeding of mares during physiologic breeding season when they have adequate body condition.
• Insemination or breeding of foal heat mares when ovulation occurs at ≥10 days postpartum and no intrauterine fluid is present.
• Progestin supplementation.
• Various forms of embryo transfer to retrieve embryos from the uterus (6–8 days after ovulation) or oviduct (≅ 2–4 days after ovulation).
• Successful in vitro fertilization is in the early stages of development.
• Primary, age-related, embryonic defects are refractory to treatment (see *Endometritis* and *Embryo Transfer*).
• Most cases can be handled in an ambulatory situation.
• Careful monitoring of embryonic development may require adequate restraint and optimal lighting in a hospital setting if such are not available in the field.

NURSING CARE

• Generally requires none.
• Minimal nursing care after more invasive diagnostic and therapeutic procedures.

ACTIVITY

• Generally no restriction of broodmare activity, unless contraindicated by concurrent maternal disease or diagnostic or therapeutic procedures.
• Preference may be to restrict activity of mares in competition.

DIET

Mare can be fed a normal diet, unless contraindicated by concurrent maternal disease.

CLIENT EDUCATION

• Emphasize age-related aspects and their refractoriness to treatment.
• Educate regarding the cause, diagnosis, and treatment of endometritis.
• Inform regarding seasonal aspects and nutritional requirements of embryonic development.
• Clients should understand the role that endophyte-infected fescue and certain heterospecific breedings might play in conception failure.

EARLY EMBRYONIC DEATH (EED)

SURGICAL CONSIDERATIONS

Surgery may be indicated in the repair of anatomic defects predisposing mares to endometritis or in certain therapeutic procedures.

MEDICATIONS

DRUGS OF CHOICE

- See *Endometritis* and *Metritis* for specific drug recommendations.
- Mares with a history of EED or moderate to severe endometrial inflammation (i.e., no active, infectious component) and/or fibrosis—Altrenogest (Regu-mate; Hoechst-Roussel Agri-Vet; 0.044–0.088 mg/kg PO q24h commencing 2–3 days after ovulation or at diagnosis of pregnancy, continued until at least day 100 of gestation [some clinicians prefer day 120], then gradually declining in daily dose over a 14-day period at the end of administration).
- Altrenogest administration may be started later in gestation, continued longer, or used for only short periods of time depending on serum progesterone levels during the first 80 days of gestation (>1 to >4 ng/mL, depending on the reference), clinical circumstances, risk factors, and clinician preference.
- If used near term, altrenogest frequently is discontinued 7–14 days before the expected foaling date, depending on the case, unless otherwise indicated by assessment of fetal maturity/viability or questions exist regarding the correct gestational age.

CONTRAINDICATIONS

Use altrenogest only to prevent EED when infectious endometritis is not present concurrently.

PRECAUTIONS

Transrectal Ultrasonography

- Used to diagnose pregnancy at 14–16 days after ovulation.
- To identify retention of intrauterine fluid or development of pyometra.
- If pregnancy is diagnosed, frequent monitoring (weekly at first) may be indicated to detect EED.

Altrenogest

Because altrenogest is absorbed through the skin, those handling this preparation should wear gloves and wash their hands.

Progestins

- Widespread use of supplemental progestins in cases of EED is supported mainly by anecdotal reports of success.
- Primary, age-related, embryonic defects do not respond to supplemental progestins.

ALTERNATIVE DRUGS

Progesterone

- Injectable progesterone (100–150 mg/day IM q24h in an oil base) can be administered instead of altrenogest.
- Variations, contraindications, and precautions in administration are similar to those associated with altrenogest.
- Other injectable and implantable progestin preparations are available commercially for use in other species, but reports of their efficacy in mares are anecdotal at present.

T_4

- Supplementation has been successful anecdotally in mares with histories of subfertility.
- Its use remains controversial, and is considered to be deleterious by some clinicians.

FOLLOW-UP

PATIENT MONITORING

- Accurate teasing records
- Re-examination of mares diagnosed and treated for endometritis before breeding.
- Early examination for pregnancy with transrectal ultrasonography.
- Monitoring of embryonic and fetal development with transrectal and/or transabdominal ultrasonography.

PREVENTION/AVOIDANCE

- Recognition of at-risk mares.
- Management of pre-existing endometritis before breeding.
- Removal of mares from fescue pasture after breeding and during early gestation.
- Prudent use of medications in bred mares.
- Avoiding exposure to known toxicants.

POSSIBLE COMPLICATIONS

Later, high-risk pregnancy or abortion

EXPECTED COURSE AND PROGNOSIS

- Young mares with resolved cases of endometritis may have a fair to good prognosis for conception and completion of pregnancy.
- Mares of >15 years with a history of EED or chronic, moderate to severe endometrial inflammation and/or fibrosis have a guarded to poor prognosis for conception and completion of pregnancy.

EARLY EMBRYONIC DEATH (EED)

MISCELLANEOUS

ASSOCIATED CONDITIONS

- Abortion
- Conception Failure
- Endometritis
- Metritis

AGE-RELATED FACTORS

- Development of chronic endometritis and endometrial fibrosis.
- Age-related embryonic defects.

ZOONOTIC POTENTIAL

N/A

PREGNANCY

- By definition, EED is associated with pregnancy.
- Increased risk of abortion.

SYNONYMS

N/A

SEE ALSO

- Abortion
- Conception Failure
- Embryo Transfer
- Endometritis
- Endometrial Biopsy
- Metritis
- Pregnancy Diagnosis

ABBREVIATIONS

- CL=Corpus luteum
- ELISA=Enzyme linked immunosorbent assay
- RIA=Radioimmunoassay
- T_3 = triiodothyronine
- T_4 = thyroxine

Suggested Reading

Ball BA, Daels PF. Early pregnancy loss in mares: application for progestin therapy. In: Robinson NE, ed. Current therapy in equine medicine 4. Philadelphia: WB Saunders, 1997:531–533.

Brendemuehl JP. Reproductive aspects of fescue toxicosis. In: Robinson NE, ed. Current therapy in equine medicine 4. Philadelphia: WB Saunders, 1997:571–573.

Ginther OJ. Reproductive biology of the mare: basic and applied aspects. 2nd ed. Cross Plains, WI: Equiservices, 1992:499–562.

LeBlanc MM. Diseases of the embryo In: Colahan PT, Mayhew IG, Merritt AM, Moore JM, eds. Equine medicine and surgery. 5th ed. St. Louis: Mosby, 1999;2:1199–1202.

Ley WB, Bowen JM, Purswell BJ, et al. Modified technique to evaluate uterine tubal patency in the mare. Proc Am Assoc Equine Pract 1998:56–59.

Author Tim J. Evans
Consulting Editor Carla L. Carleton

EASTERN (EEE), WESTERN (WEE), AND VENEZUELAN (VEE) ENCEPHALITIDES

BASICS

DEFINITION

A group of togaviral encephalitic diseases spread from wild (i.e., sylvatic) reservoirs to horses and humans, most often by mosquito species.

PATHOPHYSIOLOGY

Varying degrees of destructive encephalomyelitis associated with intraneuronal viral replication.

SYSTEMS AFFECTED

CNS, especially the cerebral cortex

SIGNALMENT

- No associated signalment
- Unvaccinated horses are at high risk.
- Old and young horses may be at greater risk.

SIGNS

Historical Findings

- Unvaccinated horses in endemic areas are at high risk.
- The proper season (spring to fall) for high vector numbers and recent history of cases in nearby areas should increase suspicion.
- Cases may occur year-round in southern latitudes.
- Geographic location can be helpful.
- WEE occurs in the western and midwestern United States.
- EEE occurs in the eastern and midwestern United States.
- VEE has been reported in southern Texas and, occasionally, in nearby locales.

Physical Examination Findings

- Signs vary in severity and lethality across the three viruses.
- Acute signs of EEE and WEE are nonspecific and include mild to severe fever, poor appetite, and stiffness. Many cases of WEE do not progress beyond this point, but with EEE, progression is more common.
- In progressive cases, fever may rise and fall sporadically.
- Cerebral signs may develop at anytime but often occur a few days after infection.
- Acute cerebral signs range from propulsive walking, depression, and somnolence to aggression and excitability. Some horses may become frenzied after any stimulation.
- Later signs are evidence of the dynamic nature of these conditions and increased severity of brain dysfunction—head-pressing, propulsive walking, blindness, circling, head tilt, and facial and appendicular muscle fasciculations.
- Paralysis of the pharynx, larynx, and tongue are common.
- Death often is preceded by recumbency for 1–7 days.
- Comatose animals rarely survive.
- Affected animals that will survive show gradual improvement of function over weeks to months.
- VEE may have a similar or different clinical presentation compared to WEE and EEE. This most likely results from the difference in strain pathogenicity.
- Diarrhea, severe depression, recumbency, and death may be prominent before neurologic deficits are evident.
- Other associated signs—abortion, oral ulceration, pulmonary hemorrhage, and epistaxis.

CAUSES

- The most common togaviral encephalitides in the western hemisphere are associated with EEE, WEE, and VEE.
- These viruses are classified as Togaviradae and are small, and lipid- and protein-enveloped, ribonucleic acid particles.
- In the past, they were referred to as Arboviruses.

RISK FACTORS

- Poor vaccination programs
- Dense populations of insects (most often mosquitoes) spreading viral particles from sylvatic reservoirs—birds, rodents, and reptiles

DIAGNOSIS

DIFFERENTIAL DIAGNOSIS

- Rabies
- Neurotoxic poisoning
- Botulism toxicity

CBC/BIOCHEMISTRY/URINALYSIS

No pathognomonic abnormalities

OTHER LABORATORY TESTS

N/A

IMAGING

N/A

DIAGNOSTIC PROCEDURES

- Complement fixation, hemagglutination inhibition, and neutralizing antibodies are present early in the disease.
- A fourfold rise in titer between acute and convalescent (7–10 days later) serum samples is considered to be positive for the diseases.
- An increased single-sample titer in an unvaccinated animal probably is sufficient to establish a diagnosis.
- Interpret a single-sample analysis cautiously in animals with a history of vaccination against the viruses.
- Vaccinal versus wild virus–induced titers can be distinguished using serum hemagglutination-inhibition titers to EEE and WEE. An EEE:WEE titer ratio of four or greater is suspicious for EEE infection. A ratio of eight or greater is highly indicative of EEE.
- ELISA can distinguish between vaccinal (i.e., IgG only) and virulent virus-induced (i.e., IgG and IgM) titers.

EASTERN (EEE), WESTERN (WEE), AND VENEZUELAN (VEE) ENCEPHALITIDES

PATHOLOGIC FINDINGS

Gross Findings

- Nonspecific findings at necropsy
- Gray discoloration with petechial hemorrhages of the brain and spinal cord, especially on formalin-fixed tissue sections.
- Often brain swelling and evidence of occipital-subtentorial herniation and brainstem compression.

Histopathologic Findings

- Strongly definitive
- Diffuse, gray matter–predominant meningoencephalomyelitis with neuronal degeneration, gliosis, perivascular and neuroparenchymal infiltrates, and meningitis are highly suggestive for this disease group.

TREATMENT

- Treatment is supportive and aimed at metabolic maintenance and care and at prophylaxis of self-induced trauma.
- No specific treatment will reduce morbidity and mortality.
- Strict mosquito control and vaccination can prevent both human and equine cases.
- Report all equine cases to state health officials.

MEDICATIONS

DRUGS OF CHOICE

- Fluid and metabolic support can be useful.
- No specific drug treatment will likely alter morbidity or mortality.

CONTRAINDICATIONS

N/A

PRECAUTIONS

N/A

POSSIBLE INTERACTIONS

N/A

ALTERNATIVE DRUGS

N/A

FOLLOW-UP

POSSIBLE COMPLICATIONS

Self-induced trauma may be severe.

EXPECTED COURSE AND PROGNOSIS

- Complete recoveries from associated neurologic deficits associated are reported but rare.
- Animals that recover from EEE often have residual neurologic deficits that commonly include clumsiness, depression, and abnormal behavior.
- Neurologic sequelae are similar, but less common, in horses that recover from WEE.
- In horses that develop neurologic disease, the mortality rate is 75%–100% for EEE, 20%–50% for WEE, and 40%–80% for VEE.
- Horses that recover from any of these diseases seem to be variably protected for up to 2 years after infection, but assume that no protection is afforded by infection itself.

MISCELLANEOUS

ASSOCIATED CONDITIONS

N/A

AGE-RELATED FACTORS

N/A

Young and old horses may be more susceptible.

ZOONOTIC POTENTIAL

- Essentially no amplification of virus from horses with EEE and WEE. Hence, they are dead-end hosts.
- Human disease most likely is associated with insect vector contact and often coincides with or is preceded by equine epidemics.
- Clinical signs of EEE in humans—acute fulminate encephalitis, headache, altered consciousness, and seizures.
- In humans, the mortality rate is ≅50%–75%.
- Clinical signs of WEE in humans occur yearly, but fatality or incomplete recovery is rare.
- Horses with VEE have sufficient circulating viral concentrations to act as amplifiers of disease. Ocular and nasal secretions from infected horses contain high concentrations of virus. Infection via entry through the respiratory tract may occur by direct contact with infected animals.
- Equine and human survivors of VEE infection and clinical disease may develop chronic, relapsing viremias and serve as chronic disease amplifiers.
- Clinical signs of VEE in humans—fever, headache, myalgia, and pharyngitis.
- Humans that contract VEE have a 1% mortality rate.

PREGNANCY

N/A

SYNONYMS

N/A

SEE ALSO

N/A

ABBREVIATIONS

ELISA = enzyme-linked immunoadsorbent assay

Suggested Reading

Hanson RP. American arboviral encephalomyelitides of equidae: virology and epidemiology of eastern and western arboviral encephalomyelitis of horses. Proc 3rd Int Conf Equine Infect Dis, 1973:100–114.

Gibbs EPJ. Equine viral encephalitis. Equine Vet J 1976;8:66–71.

Author Joseph J. Bertone

Consulting Editor Joseph J. Bertone

ECLAMPSIA (LACTATION TETANY)

BASICS

DEFINITION

- A rare, metabolic condition resulting when serum calcium levels drop below 8 mg/dL in heavily lactating mares.
- Clinical signs are progressive and relate directly to the level of serum calcium.
- The mare develops muscle fasciculations, beginning with the temporal, masseter, and triceps muscles; demonstrates a stiff, stilted gait and rear-limb ataxia; becomes anxious; and experiences tachycardia with dysrhythmias.

PATHOPHYSIOLOGY

- The cause relates to loss of calcium in the milk, particularly in mares that are heavy milkers, especially when on lush pasture.
- Also seen most often in draft mares and heavy, well-muscled mares, Quarter Horse halter-type mares, mares that are working while lactating, or lactating mares that are transported over long distances.
- Additionally recognized in heavily milking mares 1–2 days postweaning.

SYSTEMS AFFECTED

- Mammary
- Musculoskeletal
- Cardiovascular
- Neurologic

GENETICS

Draft breeds, but not exclusively.

INCIDENCE/PREVALENCE

Rare

SIGNALMENT

- Lactating mare 10 days postpartum and/or 1–2 days postweaning.
- Prolonged exercise or transport.
- On lush pasture.
- Serum calcium values in the 5–8 mg/dL range, coupled with associated clinical signs, make for a definitive diagnosis.
- Draft mares—Belgian, Percheron, and Clydesdale.
- No age predisposition.
- Unlikely in primiparous mares.

SIGNS

- Signs are varied and include muscle fasciculations involving the temporal, masseter, and triceps; generalized, increased muscle tone; stiff, stilted gait; rear-limb ataxia; *trismus*; dysphagia; salivation; profuse sweating; elevated temperature; anxiety; tachycardia with dysrhythmias; synchronous diaphragmatic flutter; convulsions; coma; and death.
- If untreated, the condition is progressive over a 24–48-hour period, and some of these mares die.
- Clinical signs relate directly to the level of serum calcium. Mares with below-normal calcium levels (range, 11–13 mg/dL) but still above 8 mg/dL commonly show increased excitability. Calcium levels of 5–8 mg/dL usually produce signs of tetanic spasms and inco-ordination. When serum calcium levels drop below 5 mg/dL, many of these mares become stuporous and recumbent.

CAUSES

- Lactation
- Exercise plus lactation
- Transport plus lactation
- Heavily lactating mare after weaning

RISK FACTORS

- Lactation
- Postpartum
- Heavier milking mares.

DIAGNOSIS

DIFFERENTIAL DIAGNOSIS

- Colic
- Laminitis
- Myositis
- Tetanus
- Other neuromuscular disorders.

CBC/BIOCHEMISTRY/URINALYSIS

Parameters should be within normal limits, except for possibly elevated muscle enzymes.

OTHER LABORATORY TESTS

- Laboratory normals for serum calcium range from 8.5–10.5 to 11–13 mg/dL. Most mares are within 11–13 mg/dL.
- In addition to abnormally low levels of serum calcium, many affected mares have abnormal serum levels of magnesium and phosphorus.
- Hypocalcemia has been associated with hyper/hypophosphatemia and hyper/hypomagnesemia.
- Reports suggest that hypomagnesemia/hypocalcemia most commonly is associated with transport of heavily lactating mares.

IMAGING

N/A

DIAGNOSTIC PROCEDURES

Serum calcium

PATHOLOGIC FINDINGS

N/A

ECLAMPSIA (LACTATION TETANY)

TREATMENT

APPROPRIATE HEALTH CARE
Because of the progressive nature of this condition, therapy is recommended in nearly all cases; however, a few mild cases recover without treatment.

NURSING CARE
None needed, other than the occasional mare that may require a second treatment if relapse occurs.

ACTIVITY
Restrict transit of heavily lactating mares during the susceptible period—the first 10–12 days postpartum.

DIET
Restrict access of heavily lactating mares to lush pasture if a history of the condition.

CLIENT EDUCATION
In addition to restricting access to lush pasture with a history of the condition, reduce nutritional intake (i.e. quality) in heavily lactating mares for 1–2 weeks before weaning to reduce milk production.

SURGICAL CONSIDERATIONS
N/A

MEDICATIONS

DRUGS OF CHOICE
- IV calcium (20% calcium borogluconate or 23% calcium gluconate at 250–500 mL per 500 kg).
- Dilute calcium solutions 1:4 with saline or dextrose.

CONTRAINDICATIONS
N/A

PRECAUTIONS
- Use caution when administering calcium solutions because of their potential cardiotoxic effects.
- Monitor the heart for any alterations in rate or rhythm; if such occur, stop the treatment immediately.
- Dilution of calcium with saline or dextrose reduces the potential for cardiotoxic effects.

POSSIBLE INTERACTIONS
N/A

ALTERNATIVE DRUGS
N/A

FOLLOW-UP

PATIENT MONITORING
- Reduction in clinical signs and positive inotropic effect indicate that therapy is effective.
- If no response is seen after the initial treatment, a second treatment may be necessary in 30 minutes.

PREVENTION/AVOIDANCE
See *Client Education* and dietary management for susceptible mares.

POSSIBLE COMPLICATIONS
Cardiovascular effects.

EXPECTED COURSE AND PROGNOSIS
- Most mares respond to treatment with full recovery, but relapses can occur, making additional therapy necessary.
- Future recurrence if mares are foaling and maintained under the same management conditions.

MISCELLANEOUS

ASSOCIATED CONDITIONS
N/A

AGE-RELATED FACTORS
N/A

ZOONOTIC POTENTIAL
N/A

PREGNANCY
The condition occurs either late during gestation or during the peripartal period.

SYNONYMS
- Hypocalcemia
- Lactation tetany
- Transit tetany

SEE ALSO
- Dystocia
- Parturition

Suggested Reading

Fenger CK. Disorders of calcium metabolism. In: Reed SM, Bayly WM, eds. Equine internal medicine. 1st ed. Toronto: WB Saunders, 1998:930–931.

Freestone JF, Melrose PA. Endocrine diseases. In: Kobluk CN, Ames TR, Geor RH, eds. The horse: diseases and clinical management. 1st ed. Philadelphia: WB Saunders, 1995:1159.

Valberg SJ, Hodgson DR. Diseases of muscle. In: Smith BP, ed. Large animal internal medicine. 2nd ed. St. Louis: Mosby, 1996:1498–1499.

Author E. Ricardo Bridges
Consulting Editor Carla L. Carleton

EHRLICHIOSIS, EQUINE GRANULOCYTIC

BASICS

DEFINITION

A seasonal, tick-borne disease caused by a granulocytotropic rickettsial organism, *Ehrlichia equi.*

PATHOPHYSIOLOGY

- *Ixodes pacificus* (the black-legged tick of the Pacific) is a vector for *E. equi* on the Pacific coast.
- *I. scapularis* (the black-legged tick) is the likely primary vector for the disease in the eastern and midwestern United States.
- Existence of a maintenance or sylvatic host is unknown but likely represents a wild reservoir; horses are considered dead-end hosts and are not directly contagious.
- Incubation period—8–25 days after experimental infection using ticks as vectors.
- The agent affects granulocytes (both neutrophils and eosinophils) and causes a vasculitis and an interstitial inflammation, leading to edema, petechial hemorrhages, ataxia, and hemolytic anemia.

SYSTEMS AFFECTED

- Behavioral—mentation alteration (i.e., lethargy) of varying degrees
- Hemic/lymphatic/immune—vasculitis, leading to edema and mucosal hemorrhages; hemolytic anemia
- Musculoskeletal—reluctance to move, limb edema
- Nervous—vasculitis in the CNS, leading to ataxia
- Cardiac—arrhythmias have been associated with myocarditis secondary to vasculitis within the myocardium.

GENETICS

N/A

INCIDENCE/PREVALENCE

- The highest prevalence is in Sierra Nevada foothills and northern coastal range of California, but individual cases have been reported in Colorado, Illinois, Florida, Washington, New Jersey, Europe, and South America.
- Seroprevalence studies in northern California show a prevalence of 3.1–10.3%, depending on geographic location, and >50% seropositivity among horses on premises known to be enzootic for *E. equi.*
- The disease is seasonal, having its highest occurrence during the late fall, winter, and spring and its peak during March in California.

SIGNALMENT

- Primarily affects horses, but asses have been experimentally infected
- No breed or sex predilections
- Horses $\geq$4 years are most severely affected.
- The disease has been reported in a foal as young as 2.5 months.

SIGNS

Historical Findings

- Lethargy
- Anorexia
- Limb edema
- Tick exposure

Physical Examination Findings

- Pyrexia
- Anorexia
- Depressed mentation
- Limb edema
- Mild petechiae and ecchymoses on mucous membranes and sclerae
- Icterus
- Ataxia
- Reluctance to move
- Arrhythmias (rare)

CAUSES

- *E. equi,* a granulocytotropic rickettsia spread by *Ixodes* ticks
- Close antigenic and genetic similarity to the agent of HGE and to European tick-borne fever (*E. phagocytophila*) affecting ruminants.

RISK FACTORS

- Geography
- Exposure to *I. ricinus* complex ticks
- Age—horses >3 years are most severely affected
- Immune status

DIAGNOSIS

DIFFERENTIAL DIAGNOSIS

- Viral encephalitis—rapid progression of disease with high mortality
- Liver disease with hepatic encephalopathy—increased serum hepatic enzyme activities and bilirubin and bile acid concentrations
- Purpura hemorrhagica—history of exposure to antigens of *Streptococcus equi* or other respiratory pathogens; usually not thrombocytopenic
- EIA—seropositive on Coggins or C-ELISA tests
- Equine viral arteritis—respiratory signs; seropositive to virus

CBC/BIOCHEMISTRY/URINALYSIS

- Leukopenia with neutropenia
- Thrombocytopenia
- Increased icteric index
- Anemia
- Hyperbilirubinemia.

OTHER LABORATORY TESTS

- Giemsa-, new methylene blue–, or Wright-stained peripheral blood smears show inclusion bodies (i.e., morula) within the cytoplasm of neutrophils and eosinophils. Inclusions are pleomorphic, blue-gray to dark blue in color, have a spoke-wheel appearance, and occur in 30–75% of circulating granulocytes within 3–5 days of the onset of fever.
- Buffy coat smears concentrate granulocytes and, therefore, increase the sensitivity of identifying inclusion bodies.
- Indirect fluorescent antibody tests are available for serology. A titer $\geq$1:10 is significant in terms of recent infections, and an increasing titer documents active infection.
- PCR amplification of DNA from buffy coats of infected horses is available experimentally.

IMAGING

N/A

DIAGNOSTIC PROCEDURES

N/A

PATHOLOGIC FINDINGS

- Mortality is rare, except for reasons of secondary complications.
- Inflammation of small arteries and veins
- Mild inflammatory vascular or interstitial lesions in the heart, CNS, kidneys, and lung

TREATMENT

APPROPRIATE HEALTH CARE

Hospitalize horses with severe ataxia or secondary complications; otherwise, uncomplicated cases can be managed in the field.

NURSING CARE

- Supportive limb bandages for edema
- NSAIDs for antipyretic purposes
- Debilitated cases may benefit from IV fluid or electrolyte therapy.
- Corticosteroids may benefit horses with severe ataxia by reducing the severity of vasculitis.

ACTIVITY

Stall confinement for ataxic animals; otherwise, hand-walking may help to reduce edema.

DIET

N/A

CLIENT EDUCATION

When entering known *Ixodes* tick–infested areas, use tick repellents, and check horses closely for ticks on their return from such areas.

SURGICAL CONSIDERATIONS

N/A

EHRLICHIOSIS, EQUINE GRANULOCYTIC

MEDICATIONS

DRUGS OF CHOICE

Oxytetracycline (7 mg/kg IV q24h for 3–7 days diluted in 5% dextrose in water)—with this treatment, a marked decrease in rectal temperature and improvement in appetite and attitude should be observed in 12–24 hours.

CONTRAINDICATIONS

N/A

PRECAUTIONS

- Tetracyclines can retard fetal skeletal development and discolor deciduous teeth; therefore, use with caution and only for a short duration during the first half of gestation, then only when the benefits outweigh the fetal risks.
- Monitor horses for signs of enterocolitis or diarrhea while on tetracycline therapy; the risk of diarrhea is greater with the oral route of administration.
- Tetracyclines have been associated with photosensitivity and nephrotoxicity.
- Corticosteroids have been associated with laminitis.
- NSAIDs have been associated with GI ulceration and nephrotoxicity.
- α_2-Agonist drugs (e.g., xylazine, detomidine) may induce tachypnea and respiratory distress in horses with pyrexia.

POSSIBLE INTERACTIONS

N/A

ALTERNATIVE DRUGS

- Enrofloxacin (5 mg/kg IV q24h for 5–7 days) has been effective in treating experimental infections.
- Do not use enrofloxacin in foals and growing horses, because it can cause arthropathies and lameness.

FOLLOW-UP

PATIENT MONITORING

- Monitor temperature, attitude, and appetite for significant improvement within 12–24 hours of treatment.
- Evaluate serial buffy coat smear for inclusion bodies.
- Monitor hydration status and renal function while on oxytetracycline.

PREVENTION/AVOIDANCE

- Minimize exposure to *Ixodes* ticks through application of topical tick repellents when entering infested areas, and carefully examine horses for ticks on their return from such areas.
- Prevention is impractical in endemic areas, and many horses may experience subclinical infections and develop subsequent immunity.

POSSIBLE COMPLICATIONS

- Secondary bacterial infections, especially bronchopneumonia.
- Horses with severe ataxia may suffer traumatic injury (e.g., fractures).
- Cardiac arrhythmias, including ventricular tachycardia, may be associated with myocarditis; treatment of myocarditis consists of corticosteroids and antiarrhythmic drugs (e.g., quinidine) along with tetracycline therapy.

EXPECTED COURSE AND PROGNOSIS

- Excellent prognosis in uncomplicated cases.
- Horses are immune to reinfection for at least 2 years; no carrier or latent state has been documented.
- With therapy, horses show rapid improvement—a decrease in rectal temperature, increase in appetite, and improvement in overall demeanor should be noted in 12–24 hours; the ataxia should resolve within 2–3 days and the edema within several days.
- Left untreated, the disease is self-limiting in 2–3 weeks; however, affected horses exhibit more severe weight loss, edema, and ataxia and are at greater risk for secondary complications than horses treated with tetracycline.

MISCELLANEOUS

ASSOCIATED CONDITIONS

N/A

AGE-RELATED FACTORS

Severity of clinical signs is associated with age—animals <1 year generally exhibit only slight lethargy and fever; animals 1–3 years of age show moderate signs; and animals ≥ 4 years are affected most severely, with ataxia, icterus, edema, and petechial hemorrhages.

ZOONOTIC POTENTIAL

- The agent of HGE may represent one or more strains of the equine pathogen; however, horses are considered dead-end hosts and do not act as a source of human infection directly.
- Ticks are required as intermediate hosts.

PREGNANCY

- Two pregnant mares are reported to have been naturally infected with *E. equi* during gestation and to have subsequently delivered live foals at full term.
- No abortions or congenital abnormalities have been described.
- Passive immunity is transferred to suckling foals but is short-lived in duration.

SYNONYMS

Equine ehrlichiosis

SEE ALSO

- EIA
- Thrombocytopenia

ABBREVIATIONS

- C-ELISA = competitive enzyme-linked immunoadsorbent assay
- EIA = equine infectious anemia
- GI = gastrointestinal
- HGE = human granulocytic ehrlichiosis
- PCR = polymerase chain reaction

Suggested Reading

Madigan JE, Gribble D. Equine ehrlichiosis in Northern California: 49 cases (1968–1981). J Am Vet Med Assoc 1987;190:445–448.

Madigan JE, Nietela S, Chalmers S, DeRock E. Seroepidemiologic survey of antibodies to *Ehrlichia equi* in horses of Northern California. J Am Vet Med Assoc 1990;196:1962–1964.

Madigan JE, Richter PJ Jr., Kimsey RB, Barlough JE, Bakken JS, Dumler JS. Transmission and passage in horses of the agent of human granulocytic ehrlichiosis. J Infect Dis 1995;172:1141–1144.

Reubel GH, Kimsey RB, Barlough JE, Madigan JE. Experimental transmission of *Ehrlichia equi* to horses through naturally infected ticks (*Ixodes pacificus*) from northern California. J Clin Microbiol 1998;36:2131–2134.

Richter PJ Jr., Kimsey RB, Madigan JE, Barlough JE, Dumler JS, Brooks DL. *Ixodes pacificus* (Acari:Ixodidae) as a vector of *Ehrlichia equi* (Rickettsiales:Ehrlichieae). J Med Entomol 1996;33:1–5.

Authors K. Gary Magdesian and John E. Madigan

Consulting Editor Debra C. Sellon

EMBRYO TRANSFER (ET)

BASICS

DEFINITION
Removal of an embryo from the uterus or oviduct of one mare (the donor) and placement into the uterus or oviduct of another (the recipient).

PATHOPHYSIOLOGY
N/A

SYSTEM AFFECTED
Reproductive

GENETICS
N/A

INCIDENCE/PREVALENCE
N/A

SIGNALMENT
- Mares of >15 years with a history of conception failure, EED, or abortion.
- Young mares in competition.
- Certain extraspecific matings—zebra into a horse.

SIGNS
N/A

CAUSES
N/A

RISK FACTORS
N/A

DIAGNOSIS

DIFFERENTIAL DIAGNOSIS
N/A

CBC/BIOCHEMISTRY/URINALYSIS
N/A

OTHER LABORATORY TESTS
- Maternal progesterone may be indicated at recipient's initial pregnancy examination to check for functional CL.
- ELISA or RIA for progesterone—acceptable levels vary from >1 to >4 ng/mL, depending on the reference lab.
- Maternal T_3/T_4 levels—anecdotal reports of lower levels in mares with a history of conception failure, EED, or abortion; significance of low T_4 levels not clear at present.

IMAGING
Transrectal Ultrasonography:
- Indicated for donor and recipient at the time of flushing and transfer, respectively, to determine the absence of intrauterine fluid and the presence of CL.
- Also used in one technique as a guide for the aspiration of oocytes.

DIAGNOSTIC PROCEDURES

Prebreeding Reproductive Evaluation
- Indicated in individuals with a history of conception failure, EED, or abortion.
- Transrectal ultrasonography, vaginal examination (both by digital manual and speculum), endometrial cytology/culture, and endometrial biopsy should detect evidence of anatomic defects, endometritis, and fibrosis, which may predispose to conception failure.

Transrectal Ultrasonography
- To monitor follicular development and more precisely monitor ovulation in both the donor and recipient.
- To time AI or breeding.
- To schedule ET for optimal success.

Embryo Collection
May be used as a diagnostic procedure to determine if embryos can enter the oviduct or uterus.

PATHOLOGIC FINDINGS
Endometrial biopsy—moderate to severe, chronic endometritis or fibrosis may be indications for ET.

TREATMENT

APPROPRIATE HEALTH CARE
Most ETs are best handled in a hospital setting with adequate facilities and personnel.

Indications
- Mares with a history of conception failure, EED, repeated abortion, or high-risk pregnancy
- Mares with chronic, moderate to severe endometritis or fibrosis
- Mares in competition

Embryo Recovery Procedures
- Nonsurgical uterine flushing 6–8 days after ovulation.
- Surgical oviductal flushing 2–4 days after ovulation.
- Laparoscopic or transvaginal ultrasound-guided recovery of oocytes

Embryo Transfer Procedures
- Nonsurgical intrauterine transfer.
- Surgical intrauterine transfer.
- Pre–embryo stage procedures.
- Laparoscopic or surgical oviductal transfer of zygotes—ZIFT.
- IVF
- Laparoscopic or surgical oviductal transfer of gametes—GIFT.

NURSING CARE
Generally required after more invasive procedures in donor and recipient mares.

ACTIVITY
Generally restricted after more invasive procedures in donor and recipient mares.

DIET
Normal diet, unless contraindicated by concurrent maternal disease or exercise restriction.

CLIENT EDUCATION
- ET procedures are not approved by all breed registries.
- Recipient mares generally need to be fairly closely synchronized with donor mares—depending on the procedure, 0–2 days
- If the number of normal, synchronized recipients is limited, embryos can be transported, and embryo-freezing procedures are improving.

SURGICAL CONSIDERATIONS
- May be indicated to repair anatomic defects predisposing to endometritis.
- Surgical oviductal recovery and implantation.

EMBRYO TRANSFER (ET)

MEDICATIONS

DRUGS OF CHOICE
Progestins, antibiotics, anti-inflammatory medications, and intrauterine therapy may or may not be used depending on the case, procedures involved, and clinician preference.

CONTRAINDICATIONS
N/A

PRECAUTIONS
N/A

POSSIBLE INTERACTIONS
N/A

ALTERNATIVE DRUGS
N/A

FOLLOW-UP

PATIENT MONITORING
- Accurate teasing records.
- Re-examination of donors diagnosed and treated for endometritis before ET.
- Early transrectal ultrasonography of recipient mare for pregnancy.
- Transrectal ultrasonography to monitor for embryonic and fetal development.

PREVENTION/AVOIDANCE
N/A

POSSIBLE COMPLICATIONS
- Recipient conception failure or EED.
- Endometritis in donor mares after the uterine flushing procedure.

EXPECTED COURSE AND PROGNOSIS
- Prognosis for successful pregnancy depends on the quality of the embryo (i.e., oocyte) and recipient mare.
- Prognosis for successful recovery of intrauterine embryo at 6–8 days after ovulation is ≅70% in normal mares (less in subfertile mares).
- Prognosis for successful surgical, intrauterine transfer of embryos is ≅70% for embryos from normal mares (less from subfertile mares).
- Nonsurgical, intrauterine transfer of embryos may be less successful (wide individual variation) than surgical transfer.
- Other embryo and early zygote procedures may have lower success rates and are still in development.

MISCELLANEOUS

ASSOCIATED CONDITIONS
- Abortion
- Conception failure
- EED
- Endometritis
- High-risk pregnancy

AGE-RELATED FACTORS
- Development of chronic endometritis and endometrial fibrosis.
- Age-related embryonic defects, especially with old mares.

ZOONOTIC POTENTIAL
N/A

PREGNANCY
By definition, the condition is associated with pregnancy.

SYNONYMS
N/A

SEE ALSO
- Abortion
- Conception failure
- EED
- Endometritis
- Endometrial biopsy
- High-risk pregnancy
- Pregnancy diagnosis

ABBREVIATIONS
- AI = artificial insemination
- CL = corpus luteum
- EED = early embryonic death
- ELISA = enzyme-linked immunoadsorbent assay
- GIFT = gamete intrafallopian transfer
- IVF = in vitro fertilization
- RIA = radioimmunoassay
- T_3 = triiodothyronine
- T_4 = thyroxine
- ZIFT = zygote intrafallopian transfer

Suggested Reading

Cochran R, Meitjes M, Reggio B, et al. Live foals produced from sperm-injected oocytes derived from pregnant mares. J Equine Vet Sci 1998;18:736–740.

Hinrichs K. Assisted reproductive techniques in the mare. In: Robinson NE, ed. Current therapy in equine medicine 4. Philadelphia: WB Saunders, 1997:565–571.

Squires EL. Maturation and fertilization of equine oocytes. Vet Clin North Am Equine Pract 1996;12(1):31–45.

Squires EL. Embryo transfer. In: McKinnon AO, Voss JL, eds. Equine reproduction Philadelphia: Lea & Febiger, 1993:357–367.

Author Tim J. Evans

Consulting Editor Carla L. Carleton

ENCEPHALITIS—EASTERN, WESTERN, VENEZUELAN, AND JAPANESE B

BASICS

DEFINITION
A nonsuppurative viral encephalitis of horses, birds, and humans that is transmitted by biting insects. The viruses are maintained in sylvatic populations of birds, small mammals, and reptiles.

PATHOPHYSIOLOGY
Biting insects, principally mosquitos, transmit viruses of the family Togaviridae from sylvatic hosts to horses. In the horse, the virus travels through the lymphatics to regional lymph nodes, where it multiplies in macrophages and neutrophils. An initial viremia results in infection of multiple organs, including the spleen and liver. A second viremia then ensues and infection of the central nervous system (CNS) occurs 3–5 days after inoculation.

SYSTEMS AFFECTED
Nervous
The viruses primarily infect the brain and spinal cord, causing associated clinical signs.

GENETICS
N/A

INCIDENCE/PREVALENCE
Western equine encephalitis (WEE) infections occur primarily in the western United States, South America, and Canada. Eastern equine encephalitis (EEE) infections occur in the eastern and southeastern United Sates and Central and South America. Venezuelan equine encephalitis (VEE) infections occur primarily in Central and South America; however, an outbreak of VEE occurred in Texas in 1971. The Japanese B and St. Louis viruses are less virulent and occur in Asia and the midwestern United States, respectively. Most cases occur during the height of the vector season; in northern temperate climates, this is between June and November. However, in warmer climates cases may be seen at any time of year. Ambient temperature and rainfall affect insect vector populations. The conditions that favor outbreaks in temperate climates (infected reservoir population, high population of vectors, and a susceptible equine population) vary from year to year; hence the incidence also varies from year to year. Some locations may go for several years with few or no cases reported, and then have a year with large numbers of cases.

SIGNALMENT
Togaviral encephalomyelitis may occur in horses of any age, breed, or sex; however, it is uncommon in foals under 3 months of age.

SIGNS
General Comments
Initial signs of fever are followed by general depression. Predominant signs are related to brain and brain stem dysfunction.

Historical Findings
The initial fever with WEE and EEE is biphasic, with fever spikes 2 and 6 days after infection. During the initial phase of infection, horses may appear dull and sleepy, spending more time in sternal recumbency. An acute onset of fever (101–106°F) may also precede signs of neurologic disease.

Physical Examination Findings
Horses infected with any of the alphaviruses may include any of the following clinical signs:
- Fever
- Dementia
- Head pressing
- Yawning
- Ataxia
- Blindness
- Circling
- Seizures
- Hypermetria
- Hyperesthesia
- Aggression
- Twitching of muzzle or appendicular musculature
- Head tilt
- Dysphagia
- Paralysis
- Convulsions
- Death

Horses with VEE may also have diarrhea, oral ulceration, and epistaxis.

CAUSES
The most pathogenic viruses of the family Togaviridae are the alphaviruses—WEE, EEE, and VEE. The less virulent flaviviruses include the Japanese B and St. Louis viruses.

RISK FACTORS
Due to exposure to the insect vectors, these diseases are more common in horses that are pastured rather than stabled.

DIAGNOSIS

DIFFERENTIAL DIAGNOSIS
Differential diagnoses include the following:
- Rabies
- Trauma
- Hepatoencephalopathy
- Herpesvirus myeloencephalopathy
- Leukoencephalomalacia
- Brain abscess
- Verminous encephalitis
- Equine protozoal myeloencephalitis

CBC/BIOCHEMISTRY/URINALYSIS
Lymphopenia and neutropenia may occur in early stages of the disease. Serum biochemistry and urinalysis are usually normal unless anorexia has led to pre-renal azotemia. Hyperglycemia may result from severe stress. Evaluation of liver enzymes (GGT, AST, and SDH) and liver function tests (blood ammonia and serum bile acids) help to rule out hepatic encephalopathy.

OTHER LABORATORY TESTS
N/A

IMAGING
Radiography of the skull may be beneficial if trauma is considered.

DIAGNOSTIC PROCEDURES
Cerebrospinal fluid (CSF) changes include pleocytosis ($\leq 700{,}000$ cells/μL) and increased protein concentration (60–200 mg/dl). Occasionally, an eosinophilic pleocytosis may occur with EEE. Virus may be isolated from CSF during the acute phase of infection. A four-fold rise in convalescent serum antibody titers may not be possible because high titers may be present at the onset of clinical signs. Hemagglutination inhibition, complement fixation, and serum neutralization assay are available. Colostral antibodies interfere with serodiagnosis in foals. Virus can be isolated from cerebral tissue post-mortem.

PATHOLOGIC FINDINGS
Gross CNS changes may be absent, or congestion and discoloration of the brain and spinal cord may be present. Microscopically, a diffuse mononuclear and neutrophilic perivascular cuffing, neuronal degeneration, and gliosis occur in the cerebral cortex. Mononuclear cell meningeal inflammation also occurs.

TREATMENT

APPROPRIATE HEALTH CARE
Hospitalization is appropriate for horses with signs of encephalitis if they can be transported safely. However, management is largely supportive, and if referral is not possible, horses can be effectively managed on the farm of origin.

NURSING CARE
Treatment is supportive because there is no specific anti-viral therapy for togaviral encephalitides. Self-trauma should be prevented by protective helmets, leg wraps, and

ENCEPHALITIS—EASTERN, WESTERN, VENEZUELAN, AND JAPANESE B

deep bedding. If possible, the horses should be placed in a padded stall. Recumbent horses should be repositioned frequently or placed in a sling. Hydration should be monitored, and balanced polyionic intravenous or oral fluids should be given as needed. Soaked pelleted feeds may be given by nasogastric tube if anorexia persists.

ACTIVITY

Activity is restricted to what the horses can safely manage. Owner should be aware of the dangers of managing horses with neurologic diseases.

CLIENT EDUCATION

Owners in endemic areas should be aware of effective preventative strategies, including vaccination and vector management (see risk factors, prevention, and zoonosis).

SURGICAL CONSIDERATIONS

N/A

MEDICATIONS

DRUG(S) OF CHOICE

Nonsteroidal anti-inflammatory drugs (phenylbutazone 2.2–4.4 mg/kg IV q12h, flunixin meglumine 1 mg/kg IV q12h) are given for analgesia and inflammation. Dimethyl sulfoxide (1mg/kg IV or by nasogastric tube as a 20% solution, once daily for 3 days) may ameliorate effects of cerebral ischemia. Seizures may be controlled by diazepam (0.1–0.4 mg/kg IV), or pentobarbital (2–10 mg/kg IV to effect). Corticosteroid administration is controversial, and if given, the horses should be monitored for signs of laminitis.

CONTRAINDICATIONS

N/A

PRECAUTIONS

N/A

POSSIBLE INTERACTIONS

N/A

ALTERNATIVE DRUGS

N/A

FOLLOW-UP

PATIENT MONITORING

The patient should be evaluated at least daily for progression of neurologic dysfunction or new signs that suggest other differential diagnoses.

PREVENTION/AVOIDANCE

- Vaccination is an effective preventive measure. Two doses of vaccine given IM 4 weeks apart should be administered for primary immunization of unvaccinated horses. Adequate titers last approximately 6–8 months, and adult horses should be vaccinated at the beginning of the vector season or twice yearly in warmer climates. Mares should be vaccinated 4–6 weeks before foaling, and foal vaccination should begin at 3 months of age. Vaccination in the face of an outbreak is recommended. Horses vaccinated against WEE and EEE have minimal protection against VEE; however, vaccination with trivalent vaccines provides enhanced antibody protection to all antigens.
- Application of repellents and avoiding pastures near mosquito habitat during dawn and dusk may reduce exposure to infected vectors during outbreaks. Management of mosquito breeding areas includes application of insecticides and drainage of standing water.

EXPECTED COURSE AND PROGNOSIS

The mortality rate for EEE is 75–100%; however, it is slightly less with WEE and VEE. Recumbent animals usually die within 5 days. Complete recovery is rare, and horses that survive often have residual neurologic deficits, such as ataxia, depression, and abnormal behavior. Mortality rates with Japanese B and St. Louis encephalitis are less than 5%.

MISCELLANEOUS

ASSOCIATED CONDITIONS

N/A

AGE-RELATED FACTORS

N/A

ZOONOTIC POTENTIAL

VEE is a reportable disease in the United States. All three equine encephalitides are transmitted from birds or rodents to humans by mosquitos. However, only VEE can produce a significant viremia in the horse such that the horse can propagate an epizootic. A brief viremia occurs in the early stages of EEE infection such that the horse may propagate the virus; however, this is unlikely due to the transient nature of the viremia. The diagnosis of any of the togaviral encephalitides in a horse suggests that there may be a sufficient sylvatic reservoir and vector population that humans may be at risk for contracting the disease.

PREGNANCY

N/A

SYNONYMS

- Arboviral encephalitis
- Equine sleeping sickness

SEE ALSO

N/A

ABBREVIATIONS

- AST = aspartate transaminase
- EEE = Eastern equine encephalitis
- GGT= γ-glutamyltransferase
- SDH = Sorbitol dehydrogenase
- VEE = Venezuelan equine encephalitis
- WEE = Western equine encephalitis

Suggested Reading

Bertone JE. Togaviral encephalitides (eastern and western) equine encephalitis. In: Robinson NE, ed. Current Therapy in Equine Medicine, 3rd ed. Philadelphia: WB Saunders, 1992:547–550.

George LW. Diseases of the nervous system. In: Smith BP, ed. Large Animal Internal Medicine, 2nd ed. St. Louis: Mosby, 1996:1018–1021.

Author Mark T. Donaldson

Consulting Editor Corinne R. Sweeney

ENDOCARDITIS

BASICS

DEFINITION

- Infective endocarditis usually is a bacterial infection of the valvular or mural endocardium.
- A platelet fibrin thrombus is attached to the endocardium and is colonized by bacteria during periods of bacteremia. The platelet fibrin thrombus forms in response to collagen exposure on a denuded endothelial surface. Proliferation of a mass of fibrin and platelets containing bacteria occurs, resulting in a vegetative mass.
- Bacterial infection is most likely to localize on a previously damaged valve. This accounts for the most common site of equine infection being the mitral valve, closely followed by the aortic valve.
- The tricuspid valve most frequently is affected in horses with septic jugular vein thrombophlebitis.

PATHOPHYSIOLOGY

- Clinical signs depend on site and severity of the intracardiac infection, embolization of vegetations to any organ, constant bacteremia, and development of immune-complex disease.
- Initially, the vegetative lesion, if large, may obstruct the outflow of blood from the chamber, resulting in a murmur of valvular stenosis.
- As vegetative lesions grow or heal, valvular damage occurs.
- Valvular incompetence and a murmur of valvular insufficiency usually develop.

SYSTEMS AFFECTED

- Cardiovascular—primary
- Respiratory—secondary
- Neurologic—secondary
- Renal—secondary
- Splenic—secondary
- Hepatic—secondary
- GI—secondary
- Musculoskeletal—secondary

GENETICS

N/A

INCIDENCE/PREVALENCE

No breed predilection

SIGNALMENT

- All ages, but horses <3 years constitute the majority of cases.
- Males may have a slightly higher risk than females.

SIGNS

General Comments

Usually associated with fever of unknown origin.

Historical Findings

- Fever
- Shifting leg lameness
- Joint or tendon sheath distention

Physical Examination Findings

- Fever
- Tachycardia
- Tachypnea
- Other, less common findings—murmur, arrhythmias, anorexia, depression, weight loss, coughing, and congestive heart failure.

CAUSES

Bacterial infection of the valvular or mural endocardium, most frequently involving *Streptococcal* or *Pasturella/Actinobacillus* sp.

RISK FACTORS

- Pre-existing valve damage
- Septic jugular vein thrombophlebitis
- Transvenous pacing catheter
- Congenital heart disease

DIAGNOSIS

DIFFERENTIAL DIAGNOSIS

- Pericarditis—heart sounds usually are muffled; friction rubs may be present; differentiate echocardiographically.
- Myocarditis—arrhythmias or murmurs usually are present; differentiate echocardiographically.
- Degenerative valve disease—fever and depression are not present; tachycardia, tachypnea, and coughing are not present unless the horse is developing congestive heart failure; differentiate echocardiographically.
- Other diseases causing fever of unknown origin (e.g., peritonitis, pleuropneumonia, abscesses, neoplasia—murmurs and shifting leg lameness usually are not present; differentiate echocardiographically and with clinicopathology, abdominocentesis or thoracocentesis, and abdominal or thoracic ultrasonography.

CBC/BIOCHEMISTRY/URINALYSIS

- CBC often reveals neutrophilic leukocytosis with hyperfibrinogenemia and nonregenerative anemia typical of chronic disease.
- BUN and creatinine may be elevated in horses with bacterial endocarditis.
- Renal azotemia may be detected in horses with left-sided vegetative lesions and renal emboli, whereas azotemia is prerenal in horses with congestive heart failure and low cardiac output.
- Urinalysis in horses with renal emboli may reveal increased bacteria, elevated protein, and WBC or renal tubular epithelial casts.

OTHER LABORATORY TESTS

- Obtain three serial blood cultures before treatment with antimicrobials, if possible. Positive bacterial growth will be obtained in ≅50% of cases.
- Previous or concurrent antimicrobial therapy inhibits the ability to obtain a positive blood culture.
- Elevated cardiac isoenzymes (e.g., cardiac troponin I, CK-MB, HBDH, LDH-1 and -2) may be present with concurrent myocardial disease.

IMAGING

Electrocardiography

- Ventricular premature depolarizations or ventricular tachycardia most frequently is detected in horses with left-sided bacterial endocarditis.
- Atrial fibrillation is most common in horses with marked atrial enlargement associated with AV valvular insufficiency.

Echocardiography

- Definitive diagnosis of bacterial endocarditis is established by identifying irregular, hypoechoic to echoic masses associated with the valve leaflet, chordae tendineae, or mural endocardium.
- Determine the number of valve leaflets affected and size of the lesions.
- Perform Doppler examination to determine if valvular insufficiency is present and, if so, to semiquantitate its severity.
- Small vegetative lesions and lesions in the atria may be difficult to detect with transthoracic echocardiography.

Thoracic Radiography

- Cardiac enlargement may be detected with severe valvular insufficiency.
- Pulmonary edema may be detected in horses with congestive heart failure.
- Pneumonia may be present in horses with right-sided endocarditis.

DIAGNOSTIC PROCEDURES

Continuous 24-hour Holter monitoring—useful in the diagnosis of horses with suspected atrial or ventricular premature depolarizations.

PATHOLOGIC FINDINGS

- Focal or diffuse thickening or distortion of one or more affected valve leaflets with vegetative masses on the leaflet, chordae tendineae, or less frequently, mural endocardium.
- Ruptured chordae tendineae and flail valve leaflets are infrequently detected.
- Jet lesions usually are detected in the preceding chamber.
- Enlargement of the respective atria and thinning of the atrial myocardium in horses with significant mitral or tricuspid regurgitation.
- Ventricular enlargement and thinning of the ventricular free wall and interventricular septum in horses with significant regurgitation.
- Pulmonary vein dilatation in horses with severe mitral regurgitation; pulmonary artery dilatation in horses with pulmonary hypertension.
- Pale areas may be seen in the atrial myocardium with areas of inflammatory cell infiltrate, necrosis, and fibrosis detected histopathologically.
- Infarcts and abscesses secondary to septic embolization of other organs, particularly the lung, kidneys, spleen, myocardium, and brain.

TREATMENT

APPROPRIATE HEALTH CARE

- Hospitalize horses with bacterial endocarditis, and treat with systemic, bacteriocidal, broad-spectrum antimicrobials that are initially empirical and subsequently based on results of blood culture and sensitivity.
- Horses with moderate to severe mitral or aortic regurgitation may benefit from long-term vasodilator therapy.
- Treat horses with severe mitral, aortic, or tricuspid regurgitation and congestive heart failure for congestive heart failure with positive inotropic drugs, vasodilators, and diuretics.
- Closely monitor response to therapy with clinical, clinicopathologic, and echocardiographic re-evaluations.

NURSING CARE

N/A

ACTIVITY

- Stall rest and hand walking only while being treated for bacterial endocarditis.
- Once a bacteriologic cure is achieved, rest with small paddock turnout for an additional month before being gradually returned to work.
- Ability of the horse to return to work successfully depends on severity of the valvular damage sustained; valvular damage associated with scarring of the affected leaflets continues for many months.
- Horses with valvular insufficiency are safe to continue in full athletic work until regurgitation becomes severe or ventricular arrhythmias develop.
- Monitor horses with moderate to severe mitral or aortic regurgitation by ECG during high-intensity exercise to ensure they are safe to compete. These horses can be used for lower-level athletic competition with frequent clinical and echocardiographic monitoring.
- Horses with significant ventricular arrhythmias or pulmonary artery dilatation are no longer safe to ride.

DIET

N/A

CLIENT EDUCATION

- Monitor the horse's temperature daily, preferably during the late afternoon or evening, during treatment of bacterial endocarditis and after discontinuation of antimicrobials.
- Regularly monitor cardiac rhythm; any irregularities other than second-degree AV block should prompt ECG.
- Carefully monitor for exercise intolerance, respiratory distress, prolonged recovery after exercise, increased resting respiratory or heart rate, cough, or edema; if detected, see cardiac re-examination.

SURGICAL CONSIDERATIONS

N/A

MEDICATIONS

DRUGS OF CHOICE

Infective Endocarditis

- To cure endocarditis requires sterilization of the vegetation.
- Bacteriocidal antimicrobials can be administered IV for 4–6 weeks.

ENDOCARDITIS

• Empirically, until blood culture and sensitivity results are available, potassium penicillin and gentocin are a good combination. Rifampin may be added to improve penetration of the antimicrobial into the lesion.
• Administer aspirin to decrease platelet adhesiveness.
• With life-threatening ventricular arrhythmias, institute appropriate antiarrhythmic drugs.

Valvular Insufficiency

• With severe mitral or aortic regurgitation, enalapril or other ACE inhibitor
• ACE inhibitors prolong the time to valve replacement in humans with moderate to severe mitral regurgitation.
• During heart failure with mitral, aortic, or tricuspid regurgitation, use digoxin, furosemide, and vasodilators.

CONTRAINDICATIONS

N/A

PRECAUTIONS

• Evaluate creatinine and BUN before starting aminoglycoside antimicrobials.
• ACE inhibitors can cause hypotension; thus, do not give as a large dose without time to accommodate to this treatment.

POSSIBLE INTERACTIONS

N/A

ALTERNATIVE DRUGS

Most other vasodilatory drugs should have some beneficial effect in horses with moderate to severe mitral and/or aortic regurgitation but may be less effective than ACE inhibitors.

FOLLOW-UP

PATIENT MONITORING

• Frequently monitor lesions echocardiographically during treatment with antimicrobials to assess the efficacy of treatment.
• Once antimicrobials have been discontinued, monitor lesions echocardiographically 2 and 4 weeks later and periodically thereafter, depending on the valve affected and the severity of the valvular regurgitation that has developed.
• With severe valvular insufficiency, echocardiographic re-evaluations are recommended at 3-month intervals.

PREVENTION/AVOIDANCE

Institute aggressive treatment of septic jugular vein thrombophlebitis to minimize seeding of the tricuspid valve from septic emboli associated with the infected jugular vein.

POSSIBLE COMPLICATIONS

• Immune-mediated synovitis or tenosynovitis
• Right-sided bacterial endocarditis—pulmonary thromboembolism, pulmonary abscess, and pneumonia
• Left-sided bacterial endocarditis—hepatic, splenic, and renal abscess; myocardial and cerebral infarction

EXPECTED COURSE AND PROGNOSIS

• Prognosis for horses with bacterial endocarditis depends on the organism(s) involved, response to antimicrobial treatment, valve(s) affected, and severity of valvular damage that develops.
• Prognosis for horses with right-sided bacterial endocarditis usually is guarded and for left-sided bacterial endocarditis is grave.
• Achieving bacteriologic cure usually is difficult, because blood culture and sensitivity blood may be nonrewarding due to previous antimicrobial treatment.
• Even when bacteriologic cure is achieved, continued damage to the affected valve occurs, because the valve heals after the infection. This usually results in worsening of the valvular insufficiency already present. These horses may develop clinical signs associated with the worsening valvular insufficiency that shorten both useful performance life and life expectancy.

ENDOCARDITIS

MISCELLANEOUS

ASSOCIATED CONDITIONS
- Septic jugular vein thrombophlebitis
- Pre-existing valve damage
- Congenital cardiac disease

AGE-RELATED FACTORS
Bacterial endocarditis is more frequent in horses <3 years of age.

ZOONOTIC POTENTIAL
N/A

PREGNANCY
- Pregnant mares with bacterial endocarditis may not experience any problems with pregnancy unless the associated valvular insufficiency is moderate to severe or clinical problems associated with dissemination of septic emboli develop.
- Pregnant mares are at risk for development of placentitis, and the fetus may become septic.
- Treating pregnant mares with IV broad-spectrum bacteriocidal antimicrobials is important. Base the antimicrobial therapy on blood culture and sensitivity, if available, and choose antimicrobials that are safe for the developing fetus.
- The volume expansion of late pregnancy places an additional load on the already volume-loaded heart and may precipitate congestive heart failure in mares with severe valvular insufficiency.
- In pregnant mares with congestive heart failure, treat for the underlying cardiac disease with positive inotropic drugs and diuretics. ACE inhibitors are contraindicated because of potential adverse effects on the fetus.

SYNONYMS
- Vegetative endocarditis
- Infective endocarditis
- Bacterial endocarditis

SEE ALSO
- Aortic regurgitation
- Mitral regurgitation
- Tricuspid regurgitation

ABBREVIATIONS
- ACE = angiotensin-converting enzyme
- AV = atrioventricular
- CK-MB = MB isoenzyme of creatine kinase
- GI = gastrointestinal
- HBDH = α-hydroxybutyrate dehydrogenase
- LDH = lactate dehydrogenase

Suggested Reading

Buergelt CD, Cooley AJ, Hines SA, Pipers FS. Endocarditis in 6 horses. Vet Pathol 1985;22:333–337.

Kasari TR, Roussel AJ. Bacterial endocarditis. Part I. Pathophysiologic, diagnostic and therapeutic considerations. Compend Contin Educ Pract Vet 1989;11:655–671.

Maxson ADM, Reef VB. Bacterial endocarditis in horses: a review of 10 cases (1984–1995). Equine Vet J 1997;29:394–399.

Roussel AJ, Kasari TR. Bacterial endocarditis in large animals. Part II. Incidence, causes, clinical signs and pathologic findings. Compend Contin Educ Pract Vet 1989;11:769–773.

Wagenaar G, Kroneman J, Breukink H. Endocarditis in the horse. Blue Book Vet Prof 1967;12:38–45.

Author Virginia B. Reef
Consulting Editor N/A

ENDOMETRIAL BIOPSY

BASICS

DEFINITION

Histopathologic evaluation of the endometrium to predict a mare's ability to carry a foal to term.

PATHOPHYSIOLOGY

Seasonal Variation

• Normal histopathologic changes of the endometrium are driven by cyclic fluctuations of ovarian steroids (estrogen and progesterone). Resultant variations reflect both stage of estrous cycle and seasonal changes.
• Winter anestrus is characterized by endometrial atrophy. The luminal and glandular epithelium becomes cuboidal, and the glands are straight, low in density, and accumulate secretions from myometrial hypotonia.
• During transition, rising levels of estrogen stimulate endometrial activity, as reflected by increasing luminal/glandular epithelial activity and glandular density.
• Spring variations in the epithelial cell layer—during the spring breeding season (mares are long-day breeders), the luminal epithelium varies in height from tall columnar in early diestrus to low/moderately columnar and cuboidal through diestrus, finally reaching maximal height/tall columnar in estrus.
• Other springtime histopathologic changes—during early estrus, edema develops in the stroma, causing "nesting" of individual branches of glands; during estrus, PMN leukocytes marginate on the sides of venules and capillaries, without migrating into the stroma; additionally, glands are straight, and some degree of edema exists.
• During diestrus (progesterone is the predominant influence), gland tortuosity increases, and edema decreases.

Assessment of Inflammation and Degenerative Changes

• Degree and extent of inflammation and degenerative changes of the endometrium—alterations caused by age, natural challenges (e.g., coitus, pregnancy), irritation/contamination by bacteria, pneumovagina, urovagina, DUC, and other unknown causes.
• Nature of change—inflammatory cell infiltration, periglandular fibrosis, cystic glandular distention and lymphangiectasia, with or without periglandular fibrosis.
• High correlation between histopathologic changes and ability of the endometrium to carry a foal to term. As duration of endometrial damage and insult increases, probability of a normal term pregnancy decreases.
• Inflammation (acute and chronic) of the endometrium is associated with repeated natural challenges.
• Degenerative changes (e.g. fibrosis, lymphangiectasia) usually are progressive, primarily associated with aging, but clearly exacerbated by factors such as parity and chronic inflammation.

SYSTEM AFFECTED

Reproductive

GENETICS

N/A

INCIDENCE/PREVALENCE

N/A

SIGNALMENT

• Degenerative changes and chronic inflammatory cellular infiltration increase with age and parity.
• Abnormal anatomic conditions, uterine insult, or history of aggressive or prolonged treatments predispose the endometrium to contamination and irritation independent of age or parity.

SIGNS

Historical Findings

Infertility/Subfertility of different degrees:
• Barren mares, from the previous or current breeding season, bred within 48 hours before ovulation with proven semen.
• Anestrus mares during the breeding season.
• Mares with reproductive tract abnormalities.
• Mares with history of EED or abortion.
• Mares with inconclusive cytologic/culture findings for the diagnosis of clinical endometritis.

Physical Examination Findings

Endometrial biopsy is advisable for a prepurchase examination to evaluate the reproductive potential of a broodmare.

CAUSES

Inflammation

• The most common endometrial abnormality.
• Neutrophils predominate in acute inflammation, whereas lymphocytes, plasma cells, and macrophages characterize chronic endometritis.
• Chronic/active inflammation is less common, and PMNs, lymphocytes, and plasma cells may be present concurrently, indicating chronic change superimposed with acute inflammation because of persistent antigenic stimulation—contamination in mares with genital abnormalities; semen in mares with DUC.
• Severity of cellular infiltration depends on severity of the insult and length of exposure and infection.
• Inflammation is described by its distribution (focal or diffuse), frequency (moderate or severe), and type of inflammatory cells present (acute, chronic, or chronic/active).
• Inflammatory cells may be in foci, scattered, or diffusely distributed within the stratum compactum (including capillaries and venules) and luminal epithelium.

- Chronic inflammation also may affect the stratum spongiosum—deeper layer.
- Other types of cells occur less frequently—macrophages, siderophages, and eosinophils.
- Macrophages are associated with irritating or poorly absorbed foreign matter.
- Siderophages (i.e., macrophages containing hemoglobin pigment from digestion of blood) indicate a previous foaling, abortion, or hemorrhagic event that may have occurred as long as 2–3 years previously.
- Eosinophils frequently indicate acute irritation caused by pneumovagina and, less commonly, by fungal endometritis.

Fibrosis

- Irreversible
- Widespread distribution, of any degree, correlates with low foaling rates.
- Stromal cells deposit collagen in response to chronic inflammation, aging, and other stimuli.
- Most collagen deposition is periglandular.
- Clusters or branches of glands surrounded by collagen are called nests.
- Periglandular fibrosis exerts pressure within the gland and decreases blood flow to the gland, leading to cystic glandular distention and epithelial atrophy.
- Mares with periglandular fibrosis can usually conceive, but the pregnancy is lost before 90 days because of impaired secretion of "uterine milk." This glandular secretion is critical nutrition for the conceptus.
- Prognosis indirectly correlates with number of collagen layers and frequency of nests per low-power, linear field—more layers indicate poorer prognosis.

Cystic Glandular Distention and Uterine Hypotonia

- When unassociated with fibrosis, may occur from impaired flow of secretions.
- Normal finding during anestrus and transition—seasonal.
- During the breeding season, associated with old, pluriparous mares having pendulous uteri and a history of repeated breeding. In this instance, clusters of cystic glands, unlike fibrotic nests, are not surrounded by collagen.
- Cystic glands may contain inspissated material and show epithelial hypertrophy.
- Cystic glandular distention has been suggested to precede periglandular fibrosis.
- In normal mares, glands are uniformly dilated after recent abortion or pregnancy.

Lymphatic Stasis

- Characterized by dilated, dysfunctional lymphatic vessels.
- Microscopically, dilated lymphatics are differentiated from widespread edema by endothelial cells lining a fluid-filled space.
- Common in mares with a pendulous uterus and DUC.
- Transrectal palpation may reveal a thickened but soft uterus with poor tone during diestrus.
- When widespread, associated with low foaling rates.
- Coalescing lymphatic lacunae may become lymphatic cysts that can be 1–15 cm in diameter.
- These cysts can be identified by ultrasonography, endoscopy, and less frequently, transrectal palpation.

Nonseasonal Glandular Atrophy or Hypoplasia

- Reduced glandular density during the breeding season is abnormal and has been associated with ovarian dysgenesis or secretory tumors—granulosa cell tumor.
- Focal glandular atrophy can develop in old, pluriparous mares.

Diagnostic/Prognostic Categories

Category I:

- Indicates the endometrium is optimal and $\geq$80% of the mares are predicted to conceive and carry the fetus to term.
- Histopathologic changes are slight, focal, and irregularly distributed—scattered.

Category IIA:

- Indicates an expected 50%–80% foaling rate with proper management.
- Chance of conception and pregnancy maintenance are reduced.
- Histopathologic changes are slight to moderate and may be improved with proper treatment.
- Individual or a combination of changes may be present, including slight to moderate, diffuse cellular infiltration of the superficial layers; scattered but frequent inflammatory or fibrotic foci; scattered but frequent periglandular fibrosis of individual branches, with one to three layers of collagen or two or less fibrotic gland nests per low-power field in at least five fields; and widespread lymphatic stasis without palpable uterine changes.

Category IIB:

- Associated with an expected 10%–50% foaling rate with proper management.
- Histopathologic changes are more extensive and severe than in category IIA but still may be reversible.
- Anticipated changes—diffuse, widespread, and moderately severe cellular infiltration of the superficial layers; widespread periglandular fibrosis of individual branches; four or more layers of collagen or two to four fibrotic gland nests per low-power field in five fields; and widespread lymphatic stasis with palpable changes in the uterus, usually detected as decreased uterine tone during diestrus.

Category III:

- Indicates greatly reduced chances of conception and pregnancy maintenance because of difficult-to-treat conditions or severe, irreversible changes in the endometrium.
- Foaling rate, even with optimal management and treatment, is $\leq$10%.
- Histopathologic changes may include widespread, severe cellular infiltration; widespread glandular fibrosis ($\geq$5 fibrotic nests per low-power field); and widespread, severe lymphatic stasis.
- Endometrial hypoplasia with gonadal dysgenesis and pyometra with severe, widespread cellular infiltration and palpable endometrial atrophy also warrant placement in category III.

RISK FACTORS

- Age
- Parity
- Genital anatomical abnormalities—pneumovagina, urovagina, DUC, and infectious endometritis.

ENDOMETRIAL BIOPSY

DIAGNOSIS

DIFFERENTIAL DIAGNOSIS

- History, physical, and behavioral findings play an important role.
- Endometrial glandular distention—seasonal and associated with the atrophy expected during anestrus/transition; nonseasonal (e.g., ovarian dysgenesis attributable to endometrial atrophy, recent abortion or pregnancy, pluriparous mares with DUC, fibrosis).
- Endometrial glandular cysts should be differentiated from endometrial lymphatic cysts by their origin and size. The former is a cystic glandular distention of ≤ 1 mm in diameter.
- Endometrial glandular nesting associated with proestrous edema is a normal, physiologic alteration; contrast with nesting secondary to irreversible, periglandular fibrosis.

CBC/BIOCHEMISTRY/URINALYSIS

N/A

OTHER LABORATORY TESTS

N/A

IMAGING

Ultrasonography—method of choice for evaluating endometrial lymphatic cysts by determining location, number, and size.

DIAGNOSTIC PROCEDURES

BSE

- During routine BSE or with suspected endometritis, samples for culture and cytology should precede biopsy to minimize contamination of the swabs.
- Perform biopsy with an equine endometrial biopsy forceps, preferably when the mare is cycling and, if convenient, during estrus.
- The forceps is carried through the cervix into the uterine body, and a sample is taken from the caudal portion of the horn or at the junction of the horn with the body (i.e., the area of attachment). Unless a gross abnormality has been detected, one sample from the uterine horn base is adequate to represent the entire endometrium; otherwise, collect a representative sample from the endometrium.
- Fix the sample in Bouin's for 4–24 hours, then move it into 70% ethanol or 10% formalin until slides are made.
- Special stains are available.
- If the sample is to be sent to a lab for slide preparation and interpretation, include a complete history, stage of cycle, and palpation findings on the day of examination.

Endoscopy

For diagnosis of intraluminal adhesions and endometrial cysts.

PATHOLOGIC FINDINGS

See interpretations by category.

TREATMENT

EPICRISIS

- Clinical evaluation of the biopsy sample includes interpretation of histopathologic findings in concert with patient history, physical examination findings, bacteriology results, and previous treatments.
- Recommendation about treatment or management and prognosis may be included.

CATEGORY I

Because mares from this group have a normal endometrium, if difficulties with conceiving or carrying a foal to term are encountered and the mare is not infected, direct your attention toward semen quality, estrus detection, and timing of breeding/insemination with respect to ovulation, anatomic, or behavioral abnormalities.

CATEGORY IIa/IIb

- Appropriate therapy may improve the mare's biopsy category.
- Inflammation decreases if the source of irritation is removed or contamination is minimized at the time of breeding.
- Pneumovagina and urovagina can be corrected surgically.
- Treat acute and chronic bacterial and fungal infections with an appropriate local or systemic antibiotic or antifungal drug.
- Treat DUC with uterine lavage and oxytocin.
- Lymphatic circulation is enhanced by administration of cloprostenol (i.e., an analogue of $PGF_{2}\alpha$) 12–24 hours after breeding.
- Fibrosis is irreversible.

CATEGORY III

- These mares often become pregnant but lose the pregnancy between 40–90 days of gestation.
- Associated histopathologic changes are either difficult to correct or irreversible.
- Therapy for inflammation, lymphangiectasia, and minimum contamination at breeding may help.
- Extensive fibrosis decreases the likelihood that a mare's category designation may improve with treatment.
- If a breed registry allows, category III mares may make suitable embryo transfer donors.
- If no improvements in endometrial architecture are possible, eliminate the mare from the breeding program.

MEDICATIONS

DRUGS OF CHOICE
Selected based on culture and sensitivity results.

CONTRAINDICATIONS
N/A

PRECAUTIONS
N/A

POSSIBLE INTERACTIONS
N/A

ALTERNATE DRUGS
N/A

FOLLOW-UP

PATIENT MONITORING
Repeat biopsy of the endometrium ≅2 weeks after the end of treatment is very important to determine effectiveness of therapy.

PREVENTION/AVOIDANCE
N/A

POSSIBLE COMPLICATIONS
- A relatively safe technique
- Possible complications—uterine perforation and excessive hemorrhage (rare).

EXPECTED COURSE AND PROGNOSIS
N/A

MISCELLANEOUS

ASSOCIATED CONDITIONS
N/A

AGE-RELATED FACTORS
- Direct correlation between category and age.
- Category I—comprised primarily by young, maiden mares.
- Category III—comprised by old, pluriparous mares with a high incidence of poor conformation, pneumovagina, urovagina, DUC, and periglandular fibrosis.

ZOONOTIC POTENTIAL
N/A

PREGNANCY
The only contraindication to endometrial biopsy.

SYNONYMS
Uterine biopsy

SEE ALSO
- Endometritis
- Metritis
- Uterine disease

ABBREVIATIONS
- BSE = breeding soundness examination
- DUC = delayed uterine clearance
- EED = early embryonic death
- PMN = polymorphonuclear

Suggested Reading

Doig PA, Waelchli RO. Endometrial biopsy. In: McKinnon AO, Voss JL, eds. Equine reproduction. Malvern: Lea & Febiger, 1993:225–233.

Kenney RM, Doig PA. Equine endometrial biopsy. In: Morrow DA, ed. Current therapy in theriogenology. Philadelphia: WB Saunders, 1986:723–729.

Author Maria E. Cadario
Consulting Editor Carla L. Carleton

ENDOMETRITIS

BASICS

DEFINITION
• Infectious/noninfectious inflammation of the endometrium.
• Major cause of infertility in mares.
• Multifactorial disease classified in four categories—infectious (active, chronic/active) endometritis, PMIE, sexually transmitted disease, and periglandular fibrosis.

PATHOPHYSIOLOGY
Infectious Endometritis
• The uterus is repeatedly exposed to contamination during breeding, parturition, and gynecologic examinations.
• Uterine mechanisms of defense against contamination are a combination of anatomic (physical) barriers, cellular phagocytosis, and physical evacuation of the uterine contents.
• Loss of anatomic integrity of the vulvar seal, vestibular sphincter, and cervix compromises their function and results in aspiration of air (pneumovagina), urine (urine pooling), or fecal material into the cranial vagina.

PMIE
• Increasing parity in old mares and incomplete cervical dilation in maiden mares predisposes to intrauterine fluid accumulation.
• Byproducts of inflammation normally are removed by uterine contractions through the open estrual cervix. When the cervix is closed, fluids within the uterine lumen are cleared by the lymphatics.
• Lymphatic stasis occurs in the endometrium when uterine contractions are abnormal or the uterus is suspended below the pelvic brim.
• Supportive structures of the genital tract stretch with each pregnancy.
Low pregnancy rate:
• *Direct*—interference with embryo survival on its arrival into the uterus
• *Indirect*: by premature luteolysis; inflammation induces release of endometrial prostaglandin.

SYSTEM AFFECTED
Reproductive

GENETICS
N/A

INCIDENCE/PREVALENCE
Frequent

SIGNALMENT
Infectious Endometritis
Predisposition to contamination is caused by an inherent or acquired anatomic defect of the vulva, vestibular sphincter, or cervix.

PMIE
• Pluriparous mares—usually > 14 years, with a pendulous uterus.
• Nulliparous mares—young or old, with incomplete cervical dilation during estrus

SIGNS
Historical Findings
• Infertility
• Accumulation of fluid in the uterus after breeding
• Failure to conceive after repeated breeding to a stallion of known fertility.
• Early embryonic loss
• Hyperemia of the cervix/vagina.
• Vaginal discharge.

Physical Examination Findings
• Can be inconclusive; in this situation, key diagnostic tools are patient history, cytology/culture, and ultrasonography.
• Guarded swab to obtain samples for endometrial cytology and uterine culture.
• Endometrial biopsy is indicated only in specific cases.

Infectious Endometritis
• Abnormal vulval conformation
• Transrectal palpation is not very diagnostic.
• Ultrasonography usually reveals fluid accumulation within the uterus.
• Vaginal and cervical mucosa is hyperemic; discharge may be observed coming through the cervix.
• Endometrial cytology and uterine culture reveals neutrophils (>5 PMNs/hpf) combined with pure bacterial growth—single organism isolated.

PMIE
• External genitalia not always abnormal
• Findings from transrectal palpation, ultrasound, and cytology/culture may be inconclusive in the spring, before the breeding season begins.
• Signs of persistent inflammation usually appear after breeding.
• Mucosa of the cranial vaginal and cervix may be hyperemic.
• Pendulous, edematous uterus
• Postbreeding ultrasonography reveals intrauterine fluid accumulation that persists for 12–24 + hours without treatment.
• Endometrial cytology reveals significant inflammation (>5 PMNs/hpf).
• Bacterial cultures—usually negative

CAUSES
See *Pathophysiology.*

RISK FACTORS
• Age of > 14 years
• Parity—multiparous and > 14 years old; nulliparous.
• Abnormal vulvar conformation.
• Excessive breeding during one or consecutive estrous periods.
• Pendulous suspension of uterus.
• Cervix that fails to relax during estrus.

DIAGNOSIS

DIFFERENTIAL DIAGNOSIS
For Vaginal Discharge:
• Pneumovagina—air irritates the mucosa, and a foamy-appearing exudate accumulates on the vaginal floor.
• Treatment-induced vaginitis and/or necrosis—may result from antiseptics used for uterine lavage; individual mares can respond quite differently to a similar treatment.
• Bacterial vaginitis secondary to pneumovagina.

ENDOMETRITIS

• Necrotizing vaginitis—secondary to excessive manipulation and inadequate lubrication during dystocias or contamination during delivery of a dead, necrotic fetus.
• Urine pooling—usually affects a population of mares similar to that affected by endometritis; presence of urine can be diagnosed during estrus with a vaginal speculum.
• Varicosities in the region of the vaginovestibular sphincter frequently are observed. These may rupture and bleed during late pregnancy or breeding. Diagnosis is established based on speculum examination of that region.
• Lochia—normal postpartum occurrence up to 5–6 days.
• Postpartum metritis.
• Pyometra
• Vaginal discharge during pregnancy may be a sign of placentitis.
• Purulent cervical discharge is associated with ascending, infectious placentitis.
• Serosanguinous discharge, with a negative bacterial swab, indicates premature placental separation.
• Premature mammary development may be present.

CBC/BIOCHEMISTRY/URINALYSIS

N/A

OTHER LABORATORY TESTS

Microbiology

Aerobes:
• *Streptococcus zooepidemicus* and *Escherichia coli* are the most common isolates.
• *E. coli*, a fecal contaminant, results from poor vulvar conformation.
• *Pseudomonas aeruginosa* and *Klebsiella pneumoniae* usually have a venereal transmission, but overgrowth may occur secondary to excessive use of intrauterine antibiotics.
• Other bacteria—*Staphylococcus, Corynebacterium, Enterobacter, Proteus,* and *Pasteurella* sp.
Anaerobes
• *Bacteroides fragilis*
• May be recovered in some cases of postpartum metritis.
Yeasts:
• *Candida sp.*
• Usually follow excessive antibiotic treatment of the uterus.
• Use slides prepared for cytology and blood agar plate to look for *Candida* and *Aspergillus* sp.

Cytology

• Sample of the endometrial cells and intraluminal content, collected by scraping the endometrial surface with the swab tip or cap (if using a Kalayjian® culture swab), gently rolling the sample onto a slide and staining with Diff Quick®.
• Neutrophils indicate active inflammation. Recent breeding or gynecologic examination results in a transient, positive cytology.
• Persistent, positive cytology without bacterial growth suggests a recurrent, noninfectious cause—pneumovagina, urine pooling, or early stages of DUC.
• Positive culture with positive cytology is diagnostic of uterine infection.
• Positive culture with negative cytology usually indicates contamination during uterine sampling.

IMAGING

Ultrasonography:
• Normal mares retain small amounts of fluid up to 12 hours after breeding.
• Mares with DUC sometimes have fluid before breeding and always retain fluid for 12–24 hours after breeding.

OTHER DIAGNOSTIC PROCEDURES

Endometrial Biopsy

• Determine the presence or absence of endometritis when clinical and bacteriologic findings are inconclusive.
• Inflammatory cells are diagnostic, if neutrophils are present, of active endometritis.
• Low numbers of lymphocytes and plasma cells (indicative of chronic endometritis) are not always associated with infertility.
• Periglandular fibrosis is associated with early abortions—gestational age, 70–90 days
• Lymphatic stasis is common in mares with a pendulous uterus and DUC.

Endoscopy

When other treatment modalities fail to define a cause for infertility—intrauterine adhesions affecting uterine drainage or uterine abscess (rare) that may not be palpable or visible at ultrasonography.

PATHOLOGIC FINDINGS

Endometritis

• Cannot predict a mare's endometrial biopsy category, which may range from IIa to III (rarely).
• Category relates to the length of sexual rest, conformational abnormalities, and age.
• Histopathology associated with endometritis—mild, diffuse lymphocytic or neutrophilic infiltration; focally moderate fibrosis (1–4 nests); lymphangiectasia.

PMIE

• Biopsy score at beginning of the breeding season is not diagnostic.
• Category may be IIa or IIb, with mild inflammation and moderate fibrosis.
• After breeding, interstitial edema, lymphatic stasis, and diffuse, acute or subacute inflammation (PMN) usually develops.
• Serial sampling may be useful.

TREATMENT

APPROPRIATE HEALTH CARE

To minimize contamination during breeding:
• Limit to one breeding per estrus.
• Breed as close to ovulation as possible.
• Infuse semen extender (100–300 mL) with antibiotics (the concentration of which is compatible with sperm viability); into the uterus before natural breeding—minimum contamination technique.

NURSING CARE

N/A

ACTIVITY

N/A

DIET

N/A

CLIENT EDUCATION

N/A

ENDOMETRITIS

SURGICAL CONSIDERATIONS

- Consider feasibility of surgical correction of predisposing causes before treating a uterine infection—Caslick's vulvoplasty for pneumovagina; urethral extension for urine pooling; repair of cervical tear.
- Rectovaginal fistulas (foaling trauma)—may be prudent to wait for endometrial biopsy results before expensive surgery if the broodmare has been barren for >1 year; chronic endometritis may have seriously diminished the mare's biopsy category in the interim.

MEDICATIONS

DRUGS OF CHOICE

General Principles

- Administer treatments during estrus, when the cervix is open; however, this issue remains a topic of some controversy.
- Organism is eliminated chemically (antibiotics, antiseptics) or mechanically (uterine lavage, ecbolic drugs).
- Local placement of antibiotics is preferred to systemic treatment, because higher concentrations are achieved in the endometrium.
- Cost of systemic treatment is higher than that of local administration.
- Most uterine infections in mares are luminal/endometrial.
- Systemic treatment is optional when access to the mare is limited (e.g., unsafe or unsanitary conditions) or when attempting to avoid further uterine contamination.
- Uterine lavage is the treatment of choice for mares with impaired uterine clearance and to evacuate debris from the uterus before antibiotic instillation. It also enhances local uterine defenses by local irritation and stimulating PMN migration to the lumen.

Endometritis

- Active endometritis—uterine lavage and oxytocin (daily or alternate day), followed by intrauterine infusion of chosen antibiotic.
- Chronic inflammation—do not breed mare until 45–60 days after treatment.
- Chronic active endometritis—surgical correction of defective anatomic barriers before intrauterine treatment; uterine lavage and oxytocin if intrauterine fluid is present.
- Uterine lavage with diluted antiseptics if no bacteria have been identified; consider postbreeding treatment.
- Yeast infection—uterine lavage and oxytocin, followed by intrauterine infusion with antifungal drugs (Nystatin, Clotrimazole); alternatively, uterine lavage with diluted 1% povidone-iodine solution (to the approximate color of light iced tea) or acetic acid (vinegar).

PMIE

Lavage and ecbolic drugs (oxytocin):

- 4–8 hours after breeding promote uterine clearance; this time ensures sperm are in the oviduct and bacteria have not yet adhered and multiplied.
- Oxytocin immediately after lavage stimulates strong uterine contractions and clears the remaining uterine contents.

$PGF_2\alpha$ and analogues (Cloprostenol):

- Sustain smoother uterine contractions longer than oxytocin (5 hours vs. 40 minutes).
- Successful in reducing persistent uterine edema by stimulating lymphatic drainage.
- Treat after each mating.

Ultrasonography:

- 4–8 hours after insemination or breeding (not ovulation), check for uterine fluid—if a diameter $\geq$3–4 cm is free fluid, lavage with 1–3 L sterile saline or lactated Ringer's solution and administer oxytocin immediately after lavage; with only a small amount of free fluid, administer oxytocin only.
- 12 hours after breeding—administer Cloprostenol if history includes dilated uterine lymphatics and poor drainage.
- 24 hours after breeding—if mare has not ovulated but has fluid, use lavage or oxytocin; if mare has ovulated but has fluid and persistent edema in the walls, lavage the uterus and administer Cloprostenol.
- 48 hours after breeding—if mare has not ovulated, she will need to be rebred; sequence begins anew.

Drugs and Fluids

Antibiotics:

- Amikacin (0.5–2 g)—Gram-negative; *Pseudomonas* and *Klebsiella* sp.
- Ampicillin (1–3 g)—Gram-positive; streptococci.
- Carbenicillin (2–6 g)—broad spectrum; persistent *Pseudomonas* sp.
- Gentamicin (0.5–2 g)—Gram-negative.
- Neomycin (3–4 g)—*E. coli* and *Klebsiella* sp.
- K-penicillin (5×10^6 U)—Gram-positive; streptococci.
- Ticarcillin (3–6 g)—broad spectrum.
- Aminoglycosides must be buffered before infusion. Mix the antibiotic with an equal volume of sodium bicarbonate (1 mL at 7.5% for every 50 mg of gentamicin or amikacin), then dilute in sterile saline.

Systemic Antibiotics:

- K-penicillin
- Procaine penicillin G
- Gentamicin
- Amikacin
- Ampicillin
- Trimethoprim-sulfamethoxazole

Antimycotics:

- Nystatin (500,000 U)—*Candida* sp.
- Clotrimazole (700 mg)—*Candida* sp.
- Amphotericin B (200 mg)—*Aspergillus, Candida* and *Mucor* sp.; tablets must be crushed and well suspended in 60–120 mL of sterile saline.

Uterotonics/Ecbolics:

- Oxytocin (10 IU IV or 20 IU IM)
- Cloprostenol (250–500 μg IM)—prostaglandin of choice because of its effectiveness and fewer adverse effects.

CONTRAINDICATIONS

Avoid administration of prostaglandin or its analogues at $\geq$72 hours after ovulation, because it could affect the CL.

PRECAUTIONS

Adverse reactions may occur when using natural or synthetic prostaglandin—transient sweating, ataxia, and increased GI motility.

POSSIBLE INTERACTIONS
N/A

ALTERNATIVE DRUGS
N/A

FOLLOW-UP

PATIENT MONITORING
• Complete gynecologic evaluation with special attention to uterine culture/cytology on first or second day of estrus after treatment.
• If no conception after several attempts, repeat the complete evaluation 45–60 days after treatment.

PREVENTION AVOIDANCE
N/A

POSSIBLE COMPLICATIONS
• Secondary bacterial/yeast overgrowth caused by excessive use of antibiotics.
• Uterine adhesions.
• Pyometra

EXPECTED COURSE AND PROGNOSIS
N/A

MISCELLANEOUS

ASSOCIATED CONDITIONS
N/A

AGE-RELATED FACTORS
See *Risk Factors.*

ZOONOTIC POTENTIAL
N/A

PREGNANCY
N/A

SYNONYMS
N/A

SEE ALSO
• Cervical lesions
• Endometrial biopsy
• Parturition
• Postpartum metritis
• Pyometra
• Urine pooling
• Venereal diseases

ABBREVIATIONS
• CL = corpus luteum
• DUC = delayed uterine clearance
• GI = gastrointestinal
• hpf = high-powered field (microscopy)
• PMIE = persistent mating-induced endometritis
• PMN = polymorphonuclear (white) cell

Suggested Reading

Asbury AC, Lyle SK. Infectious causes of infertility. In: McKinnon AO, Voss JL, eds. Equine reproduction. Philadelphia: Lea and Febiger, 1993:381–391.

Blanchard TL, Varner DD, Schumacher J. Uterine defense mechanisms in the mare. In: Manual of Equine Reproduction. St. Louis: Mosby, 1998:47–58.

LeBlanc MM. Breakdown in uterine defense mechanisms in the mare. Is a delay in physical clearance the culprit? Proc Soc Theriogenol 1994:121–129.

Author Maria E. Cadario
Consulting Editor Carla L. Carleton

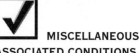

ENDOTOXEMIA

BASICS

DEFINITION

Endotoxemia is the presence of endotoxin in the blood and the sequential systemic effects that are elicited. Endotoxin (lipopolysaccharide, LPS) is a heat-stable toxin associated with the lipid portion of the outer cell membranes of certain gram-negative bacteria. Endotoxemia occurs when either gram-negative bacteria or the LPS gain access to the systemic circulation.

PATHOPHYSIOLOGY

Endotoxin is not secreted, it is only released with gram-negative bacterial cell wall disruption by rapid multiplication or bacteriolysis. It is composed of complex LPS molecules, with the phospholipid moiety (lipid A, hydrophobic) as the source of the toxicity, while the hydrophilic O-specific chain is responsible for most of the antigenic properties of the LPS.

Endotoxemia occurs through a series of events. First, LPS is absorbed systemically from gram-negative bacterial invasion (severe localized or disseminated infection) or as free LPS through damaged epithelial surfaces. The gastrointestinal tract normally contains a relatively large quantity of LPS but the mucosa must be compromised by inflammation or ischemia for it to gain access to the systemic circulation. Any gastrointestinal disorder that leads to severe mucosal inflammation and necrosis (*Salmonella* or *Clostridium* infection, strangulating and non-strangulating obstructions, toxin ingestion such as NSAIDS, heavy metals, oak, cantharidin) can result in LPS absorption. Once into the systemic circulation, the LPS complexes with plasma constituents and then directly or indirectly induces a severe inflammatory response. LPS is a potent stimulus of the host inflammation, leading to activation of defense mechanisms that initiate a series of overzealous inflammatory processes that cause the clinical manifestations seen in endotoxemia. Clinical manifestations include fever, tachycardia, hypotension, coagulopathy, vascular damage, perfusion defects leading to vital organ damage and ultimately multiple organ system failure, and death.

SYSTEMS AFFECTED

Cardiovascular

- Reduced myocardial contractility.
- Differential vasoconstriction and vasodilation in capillary beds.
- Vascular endothelial damage resulting in permeability changes, fluid leakage, and DIC.
- Compensatory responses involve increased heart rate and contractility and peripheral vasoconstriction in attempts to raise systemic blood pressure.

Gastrointestinal

Impaired mucosal perfusion may cause mucosal sloughing, allowing bacterial translocation and further LPS absorption.

Hepatobiliary

Hepatic ischemia may cause hepatocellular enzyme increases and alter hepatic function, including impaired removal of bacteria from the portal circulation.

Renal

Acute renal failure may result from reduced renal blood flow and ischemic tubular damage.

Respiratory

Pulmonary edema and pulmonary thromboembolisms may occur.

SIGNALMENT

N/A

SIGNS

Early

- Pyrexia
- Depression
- Tachycardia
- Normal or high arterial blood pressure
- Pale mucous membranes (vasoconstriction)
- Rapid capillary refill time
- Tachypnea, and/or labored respiration

Late

- Tachycardia or bradycardia
- Poor peripheral pulses
- Dark ("toxic") mucous membranes
- Prolonged capillary refill time
- Cool extremities
- Hypothermia
- Peripheral edema
- Abdominal pain
- Diarrhea
- Ileus
- Laminitis
- Abortion
- Petechial and ecchymotic hemorrhages
- Death

Neonates

Neonates can show all of the above plus decreased suckling and weakness.

ENDOTOXEMIA

CAUSES

GI Disorders

Within the gastrointestinal tract LPS normally gains access to the blood through compromised mucosa that may also allow translocation of gram-negative bacteria.

Neonatal Septicemia

• Gram-negative bacteria proliferate in the tissues and gain access to the blood.
• Localized or disseminated infectious focus causing gram-negative bacteremia or release of LPS into the circulation.

RISK FACTORS

The equine is particularly susceptible to gram-negative sepsis secondary to gastrointestinal disease, metritis, pneumonia and pleuro-pneumonia, and neonatal septicemia. Failure of passive transfer and high-risk pregnancies increase the risk of development of neonatal septicemia.

DIAGNOSIS

The diagnosis of endotoxemia is usually made based on the presence of the above mentioned clinical signs in combination with laboratory findings.

DIFFERENTIAL DIAGNOSIS

• Hypovolemic shock
• Cardiogenic shock

CBC/BIOCHEMISTRY/URINALYSIS

• Initially there is a neutropenia due to vascular margination (may be $<1000/\mu L$; 10^9 cells/L). This is followed by a neutrophilic leukocytosis with a left shift, due to induction of myeloid proliferation in the bone marrow. Toxic changes are usually present in the neutrophils.
• Hemoconcentration (increased PCV and total plasma protein)
• Hyperproteinemia initially due to hemoconcentration, but may decrease significantly with gastrointestinal losses
• High hepatocellular enzymes and bilirubin due to ischemic hepatic injury
• Azotemia may be due to renal or pre-renal azotemia associated with blood volume depletion
• Initial hyperglycemia followed by hypoglycemia.

OTHER LABORATORY TESTS

Coagulation Profile

• Prolongation of the APTT and PTT
• Increased FDPs
• Thrombocytopenia
• Decreased plasma fibrinogen
• Decreased AT-III

Blood Gas Analysis

• Hypoxemia
• Acid–base disturbances; metabolic acidosis due to decreased peripheral perfusion and hypoxemia leading to anaerobic metabolism and lactate production

IMAGING

N/A

DIAGNOSTIC PROCEDURES

Aerobic and anaerobic blood cultures

TREATMENT

Treatment should be initiated quickly and should be aimed at stabilization with aggressive symptomatic therapy, resolving the source of the gram-negative sepsis, controlling the inflammatory response, and providing supportive care while establishing tissue perfusion. If the source of sepsis can be identified, it should be addressed. This may involve surgery for intestinal compromise, peritoneal or pleural drainage, etc.

MEDICATIONS

DRUG(S) OF CHOICE

• Fluid therapy: restoration of the circulating blood volume is the most important factor in restoring peripheral perfusion.
• Balanced electrolyte solutions such as lactated Ringer's solution or 0.9% sodium chloride; in septic foals dextrose should be added to the fluid therapy.
• Rates of 10–20 mL/kg/hr to severely compromised horses.
• Use caution not to over-hydrate and cause pulmonary edema because micro-vascular alterations may be present. Foals and adults with low plasma protein levels are particularly susceptible to edema formation.

ENDOTOXEMIA

• Colloidal solutions (whole blood, plasma, hetastarch, dextrans) can be used to maintain the fluid in the vascular space.
• Colloids should be initiated when plasma proteins are <4 g/dL, 40g/L.
• Colloids should be from a commercial source or from appropriate donors (Aa and Qa isoantibody negative).
• 7.5% hypertonic saline solution for rapid volume expansion 4 mL/kg.
• Sodium bicarbonate to treat severe metabolic acidosis that does not correct with volume expansion.
• Adult: 0.5 mEq × body weight (kg) × (base deficit); give half the dose slowly intravenously over 20 min. Give the rest of the dose in crystalloid fluids over 4 hr.
• Foals: 0.7 mEq × body weight (kg) × (base deficit); then follow the same regimen as above.
• Inotropic agents can be given to increase systemic blood pressure when it drops <60 mmHg.
• Dopamine hydrochloride: 1–5 μg/kg/min by continuous IV administration.
• Dobutamine: 2–5 μg/kg/min by continuous IV administration.
• Oxygen therapy if hypoxia and respiratory distress are present.

Antimicrobials should be initiated soon after samples for culture have been obtained. Initially, broad-spectrum antimicrobials should be selected pending the results of the culture and susceptibility. Commonly used drugs include aminoglycosides, third-generation cephalosporins, potentiated sulfonamides, and expanded-spectrum penicillins. Variable pharmacokinetics of aminoglycosides in ill animals necessitate the use of therapeutic monitoring.

Corticosteroids

Controversy exists regarding the use of steroids in this condition, but they are recommended because they mediate multiple anti-inflammatory effects, including decreasing TNF synthesis, decreasing the production of arachidonic acid-derived eicosanoids, stabilizing lysosomal membranes, and decreasing vascular permeability, therefore protecting against some of the effects of endotoxin.

NSAIDs

NSAIDs (flunixin meglumine, ketoprofen, pheylbutazone, aspirin) are used for attenuation of the inflammatory cascade by inhibiting cyclooxygenase.
• Flunixin meglumine appears to have the most potent anti-endotoxic effects.
• 1.1 mg/kg q8–12 hr or 0.25 mg/kg q6–8 hr.
• Aspirin also prevents thrombus formation.
• NSAIDs inhibit vasodilator prostaglandins; therefore, care must be taken with regard to renal damage.

Immunotherapy (Hyperimmune Antisera or Plamsa)

• O-chain specific antisera works well, but due to the antigenic diversity between gram-negative bacteria in this region, it is not clinically useful.
• Different gram-negative bacteria share common core antigens; therefore, antibodies are aimed at the LPS core. These antibodies may promote opsonization and reticuloendothelial clearance and inhibit the interactions of LPS.
• J5 hyperimmune plasma 4.4 mL/kg.

CONTRAINDICATIONS

Glucocorticoids may be contraindicated in horse with severe bacterial infection or exhibiting signs of laminitis. They have only been shown to be effective when given prophylactically or very early in the course of sepsis. They cause profound immunosuppression and can induce laminitis.

PRECAUTIONS

NSAID toxicity may result in GI ulceration and renal ischemia; therefore, careful patient monitoring is required along with ensuring adequate hydration of the patient and using the lowest effective dose possible.

POSSIBLE INTERACTIONS

Sodium bicarbonate and dopamine cannot be administered in the same intravenous line.

ALTERNATIVE DRUGS

• Pentoxyphylline
• Polymyxin B
• DMSO

ENDOTOXEMIA

FOLLOW-UP

PATIENT MONITORING

Vital parameters should be closely monitored during aggressive fluid therapy (HR, pulse intensity, mucous membrane color, RR, lung sounds, urine output, mentation, rectal temperature) blood gas analysis and pulse oximetry to measure oxygenation and acid–base balance, PCV, serum total protein, serum electrolytes, hepatocellular enzymes, BUN, and serum creatinine should be monitored.

POSSIBLE COMPLICATIONS

- Laminitis
- Electrolyte and acid–base disturbances
- Pulmonary edema
- Pulmonary thromboembolism
- DIC
- Renal dysfunction
- Hepatic dysfunction
- GI ischemia and bacterial translocation
- Vasculitis and peripheral edema
- Cardiac arrest

MISCELLANEOUS

ASSOCIATED CONDITIONS

N/A

AGE-RELATED FACTORS

N/A

ZOONOTIC POTENTIAL

N/A

PREGNANCY

N/A

SYNONYMS

- Endotoxic shock
- Gram-negative sepsis

SEE ALSO

- DIC
- Hypoxemia
- Bacteremia
- Septicemia

ABBREVIATIONS

- APTT= activated partial thromboplastin time
- AT-III = antithrombin III
- BUN = blood urea nitrogen
- DIC = disseminated intravascular coagulation
- DMSO = dimethyl sulfoxide
- FDP = fibrinogen degradation products
- LPS = lipopolysaccharide
- LRS = lactated Ringers solution
- PCV = packed cell volume
- PTT = prothrombin time
- TNF = tumor necrosis factor

Suggested Reading

Kuesis B, Spier SJ. Endotoxemia. In: Reed SM, Bayly WM, eds. Equine internal medicine. Philadelphia: WB Saunders, 1998;639-651.

Morris DD. Endotoxemia in horses. J Vet Intern Med 1991;5:167-176.

Author Deborah A. Parsons

Consulting Editor Henry Stämpfli

ENTEROLITHIASIS

BASICS

DEFINITION

Calculi composed of struvite (magnesium ammonium phosphate hexahydrate) form in the ampulla of the right dorsal colon and subsequently cause partial or complete obstruction of the right dorsal, transverse, or descending colon.

PATHOPHYSIOLOGY

Enteroliths form and enlarge over a period of 1 or more years by deposition of concentric rings of struvite around a central nidus, which is usually a flint-like pebble (silicon dioxide), a piece of metal, or less commonly, fibrous material, such as nylon baling twine, rubber fencing, or hair. Enterolith formation appears to be facilitated by the relative hypomotility of the right dorsal colon, a pH of colonic contents that is more alkaline than normal, and a high dietary intake of magnesium and protein (typical of alfalfa-rich diets) or, in some cases, phosphorus (typical of diets rich in wheat bran and low in forage). The valve-like effect of the enlarging enterolith at the junction of the right dorsal and transverse colon may intermittently cause partial colonic obstruction and colic. Complete colonic obstruction and persistent colic occur when large enteroliths lodge in the narrower distal portion of the right dorsal colon, or when enteroliths migrate aborally and become lodged in the smaller diameter transverse or descending colon. Pressure from the lodged enterolith may cause necrosis and rupture of the bowel wall, or the colon may rupture secondary to distension by gas and fluid that accumulate proximal to the obstructing enterolith.

SYSTEM AFFECTED

The gastrointestinal system is the only system affected.

GENETICS

There is no known genetic basis for this disease, although breed predilections do exist (see later in this article).

INCIDENCE/PREVALENCE

Enterolithiasis has a worldwide distribution, but is much more common in certain geographic areas, particularly parts of California and Florida. In California, there has been a progressive marked increase in incidence since the early 1970s, to the extent that enterolithiasis is now one of the leading causes of colic requiring surgical correction. At the University of California, enteroliths were responsible for 15% of patients admitted for treatment of colic and almost 30% of patients undergoing celiotomy for treatment of colic between 1973 and 1996.

SIGNALMENT

Enteroliths occur in all breeds, but Arabian and Arabian crosses, Morgans, American Saddlebreds, and donkeys appear to be over-represented. In endemic areas, Thoroughbreds, Standardbreds, and warmblooded horses are underrepresented, likely because they are predominantly younger horses in active training being fed higher levels of grain. There is no apparent sex predilection, although stallions are underrepresented. Middle-age adult horses >2 years of age are at greatest risk in endemic areas. The mean age for affected horses in a recent retrospective study was approximately 11.5 yr and the age range was 1–36 yr.

SIGNS

Historical Findings

Historical feeding of a diet containing >50% alfalfa is common to almost all cases. In about one-third of cases, recurrent colic of mild to moderate severity over a period of a few weeks to as long as a year is observed. Some horses develop severe colic signs acutely without any history of recurrent colic signs. Passage of small enteroliths in the feces is a feature of the history of about 15% of affected horses. Other horses show more nonspecific signs, such as attitude changes, intermittent anorexia, lethargy, weight loss, intermittent loose manure, resentment of tightening the girth, reluctance to exercise, or reluctance to travel down hills before signs of colic appear.

Physical Examination Findings

Typical signs reflect mild to moderate abdominal discomfort and include pawing, looking at the flank, rolling, repeatedly lying down and getting up, sweating, and kicking at the abdomen. Other signs include tachycardia, anorexia, depression, intestinal hypomotility, lack of progressive peristalsis, abdominal distension, "dog-sitting" posture, prolonged capillary refill time, and tachypnea. Horses with multiple small, non-obstructing enteroliths may have progressive borborygmi resulting in a characteristic gravelly sound heard on auscultation of the colon. Signs reflecting endotoxemia may develop, particularly when the integrity of the bowel wall is compromised.

CAUSES

Enteroliths are caused by the deposition of concentric rings of struvite around a central nidus, which is usually a flintlike pebble (silicon dioxide), a piece of metal, or less commonly, fibrous material, such as nylon baling twine, rubber fencing, or hair. Enterolith formation appears to be facilitated by the relative hypomotility of the right dorsal colon, a pH of colonic contents that is more alkaline than normal, and a high dietary intake of magnesium and protein (typical of alfalfa-rich diets) or, in some cases, phosphorus (typical of diets rich in wheat bran and low in forage).

RISK FACTORS

Proved risk factors include residing in an endemic area, feeding alfalfa as the predominant or sole forage, and lack of pasture grazing. In addition, consumption of hard water, residing predominantly in a stall or paddock, limited exercise, and feeding of diets low in grain may increase risk. The high magnesium content (3–6 times the daily requirement) and high protein content of alfalfa appears to provide magnesium and nitrogen for formation of struvite as well as promoting a high colonic buffering capacity and the alkaline colonic pH necessary for precipitation of struvite. Historically, feeding of diets high in wheat bran and low in grass-based forages contributed to a problem with enterolith formation in miller's horses.

DIAGNOSIS

DIFFERENTIAL DIAGNOSIS

All other causes of colic (see relevant section), but particularly those that cause chronic or recurrent colic, including sand colic, thromboembolic colic, internal abdominal abscess, gastric ulcer, peritonitis, abdominal neoplasia, cholelithiasis, and nephrolithiasis.

CBC/BIOCHEMISTRY/URINALYSIS

Changes are non-specific for enterolithiasis. Increased hematocrit and hyperproteinemia are common secondary changes reflecting hemoconcentration and/or stress-associated splenic contraction.

OTHER LABORATORY TESTS

In uncomplicated cases, peritoneal fluid is usually of normal to increased volume, has a normal appearance, and has laboratory parameters within normal limits. Secondary bowel wall compromise leads to amber discoloration, increased turbidity, increased protein concentration, and increased cell count.

IMAGING

Abdominal radiography, preferably after fasting for 24 hr or more, is useful diagnostically in many but not all horses. The technique is most successful in smaller horses, and is more sensitive for detecting enteroliths in large colon than enteroliths that have migrated to the small colon. Enteroliths are recognized by their spherical or tetrahedral shape, homogeneously increased density, sharp borders silhouetted against gas caps in the intestinal lumen, or the presence of a metallic nidus. Equivocal radiographic findings can often be resolved by one or more repeat examinations performed after continued fasting if permitted by the clinical condition of the patient. Abdominal ultrasound is of limited utility, except to help rule out other conditions.

DIAGNOSTIC PROCEDURES

Rectal examination frequently reveals distension of the large colon and, less often, tight mesenteric bands. Enteroliths are palpable on rectal examination in about 5% of cases. Placing the horse on a ramp to elevate the front end facilitates palpation of enteroliths.

PATHOLOGIC FINDINGS

N/A

TREATMENT

Surgical intervention is the only treatment documented to be effective for formed enteroliths and is best performed via ventral celiotomy within a few hours of the onset of signs or, preferably, before signs of complete colonic obstruction are present. The preferred approach is to evacuate the colon via an enterotomy created at the pelvic flexure, after which the enterolith is gently manipulated to this site or to a second enterotomy site for removal.

APPROPRIATE HEALTH CARE

Initial evaluation and treatment of horses with enterolithiasis is handled appropriately on an outpatient basis. Horses that do not have a complete colonic obstruction frequently respond favorably to medical approaches commonly used to treat colic (i.e., withholding feed; administration of flunixin meglumine or similar NSAID; passage of a nasogastric tube; administration of fluids, laxatives, or lubricants such as mineral oil by nasogastric tube; or IV administration of polyionic fluids). Transportation to a referral center is usually necessary for radiographic confirmation of the diagnosis and surgical management.

NURSING CARE

Prevention of rolling and self-induced trauma, provision of analgesia, maintenance of an indwelling nasogastic tube and fluid therapy is indicated before referral and during transportation. Intravenous fluid therapy is often indicated before, during, and after surgery.

ENTEROLITHIASIS

ACTIVITY

As with any horse undergoing ventral celiotomy, stall rest with hand-walking is recommended for the first 4 weeks post-surgery, and the horse should not be returned to work or used for breeding for at least 6 mo.

DIET

Feed should be withheld before and immediately after surgery. Feeding of small amounts is re-introduced 24 hr after surgery and increased to full intake over the next 7 days, unless precluded by complications such as ileus or enteritis. Alfalfa should be eliminated from the diet of horses that have had enteroliths removed surgically.

CLIENT EDUCATION

Restriction of exercise in the immediate post-operative period. High likelihood of recurrence unless diet and management are not changed (see Risk Factors).

SURGICAL CONSIDERATION

If the patient shows evidence of complete colonic obstruction or has a large, non-obstructing enterolith in the large colon, surgical removal of the enterolith is the only effective treatment.

MEDICATIONS

DRUG(S) OF CHOICE

See section entitled Appropriate Health Care.

CONTRAINDICATIONS

The use of neostigmine, bethanocol, or other potent prokinetics is contraindicated. Acepromazine is contraindicated in affected horses showing evidence of shock.

PRECAUTIONS

Repeated use of potent analgesics such as flunixin meglumine or ketoprofen to control colic pain should be avoided unless appropriate diagnostic and therapeutic intervention is also pursued.

POSSIBLE INTERACTIONS

N/A

ALTERNATIVE DRUGS

N/A

FOLLOW-UP

PATIENT MONITORING

Observation for signs of colic or inappetance. Follow-up annual abdominal radiographs may be helpful in detecting recurrence.

PREVENTION/AVOIDANCE

Replace alfalfa hay in the diet with good-quality grass or oat hay. Alfalfa should make up <50%, and preferably 0%, of the diet. Supplement hay with 8 fl oz (250 mL/450 kg) of apple cider vinegar daily to help acidify colonic contents and/or mixed grain. Provide regular exercise. Eliminate hard drinking water if possible. Minimize ingestion of nidi, such as pebbles and metallic objects, by not feeding horses on the ground and by carefully screening their feed and manger for foreign material. Intermittent administration of psyllium at a dose of 16 oz (0.5 kg) orally once daily for the first 5 consecutive days of each month may help remove sand and other nidi from the large colon. Serious colic resulting from acute colonic obstruction can be avoided if large enteroliths recognized by radiographic examination or rectal examination are removed with elective surgery while horses are asymptomatic.

POSSIBLE COMPLICATIONS

Postoperative complications are uncommon. Apart from post-operative complications encountered after colic surgery (diarrhea, incisional infection, incisional hernia, laminitis, septic peritonitis, adhesions, impaction at the enterotomy site), the major complication is recurrence of enteroliths if dietary modification is not instituted.

EXPECTED COURSE AND PROGNOSIS

Horses with small enteroliths in their large colon likely remain asymptomatic for months or years and often pass the enteroliths in their manure. Prognosis for horses with small non-obstructing enteroliths is good, provided appropriate dietary modification is initiated. Prognosis for horses with large non-obstructing enteroliths in the large colon is guarded without surgical removal because there is a high likelihood that these will eventually pass aborally and cause a complete colonic obstruction. Prognosis for recovery for horses with a complete colonic obstruction detected before bowel compromise has occurred is good following surgical removal of the stone. Complete recovery can be anticipated in >90% of cases in which surgery is performed before the bowel ruptures. Without surgery, the prognosis for horses with obstructing enteroliths is virtually hopeless.

MISCELLANEOUS

ASSOCIATED CONDITIONS

Colonic rupture, colonic displacement, septic peritonitis, endotoxemia, and the post-operative complications listed previously have been recognized in association with enterolithiasis.

AGE-RELATED FACTORS

Enterolithiasis is rarely a clinical problem in horses younger than 2 yr of age. Peak incidence is in horses between 5 and 15 yr of age.

ZOONOTIC POTENTIAL

N/A

PREGNANCY

Pregnant mares are likely at increased risk for abortion, as is the case for other causes of colic requiring surgery. Prophylactic use of NSAIDs (flunixin meglumine) and progestagens such as altrenogest are indicated in pregnant mares.

SYNONYMS

- Intestinal stones
- Intestinal calculi
- Intestinal bezoars
- Stones
- Rocks

SEE ALSO

Colic

ABBREVIATIONS

N/A

Suggested Reading

Hassel, DM, Langer DL, Snyder JR, Drake CM, Goodell ML, Wyle A. Evaluation of enterolithiasis in horses: 900 cases (1973–1996). J Am Vet Med Assoc. 1999. In press.

Lloyd K, Hintz HF, Wheat JD, Schryver HF. Enteroliths in horses. Cornell Vet 1987;77:172-186.

Murray RC, Constantinescu GM, Green EM. Equine enteroliths. Compend Contin Educ Pract Vet 1992;14:1104-1113.

Hintz HF, Lowe JE, Livesay-Wilkins P, et al. Studies on equine enterolithiasis. Proc AAEP 1988;24:53-59.

Blue MG, Wittkopp RW. Clinical and structural features of equine enteroliths. J Am Vet Med Assoc 1988;179:79-82.

Author W. David Wilson and Diana M. Hassel

Consulting Editor Henry Stämpfli

EOSINOPHILIA AND BASOPHILIA

BASICS

DEFINITION

Eosinophilia is present when circulating eosinophils exceed the upper limit of the reference interval. Likewise, basophilia is defined as circulating basophils in excess of the upper limit of the reference interval. Because regional variability in peripheral eosinophil and basophil numbers is possible, readers are cautioned to use the reference interval provided by your laboratory.

Pathophysiology

Eosinophilia accompanies parasitic and allergic diseases commonly involving organs with high concentrations of mast cells (e.g., gastrointestinal tract, skin, lungs). However, eosinophilic tissue infiltration is not always accompanied by eosinophilia. Mechanisms for eosinophilia include increased production and/or release from the bone marrow, chemoattraction to specific organs, redistribution from the marginal pool, or increased intravascular survival. Movement of eosinophils into tissue is initiated by histamine release from tissue mast cells, antigen-antibody complex formation, activated complement proteins, and other inflammatory mediators. Eosinophilia occurs with parasitic disease if sensitivity to parasite-derived proteins has developed. Although helpful in controlling parasitic infections, eosinophilia and eosinophilic organ infiltration can result in tissue injury when inflammatory mediators within eosinophil granules are released. Basophilia can accompany eosinophilia particularly in hypersensitivity disorders. Basophils play a role in hypersensitivity due to secretion of vasoactive mediators such as histamine. Basophilia without eosinophilia is rare, as basophils release mediators chemotactic for eosinophils.

Systems Affected

Gastrointestinal, respiratory, skin, and hemolymphatic systems are affected in conditions associated with eosinophilia and/or basophilia.

SIGNALMENT

N/A

SIGNS

General Comments

Clinical signs are related to the organ system affected by the primary disease rather than eosinophilia and/or basophilia.

Historical Findings

The following is a list of clinical signs in horses with eosinophilia and gastrointestinal disease (e.g., colic, diarrhea, weight loss, altered appetite), respiratory disease (e.g., cough, nasal discharge), skin disease (e.g., multiple ulcerating masses, ulcerative lesions in mouth and skin adjacent to the coronary band), or hemolymphatic neoplasia (e.g., depression, altered appetite, weight loss).

Physical Exam Findings

Physical exam findings in animals with eosinophilia and/or basophilia reflect the primary disease and the involved organ systems. Abnormal physical exam findings with gastrointestinal disease include emaciation, diarrhea, abdominal pain, gastric reflux, and rectally palpable small intestine distension. Coughing, nasal discharge, increased expiratory effort, and crackles and wheezes in dorsal and caudal lung fields are indicative of respiratory disease. Physical exam abnormalities with skin disease include multiple necrotic masses containing gritty yellow material (kunkers), draining tracts, and pruritus or generalized exfoliative, exudative, ulcerative dermatitis (with involvement of the coronary bands), edema, and alopecia. Lethargy, pale mucous membranes, emaciation, and petechial hemorrhage may indicate hemolymphatic disease or neoplasia.

CAUSES

Eosinophilia

The following disease processes are associated with accumulations of eosinophils in affected tissues. Peripheral eosinophilia is a variable finding.

- Parasitism—Eosinophilia can occur in horses with *Parascaris equorum** infestations and *Strongylus vulgaris** and other large and small strongyle larval migrations and rarely with experimental or natural infections with *Strongyloides westeri.* Eosinophilia is occasionally a feature of *Dictyocaulus arnfieldi* (lungworm) infection.
- Infectious—Eosinophilia can be associated with cutaneous pythiosis.
- Neoplasia—Pronounced eosinophilia has been reported with eosinophilic myeloproliferative disease and as a paraneoplastic condition with intestinal lymphoma.
- Other Inflammatory Conditions—Eosinophilia is occasionally associated with allergic respiratory disease and rarely with multisystemic, eosinophilic, epitheliotropic disease.

Basophilia

Basophilia is rare in equine patients but can occur in conditions with peripheral eosinophilia. Mild basophilia has been reported in a single case of multisystemic, eosinophilic, epitheliotropic disease.

RISK FACTORS

Risk factors for eosinophilia include parasitism, hypersensitivity disorders, and neoplasia.

DIAGNOSIS

DIFFERENTIAL DIAGNOSIS

In animals with eosinophilia and gastrointestinal symptoms, parasitism and eosinophilic enterocolitis should be ruled out. Differential diagnoses for respiratory signs and eosinophilia include nematode larvae migration, lungworms, and hypersensitivity. Collection of a thorough deworming history can eliminate parasitism as a cause for gastrointestinal or respiratory symptoms. Lungworm infection should be considered in horses with respiratory symptoms and a history of sharing pastures or housing with donkeys. Cutaneous pythiosis should be ruled out in an animal with eosinophilia and multifocal ulcerative dermatitis. Multisystemic, eosinophilic, epitheliotropic disease should be considered in animals with generalized dermatitis, weight loss, diarrhea, and altered appetite. Although rare, profound eosinophilia with depression, lethargy, anemia, and weight loss may indicate a paraneoplastic disorder or eosinophilic myeloproliferative disease.

LABORATORY FINDINGS

Drugs That May Alter Lab Results

Eosinopenia secondary to corticosteroid administration can mask eosinophilia.

Disorders That May Alter Lab Results

N/A

Valid If Run in Human Lab?

Currently available automated methods for obtaining white cell counts and differentials in human laboratories have not been validated for use in veterinary patients. Therefore, reliable identification of equine leukocytes requires peripheral blood smear evaluation. Laboratory personnel should be informed that equine eosinophils have large red-pink granules, whereas basophils have numerous blue-purple granules.

CBC/BIOCHEMISTRY/URINALYSIS

A complete blood count (CBC) is necessary for identification of eosinophilia and basophilia. Biochemistry analysis may detect organ dysfunction resulting from eosinophilic infiltrates.

OTHER LABORATORY TESTS

Fecal flotation test is useful for identification of parasitic ova in animals with gastrointestinal symptoms. Baermann sedimentation of mucus may identify nematode larvae in horses with lungworm infection. An abnormal D-xylose absorption test and eosinophilia suggests

EOSINOPHILIA AND BASOPHILIA

malabsorption due to infiltrative enterocolitis from lymphoma or multisystemic, eosinophilic, epitheliotropic disease.

IMAGING

Endoscopic examination may reveal mucoid exudate in the trachea and bronchioles of animals with parasitic or allergic respiratory disease.

DIAGNOSTIC PROCEDURES

Cytologic evaluation of peritoneal fluid may reveal increased numbers of eosinophils, indicating parasitic migration or, rarely, eosinophilic enterocolitis. Eosinophilia and increased peritoneal fluid cellularity due to atypical lymphocytes suggests paraneoplastic eosinophilia secondary to lymphoma. Transtracheal wash (TTW) or bronchoalveolar lavage (BAL) techniques are useful in identifying eosinophilic inflammation in animals with parasitic or allergic respiratory disease. Rarely, parasitic larvae or ova are present in TTW or BAL fluid. Biopsy of skin lesions and rectal mucosa is useful in diagnosing multisystemic, eosinophilic, epitheliotropic disease in animals with generalized dermatitis, chronic weight loss, and diarrhea. Cytologic examination of necrotic tissue from cutaneous lesions may show fungal hyphae in animals with pythiosis. Confirmation of the cytologic diagnosis requires histologic examination of skin lesion biopsies. Collection of bone marrow aspirates or core biopsies from animals with profound eosinophilia can be useful in identifying paraneoplastic eosinophilia or eosinophilic myeloproliferative disorder.

TREATMENT

Because eosinophilic infiltrates are potentially damaging to organs, treatment should be directed at decreasing eosinophilic tissue infiltrates while the primary cause for eosinophilia is determined. Once identified, treatment should be directed at the primary disease. Fluid therapy should be initiated in animals with clinical dehydration from diarrhea. Animals with suspected allergic respiratory disease should be stalled to diminish exposure to environmental allergens.

MEDICATIONS

Corticosteroids diminish peripheral eosinophilia and aid in management of allergic respiratory disease. Anthelminthics should be used to treat parasitic gastroenteritis and bronchitis. Aggressive surgical excision should be performed in horses with lesions characteristic of pythiosis. Systemic, intralesional, and topical application of antifungal drugs (in association with aggressive surgical excision) can be used to treat cutaneous pythiosis; however, owners should be made aware that complete eradication of the disease is difficult and expensive. Horses with multisystemic, eosinophilic, epitheliotropic disease have been reported to respond to corticosteroid administration; however, owners should be cautioned that this is a palliative therapy only.

DRUG(S) OF CHOICE

A suggested immunosuppressive therapy with corticosteroids is 0.2 mg/kg dexamethasone intramuscularly for 5 days, followed by oral prednisolone 0.5 mg/kg twice daily for 5 days, then 1.0 mg/kg once daily for 7 days, followed by alternate day therapy.

CONTRAINDICATIONS

Corticosteroids should not be given to animals with suspected sepsis, infectious diseases, or hyperkalemic periodic paralysis.

PRECAUTIONS

Prolonged corticosteroid administration has been associated with adrenal suppression, laminitis, and opportunistic infections.

POSSIBLE INTERACTIONS

N/A

ALTERNATIVE DRUGS

N/A

FOLLOW-UP

PATIENT MONITORING

Sequential complete blood counts should be collected to monitor peripheral eosinophil and basophil counts.

POSSIBLE COMPLICATIONS

Eosinophilic infiltrates can cause organ injury and dysfunction.

MISCELLANEOUS

ASSOCIATED CONDITIONS

Basophilia often accompanies peripheral eosinophilia.

AGE-RELATED FACTORS

N/A

ZOONOTIC POTENTIAL

Although pythiosis has not been shown to be a zoonotic disease, gloves should be worn as a precaution when handling suspicious cutaneous lesions.

PREGNANCY

Corticosteroids may be contraindicated in pregnant animals.

SYNONYMS

N/A

SEE ALSO

N/A

ABBREVIATIONS

- TTW = Transtracheal wash
- BAL = Bronchoalveolar lavage

Suggested Reading

Ainsworth DM, Biller DS. Respiratory system. In: Reed SM, Bayly WM, eds. Equine internal medicine. Philadelphia: WB Saunders, 1998:251-289.

Duckett WM, Matthews HK. Hypereosinophilia in a horse with intestinal lymphosarcoma. Can Vet J 1997;38:719-720.

Jain NC. A brief review of the pathophysiology of eosinophils. Comp Cont Educ Pract Vet 1994;16: 1212-1218.

Jain NC. Essentials of veterinary hematology. Philadelphia: Lea & Febiger, 1993: 258-265.

Moriello KA, DeBoer DJ, Semrad SD. Diseases of the skin. In: Reed SM, Bayly WM, eds. Equine internal medicine. Philadelphia: WB Saunders, 1998:513-557.

Author Laura I. Boone

Contributing Editor Claire B. Andreasen

EOSINOPHILIC KERATITIS

BASICS

OVERVIEW
Eosinophilic keratoconjunctivitis is a rare disease of horses with an unknown etiology. Accumulation, mainly of eosinophils and few mast cells in the affected cornea, is characteristic.

SYSTEM AFFECTED
Ophthalmic

SIGNALMENT
All ages and breeds affected.

SIGNS
Granulation tissue, blepharospasm, chemosis, conjunctival hyperemia, mucoid discharge, and corneal ulcers covered by raised, white, necrotic plaques.

CAUSES AND RISK FACTORS
Allergic, parasitic. An allergic reaction, for example, may be an immune-mediated or inflammatory manifestation of chronic ivermectin administration for parasite control.

DIAGNOSIS

DIFFERENTIAL DIAGNOSIS
Allergic keratitis/keratoconjunctivitis; eosinophilic granuloma; bacterial, mycotic, or viral keratitis; foreign body reaction; onchocerciasis; or habronemiasis.

CBC/BIOCHEMISTRY/URINALYSIS
N/A

OTHER LABORATORY TESTS
Rule out infectious causes (bacterial or fungal) with corneal scrapings for cytology and culture. Corneal scrapings typically contain numerous eosinophils and few mast cells. Biopsy for histology helps to confirm diagnosis if corneal scrapings are not conclusive.

IMAGING
N/A

DIAGNOSTIC PROCEDURES
N/A

PATHOLOGIC FINDINGS
Histologic examination of conjunctiva adjacent to lesion reveals marked acanthosis, neutrophilic exocytosis, and scattered eosinophils. There is also thickening of the corneal epithelium.

TREATMENT

APPROPRIATE HEALTH CARE
Superficial lamellar keratectomy to remove plaques speeds healing.

EOSINOPHILIC KERATITIS

MEDICATIONS

DRUGS

Topical corticosteroids (1% prednisolone acetate or 0.1% dexamethasone) 4 to 6 times a day in early stages (in spite of corneal ulcerations). Topical antibiotics (e.g., bacitracin-neomyxin-polymyxin, chloramphenicol), 1% atropine, and 0.03% phospholine iodide BID in combination with systemic nonsteroidal antiinflammatory drugs (e.g., flunixin meglumine 0.25 to 1 mg/kg BID PO, IM, IV).

CONTRAINDICATIONS/POSSIBLE INTERACTIONS

Phospholine iodide is an acetylcholinesterase inhibitor that may be larvacidal for parasites. Its use is controversial.

FOLLOW-UP

EXPECTED COURSE AND PROGNOSIS

Slow to heal. Scarring of the cornea occurs.

MISCELLANEOUS

ASSOCIATED CONDITIONS

Uveitis.

SEE ALSO

- Equine Corneal Ulceration
- Equine Corneal Laceration
- Equine Keratomycosis
- Equine Corneal Stromal Abscessation
- Equine Nonulcerative Keratouveitis
- Equine Herpes Keratitis
- Equine Burdock Pappus Bristle Keratopathy
- Equine Limbal Keratopathy
- Equine Superficial Corneal Erosions with Anterior Stromal Sequestration
- Equine Recurrent Uveitis
- Equine Glaucoma

Suggested Reading

Brooks DE. Equine ophthalmology. In: Gelatt KN, ed. Veterinary ophthalmology. 3rd ed. Philadelphia: Lippincott Williams & Wilkins, 1999; chapter 30.

Author Andras M. Komaromy
Consulting Editor Dennis E. Brooks

EPIGLOTTIC ENTRAPMENT

BASICS

OVERVIEW
• A result of the loose, aryepiglottic mucosa, which normally is on the ventral surface of the epiglottis, enveloping part or all of the dorsal surface of the epiglottis.
• Usually, the epiglottis remains in its normal, horizontal position dorsal to the soft palate, but the condition can occur concurrently with DDSP.
• Leads to varying degrees of respiratory compromise and exercise intolerance.
• Most often diagnosed during resting endoscopy because the entrapment is persistent.
• Also can occur intermittently.

SIGNALMENT
• Affects horses participating in intensive exercise almost exclusively—Thoroughbred and Standardbred racehorses.
• Other breeds or horses engaged in other activities rarely are affected.
• Can occur at any age while in training
• No sex predilection.

SIGNS
• Exercise intolerance is the most frequent chief complaint.
• Abnormal respiratory noise also may be present during exercise.
• Other signs—coughing, dysphagia, or nasal discharge.

CAUSES AND RISK FACTORS
• The cause is unknown.
• Racing is the most significant risk factor.
• Horses with a short or small epiglottis are predisposed.
• An obscure association exists between epiglottic entrapment and DDSP.

DIAGNOSIS

DIFFERENTIAL DIAGNOSIS
• Epiglottiditis, epiglottic deformity/hypoplasia, and DDSP.
• The visual appearance of the triangular-shaped epiglottis, without a normal vascular pattern, during upper airway endoscopy should help to differentiate epiglottic entrapment from other abnormalities involving the epiglottis.

CBC/BIOCHEMISTRY/URINALYSIS
N/A

OTHER LABORATORY TEST
Arterial blood gases may reveal an exercising hypoxemia.

IMAGING
• Upper airway endoscopy at rest—the most common diagnostic technique. The triangular-shaped epiglottis above the palate remains visible, but the entrapping membrane obscures the visualization of the normal serrated edge of the epiglottis and the vascular pattern. The normal vasculature on the dorsal surface of the epiglottis consists of two longitudinal vessels that extend from the base toward the apex and that arborize into smaller vessels extending toward the edge of the epiglottis. With chronicity, the entrapping membrane becomes very thickened and, sometimes, ulcerated at the apex of the epiglottis.
• With concurrent DDSP, it is difficult to see if the epiglottis is entrapped. Close inspection over the free edge of the palate may reveal another edge of membrane, representing the epiglottic entrapment, before the dorsal surface of the epiglottis is apparent.

EPIGLOTTIC ENTRAPMENT

• Skull radiography—when the epiglottis is entrapped, the normal, convex shape of the epiglottis above the palate is obscured on lateral skull radiographs.

DIAGNOSTIC PROCEDURES

• Initiating swallowing during resting endoscopy may induce an intermittent entrapment.
• High-speed treadmill endoscopy may be required to establish the diagnosis of intermittent entrapment.

TREATMENT

• Surgical correction of the simple, nonulcerated entrapment entails axial division of the entrapping membrane in the standing horse with sedation and topical anesthetic. The division is performed with direct visualization, employing a laser fiber through the instrument portal of a videoendoscope. Axial division also can be performed with a hooked bistoury in the standing or anesthetized horse. With the hooked bistoury, general anesthesia is preferred to minimize the risk of inadvertent trauma to the pharynx or palate.
• Very thickened, ulcerated entrapping membranes often require surgical resection of the tissue, which is approached through a laryngotomy.

MEDICATIONS

DRUGS

Anti-inflammatory drugs (dexamethasone [10 mg PO SID]) and throat sprays (10 mL of a furacin-based solution with 2 mg of prednisolone in a 1 mL-solution BID) for several days postoperatively.

CONTRAINDICATIONS/POSSIBLE INTERACTIONS

N/A

FOLLOW-UP

• Perform endoscopy postoperatively and before resuming training; further examinations depend on any change in performance.
• Epiglottic entrapment has a very low recurrence rate.

MISCELLANOUS

ASSOCIATED CONDITIONS

N/A

AGE-RELATED FACTORS

N/A

ZOONOTIC POTENTIAL

N/A

PREGNANCY

N/A

SEE ALSO

• Acute epiglottiditis
• Dynamic collapse of the upper airway

ABBREVIATION

DDSP = dorsal displacement of the soft palate

Suggested Reading

Spiers VC, Tulleners EP, Ducharme NG, et al. Larynx. In: Auer JA, ed. Equine surgery. Philadelphia: WB Saunders, 1992.

Author Eric J. Parente
Consulting Editor Jean-Pierre Lavoie

ESOPHAGEAL OBSTRUCTION (CHOKE)

BASICS

DEFINITION

Choke, esophageal obstruction, refers to an inability to swallow as a sequela to partial or complete obstruction of the esophageal lumen by feed or foreign body. The disorder may occur as a single acute episode or as a chronic, intermittent problem.

PATHOPHYSIOLOGY

Intraluminal esophageal obstruction occurs with higher frequency at sites with naturally decreased esophageal distensibility. These areas are the mid-cervical region, the thoracic inlet, and the terminal esophagus. The most common type of obstruction is impaction with feed material such as beet pulp, pelleted feed, corncobs, grain, hay, and pieces of fruit or vegetable. Wood shavings and various foreign bodies can also cause obstruction of the esophagus. A frequent predisposing factor is improper mastication by older or younger horses caused by defective and erupting teeth, respectively. Improper mastication can also occur in gluttonous, sedated, or exhausted horses or in horses recovering from general anesthesia. Horses with pre-existing lesions such as external esophageal compression, megaesophagus, and esophageal diverticulum or stricture experience recurrent obstructions at the affected site. Choke can also occur secondarily to neurologic disorders (botulism, rabies, leukoencephalomalacia, and yellow star thistle poisoning).

SYSTEMS AFFECTED

Gastrointestinal

Obstruction of the esophagus causes dysphagia. Sequelae to choke, involving the gastrointestinal system, include esophageal perforation or stricture formation and mega-esophagus.

Respiratory

Aspiration of feed material and saliva frequently occurs in horses with esophageal obstruction. In some instances this can lead to aspiration pneumonia. Other less common sequela to choke are pleuritis and mediastinitis secondary to esophageal perforation.

Cardiovascular

The inability to drink water may result in dehydration. Excessive salivary loss, which occurs in some horses, can cause hyponatremia, hypochloremia, and metabolic alkalosis.

Skin/Exocrine

Esophageal perforation can result in cervical cellulitis and fistula formation.

SIGNALMENT

Age Predisposition

Younger and older horses

SIGNS

General Comments

Ptyalism and feed-containing nasal discharge are the most common clinical signs of choke. Other clinical signs vary with the duration and the degree of the obstruction. Partial obstruction might cause intermittent clinical signs depending on the diet.

Historical Findings

- Frequent, ineffectual attempts to swallow
- Retching
- Repeated extension of the head and neck
- Coughing during swallowing
- Nasal discharge of saliva mixed with feed
- Restlessness
- Sweating
- Anxiety

Physical Examination Findings

Dysphagia, coughing, ptyalism, and regurgitation of saliva and feed material through the mouth and nostrils. Sweating and halitosis. Dilation of the cervical esophagus may be palpable or visible. Patients with recurrent or chronic esophageal obstruction may demonstrate non-specific clinical signs such as weight loss, depression, and hypovolemia. The presence of subcutaneous emphysema and/or cellulitis over the cervical region may indicate esophageal rupture.

CAUSES

Obstruction of the esophagus is most frequently caused by intraluminal impaction of feed material or, less commonly, by foreign bodies. Improper mastication due to erupting or defective teeth, sedation, exhaustion, or fracture of the hyoid bone are potential predisposing factors to intraluminal feed obstruction. Dry feeds (e.g., beet pulp, pelleted feeds, oats) are most often associated with the condition. Defects in the esophageal wall (intramural lesions) such as strictures, intramural abscesses or cysts, esophageal diverticula, and neoplasia (especially squamous cell carcinoma) usually result in recurrent esophageal obstructions. Acquired lesions causing external esophageal compression are relatively rare and include abscesses, tumors, regionally enlarged lymph nodes, cervical cellulitis, and diaphragmatic hernia. Congenital disorders such as megaesophagus, achalasia, vascular ring anomalies, and right aortic arch are rare causes of esophageal obstruction. Clinical signs of dysphagia may be present from birth, but this depends on the degree of obstruction. Instead, the clinical signs may occur when soiled feeds are introduced to the diet. Esophageal motility disorders can result in esophageal obstruction and megaesophagus.

RISK FACTORS

- Poor dental care
- Rapid ingestion of feed
- Poor quality feed; pelleted or dry feeds such as beet pulp and oats
- Inadequate water intake
- Previous episode of choke

ESOPHAGEAL OBSTRUCTION (CHOKE)

DIAGNOSIS

DIFFERENTIAL DIAGNOSIS

Bilateral nasal discharge caused by pharyngeal abscessation, guttural pouch empyema, strangles, or lung edema may be mistaken for esophageal obstruction. Neurologic disorders such as rabies, botulism, leukoencephalomalacia, and yellow star thistle poisoning can cause dysphagia. Guttural pouch mycosis may cause pharyngeal dysphagia by affecting the cranial nerves IX, X, and XII. Foreign bodies in the pharynx or oral cavity may produce similar clinical signs as esophageal obstruction. In those countries where it is recognized, acute grass sickness (equine dysautonomia) should be included in the differential list.

CBC/BIOCHEMISTRY/URINALYSIS

Packed cell volume and total serum protein evaluation provide additional information on the hydration status. Leukogram and fibrinogen may give more information about inflammatory reactions and should be obtained if aspiration pneumonia is suspected as a complication. Prolonged excessive salivary loss may cause hyponatremia, hypochloremia, and metabolic alkalosis.

IMAGING

Radiography

Survey radiographic evaluation of the esophagus supplies information concerning the nature and degree of the obstruction. Single- or double-contrast esophagography is useful to identify sites of partial or complete obstructions. Esophageal perforation, diverticulum formation, strictures, and esophageal ulcers and erosions may be diagnosed by contrast esophagraphy. Esophageal motility disorders can be diagnosed by positive contrast studies.

Fluoroscopy

Fluoroscopic evaluation is particularly useful for dynamic studies of esophageal motility disorders.

DIAGNOSTIC PROCEDURES

Passage of a nasogastric tube is an important diagnostic tool. This procedure can confirm a tentative diagnosis of choke and determine the approximate location of the obstruction. Endoscopic evaluation of the esophagus gives further information about the nature of the obstruction. Predisposing factors such as strictures and diverticulum formation may also be identified by esophagoscopy.

TREATMENT

Conservative Management

Although some cases of esophageal obstruction resolve spontaneously, they should be treated as emergencies in order to limit the esophageal inflammation and receptive relaxation distal to the obstruction. The owner should be instructed to remove feed and water from the stall while waiting for the veterinarian to arrive. Most cases of esophageal obstruction can be successfully treated on the farm. Only a few cases require referral to an animal hospital.

The basic approaches to treatment of esophageal obstruction are gentle esophageal lavage in conjunction with administration of drugs (see Medication) that result in relaxation of esophageal musculature and reduced level of anxiety. In cases of mild obstruction, administration of these drugs alone may result in sufficient muscular relaxation to allow the obstruction to pass. Gentle passage of a stomach tube may also be required, but this should be attempted with great care.

If these procedures are unsuccessful, lavage of the esophagus can be done with warm water. A nasogastric tube is advanced to the level of the obstruction and warm water instilled into the tube, which allows water and ingesta to flow out of the tube. During the procedure, the patient's head should be kept at a low level to facilitate the exit of fluid and prevent aspiration. Numerous modifications of the lavage technique exist, depending on individual preferences. A cuffed nasogastric tube facilitates lavage and promotes the flow of lavaged material through the tube, thereby decreasing the risk of aspiration. Continuous lavage can be performed by passing a smaller tube through the larger cuffed esophageal tube. A small cuffed tracheal tube can be used as an alternative to a cuffed nasogastric tube as a guide for a smaller lavage tube. The procedures require patience and gentleness. If the impaction is not relieved, the lavages can be performed intermittently with the horse placed in a stall without access to feed, water, and bedding between the attempts.

ESOPHAGEAL OBSTRUCTION (CHOKE)

In most cases, the procedures described relieve the esophageal obstruction. Refractory cases can be anesthetized, intubated with an endotracheal tube, and placed in lateral recumbency with the head lowered. This procedure enhances continuous lavage and the anesthesia creates additional muscle relaxation of the esophagus. Once the choke is relieved, endoscopic evalaution of the esophagus is valauble as the extent of mucosal damage can be assessed.

Dietary Management

Dietary management after the esophageal obstruction has resolved relates to the degree of esophageal injury. If the impaction was transient and there is minimal superficial esophageal mucosal damage with no functional alteration, the horse can be fed small amounts of hay. In horses with more prolonged esophageal impactions or ulcerations, a slurry of pelleted feed, grass, or hay, pre-soaked in water, may be provided within 24–72 hr, depending on the extent of esophageal injury. If the esophageal damage is severe, the esophagus remains dilated, and the esophageal transit time is prolonged, feed should be withheld for at least 72 hr. Severe esophageal damage may require parenteral feeding.

Maintenance of Homeostasis

Intravenous isotonic fluids should be given if the horse is dehydrated or water consumption is restricted. Excessive salivary loss results in hyponatremia, hypochloremia, and, metabolic alkalosis. The type of intravenous fluids used is based on acid–base and electrolyte derangements. Patients with hypochloremic metabolic alkalosis should be treated intravenously with 0.9% sodium chloride, whereas balanced polyionic solutions such as lactated Ringer's solution may be used in metabolic acidosis. However, most cases of esophageal obstruction do not require intravenous fluid therapy.

Surgical Management

If all attempts to resolve the esophageal obstruction fail, surgical intervention is indicated. Prophylactic treatment with antibiotics should be administered before surgery and continued for several days post-surgery. Tetanus prophylaxis is necessary. Before anesthetic induction, a nasogastric tube should be placed to the level of the obstruction. Depending on the location of the obstruction, different surgical approaches are used. Thoracic esophageal surgery requires rib resection and positive pressure ventilation. Detailed descriptions of esophageal surgery are found elsewhere. Complications following esophageal surgery are a major concern and include dehydration, dehiscence of the esophageal incision, laryngeal hemiplegia, chronic esophageal obstruction due to strictures, aspiration pneumonia, pleuritis, laminitis, and Horner's syndrome.

MEDICATIONS

DRUG(S) OF CHOICE

Administration of xylazine, detomidine, or acepromazine provides sedation and muscle relaxation of the esophagus. The use of α2-adrenergic agonists has the advantage of causing lowering of the head, thereby facilitating the lavage and decreasing the likelihood of aspiration. Anti-inflammatory drugs, such as flunixine meglumine and phenylbutazone, are used to control pain and treat inflammation. There are also clinical reports of sucessful management of choke with parenteral use of oxytocin. However, the safety and value of this approach have yet to be determined.

Broad-spectrum antibiotics are indicated if esophageal perforation or aspiration pneumonia is suspected or has occurred. The antibacterial spectrum should be targeted against enteric and anaerobic bacteria. Detailed descriptions of the treatment of aspiration pneumonia are found elsewhere.

CONTRAINDICATIONS

Administration of lubricating agents, such as mineral oil or softening agents, such as dioctyl sodium sulfo-succinate (DSS) in order to facilitate the removal of an esophageal obstruction, are contraindicated because they might be aspirated.

ESOPHAGEAL OBSTRUCTION (CHOKE)

PRECAUTIONS

Non-steroidal anti-inflammatory drugs (NSAIDs) should be administered cautiously to dehydrated animals due to their potentially nephrotoxic effects.

POSSIBLE INTERACTIONS

N/A

ALTERNATIVE DRUGS

Recent reports indicate that oxytocin is capable of relaxing the equine esophagus and may be valauble in the treatment of choke. Extensive data are not yet available on the efficacy of this technique.

FOLLOW-UP

PATIENT MONITORING

Endoscopy of the esophagus should be performed after the obstruction has been relieved in order to determine the extent of any esophageal lesions, establish the prognosis, and make recommendations for additional treatments and feeding regimen. Repeated esophagoscopies are indicated if mucosal damage has occurred. Strictures most often occur 15–30 days after mucosal damage. Surgery is required in some cases of esophageal strictures.

Thoracic auscultation and monitoring of body temperature might identify aspiration pneumonia. Thoracic radiographs are indicated if aspiration pneumonia is suspected.

POSSIBLE COMPLICATIONS

- Recurrent esophageal obstructions
- Esophageal diverticulum
- Esophageal stricture
- Esophageal perforation
- Cellulitis
- Esophageal dilation
- Mediastinitis
- Aspiration pneumonia
- Pleuritis

MISCELLANEOUS

ASSOCIATED CONDITIONS

Aspiration pneumonia

AGE-RELATED FACTORS

Younger and older horses are most commonly affected.

PREGNANCY

Alpha-2-adrenergic agonists (detomidine and xylazine) may induce premature parturition if used during the last trimester of pregnancy.

SYNONYMS

Choke

Suggested Reading

Whithair KJ, Cox JH, Coyne CP, DeBowes RM. Esophageal obstruction in the horse. Compen Contin Educ 1990;1:91-96.

Author Johan T. Bröjer

Consulting Editor Henry Stämpfli

EUPATORIUM RUGOSUM (WHITE SNAKEROOT) TOXICOSIS

BASICS

OVERVIEW

- *Eupatorium rugosum* (white snakeroot) is a dark green, herbaceous, perennial plant that grows from a shallow mat of fibrous, twisting, turning roots to a height of $\cong$1.0–1.5 m.
- Numerous varieties exist and vary in their individual toxicity.
- Leaves are opposite, long to short petioled, elongated (4.5–6 cm in length), heart shaped, and three-ribbed, with characteristic coarse and sharply toothed margins and pointed tip.
- Flowers are snow-white, small, and clustered in composite heads of 10–40 flowers at the top of the plant, blooming from September through October.
- The plant is common in low, moist areas bordering streams and woodlands. It also is found in woodland areas, in great abundance in wooded ravines and open areas of recently removed timber.
- The plant grows principally in eastern North America and ranges from the eastern seaboard of the U.S. as far north as eastern Canada, west to Saskatchewan and Minnesota, and south to east Texas and the Gulf Coast.
- Toxins include tremetol (i.e., tremetone, precocenes) and high-molecular-weight alcohols (i.e., ketone, ethers) and are believed to require hepatic microsomal activation to cytotoxic metabolites to produce toxicosis.
- Toxins have their greatest abundance in the foliage of mature plants and persist in both frozen and dried leaves.
- Equine intoxication usually requires several days of continuous ingestion of pasture or hay containing significant amounts of white snakeroot.
- Cumulative ingestion of >1% of body weight can be lethal.
- Toxins are concentrated and readily passed in the milk of lactating mares, resulting in potential intoxication of nursing foals.
- White snakeroot intoxication also is referred to as trembles.

SIGNALMENT

Horses with access to white snakeroot or foals nursing mares with access to white snakeroot are at risk.

SIGNS

- Neuromuscular, GI, cardiovascular, and respiratory signs of toxicosis can occur as soon as 1–2 days or as long as 2–3 weeks after ingestion.
- Horses usually exhibit marked depression and anorexia, followed shortly by hyperpnea and dyspnea.
- A brownish-green discharge is seen from the nostrils.
- Bouts of profuse, regional sweating occur.
- Affected horses often eliminate small amounts of dark, compact feces and dark brown urine.
- Rear-limb ataxia occurs and often is characterized by crossing of the rear legs, with variable (but sometimes absent) muscle tremors in the shoulders, flanks, and rear legs.
- Affected horses also may exhibit hypersalivation and drooling and appear to have difficulty swallowing (suggestive of a choke).
- Often, a marked, pitting edema is present on the ventral mandible, abdomen, and thorax.
- Jugular veins appear distended, with very vigorous and irregular jugular pulses.
- Auscultation of the heart reveals a marked arrhythmia—heart rate >60 bpm
- Pupils are dilated and slowly responsive to light.

CAUSES AND RISK FACTORS

Equine intoxication usually occurs during late summer, autumn, or early winter, when other forage becomes less available, or during late winter or early spring, when good-quality hay is in short supply.

DIAGNOSIS

DIFFERENTIAL DIAGNOSIS

- White muscle disease—serum α-tocopherol levels <2.5 mg/mL or serum selenium levels <100 ng/mL
- Ionophore intoxication—positive feed analysis with compatible clinical signs or lesions is diagnostic.
- Gossypol intoxication—feed analysis showing >300 ppm of free gossypol
- Blister beetle intoxication—positive analysis of gastric contents or urine for cantharidin
- Botulism—detection of botulinum toxin in feed or tissues
- Organophosphate intoxication—whole-blood cholinesterase level <25% of normal reference value; analysis of feed for organophosphates

CBC/BIOCHEMISTRY/URINALYSIS

- With severe clinical signs, increasing hematocrit, neutrophilia, and lymphopenia.
- CPK—often >7000 IU/L
- AST—often >500 U/L
- LDH—often >1000 U/L
- Increased AP levels also have been consistently reported.
- Urinalysis—glucosuria, proteinuria, hemoglobinuria, and myoglobinuria.

OTHER LABORATORY TESTS

- P_{CO_2}—often >50.0 mm Hg
- pH—often <7.36
- Analysis of gastric contents for toxin is possible.

IMAGING

N/A

EUPATORIUM RUGOSUM (WHITE SNAKEROOT) TOXICOSIS

DIAGNOSTIC PROCEDURES

- ECG abnormalities characterized by marked ST-segment depression, ventricular premature beats, and occasionally, complete atrioventricular block can occur.
- ECG changes may not become evident until 7–10 days after ingestion and other clinical signs are present.

PATHOLOGIC FINDINGS

Gross Findings

- Severe pulmonary, hepatic, and renal congestion are consistently reported.
- Fatty degeneration of the liver and kidney
- Numerous prominent, pale, linear streaks on the epicardium and pale, multifocal areas of myocardium are visible on cut surfaces.
- The right heart in particular usually appears dilated and flabby.
- The pericardial sac often contains variable amounts of mildly viscous, straw-colored effusion, and areas of subcutaneous edema may be noted.

Histopathologic Findings

Lesions of the liver and heart—mild, centrilobular degeneration with multifocal areas of hepatic necrosis and fatty change and severe, multifocal myocardial degeneration and necrosis

TREATMENT

- Correct acid–base balance and electrolyte abnormalities.
- White snakeroot intoxication has no specific treatment, so therapy should be symptomatic and supportive.

MEDICATIONS

DRUGS

- AC (2–5 g/kg PO in a water slurry [1 g of AC in 5 mL of water])
- One dose of cathartic PO with AC if no diarrhea or ileus—70% sorbitol (3 mL/kg) or sodium or magnesium sulfate (250–500 mg/kg).

CONTRAINDICATIONS/POSSIBLE INTERACTIONS

- Use of drugs promoting hepatic microsomal enzymes is contraindicated—phenobarbital; rifampin
- Use of drugs inhibiting hepatic microsomal enzymes may be beneficial—chloramphenicol; cimetidine

FOLLOW-UP

- Horses have been reported to respond favorably to treatment with repeated doses of AC. This suggests the toxins involved may undergo enterohepatic recycling and, therefore, their persistence may be lessened by such treatment.
- Prevention of white snakeroot intoxication is possible—monitor for white snakeroot in pasture or hay.
- Selective use of herbicides or manual removal of plants may help to diminish a recognized potential problem.
- Horses that begin to exhibit severe signs have a grave prognosis and usually die within 48 hours; horses that recover may have permanent heart damage.

MISCELLANEOUS

ASSOCIATED CONDITIONS

N/A

AGE-RELATED FACTORS

N/A

ZOONOTIC POTENTIAL

N/A

PREGNANCY

N/A

SEE ALSO

N/A

ABBREVIATIONS

- AC = activated charcoal
- AP = alkaline phosphatase
- AST = aspartate aminotransferase
- CPK = creatine phosphokinase
- GI = gastrointestinal
- LDH = lactate dehydrogenase

Suggested Reading

Cheeke PR. Natural toxicants in feeds, forages, and poisonous plants. Danville, IL: Interstate Publishers, 1998:385–386.

Author William R. Hare
Consulting Editor Robert H. Poppenga

EXCESSIVE MATERNAL BEHAVIOR/FOAL STEALING

BASICS

DEFINITION

- Uncommon
- A mare may show maternal behavior for a foal not her own without preventing care by the foal's biologic mother by staying near the foal substantially more than expected from another herd member that is not the mother and by standing for the foal to suckle.
- Mares that are not pregnant and currently have no foals of their own occasionally produce milk for a foal they have spontaneously adopted, but this phenomenon is rare.
- Mares may prevent the foal's biologic mother from caring for it.

PATHOPHYSIOLOGY

When prepartum mares steal foals, the endocrine system changes that are preparing them to care for their own foals, combined with the social relationships that enable them to steal the foal of a subordinate mare are the cause.

SYSTEMS AFFECTED

- Behavioral—misdirected maternal behavior and increased aggressiveness.
- Neuroendocrine—maternal behavior is under neural and hormonal control, with estrogen, progesterone, and oxytocin being most significant; however, the exact neuroendocrine mechanism for mismothering is unknown.

SIGNALMENT

Subordinate mares in a herd are unlikely to be successful in stealing foals of higher-ranking mares; therefore, mares that are dominant to most other mares in the herd are the most likely to be successful.

SIGNS

- A mare other than the mother remaining near a foal and standing for the foal to suckle.
- In cases of true foal stealing, a mare remains between the foal and its biologic mother, shows aggressive behavior (e.g., biting and kicking, or threatening such) toward the mother, and may chase the mother away from the vicinity of the foal.

CAUSES

- Neuroendocrine mechanisms that prepare a prepartum mare to care for her own foal.
- Parturition by a low-ranking mare within 48 hours of parturition by a high-ranking mare provides the stimulus of a neonatal foal to the higher-ranking mare.

RISK FACTORS

- Very timid, nonaggressive, low-ranking biological mothers are most likely to have their foals stolen.
- Very aggressive nonmothers that are hormonally ready to care for a neonate are most likely to steal foals.

DIAGNOSIS

DIFFERENTIAL DIAGNOSIS

N/A

CBC/BIOCHEMISTRY/URINALYSIS

N/A

OTHER LABORATORY TESTS

N/A

IMAGING

N/A

DIAGNOSTIC PROCEDURES

- In herds that are surveyed only periodically and for which the actual birth was not observed, it may be superficially unclear which of two mares fighting over a foal is the biologic mother. Examine both mares to determine which has recently given birth and which is still pregnant.
- If the foal has been suckling a prepartum mare, it may have consumed her colostrum. Alternatively, its mother may have lost her colostrum during several hours of conflict with the foal-stealing mare, during which time the foal may have been unable to suckle. Assess the foal for dehydration and exhaustion.

EXCESSIVE MATERNAL BEHAVIOR/FOAL STEALING

TREATMENT

- Isolate the foal and its biologic mother from the mare attempting to steal the foal. Isolating the mother and foal from other herd members not attempting to steal the foal may not be necessary, unless the foal requires medical attention.
- Colostrum for the foal that was stolen and the foal of the stealing mare if the history suggests that either may be unable to get colostrum from its mother.
- Fluid therapy if dehydrated.

MEDICATIONS

DRUGS OF CHOICE
N/A

CONTRAINDICATIONS
N/A

PRECAUTIONS
N/A

POSSIBLE INTERACTIONS
N/A

ALTERNATIVE DRUGS
N/A

FOLLOW-UP

PATIENT MONITORING
Once the stealing mare has her own foal, she is unlikely to attempt to steal a foal again; nevertheless, both mares should be observed carefully once returned to the herd to ensure no resumption of conflict.

POSSIBLE COMPLICATIONS
N/A

MISCELLANEOUS

ASSOCIATED CONDITIONS
Mares that steal foals may be more likely to engage in excessive aggression toward other herd members, regardless of the presence or absence of foals.

AGE-RELATED FACTORS
N/A

ZOONOTIC POTENTIAL
N/A

PREGNANCY
Mares in late pregnancy have the greatest risk of this behavior.

SYNONYMS
- Misdirected maternal behavior
- Mismother

SEE ALSO
Aggression

Suggested Readings

Crowell-Davis SL. Normal behavior and behavior problems. In: Kobluk CN, Ames TR, Geor RJ, eds. The horse: Diseases and clinical management. Philadelphia: WB Saunders, 1995:1–21.

Crowell-Davis SL, Houpt KA. Maternal behavior. Vet Clin North Am Equine Pract 1986;2:557–571.

Author Sharon L. Crowell-Davis
Consulting Editor Daniel Q. Estep

EXERCISE-INDUCED PULMONARY HEMORRHAGE (EIPH)

BASICS

DEFINITION

Hemorrhage from the lung parenchyma associated with exertion and characterized by blood in the airways and, occasionally, by epistaxis.

PATHOPHYSIOLOGY

- Precise mechanism unknown
- Current speculation—initial bleeding associated with pulmonary capillary stress failure. Exercising horses have high cardiac outputs and high vascular pressures. High left atrial pressures (likely associated with low left ventricular compliance and, possibly, mitral valve resistance) contribute to high capillary pressures. Vascular rupture leads to pulmonary hemorrhage, and blood in the airways elicits an inflammatory reaction.
- Other factors—inhaled particles, viral respiratory disease, and air pollutants are considered to exacerbate inflammation; bronchial arterial neovascularization response to airway and parenchymal injury in concert with pulmonary capillary stress failure contributes to subsequent EIPH.

SYSTEMS AFFECTED

Respiratory—lungs

INCIDENCE/PREVALENCE

- Affects most horses exercising strenuously.
- Reported frequency ranges from 35% (Standardbreds) to >75% (racing Thoroughbreds).
- Reported for most strenuous activities—flat racing, pacing and trotting races, jumping, barrel racing, roping, steeple chase, 3-day eventing, draft-pulling competitions, polo, and endurance races
- Worldwide distribution

SIGNALMENT

- Occurs with onset of strenuous exercise and training, thus from 2 years of age.
- Males, geldings, and females are equally affected.

SIGNS

Historical Findings

- Occasionally, coughing and increased swallowing activity are found.
- Occasionally, performance is impaired.

Physical Examination Findings

- Rarely, abnormal airway sounds
- Commonly, no external clinical signs.
- <5% of affected horses have epistaxis.

CAUSES AND RISK FACTORS

- Strenuous exercise
- Less commonly, underlying parenchymal disease—pulmonary abscess

DIAGNOSIS

DIFFERENTIAL DIAGNOSIS

- Epistaxis—ethmoid hematoma, guttural pouch mycosis, and coagulopathy.
- Airway blood—pulmonary abscess, pneumonia, foreign body, and neoplasia.

CBC/BIOCHEMISTRY/URINALYSIS

Changes in CBC or biochemical panel indicate a concurrent disease process.

OTHER LABORATORY TESTS

N/A

IMAGING

- Thoracic radiography—increased homogeneous parenchymal density in dorsal caudal lung fields (not a consistent finding but, if present, usually clears in 3–5 days); increased interstitial density in the same lung region indicative of chronic EIPH.
- Endoscopy—airway endoscopy within 30–90 minutes after strenuous exercise with identification of airway blood is the definitive diagnostic method. Blood usually clears from airways by 4–6 hours.
- Scintigraphy—perfusion deficit in caudodorsal lung field; ventilation scan is often normal.

DIAGNOSTIC PROCEDURES

- Cytology of airway contents collected by transtracheal or endoscopic aspiration or bronchoalveolar lavage—identification of hemosiderophages (i.e., macrophages containing intracytoplasmic hemosiderin) is considered evidence of bleeding into the airways.
- Lung biopsy of the caudodorsal fields—characteristic hemosiderophages in the airspace or interstitial spaces.

PATHOLOGIC FINDINGS

Gross Findings

- Characteristic patchy to multifocal, symmetric, blue-brown to brown staining of the pulmonary parenchyma on the dorsal and diaphragmatic surfaces of the caudodorsal regions of the caudal lung lobe.
- Foci of subpleural scarring within discolored lung regions in association with enhanced subpleural vasculature.

Histopathologic Findings

- Small airway disease—intraluminal debris, hypertrophy of lining cells, or fibrosis
- Pleural and interlobular septa fibrosis
- Interstitial fibrosis
- Hemosiderophage sequestration in airways, airspaces, and interstitium
- Obliteration of small airways

EXERCISE-INDUCED PULMONARY HEMORRHAGE (EIPH)

TREATMENT

APPROPRIATE HEALTH CARE
No known treatment.

NURSING CARE
N/A

ACTIVITY
- Unless performance is impaired, continue athletic activity.
- Periods of rest (30 days to 1 year) help with parenchymal repair but do not prevent subsequent episodes.

DIET
N/A

CLIENT EDUCATION
N/A

SURGICAL CONSIDERATIONS
N/A

MEDICATIONS

DRUGS OF CHOICE
- The most commonly used prerace medication is furosemide (0.25–1 mg/kg). Administration in racing jurisdictions usually is limited to 4 hours prerace; in some states, other regulations guide administration. The dose is sometimes split between IV and IM administration.
- Conjugated estrogen is administered occasionally in the belief that it counters capillary fragility.
- Aspirin
- Small airway disease—systemic antibiotics, bronchodilators, or steroids

CONTRAINDICATIONS
N/A

PRECAUTIONS
Chronic furosemide administration, especially if the horse is dehydrated, may predispose electrolyte disorders.

POSSIBLE INTERACTIONS
N/A

ALTERNATIVE DRUGS
N/A

FOLLOW-UP

PATIENT MONITORING
- Repeat endoscopy examination after subsequent strenuous activities (e.g., training, racing, jumping) provides information on the frequency and severity of the condition.
- If severe bleeding, repeat examination in 24–48 hours to make sure bleeding has stopped; may indicate intercurrent disease.

PREVENTION/AVOIDANCE
N/A

POSSIBLE COMPLICATIONS
N/A

EXPECTED COURSE AND PROGNOSIS
N/A

MISCELLANEOUS

ASSOCIATED CONDITIONS
N/A

AGE-RELATED FACTORS
N/A

ZOONOTIC POTENTIAL
N/A

PREGNANCY
N/A

SYNONYMS
N/A

SEE ALSO
- Ethmoid hematoma
- Guttural pouch mycosis
- Hemorrhagic nasal discharge
- Lower airway disease
- Pleuropneumonia
- Pulmonary abscess

Suggested Reading

Pascoe JR. Exercise-induced pulmonary hemorrhage. In: Robinson NE, ed. Current therapy in equine medicine. 4th ed. Philadelphia: WB Saunders, 1997:441–443.

Pascoe JR. Exercise-induced pulmonary hemorrhage: a unifying concept. Proc Am Assoc Equine Pract 1996;42:220–226.

Author John R. Pascoe

Consulting Editor Jean-Pierre Lavoie

EXPIRATORY DYSPNEA

BASICS

DEFINITION
- A sensation of difficult breathing.
- In animals, *dyspnea* is used to describe clinical signs associated with respiratory distress, which can be present throughout the respiratory cycle or be primarily associated with either inhalation (i.e., inspiratory dyspnea) or exhalation (i.e., expiratory dyspnea).
- The lay term for expiratory dyspnea (i.e., "heaves") describes the abdominal push at end expiration.

PATHOPHYSIOLOGY
- As a primary clinical sign, usually associated with obstruction of the intrathoracic airways by mucus and bronchospasm; to move air from the lung in less time through partially obstructed airways, the horse recruits its abdominal muscles and makes a noticeable, forced abdominal exhalation.
- Can also accompany inspiratory dyspnea in any animal with severe impairment of gas exchange impairment.

SYSTEMS AFFECTED
- Respiratory
- Cardiovascular
- Hemic/lymphatic/immune

SIGNALMENT
Depends on the underlying cause, but usually occurs in mature to old animals.

SIGNS
General Comments
Expiratory dyspnea is a sign, but associated signs can indicate the source of dyspnea.

Historical Findings
- Accompanying inspiratory dyspnea and loud respiratory noises are indicative of a fixed airway obstruction—mass encroaching into the pharynx.
- A preceding or accompanying cough indicates inflammation of the tracheobronchial tree.
- Inflammation of the lower airway can result in bilateral mucopurulent nasal discharge.
- Unilateral or bilateral nasal discharge, either purulent or hemorrhagic, can be a sign of a nasal or pharyngeal mass causing severe airway obstruction.

Physical Examination Findings
- The condition is indicated by flared nostrils, increased excursions of the thorax during breathing, and a forced abdominal component to expiration, which becomes particularly obvious at end exhalation.
- The horse may rock forward during the abdominal effort.
- Careful observation reveals that the rib cage collapses rapidly at the start of exhalation and that the abdominal component is more prolonged.
- The abdominal effort raises intra-abdominal pressure and this leads to bulging of the anus.
- Fixed airway obstruction—nasal discharge, foul breath, and both inspiratory and expiratory dyspnea.
- Bronchitis/bronchiolitis—cough, wheezing audible at the nares, increased breath sounds on both inhalation and exhalation, and expiratory wheezes may be particularly evident; however, fever is unusual without a viral or bacterial cause.

CAUSES
Respiratory Causes
- Extrathoracic airway—congestion of the nasal mucosa (e.g., Horner's syndrome, inflammatory disease), deviation of the nasal septum, space-occupying lesion affecting the nasal cavity (e.g., foreign body, intraluminal mass, ethmoid hematoma, extraluminal mass or swelling), congenital pharyngeal cysts, space-occupying masses encroaching on the pharynx (e.g., enlarged lymph nodes, guttural pouch enlargement [usually by tympanites]), deformity of the larynx (e.g., edema, epiglottiditis, chondritis), and tracheal obstruction caused by trauma, masses, or foreign body
- Lower respiratory tract—severe bronchiolitis or heaves; infiltrative disease of the alveolar interstitium

Nonrespiratory Causes
See *Inspiratory Dyspnea.*

RISK FACTORS
See the individual conditions causing expiratory dyspnea.

DIAGNOSIS

DIFFERENTIAL DIAGNOSIS
Differentiating Similar Signs
- Inspiratory dyspnea is characterized by an enhanced thoracic component to inhalation.
- Tachypnea (i.e., a rapid breathing in response to severe heat stress) is not accompanied by prolonged exhalation.
- Deep breathing after strenuous exercise has a marked inspiratory and expiratory component.

Differentiating Causes
- Fixed upper airway obstructions produce severe respiratory distress on both inhalation and exhalation and are accompanied by loud respiratory noise.
- Fever, malaise, and inappetence indicate infectious inflammatory disease.
- Expiratory dyspnea of gradual onset, precipitated by an environmental cause and accompanied by cough in an afebrile mature horse, is indicative of heaves (also known as recurrent airway obstruction and COPD).
- Expiratory dyspnea of sudden onset in a febrile young horse is indicative of infectious bronchiolitis.
- Once a fixed upper airway obstruction is ruled out, heaves is the most likely cause of expiratory dyspnea.

CBC/BIOCHEMISTRY/URINALYSIS
Depends on causes.

OTHER LABORATORY TESTS
- With fixed airway obstruction, arterial blood gas analysis identifies hypoventilation (i.e., increased $PaCO_2$) and hypoxemia (i.e., low PaO_2), with the increase in $PaCO_2$ being almost equal to the decrease in PaO_2.
- Bronchitis/bronchiolitis usually is accompanied by obvious hypoxemia (i.e., $PaO_2 < 80$ torr), with only a slightly elevated $PaCO_2$ (i.e., 45–50 torr).

IMAGING
Radiography
- May identify a mass causing a fixed obstruction in the nose, pharynx, larynx, or trachea.
- Bronchitis/bronchiolitis does not produce diagnostic radiographic signs.
- Diffuse interstitial alveolar disease may be observed as a diffuse increase in density, with or without a miliary pattern.

Endoscopy
- Essential for diagnosing a fixed airway obstruction.
- Can be used to assess the presence of mucopurulent exudate in the trachea, which is a sign of inflammation of the lower airways and lung.

DIAGNOSTIC PROCEDURES
- Cytology of the lower airways, preferably by bronchoalveolar lavage, can be used to determine the presence of lower airway inflammation.
- Bacterial culture of tracheal mucus or tracheal lavage revealing a relatively pure culture of a known pathogen is suggestive of infection.

EXPIRATORY DYSPNEA

TREATMENT

APPROPRIATE HEALTH CARE

Maintain ventilation and gas exchange.

NURSING CARE

- Supplemental oxygenation via a nasotracheal or nasopharyngeal catheter relieves hypoxemia and accompanying distress when dyspnea results from lung disease.
- With fixed airway obstruction, oxygen can be life-saving until the problem is surgically corrected.
- Heaves—move horse to a low-dust environment.

ACTIVITY

N/A

DIET

Heaves—use low-dust feed.

CLIENT EDUCATION

N/A

SURGICAL CONSIDERATIONS

- Relieve a fixed upper airway obstruction sufficient to cause panic or life-threatening hypoxemia (indicated by cyanosis) by tracheotomy.
- Nasotracheal intubation also can be used to bypass the obstruction, especially if it is to be corrected surgically within a short time.
- Tracheotomy is not useful for relief of expiratory dyspnea originating in the lower airway.

MEDICATIONS

DRUGS OF CHOICE

- Depend on cause of the dyspnea.
- Heaves—dilate airways with a bronchodilator, and relieve inflammation with corticosteroids (see *Heaves*). Atropine (0.02 mg/kg IV) provides almost immediate relief from dyspnea; other bronchodilators, either oral (e.g., clenbuterol [0.8–3.2 mg/kg BID]) or inhaled (e.g., ipratropium bromide [2–3 μg/kg], albuterol [1–2 μg/kg], feneterol [2–3 μg/kg]) should be used for maintenance.

CONTRAINDICATIONS

N/A

PRECAUTIONS

N/A

POSSIBLE INTERACTIONS

N/A

ALTERNATIVE DRUGS

N/A

FOLLOW UP

PATIENT MONITORING

Heaves is a chronic problem that recurs whenever horses are exposed to the dusts and antigens that initiate the hypersensitivity response.

PREVENTION/AVOIDANCE

N/A

POSSIBLE COMPLICATIONS

N/A

EXPECTED COURSE AND PROGNOSIS

N/A

MISCELLANEOUS

ASSOCIATED CONDITIONS

N/A

AGE-RELATED FACTORS

N/A

ZOONOTIC POTENTIAL

N/A

PREGNANCY

Fetal growth retardation and fetal death may be observed in mares with severely compromised respiratory function.

SYNONYMS

N/A

SEE ALSO

- Aspiration pneumonia
- Diaphragmatic hernia
- Fungal pneumonia
- Heaves
- Inspiratory dyspnea
- Pleuropneumonia
- Pneumothorax
- Respiratory distress syndrome

ABBREVIATION

COPD = chronic obstructive pulmonary disease

Suggested Reading

Ames TR, Hmidouch A. Pathophysiology and diagnosis of respiratory disease. In: Kobluk CN, Ames TR, Geor RJ, eds. The horse: diseases and clinical management. Philadelphia: WB Saunders, 1995:199–212.

Hannas CM, Derksen FJ. Principles of emergency respiratory therapy. In: Colahan PT, Mayhew IG, Merritt AM, Moore JM, eds. Equine medicine and surgery. 4th ed. Goleta: American Veterinary Publications, 1991;1:372–374.

Lavoie J-P. Chronic obstructive pulmonary disease. In: Robinson NE, ed. Current therapy in equine medicine. 4th ed. Philadelphia: WB Saunders, 1997:431–435.

Author N. Edward Robinson

Consulting Editor Jean-Pierre Lavoie

EXUDATIVE OPTIC NEURITIS

BASICS

OVERVIEW
The optic discs are swollen with large whitish raised nodular masses spread across the surface of the optic disc. Retinal and optic disc hemorrhages may also be present.

SIGNALMENT
Occurs most often in older horses.

SIGNS
- Sudden onset of total blindness in bilateral cases.
- Dilated pupils.

CAUSES AND RISK FACTORS
- Trauma
- Acute, massive hemorrhage

DIAGNOSIS

DIFFERENTIAL DIAGNOSIS
- Blindness due to cataracts
- Equine recurrent uveitis (ERU)
- Retinal detachment
- CNS disease

CBC/BIOCHEMISTRY/URINALYSIS
N/A

OTHER LABORATORY TESTS
N/A

IMAGING
N/A

DIAGNOSTIC PROCEDURES
Diagnosed by characteristic funduscopic appearance.

TREATMENT
N/A

EXUDATIVE OPTIC NEURITIS

MEDICATION

DRUG(S) OF CHOICE

No known therapy.

CONTRAINDICATIONS/POSSIBLE INTERACTIONS

N/A

FOLLOW-UP

EXPECTED COURSE AND PROGNOSIS

Poor prognosis.

MISCELLANEOUS

ASSOCIATED CONDITIONS

Dependent on cause.

AGE-RELATED FACTORS

Occurs most often in older horses.

SEE ALSO

- Traumatic optic neuropathy
- Ischemic optic neuropathy
- Retinal detachment
- Equine recurrent uveitis (ERU)

ABBREVIATIONS

N/A

Suggested Reading

Brooks D.E., Equine ophthalmology, In: Kirk N. Gelatt, Veterinary ophthalmology, 3rd ed. Chapter 30, 1999. Philadelphia: Lippincott Williams & Wilkins.

Author Maria Källberg
Consulting Editor Dennis E. Brooks

EYELID DISEASES

BASICS

OVERVIEW

• A variety of conditions lead to abnormal function of the upper and lower eyelids, predisposing the globe to secondary diseases—conjunctivitis and keratitis
• Major categories—congenital, inflammatory, neoplastic, and traumatic; manifestation of each type depends on age, environment, duration and progression of problem, and previous treatment.
• Regardless of the cause, all types disrupt normal functions of the equine eyelids—to provide the lipid part of the tear film, to distribute the tear film across the cornea, to protect the globe from excessive exposure to UV light, and to serve as an external barrier against foreign material in the external orbit.
• Blinking should occur ≅5–25 times per minute; keratitis may be secondary to a primary blinking disorder.
• Organ systems—ophthalmic and skin

SIGNALMENT

• Eyelid melanomas are found in gray horses, with Arabians and Percherons at increased risk; entropion is predominantly found in young foals.
• Equine papillomas are common in immature horses.
• Median age in one report of ocular lymphoma was 11 years (range, 4 months to 21 years).
• Arabians may inherit juvenile Arabian leukoderma; the mechanisms are unknown.

SIGNS

• Vary according to disease process
• Acute or chronic—owners may not notice a change in the eyelids until the disease is advanced; however, trauma, usually is recognized acutely.
• Blepharospasm
• Epiphora
• Conjunctivitis
• Keratitis—acutely ulcerative and edematous, or chronic, pigmentary, and vascularized, possibly due to sicca; a mixed form also is recognized.
• Rubbing at the eye
• Blepharedema
• Periocular discharge, ranging from frank blood if traumatic to purulent or serosanguinous if inflammatory or neoplastic
• Asymmetry of the eyelids (comparing OD to OS and upper to lower) can result from raised firm or soft masses, erosive blepharitis, or overt trauma.
• Lack of palpebral reflex may stem from a neurogenic disorder or trauma.

CAUSES AND RISK FACTORS

• Entropion—an inward rolling of the eyelid margin that can be a primary problem in foals or secondary to dehydration or emaciation (e.g., "downer foals"). Previous eyelid damage that left scarring may lead to a cicatricial entropion. Acquired or blepharospastic entropion is a secondary condition resulting from chronic irritation and pain, causing spasms of the orbicularis oculi muscle. Entropion has multiple causes; therefore, the pathophysiologies of each clinical presentation must be identified.
• Some foals have eyelid abnormalities identified at birth. Microphthalmos causes a related macropalpebral fissure and, often, secondary entropion requiring intervention. Dermoids (i.e., choristomas) are aggregates of skin tissue aberrantly located within adnexal tissue, conjunctiva, and cornea, and they have been reported in the eyelids of foals. Eyelid colobomas are focal to diffuse areas of eyelid agedness leading to exposure keratitis. Faulty induction of the surface ectoderm by defective or absent neuroectoderm most likely is the cause of some of these congenital anomalies.
• Blepharitis (i.e., inflammation of the eyelids) has multiple causes—viral, fungal, parasitic, allergic, and immune-mediated.
• Traumatic blepharitis can develop into eyelid abscesses and may be associated with orbital fractures, penetrating and lacerating trauma, subpalpebral lavage system irritation, and bony sequestra.
• *Trichophyton* or *Microsporum* sp. cause blepharitis, as do *Histoplasma farciminosum* and *Cryptococcus mirandi.*
• Equine papillomas from a papovavirus cause a focal eyelid inflammation in immature horses.
• *Demodex* infestation may lead to lid alopecia, meibomianitis, and papulopustular blepharitis.
• *Thelazia lacrimalis* is a spirurid nematode and commensal parasite of the equine conjunctival fornices and nasolacrimal ducts that can cause diffuse blepharitis.
• Habronemiasis, a common cause of granulomatous blepharitis, occurs mainly during the summer months, when house- and stableflies serve as vectors. Dying microfilaria in the eyelids, conjunctiva, lacrimal caruncle, medial canthus, and nictitans are thought to incite a immune-mediated hypersensitivity.
• Fly-bite blepharitis, dermatophilus, and staphylococcal folliculitis are other causes of blepharitis, especially in young foals.
• Juvenile Arabian leukoderma (i.e., "pinky" syndrome) is a cutaneous depigmentation condition affecting 6–24-month-old Arabians and may present as several cycles of depigmentation and repigmentation.
• Allergic blepharitis, eosinophilic granuloma with collagen degeneration, pemphigus foliaceus and bullous pemphigoid, solar blepharitis of nonpigmented skin, and St. John's wort photosensitization of the lids also are reported.
• Topical chemical toxicities also can cause a caustic blepharitis.
• Eyelid lacerations are common. Upper eyelid damage is more significant, because the upper lid moves over more of the cornea than the lower lid does. Medial canthal lid trauma can involve the nasolacrimal system.
• Eyelid tumors other than squamous cell carcinoma and sarcoids include, but are not limited to, melanoma and lymphoma.

DIAGNOSIS

DIFFERENTIAL DIAGNOSIS

• Many conformational eyelid diseases are confirmed on clinical presentation and successful outcome of medical or surgical intervention. Careful examination of the eyelids and eye is essential to proper management of diseases such as entropion and microphthalmos.
• Inflammation and neoplasia can look very similar on presentation; documenting an accurate history and performing other diagnostic tests provide information and guide the choice of direct therapeutic efforts.
• Often, blepharitis is nonspecific and may mask a specific infection, parasitism, or neoplasia.
• Habronemiasis may mimic mastocytomas, nodular necrobiosis, or fungal granulomas.

CBC/BIOCHEMISTRY/URINALYSIS

Usually normal, unless there is systemic involvement.

OTHER LABORATORY TESTS

• Cytology of tissue aspirates or impressions
• Microbial culture and sensitivity if fungal or bacterial infection is suspected.
• Biopsy if neoplasia is a primary differential.

IMAGING

N/A

DIAGNOSTIC PROCEDURES

• Complete ophthalmic examination for suspected congenital lesions.
• Instillation of topical anesthesia (proparacaine) differentiates blepharospastic entropion from other causes.
• Look under the nictitans and in conjunctival fornices for signs of tumor, parasites, or foreign bodies.
• Flush the nasolacrimal duct if obstruction is suspected.
• Stain any painful eye with fluorescein.

EYELID DISEASES

PATHOLOGIC FINDINGS

Range from simple blepharitis with neutrophilic (septic or nonseptic), lymphocytic/plasmacytic, or eosinophilic infiltrates to specific descriptions of differentiated tumors.

TREATMENT

• Most eyelid diseases are treated on an outpatient basis. More severe infections may require more intensive topical or systemic therapy but can be managed by most owners/trainers. Periodic rechecks every few weeks initially are advised with tumors and severe eyelid malformations.
• If the pathology impairs vision or a protective eye covering must be worn, restrict activity to the horse's ability to navigate safely until the visual impairment resolves.
• No specific change in diet is necessary, but keep dust and debris to a minimum by feeding hay at ground level.
• If caught early, most eyelid diseases are amenable to treatment. Medication may be give two to four times per day for inflammatory causes. During treatment, a protective eye covering may be worn to keep dirt out, to prevent further self-trauma from rubbing, and to protect any sutures that may be present.
• Young foals with entropion can have temporary tacking sutures placed in a vertical mattress pattern (4-0 silk) 2–3 mm from the eyelid margin at the affected areas. They also can receive surgical staples in the affected areas until the causative mechanism has resolved. Old foals and adult horses with entropion can receive permanent reconstructive surgeries (e.g., Hotz-Celsus procedure).
• Blepharoplastic measures may be necessary in horses with primary anatomic entropion, eyelid colobomas, or severe eyelid trauma.
• Lid trauma must be corrected as soon as possible to prevent undesirable scarring and secondary corneal desiccation and ulceration.
• Papillomas may regress spontaneously or require surgery, cryotherapy, or autogenous vaccination.

MEDICATIONS

DRUGS

• With exposure keratitis or conjunctivitis, supplemental lubrication in the form of artificial tears or ophthalmic antibiotic ointment is recommended until the problem is corrected.
• With eyelid swelling from acute trauma, ophthalmic antibiotic/steroid combinations may be indicated. Therapy for severe, chronic, or aggressive bacterial blepharitis should be directed by the results of culture and sensitivity.
• Intralesional steroid injections (triamcinolone [10–40 mg]) may be effective against granulomatous diseases stemming from habronemiasis; systemic ivermectin (200 mg/kg PO) is indicated for demodex and habronemiasis.
• Topical therapy for solitary, focal habronema lesions consists of a topical mixture of 135 g of nitrofurazone ointment, 30 mL of 90% DMSO, 30 mL of 0.2% dexamethasone, and 30 mL of a 12.3% oral trichlorphon solution and is applied two to three times daily to the affected areas.
• Topical 2% miconazole or thiabendazole is effective against eyelid ringworm, whereas systemic antifungals are effective against *Histoplasma* and *Cryptococcus* sp.
• Consult a current formulary for alternatives to all types of topical medications.

CONTRAINDICATIONS/POSSIBLE INTERACTIONS

• As in all cases involving ulcerative keratitis, all steroid preparations are contraindicated.
• Antifungal drugs, antiparasitic drugs, and chemotherapy may be irritating to the local tissues; if a drug hypersensitivity is suspected, discontinue the drug temporarily and then restart with caution if necessary.
• Many topical skin antibiotic preparations can be highly irritating to the cornea; prevent ocular exposure to these drugs

FOLLOW-UP

PATIENT MONITORING

Careful monitoring of the response to therapy is critical in managing eyelid diseases, because the correct diagnosis may not be evident initially and ocular health depends on normal eyelid function.

PREVENTION/AVOIDANCE

• A clean, dust-free environment eliminates the likelihood of irritant or allergic blepharitis; however, allergies to common barn items (e.g., wood shavings) and certain types of hay are not uncommon.
• Fly repellants or insecticide strips reduce the incidence of fly-strike blepharitis.

POSSIBLE COMPLICATIONS

Loss of eyelid tissue or extreme postsurgical scarring can be extremely detrimental to corneal health and, without correction, may lead to severe keratitis and loss of vision.

EXPECTED COURSE AND PROGNOSIS

• Eyelids have a tremendous blood supply and heal readily when treated appropriately. Because this tissue is also highly mobile, sutures in the eyelids may be left for 3 to 4 weeks to ensure proper wound healing.
• Most eyelid tumors are locally invasive and will not metastasize if treated appropriately.
• Certain types of tumors, if left unchecked, are invasive and destroy adnexal tissue and the globe.

MISCELLANEOUS

ASSOCIATED CONDITIONS

• Conjunctivitis
• Nasolacrimal disease
• Nictitans disease

AGE-RELATED FACTORS

Horses with a difficult temperament or who are untrained (i.e., foals and yearlings) may be more likely to suffer eyelid trauma.

ZOONOTIC POTENTIAL

PREGNANCY

• Systemic absorption of topical medication is possible.
• General anesthesia versus sedation and local akinesia always must be contemplated in cases of eyelid surgery in pregnant mares.

SEE ALSO

• Conjunctival diseases
• Disorders of the neonate
• Keratopathies
• Nasolacrimal disease
• Ocular neoplasia

ABBREVIATIONS

• DMSO = dimethyl sulfoxide
• OD = oculus dexter
• OS = oculus sinister

Suggested Reading

Brooks DE. Equine ophthalmology. In: Gelatt KN, ed. Veterinary ophthalmology. 3rd ed. Philadelphia: Lippincott Williams & Wilkins, 1999.

Author Daniel Biros
Consulting Editor Dennis E. Brooks

FAILURE OF PASSIVE TRANSFER (FPT)

BASICS

DEFINITION

• Inadequate absorption of maternal immunoglobulins from colostrum by foals during the first 24 hours of life
• Complete FPT transfer in an 18–24-hour-old foal—serum or plasma IgG concentration <200 mg/dL
• Partial FPT—IgG concentration of 200–800 mg/dL
• Optimal passive transfer—IgG concentration >800 mg/dL

PATHOPHYSIOLOGY

• Because of diffuse epithelial chorial placentation in mares, immunoglobulins do not cross the placenta during gestation.
• Foal are born immunologically competent but naïve and dependent on absorption of immunoglobulins in colostrum.
• Immunoglobulins are concentrated by selective secretion in the mare's udder during the last 2 weeks of gestation.
• Specialized epithelial cells in the foal's small intestine pass macromolecules via pinocytosis into local lacteals and, subsequently, into the blood.
• Protein absorption is nonselective; any large molecules in the intestine are absorbed.
• Specialized epithelial cells are present at birth and are sloughed and replaced by nonspecialized intestinal epithelial cells; thus, the absorption process is both time and use dependent.
• Maximal absorption occurs after birth, decreases in efficiency by 12 hours, and is gone by 24 hours.
• Immunoglobulin composition of colostrum—primarily IgG and IgG(T), with smaller amounts of IgA and IgM; colostrum also contains factors such as cytokines, complement, and lactoferrin, which are important in up-regulation of the foal's immune system and which provide local protection to the gastrointestinal tract.
• Because of the foal's dependence on absorption of colostrum for a fully functional immune system, foals without adequate passive transfer are at increased risk for infectious disease and death.
• FPT has been reported to occur in 3–24% of otherwise normal Thoroughbreds, Standardbreds and Arabians in the United States, United Kingdom, and Australia.

SYSTEMS AFFECTED

• Hemic/lymphatic/immune—foals with FPT have low antibody levels and, thus, a higher risk of infection.
• The most common disease process associated with FPT is sepsis. Most septicemic foals have FPT, but not all FPT foals are septic, just at higher risk of developing sepsis.

SIGNALMENT

• All neonatal foals may be affected.
• Management practices that include observation of time to stand and nurse help to minimize the probability of FPT; however, inadequate quality or quantity of colostrum still may result in FPT.

SIGNS

No outward signs

HISTORICAL FINDINGS

• Foals born to mares >15 years are at increased risk.
• Because colostrum is produced only once, premature lactation may diminish the quantity of colostrum in the udder.
• Mares kept on endophyte-infected tall fescue pasture or hay may be agalactic.
• Failure, for any reason, of the foal to stand and nurse within 3–6 hours after birth may result in adequate amounts of immunoglobulin absorption.

Physical Examination Findings

• Affected foals are clinically normal unless they become infected.
• Many foals with partial FPT kept in optimal conditions do not become sick.

CAUSES

• Colostrum may not be produced in sufficient quantity, may be lost by premature lactation, or may contain insufficient amounts of immunoglobulins.
• Colostrum with a specific gravity <1.060 (as measured with a colostrometer; Equine Colostrometer, Jorgensen Laboratories, Loveland, CO; Gamma-Check-C, Veterinary Dynamics, San Luis Obispo, CA) is associated with FPT.
• Failure of the foal to nurse by 3–6 hours after birth is associated with complete or partial FPT; foals that fail to nurse by 12 hours usually have complete FPT.

RISK FACTORS

• Illness or chronic debilitating disease in the mare during gestation, mares >15 years, and mares with poor mothering behavior have an increased incidence of affected foals.
• Foals born in cold, overcast climates have an increased incidence compared to foals born in climates with more total solar radiation.
• Premature foals and foals with prolonged gestation (especially when associated with endophyte-infected fescue grass or hay) are at increased risk.
• Any foal that is weak or otherwise poorly adapted to extrauterine life, such that the time to first suckle is >3 hours, is more likely to be affected.

DIAGNOSIS

DIFFERENTIAL DIAGNOSIS

• Affected foals may be clinically normal.
• Evaluate foals with sepsis or other medical conditions (e.g., hypoxic ischemic encephalopathy, limb deformities preventing normal gait) for FPT.

CBC/BIOCHEMISTRY/URINALYSIS

Total plasma or serum protein concentration cannot be used to establish the diagnosis, because consistent correlation between foal protein and immunoglobulin concentration does not occur; however, one study found foals with total protein <4.7 g/dL at 18 hours or older were most likely to have partial or complete FPT.

OTHER LABORATORY TESTS

• The most accurate method to determine IgG concentration is the single radial immunodiffusion test (Equine RID kits, VMRD, Pullman, WA), which requires 5–24 hours to complete; thus, other, more rapid semiquantitative field tests are more commonly used.
• An ELISA kit (CITE Foal IgG Test Kit, IDEXX Laboratories, Westbrook, ME) uses serum, plasma, or whole blood and provides semiquantitative measurement of IgG that correlates well with SRID. Results are obtained in 10–15 minutes.
• The zinc sulfate turbidity test (Equi-Z, VMRD, Pullman, WA) measures total immunoglobulins based on formation of a precipitate of zinc ions and immunoglobulins. The test takes 1 hour and, in certain conditions, may overestimate the concentration of immunoglobulins.
• The gluteraldehyde clot test (Gamma-Check-E, Veterinary Dynamics, San Luis Obispo, CA) is based on formation of a clot from interaction of the glutaraldehyde with immunoglobulin.
• The latex agglutination test (Foalcheck, Centaur, Overland Park, KS) estimates the amount of IgG from the degree of agglutination of serum or blood with latex beads coated with anti-equine IgG antibody.
• Serum IgG is detectable at 6 hours of age in foals that nursed by 2 hours; however, maximal concentrations are not reached until 18–24 hours.

FAILURE OF PASSIVE TRANSFER (FPT)

TREATMENT

• If FPT is diagnosed during the first 12 hours after birth, oral administration of colostrum with a specific gravity >1.060 is the preferred treatment. In foals with complete FPT, 2–4 L of colostrum administered in 500-mL increments every 1–2 hours during the first 6–8 hours of life is desirable.
• In foals >12 hours, adequate absorption for optimal IgG concentrations is unlikely. If equine colostrum is not available, bovine colostrum may be safely used; however, immunoglobulins in bovine colostrum are catabolized faster and do not have specificity for equine pathogens.
• Concentrated equine serum and lyophilized or other concentrated equine immunoglobulins are available; however, results with these products are variable and generally not sufficient in foals with complete FPT.
• If colostrum is not available or in foals >12 hours, administer IV plasma or serum. Fresh plasma may be harvested from the mare or another horse with neither lysins nor agglutinins to equine RBC antigens. Alternatively, frozen plasma may be obtained from commercial sources (Veterinary Dynamics, San Luis Obispo, CA; Lake Immunogenics, Ontario, NY). Generally, a 45-kg, well foal with complete FPT requires two to four 900-mL bags of normal plasma for optimal IgG concentrations. In foals with partial FPT, 1–2 bags usually are sufficient. Some frozen plasma products may have higher IgG amounts (more concentrated), thus decreasing the total volume needed. Septic foals have much reduced half-life of exogenous IgG and, thus, may need multiple transfusions to maintain serum concentrations. Repeated IgG testing after each bag of plasma helps to determine the amount needed to raise IgG to acceptable levels.
• Concentrated serum (Endoserum, Immvac, Columbia, MO; Seramune, Sera, Shawnee Mission, KS) also may be used; however, serum does not contain complement and other components augmenting the neonatal immune system.
• Administer IV plasma through an in-line filter. Thaw frozen plasma slowly in a water bath at 39–45°C (102–113°F), and warm to at least 20°C before administration. The initial plasma or serum infusion should be slow and the foal observed for adverse reactions. Subsequently, the infusion may be given at 20–30 mL/kg per hour.

MEDICATIONS

DRUGS OF CHOICE

N/A

CONTRAINDICATIONS

• No contraindications to commercially available, fresh-frozen plasma.
• Use of fresh plasma from horses with agglutinins or lysins to equine RBC carries a risk for neonatal isoerythrolysis.

PRECAUTIONS

• Frozen plasma thawed at too high a temperature contains denatured proteins that subsequently may cause vasomotor reactions during administration, characterized by tachypnea, tachycardia, pyrexia, muscle fasciculations, blanching of the mucous membranes, and in severe cases, marked hypotension. Serum products made from multiple donors may contain heterologous protein aggregates that also produce such reactions.
• If adverse reactions occur during administration of plasma or serum products, discontinue the infusion until signs abate, and then continue the infusion at a slower rate. If adverse reactions continue, terminate the infusion.
• Pretreatment of foals with flunixin (0.5–1.1 mg/kg) before infusion may decrease adverse reactions, however, this strategy should not be a substitute for proper handling of frozen plasma.

POSSIBLE INTERACTIONS

N/A

ALTERNATIVE DRUGS

N/A

FOLLOW UP

PATIENT MONITORING

• Marked reductions in the immediate posttransfusion IgG concentration occur within 24 hours of administration.
• In septic patients, the serum half-life of exogenous IgG may be half that in patients treated prophylactically. Thus, determination of serum IgG concentration should be repeated after 5–7 days in foals treated prophylactically and more frequently in septic foals.

POSSIBLE COMPLICATIONS

• Exogenous IgG may be redistributed to extravascular sites, complexes may be formed with pre-existing antigens, denatured IgG may be cleared, and a change in the catabolic rate or destruction of IgG may occur, particularly in foals that are sick or receiving inadequate nutrition.
• Rapid continuous loss of exogenous IgG occurs during the first 3–7 days, such that 30–60% of the immediate posttransfusion concentration is reached by day 7.

MISCELLANEOUS

ASSOCIATED DISEASES

Neonatal sepsis

AGE-RELATED FACTORS

N/A

ZOONOTIC POTENTIAL

N/A

SEE ALSO

Neonatal septicemia

ABBREVIATIONS

• ELISA = enzyme-linked immunoadsorbent assay
• SRID =

Suggested Reading

Hines MT. Immunodeficiencies of foals. In: Robinson NE, ed. Current therapy in equine medicine 4. 1997:581–584.

McClure JJ. Failure of passive transfer. In: Smith BP, ed. Large animal internal medicine. St. Louis: Mosby, 1996:1847–1850.

Morris DD. Disorders of the immune system. In: Reed SM, Bayly WM, eds. Equine internal medicine. Philadelphia: WB Saunders, 1998:47–50.

Author Susan L. White
Consulting Editor Mary Rose Paradis

FEARS AND PHOBIAS

BASICS

DEFINITION

Fear

• An emotion of alarm and agitation caused by real or perceived danger and manifested by physiologic responses (e.g., tachycardia, trembling, elimination) and by behavioral responses (e.g., escape, immobility, defensiveness).

• Among horses, which evolved as prey in open habitat, escape behavior is the most common response to fearful stimuli and occurs as a reaction to the presence or proximity of an object, individual, or social situation.

• Horses that exhibit excessive fear or reactivity are often termed *flighty* or *spooky* by riders.

Phobia

• A psychiatric term applied to animals for a marked, persistent, and excessive fear of clearly discernible, circumscribed objects or situations.

• Exposure to a phobic stimulus almost invariably provokes an immediate fear response, which may take the form of a situationally bound or predisposed panic attack, including escape behavior or defensive aggression.

• Often leads to avoidance behavior.

PATHOPHYSIOLOGY

• In an evolutionary sense, detection by horses of unusual features in the environment (e.g., movement of a predator) followed by an avoidance reaction (e.g., running away) has been an effective strategy to ensure survival and reproductive success. Horses are anatomically and socially adapted as prey to detect and escape potential dangers. Though domesticated for thousands of years, a process that selectively has bred animals with attenuated fear responses, some ancestral characteristics remain, including heritable (i.e., genetic) tendencies to exhibit fears and phobias. The degree and method of handling by humans also can impact the expression of fears and phobias; over time, with consistent handling, horses habituate to common stimuli and learn acceptable responses to novel stimuli.

• When evaluating an individual animal, medical explanations of fearful behavior must be considered, particularly in horses showing an acute change in their behavior or with concomitant neurological abnormalities. Infectious conditions (e.g., rabies, tetanus, equine protozoal myelitis) or toxin exposure can cause animals to exhibit extreme, hyperreactive responses. Ophthalmic conditions (e.g., ERU) may cause horses to be particularly reactive to light or motion.

SYSTEMS AFFECTED

• Behavioral—pacing, attempts to escape restraint or confinement, inattentiveness during training, inadequate performance, or aggression to handlers

• Cardiovascular—tachycardia

• Respiratory—tachypnea or frequent snorting when exposed to fearful stimulus

• GI—inappetance or altered eating habits and increased defecation rate when fearful

• Endocrine/metabolic—increased metabolic rates and altered cortisol levels

• Musculoskeletal—traumatic injuries during escape attempts or restraint

SIGNALMENT

• Any age, sex, or breed, though more common in young animals, animals without positive experiences with humans, and animals of certain breeds, particularly those used for racing (i.e., escape behavior).

• Individual differences in reactivity or tendency to respond to novel stimuli by attempting to flee.

SIGNS

Historical Findings

• Vary according to the situation and reactivity of the particular horse.

• Signs indicative of a fearful response include head-up alert behavior, orientation toward the stimulus, and stiff-legged stance.

• Early handling and experience of the horse with humans and its learned associations with other horses strongly influence its reactivity level.

Physical Examination Findings

• Usually unremarkable, though horses in chronic fearful states may exhibit a low body score caused by decreased appetite or elevated metabolic rate.

• Signs of trauma may be evident secondary to attempts at escaping fearful situations.

• Very fearful horses may be difficult to examine, attempting escape or defensive/aggressive behavior when restrained; the presence of a familiar, tractable horse may be helpful.

• The veterinarian's success may be enhanced by moving slowly and avoiding jerky movement; allowing the horse time to sniff and visually inspect a new person (e.g., the veterinarian) also may help.

CAUSES

• Fearfulness is part of normal equine behavior and strongly influenced by breed, sex, early socialization history, handling, associations with conspecifics, and other variables.

• Phobic behavior, though rare, can be a manifestation of an organic condition; in all horses, medical causes of fears and phobias must be ruled out before seeking a behavioral explanation.

RISK FACTORS

• Horses that were poorly socialized as juveniles to humans and their activities

• Mismanagement, abuse, and inadequate training

• Excessive arousal or frustration

DIAGNOSIS

DIFFERENTIAL DIAGNOSIS

Identify pathologic conditions associated with fears and phobias before seeking a purely behavioral diagnosis—infectious conditions (e.g., rabies, tetanus, equine protozoal myelitis), toxins, CNS neoplasias or vascular accidents, ophthalmic conditions (e.g., ERU), and other sources of pain or tactile sensitivity.

CBC/BIOCHEMISTRY/URINALYSIS

- Usually normal
- Abnormalities may suggest metabolic or endocrine explanations.

OTHER LABORATORY TESTS

May be indicated to rule out medical explanations.

IMAGING

- May be indicated to identify sources of pain.
- CT or MR imaging if congenital abnormalities or cerebral neoplasia are suspected

DIAGNOSTIC PROCEDURES

Postmortem fluorescent antibody test for any fearfully aggressive horse in which rabies is a differential diagnosis

TREATMENT

RISK ASSESSMENT

- The importance of risk assessment in cases of equine fears and phobias cannot be overemphasized and, therefore, is considered a separate procedure to be performed before treatment is initiated.
- Risk analysis consists of historical information, observation of the animal, and supporting medical and legal data. The goal is to prevent human injury, to reduce the client's and veterinarian's liability risk, and to establish a management plan.
- The situation is considered high risk if the horse has displayed fear aggression (e.g., kicking, biting, lunging) when approached or handled, especially if the horse has caused injury to humans in the past.
- The adequacy of management and experience by the owner should be considered.
- "Flighty" horses that unpredictably exhibit fearful behavior (e.g., bolting) and horses that exhibit fear-motivated aggression can be dangerous and should be handled only by experienced personnel. Because of the heritable nature of these behaviors, such horses should not be bred.
- To prevent human injury and extensive self-trauma, consider euthanasia for high-risk cases in which all other treatment options have failed.

CASE MANAGEMENT

- First tenet—prevent human injury. Make specific suggestions to the owner regarding management and control of the horse to eliminate that animal's contact with individuals who are not familiar with safe and humane horse handling. Referral to an experienced behaviorist or trainer may be advised.
- Second tenet—prevent the horse from injuring itself. Extreme fear reactions or phobic behavior can cause a horse to run through fences or to batter itself against a fixed barrier during an escape attempt. Particularly when in a fearful state, horses cannot successfully explore and detect indirect routes of escape; therefore, they may repeatedly attempt a direct path through a sturdy barrier or narrow opening instead of seeking an alternate route.
- Horses in a chronic, high-fear state or that experience repeated phobic attacks suffer from a high level of stress. Particularly if isolated, chronically stressed horses may eat or drink poorly or exhibit stereotypic behaviors. Wild mustangs transported for long distances have died from the acidosis and dehydration associated with such a state. Thus, fears and phobias may need to be addressed as a welfare issue.
- Management success combines multiple treatment modalities—surgery, environmental control, behavior modification, and pharmacotherapy. Stallions that display fear aggression should be altered to prevent their genetic representation in the next generation and to facilitate their handling. In some cases, castration has a beneficial behavioral effect, decreasing aggression toward humans.

ENVIRONMENTAL CONTROL

- Use adequate barriers and restraint to prevent human and self-induced injury.
- Visual barriers may protect phobic horses from constant visual stimuli.
- Use well-fitting, sturdy halters and other necessary restraint devices.

BEHAVIOR MODIFICATION

- Do not punish fearful behavior; this might teach the horse that its fear is justified.
- Based on history and observations, list all situations in which the horse appears fearful or exhibits such behavior. Align these situations along a continuum from most to least fearful. Initially, avoid all these situations. Teach the horse basic obedience commands (e.g., whoa, come along), and reinforce these as control exercises under nonfearful conditions. Reward the horse for being calm and obedient with food treats, tactile massage in favored areas, or the release of constant pressure (e.g., from a lip chain or rein). Precede each reward with a kind word (e.g., good boy) that, eventually, can become a conditioned reinforcer. Practice these control exercises in a range of environmental conditions so the horse generalizes the learning to different locations and situations. Initially, a second, nonfearful horse may be used for social facilitation of the desired behavior.

FEARS AND PHOBIAS

• Next, begin to expose the horse to the least fearful stimulus on the continuum when practicing control exercises. The goal is to expose the horse to mildly fearful situations while in a nonfearful state. If the horse exhibits fearful behavior during training, do not punish but firmly insist on and reward an alternate behavior that is incompatible with a fearful response. For example, a horse that shies at paper on the ground should be turned away from the fearful stimulus and rewarded for performing a trained behavior (e.g., turning in a circle). It may be necessary to reduce the intensity of the fearful stimulus by moving it farther away and only gradually moving it closer.
• Recent techniques popularized by professional horse trainers, dubbed *horse whisperers*, use their keen observation of the horse, patience, and knowledge of equine communication to "tame" fearful horses. Such techniques avoid the confrontational and often abusive techniques previously used to "break" horses. Practitioners of these techniques usually work with individual horses in social isolation, and they commonly use a high-fenced pen to prevent the horse's escape and to focus its attention on the trainer. The practitioners are adept at shaping behavior using subtle positive and negative reinforcement as well as "learned helplessness" to produce calm, tractable horses with reduced fearful or phobic behavior.

MEDICATIONS

DRUGS OF CHOICE

• Generally, drugs are not necessary for treatment. Systematic counter-conditioning and desensitization paired with effective handling techniques reduce fearful responses; however, medication sometimes may help to decrease arousal or anxiety and, thus, to facilitate learning and safe handling.
• No drugs are approved by the FDA for treatment of fearful or phobic behavior in horses. Inform the client regarding the experimental nature of these treatments and the risk involved, and document discussion in the medical record.

Azaperones

Buspirone hydrochloride (100–250 mg/day PO)—blocks serotonin-1A receptors; side effects can include GI signs and personality changes.

Tricyclic Antidepressants

Imipramine hydrochloride (500–1000 mg PO q12h)—serotonin and norepinephrine reuptake inhibitor; side effects can include sedation and anticholinergic effects.

CONTRAINDICATIONS

Tricyclic antidepressants are contraindicated in patients with cardiac conduction disturbances, glaucoma, and fecal or urinary retention.

PRECAUTIONS

No clinical trials have been performed on these extralabel drugs; our knowledge is based on evidence from other species and anecdotal information from a few, individual cases.

POSSIBLE INTERACTIONS

• The drugs listed should not be used with monoamine oxidase inhibitors, including the drugs amitraz and deprenyl.
• Cimetidine may decrease tricyclic antidepressant clearance.
• With concurrent use of tricyclic antidepressants, absorption of phenylbutazone may be delayed to the extent that it becomes inactivated in the stomach.

ALTERNATIVE DRUGS

• Tranquilizers (e.g., phenothiazine acepromazine) and synthetic hormones (e.g., the synthetic progestin altrenogest) have been used for their behavioral effects, but they do not directly decrease anxiety or fear.
• Oral tryptophan, a serotonin precursor, is purported to have calming effects, but one controlled study showed no such clinical response.
• The Rauwolfia alkaloid reserpine and the phenothiazine fluphenazine have been used to reduce responsiveness but are not recommended because of potentially adverse side effects.

FEARS AND PHOBIAS

FOLLOW-UP

PATIENT MONITORING
• Weekly to biweekly contact during the initial phases.
• Clients frequently need feedback and assistance with behavior modification plans and medication management.

POSSIBLE COMPLICATIONS
Human injury caused by the a horse exhibiting fear-motivated or phobic behavior.

MISCELLANEOUS

ASSOCIATED CONDITIONS
N/A

AGE-RELATED FACTORS
• Fear-motivated behavior problems are common in young horses with little training.
• Adult- or acute-onset fear-motivated behavior, particularly in previously well-handled animals, suggests a medical cause; evaluate sources of pain and sensory acuity carefully.

ZOONOTIC POTENTIAL
Rabies is a potential cause of fearful behavior or fear-motivated aggression.

PREGNANCY
Chronic use of tricyclic antidepressants is contraindicated in pregnant animals and breeding stallions.

SYNONYMS
N/A

SEE ALSO
N/A

ABBREVIATIONS
• ERU = equine recurrent uveitis
• GI = gastrointestinal
• MR = magnetic resonance

Suggested Reading

Bagshaw CS, Ralston SL, Fisher H. Behavioral and physiological effect of orally administered tryptophan on horses subjected to acute isolation stress. Appl Anim Behav Sci 1994;40:1–12.
Brewer BD, Hines MT, Stewart JT. Fluphenazine induced parkinson-like syndrome in a horse. Equine Vet J 1990;22:136–137.
Budiansky S. The nature of horses: exploring equine evolution, intelligence, and behavior. New York: Simon and Schuster, 1997.
Crowell-Davis SL. Normal behavior and behavioral problems. In: Kobluk CN, Ames TR, Geor RJ, eds. The horse: diseases and clinical management. Philadelphia: WB Saunders, 1995:1–21.
Fraser AF. The behaviour of the horse. Wallingford, UK: CAB International, 1992.
Houpt KA. Domestic animal behavior for veterinarians and animal scientists. 3rd ed. Ames, IA: Iowa State University Press, 1998.
McDonnell SM. Pharmacological aids to behavior modification in horses. Proceedings of the Equine Clinical Behavior Symposium. Swiss Federation for Equine Medicine. Basel, Switzerland, June 1996.
Voith VL. Principles of learning. Vet Clin North Am Equine Pract 1986;2:485–506.

Author Barbara Sherman Simpson
Consulting Editor Daniel Q. Estep

FECAL, CYTOLOGY

BASICS

DEFINITION

The presence of more than the occasional leukocyte (>2 cells per 10 LPF) identified on a stained fecal smear.

PATHOPHYSIOLOGY

- Normally, only a few leukocytes can be found in feces.
- Pathologic processes of the intestinal mucosa attract inflammatory cells.
- If leukocytes are readily identified in the fecal smear, the source likely is the colon, because cells from further proximal in the digestive tract degenerate before being expelled in feces.
- Presence of neutrophils indicates inflammation and damage to the mucosa.
- Epithelial cells can be seen in feces from some normal horses, but their numbers may increase with invasive diseases of the colon.
- Failure to find leukocytes in feces does not eliminate the possibility of any invasive disease, because the test has poor sensitivity. Finding these cells, however, does predict some invasive process of the colon.

SYSTEM AFFECTED

GI damage is the cause, not the effect, of fecal leukocytes.

SIGNALMENT

N/A

SIGNS

- Clinical signs vary, depending on cause of the colon disease.
- Diarrhea, blood in feces, fever, and tenesmus

CAUSES

- Salmonellosis—usually neutrophils, if any cells are present.
- Acute necrotizing colitis, without *Salmonella* sp. being isolated.
- Clostridial infections of the colon—*Clostridium difficile, C. perfringens,* and others.
- Granulomatous colitis—macrophages may be present in feces.
- Ulcerative eosinophilic gastroenteritis—if the colon is involved, eosinophils may be found in feces.
- Cyanthostomiasis—small strongyle larvae embedded in the colon mucosa; mixed inflammatory cells.
- Right dorsal colitis
- Infiltrative lymphosarcoma of the colon mucosa—lymphocytes may be present.
- Colitis X
- Rectal tear.
- Other causes of colitis.

RISK FACTORS

GI parasitism, high doses of phenylbutazone, stress, and other diseases or surgery

DIAGNOSIS

DIFFERENTIAL DIAGNOSIS

- Leukocytes more often are found with acute diarrhea; if a large portion of the colon is involved, diarrhea usually is present.
- Feces with putrid odors may indicate salmonellosis.
- Blood is present in some cases of salmonellosis, acute necrotizing colitis, clostridial infections, and rectal tears.

LABORATORY FINDINGS

- Fecal leukocytes decompose and are not recognized after 3–4 days at 4°C (faster at room temperature), so perform the examination on fresh feces.
- Results are valid if run in a human lab.

CBC/BIOCHEMISTRY/URINALYSIS

- Leukopenia often is present with salmonellosis and acute necrotizing colitis.
- Hyponatremia also may be present with salmonellosis.
- A metabolic acidosis, manifested by low tCO_2, is a complication of acute diarrheal diseases.
- Low serum albumin indicates a protein-losing enteropathy (e.g., granulomatous colitis, eosinophilic gastroenteritis, lymphangiectasia, salmonellosis) once dehydration is corrected.
- Elevated BUN and creatinine could be prerenal azotemia, resulting from dehydration in acute diarrheal diseases.

OTHER LABORATORY TESTS

Fecal occult blood may be detected in salmonellosis, acute necrotizing colitis, clostridial infections, right dorsal colitis, and rectal tears.

IMAGING

N/A

DIAGNOSTIC PROCEDURES

- Rectal biopsy may be useful in detecting the cause of colon inflammation.
- Granulomatous colitis, eosinophilic colitis, cyanthostomiasis, and sometimes, salmonellosis can be detected in as many as 50% of rectal biopsy specimens from horses with diarrhea and fecal leukocytes.
- Repeated fecal cultures may reveal *Salmonella* sp. or *Clostridia* sp.

FECAL, CYTOLOGY

TREATMENT

• Leukocytes in feces are not harmful.
• The cause of the colon inflammation must be treated.
• IV fluids are needed in dehydrated horses with acute diarrhea.

MEDICATIONS

DRUGS OF CHOICE

• Medications vary, depending on the cause of colon inflammation.
• Metabolic acidosis may need to be corrected with bicarbonate.
• Inflammatory bowel diseases can, at times, be improved with corticosteroids.

CONTRAINDICATIONS

• Do not use high doses of NSAIDs if right dorsal colitis is suspected.
• Avoid drugs that irritate the intestinal mucosa.
• Corticosteroids in cases of acute colitis.

PRECAUTIONS

N/A

POSSIBLE INTERACTIONS

N/A

ALTERNATIVE DRUGS

N/A

FOLLOW-UP

PATIENT MONITORING

• Check fecal consistency and volume at each passage.
• Check fecal leukocytes and occult blood again in 2–3 days.
• Dehydration, acid–base, and serum protein status of the patient are more important than the presence of cells in feces.

POSSIBLE COMPLICATIONS

N/A

MISCELLANEOUS

ASSOCIATED CONDITIONS

N/A

AGE-RELATED FACTORS

N/A

ZOONOTIC POTENTIAL

Salmonellosis

PREGNANCY

N/A

SYNONYMS

N/A

SEE ALSO

• Diarrhea
• Fecal occult blood
• Fecal solute gap

ABBREVIATIONS

• GI = gastrointestinal
• LPF = low-power field

Suggested Reading

Deem Morris D, Whitlock RH, Palmer J. Fecal leukocytes and epithelial cells in horses with diarrhea. Cornell Vet 1983;73:265–274.

Jiang ZD, Smith MA, Kelsey KE, et al. Effect of storage time and temperature on fecal leukocytes and occult blood in the evaluation of travelers' diarrhea. J Travel Med 1994;1:184–186.

Merrit AM, Bolton JR, Cimprich R. Differential diagnosis of diarrhea in horses over six months of age. J S Afr Vet Assoc 1975;46:73–76.

Author Erwin G. Pearson
Consulting Editor Claire B. Andreasen

FECAL, ELECTROLYTES

BASICS

DEFINITION

• Measurement of electrolyte concentrations and feces osmolality could help to rule out certain diseases in cases of diarrhea—fecal solute gap, Na:K ratio, and in foals, pH may be the most useful determinations.
• Solute gap is determined by subtracting 2 × the concentration of sodium plus potassium from the osmolality; this gives an estimate of the unmeasured osmotic material in the feces.
• Na:K ratio is the concentration of sodium divided by the concentration of potassium in feces.
• Fecal pH changes after passage of feces because of continued bacterial action; thus, it is useful only in fresh feces of foals.

PATHOPHYSIOLOGY

• The equine colon helps to maintain fluid, electrolyte, and acid–base homeostasis.
• The healthy colon can absorb against an osmotic, or electrochemical, gradient. It also exchanges considerable amounts of HCO_3 in the blood with chlorine in the lumen, so the VFA produced by bacterial fermentation in the colon can be neutralized.
• The normal colon has a reserve capacity of at least fourfold to absorb excess water and solute entering from the ileum. Therefore, feces of normal horses can contain a wide range of osmolalities and electrolyte concentrations.
• The diseased colon may not be able to control fluxes of sodium and potassium to maintain homeostasis, so excretion may be inappropriate.
• With secretory diarrheas, excessive amounts of sodium, the predominant extracellular anion, are lost in the feces.
• With protein-losing enteropathies and other colon mucosal diseases, an increased amount of protein or unabsorbed but digested nutrients may be lost in feces, contributing to its osmolality.

SYSTEM AFFECTED

Gastrointestinal

SIGNALMENT

N/A

SIGNS

Diarrhea usually is present if fecal electrolyte concentrations are determined.

CAUSES

• High solute gap (>30 mEq/L)—granulomatous colitis, eosinophilic gastroenteritis, diffuse intestinal lymphosarcoma, cyanthostomiasis, overfeeding of grain, other protein-losing enteropathy, lymphangiectasia, and osmotic cathartic administration
• Low solute gap (<30 mEq/L)—salmonellosis, endotoxemia, foal heat diarrhea, and other secretory diarrheas
• High Na:K ratio (>2.0)—normal horse with high sodium load, salmonellosis, endotoxemia, peritonitis, ileal disease with bile acid–induced sodium secretion, idiopathic colitis, foal heat diarrhea, and other secretory diarrheas
• Low Na:K ratio (<1.0)—normal horse with deficient sodium, hypovolemic shock with conservation of sodium, granulomatous colitis, eosinophilic gastroenteritis, cyanthostomiasis, and chronic parasitism
• Low pH (<6.5) in foals—possible malabsorption, maldigestion, rotavirus, or cryptosporidia
• High pH (>7.5) in foals—possible secretory or foal heat diarrhea

RISK FACTORS

• Unless diarrhea is present, consider electrolyte variation to be physiologic.
• Cathartic administration (e.g., $MgSO_4$, Na_2SO_4) changes solute gap.
• Antacid administration (e.g., $Mg[OH]_2$, $NaHCO_3$, $Al[OH]_2$) changes pH and solute gap.
• Anorexia may increase the Na:K ratio because of the lack of potassium intake.
• Delay in examining feces may result in altered pH and osmolality because of continued fermentation.

DIAGNOSIS

DIFFERENTIAL DIAGNOSIS

• Chronic diarrhea with weight loss more likely is an inflammatory bowel disease—granulomatous colitis or cyanthostomiasis
• Acute diarrhea more likely is salmonellosis, equine monocytic ehrlichiosis, or clostridial disease.

LABORATORY FINDINGS

• Measuring the osmolality of some samples by freezing-point reduction may be impossible, because the fecal sample may not freeze.
• Results probably are valid if run in a human lab.

CBC/BIOCHEMISTRY/URINALYSIS

• Neutropenia may be present with salmonellosis.
• Low serum albumin might indicate a protein-losing enteropathy in cases of diarrhea with high solute gap.
• Low serum sodium concentration and high Na:K ratio indicate inadequate sodium absorption or retention by the colon.
• Low serum potassium concentration and low Na:K ratio could indicate lack of dietary potassium intake or need to conserve sodium in cases of osmotic diarrhea.

OTHER LABORATORY TESTS

• Absorption tests could incriminate small intestinal absorption along with colon disease.
• Other tests appropriate to differentiate causes of diarrhea

IMAGING

N/A

DIAGNOSTIC PROCEDURES

Rectal biopsy is useful in detecting some colon and rectal diseases—granulomatous colitis, eosinophilic gastroenteritis, cyanthostomiasis, and salmonellosis

FECAL, ELECTROLYTES

TREATMENT

- Direct treatment toward cause of the diarrhea.
- Alterations in the solute gap or Na:K ratio may be physiologic to maintain homeostasis in the normal horse and do not need treatment.

MEDICATIONS

DRUGS OF CHOICE

Medications used to treat the disease causing diarrhea and to replace lost fluids and electrolytes.

CONTRAINDICATIONS

N/A

PRECAUTIONS

N/A

POSSIBLE INTERACTIONS

N/A

ALTERNATIVE DRUGS

N/A

FOLLOW-UP

PATIENT MONITORING

Once treatment begins, it will be difficult to interpret fecal electrolyte changes, so repeated analyses may not be helpful.

POSSIBLE COMPLICATIONS

N/A

MISCELLANEOUS

ASSOCIATED CONDITIONS

N/A

AGE-RELATED FACTORS

The colon in foals may not be developed enough to absorb ingesta as efficiently as that in adults, so fecal changes could reflect small intestinal as well as colon diseases.

ZOONOTIC POTENTIAL

Salmonellosis

PREGNANCY

N/A

SYNONYMS

N/A

ABBREVIATIONS

VFA = volatile fatty acids

Suggested Reading

Argenzio RA, Stevens CE. Cyclic changes in ionic composition of digesta in the equine intestinal tract. Am J Physiol 1975;228:1224–1230.

Argenzio RA, Whipp SC. Pathophysiology of diarrhea. In: Anderson NV, ed. Veterinary gastroenterology. Philadelphia: Lea & Febiger, 1980:229–231.

Field M, Rao MC, Chang EB. Intestinal electrolyte transport and diarrheal disease. N Engl J Med 1989;321:800–806,879–893.

Masri MD, Merrit AM, Gronwall R, Burrows CF. Faecal composition in foal heat diarrhoea. Equine Vet J 1986;18:303–306.

Pearson EG. Interpretation of fecal chemistries and fecal occult blood. Proc Am Coll Vet Intern Med 1986;4:10,61–10,64.

Author Erwin G. Pearson

Consulting Editor Claire B. Andreasen

FECAL, OCCULT BLOOD

BASICS

DEFINITION

Detection of any amount of blood in feces using standard chemical (i.e., guaiac) tests (e.g., Hemoccult II-TM, which tests for peroxidase activity of intact hemoglobin) or tests for the porphyrin ring (e.g., HemoQuant).

PATHOPHYSIOLOGY

- Fecal occult blood is detected by chemical tests that react to the peroxidase activity of intact hemoglobin. Feces is added to a pad containing benzidine dye, which turns blue when oxidized by hemoglobin and hydrogen peroxide. Degraded hemoglobin does not react to these tests, so false-negative results can occur.
- A newer test used in humans is the HemoQuant, which detects the porphyrin ring remaining from degraded hemoglobin. Thus, it is more sensitive, but it is not commonly used with horses.
- Minute amounts of intact hemoglobin react to either test.
- Swallowed blood or hemorrhage from any portion of the GI tract react to the test if the amount is sufficient to leave some hemoglobin intact when it is expelled in the feces.
- Microorganisms in the cecum and colon readily degrade most of the hemoglobin, so only 4–7% of blood from the stomach reaches the feces intact.
- It takes $\cong$100 mL of blood in the stomach of an average-size horse to be detected in feces by peroxidase dye tests.
- Blood in the stomach does not appear until at least 12 hours. The peak amount occurs at $\cong$18 hours, and it is not detected after 42 hours unless hemorrhaging persists.
- Hemorrhage more distal in the GI tract takes less time to be expelled and to produce positive results on fecal occult blood tests.
- Much less blood is needed to react if hemorrhage is from the distal colon.

SYSTEMS AFFECTED

- GI
- Respiratory
- Hemic/lymphatic/immune

SIGNALMENT

Foals are more likely to have gastric ulcers that bleed.

SIGNS

- Listless
- Weakness
- Colic
- Diarrhea
- Pale mucus membranes
- Cough
- Hemoptysis
- Epistaxis

CAUSES

- Iatrogenic—nasal gastric tube, rectal examination, GI surgery, enterotomy, and phenylbutazone toxicity
- GI—gastric ulcers, stomach bots (*Gastrophilus* sp.), duodenal ulcers, right dorsal colitis, salmonellosis, clostridial infections, colon ulceration, intussusception, intestinal torsion, GI neoplasia, and polyps in the colon
- Respiratory—epistaxis, ruptured abscess in airways, guttural pouch mycosis, and neoplasia with swallowed blood
- Bleeding disorders—DIC, moldy sweet-clover poisoning, and thrombocytopenia
- Toxicity—cantharides (i.e., blister beetle), arsenic, lead, oak, and acorn

RISK FACTORS

- Stress, surgery, or diarrhea may increase the prevalence of gastric ulcers.
- Overdosing with NSAIDs may cause ulcerations throughout the GI tract.
- Diets containing GI irritants may induce hemorrhage.
- Rectal examinations and nasal gastric intubation can lead to detectable blood in feces.

DIAGNOSIS

DIFFERENTIAL DIAGNOSIS

- Colic with bruxism and gastric reflux are common in cases of gastric ulcers.
- Diarrhea may be present with salmonellosis, clostridial infections, and arsenic poisoning.
- Signs of renal failure (e.g., polydipsia/polyuria) may be present with phenylbutazone or cantharides toxicities.
- Colic with distended bowel might be seen with intussusception and intestinal torsion.
- Coughing, dyspnea, or abnormal lung sounds could indicate hemorrhage from the respiratory system, with swallowed blood.
- Epistaxis caused by trauma, ethmoid hematomas, guttural pouch mycosis, and many other conditions lead to swallowed blood that could be detected on fecal occult blood tests.

LABORATORY FINDINGS

- Oral medications with peroxidase activity could alter results and cause false positives.
- Sufficient amounts of meat or blood meal in the diet could cause false positives.
- Delayed analysis at high temperatures could lead to false negatives because of hemoglobin degradation.
- Results are valid if run in a human lab.

CBC/BIOCHEMISTRY/URINALYSIS

- Low hematocrit and hemoglobin level could indicate extensive hemorrhage.
- Low protein and hematocrit indicate recent hemorrhage.
- Neutropenia often is present with salmonellosis.
- Thrombocytopenia might be the cause of a coagulation disorder leading to GI hemorrhage.
- Azotemia could indicate concurrent renal damage that would occur with phenylbutazone toxicity.
- Nonspecific enzymes often are elevated with neoplasia.

FECAL, OCCULT BLOOD

OTHER LABORATORY TESTS

- A coagulation panel detects a bleeding disorder.
- Elevated fibrin degradation products (>40 μg/mL) indicate DIC.
- Bone marrow cytology could verify a regenerative anemia.
- Fecal culture could detect salmonellosis or clostridial infections.

IMAGING

Not applicable, unless upper respiratory signs are present.

DIAGNOSTIC PROCEDURES

- Stomach endoscopy to look for gastric ulcers.
- Respiratory tract endoscopy could locate sources of swallowed blood.

TREATMENT

- Treat the condition causing the hemorrhage.
- Blood in feces is not harmful in itself.

MEDICATIONS

DRUGS OF CHOICE

N/A

CONTRAINDICATIONS

N/A

PRECAUTIONS

N/A

POSSIBLE INTERACTIONS

N/A

ALTERNATIVE DRUGS

N/A

FOLLOW-UP

PATIENT MONITORING

- Monitoring the erythron and estimating the total blood loss are more important than monitoring the amount or presence of blood in feces.
- If the hemorrhage has stopped, blood will not be detected after 42 hours, so repeating fecal occult blood tests after 2 days may be helpful.

POSSIBLE COMPLICATIONS

- Severe anemia
- Perforating ulcers
- Dehydration
- Hypoproteinemia

MISCELLANEOUS

ASSOCIATED CONDITIONS

- Diarrhea
- Epistaxis or hemoptysis
- Hemorrhage at other locations

AGE-RELATED FACTORS

Stressed foals may be prone to gastric ulcers.

ZOONOTIC POTENTIAL

N/A

PREGNANCY

N/A

SYNONYMS

N/A

SEE ALSO

- Coagulation disorders
- Colitis
- Fecal leukocytes
- Gastric ulcers

ABBREVIATIONS

- DIC = disseminated intravascular coagulation
- GI = gastrointestinal

Suggested Reading

Ahlquist DA, McGill DB, Schwartz S, et al. Fecal blood levels in health and disease. N Engl J Med 1985;312:1422–1428.

Markman HD. Errors in the guaiac test for occult blood. J Am Vet Med Assoc 1967;202:846–847.

Pearson EG, Smith BB, McKim JM. Fecal blood determinations and interpretations. Proc Am Assoc Equine Pract 1987;33:77–83.

Simon JB. Fecal occult blood testing: clinical value and limitations. Gastroenterologist 1998;6:66–78.

Author Erwin G. Pearson

Consulting Editor Claire B. Andreasen

FECAL, PARASITE EGGS

BASICS

DEFINITION

• Negative results on fecal egg counts do not rule out parasites, because the prepatent period is long for some and because others (cyanthostomes) may be in an arrested stage.
• High fecal egg counts prove that adult nematodes are in the GI tract and that disease is likely to occur.
• Some counts (EPG) and their meanings to consider:

	Strongyle	Ascarids in foals
Possible migrating larvae	0	0
Needs anthelmintic	200–500	1–200
Disease likely	>1000	>200

PATHOPHYSIOLOGY

• Identifying a parasite egg in feces indicates an adult of that species is present and laying eggs.
• Most nematode eggs float in a hypertonic solution and are detected in feces in that manner.
• Failure to find eggs does not eliminate the possibility of infection. Embryonated eggs or infective larvae must be ingested, and larvae must molt through several stages before becoming a mature, egg-producing adult parasite.
• Many larvae migrate through other tissues before ending in the gut lumen, where they can lay eggs.
• Some small strongyle go through a hypobiotic stage, during which they are embedded in the intestinal mucosa. In this phase, they can cause damage and disease (i.e., cyanthostomiasis), but no eggs are produced. When they emerge into the intestinal lumen and become adults, they begin producing eggs that can be detected in feces.
• The fecundity varies among species of intestinal nematodes. Some strongyle females produce only a few dozen eggs/day, whereas ascarids and small strongyle may produce >100,000 eggs/day, with great daily variability. This makes interpreting the results of egg counts more difficult, especially if the species of nematode is unknown.

SYSTEM AFFECTED

GI

SIGNALMENT

Young horses may be more susceptible to GI parasites than old ones, especially if they have not been previously exposed.

SIGNS

• Unthriftiness or weight loss
• Diarrhea
• Colic

CAUSES

• *Strongylus vulgaris*—prepatent period, 6 months; fecundity, <small strongyle
• *S. edentatus*—prepatent period, 9 months; fecundity, <small strongyle
• *S. equinus*—prepatent period, 11 months; fecundity, <small strongyle
• Small strongyle—prepatent period, 6–8 weeks; fecundity, usually 95% of fecal eggs
• *Habronema* sp.—prepatent period, 10 weeks
• *Parascaris* sp.—prepatent period, 10–14 weeks; fecundity, >100,000 eggs/day per female
• *Anoplocephala* sp.—
• *Oxyuris* sp.—prepatent period, 5 months

RISK FACTORS

Overstocking pastures with horses or feeding off the ground may increase risk of internal parasites and, therefore, of increased fecal egg counts.

DIAGNOSIS

DIFFERENTIAL DIAGNOSIS

• Differentiating parasites usually is not possible on physical examination or by history alone.
• Unthriftiness, diarrhea, or colic may raise suspicion of parasites.
• With colic, *S. vulgaris* may be more likely.
• With chronic diarrhea, cyanthostomiasis from small strongyles embedded in the mucosa is possible.
• Ascarids usually cause unthriftiness and, occasionally, colic from impaction in foals.
• *Oxyuris* sp. can cause tail rubbing.
• Strongyloides, tapeworms, and habronema may not cause clinical signs.

LABORATORY FINDINGS

• Eggs may not be recognized in old fecal samples, or eggs may have hatched to first-stage larvae.
• No correlation between number of eggs and number of nematodes in the gut.
• Eggs are not uniformly distributed in the fecal mass, and number of eggs passed varies daily.
• Animals with watery diarrhea may have diluted eggs and a lower count.
• Improper mixing or weighing of samples gives inaccurate results.
• Results not valid if run in a human lab.

CBC/BIOCHEMISTRY/URINALYSIS

• Serum total protein and albumin concentrations may be low in parasitized horses, and signs of anemia (e.g., low PCV and hemoglobin) may be seen.
• Eosinophilia has been associated with parasitism but is not consistently present.

OTHER LABORATORY TESTS

• Larval cultures by a competent parasitology laboratory using 200–400 g of feces are necessary to differentiate the various species of strongyles.
• β-Globulins may be increased with parasitism.

IMAGING

N/A

DIAGNOSTIC PROCEDURES

• Trial therapy with an effective anthelmintic may help establish the diagnosis of GI parasites if improvement is noted in 2–3 weeks.
• Rectal biopsy could detect cyanthostomiasis.
• Eosinophils in a transtracheal wash indicate parasitic lung disease.

TREATMENT

• With severe clinical debility resulting from parasite burden, whole-blood, plasma, or fluid therapy may be indicated.
• Diet may need alteration to provide adequate protein for replacement and energy for weight gain.
• Prevention by reducing exposure to infective larvae.

FECAL, PARASITE EGGS

MEDICATIONS

DRUGS OF CHOICE

An appropriate anthelmintic may be indicated if a heavy parasite load is suspected.

CONTRAINDICATIONS

Ascarid impactions occasionally are seen after anthelmintic therapy in heavily infected foals, but the ascarids must be removed.

PRECAUTIONS

Some anthelmintics may be toxic to debilitated animals.

POSSIBLE INTERACTIONS

N/A

ALTERNATIVE DRUGS

N/A

FOLLOW-UP

PATIENT MONITORING

- Repeat fecal egg count 1–2 weeks after treatment to evaluate efficacy of the anthelmintic.
- Proper dosing should reduce the herd average egg count by 80%.

POSSIBLE COMPLICATIONS

- Ascarid impaction
- Colic
- Diarrhea
- Unthriftiness

MISCELLANEOUS

ASSOCIATED CONDITIONS

N/A

AGE-RELATED FACTORS

Young animals are more susceptible to parasites.

ZOONOTIC POTENTIAL

N/A

PREGNANCY

Some anthelmintics could be teratogenic or cause abortions.

SYNONYMS

N/A

SEE ALSO

- Ascarids
- Cyanthostomiasis
- Parasites
- Pinworms
- Strongyle

ABBREVIATIONS

- EPG = eggs per gram
- GI = gastrointestinal
- PCV = packed cell volume

Suggested Reading

Uhlinger CA. Parasite control programs. In: Smith BP, ed. Large animal internal medicine. 2nd ed. St Louis: Mosby, 1996:1685–1697.

Uhlinger CA. Uses of fecal egg count data in equine practice. Compend Contin Educ Pract Vet 1993;15:742–748.

Warnick LD. Daily variability of equine fecal strongyle egg counts. Cornell Vet 1992;82:453–463.

Author Erwin G. Pearson

Consulting Editor Claire B. Andreasen

FESCUE TOXICOSIS

BASICS

DEFINITION

• Toxicosis in pregnant mares associated with ingestion of endophyte-infected tall fescue (*Festuca arundinacea* Schreb.) during late gestation.
• The endophyte is a fungus (*Acremonium coenophialum*) that lives in a symbiotic relationship within the intracellular spaces of the plant. A more recently proposed name for the fungus is *Neotyphodium coenophialum*; a former name was *Epichloe typhina*.

PATHOPHYSIOLOGY

• The endophyte produces ergot peptide alkaloids, the most prominent being ergovaline.
• Ergot peptides act as dopamine agonists, binding D_2-dopamine receptors and suppressing prolactin secretion.
• Prolactin affects not only mammary development and milk production but also lipogenesis, immunity, and reproductive hormones.

SYSTEMS AFFECTED

Reproductive system and mammary gland

GENETICS

N/A

INCIDENCE/PREVALENCE

• Tall fescue occupies >35 million acres in the U.S. and is especially prominent in the Southeast.
• Most tall fescue pastures derive from a Kentucky 31 variety released in 1943 that was contaminated by an endophyte; >90% of tall fescue pastures are estimated to contain this endophyte. The ergot peptide alkaloids produced by the endophyte, therefore, are mycotoxins—secondary metabolites of a fungus.
• ≅688,000 horses are maintained on tall fescue pastures.
• One survey indicated that 53% of pregnant mares maintained on fescue pastures were agalactic, 38% had prolonged gestation, and 18% had stillborn or weak foals that died.

SIGNALMENT

Pregnant mares during late gestation, with the last 30 days of pregnancy being the most critical.

SIGNS

General Comments

• Dystocia, prolonged gestation (average, 20–27 days), thickened placenta, and agalactia in mares
• Dysmature foals that are weak or stillborn
• Lower ADG possible in yearlings

Physical Examination Findings

• Typically, mares are 3–4 weeks past their due date.
• Larger-than-normal foal may cause dystocia and be turned 90° in the pelvis.
• The placenta may be thickened enough that the foal has trouble breaking through, and the mare may retain the placenta.
• Foals are large and gangly, with long and fine hair coats, poor muscle mass, overgrown hooves, and nonerupted incisor teeth.
• Foals may be hypothyroid, with signs of inco-ordination and poor suckling reflex.
• Often, mares are agalactic; therefore, foals may suffer from failure of passive transfer of colostral antibodies.

CAUSES AND RISK FACTORS

• Any tall fescue should be considered infected by the endophyte unless the owner has purposely planted an endophyte-free variety.
• Lower percentages of fescue in mixed pastures decrease the severity or likelihood of problems; however, minimal toxic concentrations of ergovaline in endophyte-infected tall fescue have not been determined for horses.

DIAGNOSIS

DIFFERENTIAL DIAGNOSIS

• Other causes of dystocia, placentitis, and dysmature foals.
• Ergot alkaloids associated with ergot sclerotia from *Claviceps purpurea* in small grains or hay can mimic fescue toxicosis.

CBC/BIOCHEMISTRY/URINALYSIS

No major changes are likely, unless a stress leukogram caused by prolonged parturition is present.

OTHER LABORATORY TESTS

• Mares—decreased serum prolactin and progesterone concentrations; increased serum estradiol-17β
• Foals—decreased serum T_3 concentrations

IMAGING

Ultrasonography may show a thickened placenta and large foal.

DIAGNOSTIC PROCEDURES

• Pasture or hay concentrations of ergovaline likely are >200 ppb.
• Endophyte contamination can be checked qualitatively by staining plant tillers at plant pathology laboratories or by ELISA.

PATHOLOGIC FINDINGS

• Thickened, congested, and edematous placenta, with no significant bacterial cultures.
• Edema is most severe in allantochorion at the area of the cervical star.
• The amnion is edematous throughout, and the umbilical cord also may be edematous.
• Placenta may be ruptured in the uterine body rather than the typical location at the cervical star.
• Foals with overgrown hooves and nonerupted incisor teeth.
• An enlarged thyroid in a foal is not apparent grossly but, histopathologically, shows up as large, distended thyroid follicles lined by flat, cuboidal epithelial cells.
• If a mare dies from dystocia, uterine rupture may be present and the mammary gland undeveloped.

FESCUE TOXICOSIS

TREATMENT

APPROPRIATE HEALTH CARE
N/A

NURSING CARE
N/A

ACTIVITY
N/A

DIET
N/A

CLIENT EDUCATION
N/A

SURGICAL CONSIDERATIONS
N/A

MEDICATIONS

DRUGS OF CHOICE
- Oxytocin, uterine infusion of fluids, and possibly, antibiotics/anti-inflammatory drugs for retained placentas
- Stored colostrum, antiserum, or plasma as immunoglobulin sources for foals not receiving enough colostrum.
- Domperidone is an experimental drug that requires an INAD form for use.

CONTRAINDICATIONS
N/A

PRECAUTIONS
N/A

POSSIBLE INTERACTIONS
N/A

ALTERNATIVE DRUGS
N/A

FOLLOW-UP

PATIENT MONITORING
- Monitor serum IgG concentration in foals to assess adequate passive transfer.
- Keep mares away from fescue for $\cong$1 week until lactating well.
- Bottle feeding of milk replacers or a nurse mare may be needed for foals.
- Mares may have rebreeding problems.

PREVENTION/AVOIDANCE
- Prevention is much more feasible than treatment.
- Remove mares from fescue pastures and fescue hay a minimum of 3–4 weeks before their foaling date; some practitioners recommend 6–8 weeks before foaling.
- If removal from fescue pasture is not possible; domperidone, a dopamine-receptor antagonist, can be administered (1.1 mg/kg per day mixed with 0.8 lb of corn, 0.2 lb of molasses, and 1 tbsp of vinegar during the last 30 days of gestation).

POSSIBLE COMPLICATIONS
Dystocia or uterine rupture in mares

EXPECTED COURSE AND PROGNOSIS
Guarded prognosis for dysmature foals

MISCELLANEOUS

ASSOCIATED CONDITIONS
N/A

AGE-RELATED FACTORS
N/A

ZOONOTIC POTENTIAL
N/A

PREGNANCY
See above.

SEE ALSO
- Agalactia
- Dysmaturity
- Ergot alkaloids
- Failure of passive transfer
- Retained placenta

ABBREVIATIONS
- ADG = average daily gain
- ELISA = enzyme-linked immunoadsorbent assay
- INAD = investigational new animal drug
- T_3 = triiodothyronine

Suggested Reading

Boosinger TR, Brendemuehl JP, Bransby DL, et al. Prolonged gestation, decreased triiodothyronine concentration, and thyroid gland histomorphologic features in newborn foals of mares grazing *Acremonium coenophialum*–infected fescue. Am J Vet Res 1995;56:66–69.

Cross DL, Redmond LM, Strickland JR. Equine fescue toxicosis: signs and solutions. J Anim Sci 1995;73:899–908.

Green EM, Loch WE, Messer NT. Maternal and fetal effects of endophyte fungus-infected fescue. Proc Annu Convention Am Assoc Equine Pract 1992;37:29–44.

Putnam MR, Bransby DI, Schumacher J, et al. Effects of the fungal endophyte *Acremonium coenophialum* in fescue on pregnant mares and foal viability. Am J Vet Res 1991;52:2071–2074.

Redmond LM, Cross DL, Strickland JR, et al. Efficacy of domperidone and sulpiride as treatments for fescue toxicosis in horses. Am J Vet Res 1994;55:722–729.

Swerczek TW. Perinatal mortality in foals caused by fescue grass toxicosis. In: Kirkbride CA, ed. Laboratory diagnosis of livestock abortion. 3rd ed. Ames: Iowa State University Press, 1990:214–216.

Author Dennis J. Blodgett

Consulting Editor Robert H. Poppenga

FETAL STRESS/DISTRESS/VIABILITY

BASICS

DEFINITION

Parameters that indicate less-than-ideal conditions for fetal survival (often impaired placental function) that, if they progress, will lead to fetal compromise and eventual demise.

PATHOPHYSIOLOGY

- Maternal systemic disease, fetal abnormalities, and/or placental infection, insufficiency, and separation impede efficient fetal gas exchange and nutrient transfer.
- The fetus responds physiologically (or pathologically) to these alterations in oxygenation and nutrient supply and dies if the impairment is not resolved.
- In some cases, acute fetal stress may cause premature birth of a nonviable foal.

SYSTEM AFFECTED

- Maternal—reproductive
- Fetal—all organ systems

GENETICS

N/A

INCIDENCE/PREVALENCE

Sporadic

SIGNALMENT

- May be nonspecific.
- Thoroughbred or draft mares and related breeds—twins
- Mares older than 15 years
- American Miniature Horse mares

SIGNS

Historical Findings

- Maternal disease during gestation—colic, hyperlipemia, prepubic tendon rupture, uterine torsion, etc.
- Mucoid, hemorrhagic, serosanguinous, or purulent vulvar discharge
- Premature udder development and dripping of milk
- Previous examination indicating placentitis or fetal compromise
- Previous abortion, high-risk pregnancy, or dystocia
- History of delivering a small, dysmature, septicemic, and/or congenitally malformed foal
- Pre-existing maternal disease at conception—laminitis, equine Cushing's-like disease, endometrial inflammation and/or fibrosis

Physical Examination Findings

Maternal and Placental Signs:

- Anorexia, fever, or other signs of concurrent, systemic disease
- Abdominal discomfort
- Mucoid, hemorrhagic, serosanguinous, or purulent vulvar discharge
- Premature udder development and dripping of milk
- Placentitis, placental separation, or hydrops of fetal membranes by transrectal or transabdominal ultrasonography
- Excessive swelling along the ventral midline and evidence of ventral body wall weakening by palpation or transabdominal ultrasonography
- Excessive abdominal distention
- Maternal circulating levels of progestins, estrogens, and relaxin reflect fetal well-being and/or normal placental function.

Fetal Signs

- Fetal hyperactivity or inactivity (concurrent with maternal or placental abnormalities) may suggest a less-than-ideal fetal environment or fetal compromise.
- Can be assessed by visual inspection or transrectal palpation of the mare.
- Transrectal or transabdominal ultrasonography to measure directly some parameters (see *Imaging*)

CAUSES AND RISK FACTORS

Pre-existing Maternal Disease

- Equine Cushing's-like disease
- Chronic, moderate to severe endometrial inflammation and/or fibrosis
- Laminitis

Gestational Maternal Conditions

- Malnutrition
- Colic
- Endotoxemia
- Hyperlipemia
- Prepubic tendon rupture
- Uterine torsion
- Ovarian granulosa cell tumor
- Laminitis
- Musculoskeletal disease
- Equine fescue toxicosis
- Exposure to xenobiotics

Fetal Conditions

- Twins
- Fetal abnormalities—hydrocephalus
- Delayed fetal development—small for gestational age; growth retardation
- Fetal trauma

Placental Conditions

- Placentitis
- Placental insufficiency
- Placental separation
- Hydrops of fetal membranes

DIAGNOSIS

DIFFERENTIAL DIAGNOSIS

- Normal, uncomplicated, pregnancy—an active, normal fetus as assessed by transrectal palpation, transrectal or transabdominal ultrasonography, and various laboratory tests
- See sections for specific maternal, fetal, and placental conditions; historical and physical examination findings suggesting maternal, fetal, or placental disease; and laboratory tests, imaging, and other diagnostic procedures indicating maternal, fetal, or placental disease.

CBC/BIOCHEMISTRY/URINALYSIS

CBC and a serum biochemistry profile may be indicated based on physical examination findings to determine a maternal inflammatory, stress, or left shift (e.g. degenerative, regenerative) leukocyte response or other maternal organ-system involvement that may reflect primary maternal and/or fetal disease.

OTHER LABORATORY TESTS

Maternal Progesterone

- May be indicated when uterofetoplacental unit function is in question.
- After day 100 of gestation, RIA will detect both progesterone (may be very low after day 150) and cross-reacting 5α-pregnanes of uterofetoplacental origin.
- Decreased maternal 5α-pregnanes are seen in cases of equine fescue toxicosis.
- Normal ranges for levels of 5α-pregnanes may vary with gestational stage and by laboratory.

Maternal Estrogens

- Reflection of fetal estrogen production and viability, especially conjugated estrogens—estrone sulfate.
- Normal levels vary by laboratory.

Maternal Relaxin

- Decreases with placental abnormalities.
- Assay is not yet commercially available

FETAL STRESS/DISTRESS/VIABILITY

Allantoic/Amniotic Fluid Analysis

• May become a future means to assess fetal karyotype, pulmonary maturity, and to measure fetal proteins.
• Samples may reveal bacteria, meconium, or inflammatory cells.
• A higher risk technique in horses than in humans, and its utility is not yet established.

IMAGING

General Comments

• Transrectal and transabdominal ultrasonography can be useful in diagnosing twins, assessing fetal stress/distress/viability, monitoring fetal development, evaluating placental health, and diagnosing other gestational abnormalities—hydrops of fetal membranes.
• Confirmation of pregnancy and diagnosis of twins should be performed anytime serious, maternal disease occurs or surgical intervention is considered for a mare bred within the last 11 months.
• Twin pregnancy can be confirmed by identifying two fetuses (easier by transrectal ultrasonography when the mare is <90 days pregnant) or ruled out by a nonpregnant uterine horn (by transabdominal ultrasonography during late gestation).
• Fetal stress/distress/viability can be determined best by transabdominal ultrasonography during late gestation. View fetus in both active and resting states for at least 30 minutes. Note abnormal fetal presentation and position.
• Abnormally high FHR—after activity, >100 bpm; >40 bpm difference between resting and active rates reflects fetal stress rather than distress.
• Abnormal fetal heart rhythm by echocardiography—may occur immediately before, after, and during foaling; also may indicate distress from acute hypoxia.
• Abnormally low FHR—resting, <60 bpm; <50 bpm after day 330 of gestation.
• Bradycardia and absence of heart rate variation with activity indicate CNS depression, probably from acute hypoxia.
• Persistent bradycardia correlates well with poor prognosis for survival.
• Absence of fetal heart beat is a reliable sign of fetal death.
• Absence of fetal breathing movements correlates well with fetal distress.
• Alterations in fetal fluid amounts—normal range for maximal allantoic fluid depth, 4.7–22.1 cm; normal range for maximal amniotic fluid depth, 0.8–14.9 cm; increased amounts reflect hydrops; low amounts indicate fetal distress and longstanding, chronic hypoxia.
• Increased echogenicity of fetal fluids may reflect distress earlier during pregnancy; may be normal during later gestation.

DIAGNOSTIC PROCEDURES

• Fetal ECG has been used to detect twins and to assess fetal viability and distress but largely has been replaced by transabdominal ultrasonography with ECG capabilities.
• Ultrasonographically guided amnio- or allantocentesis—poses some risk to the pregnancy; utility not yet established; some interesting possible future applications.

PATHOLOGIC FINDINGS

N/A

TREATMENT

GENERAL COMMENTS

• Early diagnosis of at-risk pregnancies is essential for successful treatment. The impact of maternal disease on fetal and placental health cannot be underestimated.
• With fetal distress, maintenance of pregnancy (while attempting to treat the cause of fetal compromise) must be balanced with the need to induce parturition (with or without cesarean section) if that becomes necessary to stabilize the mare's health.
• Parturition requires close supervision in cases of fetal stress and distress. The neonatal foal will very likely require intensive treatment.
• Individual circumstances and their sequelae requiring consideration to determine nature and timing of treatment—PE findings; CBC and biochemistry profile results; stage of gestation; nature of maternal disease; hydrops of fetal membranes; evidence of fetal stress, distress, or impending demise; occurrence of complications such as dystocia or RFM; refer to individual topics for treatment recommendations.

APPROPRIATE HEALTH CARE

Monitoring/managing fetal stress/distress, including the prolonged examination times required for complete serial transabdominal fetal assessments, is best performed at a facility prepared to manage high-risk pregnancies, especially if distress is severe and parturition (induction or cesarean section) is imminent.

FETAL STRESS/DISTRESS/VIABILITY

NURSING CARE
Depending on the nature of the maternal disease, fetal distress, and necessity of surgical intervention, intensive nursing care very likely will be required for the neonatal foal and mare.

ACTIVITY
- For most cases, exercise will be somewhat limited and supervised.
- Prepubic tendon rupture, laminitis, and/or fetal hydrops may necessitate complete restriction of exercise.

DIET
Feed the mare an adequate, late-gestational diet with proper levels of energy, protein, vitamins, and minerals, unless contraindicated by concurrent maternal disease.

CLIENT EDUCATION
- Clients should be aware that early diagnosis is essential for fetal survival.
- Predisposing conditions compromising fetal well-being must be corrected and/or managed for a successful outcome.
- Induction of parturition and cesarean section are not without risk to the mare and foal.

SURGICAL CONSIDERATIONS
Cesarean section may be indicated when vaginal delivery is not possible or in dystocias not amenable to resolution by manipulation alone.

MEDICATIONS

DRUGS OF CHOICE
See recommendations in sections for specific conditions—dystocia, prepubic tendon rupture, RFM, hydrops, and so on.

CONTRAINDICATIONS
N/A

PRECAUTIONS
N/A

POSSIBLE INTERACTIONS
N/A

ALTERNATIVE DRUGS
N/A

FOLLOW-UP

PATIENT MONITORING
- Mare and fetus need frequent monitoring until termination of pregnancy.
- Specific monitoring depends on the therapy undertaken, nature of the maternal and/or fetal disease, and complications that may develop.
- Vaginal speculum examination and uterine cytology and culture (as indicated) may be performed 7–10 days after parturition.
- Endometrial biopsy may be indicated as part of the postpartum examination as a prognostic tool for future reproduction.
- Take appropriate therapeutic steps should be taken based on these findings.

PREVENTION/AVOIDANCE
- Early monitoring of mares with a history of fetal stress/distress/viability
- Correction of perineal conformation to prevent placentitis
- Complete breeding records, especially for recognition of double ovulations, early diagnosis of twins (<25 days; ideally, days 14–15), and selective embryonic or fetal reduction
- Management of pre-existing endometritis before breeding
- Removing mares from fescue pasture during last trimester (minimum of 30 days prepartum)
- Avoid breeding or using ET procedures in mares predisposed to producing stressed, distressed, or dead foals.
- Prudent use of medications in pregnant mares
- Avoid exposure to known toxicants.

FETAL STRESS/DISTRESS/VIABILITY

POSSIBLE COMPLICATIONS

- Abortion, dystocia, RFM, endometritis, metritis, laminitis, septicemia, reproductive tract trauma, and impaired fertility affect the mare's well-being and reproductive value.
- Neonatal foals that have been compromised during pregnancy are more likely to be dysmature, septicemic, and subject to angular limb deformities than foals from normal pregnancies.

EXPECTED COURSE AND PROGNOSIS

- Pregnancies in which fetal stress has been diagnosed have a guarded prognosis for successful completion if the predisposing conditions can be treated or managed.
- If evidence of fetal distress continues in the face of treating the mare and fetal viability is a concern, the prognosis for successful completion of gestation is guarded to poor.

MISCELLANEOUS

ASSOCIATED CONDITIONS

- Dystocia
- Endometritis
- Hydrops allantois and amnion
- Metritis
- Placental insufficiency
- Placentitis
- Premature placental separation
- Prepubic tendon rupture
- RFM

AGE-RELATED FACTORS

Generally a greater concern in old mares

ZOONOTIC POTENTIAL

N/A

PREGNANCY

By definition, the condition is associated with pregnancy.

SYNONYMS

- Premature placental passage/separation
- Red bag
- RFM
- Retained placenta

SEE ALSO

- Dystocia
- Embryo transfer
- Endometrial biopsy
- Endometritis
- Hydrops amnion/allantois
- Induction of parturition
- Metritis
- Placental insufficiency
- Placentitis
- Premature placental separation/passage
- Prepubic tendon rupture
- RFM
- Twin pregnancy

ABBREVIATIONS

- ET = embryo transfer
- FHR = fetal heart rate
- PE = physical examination
- RIA = radioimmunoassay
- RFM = retained fetal membranes, retained placenta

Suggested Reading

Adams-Brendemuehl C. Fetal assessment. In: Koterba AM, Drummond WH, Kosch PC, eds.

Equine clinical neonatology. Philadelphia: Lea & Febiger, 1990:16–33.

McGladdery A. Fetal ultrasonography. In: Rantanen NW, McKinnon AO, eds. Equine diagnostic ultrasonography. Baltimore: Williams & Wilkins, 1998:171–180.

Santschi EM. Prepartum conditions In: Robinson NE, ed. Current therapy in equine medicine. 4th ed. Philadelphia: WB Saunders, 1997:541–546.

Sertich PL. Fetal ultrasonography. In: Reef VB, ed. Equine diagnostic ultrasound. Philadelphia: WB Saunders, 1999:425–445.

Author Tim J. Evans

Consulting Editor Carla L. Carleton

FEVER

BASICS

DEFINITION

Fever is an elevation of the core body temperature caused by resetting the hypothalamic thermostat to a point above that at which body temperature is normally maintained. During fever, the mechanisms of heat conservation and heat production are activated in an attempt to increase and keep the body temperature to that new, desired level. Fever must be distinguished from hyperthermia, which occurs when body heat production and absorption are greater than what the body can normally dissipate as can happen during sustained exercise in hot and humid conditions. The normal rectal temperature in adult horses is 37.5–38.5°C (99.5–101.3°F), but can be as high as 39.0°C (102.2°F) in the normal, active foal.

PATHOPHYSIOLOGY

Fever is a clinical sign that can accompany infectious, inflammatory, immunologic, or neoplastic disorders that may have a beneficial role in combating some disease processes. The specific agents that can produce fever are called *exogenous pyrogens* if derived from outside of the host (bacteria, viruses, fungi, antigenic material from a non-microbial source, some drugs) or *endogenous pyrogens* if produced by the host (interleukin-1). These pyrogens apparently change the activity of thermosensitive neurons in the central nervous system (preoptic area of the anterior hypothalamus and midbrain) by increasing the firing rate of cold-sensitive neurons (which drive heat production and conservation effectors) and by decreasing the firing rate of warm-sensitive neurons (which normally drive heat loss effectors). The exact mechanism by which pyrogens alter central neuronal function is not known. Many mediators have been implicated in the mechanism of fever, and the metabolites of arachidonic acid have received most attention. The implication of these metabolites in fever would explain the antipyretic effect of cyclooxygenase inhibitors and their lack of effect on normal temperature or hyperthermic states.

SYSTEMS AFFECTED

All systems can be affected by a disease process that can induce fever. The respiratory and gastrointestinal systems are the most common source of fever in horses.

SIGNALMENT

N/A

SIGNS

Historical Findings

- Inappetance
- Lethargy

Physical Examination Findings

- Hyperthermia
- Tachycardia
- Tachypnea
- Dehydration
- Signs associated with the specific system involved

CAUSES

Infectious Causes*

- Respiratory*—upper respiratory viral disease, strangles (*Streptococcus equi*), pneumonia (viral, bacterial, or fungal), pleuropneumonia, localized abscess.
- Gastrointestinal*—parasitic infection, enteritis of unknown cause, salmonellosis, *Clostridium* enteritis, equine monocytic ehrlichiosis (Potomac horse fever), anterior enteritis, rotaviral diarrhea (foals), peritonitis, intra-abdominal abscess.
- Hepatobiliary—cholangiohepatitis, cholelithiasis, Tyzzer's disease (foals).
- Urogenital—urachal abscess*, metritis*, mastitis, pyelonephritis.
- Neurologic—tetanus, equine encephalomyelitis (flavivirus and alphavirus encephalitis, e.g., EEE, WEE), otitis media/interna, rabies.
- Cardiovascular—thrombophlebitis, endocarditis, pericarditis.
- Musculoskeletal—septic arthritis, tenosynovitis, osteomyelitis, cellulitis, *Clostridium* myositis.
- Miscellaneous/generalized—endotoxemia, septicemia (foals), equine infectious anemia, equine viral arteritis, aspergillosis, candidiasis, brucellosis, tularemia, anthrax, Lyme disease (*Borrelia burgdorferi*), nocardiosis, coccidioidomycosis, babesiosis (pyroplasmosis).

Neoplastic Causes

- Lymphosarcoma*
- Metastatic melanomas*
- Squamous cell carcinoma*
- Fibrosarcoma
- Granulosa cell tumors (mare)
- Undifferentiated reticuloendothelial cell sarcomas
- Adenocarcinomas
- Myeloproliferative disease
- Hemangiosarcoma
- Mesothelioma
- Pheochromocytoma
- Osteosarcoma
- Myeloma of gastrointestinal tract

Immunologic Causes

- Purpura hemorrhagica*
- Urticaria*
- Drug-induced fever
- Immune-mediated hemolytic anemia/thrombocytopenia
- Combined immunodeficiency in foals
- IgM deficiency
- Pemphigus foliaceous
- Chronic necrotizing vasculitis
- Neonatal isoerythrolysis
- Connective tissue disorders
- Rheumatoid arthritis
- Transient agammaglobulinemia in foals
- Bullous pemphigoid

Noninfectious Inflammatory Disorders

- Hepatic disorders—hyperlipidemia/hyperlipemia, equine hepatic lipidosis, acute hepatic necrosis (Theiler's disease), chronic active hepatitis, cholelithiasis.
- Foreign bodies—nasal, oral, pharyngeal, tracheal, bronchial.
- Ocular trauma
- Recurrent uveitis
- Burns
- Smoke inhalation
- Snake bite
- Acute renal failure

Drugs

- Penicillins
- Sulfonamides
- Antihistamines
- Procainamide
- Quinidine
- Amphotericin B
- Cephalosporins
- Cimetidine
- Iodides
- Rifampin
- Levamisole
- Furazolidone
- Chloramphenicol
- Tetracyclines

Toxins
- Blister beetles (cantharidin)
- Selenium
- Arsenic
- Mercury
- Chlorinated hydrocarbons
- Dinitrophenol
- Propylene glycol
- Trichloroethylene extracted feed
- Pyrrolidine alkaloid–containing plant
- Algae
- Castor bean (*Ricenius* spp.)
- Water hemlock (*Cicuta* spp.)
- Jimson weed (*Datura stramonium*)
- Mycotoxicosis

RISK FACTORS
- Immunosuppression
- Recent transportation
- Intense training
- Showing
- Racing

DIAGNOSIS

DIFFERENTIAL DIAGNOSIS
Most fever of unknown origin (FUO) in horses is caused by infectious disease (~43%, compared to ~22% for neoplasia and 6.5% for immune disorders). The majority of horses with FUO are not suffering from unusual disease, but are showing atypical signs of common diseases.

When a horse presents with non-specific signs such as fever, lethargy, and inappetance, the examiner should first try to localize the primary system affected and then try to identify the type of disease process involved. Obtaining a complete history and performing a thorough physical examination are the first and most important steps.

Minimal laboratory data (WBC, differential, fibrinogen, chemistry panel, urinalysis) should always be obtained in horses with FUO. A complete, chronologic history should be obtained and should include information pertaining to the past medical history of the patient; recent change in management, training, or feeding; health status of other horses on the farm; and clinical signs recognized by the owner and their evolution and response to treatment.

A thorough physical examination is absolutely essential and often rewarding, allowing the examiner to identify the primary system involved. The horse should be examined from a distance, at rest, and in motion. All body parts and articulations should be palpated. Careful auscultation of the heart from both sides as well as auscultation of the thorax using a rebreathing bag are always indicated. Oral, ophthalmic, and rectal examination are also often indicated.

CBC/BIOCHEMISTRY/URINALYSIS
The fibrinogen concentration should always be measured in horses because it tends to be a more sensitive indicator of inflammation and infection than the WBC. A blood smear should also always be submitted for cytologic examination. Toxic or non-segmented neutrophils can be present and indicate severe acute inflammation, even when the WBC is normal. It can also be useful in detecting blood-borne parasites. Low-grade anemia accompanied by an increase in total solids is indicative of chronic disease.

Chemistry

Chemistry is sometimes useful to identify the primary organ involved (e.g.: increased GGT in liver disease) or to identify hydroelectrolytic abnormalities that must be addressed while awaiting for a final diagnosis.

Urinalysis

A cheap, noninvasive laboratory test that should routinely be performed. Useful to detect urinary tract infection, neoplasia, or tubular damage.

OTHER LABORATORY TESTS
Direct Coombs' Test

Should be performed when hemolytic anemia is suspected or if RBC agglutination is detected.

Serology

A single titer for equine infectious anemia and brucellosis; paired serums for equine viral arteritis, various mycotic diseases, equine monocytic and granulocytic ehrlichiosis, and babesiosis.

Serum Protein Electrophoresis

Perform when abnormal serum protein level is detected.

Serum Immunoelectrophoresis

Perform when hypo- or hypergammaglobulinemia is detected.

IMAGING
Radiography
- Thorax—to look for evidence of pneumonia, abscesses, masses, metastasis, or pleural effusion.
- Abdomen—sometimes useful in young foals.
- Skeleton—to rule out osteomyelitis, bone tumor, or hypertrophic osteopathy.

Ultrasonography

Always useful to guide for aspiration/biopsy of masses/fluid accumulation.
- Thorax—more sensitive than radiography to detect pleural effusion. Useful to localize consolidation, superficial abscesses and masses.
- Abdomen—to look for fluid accumulation, thickening of the intestine, abnormal masses or abscesses. Allow to visualize both kidneys, the spleen, part of the liver.
- Heart—to detect pericardial effusion/pericarditis, thickening of the valves, endocarditis, vegetative lesions. Indicated in cases of heart murmur or muffled heart sounds.
- Thrombosed vein—to look for evidence of septic foci (abscess) in the thrombus.
- Any abnormal mass—to help in identifying its nature and extent.

DIAGNOSTIC PROCEDURES
Abdominocentesis

Performed when problem can be localized to the gastrointestinal system. Send for WBC, differential, total solid count, and cytologic examination. Allows differentiation among a normal fluid, a transudate, or an exudate. Abnormal, neoplastic cells can sometimes be detected. Send for culture if peritonitis is suspected.

Transtracheal Wash

Performed when pneumonia is suspected; send for culture and cytology, and do a direct Gram stain.

Thoracocentesis

Performed when important pleural effusion is present. Can be diagnostic and therapeutic. Send for culture and cytology.

Synoviocentesis

Performed to rule out septic arthritis. Send for culture (in a blood culture vial), total cell and solid count, and cytologic examination.

Fecal Sample

Perform a routine egg count for parasites. In cases of diarrhea, send for *Salmonella* and *Clostridium* culture and for *Clostridium* toxin isolation. Rotavirus isolation in young foals. Perform an occult blood test.

FEVER

Biopsy
Perform on any mass or suspected diseased organ. Usually safe, especially if ultrasound guided.

Blood Culture
Should always be performed in the sick neonate. Can sometimes be useful in adult with septic thromboplebitis, endocarditis, or FUO.

ECG
Perform to qualify any detected arrhythmia.

Gastrointestinal Absorption Tests
Perform when malabsorption is suspected (chronic weight loss, hypoproteinemia).

Exploratory Laparotomy
Perform in cases of recurrent colic for mass or intestinal biopsies.

Endoscopy
Perform on upper airways, guttural pouches, trachea, esophagus, stomach, duodenum (in foals), bladder, uterus, rectum, and sinuses.

Bone Marrow Aspiration
Perform to document anemia.

CSF Tap
Perform to determine disease of the central nervous system.

TREATMENT
Depends on the cause of the fever. The patient should be stall rested and placed in a comfortable, temperature-regulated environment. Febrile animals are catabolic and have higher energetic requirement, but are often anorectic. They should be offered a small amount of a wide variety of hay and grains frequently. Fresh water should be available, preferably from a bucket so that water consumption can be monitored. A salt block and water containing electrolytes should also be offered. Intravenous or oral fluid supplementation is sometimes necessary. Most horses with FUO require hospitalization in order to complete the thorough work-up necessary and so they can be provided with constant monitoring and care.

MEDICATIONS

DRUG(S) OF CHOICE

Antipyretics/NSAIDS
Antipyretics/NSAIDS (e.g., flunixine meglumine: 1.1 mg/kg, IV or IM) are indicated in cases of dangerously high fever (3°C or 5°F above normal) or when it is judged necessary to improve the patient's comfort and to promote feed and water intake. Fever is, however, thought to enhance the host defenses mechanisms and has been associated with favorable outcome in human medicine. Overzealous anti-inflammatory therapy should be avoided because adverse effects are associated with the use of NSAIDS.

Corticosteroids
Corticosteroids (dexamethasone: 0.05–0.2 mg/kg IV or PO, SID at a decreasing dose) should be used with caution. Their use is indicated in cases of confirmed immune-mediated diseases. However, infectious disease should be ruled out first or use appropriate antibiotics.

Antibiotics
Use of antibiotics is indicated when a bacterial infection has been identified. The clinician should always try to get a sample for cytology, culture, and sensitivity prior to instituting antimicrobial therapy. In cases of acute severe infectious process, broad-spectrum, bactericidal, intravenous antibiotics should be chosen while waiting for culture results (potassium penicillin: 22,000 IU/kg, IV QID and gentamicin sulfate: 6.6 mg/kg, IV, SID). Indiscriminate use of antibiotics should be discouraged because of their potential for inducing severe, fatal enterocolitis and to avoid promoting bacterial resistance.

DRUG(S) OF CHOICE
N/A

CONTRAINDICATIONS
N/A

PRECAUTIONS

NSAIDs
Potentially nephrotoxic and ulcerogenic, especially in dehydrated animals.

Steroids
Can potentially induce immunosuppression or iatrogenic hypoadrenocortism. Have been associated with development of laminitis in horses.

Antibiotics
Aminoglycosides are potentially nephrotoxic. Creatinine concentration should be measured before starting treatment and regularly (every other day) during treatment. Plasma level (peak and trough) should be monitored when possible.

POSSIBLE INTERACTIONS
NSAIDs + aminoglycosides + dehydration = increased risk of nephrotoxicity.

ALTERNATIVE DRUGS
N/A

FOLLOW-UP

PATIENT MONITORING
Rectal temperature, pulse, respiration, attitude, appetite, and water consumption should be monitored twice daily. When treating infectious disease, frequent monitoring of fibrinogen concentration is useful is assessing the response to treatment. This should also be monitored for a week or so after antibiotics have been discontinued. Creatinine concentration should be monitored in horses receiving NSAIDs or aminoglycosides.

POSSIBLE COMPLICATIONS
Laminitis is always a possible complication in horses affected with febrile condition. Vessels used for IV injections may thrombose. Donkeys, ponies, and miniature horses that are anorectic are particularly at risk of developing hyperlipidemia/hyperlipemia. Intravenous dextrose supplementation should be considered in these patients.

FEVER

MISCELLANEOUS

ASSOCIATED CONDITIONS
N/A

AGE-RELATED FACTORS

Neonates
Septicemia

Foals and Young Horses
Pneumonia (*Streptococcus* spp., *Rhodococcus equi*), immunodeficiencies.

Race Horses
- Viral respiratory disease
- Pleuropneumonia

Older Horses
Neoplasia

ZOONOTIC POTENTIAL
- Anthrax
- Lyme disease
- Salmonellosis
- Tetanus
- Equine encephalomyelitis
- Rabies

PREGNANCY
All drugs should be used with caution in pregnant mares, especially during the first trimester of gestation. Daily progesterone supplementation should be considered. High-risk mares should foal in a facility where constant monitoring is provided and veterinary assistance is available.

SYNONYMS
Pyrexia

SEE ALSO
See specific causes, hyperthermia.

ABBREVIATIONS
- EEE = eastern equine encephalitis
- FUO = fever of unknown origin
- WEE = western equine encephalitis

Suggested Reading

White SL. Alterations in body temperature. In: Smith, BP. Large animal internal medicine, 2nd edition. St. Louis: Mosby-Year Book Inc., 1996:35-45.

Mair TS. Fever of unknown origin in the horse: a review of 63 cases. Eq Vet J 1989:21:260-265.

Dascombe MJ. The pharmacology of fever. Prog Neurobiol 1985:25:327-373.

Author Marie-France Roy

Consulting Editor Corinne R. Sweeney

FIBRINOLYSIS, EXCESSIVE

BASICS

DEFINITION

• As a medical entity, bleeding is the primary clinical sign, but thrombosis can occur during earlier phases.
• The pathophysiologic phenomenon occurring during the late phases of DIC

PATHOPHYSIOLOGY

• Fibrinolysis is the multilevel, physiologically controlled, enzymatic breakdown of fibrin. Maintenance of vessel patency, thrombotic vessel recanalization, and fibrin removal from tissues depend on it.
• Dissolution of fibrin occurs by the action of plasmin, the only known in vivo fibrinolytic protease.
• Plasminogen, the zymogen (i.e., inactive enzyme precursor) of plasmin, is present in circulation and has at least two different in vivo activators—t-PA, found mostly in the tissues; and urinary-plasminogen activator (i.e., urokinase), found in urine
• Plasminogen is efficiently activated by t-PA in the presence of fibrin but is very inefficiently activated in plasma.
• Plasminogen-activator inhibitors (i.e., PAI-I and -II) can rapidly inactivate t-PA or urokinase in circulation.
• α_2-Antiplasmin is the primary inactivator of plasmin.
• α_2-Antiplasmin inactivation of free plasmin is one of the fastest reactions in nature. Plasmin attached to fibrin is inactivated 100–1000-fold more slowly compared with free plasmin, because the active site is occupied. This effectively confines fibrinolysis to locations where fibrin is present.
• Plasmin degradation of fibrin releases several smaller fragments collectively called FDPs. With excessive fibrinolysis (e.g., during the latter stages of DIC), fibrinogen also may get degraded because of the imbalance in hemostatic factors.
• Assays for plasminogen, α_2-antiplasmin, and t-PA are not readily available to practitioners but have been used by researchers investigating various hemostatic abnormalities related to colic, jugular thrombosis, and laminitis. Therefore, being able to diagnose the cause of a suspected thrombotic event as a lack of plasminogen, lack of t-PA, or excess of α_2-antiplasmin is not practical.
• With excessive hemorrhage (e.g., DIC), FDPs, as measured by several different commercial assays, may be increased. Controversy exists concerning the validity of the test results from some manufacturers' products, and all results are subject to question if no other hemostatic abnormality (e.g., thrombocytopenia) is concurrent.

SYSTEMS AFFECTED

• Vascular
• GI
• Musculoskeletal
• Nervous

SIGNALMENT

• No breed, sex, or age predilections
• Any horse with severe systemic disease is at potential risk of excessive fibrinolysis/DIC.

SIGNS

• DIC/excessive fibrinolysis is never a primary problem; it is always a secondary complication.
• Any animal with severe systemic disease is at risk
• Equine situations serious enough to result in DIC—severe diarrhea, usually of infectious origin (e.g., salmonellosis); severe colic, usually resulting from bowel strangulation or other causes of bowel devitalization; severe pleuritis; severe peritonitis; or severe metritis
• Horses have variable clinical signs that reflect the underlying systemic disease and no clinical signs directly resulting from excessive fibrinolysis/DIC. This is a laboratory diagnosis mainly. Horses usually do not develop overt evidence of excessive fibrinolysis, as might be seen in dogs and cats such as—bleeding from body orifices, petechiation, excessive hemorrhage from venipuncture sites, or bruising

CAUSES

• No consistent, specific causes of excessive fibrinolysis/DIC
• Several conditions are associated with development of secondary excessive fibrinolysis/DIC.

RISK FACTORS

• Severe systemic diseases—GI disease (e.g., colic, acute diarrhea)
• Severe infectious diseases—septicemia, pneumonia, pleuritis, peritonitis, and metritis

DIAGNOSIS

DIFFERENTIAL DIAGNOSIS

• Clinical signs in affected horses are those of the underlying disease.
• Jugular thrombosis, laminitis, or renal disease may be present as evidence that DIC/excessive fibrinolysis are occurring.
• Endotoxemia secondary to severe GI disease is an important factor in the pathogenesis of all these lesions.
• Endothelial cells are injured by endotoxin, cells of the mononuclear phagocytic system are induced to produce procoagulant factors, and the resultant microthrombi cause stasis of blood flow.

LABORATORY FINDINGS

• Thrombocytopenia ($<100{,}000$ cells/μL) and increased FDPs (>40 μg/mL), with or without prolonged APTT and PT, are the usual laboratory findings.
• Heparin, which sometimes is used in treatment of DIC/excessive fibrinolysis, may cause prolongation of coagulation screening tests.
• Significant hemolysis can interfere with interpretation of the FDP test. Thrombo-Wellcotest (the most commonly used FDP kit) blood collection tubes contain soybean trypsin inhibitor as an inhibitor of in vitro fibrinolysis and a snake venom (*Bothrops atrox*) that initiates rapid in vitro clotting. The snake venom is claimed to cause rapid and complete clot formation, even in the presence of heparin; however, it causes massive hemolysis of equine erythrocytes. A few laboratories report minimal interference with test interpretation; others report total inability to read results. Blood collection tubes containing thrombin (rather than snake venom) and soybean trypsin inhibitor are commercially available separate from the Thrombo-Wellcotest.
• Several different laboratory assays are available for the detection of human FDPs. Several use monoclonal antibodies in the detection of specific components in the fibrin degradation cascade (e.g., D-dimer). D-Dimer assays need further evaluation in the horse. The Thrombo-Wellcotest has been used most extensively in veterinary medicine and contains antibodies capable of detecting fragments D and E of fibrinogen.

FIBRINOLYSIS, EXCESSIVE

CBC/BIOCHEMISTRY/URINALYSIS
Results reflect the underlying disease.

OTHER LABORATORY TESTS
- Interpretation of FDP results should be accompanied by evaluation of platelet count and, usually, other coagulation screening tests—APTT, PT, thrombin time, and fibrinogen concentration.
- In horses, prolonged APTT and PT are inconsistent findings, but thrombocytopenia (<100,000 cells/μL) often accompanies excessive fibrinolysis/DIC.
- Hypofibrinogenemia and prolonged thrombin time are not seen in equine DIC, unlike in dogs and humans.
- Fibrinogen, an acute-phase reactant, often is increased because of rapid production by the liver during severe systemic disease.

IMAGING
N/A

DIAGNOSTIC PROCEDURES
N/A

TREATMENT
- Excessive fibrinolysis/DIC is associated with severe systemic diseases; treat these horses on an in-patient basis for the underlying disease.
- Fluid therapy to maintain adequate tissue perfusion with dilution of activated coagulation factors and delivery of activated coagulation factors and FDPs to the monocyte/macrophage system for phagocytosis and inactivation is critical.
- Inform owners that the underlying disease is potentially life threatening, and that secondary DIC/excessive fibrinolysis is added information that the prognosis is poor.

MEDICATIONS

DRUGS OF CHOICE

Heparin
- Sometimes administered to decrease the excessive activation of coagulation factors that results in DIC/excessive fibrinolysis.
- If administered, a loading dose of 150 U/kg SC is followed by 125 U/kg SC q12h, then further decreased to 100 U/kg q12h after the seventh dose.
- Heparin depends on the presence of antithrombin III for its function. If the horse has a protein-losing disease (e.g., protein-losing enteropathy such as severe diarrhea or protein-losing nephropathy), serum or plasma protein concentration may be decreased, and antithrombin III activity may be decreased as well. Many laboratories can measure antithrombin III activity in citrated plasma.

Transfusions
Fresh plasma or whole-blood transfusions containing normal coagulation factors often are not feasible in horses; to be effective, the quantity and cost may be prohibitive.

CONTRAINDICATIONS
N/A

PRECAUTIONS
- Heparin causes an anemia that results from agglutination of erythrocytes and possible trapping in the microvasculature, but no clinical signs or histopathologic evidence of microagglutination have been found.
- Heparin added to equine blood in vitro does not cause erythrocyte agglutination; therefore, the agglutination is thought to be heparin-mediated but not caused by heparin itself.
- Hematocrit returns to normal within 96 hours of heparin therapy cessation, which is far more rapid than physiologically possible by bone marrow production.
- Excessive heparin can lead to life-threatening hemorrhage.
- Subsequent coagulation test results usually are abnormal because of heparin administration
- Thrombocytopenia and painful swellings at the injection sites are complications of heparin administration.

POSSIBLE INTERACTIONS
See *Precautions.*

ALTERNATIVE DRUGS
N/A

FOLLOW-UP

PATIENT MONITORING
Evaluate physical and laboratory findings of the underling disease process to assess improvement or worsening of the patient's condition.

POSSIBLE COMPLICATIONS
DIC/excessive fibrinolysis accompany serious systemic illnesses that often result in death.

MISCELLANEOUS

ASSOCIATED CONDITIONS
N/A

AGE-RELATED FACTORS
N/A

ZOONOTIC POTENTIAL
N/A

PREGNANCY
N/A

SYNONYMS
DIC

SEE ALSO
Clotting factors

ABBREVIATIONS
- APTT = activated partial thromboplastin time
- DIC = disseminated intravascular coagulation
- FDP = fibrinogen degradation product
- GI = gastrointestinal
- PAI = plasminogen-activator inhibitor
- PT = prothrombin time
- t-PA = tissue-plasminogen activator

Suggested Reading

Meyers KM, Menard M, Wardrop KJ. Equine hemostasis. Description, evaluation, and alteration. Vet Clin North Am Equine Pract 1987;3:485–505.

Morris DD, Beech J. Disseminated intravascular coagulation in 6 horses. J Am Vet Med Assoc 1983;183:1067–1071.

Author Elizabeth G. Welles

Consulting Editor Claire B. Andreasen

FLEXURAL LIMB DEFORMITY (FLD)

BASICS

DEFINITION
• A conformational limb abnormality that deals with laxity or contracture of the fore or hind limbs in foals
• Can be described as the appearance of the limbs when observed from the side.
• May be present at birth or develop as the foal grows.

PATHOPHYSIOLOGY
Congenital Deformities
• Incompletely understood pathophysiology, but may be multifactorial in origin—intrauterine positioning, genetic predisposition, and teratogenic factors
• Generally a soft-tissue problem that may involve the flexure tendons, muscles, ligaments, and joint capsules

Acquired Deformities
• Excessive grain intake or sudden increases in quality and quantity of feed may lead to accelerated growth during the first several months of life. During this period, the longitudinal growth rate of the bone is postulated to be greater than the potential for the tendons to elongate accordingly, which results in a length discrepancy between that of the bone and that of the tendon–muscle unit.
• Polyarthritis and trauma have also been suggested as possible causes. These result in painful limbs, which may cause an inability to bear weight on the affected limbs or a prolonged overload of the nonaffected limbs, resulting in FLD.

SYSTEMS AFFECTED
Musculoskeletal
• Most often disorders of soft-tissue structures (i.e., tendons and ligaments) that result in some degree of flexion or laxity of a joint.
• Congenital contracture FLD usually is bilateral and involves the metacarpophalangeal joint, metatarsophalangeal joint, or carpi.
• Degree of flexure varies from slight, in which the foal can stand on its own unassisted, to severe, in which the foal cannot stand or walks on the dorsal surface of the fetlock.

Reproductive
Severe cases of congenital contractural FLD may result in dystocia.

SIGNALMENT
N/A

SIGNS
General Comments
In acquired FLD, severity of signs usually relates to chronicity of the underlying cause and how long the condition is left unattended.

Historical Findings
• Congenital deformities usually are noticed at birth or shortly thereafter.
• Foals may fail to stand and nurse after birth.
• Foals with acquired deformities may have a history of chronic, severe tendonitis; crib feeding and excessive protein diets also are reported.

Physical Examination Findings
Congenital Deformities:
• Digital hyperextension—foals walk on the bulbs of their heels and cannot keep the toe on the ground; in severe cases, foals walk on the palmar/plantar phalangeal surfaces; if chronic and untreated, foals may have skin sores or damage to tendinous structures or proximal sesamoid bones.
• Contractural deformities—foals with contractural deformity of the distal interphalangeal joint (i.e., "club foot") walk on the toes; the dorsal hoof wall is abnormally straight or concave in appearance; heel length is similar to dorsal hoof wall, giving the foot a boxy appearance; a straight to "knuckling over" appearance of the fetlock is characteristic of metacarpophalangeal/tarsophalangeal joint deformity; foals with carpal deformities buckle over at the carpus or may be unable to stand.
Acquired Deformities:
• Contractural deformities of the distal interphalangeal joint—steep dorsal hoof wall angle and relatively short toe early on, then progressing to a "boxy" foot, in which the hoof wall length at the toe is as long as the heel; classified as type I (i.e., angle formed by the dorsal hoof wall and the sole $<90^\circ$) or type II (i.e., angle $<90^\circ$); the DDFT may feel tighter on palpation than the SDFT.
• Contractural deformities of the metacarpophalangeal or tarsophalangeal joint—recognized by a straight to "knuckled over" appearance of the fetlock joint; SDFT may feel tighter than DDFT on palpation, but in severe cases, both may be equally taut.

CAUSES
• Congenital—for the most part, the cause is unknown; uterine malpositioning, toxin ingestion during gestation (e.g., *Astralgalus* sp., Sudan grass), hyperplastic goiter (i.e., hypothyroidism), and genetic influences have been suggested.
• Acquired—excessive grain intake, epiphysitis, polyarthritis, and trauma have been implicated.

RISK FACTORS
• Thought to be multifactorial.
• High-protein diets are at least partially responsible.

DIAGNOSIS

DIFFERENTIAL DIAGNOSIS
• Digital hyperextension FLD—consider rupture of the SDFT or DDFT, fracture of the proximal sesamoid bones with avulsion of the suspensory ligament, and avulsion of the distal sesamoid ligaments.
• Carpal contractural FLD—consider rupture of the common digital extensor tendon.

CBC/BIOCHEMISTRY/URINALYSIS
N/A

OTHER LABORATORY TESTS
N/A

IMAGING
• Radiography—obtain radiographs of affected joints to evaluate for degenerative joint disease and osteochondrosis; severe cases may have subluxation of the joint.
• Ultrasonography—some chronic cases may have evidence for tendonitis of the DDFT and SDFT or suspensory ligament desmitis.

DIAGNOSITIC PROCEDURES
Examine the animal for signs of lameness.

TREATMENT

MEDICAL
Congenital Deformities
Digital Hyperextension Deformities:
• Adopt a moderate exercise plan to strengthen the flexor tendons.
• Corrective shoeing using glue-on shoes with palmar/plantar extension in moderate to severe cases.
• Minimally bandage legs to prevent further damage to the heel bulbs and posterior fetlock joint during exercise.
Contractural Deformities:
• Corrective shoeing with use of toe extensions protects the toe from excessive wear and increases the breakover time of the foot, thereby resulting in tendon stretching.
• Splints and casts can be used to relax the tendon–muscle unit, either alone or in conjunction with other treatments; these should be changed frequently, however, because of the fast growth of foals and potential for pressure sores.

Acquired Deformities
Contractural Deformities of the Distal Interphalangeal Joint:
• Evaluate nutritional program to ensure the foal is properly fed.
• NSAIDs may help to alleviate musculoskeletal pain and encourage foals to remain active.

FLEXURAL LIMB DEFORMITY (FLD)

• Exercise, toe extensions, and cast application also may be used.
Contractural Deformities of the Metacarpophalangeal and Tarsophalangeal Joints:
• Therapy is aimed at correcting nutritional imbalance.
• Begin corrective shoeing—wedge pads may result in improvement.
• NSAIDs to reduce pain
• Placement of bandages and splints
• Physical therapy
Deformities of the Carpal Region:
Recommended treatment includes physical therapy and bandaging, with or without use of a splint.

SURGICAL

Congenital Deformities

Digital Hyperextension Deformities:
• Flexor tendon tenoplasty (i.e., z-plasty) has been reported as a surgical salvage procedure, but results have been variable.
• This surgery rarely is required, because excellent results usually are achieved with conservative management.
Contractural Deformities:
See *Acquired Deformities.*

Acquired Deformities

Contractural Deformities of the Distal Interphalangeal Joint:
• Desmotomy of the accessory (i.e., inferior check) ligament of the DDFT is recommended for type I deformities. Apply a pressure bandage at the surgical site, and maintain for 2–3 weeks after surgery. Hand walking on a firm surface is started after 7 days, followed by pasture turnout in 3–4 weeks. Trim the heels regularly to restore a more normal hoof conformation.
• Desmotomy of the accessory (i.e., superior check) ligament of the SDFT may be indicated in conjunction with an inferior check ligament desmotomy for some severe, type II deformities.
• Tenotomy of the DDFT may be required for severe, type II deformities.
Contractural Deformity of the Metacarpophalangeal and Tarsophalangeal Joint:
• When the DDFT is tighter than the SDFT on limb palpation, inferior check ligament desmotomy is the recommended surgery.
• When the SDFT is tighter than the DDFT, desmotomy of the accessory (i.e., superior check) ligament of the SDFT should be performed.
• In severe cases, both superior and inferior check ligament desmotomies must be performed simultaneously to achieve results.
Deformities of the Carpal Region:
In the absence of response to conservative therapy, tenotomy of the ulnaris lateralis and flexor carpi ulnaris may be pursued.

MEDICATIONS

DRUGS OF CHOICE

NSAIDs

Phenylbutazone (2–4 mg/kg PO or IV SID–BID), flunixin meglumine (1 mg/kg PO or IV SID–BID), and ketoprofen (2.2 mg/kg IV SID) may be indicated to provide comfort in foals with acquired FLD.

Oxytetracycline

• This therapy (66 mg/kg, diluted in 250–500 mL of physiologic saline, IV SID for 2–3 doses) can be used in newborn foals with contractural FLD and results in passive relaxation and lengthening of the muscle as well as subsequent correction of the deformity.
• The mode of action is not understood, and this use of tetracycline is considered to be extralabel.
• The leg should also be bandaged and splinted during treatment.

CONTRAINDICATIONS

Use of splints and casts in digital hyperextension forms of FLD, because they promote tendon laxity.

PRECAUTIONS

• NSAIDs can be ulcerogenic at high concentrations or over a prolonged period of time.
• High-dosage oxytetracycline can be nephrotoxic. The foal should be well hydrated and its renal status evaluated before administration.

POSSIBLE INTERACTIONS

N/A

ALTERNATIVE DRUGS

N/A

FOLLOW-UP

PATIENT MONITORING

• Close monitoring of foals with bandage or splints/casts to minimize occurrence of pressure sores
• Monitor both creatinine and BUN closely when using oxytetracycline in neonates.

POSSIBLE COMPLICATIONS

Surgical complications—hematoma formation after superior or inferior check ligament desmotomies, septic tendon sheath (i.e., superior check ligament desmotomy), or carpal canal and scar formation, resulting in cosmetic blemish.

MISCELLANEOUS

ASSOCIATED CONDITIONS

• Dystocia commonly is associated with severe congenital contracture.
• Failure of passive transfer of colostrum may occur in newborn foals that cannot stand and nurse on their own.

AGE-RELATED FACTORS

N/A

ZOONOTIC POTENTIAL

N/A

PREGNANCY

Mares carrying severely contracted foals may experience dystocia.

SYNONYMS

• Arthrogryposis
• Contracted tendons

SEE ALSO

• Angular limb deformities
• Failure of passive transfer

ABBREVIATIONS

• DDFT = deep digital flexor tendon
• SDFT= superficial digital flexor tendon

Suggested Reading

Auer JA. Flexural deformities. Equine Surg 1992;88:957–970.
Kelly, et al. Comparison of splinting and casting on the degree of laxity induced in thoracic limbs in young horses. Equine Pract 1987;9:10–18.
Wagner PC. Chapters 93–95. Current practice of equine surgery. 1990:472–481.

Author Jose M. Garcia-Lopez
Consulting Editor Mary Rose Paradis

FOREBRAIN DISEASE AND SEIZURE DISORDERS

BASICS

DEFINITION

Disease associated with the cerebral hemispheres that often presents as behavioral changes, altered states of consciousness, central blindness, and seizures

PATHOPHYSIOLOGY

- Disease processes that alter cortical brain function can be associated with neuroanatomically related clinical signs—behavioral changes, altered states of consciousness, central blindness, and seizures
- Seizures are associated with a sudden, abnormal discharge of neurons in a portion (or all) of the cerebral cortex.
- Diseases that lower the seizure threshold are likely to induce this clinical syndrome. In this situation, a self-replicating wave of depolarization of CNS tissue progresses until a portion (or all) of the cerebral cortex is refractory.

SYSTEMS AFFECTED

- CNS
- Trauma to other systems from seizure
- Systems affected by the initiating disease

SIGNALMENT

- No associated signalment for seizures in general
- Juvenile epilepsy occurs in young foals and seems to be more common in Arabian foals.
- Estrus-associated seizures occasionally occur.

SIGNS

Historical Findings

A history of trauma or toxin exposure can be present, but often, no historical associations can be made.

Physical Examination Findings

- Bursts of cerebrocortical activity are associated with paroxysmal skeletal muscle motion and profound behavioral changes. Under these circumstances, neuroanatomically related clinical signs can include behavioral changes, altered states of consciousness, central blindness, and seizures.
- Seizures are classified as generalized, partial, or partial with secondary generalization. The type of seizure that occurs often is associated the extent of the lesion.
- Diffuse cortical disturbances often are associated with generalized disease processes.
- The onset of a generalized seizure often is preceded by a short period of restlessness and disorientation (i.e., preictal period). Inappropriate chewing, teeth grinding, and other bizarre behavior also may occur during this period. Subsequently, generalized muscular rigidity, recumbency, and unconsciousness can occur.
- Dorsocaudal positioning of the pupils (i.e., rolled back eyes), tonic/clonic paddling movements, and signs of autonomic activity (e.g., salivation, urination, defecation) are common.
- Seizure foci in other parts of the brain (e.g., thalamus, hypothalamus) may result in such behavioral abnormalities as exaggerated gulping of air, apparent blindness, confusion, viciousness, unprovoked excitement, or unconsciousness.
- Between seizures, other localizing neurologic deficits may be evident.
- Signs of a partial seizure depend on the portion of the cerebral cortex that is discharging and on the site of the seizure focus (i.e., the origin of the abnormal electrical activity). For example, if the seizure focus is in the left motor cortex, tremors and involuntary activity are more likely to be present and to be more severe on the right (i.e., contralateral) side of the head or body.
- If the electrical discharge spreads through the entire cerebral cortex, a partial seizure may progress to a generalized form.

CAUSES

- Many disease processes can be associated with seizures—trauma; neoplasm; cholesterol granuloma; hydrocephalus; bacterial, viral, verminous, and protozoal encephalitides; cerebral abscess; thromboembolism; intracarotid injection; neonatal maladjustment syndrome; hypoxemia; moldy corn poisoning; hepatoencephalopathy; hypoglycemia; hyposmolality; hyperosmolality
- In juvenile epilepsy, no other disease process is evident.

RISK FACTORS

Exposure to infectious diseases, toxins, etc. associated with seizure.

DIAGNOSIS

DIFFERENTIAL DIAGNOSIS

Any disease syndrome that affects the cerebral cortex or other portions of the forebrain

CBC/BIOCHEMISTRY/URINALYSIS

No pathognomonic abnormalities

OTHER LABORATORY TESTS

Depend on the associated disease

IMAGING

Magnetic resonance imaging may be useful.

DIAGNOSTIC PROCEDURES

- Neuroanatomic diagnostic examination may help to localize the site of a seizure focus.
- CSF may be useful.
- Disease-specific tests may be useful.
- Ancillary diagnostic aids (e.g., electroencephalography) may be useful in identifying seizure foci and monitoring those that may, over time, become quiescent.

PATHOLOGIC FINDINGS

Depend on the associated disease

FOREBRAIN DISEASE AND SEIZURE DISORDERS

TREATMENT

• The goal of treatment is to reduce harm to the patient and to protect those surrounding the animal.
• Horses may require supportive care until the seizures are controlled.

MEDICATIONS

DRUGS OF CHOICE

• Choice of drug therapies depends on the initiating disease.
• Altrenogest may be useful to control estrus-associated seizures.
• See Table 1.

CONTRAINDICATIONS

Drugs that reduce seizure threshold—acetylpromazine

PRECAUTIONS

N/A

POSSIBLE INTERACTIONS

N/A

ALTERNATIVE DRUGS

N/A

FOLLOW-UP

POSSIBLE COMPLICATIONS

• Trauma associated with the seizure episode
• Complications associated with other concurrent or initiating diseases

PREVENTION/AVOIDANCE

Depends on the initiating disease process

EXPECTED COURSE AND PROGNOSIS

• For most seizure conditions, the prognosis is fair for long-term management.
• Most foals with juvenile epilepsy experience a reduction in frequency, even to cessation, of seizures.

MISCELLANEOUS

ASSOCIATED CONDITIONS

See above.

AGE-RELATED FACTORS

• Seizures can occur at any age.
• Juvenile epilepsy occurs in foals often <5 months of age.

ZOONOTIC POTENTIAL

See specific related diseases.

PREGNANCY

See specific related diseases.

SYNONYMS

N/A

ABBREVIATIONS

CSF = cerebrospinal fluid

Suggested Reading

Hahn CN, Mayhew IG, Mackay RJ. Diseases of the forebrain. In: Colohan PT, Mayhew IG, Merritt, AM, Moore JN, eds. Equine medicine and surgery. 5th ed. St. Louis: Mosby, 1999:904–913.

Sweeney CR, Hansen TO. Narcolepsy and epilepsy. In: Robinson NE, ed. Current therapy in equine medicine 2. Philadelphia: WB Saunders, 1987:349–353.

Author Joseph J. Bertone
Consulting Editor Joseph J. Bertone

Table 1

Drugs for Controlling Seizures in Horses

Drug	*Foal (50 kg)*	*Adult (500 kg)*
Acute treatment		
Diazepam	0.1–0.3 mg IV as needed	0.1–0.3 mg IV as needed
Pentobarbital	2–3 mg/kg IV to effect	To effect
Phenobarbital	5–20 mg/kg IV slowly	4 mg/kg IV slowly
Phenytoin	4–10 mg/kg IV slowly	
Xylazine	0.5–1 mg/kg IV	0.2–1 mg/kg IV
Detomidine	0.01–0.08 mg/kg IV	
Maintenance		
Phenobarbital[a]	2–10 mg/kg PO q12h	2–6 mg/kg PO q12h
Potassium bromide[b]	10–60 mg/kg PO q24h	10–60 mg/kg PO q24h

[a]Blood concentrations should be assessed initially after 3 days. Once effective plasma concentrations (8–12 μg/mL) have been reached, assessment may occur at longer intervals, depending on the patient.
[b]Blood concentrations should be assessed initially after 14 days. Once effective plasma concentrations (8–12 μg/mL) have been reached, assessment may occur at longer intervals, depending on the patient.

γ-GLUTAMYLTRANSFERASE (GGT)

BASICS

DEFINITION

• Serum GGT is a marker for both cholestasis and hepatocellular injury and is one of the most sensitive measures of hepatobiliary disease.
• Some studies indicate serum increases may be associated with training, particularly overtraining or poor racing performance.
• Urine GGT can be used as a marker for renal tubular degeneration or necrosis.

PATHOPHYSIOLOGY

• GGT is a membrane-bound carboxypeptidase involved in amino acid absorption. It catalyzes amino acid transfers between peptides and plays a major role in glutathione metabolism.
• High tissue concentrations are found in kidney, liver, and pancreas. Lower concentrations are found in many other tissues, but these generally do not appear to affect serum activity appreciably.
• With renal injury, GGT is released into urine, not blood.
• Equine pancreatitis is uncommon, and its contribution to increased serum GGT, apart from associated hepatobiliary alterations, is unclear. However, it may result from local inflammation of both the pancreatic and bile ducts. Thus, increases in serum GGT are considered relatively specific for hepatobiliary disease.
• Liver GGT activity is greatest along the brush border of biliary epithelial cells.
• Increased membrane release or increased synthesis (i.e., induction) contribute to increased serum activity.
• The mechanism of release into the blood is unclear but is proposed to involve membrane solubilization by bile salts, release of membrane fragments/vesicles, or biliary regurgitation.
• The serum half-life is $\cong$3 days.
• The greatest serum GGT elevations are associated with cholestasis or chronic liver disease, but hepatocellular injury also increases serum activity. Experimentally, bile duct ligation causes 8–10-fold increases by 10 days; cellular injury induced by carbon tetrachloride is associated with peak increases (4–5-fold) within 2 days. In acute cholestasis, bile salts and possibly conjugated bilirubin may precede serum GGT elevations, because it depends, to some extent, on enzyme induction. Serum GGT also increases in association with biliary epithelial proliferation which, in chronic diseases, can be marked.
• The mechanism for increased serum GGT associated with training (i.e., overtraining) is unclear, but GGT values >100 U/L tend to be associated with compromised performance. Standard muscle injury markers (e.g., CK, AST, LDH-5) also may be elevated with overtraining. Affected horses often are observed to be recovering from viral infections, upper respiratory disease, or mild lameness; however, they typically do not have elevations in other hepatobiliary parameters (except possibly AST, an ambiguous marker for both liver and muscle injury).
• Unlike many species, horses do have some muscle GGT activity that, given their large muscle mass, might contribute to increased serum activity. Because increased GGT activity typically is not reported with more severe muscle injury, however, its source in association with lesser injury remains equivocal.

SYSTEMS AFFECTED

• Hepatobiliary—increases are associated with cholestasis (with or without biliary hyperplasia) and cell injury.
• Renal—tubular epithelial injury increases urinary, but not serum, GGT.
• Musculoskeletal—increases reportedly are associated with overtraining; GGT source is equivocal.
• Pancreas—pancreatitis (uncommon) is a potential source of increased serum GGT.

SIGNALMENT

Neonates—healthy neonatal values during the first 2–3 weeks of life may exceed adult values by 2–3-fold. The mechanism is unclear but may reflect biliary proliferation. In foals, GGT is not absorbed with colostrum, as it is in ruminants.

SIGNS

General Comments

Signs do not directly result from increased serum GGT activity but from the underlying disease process.

Historical Findings

• Owners may report icterus, dark-yellow/orange urine, anorexia, weight loss, listlessness, and behavioral changes associated with hepatic failure in conditions associated with cholestasis or hepatocellular injury.
• Abdominal pain (e.g., sweating, rolling) may occur with acute hepatopathies (i.e., capsular swelling) or biliary obstructions.

Physical Examination Findings

• Icterus is frequently observed.
• Increased pulse and respiratory rates, fever, photosensitization, weight loss, and obesity vary and depend on the underlying disease process.

CAUSES

Hepatobiliary System

• Metabolic—secondary to severe anemia (see *Hematopoietic System*), hyperlipemia, fasting (<50% increase by 2–3 days), or diabetes mellitus
• Immune-mediated, infectious—chronic active hepatitis, Theiler's disease (i.e., serum hepatitis), amyloidosis, endotoxemia, viral (e.g., EIA, EVA, EHV in perinatal foals), bacterial (e.g., Tyzzer's disease, salmonellosis), fungal, protozoal, and parasitic (e.g., liver flukes, with or without strongyle larval migrans)
• Nutritional—hepatic lipidosis; ferrous fumarate toxicity in neonates
• Degenerative—cirrhosis; cholelithiasis

- Toxic—pyrrolizidine alkaloid–containing plants (e.g., senecio, crotalaria), alsike clover, kleingrass, aflatoxin, rubratoxin; chemical toxins (e.g., arsenic, chlorinated hydrocarbons, monesin, phenol, paraquat); mild increases are inconsistently reported with halothane anesthesia.
- Anomaly—biliary atresia; portovascular shunts
- Neoplastic—primary liver tumors (rare); metastatic neoplasia (uncommon)

Musculoskeletal System

Possibly associated with overtraining

GI System

Potentially associated with pancreatitis

Hematopoietic System

- Severe anemia (e.g., acute EIA, red maple leaf toxicity, onion toxicity, postparturient hemorrhage) leads to hypoxic injury and hepatocellular swelling, with subsequent cholestasis.
- Hepatic lymphosarcoma, leukemias, and so on

RISK FACTORS

- Pregnancy—some liver diseases causing increased GGT are seen with higher frequency in pregnant mares (e.g., hyperlipemia, Theiler's disease associated with receiving tetanus toxoid, etc.).
- Ponies and donkeys—particularly susceptible to developing hyperlipemia and hepatic lipidosis if subjected to negative nitrogen balance
- Antisera donors—horses used long term as hyperimmunized serum donors (e.g., for *Escherichia coli, P. multocida*) tend to develop amyloidosis; sustained GGT increases ($\leq$10-fold) in horses used for $\geq$6–7 years correlate well with histopathologically confirmed amyloidosis.
- Fasting—increases of <50% may be seen with 2–3 days of fasting (presumably nonpathologic).
- Other factors—those associated with any disease leading to cholestasis or hepatocellular injury.

DIAGNOSIS

DIFFERENTIAL DIAGNOSIS

- Other than potential increases associated with pancreatitis and training, increased serum GGT is considered specific for hepatobiliary disease; however, it is not specific for the type of hepatobiliary condition.
- Highest elevations generally are associated with long-standing conditions with severe cholestasis or biliary hyperplasia—chronic active hepatitis, cirrhosis, cholelithiasis, and lipidosis
- Concurrent obesity and high enzyme activities suggest hyperlipemia/lipidosis; anorexia and weight loss are typical of most other differentials.

LABORATORY FINDINGS

Drugs That May Alter Lab Results

N/A

Disorders That May Alter Lab Results

- Very high bilirubin values, severe lipemia, and marked hemolysis may cause falsely elevated values.
- Serum is the preferred sample type, but heparin or EDTA plasma can be used. Other anticoagulants (e.g., citrate, oxalate, fluoride) depress human GGT activity by 10–15%.
- Serum samples are stable for 3 days at 4°C or for at least 1 month at −20°C.

Valid If Run in Human Lab?

Yes, but equine reference intervals should be generated in-house or based on literature values using the same methodology.

CBC/BIOCHEMISTRY/URINALYSIS

- No routine lab tests provide a causative or specific diagnosis for increased GGT.
- Most suggest a type of alteration (e.g., injury, cholestasis, insufficiency/vascular shunt) rather than a cause for the alteration.

Erythrocytes

- Nonregenerative anemia may be seen with liver disease.
- Morphologic changes may be reported—poikilocytosis; acanthocytosis
- Some morphologic changes induced by liver disease (e.g., acanthocytes, schistocytes from microvascular disease in the liver) are associated with decreased RBC survival and may contribute to mild hemolytic (i.e., regenerative) anemia.
- Severe hemolytic anemia from any cause (e.g., oxidation injuries manifested by Heinz bodies or eccentrocytes, immune-mediated anemia) can cause hypoxic injury, leading to hepatocellular swelling and secondary cholestasis.

Leukocytes

- Neutrophilia or neutropenia and monocytosis may occur with inflammatory liver disease—bacterial cholangiohepatitis
- Evidence of antigenic stimulation may be seen—lymphocytosis or reactive lymphoid cells

Glucose

- Postprandial or fasting hypoglycemia may occur with hepatic insufficiency/shunts.
- Hypoglycemia with liver disease carries a guarded prognosis.

Albumin

- Decreased production with hepatic insufficiency may decrease serum concentrations, but this usually occurs very late in equine hepatic failure.
- Albumin is a negative acute-phase reactant; mild decreases may occur in inflammatory liver disease.

BUN

Decreased BUN (especially relative to creatinine) with hepatic insufficiency/shunts because of conversion of ammonia to urea

γ-GLUTAMYLTRANSFERASE (GGT)

SDH

- Increases specifically with hepatocellular injury.
- May occur concurrent with or independent of cholestasis.

AST

Increases with hepatocellular or muscle injury.

ALP

- Increases primarily with cholestasis.
- Other causes—proliferative bone disease or rapid growth (i.e., bone isoform); severe GI disease (i.e., mild increases only).

Bilirubin

- Conjugated—increases with cholestasis; seen with hepatocellular injury, presumably related to cell swelling and secondary cholestasis.
- Unconjugated—increases with increased RBC destruction (i.e., hemolysis) and defective hepatocellular uptake (e.g., injured hepatocytes, hepatic insufficiency, vascular shunting); increases with fasting because of a nonpathologic decrease in uptake.

Cholesterol

- May be decreased with hepatic insufficiency/shunts.
- Commonly increased with cholestasis and lipid metabolism disorders—hyperlipemia

Triglycerides

Increased with hyperlipemia.

Urinalysis

- Bilirubinuria supports the presence of cholestasis.
- Ammonia urates may be observed with hepatic insufficiency/shunt.

OTHER LABORATORY TESTS

Bile Acids

- Sensitive indicator of decreased hepatobiliary function, but not specific for the type of process
- Concentrations depend on adequate enterohepatic circulation, hepatobiliary function, and hepatocellular perfusion.
- More sensitive than GGT for acute cholestasis.

Ammonia

Serum concentrations are affected by hepatic uptake and correlate inversely with hepatic functional mass.

Clearance Tests (BSP, ICG)

- Prolonged clearance intervals with decreased functional mass or cholestasis
- Accelerated clearance (possibly masking insufficiency) with hypoalbuminemia

Serology

Depends on degree of suspicion for specific diseases—viral, fungal, and so on

Coagulation Tests

May be prolonged with hepatic insufficiency/shunting—prothrombin time; activated partial thromboplastin time

IMAGING

Ultrasonography—useful for assessing liver size, shape, position and parenchymal texture; may help to detect focal parenchymal lesions (e.g., abscesses, neoplasms) and abnormalities in the biliary tree (e.g., dilatations, obstructions) or large vessels (e.g., shunts, thrombosis).

DIAGNOSTIC PROCEDURES

Aspiration cytology or use of biopsied tissue for microbiologic testing, cytologic imprints, and histopathologic evaluation may provide specific diagnostic information.

TREATMENT

- Decision regarding outpatient vs. inpatient treatment depends on severity of disease, intensity of supportive care required, and need for isolation of infectious conditions.
- Fluid and nutritional support may be needed.
- Anorexic and hypoglycemic cases may benefit from IV dextrose (5%, 2 mL/kg per hour). Otherwise, fluid support depends on specific electrolyte and acid–base abnormalities.
- Avoid negative energy balance, especially in ponies and donkeys, to avoid/treat hyperlipemia and hepatic lipidosis.
- Toxicities or hepatic insufficiency may warrant efforts to reduce production/absorption of toxins.
- Mineral oil given by nasogastric tube helps to reduce toxin absorption.
- Lactulose (0.3 mL/kg q6h by nasogastric tube) is suggested to combat GI ammonia production/absorption but causes diarrhea.
- A high-carbohydrate, low-protein diet reduces ammonia production.
- Specific therapy, including surgery, depends on the specific underlying cause.

γ-GLUTAMYLTRANSFERASE (GGT)

MEDICATIONS

DRUGS OF CHOICE

Depend on the suspected cause and observed complications.

CONTRAINDICATIONS

Depend on the suspected cause and observed complications.

PRECAUTIONS

- Depend on the suspected caused.
- With suspected hepatic insufficiency, assess coagulation profiles before invasive procedures.

POSSIBLE INTERACTIONS

Depend on the underlying cause.

ALTERNATIVE DRUGS

Depend on the underlying cause.

FOLLOW-UP

PATIENT MONITORING

- Serial chemistries can help to establish a prognosis by characterizing disease progression and identifying evidence of improvement.
- Initial evaluation at 1–2 day intervals helps to establish disease course.
- Subsequent testing can be at increasing intervals, depending on signs and severity.

POSSIBLE COMPLICATIONS

Depend on the underlying cause.

MISCELLANEOUS

ASSOCIATED CONDITIONS

Depend on the underlying cause.

AGE-RELATED FACTORS

See *Signalment.*

ZOONOTIC POTENTIAL

Depends on the underlying cause.

PREGNANCY

See *Risk Factors.*

SYNONYMS

γ-Glutamyltranspeptidase

SEE ALSO

See *Causes.*

ABBREVIATIONS

- ALP = alkaline phosphatase
- AST = aspartate aminotransferase
- BSP = sulfobromophthalein
- CK = creatine kinase
- EIA = equine infectious anemia
- EHV = equine herpes virus
- EVA = equine viral arteritis
- GI = gastrointestinal
- ICG = indocyanine green
- LDH = lactate dehydrogenase
- SDH = sorbitol dehydrogenase

Suggested Reading

Barton MH, Morris DD. Diseases of the liver. In: Reed S, Bayly W, eds. Equine internal medicine. Philadelphia: WB Saunders, 1998.

Hoffmann W, Baker G, Rieser S, Dorner J. Alterations in selected biochemical constituents in equids after induced hepatic disease. Am J Vet Res 1987;48:1343–1347.

Snow DH, Harris P. Enzymes as markers for the evaluation of physical fitness and training of racing horses. Adv Clin Enzymol 1988;6:251–258.

West HJ. Clinical and pathological studies in horses with hepatic disease. Equine Vet J 1996;28:146–156.

Authors John A. Christian and Armando Irizarry-Rovira

Consulting Editor Claire B. Andreasen

GASTRIC DILATION/DISTENSION

BASICS

DEFINITION

Accumulation of excessive amounts of gas, fluid, or solid material in the stomach, resulting in dilatation.

PATHOPHYSIOLOGY

Horses are not able to regurgitate; therefore, horses are predisposed to excessive distension of the stomach followed by possible rupture. Causes of gastric dilation can be primary, secondary, or idiopathic. Primary causes of gastric dilation include diseases of the stomach, feed engorgement, and rapid intake of water. The dilation results in decreased motility and a failure to discharge the stomach contents into the proximal duodenum. Overeating of easily fermentable food such as grain, fresh grass, beets, or beet-pulp leads to production of lactic acid and volatile fatty acids by the gastric flora. Gastric emptying is inhibited by increased concentrations of volatile fatty acids, resulting in further fermentation and production of gas. Primary gastric dilation may also result from local infestation of *Gasterophilus* larvae or habronemiasis, especially in the area of the pylorus. Primary gastric distension can also be caused iatrogenically following passage of a nasogastric tube and overloading the stomach with liquids. Gastric dilation can be secondary to an obstructive lesion of the small intestine, resulting in retrograde movement of intestinal fluid and bile, or non-obstructive small intestinal ileus (e.g., proximal duodeno-jejunitis).

SYSTEMS AFFECTED

Gastrointestinal

The cardiovascular system can be affected if the gastric dilation results in dehydration or rupture. Gastric rupture results in endotoxemia, shock, and death.

Respiratory

Abdominal distension and pressure on the diaphragm may affect breathing.

INCIDENCE/PREVALENCE

No data available.

SIGNALMENT

No sex or breed disposition, but the age might assist in the identification of a primary cause. For example, foals are more predisposed to gastric ulceration.

SIGNS

General Comments

A gastric dilation/distension can lead to gastric rupture.

Historical Findings

Depend on the severity of the dilation/distension. Signs of abdominal pain may occur abruptly following excessive or rapid consumption of large amount of liquid or food. There may be a history of ingestion of highly fermentable food. If secondary to a distal obstruction, the clinical signs are initially related to the primary problem. Mild to severe signs of abdominal pain (see Acute Abdominal Pain) may be observed. The animal may assume a dog-sitting position and present with retching or gurgling sounds.

Physical Examination Findings

The following findings may accompany the clinical signs of abdominal pain. Increase in heart and respiratory rates, may have sour smell to the breath, and possibly some ingesta at the nares. Cyanosis and pale mucous membranes may be present, likely due to the local increase in gastric space occupation, thus reducing venous return. There may be signs of dehydration or toxic shock as the disease progresses. Rectal examination may reveal the spleen to be displaced caudally. If the condition is secondary to an obstruction aborally, other abnormalities such as distension of the small intestines may be palpated. On passage of the nasogastric tube, large amounts of gas, fluid, or ingesta may escape. Gastric reflux of more than two liters is considered significant.
Spontaneous reflux may also be present. If gastric rupture occurs, the signs of colic will initially subside. Depression and severe signs of shock will develop, and once endotoxemic shock occurs, the signs of colic may return.

CAUSES

See Pathophysiology.

RISK FACTORS

- Overeating
- Intestinal obstructions

DIFFERENTIAL DIAGNOSIS

Any other cause of colic.

CBC/BIOCHEMISTRY/URINALYSIS

May have an elevated PCV and TP in relation to dehydration or endotoxemic shock. There may be hypoproteinemia secondary to protein loss in the abdominal cavity. There may be mild to moderate hypochloremia if gastric reflux is present, resulting in metabolic alkalosis. Metabolic acidosis may develop secondary to severe endotoxemic shock. If gastric rupture occurs, a moderate to severe leukopenia will be noticed secondary to the acute peritonitis. Horses with severe dehydration may have azotemia.

OTHER LABORATORY TESTS

pH

pH of reflux might help determine the origin of the problem. Normal gastric pH varies between 3 and 6. pH of fluid originating from the small intestine is between 5 and 7 and has a bilious color.

Abdominocentesis

Abdominocentesis is usually normal if there is a primary gastric dilation without rupture. There may be an increase in protein, and WBC may be present if there is some devitalized bowel (stomach or small intestine). Sanguineous fluid may be indicative of a strangulated obstructive lesion of the small intestine or devitalization of the stomach. Plant material in the sample in the absence of an enterocentesis suggests intestinal rupture. No leukocytes or cells should be present if an enterocentesis was performed.

IMAGING

Radiology

Radiology may be useful in foals. A contrast study can help in outlining the gastric wall for detection of gastric ulcers and possibly strictures and determining the gastric emptying time.

Gastroscopy

Gastroscopy is useful for identification of impacted stomach, gastric ulcer, and neoplasm. In small horses, the duodenum also may be inspected for presence of ulceration and strictures.

GASTRIC DILATION/DISTENSION

Abdominal Laparoscopy

Abdominal laparoscopy is useful for visual inspection of the visceral part of stomach and small intestine for serosal lesions.

Ultrasonography

May be useful to identify a primary lesion in the small intestine by evaluation of its wall thickness and diameter. Abnormal findings such as intussusception, abscess, and adhesions may sometimes be identified. The evaluation of the amount, quality, and characteristics of abdominal fluid is also possible.

DIAGNOSTIC PROCEDURES

Exploratory laparotomy is useful to treat small intestinal lesions and possibly some gastric problems.

TREATMENT

Supportive therapy for treatment of shock.

Primary Gastric Dilatation

Primary gastric dilatation consists of deflating the stomach by passage of the nasogastric tube. If impaction is present, lavage of the stomach followed by administration of dioctyl sodium succinate (DSS) (10–30 mg/kg of a 10% solution), acts as a surfactant and allows water to penetrate the impaction. It is possible that it may be necessary to repeat this procedure. Care should be taken not to give too much DSS.

Secondary Gastric Dilatation

Secondary gastric dilatation consists of leaving the nasogastric tube in place and performing periodic decompression until resolution of the primary problem by medical or surgical treatment (see Small Intestinal Obstruction).

Fluidotherapy

Fluidotherapy may be necessary to treat the dehydration.

MEDICATIONS

DRUG(S) OF CHOICE

Analgesics may be necessary to control the abdominal pain. They include:

- Non-steroidal anti-inflammatory drugs—flunixin meglumine (0.5–1.1 mg/kg IV, IM q8 or 12 hr); and alpha-2-blockers, such as xylazine (0.25–0.5 mg/kg IV or IM), detomidine (5–10 μg/kg IV or IM), or romifidine (0.02–0.05 mg/kg IV or IM)
- Narcotic or narcotic-derivative analgesics such as butorphanol (0.02–0.04 mg/kg IV), which can be given alone or in combination with xylazine. There is potentiation of these two drugs. Analgesics should be used judiciously as they may mask clinical signs and may lead to postponement of a needed surgery.

Parenteral fluid treatments (100–200 mL/kg/day)

- In cases of dehydration or endotoxemic shock. In cases where cardiovascular shock is present, hypertonic saline IV (in the adult horse, 2 L of 7% NaCl; 4 mL/kg) prior to balanced electrolyte solutions (e.g., LRS)

In case of grain overload, secondary endotoxemia may result in laminitis. See Preventive Treatment or Treatment of Acute Laminitis.

PRECAUTIONS

The nasogastric tube should be manipulated gently; avoid overloading the stomach.

FOLLOW-UP

PATIENT MONITORING

The patient should be monitored for any increase in heart rate or discomfort indicating that the stomach may need to be further decompressed. If the condition is secondary to gastric ulcer, the use of NSAIDs may aggravate the problem.

POSSIBLE COMPLICATIONS

- Gastric rupture
- Endotoxemic shock

ASSOCIATED CONDITIONS

Primary Condition

- Gastric ulceration
- Parasitism
- Neoplasia

Secondary Condition

- Small intestinal obstruction (strangulated or non-strangulated)
- Anterior duodeno-jejunitis

AGE-RELATED FACTORS

Gastric ulceration is often the primary cause of gastric dilatation/distension in young foals.

ZOONOTIC POTENTIAL

N/A

PREGNANCY

N/A

ABBREVIATIONS

N/A

Suggested Reading

Kiper ML, Traub-Dargatz J, Curtis CR. Gastric rupture in horses: 50 cases (1979–1987). J Am Vet Med Assoc. 1990:196:333-336.

Todhunter RJ, Erb HN, Roth L. Gastric rupture in horses: a review of 54 cases. Eq Vet J 1986:18:288-293.

Carter GK. Gastric diseases. In: Robinson NE. Current therapy in equine medicine, 2nd ed. Philadelphia: WB Saunders Co., 1987:41–44.

Author Nathalie Coté

Consulting Editor Henry Stämpfli

GASTRIC EROSIONS AND ULCERS

BASICS

DEFINITION
Gastric ulcers are defects in the gastric mucosa that extend into the muscularis mucosa. Erosions are less severe and do not extend into the muscularis mucosa. Endoscopically, it can be difficult to distinguish erosions from ulcers in some cases. The equine stomach consists of a dorsal portion lined with stratified squamous epithelium and a ventral portion lined with a glandular epithelial mucosa.

PATHOPHYSIOLOGY
The pathophysiology of equine gastric ulcers is poorly understood. In general, gastric ulcers are thought to occur when there is an imbalance of aggressive and protective factors. The aggressive factors are primarily hydrochloric acid and pepsin. Protective factors include the gastric mucosal barrier (mucus, bicarbonate), prostaglandins, mucosal blood flow, and mucosal restitution. Restitution is the process in which existing mucosal cells migrate rapidly to replace damaged mucosal cells and occurs in minutes to hours. Mucosal protective factors are important primarily in the glandular mucosa. The stratified squamous mucosa has less-advanced protective properties.

SYSTEMS AFFECTED
Gastrointestinal

Primarily, the gastric stratified squamous mucosa and a smaller number in the glandular mucosa. Esophageal mucosal inflammation and erosions/ulcers when gastroesophageal reflux is present (primarily foals).

Cardiovascular

Although hemorrhage is often visible on gastroscopic examination, blood loss sufficient to affect the cardiovascular system is rare.

Respiratory

Foals with gastroesophageal reflux may develop aspiration pneumonia.

Hepatobiliary

Ascending cholangitis possible with duodenal ulceration.

INCIDENCE/PREVALENCE
Equine gastric ulcers have been reported from most parts of the world. The reported prevalence is 25–50% of foals, 80–90% of racehorses in training, and >90% of weanlings after housing in stalls and halter breaking. Ulcers identified endoscopically are primarily in the stratified squamous mucosa. However, it is often difficult to visualize large portions of the glandular mucosa in the standing horse, and therefore the true frequency of glandular ulcers may be underestimated. Necropsy results in racehorses indicate a 10% prevalence of glandular mucosal ulcers, and as many as 40% of foals 2–90 days old may have glandular mucosal lesions. Ninety-two percent (92%) of horses showing clinical signs had visible gastric ulceration. Approximately 5% of foals necropsied had duodenal ulceration.

SIGNALMENT
Breed Predilections

Although Thoroughbred racehorses in training appear to be over-represented, all breeds appear to be affected.

Mean Age and Range

Horses of all ages are affected.

Predominant Sex

N/A

SIGNS
General Comments

Asymptomatic in many animals. Signs may vary with the age group involved and are not specific for the condition.

Historical Findings

- Poor appetite
- Decrease in performance
- Weight loss

Physical Examination Findings

- Foals—Many are asymptomatic, poor appetite, intermittent nursing (may nurse for short period and then act mildly uncomfortable), episodes of mild colic, diarrhea, pot-bellied appearance, bruxism, salivation, and dorsal recumbency. Salivation and bruxism are usually indicative of severe glandular or duodenal ulcers with concurrent gastroesophageal reflux and delayed gastric emptying.
- Adults—Many are asymptomatic, poor appetite, lethargy, poor body condition, rough hair coat, low-grade colic, and weight loss.

CAUSES
Probably multifactorial, any illness, surgery, intense training, halter breaking, confining and handling young horses, nonsteroidal anti-inflammatory drugs (NSAIDs), fasting, lack of roughage in diet in racehorses.

RISK FACTORS
- Significant illness
- Intense training
- Administration of NSAIDs
- Halter breaking and confinement
- Fasting

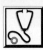

DIAGNOSIS
Although a definitive diagnosis can be reached with gastroscopic examination, a tentative diagnosis can be made based on clinical signs and response to therapy.

DIFFERENTIAL DIAGNOSIS
The clinical signs and physical examination findings with gastric ulcers are not pathognomonic and can be associated with many other conditions. In addition, gastric ulcers are often secondary to other diseases.

CBC/BIOCHEMISTRY/URINALYSIS
There are no changes in CBC/biochemistry/urinalysis associated with equine gastric ulcers. Anemia and hypoproteinemia are not associated with gastric ulcers and when present, other causes should be pursued.

OTHER LABORATORY TESTS
Fecal occult blood tests are usually negative because colonic microflora digest hemoglobin.

IMAGING
Abdominal Radiography

Abdominal radiographs usually do not demonstrate gastric ulcerations. In foals, positive contrast studies might outline gastric ulcers but more effective methods should be used.

DIAGNOSTIC PROCEDURES
Gastroscopic Examination

Gastroscopic examination is the most effective diagnostic procedure. For foals, a 10-mm diameter, 1-m gastroscope is adequate. However, for optimum gastroscopic examination in the adult horse, a 2- to 3-m gastroscope is necessary. Fasting is necessary to ensure gastric emptying for adequate visualization. Young foals may require minimum fasting. However, older foals and adults eating roughage require a fasting period of 4–18 hr. Lesions in the stratified squamous mucosa are easily identified. Glandular mucosal lesions are frequently not visible because they are covered by ingesta and gastric secretions remaining in the stomach.

TREATMENT

APPROPRIATE HEALTH CARE
Treat as outpatient if stable and any underlying conditions have been corrected.

GASTRIC EROSIONS AND ULCERS

NURSING CARE
Treat any underlying medical conditions. Use NSAIDs with caution.

ACTIVITY
Decrease level of intense training if possible.

DIET
Turn out on pasture if practical.

CLIENT EDUCATION
- Decrease intensity of training
- Allow as much pasture time as possible
- Minimize NSAID administration
- Minimize periods of fasting
- Ulcers will likely recur when intense training is resumed

SURGICAL CONSIDERATION
Surgical intervention not indicated in uncomplicated cases. Foals with chronic gastric outflow disease caused by stricture of the pylorus or duodenum post-ulcer healing may require gastrojejunostomy.

DRUG(S) OF CHOICE
- Proton pump inhibitors (omeprazole and lansoprazole)—significantly inhibit gastric acid secretion by the inhibition of hydrogen–potassium adenosine triphosphatase (H^+, K^+–ATPase). This enzyme in gastric parietal cells is believed to be the terminal step in the acid secretory pathway. These compounds have a long-term antisecretory effect that lasts for at least 24 hr. Omeprazole is administered 1–4 mg/kg PO once daily. Omeprazole has a time- and dose-related effect on healing of gastric ulcers. Therefore, higher doses result in more rapid and complete healing. However, lower doses are frequently effective in relieving clinical signs and promoting healing. Omeprazole requires 3–5 days treatment for maximum antisecretory effect to occur. There are currently no data available on the use of lansoprazole in horses.
- Histamine H_2 receptor antagonists (cimetidine, ranitidine, and famotidine)—inhibit gastric acid secretion by blocking the effect of histamine on the parietal cell. These compounds rapidly inhibit secretion after oral or intravenous administration. However, the effect is short-lived and they must be administered q6–8hr. Cimetidine is administered at 20–25 mg/kg PO or at 4–6 mg/kg IV bwt q6–8hr. Ranitidine is administered at 6–8 mg/kg PO or 1.5–2.0 mg/kg IV every q6–8hr.

CONTRAINDICATIONS
Use NSAIDs with caution. These compounds may increase the severity of squamous mucosal lesions and cause lesions in the glandular mucosa.

PRECAUTIONS
Clinical signs of gastric ulcers usually diminish quickly with appropriate therapy. If signs or condition worsen while on appropriate treatment, pursue an alternate diagnosis or concurrent disease.

POSSIBLE INTERACTIONS
Cimetidine and, to a lesser extent, omeprazole are hepatic cytochrome P450 inhibitors and might slow the metabolism of concurrently administered compounds that require this enzyme for metabolism and elimination. Drugs whose metabolism might be inhibited include phenylbutazone, diazepam, phenytoin, theophylline, and others.

ALTERNATIVE DRUGS
Antacid Compounds
Antacid compounds buffer gastric acid and are impractical to use in most instances. They must be administered 4–6 times daily and at approximately 250 mL/450 kg horse.

Sucralfate
Likely to be ineffective for treatment of stratified squamous lesions, but possibly effective in glandular lesions. Administered as crushed tablets in syrup at 1 g/100 lbs bwt PO q6–8hr.

FOLLOW-UP

PATIENT MONITORING
Clinical Signs
- Diminished appetite
- Interrupted nursing
- Mild colic
- Teeth grinding

Signs of colic should be monitored frequently. If colic is more than low-grade or persists for >24–48 hr, an alternate diagnsis should be pursued. Endoscopic examination should be repeated after 14 days of treatment and, if not healed, again at 28 days.

PREVENTION/AVOIDANCE
May require prophylactic treatment with omeprazole or histamine H_2 receptor antagonists during periods of intense training/racing. Horses with access to pasture have fewer gastric ulcers than horses in confinement. Avoid chronic administration of NSAIDs and minimize periods of fasting.

POSSIBLE COMPLICATIONS
Pyloric or duodenal stricture in foals; gastric or duodenal perforation (rare). Severe hemorrhage is rare but has been reported in one foal. Recurrence is frequent when intense training resumes.

EXPECTED COURSE AND PROGNOSIS
Most uncomplicated gastric ulcers heal after 14–28 days of treatment. The prognosis is generally good for uncomplicated cases. However, recurrence is frequent when intense training is resumed. Foals that develop pyloric or duodenal strictures and require surgical intervention have a guarded prognosis.

MISCELLANEOUS

ASSOCIATED CONDITIONS
Any disease process has the potential to have secondary gastric ulceration.

AGE-RELATED FACTORS
Foals have a higher incidence of glandular mucosal and duodenal ulcers.

ZOONOTIC POTENTIAL
N/A

PREGNANCY
There are not adequate data on the use of histamine H_2 receptor antagonists or omeprazole in pregnant mares. However, clinical cases of gastric ulcers in pregnant mares have been treated successfully with these compounds with no apparent adverse effects on the mare or the fetus.

SYNONYMS
N/A

SEE ALSO
N/A

ABBREVIATIONS
N/A

Suggested Reading

Andrews FM, MacAllister CG, Jenkins CC, Blackford JT. Omeprazole: A promising antiulcer drug in horses. Compend Cont Edu 1996;18:1228-1240.

MacAllister CG. Medical therapy for equine gastric ulcers. Vet Med 1995:168-176.

Murray MJ. Gastroduodenal ulceration. In: Reed SM, Bayly WM, eds. Equine internal medicine. Philadelphia: WB Saunders, 1998.

Author Charles G. MacAllister

Consulting Editor Henry Stämpfli

GASTRIC NEOPLASIA

BASICS

DEFINITION

Neoplasms of the stomach include squamous cell carcinoma (SCC), adenocarcinoma, lymphosarcoma, leiomyoma, and fibrosarcoma. SCC usually originates in the non-glandular portion of the stomach, infiltrates the wall, and projects into the lumen. Adenocarcinoma of the glandular part of the stomach may affect the pylorus and the fundic region. Tumors of the gastrointestinal tract of horses are rare. Although SCC is the most common gastric neoplasm, only 3% of carcinomas in horses are of gastric origin, which is in marked contrast to the incidence in humans. The tumors may cause physical obstruction within the stomach, and may occasionally be associated with severe intraluminal hemmorrhage. Other signs may be related to the effects of metastases (e.g., pleural effusion). SCC lesions of the stomach may reach a considerable size and have an invasive proliferative appearance. They are often ulcerated and secondarily infected. In these circumstances, the surface may have a grayish-white and hemorrhagic appearance. There may be adhesions of stomach to adjacent liver, spleen, or diaphragm and there are frequently metastatic nodules in the abdominal and thoracic cavities. Although adenocarcinomas may project into the gut lumen, the predominant feature is growth from the mucosa into the submucosa and the muscularis to the serosa.

SIGNALMENT

Horses of middle-age and older (range 6–10 yr) are susceptible to SCC and a 4:1 male:female ratio has been reported. No breed susceptibility has been suggested of this or any other gastric neoplasm. Adenocarcinoma and lymphosarcoma have a similar age distribution.

SIGNS

Affected horses have a history of gradual weight loss, anorexia, and lethargy extending over a period of 2–6 weeks. Abdominal pain and difficulty in eating or swallowing are not usually features of gastric carcinoma or the other neoplasms listed. Pallor of mucous membranes and an increase in heart rate may be seen due to anemia resulting from hemorrhage to the stomach or depressed erythrogenesis. Recurrent episodic pyrexia up to 40°C may occur as the result of necrosis in the neoplasm, and the respiratory rate may be raised in response to metastatic masses in the thorax. Ascites and ventral edema may be primary signs in a few horses, so that despite the weight loss the abdomen appears distended.

CAUSES/RISK FACTORS

None known

DIAGNOSIS

A definitive diagnosis is made on histologic examination of tissue obtained at autopsy or by biopsy.

DIFFERENTIAL DIAGNOSIS

See Chronic Weight Loss 1. Inadequate or poor-quality feed or failure to eat the food offered.

GASTRIC NEOPLASIA

CBC/BIOCHEMISTRY/URINALYSIS

The PCV may be as low as 12–28% in horses with anemia, secondary to gastric carcinoma.

OTHER LABORATORY TESTS

- Feces may test positive for occult blood.
- Neoplastic cells may be found in fluid recovered by gastric lavage or in peritoneal fluid.

IMAGING

- Endoscopy using a video or fiber endoscope at least 2 m in length enables a positive diagnosis by direct visualization and biopsy of the tumor.
- Exploratory laparotomy or standing laparoscopy allows a more complete examination of the stomach and valuation of the extent of spread and allows biopsy of primary tumor mass or metastatic nodules.
- Radiographs of the thorax may reveal fluid, and a pneumo-gastrogram may be of value in delineating the intraluminal portion of the tumor.
- Ultrasonography from the left cranial abdomen may show thickening and abnormal echogenicity of the stomach wall.

DIAGNOSTIC PROCEDURES

Rectal examination may indicate metastatic masses or increased abdominal fluid.

TREATMENT

By the time a diagnosis is made the tumors have progressed beyond the point where any treatment is feasible, and euthanasia is the only option.

MEDICATIONS

N/A

CONTRAINDICATIONS/POSSIBLE INTERACTIONS

N/A

FOLLOW-UP

N/A

Suggested Reading

Meagher DM, Wheat JD, Tennant B, Osburn BI. Squamous cell carcinoma of the equine stomach. J Am Vet Med Assoc. 1974;164:81-84.

Author Garry B. Edwards
Consulting Editor Henry Stämpfli

GASTRIC ULCERS IN FOALS

BASICS

DEFINITION

Erosive lesions in the squamous or glandular mucosal lining of the stomach

PATHOPHYSIOLOGY

• Stomach ulceration is considered to result from an imbalance of gastric acidic factors (i.e., hydrochloric acid, pepsin) and protective factors (i.e., mucus/bicarbonate barrier, PGE_2, mucosal blood flow, cellular restitution, and growth factors promoting angiogenesis and mucosal proliferation).
• Foals have significant gastric acid secretion as early as 2 days of age.
• The squamous mucosa of the equine stomach lacks a mucus/bicarbonate layer and has minimal resistance to exposure to hydrochloric acid. Ulceration may result primarily from excessive exposure to hydrochloric acid and pepsin, as seen during fasting.
• Excessive administration of nonsteroidal drugs results in inhibition of PGE_2 synthesis, increased acid secretion, diminished mucosal blood flow, local vasoconstriction, ischemic injury, and ulcer development.
• Stress impairs epithelial cell replication and can result in development of gastric mucosal ischemia.

SYSTEMS AFFECTED

GI—primary site of gastric ulceration is in the squamous mucosa at the margo plicatus; ulcers in the glandular mucosa of the stomach and duodenum are less commonly seen.

GENETICS

N/A

INCIDENCE/PREVALENCE

• The overall prevalence of gastric ulcers in foals is reportedly as high as 25–50%.
• Endoscopic surveys of normal foals 2–85 days of age revealed that 50% had ulcers in the squamous mucosa and 4–9% had ulcers in the glandular mucosa.

SIGNALMENT

No breed or sex predispositions

SIGNS

General Comments

• Endoscopic studies have revealed a 50% prevalence of gastric lesions in asymptomatic foals
• Clinical signs are observed in the minority of foals with ulcers and usually reflect severe gastric lesions.

Historical Findings

Owners may report poor growth, rough hair coat, and pot-belly appearance.

Physical Examination Findings

• Bruxism, dorsal recumbency, excessive salivation, interrupted nursing, colic, and diarrhea are all clinical signs of gastric ulceration in foals.
• Esophageal reflux indicates gastric outlet obstruction or pseudo-obstruction, reflecting significant ulceration associated with the pylorus and duodenum.

CAUSES

Excessive stomach acidity

RISK FACTORS

• Feed deprivation—gastric acidity is considerably greater in horses during feed deprivation than when feed is available, and repeated periods of feed deprivation result in erosion and ulceration of the gastric squamous mucosa.
• Excessive administration of nonsteroidal drugs—foals are exceptionally susceptible to the toxic affects of phenylbutazone and flunixin meglumine.
• Stress—restraint, severe illness, sepsis, surgery, shock, and hypotension

DIAGNOSIS

DIFFERENTIAL DIAGNOSIS

Any disorder resulting in signs of colic—small intestinal intussusceptions, small intestinal volvulus, peritonitis, pyloric hypertrophy, large colon impaction, diaphragmatic hernia, abdominal abscess, and enterocolitis

CBC/BIOCHEMISTRY/URINALYSIS:

• Hematologic values usually are normal.
• Anemia may be present if blood loss is substantial.
• Leukogram might show increased WBC count and fibrinogen with peritonitis or severe pain.

OTHER LABORATORY TESTS

Evaluation of Gastric Reflux for pH

• An acidic pH (<4) suggests that accumulated fluid is gastric in origin.
• A pH >6 should raise concern that fluid from the small intestine is backflowing into the stomach because of intestinal ileus or obstruction.

Presence of Blood on Gastric Reflux/Fecal Occult Blood Testing

• A strongly positive result without rectal trauma supports the diagnosis of GI tract bleeding but does not determine the source—stomach versus intestine
• A negative result does not rule out gastric or duodenal ulceration.

Acid–Base Status

May be normal or show metabolic alkalosis with significant HCl sequestration in the stomach.

IMAGING

Radiography—barium contrast may outline filling defects in the esophagus, stomach, or duodenum and provide a marker for determining gastric emptying time (30% [w/v] barium sulfate at a dose of mL/kg via nasogastric tube); most of the barium should have left the stomach within 2 hours of administration.

DIAGNOSTIC PROCEDURES

Gastroscopy—a 1-m endoscope is sufficient to examine the gastric mucosa of a 45-kg neonatal foal; withholding milk for 2 hours may be necessary to visualize both the squamous and glandular portions of the stomach.

TREATMENT

Foals with mild to moderately severe gastric ulcers should respond to treatment within 24–48 hours.

APPROPRIATE HEALTH CARE

• Patient with gastric ulcers can be treated in the field.
• With dehydration or electrolyte imbalance, peritonitis, toxic clinical signs, esophageal reflux, and uncontrolled pain, the animal should be hospitalized.

NURSING CARE

Fluid therapy may be necessary in foals showing signs of dehydration.

ACTIVITY

Normal activity

GASTRIC ULCERS IN FOALS

DIET

- Normal diet in cases without esophageal reflux.
- In case with esophageal reflux, parenteral nutrition sometimes is necessary.

CLIENT EDUCATION

- Avoid the use of NSAIDs without veterinary supervision.
- Ensure the animal has a regular feeding program.

SURGICAL CONSIDERATIONS

Persistent gastric emptying problems or signs of duodenal or pyloric obstruction should evoke strong considerations of surgery to bypass the strictured area.

MEDICATIONS

DRUGS OF CHOICE

- The primary objective in treatment of gastric ulcers is to reduce or neutralize acid secretion so the gastric mucosal epithelium can heal.
- Antacids—the common antacids are bases of aluminum, magnesium, or calcium (i.e., magnesium/aluminum hydroxide antacid [200–250 mL QID]).
- H_2-antagonists—cimetidine (6–20 mg/kg PO TID or 6.6 mg/kg IV QID) or ranitidine (6.6 mg/kg PO TID or 1.5 mg/kg IV TID); treatment should continue for 14–21 days.
- Sucralfate has a cytoprotective effect on the GI mucosa. Administer 1–2 hours before administering an H_2-antagonist; dosage ranges from 1–2 g per 100 kg BID or TID.
- Proton-pump inhibitor—omeprazole (0.7 mg/kg once a day) administered by nasogastric tube or as an oral paste.
- Prokinetic drugs may be required to inhibit gastroesophageal reflux and to enhance gastric emptying—metoclopramide (0.1–0.25 mg/kg TID or QID).
- Bethanechol (0.025 mg/kg SC q4–6h, followed by maintenance dosages of 0.35–0.40 mg/kg PO TID or QID) has been effective in promoting gastric motility and emptying.

CONTRAINDICATIONS

Metoclopramide in patients with GI hemorrhage.

PRECAUTIONS

Neurologic excitation and possible seizure activity have been noted as side effects of metoclopramide in some horses.

POSSIBLE INTERACTIONS

- Cimetidine may inhibit the hepatic microsomal enzyme system and, thereby, reduce metabolism, prolong serum half-lives, and increase serum levels of some drugs—metronidazole.
- Do not use bethanechol concomitantly with other cholinergic or anticholinesterase agents.

ALTERNATIVE DRUGS

N/A

FOLLOW-UP

PATIENT MONITORING

- Look for signs of colic or bruxism.
- Repeat gastroscopy in 3–4 weeks to evaluate ulcer healing.

PREVENTION/AVOIDANCE

Avoid NSAIDs in foals.

POSSIBLE COMPLICATIONS

- Ulcer perforation and peritonitis
- Anemia
- Pyloric and duodenal stenosis

EXPECTED COURSE AND PROGNOSIS

- Ulcers may take 2–3 weeks to heal.
- Peritonitis and duodenal stenosis have a poor prognosis.

MISCELLANEOUS

ASSOCIATED CONDITIONS

- Septicemia
- Septic arthritis
- Hypoxic ischemic encephalopathy

AGE-RELATED FACTORS

Frequently seen in neonatal foals with concomitant disease.

ZOONOTIC POTENTIAL

N/A

PREGNANCY

N/A

SYNONYMS

N/A

SEE ALSO

- Adult gastric ulceration
- NSAID toxicity

ABBREVIATION

GI = gastrointestinal

Suggested Reading

Murray MJ. Current concepts in healing of equine gastric ulcers. Proc Am Coll Vet Intern Med 1995;13:1072–1078.

Murray MJ. The pathogenesis and prevalence of gastric ulceration in foals and horses. Vet Med 1991:815–819.

Nappert G, Vrins A, Larybyere M. Gastroduodenal ulceration in foals. Compend Contin Educ 1989;11:338–344.

Rebhun WC, Dill SG, Power HT. Gastric ulcers in foals. J Am Vet Med Assoc 1982;180:404–407.

Sanchez LC, Lester, GD, Merritt AM. Effect of ranitidine on intragastric pH in clinically normal neonatal foals. J Am Vet Med Assoc 1998;212:1407–1411.

Author Gabriel Ramirez

Consulting Editor Mary Rose Paradis

GETAH VIRUS INFECTION

BASICS

OVERVIEW

Getah virus is an RNA alphavirus of the family Togaviridae. It is widely distributed throughout Southeast Asia and surrounding areas.

It is maintained in a cycle between mosquitoes and various vertebrate hosts. Clinical signs associated with infection with the virus have been described only in horses and occasionally pigs. Although serologic evidence indicates equine exposure to the virus in Hong Kong, Korea, Japan, and India, and in other mammals throughout the area, clinical signs associated with infection in horses have only been reported from Japan and India. There have been two significant outbreaks in Japan (1978 and 1983) and one localized outbreak in India (1990).

SIGNALMENT

Horses of any breed can be infected experimentally, but reported outbreaks have been mostly in thoroughbreds. Few cases have been reported in foals.

SIGNS

- Anorexia
- Fever
- Limb and preputial edema
- Urticarial rash
- Serous nasal discharge
- Submandibular lymphadenopathy
- Stiff gait

Not all horses have all clinical signs, and in the Indian outbreak the rash and lyphadenopathy were absent. Fever usually develops 2–6 days after infection and lasts 3–4 days. Clinical signs resolve within 7–10 days after onset.

CAUSES AND RISK FACTORS

Getah virus is transmitted by mosquitoes, and hence is prevalent in areas with a mosquito population and a reservoir host population. However, some cases in Japan have been reported when the mosquito population is very low, suggesting other means of transmission, such as fomites or direct contact.

DIAGNOSIS

DIFFERENTIAL DIAGNOSIS

Equine viral arteritis is clinically very similar in some cases, although abortions are not reported as a feature of Getah virus infection. The two diseases can be distinguished based on acute and convalescent serology and virus isolation. Mild forms of African horse sickness can appear with similar signs, although the geographic distribution of the two etiologic agents is very different.

CBC/BIOCHEMISTRY/URINALYSIS

The only consistent laboratory finding has been a lymphopenia in the early phase of the disease. Chemistries are usually normal.

GETAH VIRUS INFECTION

OTHER LABORATORY TESTS
Acute and convalescent serology for neutralizing antibodies to Getah virus can confirm recent exposure to the virus.
In the acute phase, virus can be isolated from blood and, in some horses, from nasal swabs.

IMAGING
N/A

DIAGNOSTIC PROCEDURES
N/A

PATHOLOGIC FINDINGS
Moderate enlargement of lymph nodes and scattered maculae in the dermis and subcutaneous edema. Histologically, there is lymphoid hyperplasia in the lymph nodes and spleen. In the dermal maculae there is perivascular infiltration of lymphocytes, histiocytes, and eosinophils, with edema of blood vessel walls and hemorrhagic foci.

TREATMENT
N/A

MEDICATIONS

DRUG(S) OF CHOICE
Not usually necessary. Non-steroidal anti-inflammatory agents may be helpful in anorexic horses during the febrile period.

CONTRAINDICATIONS/POSSIBLE INTERACTIONS
N/A

FOLLOW-UP

PREVENTION/AVOIDANCE
The killed vaccine is available in Japan and should be used prior to the onset of the mosquito season.

EXPECTED COURSE AND PROGNOSIS
Clinical signs last about 6–10 days and resolve without any reported sequelae.

MISCELLANEOUS
Suggested Reading

Brown CM, Timoney PJ. Getah virus infection of Indian horses. Trop An Hlth Prod 1998;30:241-252.

Authors Christopher M. Brown and Peter J. Timoney
Consulting Editor Corinne R. Sweeney

GLANDERS

BASICS

OVERVIEW

Glanders, a zoonosis, is a contagious disease of equids caused by *Pseudomonas mallei* and is characterized by pneumonia and ulcerative nodules of the skin and upper respiratory tract. The mortality rate is high, although some animals remain asymptomatic and serve as a source of infection. The disease has been eradicated from North America and Western Europe, but still occurs in parts of Asia, the Middle East, Eastern Europe, and North Africa.

SIGNALMENT

Horses, donkeys, and mules of all ages are susceptible to glanders.

SIGNS

- Acute cases develop fever, depression, weight loss, cough, a mucopurulent or sanguinous nasal discharge, enlarged submandibular lymph nodes, ulceration of the nasal septum, and death within a few days. This form is most common in donkeys and mules.
- Chronic glanders is typically seen in horses and is marked by intermittent fever, cough, weight loss, purulent nasal discharge, and epistaxis. Submucosal nodules of the nasal septum and turbinates open and form ulcers that heal with a characteristic stellate scar.
- Some cases are asymptomatic.
- The cutaneous form, known as *farcy,* is characterized by nodules and thickened lymphatic vessels. The nodules frequently ulcerate and drain a honey-like fluid. The medial hock and thigh are the most common sites of cutaneous infection, and edema of the lower limb is a common sequela. Cases may have both respiratory and cutaneous involvement.

CAUSES AND RISK FACTORS

- The source of infection is nasal and cutaneous discharges from infected equids. Ingestion of feed or water contaminated by *P. mallei* is believed to be the primary route of infection, although inhalation and cutaneous exposure may occur.
- *Pseudomonas mallei* does not survive in the environment more than a few weeks.
- Stresses including hard work, extreme weather, and gathering of animals (such as during wars) increase the severity of the disease.
- *Pseudomonas mallei* causes nodules in the lymph nodes and lungs. The upper airway, skin, liver, and other organs may also be involved.

DIAGNOSIS

DIFFERENTIAL DIAGNOSIS

- Melioidosis, caused by *Pseudomonas pseudomallei,* has similar signs. Identification of the organism is necessary to confirm the diagnosis because melioidosis patients may be positive on mallein test or serology for glanders.
- Lymphangitis caused by *Histoplasma farcimosum, Corynebacterium pseudotuberculosis,* or *Sporothrix schenkii* may have similar cutaneous lesions. Pneumonia and nasal lesions do not occur, however, and the causative agent is usually readily identified by culture or microscopic examination of exudate or tissue.
- Strangles (*Streptococcus equi*) is usually marked by abscessation and drainage of submandibular or retropharyngeal lymph nodes in contrast to glanders in which the submandibular lymph nodes rarely open. Culture of the nasopharynx or abscess should yield *S. equi.*

CBC/BIOCHEMISTRY/URINALYSIS

- Leukocytosis with neutrophilia
- Hyperfibrinogenemia
- Anemia in chronic cases

GLANDERS

OTHER LABORATORY TESTS

• Bacterial culture of material from exudates, nodules, ulcers, or blood may yield *P. mallei,* especially in acute cases. *Pseudomonas mallei* is a gram-negative, nonencapsulated, nonmotile rod. Precautions should be taken to prevent exposure of laboratory personnel to infective material.
• Complement fixation (CF) is considered the most reliable serologic test, although animals may not seroconvert until 4–12 weeks post-infection. False-positive CF may result from mallein testing or *P. pseudomallei* infection.

IMAGING

N/A

OTHER DIAGNOSTIC PROCEDURES

The mallein test is commonly used to diagnose glanders. An injection of 0.1 mL of mallein (*P. mallei* purified protein derivative) is made intradermally in the lower eyelid. A positive test is characterized by pain, swelling, or purulent conjunctivitis 48 hr post-injection.

PATHOLOGIC FINDINGS

• The acute form is characterized by severe bronchopneumonia, enlarged bronchial lymph nodes, and widespread petechial hemorrhage.
• The chronic form is marked by miliary nodules in the lungs as well as lymphadenopathy and ulcerative nodules in the skin and upper respiratory tract.

TREATMENT

Regulatory officials should be notified if glanders is suspected. Affected animals should be destroyed and all exposed animals quarantined for further testing. Treatment of animals should not be attempted.

MEDICATIONS

DRUG(S) OF CHOICE

Sodium sulfadiazine may be effective; however, treatment is not usually permitted.

CONTRAINDICATIONS/POSSIBLE INTERACTIONS

N/A

FOLLOW-UP

• Management of an outbreak includes destruction of clinical cases, mallein testing of all exposed horses with destruction of reactors, and destruction or disinfection of bedding and equipment associated with infected horses.
• No vaccine for glanders is available.
• All equids should be tested prior to entering a glanders-free area.

MISCELLANEOUS

ZOONOTIC POTENTIAL

People who handle infected horses and laboratory personnel working with *P. mallei* may be infected via breaks in skin or inhalation. Gloves and masks should be worn when handling clinical cases, and special biosecurity procedures should be followed in the laboratory.

SYNONYMS

• Farcy is often used to indicate the cutaneous form of glanders.
• *Pseudomonas mallei* was formerly classified as *Actinobacillus* and *Malleomyces mallei.*

Suggested Reading

Pritchard DG. Glanders. Equine Vet Educ 1995;XX:29-32.

Radostitis OM, Blood DC, Gay CC, et al. Veterinary medicine. Philadelphia: Balliere Tindall. 1994:854-856.

Schlater LK. Glanders. In: Robinson NE, ed. Current therapy in equine medicine. Philadelphia: Saunders. 1992:761-762.

Author Laura K. Reilly
Consulting Editor Corinne R. Sweeney

GLAUCOMA

BASICS

OVERVIEW

• A group of diseases resulting from alterations of aqueous humor dynamics that increase the IOP more than is compatible with normal function of the retinal ganglion cells and optic nerve.
• Recognized with increased frequency in horses, but the prevalence is surprisingly low given the equine propensity for ocular injury and marked intraocular inflammatory responses.
• Five stages—an initial event (or series of events) that influences the aqueous humor outflow system, morphologic alterations of the aqueous outflow system that eventually lead to aqueous outflow obstruction and elevated IOP, elevated IOP or ocular hypertension that severely reduces retinal ganglion cell sensitivity and function, subsequent retinal ganglion cell and optic nerve axon degeneration, and progressive visual deterioration that eventually leads to blindness.
• Frequently categorized as primary, secondary, and congenital.
• All types have a causative mechanism.
• Primary glaucomas possess no overt ocular abnormality to account for the increased IOP.
• Secondary glaucomas have an identifiable cause—intraocular inflammation, neoplasia, or lens luxation
• Primary bilateral glaucoma—rarely reported
• Secondary glaucomas from anterior uveitis and intraocular neoplasia are most commonly recognized.
• Congenital glaucoma—reported in foals and associated with developmental anomalies of the iridocorneal angle.

SIGNALMENT

• Reported in the Appaloosa, Paso Fino, Thoroughbred, and warmbloods, but all ages and breeds are at risk.
• Increased incidence in horses with previous or concurrent ERU, those >15 years, and Appaloosas

SIGNS

• May not be easily recognized during the early stages because of the subtle clinical signs—generally a low index of suspicion, pupils often are only slightly dilated, and overt discomfort is uncommon; afferent PLR deficits, corneal striae, decreased vision, lens luxations, mild iridocyclitis, and optic nerve atrophy/cupping also may be found.
• Corneal striae, or corneal endothelial "band opacities," in nonbuphthalmic eyes warrant a high degree of suspicion for elevated IOP but also may be found in normotensive eyes at the time of examination. Corneal striae are linear, often interconnecting, white opacities deep in the cornea that result from stretching or rupture of Descemet's membrane, and they may be associated with increased IOP.

CAUSES AND RISK FACTORS

• Aqueous humor is produced in the ciliary body by energy-dependent and -independent mechanisms. The ciliary enzyme carbonic anhydrase plays an important role in this production. Aqueous humor passes into the posterior chamber, through the pupil into the anterior chamber, then exits through the iridocorneal angle (i.e., conventional) outflow pathway or the uveovortex and uveoscleral (i.e., unconventional) outflow pathways.
• Perfusion and morphologic studies indicate potentially extensive unconventional aqueous humor outflow pathway involvement in horses. The extensive, low-resistance equine conventional aqueous humor outflow pathway and the prominent unconventional outflow pathways may minimize development of glaucoma in many cases of anterior uveitis.
• Anterior uveitis can, however, lead to formation of preiridal fibrovascular membranes that limit aqueous absorption by the iris and to physical and functional obstruction of the iridocorneal angles with inflammatory cells and debris.
• Iridal and ciliary body neoplasms can cause secondary glaucoma by infiltration of the outflow pathways.

DIAGNOSIS

DIFFERENTIAL DIAGNOSIS

ERU and corneal ulceration may be associated with corneal edema, ocular pain, and blindness.

CBC/BIOCHEMISTRY/URINALYSIS

N/A

OTHER LABORATORY TESTS

Serologic tests for infectious diseases causing anterior uveitis in horses with glaucoma may identify the causative organism.

IMAGING

B-scan ultrasonography can demonstrate intraocular tumors associated with glaucoma.

DIAGNOSTIC PROCEDURES

• The diagnosis is established with the tonometric documentation of elevated IOP and the presence of clinical signs specific to glaucoma—a mydriatic pupil and buphthalmia
• ERU, in contrast, has a low IOP and a miotic pupil.
• Accurate measurement of equine IOP requires applanation tonometry; mean equine IOP ranges from 17–28 mm Hg.

PATHOLOGIC FINDINGS

• Preiridal fibrovascular membrane formation with secondary iridocorneal angle closure
• Trabecular meshwork sclerosis and collapse

TREATMENT

• Various combinations of drugs and surgery may be necessary to reduce IOP to levels compatible with preservation of vision.
• Glaucoma is particularly aggressive and difficult to control in Appaloosas.

GLAUCOMA

MEDICATIONS

DRUGS

- The systemically administered carbonic anhydrase inhibitors (acetazolamide [1–3 mg/kg PO QID] and dichlorphenamide [1 mg/kg PO BID], topical miotics (phospholine iodide [0.12–0.25% BID] and pilocarpine [2% QID]), and the β-blocker timolol maleate (0.5% BID) have been used to lower IOP with varying degrees of success.
- Anti-inflammatory therapy consisting of topically and systemically administered corticosteroids and/or topically and systemically administered NSAIDs (phenylbutazone [1 mg/kg PO BID] or flunixin meglumine [250 mg PO BID]) also appear beneficial in the control of IOP.
- When medical therapy is inadequate, Nd:YAG laser cyclophotoablation may be a viable alternative for long-term IOP control; such laser cyclophotoablation is very effective at controlling IOP and maintaining vision in the horse. Use 55 laser sites per eye for contact Nd:YAG laser cyclophotoablation, 5–6 mm posterior to the limbus, at a power setting of 12 W at 0.3 sec per site. Diode lasers may be used at 55–60 sites for 1500 mW at 1500 msec per site.

CONTRAINDICATIONS/POSSIBLE INTERACTIONS

- Conventional glaucoma treatment with miotics may provide varying amounts of IOP reduction, and a number of horses have had increased IOP when administered topical miotics.
- Because miotics can potentiate clinical signs of uveitis, miotic therapy generally is considered contraindicated in glaucoma secondary to uveitis and should be used cautiously, with careful IOP monitoring, in horses with mild or quiescent anterior uveitis.

FOLLOW-UP

PATIENT MONITORING

- Serial tonometry is required to document IOP spikes in horses with anterior uveitis and secondary glaucoma.
- Continued pupillary dilation is a sign of continued IOP elevation and optic nerve damage.
- Stall rest horses until the condition is under control; intraocular hemorrhage and increased severity of uveitis are sequela to overexertion.
- Diet should be consistent with the training level.
- Protect the horse from self-trauma by using of hard or soft cup hoods.

PREVENTION/AVOIDANCE

Do not breed horses with glaucoma.

POSSIBLE COMPLICATIONS

- Chronic pain
- Blindness

EXPECTED COURSE AND PROGNOSIS

- The equine eye seems to tolerate an elevated IOP for many months to years that would blind a dog; however, blindness is still the end result.
- Buphthalmia can be associated with exposure keratitis.

MISCELLANEOUS

ASSOCIATED CONDITIONS

- ERU
- Exposure keratitis and persistent corneal ulcerations

AGE-RELATED FACTORS

Old horses are at risk.

ZOONOTIC POTENTIAL

N/A

PREGNANCY

N/A

SEE ALSO

ERU

ABBREVIATIONS

- ERU = equine recurrent uveitis
- IOP = intraocular pressure
- Nd:YAG = neodymium:yttrium-aluminum-garnet
- PLR = pupillary light reflex

Suggested Reading

Brooks DE. Equine ophthalmology. In Gelatt KN, ed. Veterinary ophthalmology. 3rd ed. Philadelphia: Lippincott, Williams and Wilkins, 1999.

Miller TR, Brooks DE, Smith PJ, et al.: Equine glaucoma: clinical findings and response to treatment in 14 horses. Vet Comp Ophthalmol 1995;5(3):170–182.

Author Dennis E. Brooks

Consulting Editor Dennis E. Brooks

GLUCOSE, HYPERGLYCEMIA

BASICS

DEFINITION

Glucose concentration > the laboratory reference interval

PATHOPHYSIOLOGY

- Serum glucose concentration depends on a variety of factors, with a net result from rate of entry and removal as influenced by intestinal absorption, hepatic production, hormonal regulation, and tissue utilization.
- Hyperglycemia may result from an absolute (rare) or relative insulin deficiency, reduced utilization of glucose in peripheral tissue, increased gluconeogenesis, or increased glycogenolysis. Glucocorticoids, catecholamines, glucagon, growth hormone, and thyroid hormone can increase gluconeogenesis and glycogenolysis.
- During cortisol release, cellular insulin receptors are down-regulated (i.e., insulin resistance); this can result from a marked endogenous cortisol release "stress response" or hypercortisolemia from pituitary adenomas.
- Epinephrine can mediate hyperglycemia during the "fight or flight" response.
- Physiologic, transient, postprandial hyperglycemia may be seen.

SYSTEMS AFFECTED

- Endocrine/metabolic—hormonal regulation of gluconeogenesis and glycogenolysis
- Renal/urologic—PU/PD caused by glucosuria, resulting in osmotic diuresis
- Nervous—severe hyperglycemia may result in CNS dysfunction because of increased osmolality.

SIGNALMENT

Any horse, but old horses are candidates for pituitary adenomas.

SIGNS

Historical Findings

- Variable
- PU/PD, depression, weight loss, obesity, polyphagia, hirsutism (i.e., pituitary adenoma), and underlying disease resulting in severe stress
- Asymptomatic if transient physiologic or stress response

Physical Examination Findings

Depend on the underlying cause—obesity, hirsutism, weight loss, muscle wasting, pendulous abdomen, hyperhidrosis, or laminitis

CAUSES

- Hypercortisolemia can result in increased gluconeogenesis, decreased peripheral glucose utilization, sparing of glucose because of increased mobilization of free fatty acids, and insulin resistance.
- Insulin resistance because of cortisol release and down-regulation of insulin receptors; usually, significant glucose concentrations result from functional pituitary adenomas, with release of pituitary ACTH and POMC and subsequent cortisol release.
- Absolute insulin deficiency (i.e., hypoinsulinemia) from diabetes mellitus, but this is uncommon in horses and thought to be secondary to chronic pancreatitis that destroys pancreatic islets.
- Physiologic—postprandial, exertion or excitement that is epinephrine-mediated, or stress response that is cortisol-mediated; can be from a severe disease process (e.g., painful colic).
- When giving parenteral nutrition, concurrent sepsis, shock, and major trauma can lead to insulin resistance and reduced glucose utilization.
- Iatrogenic because of dextrose-fluid administration or parenteral nutrition
- Acquired non–insulin-dependent diabetes mellitus (type II) in obese ponies
- Administration of corticosteroids, xylazine, or detomidine

RISK FACTORS

- Obesity
- Pancreatitis
- Old age
- Severe disease
- Colic

DIAGNOSIS

DIFFERENTIAL DIAGNOSIS

- Physiologic—mild, transient hyperglycemia can be associated with cortisol or epinephrine release or postprandial fluctuations.
- Colic—hyperglycemia has been reported in colic, with concentrations >300 mg/dL indicating a poorer prognosis.

LABORATORY FINDINGS

Drugs that May Alter Lab Results

- Glucocorticoids
- ACTH
- Dextrose-containing fluids
- Epinephrine
- Xylazine
- Detomidine

Disorders that May Alter Lab Results

- Lipemia, hemolysis, and icterus may alter results depending on the assay used.
- Delayed serum separation can result in decreased serum glucose concentration because of cellular utilization of glucose; sodium fluoride collection tubes can stabilize glucose concentrations for analysis.

Valid If Run in Human Lab?

Yes

CBC/BIOCHEMISTRY/URINALYSIS

Hyperglycemia may be the only laboratory finding.

CBC

- Inflammatory leukogram if underlying inflammatory disease
- Stress leukogram with neutrophilia and lymphopenia if cortisol mediated
- Mature neutrophilia if epinephrine induced.

Biochemistry/Urinalysis

- Dependent on the underlying disease
- Functional pituitary adenoma—possible hyperglycemia, azotemia, elevated CK and AST because of muscle catabolism, and electrolyte abnormalities because of PU/PD or anorexia; decreased urine specific gravity; glucosuria if renal threshold (180–200 mg/dL) is exceeded.
- Diabetes mellitus—hyperglycemia; glucosuria

OTHER LABORATORY TESTS

- ACTH stimulation test—often an exaggerated response in pituitary-dependent hypercortisolemia, but not completely reliable; plasma ACTH measurement may be more useful.
- Dexamethasone suppression test—the cortisol concentration will be suppressed (80% after 1 hour) in normal horses, but will not suppress or have only modest suppression in horses with functional pituitary adenomas; not completely reliable because of the complexity of pituitary adenoma secretion.

GLUCOSE, HYPERGLYCEMIA

• Glucose tolerance test—used after pituitary adenoma is ruled out. Recommended method is to give IV glucose versus the oral route to prevent confounding effects of GI motility. Published recommendation is a 50% glucose solution (0.5 g/kg IV), and serum concentrations of glucose and insulin are then measured. In cases of primary insulin-dependent diabetes mellitus, sustained, elevated glucose concentrations are found, with no rise in insulin. In cases of insulin resistance, the insulin concentration rises, but return of the glucose concentration to normal is delayed more than 3 hours.
• Measurement of plasma insulin—low in diabetes; high-normal or high in hypercortisolemia (i.e., insulin resistance)
• Insulin tolerance test—published recommendation is soluble regular insulin (1–8 IU/kg IV), with assay of the glucose concentration every 15 minutes for 3 hours; failure of insulin to lower the glucose concentration to normal suggests insulin-resistant diabetes.

IMAGING

Ultrasonography or radiology can be used to detect underlying diseases.

DIAGNOSTIC PROCEDURES

N/A

TREATMENT

• Manage stress or the situation inducing epinephrine release—sample when calm.
• Resolve the underlying disease condition.
• Medical management of pituitary adenomas—correct any biochemical abnormalities with appropriate fluid therapy and diet supplementation (see the section on pituitary adenomas).
• Medical management of diabetes mellitus

MEDICATIONS

DRUGS OF CHOICE

• Diabetes mellitus—insulin, but long-term therapy currently is not documented.
• Functional pituitary adenomas—dopamine agonists or serotonin antagonists

CONTRAINDICATIONS

• Corticosteroids
• Dextrose-containing fluids

PRECAUTIONS

• Hyperglycemia may lead to laminitis and other complications depending on the underlying disease.
• Avoid abruptly decreasing serum glucose concentrations.
• High glucose concentrations above the renal threshold from severe disease can lead to cell deprivation of glucose for energy and may indicate a poorer prognosis for recovery.
• Ketosis may develop during diabetes mellitus.

POSSIBLE INTERACTIONS

N/A

ALTERNATIVE DRUGS

N/A

FOLLOW-UP

PATIENT MONITORING

• Monitor blood glucose concentrations after treatment.
• Monitor for signs associated with the underlying disease.
• Monitor urine specific gravity, glucosuria, ketonuria or other abnormalities, and electrolytes if PU/PD.

POSSIBLE COMPLICATIONS

• Hypercortisolemia and diabetes mellitus can predispose to secondary infections.
• Severe hyperglycemia can result in hyperosmolality and possible CNS depression.

MISCELLANEOUS

ASSOCIATED CONDITIONS

• Electrolyte concentration abnormalities
• Complications of diabetes mellitus—cataracts, glomerulopathies, ketosis, and acidosis

AGE-RELATED FACTORS

Young foals can be prone to transient, increased glucose concentrations because of excitability and epinephrine release.

ZOONOTIC POTENTIAL

N/A

PREGNANCY

N/A

SYNONYMS

N/A

SEE ALSO

• Diabetes mellitus
• Hypercortisolemia
• Pituitary adenoma

ABBREVIATIONS

• AST = aspartate aminotransferase
• CK = creatine kinase
• GI = gastrointestinal
• POMC = pro-opiolipomelanocortin
• PU/PD = polyuria/polydipsia

Suggested Reading

Kaneko JJ. Carbohydrate metabolism and its diseases. In: Kaneko JJ, Harvey JW, Bruss ML, eds. Clinical biochemistry of domestic animals. San Diego: Academic Press, 1997:61–75.

Parry BW. Prognostic evaluation of equine colic cases. Compend Contin Educ Pract Vet 1986;8:S98–S104.

Reed SM. Pituitary adenomas: equine Cushing's disease. In: Reed SM, Bayly WM, eds. Equine internal medicine. Philadelphia: WB Saunders, 1998:912–915.

Rivas L. Endocrine pancreas. In: Reed SM, Bayly WM, eds. Equine internal medicine. Philadelphia: WB Saunders, 1998:936–937.

Author Claire B. Andreasen
Consulting Editor Claire B. Andreasen

GLUCOSE, HYPOGLYCEMIA

BASICS

DEFINITION

Serum or plasma glucose concentration < the laboratory reference interval

PATHOPHYSIOLOGY

- Serum glucose concentration depends on a variety of factors, with a net result from the rate of entry and removal as influenced by intestinal absorption, hepatic production, hormonal regulation, and tissue utilization.
- Hypoglycemia may result from an absolute insulin excess (e.g., insulinomas [rare], iatrogenic insulin overdose), increased utilization of glucose in peripheral tissue, decreased gluconeogenesis, or decreased glycogenolysis caused by hepatic failure or altered hormonal regulation.
- Increased utilization occurs in septicemia/bacteremia, extreme exercise, pregnancy, and some systemic diseases—neoplasia/leukemias
- Hypoglycemia from reduced intake results from starvation/malnutrition.
- When the cells are not separated from the plasma/serum, continued utilization of glucose results in artifactually low glucose concentrations.

SYSTEMS AFFECTED

- Endocrine/metabolic—hormonal regulation of gluconeogenesis and glycogenolysis
- Musculoskeletal—weakness; exercise intolerance
- Nervous—seizures; altered behavior

SIGNALMENT

Any horse, but foals may have a higher incidence of septicemia with failure of passive transfer.

SIGNS

Historical Findings

- Variable
- Anorexia
- Weakness
- Exercise intolerance
- Coma
- Seizures
- Collapse
- Abnormal behavior
- Hepatic encephalopathy

Physical Examination Findings

- Depend on the underlying cause
- Pyrexia or hypothermia if septic
- Tachycardia or hyperemic mucous membranes if endotoxemic
- Coma
- Muscle fasciculations
- Weakness
- Exercise intolerance
- Icterus or encephalopathy if hepatic disease

CAUSES

- Hepatic disease—uncommonly seen in liver insufficiency; can be seen in severe hepatic failure with decreased functional mass that impairs gluconeogenesis and glycogenolysis; worsened by anorexia.
- Septicemia/bacteremia—endotoxemia that depresses hepatic gluconeogenesis; hypoglycemia may be profound in foals that fail to nurse, because they have minimal glycogen stores and endotoxemia/bacteremia compounds the hypoglycemia.
- Absolute insulin increase—insulinoma (rare); therapeutic or malicious administration of excessive insulin
- Hypoadrenocorticism—rare; horses could lack glucocorticoids, mineralocorticoids, or both.
- Malnutrition/starvation—could be lack of intake or maldigestion/malabsorption related to the GI tract.
- Overutilization—more often increased utilization with decreased intake
- Hyperlipemia of obese ponies, especially during pregnancy and lactation
- Rebound hypoglycemia resulting from parenteral nutrition, when glucose delivery is suddenly ceased without providing an alternative source of enteral carbohydrates

RISK FACTORS

- Poor-quality foodstuffs
- Failure of passive transfer
- Obesity

DIAGNOSIS

DIFFERENTIAL DIAGNOSIS

- See *Causes.*
- Laboratory artifact (see below)

LABORATORY FINDINGS

Drugs that May Alter Lab Results

N/A

Disorders that May Alter Lab Results

- Lipemia, hemolysis, and icterus may alter results depending on the assay used.
- Delayed separation of serum can decrease serum glucose concentration because of cellular utilization of glucose; sodium fluoride collection tubes can stabilize glucose concentrations for analysis.

Valid If Run in Human Lab?

Yes

CBC/BIOCHEMISTRY/URINALYSIS

- Dependent on the underlying disease

CBC

- With possible anemia, inflammatory leukogram if underlying inflammatory disease
- With sepsis/endotoxemia, may see neutropenia with left shift and toxic change, including Döhle bodies, in neutrophils.
- May have concurrent stress leukogram, with variable neutrophil numbers and lymphopenia.

Biochemistry/Urinalysis

- Liver failure—may have elevations in SDH, AST, bile acids, ammonia, and GGT, as well as decreased BUN, coagulation factor production, and late in disease, albumin.
- Septicemia—possible azotemia and electrolyte imbalances.
- Hypoglycemia may be very profound in neonates.

OTHER LABORATORY TESTS

- ACTH stimulation test—variable results, but cortisol concentration often is not increased by ACTH in hypoadrenocorticism.
- IgG concentrations to detect failure of passive transfer
- Blood culture in cases with suspected septicemia
- Measurement of plasma insulin—insulinomas increase insulin concentrations.
- Intestinal absorption tests—D-xylose absorption; glucose absorption

IMAGING

Ultrasonography or radiology can be used to detect underlying diseases.

DIAGNOSTIC PROCEDURES

N/A

GLUCOSE, HYPOGLYCEMIA

TREATMENT

- Treatment with dextrose-containing fluids
- Resolve underlying disease condition
- Medical management of septicemia, with appropriate antibiotics and supportive care
- In foals, hypoglycemia, especially with septicemia, is life-threatening and requires emergency therapy.

MEDICATIONS

DRUGS OF CHOICE

Those for treatment of the underlying disease

CONTRAINDICATIONS

Insulin

PRECAUTIONS

- Proper hydration of hypovolemic/azotemic patients is needed before use of aminoglycoside antibiotics and NSAIDs.

POSSIBLE INTERACTIONS

N/A

ALTERNATIVE DRUGS

N/A

FOLLOW-UP

PATIENT MONITORING

- Monitor blood glucose concentrations after treatment.
- Monitor for signs associated with the underlying disease.

POSSIBLE COMPLICATIONS

Multiple complications can occur with neonatal septicemia/endotoxemia, including DIC, cardiovascular collapse, and multiple organ failure.

MISCELLANEOUS

ASSOCIATED CONDITIONS

Electrolyte concentration abnormalities.

AGE-RELATED FACTORS

- Neonates can be prone to failure of passive transfer.
- Obese ponies may develop hyperlipidemia and hypoglycemia.

ZOONOTIC POTENTIAL

N/A

PREGNANCY

- In obese ponies, pregnancy is a risk factor for hyperlipidemia.
- If hypoglycemic, pregnancy can lead to weakness and dystocia.

SYNONYMS

N/A

SEE ALSO

- Hepatic failure
- Insulinoma
- Septicemia

ABBREVIATIONS

- AST = aspartate aminotransferase
- DIC = disseminated intravascular coagulation
- GGT = γ-glutamyltransferase
- GI = gastrointestinal
- SDH = sorbitol dehydrogenase

Suggested Reading

Eades SC, Bounous DI. Laboratory profiles of equine diseases. 1st ed. St. Louis: Mosby, 1997.

Fenger CK. Neonatal and perinatal diseases. In: Reed SM, Bayly WM, eds. Equine internal medicine. Philadelphia: WB Saunders, 1998:950–956.

Kaneko JJ. Carbohydrate metabolism and its diseases. In: Kaneko JJ, Harvey JW, Bruss ML, eds. Clinical biochemistry of domestic animals. San Diego: Academic Press, 1997:61–75.

Rivas L. Endocrine pancreas. In: Reed SM, Bayly WM, eds. Equine internal medicine. Philadelphia: WB Saunders, 1998:936–937.

Author Claire B. Andreasen
Consulting Editor Claire B. Andreasen

GLUCOSE TOLERANCE TEST

BASICS

DEFINITION

- Performed to evaluate a horse's ability to metabolize glucose appropriately.
- In normal horses, insulin secretion is closely tied to blood glucose concentrations. Fasted insulin concentrations are quite low but increase rapidly when the horse receives glucose. In turn, this rapidly causes blood glucose to return to the normal range.
- Administer dextrose (0.5 gm/kg as a 50% solution IV). Either blood glucose alone or glucose and insulin are determined before and every 30 minutes after administration for 4 hours. Glucose is not given orally to remove the confounding effects of poor intestinal absorption or delayed gastric emptying. Serum glucose should be normal within 3 hours of administration.
- The most common pathologic process causing abnormal results is insulin resistance in horses with pars intermedia tumors or hyperplasia (i.e., equine Cushing's disease), leading to prolonged elevation in blood glucose levels. Blood glucose also will be elevated longer than 3 hours in horses with diabetes mellitus caused by insulin deficiency.
- Also advocated as a means to assess maturity in neonatal foals. An insulin response of 250% over baseline at 5 minutes is associated with a good prognosis for life; a response of 100% or less at 15 minutes is associated with prematurity and a poor prognosis for life.

PATHOPHYSIOLOGY

- Pancreatitis leading to destruction of beta cells and development of type 1 diabetes mellitus leads to low insulin and increased glucose tolerance test times.
- Increased serum insulin levels in euglycemic or hyperglycemic horses may result from peripheral insulin resistance caused by type II diabetes mellitus or an insulin antagonist (e.g., cortisol) in horses with equine Cushing's disease, stressed horses, or those receiving glucocorticoid therapy.
- Poor response to insulin in premature foals reflects immaturity of the pancreatic beta cells and poor homeostatic mechanisms.

SYSTEM AFFECTED

The endocrine system is primarily affected by abnormal blood glucose response tests—slow return of blood glucose to the normal range indicates either insulin deficiency or resistance.

SIGNALMENT

- Ponies tend to have a physiologic degree of insulin resistance; thus, blood glucose returns to normal levels more slowly than in adults.
- No sex differences
- Obese animals, particularly ponies, are more insulin resistant than thinner animals.
- Cushing's disease tends to occur in old horses (>10 years).
- Premature foals are those born before 320 days of gestation.
- Dysmature foals are those born after 320 days of gestation but with signs of prematurity.

SIGNS

- In horses with an abnormal test, most commonly those of equine Cushing's disease—hirsutism and failure to shed winter coat
- Also common—abnormal fat distribution, pendulous abdomen, weight loss, polyuria and polydipsia, laminitis, and tendency to chronic infections
- The eyelids can look swollen, and the supraorbital fat pad may look bulged.
- The owner may report the horse is dull or depressed.
- Similar clinical signs, but without hirsutism or abnormal hair coat, are seen in horses with type II diabetes mellitus.
- In horses with type I diabetes mellitus—weight loss, polyuria and polydipsia, and lethargy or depression
- Prematurity—low body weight, weakness, short or silky hair coat, increased joint range of motion, bulging forehead, incomplete cartilage formation of the ears, and incomplete ossification of the tarsal and carpal bones

CAUSES

- The primary cause for abnormal results is insulin antagonist. Exogenous or endogenous corticosteroids are the most common, although other hormones (e.g., growth hormone) also may have this effect.
- When insulin resistance occurs without a predisposing cause, type II diabetes mellitus is diagnosed.
- The most common reason for type I diabetes mellitus is pancreatic damage secondary to parasite migration.
- The most common reason for prematurity is an adverse uterine environment, often placentitis or placental insufficiency.
- Some sedatives, particularly xylazine and detomidine, can cause a transient hyperglycemia that confounds results; thus, avoid these sedatives when performing these tests.
- High-carbohydrate diets may increase serum glucose; thus, perform the test on fasting horses.

RISK FACTORS

- A pituitary tumor is the most common risk factor for abnormal test results.
- Glucocorticoid administration or increased cortisol from a stress response also leads to insulin resistance and hyperglycemia.
- Obesity, particularly in ponies, is associated with insulin resistance, as is hyperlipidemia.

DIAGNOSIS

DIFFERENTIAL DIAGNOSIS

- Polyuria, polydipsia, and glucosuria in horses with suspected endocrine disorders indicate a disorder in glucose homeostasis.
- Weak foal—sepsis and neonatal maladjustment syndrome.
- History of gestational length allows a diagnosis of prematurity to be established. Premature foals also often are septic and have other medical conditions, so this diagnosis of prematurity does not preclude others.

LABORATORY FINDINGS

Drugs That May Alter Laboratory Results

N/A

Disorders That May Alter Laboratory Results

Delayed separation of serum from cells falsely lowers blood glucose values.

Valid If Run in a Human Lab?

Yes

CBC/BIOCHEMISTRY/URINALYSIS

- Horses with abnormal glucose response caused by Cushing's disease exhibit a stress response with mature neutrophilia, lymphopenia, and eosinopenia. They also may have glucosuria.
- Horses with type I or II diabetes mellitus have hyperglycemia.
- Premature foals have variable leukogram results. Good prognosis for life is associated with WBC counts >5000 cells/μL and fibrinogen levels <400 mg/dL.

OTHER LABORATORY TESTS

- Pituitary function—endogenous ACTH determination and dexamethasone suppression tests. If these results are consistent with equine Cushing's disease, that diagnosis is supported; if these results do not indicate Cushing's disease, suspect either a stress response or type II diabetes mellitus.
- Check IgG levels in all neonatal foals; give plasma if <600 mg/dL.
- Arterial blood gas determination to assess the foal's ability to ventilate and oxygenate its tissues

IMAGING

- Increased pituitary gland size may be visualized with specialized modalities—CT or venous contrast
- Lung maturity may be partially assessed in premature foals by thoracic radiography.

DIAGNOSTIC PROCEDURES

Exploratory laparotomy or abdominocentesis may reveal a damaged pancreas. However, these tests should be considered extremely low yield, because the pancreas normally is difficult to visualize and pancreatic tumors are too small to distort the pancreas so that they can be localized.

TREATMENT

APPROPRIATE HEALTH CARE

- Premature foals require inpatient treatment if severely affected, IV fluids, and nutritional support to maintain blood glucose at adequate levels. They also often require insufflation with oxygen or ventilatory support.
- Horses with hyperlipemia require inpatient treatment with IV dextrose, balanced electrolyte solutions, caloric replacement, heparin, and exogenous insulin.
- All other horses with abnormal test results can be treated as outpatients.

NURSING CARE

- Premature foals need extensive nursing care. They are prone to complications such as corneal ulcers, gastric ulcers, and pressure sores, and they need aggressive, proactive care to minimize such occurrences.
- Horses with laminitis need corrective hoof trimming and shoeing.

ACTIVITY

- Limit the activity of horses with laminitis.
- Increase the activity of sound, obese horses in an effort to lose weight.

DIET

- Horses with laminitis generally benefit from a low-carbohydrate, high-fiber diet—grass hay
- Keep horses with insulin resistance on a low-carbohydrate diet.
- Restrict or increase caloric intake in all horses until a condition score of 4–6 out of 10 is achieved.

CLIENT EDUCATION

- Long-term prognosis for life and work is good in premature foals if they can survive and develop to the point of no longer needing nursing care.
- Horses with Cushing's disease may be managed with medication and nursing care, but their prognosis is quite variable. Some do well for several years; others are refractory to treatment. Inform owners that treatment of such horses is palliative and required for life.
- Encourage clients to maintain horses at condition scores of 4–6 out of 10 and to prevent obesity.

SURGICAL CONSIDERATIONS

N/A

MEDICATIONS

DRUGS OF CHOICE

- The two agents most commonly used to alter symptoms of Cushing's disease are cyproheptadine (0.25–1.2 mg/kg PO SID) and pergolide (0.50–2 mg/day). These drugs also have been used with some success in horses with suspected type II diabetes.
- Horses with insulin deficiency (i.e., type I diabetes mellitus) require insulin supplementation. Protamine zinc insulin (0.5 IU IM BID) was reported to normalize blood glucose in a case report of a pony.
- Hyperlipemia—protamine zinc insulin (0.075–0.4 IU/kg SQ or IM BID or SID). Regular insulin (0.4 IU/kg) also has been recommended.
- Regard these doses as starting points that should be changed in response to blood glucose levels.

CONTRAINDICATIONS

N/A

PRECAUTIONS

- Dextrose for injection should always be available when administering insulin to any horse. If signs of hypoglycemia occur, treat immediately with IV dextrose.
- Horses that receive overdoses of cyproheptadine or pergolide may exhibit lethargy and ataxia.

POSSIBLE INTERACTIONS

N/A

ALTERNATIVE DRUGS

N/A

FOLLOW-UP

PATIENT MONITORING

- Test horses with Cushing's disease every 6–12 weeks by endogenous ACTH determination or dexamethasone response testing. Abnormal results indicate the need for an increased dose of the compound the horse is receiving or change in medication.
- Check the blood glucose level of horses with diabetes mellitus on insulin therapy twice a day. Increase or decrease insulin doses in response to blood glucose values outside the normal range.

POSSIBLE COMPLICATIONS

N/A

MISCELLANEOUS

ASSOCIATED CONDITIONS

- Hirsutism, chronic infections, and laminitis are commonly associated with equine Cushing's disease.
- Obesity and hyperlipemia are commonly associated with insulin resistance.
- Sepsis is common in premature foals.

AGE-RELATED FACTORS

N/A

ZOONOTIC POTENTIAL

N/A

PREGNANCY

N/A

SYNONYMS

N/A

SEE ALSO

- Insulin response test
- Pituitary tumors
- Premature foals

Suggested Reading

Beech J. Endocrine System. In: Colahan PT, Mayhew IG, Merritt AM, Moore JN, eds. Equine medicine and surgery. 5th ed. St. Louis: Mosby, 1999:1947–1968.

Fowden AL, Silver M, Ellis L, et al. Studies on equine prematurity: III. Insulin secretion in the foal during the perinatal period. Equine Vet J 1984;16:286–291.

Freestone JF, et al. Insulin and glucose response following oral glucose administration in well conditioned ponies. Equine Vet J 1992;11;13–17.

Riggs WL. Diabetes mellitus secondary to necrotizing pancreatitis in a pony. Southwest Vet 1972;25:149–152.

Author Janice Sojka
Consulting Editor Michel Levy

GOITER

BASICS

OVERVIEW

• Enlargement of the thyroid gland to as much as twice its normal size
• Diffuse or nodular
• Nodular cases—either uninodular or multinodular, functional or nonfunctional, and usually caused by thyroid adenomas that are nonfunctioning and not associated with clinical signs.
• Diffuse cases—caused by either excess or deficient iodine in the diet or by ingestion of goitrogens that make ingested iodine unavailable; horses with diffuse goiters generally are hypothyroid.
• Most frequently congenital and seen in foals born to mares ingesting excess amounts of iodine during pregnancy.
• Organ system—endocrine

SIGNALMENT

• No breed or sex predilections
• Most cases involve foals born with congenital goiters resulting from ingestion of goitrogens or unbalanced amounts of iodine by the dam.
• No genetic basis

SIGNS

Defining characteristic—a thyroid gland enlarged to as much as twice its normal size.

CAUSES AND RISK FACTORS

• Diffuse goiters—caused by ingestion of too much or too little iodine. Pregnant mares that receive high-iodine diets will be clinically normal, but their offspring will have enlarged thyroid glands.
• Nodular goiters—most often caused by thyroid adenoma or adenocarcinoma.
• Uncommon in horses
• Endemic goiters may occur on broodmare farms if dietary iodine is unbalanced.
• Idiopathic hypothyroidism and goiters occur in foals born to mares pastured in the northwestern portion of the North American continent. The cause of this syndrome is not known, but an ingested goitrogen is suspected.

DIAGNOSIS

DIFFERENTIAL DIAGNOSIS

• The diagnosis can be established at physical examination by observing and palpating a grossly enlarged thyroid gland.
• Differential diagnosis includes other structures that might cause swelling in the proximal neck—abscesses, enlarged lymph nodes, guttural pouches, and generalized edema or cellulitis

CBC/BIOCHEMISTRY/URINALYSIS

Usually normal

OTHER LABORATORY TESTS

Serum T_3 and T_4 levels may be low if the animal is hypothyroid.

IMAGING

• An enlarged thyroid gland may be seen as a soft-tissue mass on proximal neck radiographs.
• An enlarged thyroid also can be seen via ultrasonography.

DIAGNOSTIC PROCEDURES

Fine-needle biopsy or aspiration of the goiter to confirm that the structure in question is, indeed, the thyroid gland.

PATHOLOGIC FINDINGS

• Nodular goiters—a tumor in the thyroid gland often is found.
• Diffuse goiters—enlarged follicles filled with colloid, with or without a few resorption vesicles, can be seen.

GOITER

TREATMENT

- Determine the dietary iodine concentration of affected horses or of dams with affected foals; 35–40 mg/day in a pregnant mare's diet may cause congenital goiters in her foal (NRC recommendations for daily iodine intake, 1–2 mg/day.
- Once the diet is corrected to a proper iodine level, the goiter generally resolves.
- Recommend that broodmare owners not feed supplements containing excessive amounts of iodine to pregnant mares.
- Nodular goiter—removal of a thyroid tumor is curative.

MEDICATIONS

DRUGS

- If the horse is hypothyroid, supplementation with T_4 is curative.
- Synthetic T_4 (20 μg/kg) maintains normal thyroid hormone levels for 24 hours.

CONTRAINDICATIONS/POSSIBLE INTERACTIONS

N/A

FOLLOW-UP

- If the goiter is caused by a benign tumor, removal of the tumor should be curative.
- If the goiter is caused by excess or deficient iodine, dietary correction to an acceptable level should result in resolution of the symptoms.
- Monitor foals with goiters to ensure that skeletal abnormalities associated with hypothyroidism (e.g., angular limb deformities) do not develop.
- Expected course—resolution of the goiter; return to normal size of the thyroid gland once the goiter has been removed.

MISCELLANEOUS

ASSOCIATED CONDITIONS

N/A

AGE-RELATED FACTORS

N/A

ZOONOTIC POTENTIAL

N/A

PREGNANCY

N/A

SEE ALSO

- Hypothyroidism
- Thyroid tumors
- T_3/T_4 determination

ABBREVIATIONS

- NRC = National Research Council
- T3 = triiodothyronine
- T4 = thyroxine

Suggested Reading

Driscoll J, Hintz HF, Schryer HF. Goiter in foals caused by excessive iodine. J Am Vet Med Assoc 1968;153:1618–1630.

Author Janice Sojka
Consulting Editor Michel Levy

GRANULOMATOUS ENTERITIS

BASICS

DEFINITION

Granulomatous enteritis (GE) represents one of several types of chronic inflammatory bowel diseases affecting the mature horse. The disease is characterized by a diffuse and circumscribed infiltration of the lamina propria and submucosa of the gastrointestinal tract with lymphocytes, macrophages, and epithelioid cells with occasional plasma cells and multinucleated giant cells. The ileum is the most consistently and most severely affected site, whereas the large colon is the least commonly affected. Granulomatous changes are also found in the mesenteric lymph nodes of most affected horses. Marked villus atrophy and clubbing is present and contributes to the malabsorption due to loss of absorptive surface area and the loss of absorptive epithelial cells at the tips of the villi. Other features of the small bowel mucosa include ulceration, lymphoid hyperplasia, crypt abscesses, and lymphangiectasia. Clinically, this condition is associated with carbohydrate malabsorption and excessive protein loss into the gastrointestinal tract.

SIGNALMENT

Young adult horses (mean 2.2 yr; range 1–5 yr). May affect any breed of horse; however, Standardbreds have been the most commonly affected. A familial tendency for the development of GE has been suggested in Standardbreds. There is no sex predilection.

SIGNS

- Chronic, insidious weight loss over several months' duration is the most common presenting sign. Horses present in thin or emaciated body condition.
- Appetite variable; may be increased, normal, or decreased. Initially, appetite is usually increased.
- Edema of the ventral thorax, ventral abdomen, and distal extremities may develop as animal becomes hypoproteinemic.
- Multiple, firm nodules or masses (5- to 10-cm diameter) within the mesentery or small intestine may be palpated consistently on rectal examination.
- Roughened hair coat; alopecia; skin dry and flaky.
- Diarrhea is not usually present unless there is involvement of large intestine and rectum. Intermittent diarrhea with semi-formed feces recorded in 24% (4/17) of cases.
- Bright and alert initially, but become depressed with debilitation.
- Decreased exercise tolerance may be the first clinical sign observed.

CAUSES AND RISK FACTORS

The etiologic agent or the initiating pathophysiologic mechanism is currently unknown. It has been hypothesized that the granulomatous lesions may result from an aberrant host immune-mediated response to dietary, parasitic, or bacterial antigens.

DIAGNOSIS

DIFFERENTIAL DIAGNOSIS

Rule out other diseases that cause significant protein loss into the pleural or peritoneal cavities or urinary system, and other causes of chronic weight loss.

- Chronic eosinophilic gastroenteritis
- Intestinal lymphosarcoma
- Abdominal abscessation
- Lymphocytic–plasmacytic enteritis

CBC/BIOCHEMISTRY/URINALYSIS

- Hypoalbuminemia (moderate to severe) (8–22 g/L; normal 26–35 g/L) is the most consistent laboratory finding. In the initial stages of GE, intestinal protein loss involves relatively larger quantities of albumin than globulins.
- Total plasma or serum protein concentration may be low or normal, depending on serum globulin values.
- Mild to moderate hypoglobulinemia. Varying serum gamma-globulin levels.
- Normal complete blood counts or anemia (11/17)
- Moderate neutrophilia with mild left shift
- Urinalysis normal

DIAGNOSTIC PROCEDURES

- Decreased d-xylose and glucose absorption tests if there is significant small intestine involvement.
- Abdominocentesis is usually normal, except occasionally peritoneal macrophages may exhibit evidence of decreased phagocytic activity.
- Rectal mucosal biopsy may provide a diagnosis if the rectum is involved. Granulomatous changes in rectal mucosa.
- Intravenous administration of $[^{51}Cr]$ albumin documents increased fecal radioactivity due to gastrointestinal protein loss.
- Ileal biopsy through a standing left-flank laparotomy is necessary for a definitive diagnosis; however, surgery on a debilitated, hypoproteinemic animal is not without risk.

MEDICATIONS

DRUG(S) OF CHOICE

- Medical therapies have been generally unsuccessful in resolving the chronic inflammatory lesions.
- Prednisolone 0.5–2.0 mg/kg PO q24hr has been ineffective. As malabsorption is a feature of this disease, parenteral administration should be considered.
- Long-term parenteral dexamethasone sodium phosphate administration—40 mg IM q96hr for 4 weeks; 35 mg IM q96hr for 4 weeks; 30 mg IM q96hr for 4 weeks; 20 mg IM q96hr for 2 weeks; 10 mg IM q96hr for 2 weeks has been used successfully in one case reported in the literature.
- Total parenteral nutrition may be indicated in very valuable patients.

CONTRAINDICATIONS/POSSIBLE INTERACTIONS

Alleged risk of laminitis following parenteral dexamethasone administration.

FOLLOW-UP

- Monitor body weight, total serum protein, and serum albumin levels following dexamethasone therapy.
- Repeat rectal examinations and d-xylose absorption test.
- Feed free-choice, high-quality ration.
- Guarded long-term prognosis.

MISCELLANEOUS

ABBREVIATION

- GE = granulomatous enteritis

Suggested Reading

Cimprich RE. Equine granulomatous enteritis. Vet Pathol 1974;11:535-547.

Duryea JH, Ainsworth DM, Mauldin EA, Cooper BJ, Edwards RB. Clinical remission of granulomatous enteritis in a Standardbred gelding following long term dexamethasone administration. Eq Vet J 1997;29:164-167.

Lindberg R, Persson SGB, Jones B, Thoren-Tolling K, Ederoth M. Clinical and pathophysiological features of granulomatous enteritis and eosinophilic granulomatosis in the horse. Zbl Vet Med A 1985;32:526-539.

Sweeney RW, Sweeney CR, Saik J, Lichtensteiger CA. Chronic granulomatous bowel disease in three sibling horses. J Am Vet Med Assoc. 1986;188;1192-1194.

Author John D. Baird

Consulting Editor Henry Stämpfli

GRASS SICKNESS

BASICS

DEFINITION

Grass sickness is a dysautonomia, of unknown etiology that causes severe alterations of the alimentary tract and is characterized by high mortality. The condition is associated with severe changes in neurons of the autonomic nervous system, enteric nervous system, and in certain selected somatic ganglia and nuclei of the central nervous system. Recent reports suggest that *Clostridium botulinum* toxins may play a role in the etiology of some cases of the disease.

PATHOPHYSIOLOGY

There are widespread changes in autonomic neurons, the enteric plexuses, and some central neurons. The major clinical signs are related to alimentary dysfunction, athough dysphagia and muscular tremors may reflect central involvement.

SYSTEM AFFECTED

Gastrointestinal

Autonomic, enteric, and central nervous systems

INCIDENCE/PREVALENCE

The disease is currently recognized in many European countries, including Great Britain, Norway, Sweden, Denmark, France, Switzerland, and Germany. In the Southern Hemisphere of the Americas, mal seco has been reported in the Patagonian region of Argentina and the Falkland Islands. Mal seco is a syndrome indistinguishable from grass sickness. A similar clinical disease has been reported in Colombia and is called "Tambora," but there has not been adequate histopathologic documentation to establish a final diagnosis. Different studies from Scotland have indicated that grass sickness affects from 0.5% to 4% of the local horse population. This accounts for 18.3% of all fatal colics and it has been estimated that up to 1% of horses die of grass sickness annually in some areas of Scotland. In a telephone-based case-controlled study in Wales, it was determined that 1.3% of all colic cases examined were due to grass sickness.

SIGNALMENT

Grass sickness is a disease of young adult horses with a peak range of 2–7 yr. However, horses may be affected at an early age of 4 months. There does not seem to be any breed or gender predisposition.

SIGNS

Grass sickness seems to have three typical clinical presentations that may overlap. The acute form has a survival <2 days, the subacute with a duration between 2 and 7 days, and the chronic presentation with a duration of >7 days.

Acute

The clinical signs in the acute form are dullness and anorexia as well as different degrees of colic. At presentation, the horses are usually in good physical condition. Depression is more common in this clinical form and can be marked. Abdominal distension becomes very evident and is accompanied by reduced or absent abdominal sounds. Muscle tremors occur in approximately 74% of the cases, may vary from mild to severe, and occur more commonly over the shoulders, triceps, and flank areas. Sweating is also very evident. Heart rate is elevated, frequently reaching 100 bpm; the heart rate seems to be more elevated than would be expected for the degree of abdominal pain observed. Rectal temperature may be normal or occasionally elevated (up to 39.5°C/103.5°F).

Affected horses may show different degrees of dehydration, and the mucous membranes are usually injected. Ptyalism is frequently observed. Spontaneous gastric reflux may occur and is often manifested by green or brown malodorous regurgitation on the nares. Naso-gastric intubation yields moderate to abundant amounts of gastric reflux. If not relieved, rupture of the stomach may follow. Dysphagia is frequent, but is not very obvious at the beginning of the disease due to lack of appetite.

On rectal examination, there usually are small dry fecal balls present covered with abundant mucus. The rectal wall feels dry. In most cases, an impaction of the large left ventral and dorsal colon may be palpated. In some cases, distended loops of small intestine are present.

Subacute

Findings are very similar to those observed in the acute form but the signs are less severe. Heart rate is usually high, but the animal does not appear to be distressed. Dry feces are commonly found. Some animals have slow mastication, and usually gastric reflux is absent in this form.

Chronic

In the chronic form, the onset of clinical signs is more protracted and may be a progression from the subacute form. The animals lose physical condition to the point of emaciation, have a sleepy appearance, a "tucked up" abdomen, a weak gait, and a tendency to stand with all four feet together. In males, the penis may be flaccid and pendulous. As in the acute form, there are different degrees of muscular tremors, colic signs, sweating, dysphagia, and decrease in intestinal sounds. Heart rate can be normal to increased. Horses are hungry, but are dysphagic. Mastication is slow, and swallowing may be followed by an observable esophageal spasm. There may be intermittent diarrhea, chronic rhinitis, and bilateral nasal discharge. Rectal examination reveals empty intestines and possibly splenomegaly.

CAUSES

So far, definitive common etiologic factors have not been identified. There is epidemiologic evidence that a possible agent is related to pasture. A neurotoxin of 30 kD has been detected in serum of affected horses that may reach the ganglions through retrograde ascension from the intestines.

RISK FACTORS

Grass sickness occurs mainly in grazing horses, but there have been case reports in horses housed full time. Grass sickness occurs all year round, but in Europe it peaks in May, with a high incidence between April and July. However, in the Southern Hemisphere, mal seco tends to occur mainly from October to February.

The condition usually affects animals in good body condition. Mares seem to be at a slightly reduced risk, as animals with a history of contact with previous cases of the disease and increasing frequency of anthelmintic therapy seems to increase the risk of the disease. Moving animals to new pastures favors the occurrence of the disease. There are premises with observed greater incidence, but it has not been possible to associate it to a specific type of pasture.

In east Scotland, dry and cool weather with mean average temperatures of 7–11°C that lasts for at least 10 days and irregular ground frosts are conditions favoring the outbreak of grass sickness.

GRASS SICKNESS

DIAGNOSIS

DIFFERENTIAL DIAGNOSIS

The most important differential diagnosis is to determine whether the colic is surgical (see Acute Colic and Chronic Colic). A horse presenting with changing degrees of colic pain and dysphagia is very suggestive of acute grass sickness. In the chronic cases, the rapid weight loss accompanied with dysphagia, rhinitis, colic, and abnormal sweating indicates the possible diagnosis of the disease.

CBC/BIOCHEMISTRY/URINALYSIS

The CBC and biochemical profile alterations are the same as those seen in moderate to severe colic. There are no singular alterations in these parameters permitting differentiation of grass sickness from other colics.

Haptoglobin and orosomucoid are elevated in horses with grass sickness but not in usual colic cases. However, these two acute-phase proteins are elevated in other inflammatory processes. Ceruloplasmin and alpha-2-macroglobulin are increases in acute cases of grass sickness, but are not different from other colic cases.

Peritoneal fluid analysis is very similar to other colic cases; the difference detected is the higher increase in protein levels.

OTHER LABORATORY TESTS

The final diagnosis in grass sickness is provided by the demonstration of the pathologic changes in the autonomic or enteric nervous system. This has prompted the use of full-thickness ileal biopsies for making an antemorten diagnosis. As an alternative, rectal biopsy has been proposed, but the neuronal lesion is not very evident in the rectum, and at this time is not a reliable diagnostic tool.

Pathologic Changes

The gross pathologic and histopathologic changes described for grass sickness, mal-seco, and the Colombian grass sickness-like disease are indistinguishable. The gross pathologic findings are most obvious in the alimentary tract. The esophageal wall may be edematous and the mucosa may show longitudinal bands of congestion. If the stomach has not ruptured, it may be severely distended with fluids. There is excess fluid in the small intestine, which may have hemorrhage and edema. The large intestine is impacted with very dry contents. The intestinal wall may have a blackened surface. The small colon and rectum have small dry balls of fecal material. Chronic cases show lack of intestinal content, and in some cases of chronic mal seco there can be large colon impactions. Histologic lesions are located mainly in the neurons of the enteric nervous system; the autonomic ganglia, especially the celiacomesenteric; and brain stem nuclei. The morphologic neuronal changes include chromatolysis resulting in cytoplasmic eosinophilia, cytoplasmic vacuolization, pyknosis, karyorrhexis, or apparent loss of nuclei. In the enteric nervous system, the typical neuronal lesion is observed in the stomach and intestine. However, it is the ileum where the most severe changes occur. The ileum is affected in both acute and chronic grass sicknesses. This is the only area that is usually affected in chronic cases. Brain lesions occur in several nuclei, but these lesions do not seem to be specific for grass sickness.

TREATMENT

It has always been accepted that therapy for grass sickness cases was hopeless. However, reports from Scotland suggest that therapy could be warranted in some selected chronic cases. In the Colombian form there are reports of recovery.

It has been reported that in acute and subacute cases, the mortality is 100%, and in chronic cases slightly lower. The probability of success has been improved by case selection; it has been pointed out that the success rate may reach 70% when certain case selection criteria are used. For chronic cases, they include that the horse be able to swallow some of the feed offered, be alert, and has not become cachectic.

DIET

Scottish researchers have suggested the following management regimen. Housing is advisable, and there should be short hand-walks daily. High-energy, high-protein diets should be provided. The recommended feeds are sweet feed, crushed oats, and high-energy cubes fed wet or dry. Providing up to 500 mL of cotton oil could increase dietary fat content. Feeding by nasogastric tube has not been successful.

MEDICATION

Cisapride at a dose of 0.5–0.8 mg/kg PO three times a day for 7 days has been found to increase intestinal motility in chronic cases. It has been observed that administration causes mild colic, which may occur during feeding. There are no reports of recovery in animals with mal seco. However, in the Colombian disease there are reports of cases that have recovered. Treatment is usually prolonged, and signs of recovery are detected when the patient starts gaining weight 2–5 weeks from the onset of the disease process. However, in a recent study on long-term prospects for horses with chronic grass sickness, the owners thought that the treated animals were capable of strenuous work, regained weight they had lost, had returned to normal life, apart from few residual problems such as difficulty in ingesting dry, fibrous food.

PREVENTION

In areas with high prevalence, the only method known that may work is to keep the horses stabled during dry cool days as well as during the time of high incidence of the disease, and if possible, to not use pastures where the disease is known to occur.

Suggested Reading

Doxey DL, Milne EM, Gilmour JS, Pogson DM. Clinical and biochemical features of grass sickness (equine dysautonomia). Eq Vet J. 1991;23:360-364.

Doxey DL, Milne EM, Ellison J, Curry PJ. Long-term prospects for horses with grass sickness. Vet Rec 1998;142:207-209.

Hahn C, Gerber V, Herholz C, Mayhew IG. Proceedings of the First International Workshop on Grass Sickness, Equine Motor Neuron Disease and Related Disorders. Bern, Switzerland. October 26–27, 1995.

Ochoa R, Velandia S. Equine grass sickness: serologic evidence of association with *Clostridium perfringens* type A enterotoxin. Am J Vet Res. 1978;39:1049-1051.

Uzal FA, Robles CA. Mal seco, a grass sickness-like syndrome of horses in Argentina. Vet Res Comm. 1993;17:449-457.

Author Oliver Olimpo

Consulting Editor Henry Stampfli

GUTTURAL POUCH EMPYEMA

BASICS

OVERVIEW

Definition

- Guttural pouches are diverticula of the auditory tubes that communicate with the pharynx through the pharyngeal orifice of the auditory tube.
- Accumulation of mucopurulent material within the guttural pouch usually results from a secondary bacterial infection of the upper respiratory tract.

Pathophysiology

- Upper respiratory tract infection associated with β-hemolytic streptococci invading the guttural pouch often follows abscessation of the retropharyngeal lymph nodes.
- The guttural pouch opening to the pharynx is situated somewhat dorsally; therefore, the condition is exacerbated by poor drainage.
- Uni- or bilateral
- Any condition of the upper airways causing stenosis or occlusion of the guttural pouch pharyngeal opening predisposes.

System Affected

Upper respiratory tract

Incidence/Prevalence

Worldwide

SIGNALMENT

- Guttural pouch infection occurs in horses of any breed or age.
- Retropharyngeal lymph node abscessation caused by strangles draining into the guttural pouches is reportedly more frequent in foals and yearlings than in adults.

SIGNS

Historical Findings

- Commonly associated as a complication of strangles infection.
- Chronic, unilateral, mucopurulent nasal discharge of unknown cause

Physical Examination Findings

- Intermittent nasal discharge
- Swelling of adjacent lymph nodes; painful lymph nodes on palpation
- Occasional difficulty in swallowing (i.e., dysphagia) or breathing (i.e., stertorous noise)

CAUSES AND RISK FACTORS

- Most frequently *Streptococcus equi* var *equi* and var *zooepidemicus*
- Outbreaks of strangles
- Congenital stenosis of the pharyngeal orifice of the auditory tube

DIAGNOSIS

DIFFERENTIAL DIAGNOSIS

- Guttural pouch mycosis
- Trauma to the guttural pouch

CBC/BIOCHEMISTRY/URINALYSIS

- If associated with an upper respiratory bacterial infection (e.g., *S. equi* var *equi*), the leukogram shows a leukocytosis, and the fibrinogen level is elevated.
- If the guttural pouch infection is without systemic effect, the leukogram is in the normal range.

OTHER LABORATORY TESTS

Bacterial culture and sensitivity as well as cytology of purulent material are obtained through a catheter.

IMAGING

- Radiography—a standing, lateral projection is useful to identify a distinct fluid line representing the exudate within the pouch.
- Ultrasonography—potential diagnostic value if fluid can be identified in the dependent area of the guttural pouch; however, the scientific literature supporting the comparison is very limited.

DIAGNOSTIC PROCEDURES

- Pharyngeal endoscopy identifies a purulent discharge from the orifice of the affected guttural pouch; however, direct visualization of the guttural pouch itself confirms the presence of mucopurulent debris and the formation of chondroids.
- During endoscopy of the guttural pouch, a polyethylene catheter can be passed through the biopsy channel of the endoscope and mucopurulent debris collected for cytology and bacterial culture.

PATHOLOGIC FINDINGS

If related to strangles, possible abscessation of the retropharyngeal lymph nodes draining directly into the guttural pouches; these lesions are frequently observed in foals and yearlings infected with *S. equi* var *equi.*

TREATMENT

APPRORIATE HEALTH CARE

- Placement of an indwelling catheter to facilitate irrigation of the guttural pouch is paramount to successful treatment.
- During the first 2 days, irrigate the affected pouch with a weak solution (1–3%) of povidone iodine (500 mL) twice daily, then continue irrigation with sterile saline twice a day until mucopurulent debris no longer is visible during the irrigation procedure.

NURSING CARE

Unless the affected horse is dysphagic or dyspneic, no particular care is needed.

ACTIVITY

- Rest is advised until the condition resolves.
- Activity is not recommended during therapeutic flushing of the guttural pouches.

GUTTURAL POUCH EMPYEMA

CLIENT EDUCATION

If the cause was strangles, provide specific advice relating to the condition (see the section on *S. equi* var *equi*).

SURGICAL CONSIDERATIONS

• When treatment involves combination systemic antibiotic, local irrigation of the guttural pouch has been unsuccessful, and if chondroids have formed, surgical drainage of the guttural pouch is the intervention of choice.
• The hyovertebrotomy approach, which is a lateral approach to the guttural pouch combined with a ventral approach through the Viborg's triangle, assures maximal drainage of the guttural pouch.

MEDICATIONS

DRUGS

• Antibiotics, depending on bacterial culture and sensitivity results.
• Affected horses usually respond to most β-lactam antibiotics (e.g., penicillin, cephalosporins, etc.) administered for a period of 10 days.

CONTRAINDICATIONS/POSSIBLE INTERACTIONS

Avoid irrigation with irritating solutions (e.g., strong iodine solution) and placement of traumatic catheter. This may damage several cranial nerves that course through the pouch wall, leading to a variety of signs—dysphagia, dorsal displacement of the soft palate, and occasionally, head tilt.

FOLLOW-UP

PATIENT MONITORING

• Repeat endoscopy 1–2 weeks after the last irrigation therapy.
• Ground feeding to encourage natural drainage

PREVENTION/AVOIDANCE

Encourage annual strangles vaccination in foals, yearlings, and mature horses in forms where the infection is endemic.

POSSIBLE COMPLICATIONS

• Chondroid formation necessitating surgical removal
• Neurologic injury to the glossopharyngeal, vagus, accessory, and hypoglossal nerves, leading to pharyngeal paralysis, dysphagia, and dyspnea

EXPECTED COURSE AND PROGNOSIS

• Duration of the condition depends on the causal agent if empyema results from abscessation of retropharyngeal lymph nodes or simple infection of the guttural pouch mucosa.
• Prognosis is favorable with early diagnosis and treatment.
• Chondroid formation with neurologic injury carries a poor prognosis.

MISCELLANEOUS

ASSOCIATED CONDITIONS

• Strangles
• *S. zooepidemicus* infection of the upper respiratory tract

AGE-RELATED FACTORS

Retropharyngeal lymph node abscessation caused by strangles draining in the guttural pouches is reportedly more frequent in foals and yearlings than in adults.

ZOONOTIC POTENTIAL

N/A

PREGNANCY

N/A

SEE ALSO

• Guttural pouch mycosis
• Purulent nasal discharge
• Strangles

Suggested Reading

DE Freeman. Diagnosis and treatment of diseases of the guttural pouch (part 1). Compend Contin Educ Large Anim Suppl 1980;II:S3–S11.

Author Laurent Viel
Consulting Editor Jean-Pierre Lavoie

GUTTURAL POUCH MYCOSIS

BASICS

OVERVIEW

- A fungal disease of the auditory tube diverticulum
- Usually affects one guttural pouch, but bilateral lesions are possible.
- Clinical signs relate to damage to the arteries and nerves.
- Spontaneous epistaxis in a resting horse usually is the first sign of this life-threatening condition.
- Organ systems—respiratory, nervous, hemic/lymphatic/immune, and cardiovascular

SIGNALMENT

- Uncommon in foals and young horses.
- No breed or sex predilection.
- Believed to be more common in stabled horses during the warmer months of the year.

SIGNS

- May be asymptomatic.
- Epistaxis—the most frequent clinical sign; not related to exercise; severity varies from a mild, blood-tinged nasal secretion to fatal hemorrhage. Bleeding usually is unilateral but may be bilateral with severe hemorrhage; bleeding can stop spontaneously but, in most untreated cases, recurs in the following days or weeks. Premonitory bleeding often, but not always, precedes fatal hemorrhage.
- Ingesta in nasal discharge—the second most common clinical sign
- Dysphagia results from lesions involving the vagus and glossopharyngeal nerves and may lead to aspiration pneumonia.
- Other neurologic deficits—laryngeal hemiplegia, facial paralysis, and Horner's syndrome
- Less commonly seen—nasal discharge, head shaking, abnormal head posture, visual disturbances, and parotid pain

CAUSES AND RISK FACTORS

- An initiating factor that predisposes to growth of opportunistic fungi in the affected guttural pouch has not been determined.
- Different fungal species have been incriminated, with *Asperigillus nidulans* the most frequently isolated.
- Major blood vessels in the guttural pouch wall include internal and external carotids, maxillary, caudal auricular, and superficial temporal arteries. Mycotic diphtheritic membranes usually are in the caudodorsal part of the medial compartment of the guttural pouch, involving the internal carotid artery more frequently.
- Cranial nerves (IX, X, XI, XII), cranial cervical ganglion, and sympathetic trunk are in a mucous membrane fold in the caudal aspect of the medial compartment, and a small portion of the facial nerve (VII) crosses the dorsal aspect of the guttural pouch. The fungal plaque may invade one or more of these structures.

DIAGNOSIS

DIFFERENTIAL DIAGNOSIS

- Epistaxis—exercise-induced pulmonary hemorrhage, ethmoid hematoma, head trauma, foreign bodies, upper airway neoplasia, abscess rupture, longus capitis muscle rupture, and coagulopathy. Longus capitis muscle rupture usually is associated with a recent history of trauma. Epistaxis caused by coagulopathy is rare in horses and usually associated with other clinical signs and hemorrhages at other sites.
- Guttural pouch hemorrhage—longus capitis muscle rupture, iatrogenic trauma, and neoplasia
- Dysphagia—esophageal obstruction, megaesophagus, fracture of the hyoid apparatus, inflammatory reaction, cyst or neoplasia in the pharyngeal area, and cleft palate. Empyema or tympanism of the guttural pouch may lead to dysphagia in severe cases.
- Dysphagia of neurologic origin—bacterial, viral, or mycotic infection of the CNS: neuritis of cranial nerves IX, X, and XI; botulism; lead or plant poisoning; hepatic encephalopathy; and leukoencephalopathy

CBC/BIOCHEMISTRY/URINALYSIS

- Anemia is observed 12–24 hours after severe blood loss, but PCV may remain within normal ranges initially because of a loss of RBCs and plasma in equal proportions.
- Leukocytosis suggests concurrent aspiration pneumonia.
- Biochemistry profile and urinalysis—unremarkable unless the affected horse is dehydrated because of an inability to drink.

OTHER LABORATORY TESTS

Fungal cultures, but these are not routinely done.

IMAGING

- Endoscopy—mycotic lesions of affected guttural pouches appear as a white, black, and yellow paste on the surface of the mucosa. Perform a thorough examination of both guttural pouches to determine which vessels are affected, and take care to avoid dislodging a thrombus on the affected artery. No relationship exists between lesion size and severity of the clinical signs. Large quantities of blood in the guttural pouch may be present, precluding visualization of affected nerves and arteries. Blood may flow back into the trachea and must not be misinterpreted as coming from the lung.
- Radiography of head has little value when endoscopy is available.

DIAGNOSTIC PROCEDURES

N/A

PATHOLOGIC FINDING

Involvement of deeper structures (e.g., hyoid apparatus, petrous temporal bones, and atlanto-occipital joint) have been described in severe cases.

GUTTURAL POUCH MYCOSIS

TREATMENT

• The first goal is to prevent spontaneous fatal hemorrhage. Perform arterial occlusion as soon as possible. Proximal ligation of the artery does not immediately negate the blood pressure distally because of retrograde flux from the circle of Willis. Because distal ligation is very difficult, balloon catheter–occlusion techniques have been developed to stop the blood flow proximal and distal to the lesion. The artery is ligated proximally, and a balloon-tipped catheter is inserted into the artery and driven beyond the lesion. The balloon is inflated to stop retrograde flow and cause thrombosis, and the catheter is secured and left in place. Mycotic lesions usually resolve without specific treatment after arterial occlusion.
• IV administration of polyionic fluids and blood transfusion from an appropriate donor may be required before surgery in horses with profuse bleeding.

MEDICATIONS

DRUGS

• Medical treatment has been used with variable results.
• Topical treatment with ketoconazole, enilconazole, nystatin, and iodine, used alone or in combination with systemic drugs such as itraconazole (5 mg/kg PO SID) and amphotericin B (0.05 mg/kg IV q48h).
• In most cases, the risk of fatal hemorrhage is still present during long-term medical treatment.

CONTRAINDICATIONS/POSSIBLE INTERACTIONS

Development of dysphagia during apparently successful medical treatment suggests that topical drugs may have an irritating or neurotoxic effect.

FOLLOW-UP

• 50% of horses with guttural pouch mycosis left untreated die from fatal hemorrhage.
• Surgical treatment provides a favorable prognosis.
• Dysphagia suggests a poor prognosis for recovery.

MISCELLANOUS

ASSOCIATED CONDITIONS

N/A

AGE-RELATED FACTORS

N/A

ZOONOTIC POTENTIAL

N/A

PREGNANCY

N/A

SEE ALSO

Hemorrhagic nasal discharge

ABBREVIATION

PCV = packed cell volume

Suggested Reading

Freeman DE. Guttural pouch. In: Auer JA, ed. Equine surgery. Philadelphia: WB Saunders, 1992.

Author Vincent J. Ammann
Consulting Editor Jean-Pierre Lavoie

GUTTURAL POUCH TYMPANY

BASICS

OVERVIEW

• A nonpainful, tympanic swelling in the parotid region caused by distention of one or both guttural pouches with air.
• The enlarged guttural pouch may displace the pharynx, larynx, and trachea ventrally or contralaterally.

SIGNALMENT

• Foals and weanlings, predominantly fillies.
• No breed predilection.

SIGNS

Historical Findings

• Foals usually appear normal at birth; the swelling develops over several days.
• Spontaneous cases may develop in old foals.

Physical Examination Findings

• Unilateral guttural pouch involvement is most frequent.
• Nonpainful, tympanic swelling over the parotid region is found.
• In severe cases, stertorous breathing and dysphagia may develop.
• Secondary guttural pouch empyema and aspiration pneumonia may be present.

CAUSES AND RISK FACTORS

The exact cause is unknown but is considered to be a congenital dysfunction of the pharyngeal orifice of the affected guttural pouch. During respiration, the ingress of air into the guttural pouch occurs, but because of the defective orifice, the air cannot escape. Thus, a progressive distension of the guttural pouch arises.

DIAGNOSIS

DIFFERENTIAL DIAGNOSIS

• *Streptococcus equi* infection (i.e., strangles), which causes severe swelling of the submandibular or retropharyngeal lymph nodes, retropharyngeal abscesses, and cellulitis, is easily distinguished from uncomplicated guttural pouch tympany, because the former is associated with pain, fever, leukocytosis, and hyperfibrinogenemia.
• Primary guttural pouch empyema is differentiated by the presence of nasal discharge and by fluid in the guttural pouch on standing lateral radiography and endoscopy. In addition, it rarely causes tympanic swelling in the parotid region.

CBC/BIOCHEMISTRY/URINALYSIS

• A stress leukogram may be present with significant respiratory distress.
• Leukocytosis and hyperfibrinogenemia may be found with aspiration pneumonia.

OTHER LABORATORY TESTS

N/A

IMAGING

Endoscopy

• Decreased pharyngeal lumen caused by a collapse of both the roof and the pharyngeal walls.
• Introduction of the endoscope into the affected guttural pouch deflates it and helps to distinguish between unilateral and bilateral tympany.
• Secondary guttural pouch empyema may be observed.

RADIOGRAPHY

• The normal guttural pouch extends as far caudally as the ventral tubercle of the atlas; in guttural pouch tympany, the limit of this extension is further caudally.
• Collapse of the pharynx may be noted, and large, air-filled guttural pouches with evidence of a fluid line may be observed. A ventrodorsal radiograph of the area may help to distinguish between unilateral and bilateral tympany in some cases.
• Standing lateral thoracic radiography to rule out aspiration pneumonia.

DIAGNOSTIC PROCEDURES

Bacterial culture and antimicrobial sensitivity of fluid from guttural pouch in cases of secondary empyema.

TREATMENT

• External deflation of the guttural pouch by needle aspiration is not recommended because of the possibility of causing hemorrhage or damaging the nerves traversing the pouch walls.
• Temporary alleviation of airway obstruction can be achieved by applying gentle pressure bilaterally on the parotid area or through an indwelling catheter placed in the pharyngeal orifice of the affected pouch.
• Definitive treatment is surgery with general anesthesia—fenestration of the median septum that separates the two guttural pouches, or resection of a small segment of the medial lamina of the eustachian tube and its associated mucosal fold to create a larger opening of the affected guttural pouch into the pharynx.

• Fenestration of the median septum is used in unilateral guttural pouch tympany; both procedures are performed in bilateral involvement.
• Creation of a fistula between the pharynx and the eustachian tube with laser equipment or electrosurgery can be performed under sedation and endoscopic guidance.

MEDICATIONS

DRUGS

• Pre- and postoperative medication—systemic antibiotics (procaine penicillin G [20,000 U/kg IM BID], trimethoprim sulfamethoxazole [5 mg/kg IV BID], ceftiofur [2.2 mg/kg SID or BID]) and NSAIDs (flunixin meglumine [1 mg/kg IV or IM BID]).
• In cases complicated by aspiration pneumonia or guttural pouch empyema, broad-spectrum antibiotics based on sensitivity tests are required.
• Resolution of aspiration pneumonia symptoms is recommended before attempting surgical correction under general anesthesia.

CONTRAINDICATIONS/POSSIBLE INTERACTIONS

Use α_2 adrenergic agonist agents (e.g., xylazine, detomidine) with caution, because they may worsen upper airway obstruction by relaxing the pharyngeal and laryngeal muscles.

FOLLOW-UP

• In the absence of aspiration pneumonia or guttural pouch empyema, the prognosis for unilateral guttural pouch tympany is favorable.
• The recurrence rate following a surgical correction is 30%.
• Aspiration pneumonia warrants a guarded prognosis.

MISCELLANEOUS

ASSOCIATED CONDITIONS

N/A

AGE-RELATED FACTORS

N/A

ZOONOTIC POTENTIAL

N/A

PREGNANCY

N/A

SEE ALSO

N/A

Suggested Reading

McCue PM, Freeman DE, Donawick WJ. Guttural pouch tympany: 15 cases (1977–1986). J Am Vet Med Assoc 1989;194:1761–1763.

Author Ludovic Bouré
Consulting Editor Jean-Pierre Lavoie

HEAD TRAUMA

BASICS

DEFINITION

• Trauma to the skull or associated soft tissues, resulting in primary damage to the brain
• Secondary brain injury results from the primary injury and causes physiologic changes in brain tissue.
• Secondary brain injury can be prevented or lessened; primary injury cannot.

PATHOPHYSIOLOGY

• After traumatic insult to the brain, a cycle of cellular events occurs, including membrane disruption, ischemia, hypoxia, edema, and hemorrhage.
• Severity of these abnormalities depends on the type and extent of the initial primary injury.
• The traumatic insult also is responsible for increased permeability of brain capillary endothelial cells, resulting in vasogenic edema. This is the most common type of edema found after head trauma, and white matter is especially prone.
• Vasogenic edema results in displacement of cerebral tissue and increased ICP. Ultimately, these changes may produce brain herniation.
• Cytotoxic edema results from swelling of the cellular elements of the brain. This type of edema occurs in gray and white matter and often results in decreased cerebral function, with stupor and coma as signs.
• A cycle occurs in which increased ICP leads to decreased cerebral blood flow, resulting in further ischemia and brain swelling.
• Types of cranial trauma (from least to most severe)—concussion, contusion, laceration, and hemorrhage
• Concussion is short-term loss of consciousness, often is reversible, and occurs without anatomic lesions.
• Contusion is associated with vascular and neural tissue damage without major structural disruption.
• Laceration and hemorrhage result from penetrating wounds, fractures, or direct blunt trauma.
• Cerebral hemorrhage in horses may be epidural, subdural (rare), intracerebral, or subarachnoid (common).
• Hematoma formation is potentially devastating, because hemorrhage results in expansion within the rigid skull, with possible herniation, pressure necrosis, and brainstem compression.

SYSTEMS AFFECTED

• Behavioral—altered mentation
• Cardiovascular—arrthymias/bradycardia due to dysfunction of central cardiovascular centers
• Musculoskeletal—skull fracture(s); postural/gait abnormalities due to disruption of central motor pathways; other lacerations/fractures from the traumatic episode
• Nervous—disruption of neural pathways, resulting in changes in behavior, heart rate and rhythm, respiratory rate and rhythm, and neurologic testing
• Ophthalmic—abnormal eye position, movements, and reflexes; changes in vision
• Respiratory—apneustic or erratic breathing due to dysfunction of the respiratory regulatory center in the caudal medulla oblongata

GENETICS

N/A

INCIDENCE/PREVALENCE

N/A

SIGNALMENT

Species

Equine

Breed Predilections

N/A

Mean Age Range

N/A

Predominant Sex

N/A

SIGNS

Historical Findings

• Ascertain any known episode of trauma or physical evidence of trauma to the horse or its environment.
• Sometimes abnormal behavior, gait changes, sudden blindness, or recumbency.

Physical Examination Findings

• Direct initial evaluation toward identification and stabilization of life-threatening problems—open skull fractures, airway obstruction, hemorrhage, cardiovascular collapse, pneumothorax, and other fractures
• Look for evidence of head trauma.
• Palpation of the skull may reveal fractures.
• Blood from the ears, mouth, or nostrils suggest potential basisphenoid or basioccipital fractures.
• Occasionally, CSF may be seen draining from the ears with basilar fractures.
• Bradycardia or arrhythmias may be present, with apneustic or erratic breathing, with injury to the central cardiac and respiratory centers.

Neurologic Examination Findings

• Neurologic deficits may range from inapparent to recumbency with profound depression, dementia, and tetraparesis.
• Injury to the cerebrum may manifest as behavioral changes, depression, coma, circling or wandering, seizures, and blindness with normal pupillary reflexes.
• Injury to the cerebellum may manifest as altered behavior, ataxia, hypermetria, intention tremor, hypertonicity, and lack of menace without blindness.
• Injury to the diencephalons (i.e., thalamus) may manifest as depression to stupor, normal to mild tetraparesis, deviation of the head and eyes with circling toward the side of a unilateral lesion, and bilateral nonreactive pupils with blindness.
• Midbrain trauma may demonstrate stupor to coma with hemiparesis, tetraparesis, or tetraplegia and nonreactive pupils with mydriasis, anisocoria, and ventrolateral strabismus.
• Trauma to the pons and rostral medulla oblongata (including the inner ear) often manifests as depression, ataxia with tetraparesis or tetraplegia, head tilt, nystagmus, facial paralysis, and medial strabismus.
• Trauma to the caudal medulla oblongata may manifest as depression, ataxia with hemiparesis to tetraparesis, abnormal respiratory patterns, and dysphagia with a flaccid tongue.

HEAD TRAUMA

CAUSES

Head trauma

RISK FACTORS

- Young age
- Fractious behavior
- Unsafe environment

DIAGNOSIS

DIFFERENTIAL DIAGNOSIS

- Consider other primary brain disorders—seizures, infection, inflammation, neoplasia, degenerative disease, and congenital problems
- Syncope from cardiovascular disease, metabolic diseases, toxin exposure, adverse drug reactions, and nutritional deficiencies also may affect brain function.

CBC/BIOCHEMISTRY/URINALYSIS

- Changes in any of these tests may reflect changes in other organ systems secondary to the effects of trauma or due to other underlying disease processes.
- No specific changes in any of these tests for head trauma.

OTHER LABORATORY TESTS

N/A

IMAGING

- Skull radiographs may reveal fractures, luxations, and subluxations. Radiographs of other areas (e.g., long bones, chest) that have evidence of trauma is warranted.
- CT or magnetic resonance imaging of the head may reveal fractures, hemorrhage, or foreign bodies lodged in the skull or brain.
- Scintigraphy is useful for diagnosis of nondisplaced and occult fractures and soft-tissue lesions.

DIAGNOSTIC PROCEDURES

- CSF analysis in cases of trauma may show xanthochromia, with mild to moderate increases in protein. In acute or chronic cases, CSF may be normal. A cisternal CSF tap is contraindicated if increased ICP is suspected due to the possibility of brain herniation.
- EEG may show diminished brain-wave activity.
- Brainstem auditory-evoked potentials are evaluated to determine brainstem function.
- ECG aids in determining cardiac rhythm dysfunction.

PATHOLOGIC FINDINGS

- Gross and histopathologic findings may include skull fractures, brain laceration/foreign body, hemorrhage, edema, and evidence of hypoxia.
- Contusion and concussion may be seen.

TREATMENT

APPROPRIATE HEALTH CARE

Usually requires intensive inpatient care, often on an emergency basis.

NURSING CARE

- Treat shock first, because neurologic status may improve once the shock is corrected.
- Adhere to the ABCs of trauma management.
- Monitor oxygenation with pulse oximetry, and supplement oxygen as necessary.
- Consider controlled ventilation if the horse is stuporous, comatose, or experiencing rapid neurologic deterioration.
- Maintain CO_2 between 30–35 mm Hg.
- Elevate the head up to an angle of 20° to help prevent increased ICP. Do not put the head at a greater angle to avoid pressure on the jugular vein, because this increases ICP.
- Institute fluid therapy to avoid hypotension.
- Overzealous administration of crystalloids (shock doses of 40–90 mL/kg per hour) may exacerbate increased ICP. Possibly, the use of colloids (e.g., hetastarch, dextran 70, or hypertonic saline) is preferable to restore normal blood volume while preventing increases in ICP. Use of colloids is contraindicated if intracranial hemorrhage is ongoing.

HEAD TRAUMA

• Hypertonic saline (4–6 mL/kg IV over 15 minutes) is the preferred fluid choice for head trauma horses in shock. Isotonic fluids then may be used for maintenance requirements (60 mL/kg per day).
• In recumbent horses, physical therapy is critical to prevent myositis, decubital sores, and hypostatic pulmonary congestion.
• Lubricate the eyes, and turn the horse every 2–4 hours.
• Use deep bedding.
• Hydro/massage therapy and therapeutic ultrasound are useful for maintaining circulation to the large muscle groups.
• Ensure normothermia, and especially avoid hyperthermia.

ACTIVITY

• Restricted, with strict stall confinement.
• Once stable, controlled exercise is useful for physical therapy/rehabilitation.

DIET

• Allow access to food and water if mental status allows.
• Provide supplemental tube feedings or parenteral nutrition if the horse is unable/unwilling to eat and drink.
• Adequate nutrition must be maintained to provide for the increased metabolic demands of the recovery period.

CLIENT EDUCATION

• True neurologic status may not be evident for several days, and intensive and potentially costly care may be required.
• Full recovery may take months, and residual deficits may persist.
• An ataxic and demented horse is a potential hazard to humans.

SURGICAL CONSIDERATIONS

• Consider intervention of open or depressed skull fractures and for retrieval of foreign bodies.
• Craniectomy is possibly useful for decompression if increased ICP is suspected despite medical treatment and for midbrain signs with a history of cerebral trauma or bleed. The practicality of this in the horse, however, is suspect.

MEDICATIONS

DRUGS OF CHOICE

• Reduce inflammation with corticosteroids.
• Dexamethasone may be used (0.1–0.25 mg/kg IV q6–24h for 24–48 hours).
• Currently, high-dose methylprednisolone treatment has limited evidence of efficacy in head trauma.
• Dimethyl sulfoxide (1 g/kg IV as a 10%–20% solution) for 3 days may help to improve blood flow and decrease edema.
• Cerebral edema may be treated with 20% mannitol (0.25–2.0 mg/kg IV over 20 minutes) or glycerol (1 g/kg PO QID) once adequately hydrated.
• Furosemide (1–3 mg/kg IV up to four times daily) also may decrease ICP and interacts synergistically with mannitol.
• If all the above measures to lower ICP fail, induction of a barbiturate coma may be considered.
• A 5–10 mg/kg bolus IV to effect can be used, but severe hypotension may occur. Therefore, adequate blood pressure monitoring is imperative.
• Seizures should be controlled with diazepam (0.03–0.5 mg/kg IV to effect). If seizures are not controllable with diazepam, consider general anesthesia.
• Use of broad-spectrum antimicrobials (e.g., trimethoprim-sulfa [30 mg/kg]) is warranted if skull fractures are present, because hemorrhage increases the possibility of septic meningitis.
• Management of pain should be undertaken with appropriate medications (e.g., phenylbutazone [2.2–4.4 mg/kg IV or PO], ketoprofen [2.2 mg/kg IV or IM QID], butorphanol [0.1 mg/kg IV or IM PRN]).
• Thiamine (1 g IM QID for 5 days) may be administered to aid breakdown of lactic acid and for its action as a necessary coenzyme in neural energy pathways.
• Selenium (0.055 mg/kg IM weekly) may be useful for its antioxidant effects.

CONTRAINDICATIONS

Avoid drugs that may increase ICP such as ketamine or cause hypertension.

PRECAUTIONS

• Avoid overzealous fluid administration, which may cause hypertension.
• Hypertonic saline may increase ICP due to its high salt content. Hypertonic saline and mannitol may worsen neurologic signs if used when intracranial hemorrhage is ongoing.
• Corticosteroids may increase the possibility of laminitis.
• Ulcer disease may occur with use of NSAIDs.

POSSIBLE INTERACTIONS

N/A

ALTERNATIVE DRUGS

N/A

HEAD TRAUMA

FOLLOW-UP

PATIENT MONITORING

Evaluate progress with serial neurologic examinations. Perform examinations several times a day initially, then taper the frequency based on stability of the horse.

PREVENTION/AVOIDANCE

- Keep the area in which horses are housed free of clutter.
- Tranquilize fractious horses as necessary to perform procedures.

POSSIBLE COMPLICATIONS

- Increases in ICP may lead to further hemorrhage and, ultimately, herniation.
- Problems associated with recumbent horses—myositis; decubital sores; corneal lacerations; hypostatic pulmonary congestion leading to pneumonia; fecal and urine scalding
- Malnutrition, seizures, cardiac and respiratory abnormalities, and death

EXPECTED COURSE AND PROGNOSIS

- The best prognosis is with minimal injury identified early after its occurrence and for which prompt treatment is sought.
- Horses that show rapid improvement with stabilization of signs have a better prognosis.

MISCELLANEOUS

ASSOCIATED CONDITIONS

N/A

AGE-RELATED FACTORS

N/A

ZOONOTIC POTENTIAL

N/A

PREGNANCY

N/A

SYNONYMS

- Brain trauma
- Brain injury
- Traumatic brain injury

SEE ALSO

- Basisphenoid-basioccipital fracture
- Coma and stupor
- Recumbency
- Weakness

ABBREVIATIONS

- CSF = cerebrospinal fluid
- ECG = electrocardiography
- EEG = electroencephalography
- ICP = intracranial pressure

Suggested Reading

Matthews HK. Spinal cord, vertebral, and intracranial trauma. In: Reed SM, Bayly WM, eds. Equine internal medicine. Philadelphia: WB Saunders, 1998:457–466.

Proulx J, Dhupa N. Severe brain injury. Part I. Pathophysiology. Compend Contin Educ 1998;20:897–905.

Proulx J, Dhupa N. Severe brain injury. Part II. Therapy. Compend Contin Educ 1998;20:993–1005.

Author Hilary K. Matthews

Consulting Editor Joseph J. Bertone

HEAVES

BASICS

DEFINITION

A reversible, inflammatory condition of the lower airways characterized by bronchospasm, excess mucus production, exudate, and pathologic changes of the bronchiolar walls, leading to airway obstruction.

PATHOPHYSIOLOGY

- Inhaled, dusty hay leads to inflammation and obstruction of the lower airways.
- Hypoxemia, presumably resulting from ventilation and perfusion inequalities, is common.
- Strong evidence implicates hypersensitivity reaction to thermophilic molds and actinomyces antigens in dusty hay.
- The role of viral infections and nonspecific environmental dust particles (e.g., endotoxins) on the induction and maintenance of heaves is ill-defined.

SYSTEMS AFFECTED

Respiratory

GENETIC

Unknown, but a genetic susceptibility has been reported.

INCIDENCE/PREVALENCE

- Worldwide
- Common in countries with temperate and cold climates, where horses are stabled for prolonged periods.

SIGNALMENT

- No sex or breed predilections
- Incidence increases with age; uncommonly diagnosed in horses <7 years.

SIGNS

- Affected horses are alert and afebrile.
- Anorexia may occur with respiratory distress.
- Initial signs may be limited to exercise intolerance, with an occasional cough at the onset of exercise or when eating. The frequency and severity of coughing episodes increase as the disease progresses, finally becoming paroxysmal bouts of deep, nonproductive coughs.
- In severe cases, increased respiratory rate, flared nostrils, and double expiratory effort may be present, and emaciation and a "heave line," caused by hypertrophy of the external abdominal oblique muscles, may develop.
- Appearance and severity of the clinical signs wax and wane. The duration of attacks varies from days to weeks, and some horses are asymptomatic between attacks.
- Thoracic auscultation may be normal in mild cases.
- Increased breath sounds, wheezes throughout the lung fields, and expiratory crackles are common findings during forced breathing using a rebreathing bag or after exercise.
- Bronchovesicular lung sounds may be decreased during severe episodes.
- Thoracic percussion may reveal hyperresonance of the ventral and caudal borders of the lung fields because of air trapping.

CAUSES

- Unknown
- Inhalation of environmental dust particles, particularly moldy hay and straw, has been incriminated as the inciting cause.
- Close contact between horses and chickens has been associated with clinical signs closely resembling those of heaves.

RISK FACTORS

- Moldy hay and straw.
- Prolonged stabling.

DIAGNOSIS

DIFFERENTIAL DIAGNOSIS

- Pharyngitis and mild dysphagia may cause chronic cough. Pharyngitis usually affects young horses and is associated with normal lung sounds; dysphagia is diagnosed on the basis of food particles in the airways and nasal secretions.
- Viral and bacterial airway infections may lead to cough and increased respiratory effort. These conditions can be differentiated from heaves on the basis of febrile episodes and other signs of infection.

CBC/BIOCHEMISTRY/URINALYSIS

No consistent changes

OTHER LABORATORY TESTS

- The most consistent finding in BAL cell cytology is an increased percentage of neutrophils (>10%).
- Presence of bacteria and fungal elements are common but believed to indicate impaired mucociliary clearance rather than an ongoing intrapulmonary septic process.
- Cytology of transtracheal washes or tracheal aspirates also reveals neutrophilia, but this is less specific than similar findings in BAL cell cytology.
- Bacterial culture of tracheal secretions commonly yields bacterial growth, but without other signs of infection, this may represent colonization of the lower airways because of impaired mucociliary clearance.
- Arterial blood gases provide an easy assessment of the degree of respiratory dysfunction in affected horses—PaO_2 values often are <80 and may be as low as 40 mm Hg in horses with labored breathing; $PaCO_2$ values may be slightly elevated.
- Routine lung biopsy for diagnosis of heaves is not recommended because of the uncommon but severe bleeding that may occur with this test.

IMAGING

- Endoscopy usually reveals copious mucopurulent exudate in lower airways.
- Thoracic radiography often is unremarkable but may reveal an increased bronchointerstitial pattern.

DIAGNOSTIC PROCEDURES

- The diagnosis is established on the basis of signalment, history, and clinical findings combined with exclusion of other common diseases affecting the respiratory tract and response to therapy.
- The diagnosis is confirmed by >10% neutrophils in BAL fluid.

PATHOLOGIC FINDINGS

- Histologic lesions are of a chronic active bronchiolitis, with accumulation of mucus and often neutrophils, epithelial hyperplasia with goblet cell metaplasia, and peribronchiolar fibrosis with lymphocyte and plasma cell infiltration.
- Interstitial emphysema, mostly in the cranial regions, and patchy areas of alveolar hyperinflation (i.e., alveolar emphysema) may be seen.

TREATMENT

APPROPRIATE HEALTH CARE

In- or outpatient medical management

NURSING CARE

- The disease is reversible with proper control of environmental dust, which is best achieved by keeping horses outdoors, preferably on pasture. If horses remains indoors, replace hay with cubed or pelleted food, haylage, or hydroponic hay, and use shredded paper or good-quality wood shavings instead of straw.
- Respiratory signs usually recur within days of re-exposure to dusty hay and bedding.
- Without drug therapy, a few weeks to months of environmental dust control may be required before affected horses become free of respiratory signs.
- In horses with profound hypoxemia (PaO_2 <60 mm Hg), inhaled oxygen supplementation may be required until ventilation is improved by environmental dust control and medication.

ACTIVITY

- Adjust exercise level according to the degree of respiratory dysfunction.
- Rest is indicated in horses with severely compromised respiratory function.

DIET

- Cubed or pelleted food or haylage is preferred.
- Hay soaked in water for 2–3 hours may be an adequate alternative for some horses.

CLIENT EDUCATION

- Maintain affected horses in a dust free environment.
- Place susceptible horses stabled in barns in paddocks when other horses are fed, the boxstalls are cleaned, or the aisles are brushed.
- Never feed moldy hay to horses.

SURGICAL CONSIDERATIONS

N/A

MEDICATIONS

DRUGS OF CHOICE

Corticosteroids

- Systemic corticosteroids allow effective control.
- Expect a delay of a few days between initiation of therapy and maximal clinical response.
- For severe attacks, dexamethasone (initial dose of 0.05 mg/kg, then decrease and administer on alternate days) and isoflupredone acetate (0.02 mg/kg IM daily for 5 days, then decrease and administer on alternate days for 10–20 days) may be used.
- A single dose of triamcinolone acetonide (20–40 mg IM) also reverses clinical signs of airway obstruction for as long as 5 weeks.
- For mild cases, oral prednisone (1–4 mg/kg) often is recommended, but its efficacy in affected horses has not been documented.
- Inhaled corticosteroids allow maximal concentration of drug at the effector sites and minimize side effects.
- Inhaled drugs can be delivered using nebulization, MDIs, and dry-powder inhalers. Masks have been designed for use of MDIs (Equine Aeromask) and dry-powder inhalers (EquiPoudre).
- Short-term administration of inhaled beclomethasone diproprionate (initial dose of 3500 μg per 500 kg q12h) and fluticasone propionate (2000 μg per 500 kg q12h) are both efficacious and well tolerated but have few residual effects once treatment is discontinued.
- A delay in response of 4 days or longer should be expected with inhaled corticosteroids, however, so combination with faster-acting drugs (e.g., bronchodilators, systemic corticosteroids) in horses with respiratory distress may be beneficial.

Bronchodilators

- Bronchodilators are used to relieve small airway obstruction caused by the airway smooth muscle contraction.
- May be life-saving dyspnea.
- Long term administration of bronchodilators should be combined with strict environmental dust control and corticosteroid, because inflammation of the lower airways may progress despite the improvement of clinical signs observed with these drugs.
- Clenbuterol (0.8–3.2 μg/kg BID), a β_2-adrenergic agonist, has bronchodilator effects and increases mucociliary transport. Clinical efficacy at the lower recommended dosage (0.8 μg/kg BID), however, is inconsistent if exposure to dusty hay and bedding is maintained.
- Terbutaline sulfate, another β_2-adrenergic agonist, may be used orally or by inhalation in countries where clenbuterol is unavailable.
- Ipratropium bromide (2–3 μg/kg), albuterol (1–2 μg/kg), and feneterol (2–3 μg/kg) are bronchodilators that can be used by inhalation with MDIs.
- Aminophylline (5–10 mg/kg), a xanthine derivative, is used as a bronchodilator in horses. Because of its low therapeutic index, aminophylline and other theophylline salts are used when bronchodilation is not achieved with other therapeutic agents or in horses with hypoventilation.

Expectorant, Mucolytic, and Mucokinetic Agents

- Evidence of efficacy for these agents in improving clinical signs is sparse.
- Clenbuterol, because of its bronchodilatory and mucokinetic properties, may be preferred to clear mucus from the airways.

CONTRAINDICATIONS

Corticosteroid administration in the face of sepsis

PRECAUTIONS

- Administration of bronchodilators initially may be associated with temporary worsening of hypoxemia.
- Administration of methylxanthine derivatives may lead to excitability, tachycardia, muscular tremors, and sweating.
- Administer potassium iodide with caution in affected horses, because it irritates the respiratory tract and can induce or worsen bronchospasm.

POSSIBLE INTERACTIONS

N/A

ALTERNATIVE DRUGS

- Inhaled sodium cromoglycate (80–200 mg q12–24h) in horses in clinical remission prevents the appearance of clinical signs for as long as 3 weeks after introduction to a dusty environment.
- Nedocromil sodium (24 mg q12h), another cromone, may be used by inhalation.

FOLLOW-UP

PATIENT MONITORING

Sequential PaO_2 determination to monitor response to therapy in horses with severely compromised respiratory function

PREVENTION/AVOIDANCE

Dust-free environment

POSSIBLE COMPLICATIONS

- Heaves is a wasting disease that may lead to death in severe cases if proper environmental control and effective medication are not provided.
- Right heart failure is a rare complication in severe cases.

EXPECTED COURSE AND PROGNOSIS

- The condition is reversible with prolonged environmental control and therapy.
- In some horses, pulmonary neutrophilia persists after therapy even if the horse is clinically asymptomatic.

MISCELLANEOUS

ASSOCIATED CONDITIONS

N/A

AGE-RELATED FACTORS

- Rarely seen in horses <7 years.
- Incidence increases with age.

ZOONOTIC POTENTIAL

None

PREGNANCY

- Anecdotal reports suggest clinical signs may improve in some mares during pregnancy.
- Fetal growth retardation and death may occur in mares with severely compromised respiratory function.

SYNONYMS

- Broken wind
- Chronic bronchitis
- Chronic bronchiolitis
- COPD
- Equine asthma
- Recurrent airway disease
- Small airway disease

SEE ALSO

- Expiratory dyspnea
- Summer pasture-associated COPD

ABBREVIATIONS

- BAL = bronchoalveolar lavage
- COPD = chronic obstructive pulmonary disease
- MDI = metered dose inhaler

Suggested Reading

Lavoie JP. Chronic obstructive pulmonary diseases. In: Robinson NE, ed. Current therapy in equine medicine. 4th ed. Philadelphia: WB Saunders, 1997:431–435.

Robinson NE, Derksen FJ, Olszewski MA, et al. The pathogenesis of chronic obstructive pulmonary disease of horses. Br Vet J 1996;152:283–306.

Author Jean-Pierre Lavoie

Consulting Editor Jean-Pierre Lavoie

HEMANGIOSARCOMA

BASICS

OVERVIEW

• Malignant neoplasm originating from vascular endothelium; any organ system may be affected.
• Cutaneous, locally invasive (vertebrae and spinal cord, oral cavity, eye, tarsal sheath, frontal sinus), and disseminated forms
• 0.9% reported incidence

SIGNALMENT

• All forms appear to be most common in middle-aged horses (mean age for disseminated hemangiosarcoma, 12 years; age range, 3–27 years).
• No apparent breed or sex predilection

SIGNS

• Vary depending on location
• Cutaneous—dermal or subcutaneous lesions with no site predilection; typically solitary, rapidly growing, and poorly circumscribed; firm or friable; necrosis, ulceration, and bleeding are common.
• Disseminated—respiratory and musculoskeletal systems most often affected; dyspnea, epistaxis, subcutaneous or muscular swelling, lameness, tachycardia, tachypnea, and pale or icteric mucous membranes are common.
• Rectal palpation may reveal an abdominal mass or splenomegaly.

CAUSES AND RISK FACTORS

No identified specific causes or risk factors

DIAGNOSIS

DIFFERENTIAL DIAGNOSIS

• Hemangiomas—generally seen in horses <1 year of age; predilection for distal limbs
• Dyspnea—infectious respiratory tract disease, chronic obstructive pulmonary disease, and nasal or thoracic tumors. Thoracic radiography or ultrasonography may be useful to differentiate these conditions.
• Epistaxis—trauma, infection, exercise-induced pulmonary hemorrhage, ethmoid hematoma, guttural pouch mycosis, and neoplasia. Endoscopy often is useful to differentiate these conditions.
• Intramuscular swelling and lameness—trauma, hematoma, abscessation, neoplasia, and vascular anomalies (varicocele)

CBC/BIOCHEMISTRY/URINALYSIS

• Anemia is the most common laboratory abnormality.
• Neutrophilic leukocytosis and thrombocytopenia also are common.
• Variable total protein
• Typically normal or mildly elevated fibrinogen
• Biochemistry—variable, mild to moderate azotemia, and hyperbilirubinemia recognized in approximately 50% of cases.
• Urinalysis—normal in most cases; may have increased red blood cells.

OTHER LABORATORY TESTS

Clotting times—most often normal; prolonged PTT in one case

IMAGING

Radiography and ultrasonography may confirm abnormalities (e.g., effusion, mass, or hematoma depending on location) but typically are not specifically diagnostic.

DIAGNOSTIC PROCEDURES

• Cytologic analysis of various samples (e.g., pleural fluid, peritoneal fluid, transtracheal wash or bronchoalveolar lavage fluid, cerebrospinal fluid, tissue aspirates) often demonstrates hemorrhage or inflammation but infrequently confirms neoplasia.
• Bone marrow aspiration—erythroid hyperplasia
• Depending on the localizing signs, endoscopy of the bladder, airways, or pleural space may identify the source of hemorrhage or nodules; laparoscopy or laparotomy may identify abdominal involvement.
• Biopsy or fine-needle aspiration can be diagnostic, demonstrating endothelial cells with mitotic figures; however, differentiating hemangiosarcoma from hemorrhage and inflammation often is difficult.
• Diagnosis is established at postmortem examination in many cases.

HEMANGIOSARCOMA

PATHOLOGIC FINDINGS

• Most common sites for disseminated hemangiosarcoma—lung and pleura, skeletal muscle, spleen, heart, kidney, and brain; primary tumor site often not identified
• Gross findings—hemorrhagic, friable, red-black masses; blood in the thoracic and abdominal cavities, pericardium, or muscle associated with hemorrhage from tumor sites is a common finding at necropsy.
• Histologic findings—multiple, variably sized, poorly organized vascular channels lined by plump, spindle-shaped cells; neoplastic endothelial cells have large, round to oval, vesicular hyperchromatic nuclei and prominent nucleoli; mitotic figures are common.
• Neutrophils, lymphocytes, hemosiderin-filled macrophages, or free hemosiderin pigment in some tumors

TREATMENT

• Treatment largely supportive—nonsteroidal and steroidal anti-inflammatory drugs, blood transfusions, intravenous fluid therapy, plasma, and antibiotics
• Surgical excision may be beneficial for cutaneous or localized lesions.

MEDICATIONS

DRUGS

No established protocols for medical treatment of hemangiosarcoma in horses. In dogs, treatment typically involves surgical excision followed by chemotherapy, immunotherapy, or both, with a guarded prognosis.

CONTRAINDICATIONS/POSSIBLE INTERACTIONS

N/A

FOLLOW-UP

• Monitor for recurrence after surgical removal of cutaneous or localized lesions.
• Long-term prognosis with disseminated form is poor (median time from onset of clinical signs to euthanasia/death, 17 days; range, 0 days to 4 years).

MISCELLANEOUS

ASSOCIATED CONDITIONS

N/A

AGE-RELATED FACTORS

N/A

ZOONOTIC POTENTIAL

N/A

PREGNANCY

N/A

ABBREVIATION

• PTT = partial thromboplastin time

Suggested Reading

Schott HC, Southwood LL. Disseminated hemangiosarcoma in horses. Proc Am Coll Vet Intern Med 1996;14:568.

Author Melissa T. Hines
Consulting Editor Debra C. Sellon

HEMORRHAGE, ACUTE

BASICS

DEFINITION

• Rapid loss of blood from the vasculature within a short time period (usually <24 hours)
• May be internal (into body cavities) or external (including hemorrhage into the GI tract).

PATHOPHYSIOLOGY

• Acute loss of >20–25% of circulating blood volume results in severe hypovolemic shock—tachycardia, polypnea, pale mucous membranes, prolongation of capillary refill time, poor venous distension, and generalized weakness
• Rapid loss of >50% of circulating blood volume results in death.
• After acute hemorrhagic event, indices of red cell mass are within normal limits, because all blood components have been lost in equal volumes; evaluation of the erythron may be complicated further by release of splenic red cells into the circulation.
• Fluid moves from the extravascular compartment into the vasculature during the first 24–48 hours, with a gradual decrease in red cell mass and plasma protein concentrations.
• With internal hemorrhage, approximately two-thirds of the erythrocytes are autotransfused back into circulation within 24–72 hours.
• Decreased oxygen delivery associated with loss of red cell mass can result in CNS dysfunction and injury to other organs (e.g., kidneys).

SYSTEMS AFFECTED

• Cardiovascular—loss of circulating blood volume, reduction in systemic blood pressure, and compensatory increase in heart rate and peripheral resistance
• Hemic/lymphatic/immune—decrease in circulating red cell mass and plasma protein concentrations (after redistribution of fluid volumes)
• Renal—ischemic injury
• Nervous—ischemic impairment of function and altered behavior

SIGNALMENT

• Old breeding stallions—acute aortic rupture
• Old, multiparous, peripartum mares—hemorrhage involving the reproductive tract (e.g., uterine or ovarian arterial ruptures)
• Neonatal foals—rib fractures and umbilical cord hemorrhage
• Exercising horses—pulmonary hemorrhage

SIGNS

General Comments

Vary with the duration and severity of blood loss, site of hemorrhage (i.e., internal vs. external), and accompanying or underlying diseases.

Historical Findings

• Respiratory distress, dystocia, or trauma in neonatal foals with hemothorax
• Mild signs of colic in adult horses with intra-abdominal hemorrhage
• Sudden collapse or distress in stallions after breeding with aortic root rupture
• Epistaxis and respiratory distress in horses after intense exercise with pulmonary hemorrhage
• Other historical findings reflect the underlying cause of hemorrhage (e.g., hemorrhage associated with DIC in patients with colitis or colic).

Physical Examination Findings

• Tachycardia, polypnea, pale mucous membranes, trembling, sweating, mild colic signs, decreased GI motility, or systolic heart murmur
• Alterations in neurologic function, including behavioral abnormalities; ataxia and collapse with >40% blood loss
• Sudden death
• Intra-abdominal hemorrhage—colic
• Intrathoracic hemorrhage—tachycardia, dyspnea, and decreased or absent ventral lung sounds

CAUSES

Internal Hemorrhage

Abdominal
• Splenic rupture
• Hepatic rupture
• Rupture of the middle uterine artery
• Rupture of the caudal vena cava associated with incarceration of the small intestine in the epiploic foramen
• Mesenteric arterial hemorrhage secondary to verminous arteritis, strangulating lipoma, coagulopathy, or previous GI surgery
• Uterine bleeding secondary to birth trauma
• Hemorrhage from ovarian arteries or tumors
• Iliac arterial rupture secondary to a displaced pelvic fracture
• After surgery or biopsy

Thoracic
• Rib fractures
• Aortic root rupture
• Diaphragmatic hernia with vascular tearing
• Chest and lung trauma, including vessel rupture during lung biopsy
• Pulmonary hemorrhage—rarely, hemothorax can develop after exercise and massive pulmonary hemorrhage
• Coagulopathy

External Hemorrhage

General
• Trauma
• Gunshot wounds
• Cellulitis—erosion through a major vessel
• Umbilical hemorrhage
• Surgical complications
• Coagulopathy

Respiratory
• Guttural pouch mycosis
• Ethmoid hematoma—usually chronic rather than acute hemorrhage
• Coagulopathy
• Exercise-induced pulmonary hemorrhage

GI
• Coagulopathy
• Neoplasia

RISK FACTORS

Mares with a history of periparturient hemorrhage are likely to bleed during future pregnancies.

HEMORRHAGE, ACUTE

DIAGNOSIS

DIFFERENTIAL DIAGNOSIS

• Colic—consider internal hemorrhage (particularly intra-abdominal) and other causes of colic; differentiate by rectal examination, abdominal sonography, and abdominocentesis.
• Intra-abdominal hemorrhage—differentiated from inadvertent splenic puncture or subcutaneous vessel laceration during abdominocentesis by erythrophagocytosis
• Recent hemorrhage—differentiated from old hemorrhage by platelets in the abdominal aspirate
• Epistaxis—endoscopy, thoracic radiography, and sonography to differentiate causes

CBC/BIOCHEMISTRY/URINALYSIS

• PCV and plasma protein concentration—little or no change during the first 24 hours; thereafter, a variable decrease in red cell mass (i.e., hematocrit, red cell count), with no change in MCV, MCH, and MCHC
• Transient thrombocytopenia
• Leukocytosis with neutrophilia
• Increased serum creatinine and urea nitrogen concentrations reflecting prerenal or renal azotemia
• Increased AST and CK activities with significant trauma
• Oliguria and increased urine specific gravity (>1.040) with hypovolemic shock; inappropriately low urine specific gravity may indicate acute renal failure.

OTHER LABORATORY TESTS

• Coagulation tests (i.e., PT, PTT, FDP, ATIII, platelet count) if a coagulopathy is suspected
• With hemothorax, arterial blood gas analysis to assess ventilatory function

IMAGING

Radiography

Thoracic radiography to demonstrate accumulation of fluid in cases of hemothorax and, possibly, to reveal rib fractures and pneumothorax.

Ultrasonography

• Thoracic and abdominal ultrasonography to demonstrate fluid accumulation
• Splenic ultrasonography to identify masses—hematomas, abscesses, tumors
• Transrectal ultrasonography to examine abnormalities of the caudal abdomen (e.g. swelling of the broad ligament)
• Echocardiography in stallions with suspected aortic root rupture

DIAGNOSTIC PROCEDURES

• Abdominocentesis and thoracocentesis to demonstrate blood; evidence of erythrophagocytosis aids in differentiating inadvertent splenic aspiration from subcutaneous vessel puncture.
• Comprehensive and systematic palpation per rectum with suspected intra-abdominal hemorrhage.
• Airway endoscopy to localize the source of hemorrhage in patients with epistaxis
• Laparoscopy to differentiate causes of intra-abdominal hemorrhage
• Measurement of blood pressure (e.g., Doppler tail cuff)—systolic pressure <80 mm Hg indicates hypotension.

TREATMENT

• Acute hemorrhage constitutes a medical or surgical emergency; perform life-saving procedures immediately.
• External hemorrhage is controlled by application of pressure bandages or surgical ligation of ruptured vessels.
• After stabilization, move the patient to a hospital for further diagnostic evaluation, treatment, and intensive care.
• Keep the patient as quiet as possible.
• After stabilization, further diagnostic evaluation may be required to establish a definitive diagnosis and prognosis.
• Minor (e.g., repair of ruptured superficial vessels) or major (e.g., occlusion of the arterial supply to the guttural pouches, exploratory celiotomy for suspected splenic tear) surgery may be indicated.

Fluid Therapy

• IV fluid therapy is indicated if the patient exhibits tachycardia, poor pulse quality, cool extremities, and low blood pressure.
• Administer isotonic crystalloid solutions (total volume $\cong$3 estimated blood loss).
• Resuscitation with hypertonic saline (7%) solution may be indicated in life-threatening circumstances to stabilize the patient and to allow time for other medical and surgical procedures to be initiated.
• Administration of isotonic crystalloid solutions must follow treatment with hypertonic saline solutions.

HEMORRHAGE, ACUTE

Blood Transfusions

- Indications for blood transfusion therapy—severe blood loss and hypotension (heart rate >80–100 bpm, white to gray mucous membranes; in peracute hemorrhage, death from blood loss and hypovolemic shock can occur without decreased hematocrit); hematocrit decreases to <20% within a 12-hour period and hemorrhage is ongoing; hematocrit falls to <10–12% during a 24–48 hour period; and signs of altered neurologic function indicative of impaired oxygen delivery.
- Ideally, the choice of donor is based on cross-match testing; however, during an emergency, a gelding or stallion that has not had previous transfusions is acceptable.
- A total of 5–10 L of blood may be safely collected from adult horses (450–550 kg).
- Collect blood into ACD anticoagulant (one part ACD to nine parts blood).
- Hematocrit is an unreliable indicator for the extent of blood loss after acute hemorrhage. The volume of blood administered should be based on the degree of hypovolemia and estimates of blood loss. For adult horses, at least 6–8 L usually is required, with additional volume replacement from isotonic crystalloid fluids. Transfusion volume should not exceed 20% of blood volume (blood volume [L] = 0.08 × body weight [kg]).
- Transfused red cells have a life span of only 4–6 days.
- Administer blood through an IV system with an in-line filter, and replace the filter regularly during the transfusion (every 3–4 L). The blood should be mixed gently and frequently during administration.

Respiratory Therapy

- If ventilation is mechanically limited by hemothorax (e.g., severe dyspnea, hypercarbia), remove blood by thoracocentesis. Monitor the patient closely, because the pleural cavity can refill rapidly. With evidence of pneumothorax and labored respiration, insert a Heimlich chest drain.
- Nasal administration of oxygen is indicated in hypoxemic patients.

MEDICATIONS

DRUGS OF CHOICE

- Several drugs have been advocated to control hemorrhage, but their efficacy in horses has not been demonstrated.
- Aminocaproic acid (20–80 mg/kg IV diluted in 0.9% saline and administered over 30–60 minutes)—purported to stabilize fibrin clots by inhibiting activity of plasminogen activator
- Naloxone (0.01–0.02 mg/kg IV)—antifibrinolytic.
- Oxytocin (20 IU IM q30min)—for hemorrhage in postpartum mares; decreases bleeding from the myometrium but has no effect on hemorrhage from the uterine arteries; contraindicated with a hematoma of the broad ligament
- Pain relief—flunixin meglumine (0.5–1.0 mg/kg q8–12 h)
- Broad-spectrum antibiotics—patients with open wounds or foals with rib fractures or pneumothorax

CONTRAINDICATIONS

- Synthetic colloidal products (e.g., dextrans, hetastarch) may inhibit platelet aggregation and alter coagulation protein function.
- Parenteral iron dextran preparations have resulted in fatalities among horses.

PRECAUTIONS

Acepromazine (0.02 mg/kg)—indicated for its anxiolytic properties, but use with extreme caution in hypotensive animals.

POSSIBLE INTERACTIONS

N/A

ALTERNATIVE DRUGS

Bovine hemoglobin (Biopure Corp., Boston, MA)—an alternative to whole-blood transfusion (30 mL/kg), but only one report of this product being used in horses.

FOLLOW-UP

PATIENT MONITORING

- Monitor circulating volume status (i.e., heart rate, pulse quality, blood pressure) frequently during the initial 12–24 hours of treatment.
- Determine hematocrit at 12-hour intervals for 1–3 days after acute hemorrhage to assess red cell mass, especially if hemorrhage may be ongoing.

POSSIBLE COMPLICATIONS

- Blood transfusion reactions—signs of immediate transfusion reaction include restlessness, trembling, tachycardia, tachypnea, urticaria, and collapse; if these signs occur, stop the transfusion.
- For severe transfusion reactions, treatments may include epinephrine (0.01–0.02 mg/kg at 1:1000 IM), isotonic IV Fluids, and short-acting corticosteroids such as prednisolone sodium succinate (4.5 mg/kg IV).
- For mild transfusion reactions, administer flunixin meglumine (1.1 mg/kg IV) and wait 15–30 minutes before proceeding with the transfusion.
- Bacterial sepsis
- Laminitis

MISCELLANEOUS

ASSOCIATED CONDITIONS

N/A

AGE-RELATED FACTORS

N/A

ZOONOTIC POTENTIAL

N/A

PREGNANCY

Severe hypovolemic shock may compromise the fetus, particularly during the last trimester; follow-up monitoring should include an evaluation of fetal viability.

SYNONYMS

N/A

SEE ALSO

- Anemia
- Coagulation defects, acquired/induced
- Coagulation defects, inherited
- Hemorrhage, chronic
- Transfusion reactions
- Thrombocytopenia

ABBREVIATIONS

- AST = aspartate aminotransferase
- ATIII = antithrombin III
- CK = creatine kinase
- DIC = disseminated intravascular coagulation
- FDP = fibrin degradation products
- GI = gastrointestinal
- MCV = mean cell volume
- MCHC = mean cell hemoglobin concentration
- MCH = mean cell hemoglobin
- PCV = packed cell volume
- PT = prothrombin time
- PTT = partial thromboplastin time

Suggested Reading

Collatos C. Blood and blood component therapy. In: Current therapy in equine medicine 4. Philadelphia: WB Saunders, 1996:290–292.

Maxson AD, Giger U, Sweeney CR, et al. Use of bovine hemoglobin preparation in the treatment of cyclic ovarian hemorrhage in a miniature horse. J Am Vet Med Assoc 1993;203:1308–1311.

Mehl ML, Ragle CA, Mealey RH, Whooten TL. Laparoscopic diagnosis of subcapsular splenic hematoma in a horse. J Am Vet Med Assoc 1998;213:1171–1173.

Schmall LM, Muir WW, Robertson JT. Haemodynamic effects of small volume hypertonic saline in experimentally induced haemorrhagic shock. Equine Vet J 1990;22:273–277.

Author Raymond J. Geor
Consulting Editor Debra C. Sellon

HEMORRHAGE, CHRONIC

BASICS

OVERVIEW
Low-grade, ongoing blood loss, most commonly GI in origin

SIGNALMENT
N/A

SIGNS
- Overt signs of anemia (tachycardia, tachypnea, weakness) may not be seen until PCV < 12%.
- Pale mucous membranes
- Signs of underlying disease process (e.g. weight loss for neoplasia, diarrhea for parasitism)

CAUSES AND RISK FACTORS
Secondary to an underlying disease process

Gastrointestinal
- Parasitism
- Ulceration
- Gastric ulcers—foals
- NSAID toxicity
- Neoplasia (e.g., gastric squamous cell carcinoma)

Renal/Urologic
- Hemorrhagic or erosive cystitis
- Renal or bladder neoplasia
- Vascular anomaly—idiopathic urethral hemorrhage in geldings

Respiratory
- Guttural pouch mycosis
- Ethmoid hematoma
- Fungal rhinitis
- Upper respiratory neoplasia
- Pulmonary abscess
- Pulmonary neoplasia
- Exercise-induced pulmonary hemorrhage

Miscellaneous
- Thrombocytopenia
- Hemostatic dysfunction

DIAGNOSIS

DIFFERENTIAL DIAGNOSIS
- Anemia of chronic disease—differentiated by evidence of nonregenerative anemia and clinical identification of primary, chronic disease process
- Causes of low-grade hemolysis—differentiated by Coombs' test, Coggins test, blood smear examination, and evaluation of history and clinical signs

CBC/BIOCHEMISTRY/URINALYSIS
- Hemogram findings are inconsistent; diagnosis should be based primarily on clinical signs and evidence of underlying disease process.
- Microcytic, hypochromic anemia with low serum iron, low marrow iron stores, and increased TIBC may be present.
- Hypoproteinemia suggests extracorporeal blood loss (GI, urogenital, respiratory).
- Hyperbilirubinemia suggests hemolysis or intracorporeal blood loss.
- Chronic tissue hypoxia (PCV < 12%) may cause increased serum hepatic enzymes and increased serum creatinine.
- Microscopic or gross hematuria may indicate primary renal/urologic problem.

OTHER LABORATORY TESTS
Chronic blood loss may deplete iron stores, resulting in low serum iron, low marrow iron stores, and increased TIBC.

IMAGING
- Ultrasonography may be useful in identifying NSAID-induced, right dorsal colitis or may identify intra-abdominal or intrathoracic masses
- Upper airway radiography may reveal sinus or ethmoidal masses.

OTHER DIAGNOSTIC PROCEDURES
- After characterizing the anemia and ruling out causes other than hemorrhage, diagnostic procedures should aim at identifying the source of blood loss.
- Positive fecal occult blood indicates significant GI hemorrhage or swallowed blood from the respiratory tract.
- Positive fecal examination for parasitic ova supports the diagnosis of parasitism when accompanied by positive fecal occult blood test, weight loss, diarrhea, or poor deworming history.
- Endoscopy—gastroscopy may reveal gastroduodenal ulceration or gastric squamous cell carcinoma; cystoscopy may identify urethral, bladder, or ureteral hemorrhage; upper airway endoscopy may reveal rhinitis, neoplasia, guttural pouch mycosis, ethmoid hematoma, or blood in the trachea.
- Erythrocytophagia and hemosiderophages may be identified in abdominal fluid, transtracheal aspirate, or bronchoalveolar lavage fluid.

HEMORRHAGE, CHRONIC

- Ultrasound-guided mass biopsies may characterize the primary disease process as infectious or neoplastic, guiding treatment and prognosis.

TREATMENT

- Appropriate treatment and level of care (inpatient vs. outpatient) depends on the primary disease process.
- Identification and resolution of the underlying disease is essential.
- Transfusion indicated if PCV < 12% and clinical and laboratory signs of tissue hypoxia (tachypnea, tachycardia, weakness, increased serum creatinine or SDH concentration) are present.
- If signs of iron-store depletion are present, ferrous sulfate can be supplemented at 2 mg/kg PO daily.
- Discontinue forced activity, and provide a balanced maintenance diet until the hematocrit is within the normal range.
- If possible, provide access to pasture.

MEDICATIONS

DRUGS

Only medications to treat the underlying disease are indicated.

CONTRAINDICATIONS/POSSIBLE INTERACTIONS

Do not administer parenteral iron dextran solutions because of the possibility of fatal reactions.

FOLLOW-UP

- In addition to follow-up care and evaluation related to the underlying disease process, measure the PCV weekly, and expect a gradual increase to a normal value over 6–12 weeks.
- Serial bone marrow aspiration is not recommended, because the equine regenerative response is difficult to assess.
- If GI parasitism was the underlying disease, client education regarding parasite control is essential.
- Prognosis depends on accurately identifying the underlying disease; persistence with diagnostic evaluation is important, particularly in light of the number of neoplastic conditions responsible for chronic blood loss in horses.

MISCELLANEOUS

ASSOCIATED CONDITIONS

N/A

AGE-RELATED FACTORS

N/A

ZOONOTIC POTENTIAL

N/A

PREGNANCY

N/A

SEE ALSO

- Anemia
- Hemorrhage, acute

ABBREVIATIONS

- GI = gastrointestinal
- PCV = packed cell volume
- SDH = sorbitol dehydrogenase
- TIBC = total iron-binding capacity

Suggested Reading

Morris DD. Diseases of the hemolymphatic system. In: Reed SM, Bayly WM, eds. Equine internal medicine. Philadelphia: WB Saunders, 1998:558–602.

Author Chrysann Collatos
Consulting Editor Debra C. Sellon

HEMORRHAGIC NASAL DISCHARGE

BASICS

OVERVIEW

- May be composed of frank blood or blood mixed with secretions—mucous, pus, froth, and necrotic debris
- May be caused by lesions within the respiratory tract or adjacent structures and by hemostatic dysfunctions; the latter, particularly thrombocytopenia and disseminated intravascular coagulopathies, often are associated with mucosal petechia or ecchymotic hemorrhage.
- Unilateral discharge usually results from lesions rostral to the nasopharynx (e.g., nasal passage, nasolacrimal duct, paranasal sinuses).
- Bilateral discharge usually results from lesions caudal to the nasopharynx or from hemostatic dysfunctions.
- Organ systems—hemic and respiratory

SIGNALMENT

N/A

SIGNS

- Bleeding—acute or chronic
- Discharge may be composed of blood only (i.e., epistaxis) or blood mixed with seromucoid, mucopurulent, or frothy nasal discharge.
- Mucopurulent discharge suggests an infectious or necrotic origin.
- Bilateral frothy discharge is consistent with pulmonary edema.
- Hemorrhage from the nasal passage, turbinates, or paranasal sinuses manifests as an ipsilateral discharge; hemorrhage originating caudal to the nasal septum, including the nasopharynx, auditory tube diverticulum (i.e., guttural pouch), larynx, trachea, and lower respiratory tract, usually causes bilateral discharge.
- Hemostatic disorders may also result in bleeding diatheses from other organs.
- Thrombocytopenia and DIC often are associated with mucosal petechiation, ecchymotic hemorrhages, and occult blood from the GI or urinary tracts.
- DIC frequently leads to thrombophlebitis; spontaneous epistaxis is less common.
- Coagulation factor deficiencies tend to result in hemorrhages into body cavities (e.g., joints, abdomen, thorax), epistaxis, melena, and excessive bleeding and hematoma formation after trauma, injection, venipuncture, or surgery.

CAUSES AND RISK FACTORS

- Hemostatic dysfunction—thrombocytopenia (e.g., immune-mediated, DIC, myelophthisic disease, bone marrow aplasia), DIC (e.g., sepsis, GI and renal disease, hemolytic anemia, neoplasia), coagulation factor deficiency (e.g., inherited coagulopathies, warfarin and sweet-clover toxicosis), or envenomation (e.g., rattlesnake venom poisoning).
- Respiratory tract disease—upper respiratory disease may result from bacterial or fungal infections (e.g., guttural pouch mycosis, sinusitis), tumors (e.g., carcinomas, mesenchymal neoplasms), or idiopathic diseases (e.g. nasal polyp, nasal amyloidosis, ethmoid hematoma, paranasal sinus cyst); relevant lower respiratory diseases include exercise-induced pulmonary hemorrhage, pleuropneumonia, pulmonary edema, primary lung tumors (e.g., myoblastoma, pulmonary carcinoma, bronchial myxoma), and metastatic neoplasms (e.g., hemangiosarcoma, adenocarcinoma).
- Trauma—nasal intubation, facial bone and skull base fractures, longus capitis muscle rupture secondary to falling backward, transtracheal puncture, and lung biopsy
- Other—vasculitis (e.g., purpura hemorrhagica), myeloid neoplasia, fibrous dysplasia, periocular bleeding, and dacryohemorrhea

DIAGNOSIS

DIFFERENTIAL DIAGNOSIS

N/A

CBC/BIOCHEMISTRY/URINALYSIS

- Anemia may result from blood loss.
- Neutrophilia or neutropenia may accompany inflammatory diseases.
- Leukemia may be evident with myeloid neoplasia.
- Occult blood in the feces and urine may result from a bleeding diathesis.

OTHER LABORATORY TESTS

Assessment of hemostasis requires platelet count (reference range, 100,000–600,000 cells/μL), plasma fibrinogen (reference range, 200–400 mg/dL), prothrombin time (reference range, 75–125% of control values), activated partial thromboplastin time (reference range, 75–125% of control values), and fibrin/fibrinogen degradation products (reference range, $<$10–32 μg/mL).

IMAGING

- Skull radiography may reveal bone fracture, mass (e.g., tumor, sinus cyst, ethmoid hematoma), or fluid accumulation in the sinuses or guttural pouches.
- Thoracic radiography may help to identify pleuropneumonia, exercise-induced pulmonary hemorrhage, pulmonary edema, and primary or metastatic lung tumors.
- Thoracic ultrasonography is a sensitive means to detect fluid accumulation in the pleural space—blood or purulent effusion.

DIAGNOSTIC PROCEDURES

- Endoscopy of the respiratory tract may help to identify the cause; trephination provides access to paranasal sinuses using a flexible or rigid endoscope and may help to characterize the disease process.

HEMORRHAGIC NASAL DISCHARGE

• Fluid cytology from tracheobronchial aspirates, bronchoalveolar lavage, or thoracocentesis may reveal the source or cause of bleeding.
• Percutaneous centesis of the paranasal sinuses is helpful when the condition is suspected to originate from them.
• Biopsy should help to identify the nature of a mass; full-thickness punch biopsies of the skin in the affected areas may confirm a diagnosis of vasculitis.
• Surgical exploration of paranasal sinuses for diagnostic purposes should be used only as a last resort.

PATHOLOGIC FINDINGS

• Depend on the primary disease process.
• Nasal and paranasal neoplasms are malignant in 68% of cases.

TREATMENT

• Treat the primary disease.
• Stall rest is recommended.
• Treat severe blood loss with IV administration of sodium-containing crystalloid solutions to maintain the circulating blood volume. Perform blood transfusion when the RBC mass is insufficient to maintain tissue oxygenation.
• Patients with hemostatic disorders (e.g., DIC, thrombocytopenia) may benefit from fresh plasma administration.
• Surgical treatment may consist of resecting a nasal or paranasal neoplasm, mass, ethmoid hematoma, sinus cyst, or polyp.
• Radiation therapy may be useful with paranasal neoplasm.
• If the condition is secondary to guttural pouch mycosis, treated surgically by ligation of the affected arteries.

MEDICATIONS

DRUGS

• Immunosuppressive therapy with corticoids (e.g., dexamethasone [0.05–0.2 mg/kg IM or IV q24h]) is useful in cases of immune-mediated coagulopathy or vasculitis.
• Heparin (20–80 IU/kg SQ or IV q6–12h) and low-dose aspirin (15 mg/kg PO q24–48h) may reduce complications of DIC.
• Warfarin and sweet-clover toxicosis—treat with vitamin K_1 (1/kg SC q6h) until the clinical signs resolve and the prothrombin time is normal for at least 2 days.
• Institute appropriate antimicrobial or antifungal therapy for underlying infectious diseases. Local antifungal therapy has limited value in cases of guttural pouch mycosis associated with hemorrhage.
• Pulmonary edema—treat with furosemide (1 mg/kg IV) and respiratory support.
• Head trauma—corticosteroids (e.g., dexamethasone [0.1–0.25 mg/kg IV q6–24h for 24–48 hours]), DMSO (1 g/kg IV as a 10–20% solution for 3 days, followed by three every-other-day treatments), and mannitol (0.25–2.0 mg/kg IV over 20 minutes using a 20% solution) are beneficial.

CONTRAINDICATIONS/POSSIBLE INTERACTIONS

N/A

FOLLOW-UP

PATIENT MONITORING

• Monitor hematocrit and hydration status.
• Monitor the condition both qualitatively and quantitatively.

PREVENTION/AVOIDANCE

N/A

POSSIBLE COMPLICATIONS

Severe, fatal bleeding may occur if a major artery is involved.

EXPECTED COURSE AND PROGNOSIS

Depends on the underlying cause.

MISCELLANEOUS

ASSOCIATED CONDITIONS

N/A

AGE-RELATED FACTORS

N/A

ZOONOTIC POTENTIAL

N/A

PREGNANCY

N/A

SEE ALSO

• Exercise-induced pulmonary hemorrhage
• Guttural pouch mycosis
• Pleuropneumonia
• Sinusitis

ABBREVIATIONS

• DIC = disseminated intravascular coagulation
• DMSO = dimethyl sulfoxide
• GI = gastrointestinal

Suggested Reading

Ainsworth DM, Biller DS. Diseases of specific body systems: respiratory tract. In: Reed SM, Bayly WM, eds. Equine internal medicine. Philadelphia: WB Saunders, 1998:251–289.

Author Laurent Couëtil
Consulting Editor Jean-Pierre Lavoie

HEMOSPERMIA

BASICS

OVERVIEW

• Contamination of an ejaculate with blood.
• Causes of such blood contamination include injury to the urethral process (e.g., lacerations by tail hair, cutaneous habronemiasis, squamous cell carcinoma), lacerations to the glans or body of the penis, tears in the urethral mucosa, and infection/inflammation of the accessory sex glands.

SIGNALMENT

N/A

SIGNS

• General physical examination of the stallion at rest usually is unremarkable.
• Semen discoloration, ranging from pink-tinged to frank hemorrhage, is the most common sign.
• In natural breeding situations, blood may be seen dripping from the penis on dismount or at the vulvar lips of the mare after breeding; mares may not become pregnant after breeding.
• Some horses have concurrent hematuria.

CAUSES AND RISK FACTORS

• Trauma—laceration of the urethral process, glans penis, or body of penis (usually from tail hair); urethral stricture from a stallion ring.
• Urethral defects.
• Urethritis.
• Infection/inflammation of the accessory sex glands.
• Neoplasia—squamous cell carcinoma; papilloma.
• Cutaneous habronemiasis.

DIAGNOSIS

DIFFERENTIAL DIAGNOSIS

• Semen collected with an artificial vagina permits visualization of hemorrhage within the ejaculate.
• Fractionation of the ejaculate, using an open-ended artificial vagina, allows direct visualization of the source of hemorrhage in some cases (e.g., penile laceration); fractionation also may aid in determining from which portion of the ejaculate hemorrhage originates (e.g., blood in the gel fraction likely originates from the seminal vesicle).
• WBCs predominate over RBCs with infections of the accessory sex glands.

CBC/BIOCHEMISTRY/URINALYSIS

• CBC and chemistry panel generally are unaffected.
• Urinalysis might reveal RBCs.

OTHER LABORATORY TESTS

N/A

IMAGING

Ultrasonography:
• Transrectal ultrasonography may be useful in diagnosing seminal vesicle abnormalities.
• Normal seminal vesicle can vary significantly in appearance, ranging from flat in the non-aroused state to enlarged and filled with hypoechoic fluid after sexual stimulation.
• Inflamed seminal vesicle may be thickened and filled with echogenic fluid. Echogenic luminal contents do not always indicate pathology of the glands, however, because some stallions produce normal gel that is ultrasonographically echogenic.
• Consider ancillary tests (e.g., culture, cytology, endoscopy) for a definitive diagnosis of accessory sex gland infection/inflammation.

DIAGNOSTIC PROCEDURES

• Endoscopy—very useful in diagnosing urethral abnormalities (e.g., urethritis, rents) and seminal vesicle inflammation.
• Bacterial culture and cytology of semen—beneficial in determining accessory sex gland infection.
• Biopsy and histopathology—can be used to diagnose neoplasia or cutaneous habronemiasis.

TREATMENT

• All conditions warrant sexual rest.
• Trauma—usually outpatient care; palliative therapy aimed at hygiene and parasite control.
• Urethral defects—conservative approach: sexual rest (limited success); surgical approach: ischial urethrotomy and $\geq$2 months of sexual rest.
• Urethritis—antibiotic therapy.
• Infection/inflammation of the accessory sex glands—antibiotic therapy (e.g., local, systemic); endoscopic lavage of the seminal vesicles; intrauterine infusion of semen extender containing appropriate antibiotics.
• Neoplasia—cryotherapy, hyperthermia, local excision, reefing operation, or phallectomy.
• Cutaneous habronemiasis—parasite control; cryotherapy or surgical removal of affected sites.

MEDICATIONS

DRUGS

- Anti-inflammatory therapy is indicated in most cases—phenylbutazone; flunixin meglumine.
- Antibiotic therapy is directed at the organism causing bacterial urethritis. Systemic antibiotic therapy for seminal vesicle infection often is ineffective because of poor drug diffusion into the affected area. Antibiotic of choice for systemic treatment is trimethoprim-sulfamethoxazole (15–30 mg/kg PO BID) if the identified organism is susceptible. Lavage of the vesicles and infusion of an antibiotic directly into the seminal vesicles may be more effective.
- Antiparasitic therapy for cutaneous habronemiasis—ivermectin (0.2 mg/kg PO q30d until resolution of lesions).

CONTRAINDICATIONS/POSSIBLE INTERACTIONS

Trimethoprim-sulfamethoxazole at higher doses may cause colitis; the dosage can be lowered or the drug discontinued if the horse shows signs of colitis (e.g., diarrhea).

FOLLOW-UP

PATIENT MONITORING

Semen collection for identification of RBCs and/or WBCs in the ejaculate.

PREVENTION/AVOIDANCE

N/A

POSSIBLE COMPLICATIONS

- Infertility
- Urethral stricture or adhesions.
- Adhesions of the seminal vesicles.
- Ruptured urinary bladder.

EXPECTED COURSE AND PROGNOSIS

N/A

MISCELLANEOUS

ASSOCIATED CONDITIONS

Hematuria

AGE-RELATED FACTORS

N/A

ZOONOTIC POTENTIAL

N/A

PREGNANCY

N/A

SEE ALSO

N/A

Suggested Reading

Varner DD, Schumacher J, Blanchard T, Johnson L. Diseases and management of breeding stallions. Goleta: American Veterinary Publications, 1991:257–340.

Author Margo L. Macpherson

Contributing Editor Carla L. Carleton

HEPATIC ABSCESS (SEPTIC CHOLANGIOHEPATITIS)

BASICS

OVERVIEW

• Discrete hepatic abscesses are not common in horses, but ascending septic cholangiohepatitis is.
• Rarely, discrete abscesses may occur from intestinal-hepatic adhesions with necrosis, parasite migration, *Rhodococcus* or *Streptococcal* sp.–disseminated infections in younger horses, neoplastic abscessation, septic portal vein thrombosis, or extension of umbilical vein abscess into the liver.

SIGNALMENT

• Cholangiohepatitis most commonly is diagnosed in adult horses without any age predilection.
• No sex predilection
• Focal abscesses are sporadic and, rarely, may affect foals (e.g., *Rhodococcus* sp. or umbilical vein infection) or adults (e.g., tumor necrosis).

SIGNS

• Cholangiohepatitis—weight loss, icterus, abdominal pain, fever, and dermatitis
• Focal hepatic abscesses—ill thrift

CAUSES AND RISK FACTORS

• Cholangiohepatitis is thought to result from ascending infection by enteric gram-negative bacteria.
• Generally no historical intestinal crisis to explain the ascending infection.
• Inflammation of the bile epithelium and enzymes released from the bacteria may cause calcium bilirubinate calculi to form.

DIAGNOSIS

DIFFERENTIAL DIAGNOSIS

• The differential diagnosis for chronic colic is extensive, but colic with marked jaundice and moderately to markedly elevated liver enzymes has a short differential—cholangiohepatitis, chronic displacement of the large colon, and neoplasia
• Presence of fever, leukocytosis, and elevated serum globulins in addition to the above is nearly pathognomonic for cholangiohepatitis.

CBC/BIOCHEMISTRY/URINALYSIS

CBC generally reveals a mature neutrophilia, with mildly elevated plasma fibrinogen

OTHER LABORATORY TESTS

• Serum laboratory abnormalities with cholangiohepatitis—marked elevation in GGT (generally >300 U/L), less dramatic elevation in hepatocellular enzymes, elevations in total bilirubin that may, on occasion, approach 50% or more of the total bilirubin and elevated serum globulins
• Foals and horses with discrete hepatic abscess may have mildly elevated GGT without increases in hepatocellular enzymes or bilirubin.
• Neutrophil counts generally are increased and may be dramatic with *R. equi*–associated abscesses.
• Fibrinogen and globulins generally are increased with any abscess, but these levels may be normal with neoplasia-related abscess and *R. equi* infection.

IMAGING

• Ultrasonography of the liver (right and left side) is the imaging procedure of choice.
• Cholangitis may cause distended bile ducts (≅60% of cases), calculi with acoustic shadowing, sludge with acoustic enhancement, and a subjective hepatomegaly.
• In more long-standing cases, increased echogenicity (i.e., fibrosis) may be apparent.
• In cases of focal abscesses, the echogenicity of the abscess is variable.
• Only a small percentage of the liver can be visualized at abdominal ultrasonography in adults; a greater percentage can be visualized in foals. CT scanning can be used to image the foal's liver if discrete lesions are suspected.

DIAGNOSTIC PROCEDURES

• The most important invasive diagnostic procedure is needle aspiration or biopsy for aerobic/anaerobic culture and sensitivity and microscopic examination of the liver.
• This can be performed safely using a biopsy needle after outlining the location of the liver via ultrasonography.

TREATMENT

• Hospitalization may not be required unless IV fluids are necessary.
• Do not expose icteric horses to sunlight.
• Hepatoencephalopathy rarely occurs, so a normal diet can be fed. Exposure to sunlight, however, should not occur until the bilirubin has returned to a normal range.
• If obstructing calculi are observed or no response occurs to medical therapy, surgery might be necessary to remove an obstructing stone; this has been successfully accomplished with full recovery in a few cases.
• Horses with marked hepatic fibrosis are not surgical candidates.
• Large abscess or infected umbilical veins should be drained or removed.

MEDICATIONS

DRUGS

• The primary treatment for septic cholangiohepatitis is long-term treatment with appropriate (based on culture and sensitivity) antibiotics. Several drugs have been used successfully—trimethoprim/sulfa (30 mg/kg q12h; >50% of organisms may be resistant), enrofloxacin (3.3 mg/kg q12h), and a ceftiofur (3 mg/kg q12h), and gentamicin (6 mg/kg q24h) combination. Antimicrobials that can be given PO are preferred, because long-term (3 weeks to 6 months) treatment generally is required.
• Parenterally administered antibiotics, fluids, and DMSO may be required for some cases with biliary sludge and persistent fevers.
• Use NSAIDs (e.g., flunixin meglumine) at routine dosages for abdominal pain and during the first 3–5 days of antimicrobial therapy.
• Treat discrete or focal abscess with appropriate antibiotics (based on culture and sensitivity of aspirated fluid or knowledge of suspected pathogen).

CONTRAINDICATIONS/POSSIBLE INTERACTIONS

N/A

HEPATIC ABSCESS (SEPTIC CHOLANGIOHEPATITIS)

FOLLOW-UP

- Ideally, antimicrobial therapy is continued until GGT returns to normal (or at least <100 U/L).
- After discontinuing antimicrobials, perform a follow-up measurement of GGT.
- The prognosis of septic suppurative cholangitis is good with medical therapy if no obstructing calculi are found and the liver echogenicity is normal.
- Horses with GGT > 2500 U/L have recovered.

MISCELLANEOUS

ASSOCIATED CONDITIONS
N/A

AGE-RELATED FACTORS
N/A

ZOONOTIC POTENTIAL
N/A

PREGNANCY
N/A

SEE ALSO
N/A

ABBREVIATIONS
- DMSO = dimethyl sulfoxide
- GGT = gamma-glutamyl transferase

Suggested Reading

Johnston JK, Divers TJ, Reef VB, Acland H. Cholelithiasis in horses: ten cases (1982–1986). J Am Vet Med Assoc 1989; 194:405–409.

Author Thomas J. Divers
Consulting Editor Michel Levy

HEPATIC ABSCESS (SEPTIC CHOLANGIOHEPATITIS)

BASICS

OVERVIEW

- Discrete hepatic abscesses are not common in horses, but ascending septic cholangiohepatitis is.
- Discrete abscesses may (rarely) occur from intestinal hepatic adhesions with necrosis, parasite migration, *Rhodococcus* or *Streptococcal* sp.–disseminated infections in young horses, neoplastic abscessation, septic portal vein thrombosis, or extension of an umbilical vein abscess into the liver.

SIGNALMENT

- Cholangiohepatitis most commonly is diagnosed in adult horses without any age predilection.
- No sex predilection
- Focal abscesses are sporadic and may (rarely) affect foals (e.g., *Rhodococcus* sp., umbilical vein infection) or adults (e.g. tumor necrosis).

SIGNS

- Signs of cholangiohepatitis may include weight loss, icterus, abdominal pain, fever, and dermatitis.
- Focal hepatic abscesses may cause ill thrift.

CAUSES AND RISK FACTORS

- Cholangiohepatitis is thought to result from ascending infection by enteric, Gram-negative bacteria.
- Generally no historical intestinal crisis to explain the ascending infection
- Inflammation of bile epithelium and enzymes released from bacteria may cause calcium bilirubinate calculi to form.

DIAGNOSIS

DIFFERENTIAL DIAGNOSIS

- The differential diagnosis for chronic colic would be extensive, but colic with marked jaundice and moderately to markedly elevated liver enzymes would have a short list—cholangiohepatitis, chronic displacement of the large colon, and neoplasia
- Fever, leukocytosis, and elevated serum globulins (in addition to the above) would be nearly pathognomonic for cholangiohepatitis.

CBC/BIOCHEMISTRY/URINALYSIS

CBC generally reveals a mature neutrophilia with mild elevation in plasma fibrinogen.

OTHER LABORATORY TESTS

- Serum laboratory abnormalities in horses with cholangiohepatitis include marked elevation in GGT (generally >300 U/L), less dramatic elevation in hepatocellular enzymes, elevations in total bilirubin, which may, on occasion, approach 50% or more of the total bilirubin and elevated serum globulins.
- Foals and adults with discrete hepatic abscesses may have mild elevations in only GGT without increases in hepatocellular enzymes or bilirubin.
- Neutrophil counts generally are increased and may be dramatic with *Rhodococcus equi* abscesses.
- Fibrinogen and globulins generally are increased with any abscess, but they may not be abnormal with neoplasia-related abscess and *R. equi* infection.

IMAGING

- Ultrasonography of the liver (right and left sides) is the procedure of choice.
- Cholangitis may cause distended bile ducts ($\cong$60% of cases), calculi with acoustic shadowing, sludge with acoustic enhancement, and a subjective hepatomegaly.
- In more long-standing cases, increased echogenicity (i.e., fibrosis) may be apparent.
- In adults or foals with focal abscesses, echogenicity of the abscess is variable.
- Only a small percentage of the liver can be visualized on abdominal ultrasonography in adults; a greater percentage can be visualized in foals.
- CT scan can be used in foals with suspected discrete lesions to visualize the liver.

DIAGNOSTIC PROCEDURES

- The most important invasive diagnostic procedure is needle aspiration or biopsy for aerobic/anaerobic culture and sensitivity and microscopic examination of the liver.
- This procedure can be performed safely using a biopsy needle after outlining the location of the liver at ultrasonography.

HEPATIC ABSCESS (SEPTIC CHOLANGIOHEPATITIS)

TREATMENT

• Hospitalization may not be necessary unless IV fluids are required.
• Do not expose icteric horses to sunlight.
• If obstructing calculi are observed or no response to medical therapy occurs, surgery might be indicated to remove an obstructing stone. This has been successfully accomplished, with full recovery in a few cases. Horses with marked hepatic fibrosis are not surgical candidates.
• Large abscesses or infected umbilical veins should be drained or removed.

MEDICATIONS

DRUGS

• Primary treatment for septic cholangiohepatitis is long-term, appropriate (based on culture and sensitivity results) antibiotic therapy.
• Several drugs have been used successfully—trimethoprim/sulfa (30 mg/kg q12h; >50% of organisms may be resistant), enrofloxacin (3.3 mg/kg q12h), ceftiofur (3 mg/kg q12h), and gentamicin (6 mg/kg q24h) combination.
• Oral antimicrobials are preferred, because long-term treatment (3 weeks to 6 months) generally is required.
• Parenteral antibiotics, fluids, and DMSO may be required for some cases with biliary sludge and persistent fevers.
• Use NSAIDs (e.g., flunixin meglumine) at routine dosages for abdominal pain and during the first 3–5 days of antimicrobial therapy.
• Because hepatoencephalopathy rarely occurs, a normal diet can be fed, but exposure to sunlight should not occur until bilirubin has returned to a normal range.
• Discrete or focal abscesses should be treated with appropriate antibiotics (based on culture and sensitivity results of aspirated fluid or knowledge of suspected pathogen).

CONTRAINDICATIONS/POSSIBLE INTERACTIONS

N/A

FOLLOW-UP

PATIENT MONITORING

• Antimicrobial therapy is ideally continued until GGT has returned to normal range, or at least <100 U/L.
• After discontinuing antimicrobials, perform a follow-up measurement of GGT.

EXPECTED COURSE AND PROGNOSIS

• The prognosis of horses with septic suppurative cholangitis is good with medical therapy if no obstructing calculi are found and liver echogenicity is normal.
• Horses with GGT levels >2500 U/L have recovered.

MISCELLANEOUS

ASSOCIATED CONDITIONS

N/A

AGE-RELATED FACTORS

N/A

ZOONOTIC POTENTIAL

N/A

PREGNANCY

N/A

SEE ALSO

N/A

ABBREVIATIONS

• DMSO = dimethyl sulfoxide
• GGT = γ-glutamyltransferase

Suggested Reading

Johnston JK, Divers TJ, Reef VB, Acland H. Cholelithiasis in horses: ten cases (1982–1986). J Am Vet Med Assoc 1989;194:405–409.

Author Thomas J. Divers
Consulting Editor Joseph J. Bertone

HEPATIC CLEARANCE TESTS: BROMOSULFOPHTHALEIN (BSP) AND INDOCYANINE GREEN (ICG)

BASICS

DEFINITION

- BSP and ICG are synthetic IV dyes used to assess blood flow to the liver (e.g., for evidence of vascular shunting) and/or liver function (e.g., hepatic insufficiency/failure), though both tests are not specific for these conditions. These two types of conditions are not effectively distinguished by these assays and are collectively described as *decreased hepatic functional mass.* Interpretations relative to functional mass depend on careful selection of patients subjected to testing.
- After IV injection, the dyes are rapidly removed from circulation by the liver. The amount of dye in circulation is quantified colorimetrically and expressed as the amount remaining at a certain time (i.e., % retention) or as a clearance rate. The clearance rate often is expressed as the circulating half-life, and half-life estimation is the recommended procedure in horses because of their very rapid clearance rates. Decreased hepatic functional mass results in longer half-life (i.e., slower clearance).
- Factors such as availability of dye (BSP), expense (ICG), cumbersome procedures, lack of specificity, and availability of alternative tests (e.g., ammonia, bile salts) currently limit widespread use of these assays.

PATHOPHYSIOLOGY

- In general, BSP and ICG have similar biologic handling.
- Disadvantages of BSP—severe tissue reactions on perivascular injection, occasional severe idiosyncratic hypersensitivity reactions, very short half-life, and lack of commercial availability
- ICG is essentially free of side effects, has a slightly longer circulating half-life, is more expensive than BSP, and requires specialized equipment for analysis (i.e., infrared spectrophotometry).
- Proper interpretation of dye clearance tests depends on understanding several factors—injected dye initially is protein bound (primarily to albumin) and distributed throughout the vasculature; liver handling involves receptor-mediated uptake, conjugation (BSP only) with glutathione, and excretion in bile; and competition with bilirubin occurs at some hepatocellular processing steps (e.g., binding to ligandin as an intracellular carrier protein).
- Causes of prolonged circulating half-life (i.e., decreased clearance)—decreased functional hepatocytes, decreased blood flow to the liver (e.g., portovascular shunting, congestive heart failure, severe dehydration, etc.), decreased bile flow, high bilirubin concentrations ($\geq$5—6 mg/dL), and fasting (3–4 days) via decreased uptake by hepatocytes.
- A shortened circulating half-life primarily occurs from hypoalbuminemia. Decreased availability of protein results in increased free dye, which is lost through renal excretion or leakage into extravascular fluids. Hypoalbuminemic cases have more dye molecules per albumin, which facilitates rapid hepatic clearance of the protein-bound fraction.

SYSTEMS AFFECTED

Hepatobiliary

- Decreased clearance (i.e., prolonged half-life) occurs with decreased functional hepatocytes and with cholestasis.
- Hypoalbuminemia, which may result from hepatic insufficiency, tends to increase clearance and may mask the effect of hepatic insufficiency on clearance.

CNS

Hepatic insufficiency and vascular shunts (associated with decreased clearance) can lead to hepatic encephalopathy.

Cardiovascular

Portosystemic shunts, congestive heart failure, severe dehydration, shock, and so on decrease clearance through decreased hepatic perfusion.

GI/Renal

As potential sources of severe hypoalbuminemia, abnormalities in these systems may increase clearance rates and mask the effects of hepatic insufficiency or vascular shunting.

Skin

Concurrent photosensitization is possible with hepatic insufficiency.

Hematopoietic

- Hepatic insufficiency and vascular shunts can be associated with microcytosis.
- Mild nonregenerative anemia and coagulation abnormalities associated with deficiency of vitamin K–dependent factors (among others) may be present.

SIGNALMENT

- Age—portosystemic vascular shunts are more likely to manifest at earlier ages.
- Pregnancy—some liver diseases that may culminate in hepatic insufficiency occur more frequently in pregnant mares (e.g., hyperlipemia and hepatic lipidosis, Theiler's disease associated with receiving tetanus toxoid, etc.).
- Ponies/donkeys—particularly susceptible to hyperlipemia and hepatic lipidosis if subjected to negative nitrogen balance; most common in obese animals.

SIGNS

General Comments

Signs do not result directly from the altered dye clearance but rather from the underlying disease process.

Historical Findings

- Icterus, dark-yellow/orange urine, anorexia, weight loss, diarrhea, and listlessness may accompany cholestasis or decreased hepatic functional mass.
- Behavioral changes (e.g., circling, head pressing, etc.) may accompany hepatic encephalopathy.
- Abdominal pain (e.g., sweating, rolling, etc.) may occur with acute hepatopathies (i.e., capsular swelling) or biliary obstructions.
- Photosensitization may be associated with pruritus, avoidance of direct sunlight, lacrimation, and skin lesions.

Physical Examination Findings

- Vary, depending on the underlying disease process and pathogenesis.
- Weight loss, icterus, increased pulse and respiratory rate, fever, photosensitization, diarrhea, and constipation may be observed.
- Abnormal bleeding tendencies may be observed and most commonly represent abnormal secondary hemostasis—epistaxis, hematomas from venipuncture, hemarthrosis
- With DIC, abnormal primary hemostasis may be observed—petechiation

CAUSES

Sources of acute, generalized hepatic injury may lead to transient, potentially reversible hepatic failure; however, chronic and recurrent insults often initiate fibrosis that may lead to irreversible failure.

HEPATIC CLEARANCE TESTS: BROMOSULFOPHTHALEIN (BSP) AND INDOCYANINE GREEN (ICG)

Hepatobiliary System

- Toxic—pyrrolizidine alkaloid–containing plants (e.g., senecio, crotalaria, etc.), alsike clover, kleingrass, aflatoxin, rubratoxin; chemical toxins (e.g., arsenic, chlorinated hydrocarbons, monensin, phenol, paraquat and ferrous fumarate toxicity in neonates)
- Nutritional—hepatic lipidosis
- Degenerative—cirrhosis and cholelithiasis
- Metabolic—secondary to severe anemia, hyperlipemia, fasting (i.e., delayed clearance secondary to hyperbilirubinemia), secondary to diabetes mellitus (i.e., hepatic lipidosis), and hyperadrenocorticism (i.e., steroid hepatopathy).
- Immune-mediated, infectious—chronic active hepatitis, chronic cholangitis (i.e., biliary cirrhosis), Theiler's disease (i.e., serum hepatitis), amyloidosis, endotoxemia, viral (e.g., EIA, EVA, EHV in perinatal foals), bacterial (e.g., Tyzzer's disease, salmonellosis, etc.), fungal, protozoal, and parasitic (e.g., liver flukes, strongyle larval migrans).
- Anomaly—biliary atresia and portosystemic vascular shunts (mostly congenital)
- Neoplastic—primary liver tumors (rare) and metastatic neoplasia (uncommon).

Cardiovascular System

- Congestive heart failure—congested hepatic blood flow decreases clearance; chronic hypoxia leads to secondary hepatic parenchymal lesions.
- Severe dehydration
- Shock

Hematopoietic System

- Severe anemia (e.g., neonatal isoerythrolysis, acute EIA, red maple-leaf toxicity, onion toxicity, postparturient hemorrhage) leads to hypoxic injury and hepatocellular swelling, with subsequent cholestasis.
- Chronic, severe anemia may lead to centrolobular necrosis and subsequent fibrosis.
- Hepatic lymphosarcoma, leukemias, and so on can replace hepatic parenchyma.

RISK FACTORS

- Exposure to toxins/plants
- Inadequate vaccination protocol—viral diseases
- Use as antisera donor—amyloidosis

DIAGNOSIS

DIFFERENTIAL DIAGNOSIS

- Dye clearance tests are expensive and cumbersome compared to routine tests for liver disease and cholestasis; thus, use them only when interpretation will provide specific evidence of decreased hepatic functional mass.
- Dye clearance tests are altered by several conditions (e.g., high serum bilirubin, cholestasis, chronic passive congestion, etc.), so the specificity of results is obtained by testing only patients free of these confounding variables. Appropriate candidates include those with suspected decreased hepatic functional mass (based on history, signs, and laboratory data) but with minimal or no evidence of active hepatic disease—hepatocellular injury and cholestasis

LABORATORY FINDINGS

Drugs that May Alter Lab Results

N/A

Disorders that May Alter Lab Results

- Collect samples for analysis from a vein other than that used for injection. Same-day analysis is recommended for BSP because of serum instability.
- Do not run routine chemistries or urinalyses on samples containing BSP because of potential interferences, which are especially noted for serum creatinine, urine ketones, and urobilinogen.

Valid If Run in Human Lab?

Yes

CBC/BIOCHEMISTRY/URINALYSIS

- No routine laboratory test provides a causative or specific diagnosis for prolonged dye clearance (or decreased hepatic functional mass). Most suggest a type of hepatic alteration (e.g., hepatocellular injury, cholestasis, insufficiency/vascular shunt) rather than the cause of that alteration.
- Key abnormalities identified on routine blood work suggestive of (but not specific for) decreased hepatic functional mass—microcytosis, abnormal glucose values, low BUN (relative to creatinine), hypoalbuminemia, hyperglobulinemia, hypocholesterolemia, and ammonia biurate crystalluria. These parameters are insensitive markers that typically become abnormal only after a 75–80% decrease in functional capacity. Dye clearance tests are more sensitive with changes occurring after a 50–55% reduction in functional capacity.

Erythrocytes

- Microcytosis (low MCV), often (but not always) without hypochromasia or anemia is reported to occur with portosystemic shunts.
- Nonregenerative anemia may be seen with liver disease.
- Morphologic changes may also be reported—poikilocytosis, acanthocytosis, target cells. Some morphologic changes induced by liver disease (i.e., acanthocytes, schistocytes from microvascular disease in the liver) are associated with decreased RBC survival and may contribute to mild hemolytic (regenerative) anemia.
- Severe hemolytic anemia from any cause (e.g., oxidation injuries manifested by Heinz bodies or eccentrocytes, immune-mediated anemia) can cause hypoxic injury leading to hepatocellular swelling and secondary cholestasis.
- A hemolytic crisis (unclear mechanism) occasionally occurs associated with severe hepatic disease/failure and carries a poor prognosis.

Leukocytes

- Neutrophilia or neutropenia and monocytosis may occur with inflammatory liver disease—bacterial cholangiohepatitis.
- Evidence of antigenic stimulation (lymphocytosis or reactive lymphoid cells) also may be seen.

HEPATIC CLEARANCE TESTS: BROMOSULFOPHTHALEIN (BSP) AND INDOCYANINE GREEN (ICG)

Glucose

• Postprandial hyperglycemia or fasting hypoglycemia may occur with hepatic insufficiency/shunts.
• Hypoglycemia with liver disease carries a guarded prognosis.

Albumin

• Decreased production with hepatic insufficiency may decrease serum concentrations.
• Albumin is also a negative acute-phase reactant. Mild decreases may occur in inflammatory liver disease. Albumin's long half-life in horses (20 days) often masks decreased production.

BUN

Decreased (especially relative to creatinine) with hepatic insufficiency/shunts because of decreased conversion of ammonia to urea.

SDH

• Increases specifically with hepatocellular injury.
• May increase concurrently with or independent of cholestasis or decreased functional mass.

AST

Increased with hepatocellular or muscle injury

ALP

• Increases primarily with cholestasis.
• Other causes—proliferative bone disease or rapid growth (bone isoform) and severe GI disease (mild increases only)

Bilirubin

• Conjugated—increased with cholestasis and with hepatocellular injury, presumably related to cell swelling and secondary cholestasis
• Unconjugated—increased with increased RBC destruction (i.e., hemolysis) or defective hepatocellular uptake (e.g., injured hepatocytes, hepatic insufficiency, vascular shunting) and with fasting because of a nonpathologic decrease in uptake.

Cholesterol

• May be decreased with hepatic insufficiency/shunts.
• Commonly increased with cholestasis and lipid metabolism disorders—e.g., hyperlipemia

Triglycerides

Increased with hyperlipemia

Urinalysis

• Bilirubinuria indicates intra- or posthepatic cholestasis.
• Ammonia urate crystals may be observed with hepatic insufficiency/shunt but are not pathognomonic.

OTHER LABORATORY TESTS

Bile Acids

• A sensitive indicator of hepatobiliary disease, but not specific for the type process
• Concentrations depend on adequate enterohepatic circulation, hepatobiliary function, and hepatocellular perfusion; are very sensitive in detecting acute cholestasis; and typically increase with decreased hepatic functional mass.

Ammonia

• Serum concentrations represent a balance between production (i.e., protein catabolism) and hepatic uptake.
• Fasting ammonia levels increase when 60–70% of functional mass is lost.

Serology

Depends on the degree of suspicion for specific diseases—viral and fungal

Coagulation Tests

• May be prolonged (e.g., prothrombin time, activated partial thromboplastin time) with hepatic insufficiency/shunting.
• Hypofibrinogenemia may be observed, but is uncommon.

IMAGING

Ultrasonography may be useful for assessing liver size, shape, position, and parenchymal texture; for detecting focal parenchymal lesions (i.e., abscesses, neoplasms) and abnormalities in the biliary tree (i.e., dilatations, obstructions) or large vessels (i.e., shunts, thrombosis); and increases the safety and accuracy of biopsy.

DIAGNOSTIC PROCEDURES

Aspiration cytology or use of biopsied tissue for microbiologic testing, cytologic imprints, and histopathologic evaluation may provide specific diagnostic information.

HEPATIC CLEARANCE TESTS: BROMOSULFOPHTHALEIN (BSP) AND INDOCYANINE GREEN (ICG)

TREATMENT

Decision regarding outpatient vs. inpatient treatment depends on severity of disease, intensity of supportive care required, need for isolation of infectious conditions, and so on.

MEDICATIONS

DRUGS OF CHOICE

Depend on suspected cause and observed complications.

CONTRAINDICATIONS

Depend on suspected cause and observed complications.

PRECAUTIONS

- Depend on suspected cause.
- If hepatic insufficiency is suspected, assess coagulation profiles before invasive procedures.

POSSIBLE INTERACTIONS

Depend on underlying cause.

ALTERNATIVE DRUGS

Depend on underlying cause.

FOLLOW UP

PATIENT MONITORING

Serial blood chemistries can help to establish a prognosis by characterizing disease progression and identifying evidence of improvement. Initial evaluation (at 1–2 day intervals) helps to establish disease course; subsequent testing can be performed at increasing intervals, depending on signs and disease severity.

POSSIBLE COMPLICATIONS

Depend on underlying cause

MISCELLANEOUS

ASSOCIATED CONDITIONS

Depend on underlying cause

AGE-RELATED FACTORS

See *Signalment.*

ZOONOTIC POTENTIAL

Depends on underlying cause

PREGNANCY

See *Signalment.*

SYNONYMS

BSP—bromsulphthalein, bromsulfalein, bromsulphalein, sulfobromophthalein

SEE ALSO

N/A

ABBREVIATIONS

- ALP = alkaline phosphatase
- AST = aspartate aminotransferase
- DIC = disseminated intravascular coagulation
- EHV = equine herpes virus
- EIA = equine infectious anemia
- EVA = equine viral arteritis
- GI = gastrointestinal
- MCV = mean cell volume
- SDH = sorbitol dehydrogenase

Suggested Reading

Barton MH, Morris DD. Diseases of the liver. In: Reed S, Bayly W, eds. Equine internal medicine. Philadelphia: WB Saunders, 1998:707–738.

Savage CJ. Diseases of the liver. In: Colahan PT, Merritt AM, Moore JN, Mayhew IG, eds. Equine medicine and surgery. 5th ed. St. Louis: Mosby, 1999:816–833.

VET-BSP Solution (sulfobromophthalein sodium injection, USP) 50 mg/ml. Manufacturer's package insert. Mt. Pleasant, MI: Ventec Laboratories, 1984.

Author John A. Christian
Consulting Editor Michel Levy

HEPATIC ENCEPHALOPATHY

BASICS

OVERVIEW
- Clinical syndrome in which animals have altered mentation caused by hepatic insufficiency.
- Animals may have inappropriate behavior and impaired motor status
- Thought to involve changes in neurotransmission in the CNS caused by agents accumulating as a result of hepatic insufficiency.
- Toxic metabolites may act as false neurotransmitters.
- There may be an imbalance between excitatory (i.e., glutamate) and inhibitory (i.e., GABA) neurotransmission, ammonia may act as neurotoxin, or increased levels of endogenous benzodiazepine-like substance may be present.

SIGNALMENT
No breed or sex predilections

SIGNS
- Depression
- Head-pressing
- Circling
- Ataxia
- Wandering/aimless movements
- Recumbency
- Icterus
- Photosensitization
- Pyrexia
- Weight loss
- Colic—chronic
- Coagulopathy

CAUSES AND RISK FACTORS
- Toxic hepatopathy, including pyrrolizidine alkaloids
- Acute necrotizing hepatitis—Theiler's disease
- Cholelithiasis
- Chronic active hepatitis
- Tyzzer's disease
- Hyperlipemia—ponies; miniature horses
- Neoplasia

DIAGNOSIS

DIFFERENTIAL DIAGNOSIS
- Viral encephalitis (e.g., EEE, WEE)—ruled out by virology or CSF tap cytology.
- Rabies—rule out by IFA on tactile hairs.
- Trauma—rule out based on history, palpation, radiographs, and CSF tap.
- Botulism—more likely if dysphagic
- Equine protozoal myelitis—ruled out by CSF and Western blot analyses.
- Aberrant parasite migration
- Electrolyte abnormalities

CBC/BIOCHEMISTRY/URINALYSIS
- Azotemia—may be secondary to changes in mentation/appetite/drinking.
- BUN—may be decreased in liver failure.
- Glucose—may be decreased in advanced liver failure.
- Liver-specific changes—elevated bilirubin, increased GGT, SDH, hypoalbuminemia, hypoproteinemia, elevated resting ammonia levels, and elevated bile acids
- Animals with encephalopathy from hyperlipemia—may have increased cholesterol, elevated triglycerides, and be hyperlipemic.
- Secondary hypocalcemia, hypokalemia, and metabolic acidosis

OTHER LABORATORY TESTS
Coagulation profiles—may or may not be prolonged.

IMAGING
Ultrasonography may help to assess size, changes in the parenchyma, scan for abscesses and masses, and assist with biopsy.

DIAGNOSTIC PROCEDURES
CSF tap to rule out other infectious causes of abnormal neurological behavior, including cytology, culture, viral titers and possibly, EPM by Western blot analysis.

TREATMENT
- For dysphoric or demented animals, some sedation may be necessary.
- Correction of fluid deficits caused by dehydration, and then correction of acid–base deficits if still necessary, also will help to decrease absorption of ammonia.
- For anorectic or hypoglycemic animals, give 5% dextrose (2 mL/kg per hour) to start, then 2.5%–5% in half-strength saline.
- High-carbohydrate, low-protein diet with branched chain amino acids
- Feed small amounts frequently.

HEPATIC ENCEPHALOPATHY

MEDICATIONS

DRUGS
- Lactulose (0.3 mL/kg q6h)
- Hyperlipemic horses can be given insulin, steroids, and heparin.
- Metronidazole

CONTRAINDICATIONS/POSSIBLE INTERACTIONS
N/A

FOLLOW-UP
- Prognosis depends on the primary cause.
- Animals with hyperlipidemia/hyperlipemia may respond well to aggressive treatment. For these animals, monitor cholesterol and triglycerides.
- Animals with hepatic encephalopathy from toxins probably experienced the initial insult several weeks/months before presentation; determine if signs are still progressing. These animals may be stabilized, but if signs continue to progress or recur shortly after discharged, a poor prognosis is indicated.
- Poor prognosis for recumbent animals

MISCELLANEOUS

ASSOCIATED CONDITIONS
N/A

AGE-RELATED FACTORS
N/A

ZOONOTIC POTENTIAL
N/A

PREGNANCY
N/A

SEE ALSO
N/A

ABBREVIATIONS
- CSF = cerebrospinal fluid
- EEE = eastern encephalitides
- EPM = equine protozoal myelitis
- GABA = γ-aminobutyric acid
- GGT = γ-glutamyltransferase
- IFA = indirect fluorescent antibody
- SDH = sorbitol dehydrogenase
- WEE = western encephalitides

Suggested Reading

Tyler JW. Hepatoencephalopathy. Part II. Pathophysiology and Treatment. Compendium 1990;12:1260–1270.

Author S.G. Witonsky
Consulting Editor Joseph J. Bertone

HERNIAS

BASICS

OVERVIEW

- Generally congenital defects in the body wall
- Classified by location, reducibility, and condition of the hernial contents
- Most congenital hernias in foals are umbilical or inguinal/scrotal.
- Umbilical hernias—incidence, 0.5–2%.
- Inguinal hernias—when the bowel remains in the inguinal canal; becomes a scrotal hernia when the hernial contents pass through the inguinal rings and lie next to the testicle. Generally, the bowel remains within the vaginal tunic; occasionally, it breaks through and herniates SC down the medial thigh.
- Reducible or not reducible
- Usually contain bowel, but can contain fat and omentum as well.
- Strangulated hernias—when the bowel becomes incarcerated and cannot be reduced
- Intestinal obstruction and colic accompany strangulating hernias.

SIGNALMENT

- In the newborn foal, usually evident at birth, but may not be observed until the foal is standing and active.
- Inguinal hernias—considered an inheritable trait in certain breeds
- Umbilical hernias are seen in both males and females; inguinal hernias are seen predominantly in males.

SIGNS

- Physical examination—found through palpation of and observation of swelling in the umbilical and inguinal areas; most hernias are manually reducible.
- Colic may be a sign that bowel is becoming incarcerated in the hernial sac.
- Swelling may increase and become painful to palpation.

CAUSES AND RISK FACTORS

- May have a genetic predisposition.
- Increased abdominal pressure at birth, umbilical infections, and excessive straining

DIAGNOSIS

DIFFERENTIAL DIAGNOSIS

- Distinguish umbilical hernias from umbilical swelling secondary to hematoma formation due to birth trauma or umbilical infection.
- Occasionally, swelling in the umbilical region can occur in response to irritating navel dips (e.g., tincture of iodine).
- Differentiate inguinal hernias from swelling due to trauma or testicular problems.

CBC/BIOCHEMISTRY/URINALYSIS

N/A

OTHER LABORATORY TESTS

N/A

IMAGING

- Ultrasound of the hernia may help in determining whether the swelling contains intestine.
- Ultrasound of the umbilical stalk, arteries, and veins may helps in ruling out omphalophlebitis.

DIAGNOSTIC PROCEDURES

N/A

TREATMENT

- Many simple hernias resolve within the first 6 months of life. The foal continues to grow, and the body wall defect becomes smaller. If the hernia is reducible, daily reduction is helpful.
- Umbilical hernias have been treated with local injection into the hernial ring of an irritating substance (e.g., iodine). Abdominal wraps, applying pressure to the reduced hernia, also may help.
- Hernial clamps have been used to create inflammation in the underlying tissues and reduce the hernial sac.
- A figure 8–type bandage or truss can be applied to foals with scrotal hernias after the hernia has been reduced; take care that the penis is not incorporated into the bandage.
- If a hernia has not resolved by 6 months of age, surgery may be needed.
- Incarcerated hernias require immediate emergency surgery; strangulated bowel can lead to abdominal pain, ischemic bowel, endotoxin release, and shock.

HERNIAS

MEDICATIONS

DRUGS

• No drug therapy needed for nonsurgical hernias
• Perioperative antibiotics can be used as a prophylactic measure.

CONTRAINDICATIONS/POSSIBLE INTERACTIONS

N/A

FOLLOW-UP

PATIENT MONITORING

• Check foals daily with palpation and hernia reduction; owners should be aware of any increased size or heat in the hernial swelling.
• If colic occurs, consider the hernia as a possible cause.

EXPECTED COURSE AND PROGNOSIS

• Most foals with small hernias have a good prognosis for resolution, which generally occurs within the first 6 months of life.
• Larger hernias have a greater chance of not fully resolving and of requiring surgical correction.

MISCELLANEOUS

ASSOCIATED CONDITIONS

N/A

AGE-RELATED FACTORS

N/A

ZOONOTIC POTENTIAL

N/A

PREGNANCY

N/A

SEE ALSO

Omphalophlebitis

Suggested Readings

Adams R. The urogenital system. In: Koterba AM, Drummond WH, Kosch PC, eds. Equine clinical neonatology. 1990:491–494.

Tulleners EP. Diseases of the abdominal wall: congenital and familial diseases. In: Colahan PT, Mayhew IG, Merritt AM, Moore JN, eds. Equine medicine and surgery. 1999:808–811.

Author Mary Rose Paradis
Consulting Editor Mary Rose Paradis

HERPES KERATITIS

BASICS

OVERVIEW

- Keratopathy with associated conjunctivitis and epiphora caused by EHV-2.
- Organ system—ophthalmic

SIGNALMENT

All ages and breeds

SIGNS

- Multiple superficial white, punctate, or linear corneal opacities, with or without fluorescein dye retention
- Varying amounts of ocular pain, conjunctivitis, corneal edema, epiphora, and iridocyclitis
- May stain with rose bengal
- Drooping of upper lid eyelashes

CAUSES AND RISK FACTORS

EHV-2

DIAGNOSIS

DIFFERENTIAL DIAGNOSIS

- Corneal ulcers
- ERU
- Glaucoma
- Blepharitis
- Conjunctivitis
- Dacryocystitis

CBC/BIOCHEMISTRY/URINALYSIS

N/A

OTHER LABORATORY TESTS

- Rule out other infectious causes (bacterial or fungal) with corneal scrapings for cytology and culture.
- Culture virus from ocular specimens and identify viral isolates with electron microscopy, restriction endonuclease DNA fingerprinting, and Southern blot analysis.

IMAGING

N/A

DIAGNOSTIC PROCEDURES

N/A

TREATMENT

N/A

MEDICATIONS

DRUGS

- Topical idoxuridine or trifluorothymidine (initially q2h, then q4–6h)
- Topical NSAIDs may be beneficial—diclofenamic acid (BID) or flurbiprofen (BID).

CONTRAINDICATIONS/POSSIBLE INTERACTIONS

N/A

HERPES KERATITIS

FOLLOW-UP

EXPECTED COURSE AND PROGNOSIS
Treatment often is successful, but recurrence is common.

MISCELLANEOUS

ASSOCIATED CONDITIONS
Secondary bacterial infection

AGE-RELATED FACTORS
Multiple foals in a herd may be affected.

ZOONOTIC POTENTIAL
N/A

PREGNANCY
N/A

SEE ALSO
- Burdock pappus bristle keratopathy
- Calcific band keratopathy
- Corneal laceration
- Corneal stromal abscessation
- Corneal ulceration
- Eosinophilic keratitis
- ERU
- Glaucoma
- Keratomycosis
- Nonulcerative keratouveitis
- Superficial corneal erosions with anterior stromal sequestration

ABREVIATIONS
- EHV-2 = equine herpesvirus type 2
- ERU = equine recurrent uveitis

Suggested Reading

Brooks DE. Equine ophthalmology. In: Gelatt KN, ed. Veterinary ophthalmology. 3rd ed. Philadelphia: Lippincott Williams & Wilkins, 1999.

Author Andras M. Komaromy
Consulting Editor Dennis E. Brooks

HERPESVIRUS (EHV) MYELOENCEPHALOPATHY

BASICS

DEFINITION

A spinal-cord disorder associated with EHV-1 and vasculitis with neural parenchyma affected by secondary hemorrhagic and ischemic infarction

PATHOPHYSIOLOGY

- EHV-1 can spread directly from cell to cell without an extracellular phase; thus, neutralizing antibody has little protective potential.
- Virus-bearing leukocytes may infect endothelial cells in the CNS.
- Like other herpes viruses, EHV-l likely is neurotropic and can establish reservoirs in sensory ganglia.
- Clinical signs relate to ischemia of nervous tissue secondary to vasculitis. The vasculitis may be a direct effect of the virus or secondary to immune-mediated disease.
- Immunoperoxidase staining has identified EHV-1 in astrocytes and neurons of horses during early disease. This suggests viral infection. The lesions of EHV-1 cannot be distinguished from experimentally induced Arthus reactions, however, and the neurologic form of EHV-1 infection frequently is seen in adult horses with elevated levels of circulating antibodies. This would support the hypothesis that CNS vasculitis associated with EHV-1 may be associated with an immunologic reaction to the virus on the surface of infected endothelial cells.

SYSTEMS AFFECTED

- CNS
- Lower urinary tract

SIGNALMENT

- No breed or sex predilection
- Adult horses seem more likely than very young horses to be affected.

SIGNS

Historical Findings

- Horses may or may not have a current vaccination record.
- Respiratory disease or abortion may or may not be evident in exposed horses and herdmates.

Physical Examination Findings

- The latent period is ≅7 days in experimental studies of EHV-1 infection.
- Pyrexia (≤41.1°C or 105.8°F) and mild respiratory tract signs (e.g., cough, serous nasal discharge) often precede neurologic signs by several days and may or may not be present at the onset of neurologic disease. These signs can be subtle and often are missed.
- Pregnant mares may abort immediately before, during, or sometime after development of neurologic signs.
- Peracute onset of paresis and ataxia of the trunk and limbs that commonly is most severe at 40–60 hours. Signs stabilize quickly, and improvement occurs rapidly during the next few days. In some cases, however, signs may worsen over the course of several days.
- Gait abnormalities initially may manifest asymmetrically or symmetrically in one or more limbs. Thoracolumbar lesions tend to be most common, so pelvic limb signs tend to be most severe. Early signs can vary from subtle clumsiness or stiffness to "dog-sitting" and recumbency.
- Affected horses often have paralytic bladders that present distended. In many cases, urinary incontinence also is seen.
- Decreased tail tone and perineal hypalgesia are variably seen.
- Brainstem signs are seen in rare cases.
- Horses tend to have normal mentation, but depression occurs in rare cases.
- The prognosis is poor if horses become recumbent, but many affected horses recover completely. Time to recovery depends on severity of the lesion signs, ranging from several days to >1 year.
- Urinary tract function returns before gait abnormalities resolve.
- Enteritis and chorioretinitis associated with EHV-1 have been described.

CAUSES

EHV-1

RISK FACTORS

None identified

DIAGNOSIS

DIFFERENTIAL DIAGNOSIS

- Trauma
- Equine protozoal myeloencephalitis
- Space-occupying lesions

CBC/BIOCHEMISTRY/URINALYSIS

No consistent abnormalities

OTHER LABORATORY TESTS

No consistent abnormalities

IMAGING

N/A

HERPESVIRUS (EHV) MYELOENCEPHALOPATHY

DIAGNOSTIC PROCEDURES

- A presumptive diagnosis of EHV-1 myeloencephalitis can be made in horses with peracute spinal-cord deficits, incontinence, and bladder distention.
- The diagnosis can be supported with isolation of viral particles from nasopharyngeal swabs and blood buffy coat and or a fourfold rise in virus-neutralizing or complement-fixing antibody titers between acute and convalescent serum samples obtained 7–10 days apart.
- Differentiating between antibodies to EHV-l and antibodies to EHV-4 is difficult, as is isolating virus from CNS tissue. Therefore, a definitive diagnosis is difficult to establish.
- At the onset of clinical signs, >95% of horses have increased levels of complement-fixing antibodies (>1:160).
- Analysis of complement-fixing antibody titers is preferable, because many normal horses have persistent, high levels of virus-neutralizing antibody.
- Supportive evidence also includes xanthochromia and marked elevation of protein content (100–500 mg/dL) in CSF. Serum-neutralizing titers in CSF have not been consistently elevated in cases of EHV-1 myeloencephalitis, but when positive, this finding can be supportive.

PATHOLOGIC FINDINGS

Gross Findings

A brown discoloration may be seen in the spinal cord.

Histopathologic Findings

- Areas of ischemic and hemorrhagic infarction, with perivascular edema and necrosis
- Perivascular cuffs of lymphocytes, plasma cells, and macrophages in the meninges and parenchyma
- Intranuclear inclusions may occur in other areas—respiratory tract, fetus
- Immunologic staining with EHV polyclonal antiserum may be useful.

TREATMENT

- Many affected horses can recover if given time and any necessary supportive treatment.
- Recumbent horses also may recover.

MEDICATIONS

DRUGS OF CHOICE

- Glucocorticoids during very early disease may be useful, but this is debatable.
- Dexamethasone (0.05–0.1 mg/kg q12–6h) may be useful.

CONTRAINDICTIONS

N/A

PRECAUTIONS

N/A

POSSIBLE INTERACTIONS

N/A

ALTERNATIVE DRUGS

N/A

FOLLOW-UP

POSSIBLE COMPLICATIONS

Trauma associated from weakness and attempts at rising, decubital sores, paralyzed bladder, and urinary tract infection.

PREVENTION/AVOIDANCE

Clinical evidence suggests that vaccines are not protective and actually may increase the risk of neurologic disease. Thus, it can be argued that vaccination should not be used during an outbreak.

MISCELLANEOUS

ASSOCIATED CONDITIONS

N/A

AGE-RELATED FACTORS

Mature horses

ZOONOTIC POTENTIAL

N/A

PREGNANCY

Mares may coincidentally abort.

SYNONYMS

N/A

SEE ALSO

N/A

ABBREVIATIONS

CSF = cerebrospinal fluid

Suggested Reading

Little PB, Thorsen J. Disseminated necrotizing myeloencephalitis: a herpes-associated neurological disease of horses. Vet Pathol 1976;13:161–171.

Ostlund EN. The equine herpesviruses. Vet Clin North Am Equine Pract 1993;9:283–294.

Author Joseph J. Bertone

Consulting Editor Joseph J. Bertone

HERPESVIRUS TYPES-1 AND 4

BASICS

DEFINITION

A ubiquitous, contagious viral equine pathogen that most frequently causes respiratory tract disease but may also cause abortion, fatal neonatal illness, or neurologic disease.

PATHOPHYSIOLOGY

Equine herpesvirus 1 (EHV-1) and equine herpesvirus 4 (EHV-4) infect the respiratory tract; however, EHV-1 may also infect white blood cells, subsequently causing a viremia and dissemination of the virus to the reproductive tract or central nervous system (CNS). EHV-4 infections are usually limited to the upper respiratory tract and are a common cause of respiratory disease in young horses. Following resolution of clinical signs, either virus may become dormant, only to recrudesce during periods of stress, such as shipping, weaning, training, or competition. The ability of the virus to evade the immune system and establish latent infection is important in the propagation of the disease and has made control by immunization difficult. It is unknown why EHV-1 periodically induces reproductive tract or CNS disease; infectious dose, immune status of the horse, and viral strain are likely factors.

SYSTEMS AFFECTED

Respiratory

Infection of the respiratory epithelium leads to fever (102–106°F), cough, depression, nasal discharge (serous to mucopurulent), and abnormal lung sounds.

Reproductive

Following infection of the upper respiratory tract and subsequent viremia, EHV-1 may infect endometrium and fetal tissues, resulting in fetal death and abortion.

Nervous

Both isolated cases and outbreaks of CNS disease occur. Viremic spread of EHV-1 to the CNS endothelium leads to thrombosis, ischemic neural damage, and characteristic clinical signs.

GENETICS

No known genetic predisposition.

INCIDENCE/PREVALENCE

Equine herpesvirus-related disease has been reported worldwide wherever large groups of horses are present.

SIGNALMENT

The median age of horses hospitalized for the neurologic form of EHV-1 infection is 3 years. However, horses of any age or breed are susceptible to EHV-related diseases. Respiratory tract disease due to EHV-4 is extremely common in young horses.

SIGNS

In horses with partial immunity to EHV, silent infections occur in which the only signs are fever and depression. Distal limb edema may accompany EHV-1 infection due to associated vasculitis and decreased ambulation.

Respiratory Disease

Respiratory tract disease, manifested by cough, mucopurulent nasal discharge, fever (102–106°F, 38.9–41°C), depression, and abnormal lung sounds is the most common form of EHV-1 and 4 infection.

Reproductive Tract Disease

Abortions usually occur late in gestation (7–11 months) with or without other signs of EHV-related disease. Abortions may be either sporadic or multiple mares may be affected. The lesions in the infected aborted fetus include pulmonary edema, pleural and peritoneal effusions, multifocal hepatic necrosis, icterus, and petechiation.

Neurologic Disease

Neurologic deficits may be symmetric or asymmetric. Fever usually precedes an acute onset of hindlimb ataxia, proprioceptive deficits, and weakness. In the most severe form, hindlimb paralysis leads to a dog-sitting posture or recumbency. Although the hindlimbs are most commonly affected, cranial nerve abnormalities (head tilt, tongue weakness, nystagmus, blindness) also occur. Bladder atony, fecal retention, perineal sensory deficits, and decreased tail tone are common. Ophthalmologic examination may reveal retinal hemorrhages due to optic neuritis.

CAUSES

Equine herpesvirus types 1 and 4

RISK FACTORS

Outbreaks and isolated cases of EHV-related disease are frequently associated with stress, such as transportation, weaning, overcrowding, surgery, other illnesses, or competition. The risk of infection may be increased by poor ventilation, which increases the concentration of viral particles and causes the accumulation of noxious gases, thus impairing respiratory immune function.

DIAGNOSIS

DIFFERENTIAL DIAGNOSIS

Respiratory Disease

- Influenza
- Equine viral arteritis
- Adenovirus
- Bacterial pneumonia
- COPD

Reproductive Tract Disease

Abortion—Equine viral arteritis, bacterial or fungal placentitis

Neurologic Disease

Equine protozoal myeloencephalitis, aberrant parasite migration, trauma, or cauda equina syndrome. Fever is a unique aspect of herpesvirus myeloencephalopathy that is uncommon in other equine neurologic diseases.

CBC/BIOCHEMISTRY

CBC and serum biochemistry are frequently normal at the onset of clinical signs.

OTHER LABORATORY TESTS

A four-fold increase in convalescent serum neutralizing antibody titer to EHV-1/4 collected over a 2-week period is diagnostic. Because most horses have been exposed to, or vaccinated against, EHV-1/4, positive titers are common, making interpretation of a single sample difficult. Natural infection usually causes a rapid and dramatic increase in titer such that serum must be collected early in the course of the disease to demonstrate an increasing titer.

IMAGING

Thoracic ultrasonography or radiology may be indicated in cases of EHV-1 respiratory disease complicated by secondary bacterial pneumonia.

DIAGNOSTIC PROCEDURES

Virus Isolation

Virus can be isolated from nasopharyngeal swabs. Because herpesviruses are sensitive to chemicals and variations in temperature and humidity, veterinarians should contact their diagnostic laboratory for transport media and specific collection and transportation procedures. One method is to use a sterile gauze swab attached to a flexible metal wire placed in the nasal passages and pharynx to obtain material for virus isolation. Swabs should be placed immediately in media and refrigerated or frozen until transported to the laboratory. Virus may also be isolated from citrated or heparinized whole blood. Viremia frequently occurs during clinical signs of respiratory tract, CNS, or reproductive tract disease. Nasopharyngeal secretions may be evaluated by immunoperoxidase staining for EHV-1/4 antigen.

Cerebrospinal Fluid Aspirate

Cerebrospinal fluid from horses with herpesvirus myeloencephalopathy typically reveals a dramatic increase in protein concentration and normal or only mildly increased nucleated cell concentration. Xanthochromia, a yellow discoloration of CSF due to breakdown of red blood cells, is common. Virus is rarely isolated from CSF.

PATHOLOGIC FINDINGS

EHV-1/4 infection of the respiratory epithelium can be inapparent or cause epithelial necrosis, thrombi formation, and petechiation. If viremia occurs and the reproductive tract is affected, lesions may be present in the endometrium. The virus may also infect the fetus, resulting in abortion, and an aborted fetus typically shows evidence of vasculitis. In the neurologic syndrome, characteristic lesions secondary to EHV-1 infection of CNS endothelium include vasculitis of the small arteries and veins of the white matter of the spinal cord resulting in hemorrhage, thrombosis, and secondary ischemic degeneration.

TREATMENT

APPROPRIATE HEALTH CARE

Rhinopneumonitis

If fevers persist more than 3 days, careful thoracic auscultation should be performed. Dull areas in the ventral lung fields may reveal consolidation associated with a secondary bacterial bronchopneumonia. Persistent diffuse crackles and wheezes may indicate chronic bronchitis. Transendoscopic or transtracheal aspirates for cytologic evaluation and culture of respiratory secretions are helpful in evaluating if a secondary bacterial infection is present.

HERPESVIRUS TYPES-1 AND 4

Horses recovering from respiratory tract disease should not be trained and should be maintained in well-ventilated areas. Caution should also be used when transporting horses for long distances following viral respiratory tract infection due to the possibility of severe pleuropneumonia associated with impaired respiratory tract immune function.

Abortion
Mares that abort due to herpesvirus infection should have a reproductive tract examination to rule out retained fetal membranes or trauma.

Neurologic Disease
Recumbent horses should be placed in a well-bedded stall, kept sternal, and repositioned frequently. Many horses remain standing or can stand with the assistance of a sling. Horses should be monitored for urinary incontinence, and if bladder atony is suspected, abdominal palpation per rectum may reveal a distended bladder. Urinary catheterization should then be performed at least twice daily by aseptic technique or an indwelling urinary catheter may be placed. If fecal incontinence is present, feces should be evacuated manually. If dysphagia is present, hydration should be monitored and fluids given intravenously or by nasogastric tube as needed.

ACTIVITY
With severe infections it may take the respiratory epithelium as long as 1 month to regain normal function. Mucociliary clearance is impaired during this time, leading to accumulation of respiratory secretions and inhaled antigens in the lower airways. Persistent airway inflammation may occur when training is resumed prematurely. Lung sounds should be normal, and spontaneous cough should have resolved prior to training. Many horses require 2–4 weeks of rest to recover from uncomplicated rhinopneumonitis.

DIET
N/A

CLIENT EDUCATION
Owners should be advised about sources of EHV-1/4 (other horses) and risk factors for infection. Vaccination of horses at risk is effective in reducing severity and frequency of EHV-1/4–associated respiratory and reproductive tract disease.

SURGICAL CONSIDERATIONS
N/A

MEDICATIONS

DRUG(S) OF CHOICE
Respiratory Disease
No specific antiviral therapy has been proven effective in the treatment of rhinopneumonitis. Nonsteroidal anti-inflammatory drugs (flunixin meglumine 1 mg/kg, IV or PO, q24h) can be given to combat inflammation and fever. Antimicrobials (trimethoprim–sulfamethoxazole 30 mg/kg, PO, q12h) should be administered if secondary bacterial infections are suspected. Immunostimulants (Eqstim) that increase cell-mediated immunity necessary for resolution of herpesvirus infections have had anecdotal success.

Abortion
No specific drug therapy.

Neurologic Diseases
Corticosteroids (dexamethasone, 0.05–0.25 mg/kg, IV or IM, q12h in decreasing doses for 7–14 days) may be necessary for severely affected horses due to the immune-mediated nature of this disease. Dimethyl sulfoxide (1 g/kg IV diluted in saline to a concentration of 10%, daily for 3 days), nonsteroidal anti-inflammatory drugs (flunixin meglumine 1 mg/kg PO or IV q12h), broad-spectrum antimicrobials (ceftiofur 5 mg/kg IV or IM q12h) are indicated in recumbent horses due to potential for pneumonia, cystitis, and decubital ulceration.

CONTRAINDICATIONS
N/A

PRECAUTIONS
Laminitis is a rare complication of corticosteroid administration in horses.

POSSIBLE INTERACTIONS
N/A

ALTERNATIVE DRUGS
Although the efficacy of acyclovir has not been evaluated, administration at 10 mg/kg, PO, 5 times daily appears to be safe.

FOLLOW-UP

PATIENT MONITORING
Most horses recover from rhinopneumonitis uneventfully. Fever lasting more than 3 days, persistent cough, abnormal lung sounds, depression, or anorexia may indicate secondary bacterial infections. Aborting mares should be isolated for at least 2 weeks but may be bred 1 month following abortion. Recumbent horses with the neurologic form should be monitored for dehydration, decubital ulcers, pneumonia, bladder atony, cystitis, fecal incontinence, and self-trauma.

PREVENTION/AVOIDANCE
Vaccination of animals at risk every 3 months is effective at reducing the severity and frequency of respiratory disease and decreases the chances of abortion. Currently available vaccines do not claim protection against neurologic disease. Providing adequate ventilation, decreasing stress, and ensuring quarantine of new horses may prevent herpesvirus disease in horses. Broodmares should be vaccinated during their fifth, seventh, and ninth months of pregnancy with a vaccine specifically designed for pregnant mares. Horses recovering from herpesvirus infections may shed the virus from nasal secretions for 2 weeks after infection and therefore should remaine quarantined. The aborted fetus and fetal membranes are major sources of virus and therefore should be placed in a sealed container and removed to decrease contamination of the environment.
Vaccination of unexposed horses in the face of the outbreak may decrease the spread of disease. Vaccination of animals with the neurologic syndrome is contraindicated; however, horses that are not yet exposed may benefit from vaccination.

HERPESVIRUS TYPES-1 AND 4

POSSIBLE COMPLICATIONS
N/A

EXPECTED COURSE AND PROGNOSIS

Respiratory Disease
Most horses recover from an uncomplicated infection in 2–4 weeks.

Reproductive Tract Disease
Mares recover readily and subsequent fertility is not impaired.

Neurologic Disease
Following acute onset of previously described signs, many horses stabilize in 24–48 hr, and if they remain standing, slow improvement usually occurs over a period of weeks to months. Horses that become recumbent and cannot rise with assistance have a poor prognosis. There is no apparent correlation between outcome and CSF characteristics.

MISCELLANEOUS

ASSOCIATED CONDITIONS
N/A

AGE-RELATED FACTORS
N/A

ZOONOTIC POTENTIAL
N/A

PREGNANCY
High doses of corticosteroids are necessary to induce parturition in late gestation mares; however, caution should be used when administering corticosteroids to pregnant mares with herpesvirus myeloencephalopathy.

SYNONYMS
Rhinopneumonitis

SEE ALSO
N/A

ABBREVIATIONS
N/A

Suggested Reading

Ostlund EN. The equine herpesviruses. Vet Clin North Am-Equine Practice 1993;9: 283-294.

Donaldson MT, Sweeney CR. Equine herpes myeloencephalopathy. Compendium on continuing education for the practicing veterinarian. 1997;19:864-871.

Author Mark T. Donaldson

Consulting Editor Corinne R. Sweeney

HERPESVIRUS-3

BASICS

OVERVIEW

Equine herpesvirus-3 (EHV-3) causes equine coital exanthema, a highly contagious venereal disease resulting in vesicular lesions on the penis and prepuce of stallions and on the vulva of mares. The disease is limited to the reproductive tract, and infection does not appear to affect fertility. Although coital exanthema is uncommon and resolves spontaneously, some stallions may not be willing to breed mares when affected, leading to economic losses. Like other herpesviruses, a short-lived immunity develops after infection. The disease occurs sporadically worldwide.

SIGNALMENT

The primary route of infection is by genital contact; thus, horses most frequently affected are of breeding age.

SIGNS

Occasionally, stallions are more severely affected than mares and become dull, anorectic, and febrile. Vesicles appear within 2–5 days on the penis and later on the prepuce. Vesicles become pustules, which then slough, leaving ulcerated areas up to 1.5 cm in diameter. Ulcers heal within a few weeks, leaving depigmented areas. Mares develop multifocal areas of sharply demarcated vulval erosions that subsequently develop scabs that heal in a similar manner. Aged broodmares may develop recurrent coital exanthema during late gestation or in the early post-parturient period, but a relationship with viral recrudescence has not been established. Lesions rarely occur on the oral and nasal mucosa.

CAUSES AND RISK FACTORS

Coital exanthema is caused by EHV-3. Horses of breeding age are at risk due to viral transmission by genital contact. Iatrogenic transmission by contaminated instruments is also possible.

DIAGNOSIS

DIFFERENTIAL DIAGNOSIS

Coital exanthema lesions are characteristic; however, inflammation of the penis or vulva may also occur due to trauma, bacterial infection, or contact hypersensitivities.

CBC/BIOCHEMISTRY/URINALYSIS

N/A

OTHER LABORATORY TESTS

Diagnosis can be made based on clinical signs. Serum neutralizing antibodies peak 2–3 weeks after infection and may remain detectable for up to 1 year later; however, complement fixing antibodies are not present beyond 60 days after infection.

IMAGING

N/A

DIAGNOSTIC PROCEDURES

Virus can be isolated from erosions and characteristic herpesvirus inclusions can be seen during histologic evaluation of biopsies.

HERPESVIRUS-3

TREATMENT

Specific treatment is not necessary, as lesions are self-limiting. Application of topical antibiotic ointments to affected areas may reduce chances of secondary bacterial infections.

MEDICATIONS

No specific anti-viral therapy has been evaluated for the treatment of EHV-3 infections. The use of topical antibiotic ointments may decrease secondary bacterial infections.

FOLLOW-UP

Sexual rest of infected stallions for at least 3 weeks after infection decreases spread of the EHV-3. If the breed registry permits, semen may be collected directly from the urethra through an open-ended artificial vagina and artificially inseminated, so as to reduce the chance of viral transmission to the mare. Silent recrudescence of the virus in stallions is likely, and may contribute to propagation of the disease. Iatrogenic transmission is possible; therefore, instruments that are disposable or easily cleaned should be used when working with affected horses.

MISCELLANEOUS

ABBREVIATION

- EHV-3 = Equine herpesvirus-3

Suggested Reading

Blanchard TL, Kenney RM, Timoney PJ. Venereal disease. Vet Clin North Am: Equine Practice 1992;8:191-203.

Author Mark T. Donaldson

Consulting Editor Corinne R. Sweeney

HIGH-RISK PREGNANCY, NEONATES

BASICS

DEFINITION

• Any combination of circumstances affecting the pregnant mare or fetus that may increase the likelihood of an unfavorable outcome for the pregnancy.
• The condition may lead directly or indirectly to dystocia, fetal loss, maternal death, or significant perinatal insults to the fetus, resulting in a compromised foal.

PATHOPHYSIOLOGY

• Mares with historical or current problems can be classified as being at high risk of periparturient problems.
• Except when evaluating problems that may predispose to dystocia, the most useful approach is considering the threat to the fetus rather than the individual problem affecting the mare.
• The fetal environment is under the mare's complete control. If the condition affecting the mare does not threaten this environment, the pregnancy is not at risk; however, if the fetal environment is threatened, fetal well-being is threatened.
• The fetus may be able to compensate for some changes in the maternally derived environment, but this ability is limited.
• Important threats to the fetal environment—lack of perfusion of the placenta, decreased oxygen delivery to the placenta, decreased delivery of sufficient substrates to the placenta, placentitis, failure to maintain fetal/maternal co-ordination of readiness for parturition, and presence of a twin.
• Once the threat has been identified, specific interventions may be instituted.

SYSTEM AFFECTED

• Reproductive—placentitis, placental insufficiency, and twinning put a pregnancy at risk.
• Underlying problems in the dam (e.g., endotoxemia from diarrhea, septicemia from pleuropneumonia) often involve other body systems.

SIGNALMENT

Any pregnant mare

SIGNS

General Comments

• Risk factors may be identified.
• With dystocia, usually no premonitory signs
• Fetal distress often is subclinical.

Historical Findings

• Inciting incident adversely affecting the mare—colic; diarrhea
• Precocious udder development
• Vaginal discharge
• Problems with previous pregnancies

Physical Examination Findings

• Early udder development, udder secretions, or waxing
• Vaginal discharge
• Perineal, tail base, and pelvic relaxation
• Unexpectedly large abdominal size for stage of gestation
• Stage 1 labor

CAUSES

Historical Maternal Problems

• Recurrent, premature placental separation
• Recurrent dystocia
• Recurrent, premature termination of pregnancy—abortion or premature birth
• Previous prolonged pregnancies
• Previous uterine artery hemorrhage
• History of producing foals with neonatal isoerythrolysis

Current Maternal Problems

• Placentitis
• Twins
• Premature placental separation in progress
• Over term
• Fescue toxicity
• Muscular skeletal problems—fractured pelvis, severe lameness, or laminitis
• Endotoxemia—colic, enteritis, or other infections
• Recent surgery resulting in hypotension/hypoxemia
• Abdominal surgical incisions
• Hernias—body wall; diaphragmatic
• Neurologic disease
• Hydrops allantois
• Hydrops amnion
• Pituitary hyperplasia
• Granulomatous diseases
• Lymphosarcoma
• Melanomas
• Primary hypoparathyroidism
• Recent hemorrhage—uterine artery or other source
• Starvation (for any reason)
• Fetal malposition

RISK FACTORS

• Similar problem during previous gestation
• Compromised perfusion
• Anemia
• Complete anorexia/starvation/withholding of food
• Poor perineal conformation, leading to ascending placentitis
• Vaginal examination
• Grazing fescue pasture during late gestation
• Pergolide therapy

DIAGNOSIS

DIFFERENTIAL DIAGNOSIS

• Incorrect breeding dates
• Normal, short gestation (as early as 310 days)
• Normal, long gestation (may be longer than 390 days)

CBC/BIOCHEMISTRY/URINALYSIS

N/A

OTHER LABORATORY TESTS

N/A

IMAGING

• Transabdominal and transrectal fetal ultrasonography, with special attention to detectable placental diseases, presence of twins, excessive or deficient fetal fluids, and fetal position
• Transabdominal ultrasonography-derived biophysical profile has been described but not widely used.

DIAGNOSTIC PROCEDURES

Fetal heart rate measurements through ECG—persistent fetal tachycardia, persistent fetal bradycardia, and lack of beat-to-beat variation may imply fetal distress.

TREATMENT

ALL HIGH-RISK MARES

• Monitor closely for parturition, and be prepared to intervene and resuscitate the neonate.
• With precocious udder development, monitoring of milk electrolytes can be misleading in predicting parturition in these mares.

MARES WITH COMPROMISED PERFUSION

• IV fluid therapy
• Consider inotropes.
• If pressors are used, based on experience in other species, ephedrine (0.7 mg/kg PO) is most likely to increase uterine blood flow.

ANEMIC MARES

Blood transfusion with compatible blood increases the risk of producing foals with neonatal isoerythrolysis in subsequent pregnancies.

HIGH-RISK PREGNANCY, NEONATES

COMPROMISED FETAL OXYGEN DELIVERY

- Maternal pulmonary disease—treat aggressively
- Maternal anemia or poor perfusion—treat as indicated above
- Placental transport deficiencies—place mare on intranasal oxygen (10–15 L/min) to increase maternal PaO_2 to 130-150 torr, which increases oxygen delivery to the fetus aided by the well-developed, placental countercurrent circulatory pattern.

PLACENTITIS

Therapeutic triad of an antimicrobial, NSAID, and progesterone

MARES WITH ABDOMINAL WALL HERNIAS

Support body wall with external bandaging.

INDUCTION

- Avoid, unless absolutely clear the fetus would be better off if treated outside the uterine environment.
- Perform only with colostrum in the mammary gland, a dilated cervix, pelvic relaxation, and the foal near term (based on other gestational lengths for that mare).

CESAREAN SECTION

- Avoid, unless absolutely clear the fetus would be better off if treated outside the uterine environment and vaginal delivery is not possible; a physical or physiologic pelvic obstruction contraindicates vaginal extraction; to relieve a dystocia; or to extract a dead fetus when vaginal extraction is impossible or contraindicated.
- Most likely to be successful when delayed until after the onset of stage 1 labor, performed within 30 minutes of onset of stage 2 labor, performed by a well–co-ordinated team so that time between induction of anesthesia and delivery is minimized, and a separate team is available and prepared to resuscitate the foal.

MEDICATIONS

DRUGS OF CHOICE

Antimicrobials

- Trimethoprim-potentiated sulfa drugs (15–30 mg/kg PO BID) cross the placental membranes.
- If the pathogen is identified, therapy is directed by sensitivity.
- Penicillin and gentamicin do not pass through the normal equine placenta, whereas trimethoprim-potentiated sulfa drugs do.

NSAIDs

- Flunixin meglumine (0.5–1 mg/kg IV, IM, or PO BID) appears to be safe and efficacious.
- Phenylbutazone (4.4–8.8 mg/kg PO divided BID) is safe.
- Use new NSAIDs with caution, because both uterine and fetal placenta contain high levels of numerous prostaglandins, which are important during normal pregnancy. New NSAIDs also may have very different local effects.

Progesterone

Altrenogest (0.044 mg/kg per day PO)

Corticosteroids

Dexamethasone (0.08–0.1 mg/kg SID for 4 days) when early delivery is necessary to help increase maturity of body systems.

CONTRAINDICATIONS

- Pergolide
- Corticosteroids, but only near term and when given in very large doses (e.g., 0.15–0.2 mg/kg of dexamethasone for >3 days).

PRECAUTIONS

Corticosteriods—because the exact delivery date often is not known due to normal variations in gestation length, take precautions during the last 30 days of gestation.

POSSIBLE INTERACTIONS

N/A

ALTERNATIVE DRUGS

N/A

FOLLOW-UP

PATIENT MONITORING

Until parturition, examine the mare every 0.5–1 hour for signs of labor.

POSSIBLE COMPLICATIONS

- Dystocia
- Ruptured uterus
- Uterine bleeding
- Fetal death
- Fetal compromise
- Others, depending on the underlying problem

MISCELLANEOUS

ASSOCIATED CONDITIONS

N/A

AGE-RELATED CONDITIONS

- Many underlying conditions are age-related.
- Mares that have been accidentally bred at a young age, or elderly mares with poor condition or perineal conformation, may be at a higher risk.

ZOONOTIC POTENTIAL

N/A

PREGNANCY

N/A

SYNONYMS

N/A

SEE ALSO

N/A

Suggested Reading

Vaala WE, Sertich PL. Management strategies for mares at risk for periparturient complications. Vet Clin North Am Equine Pract 1994;10:237–265.

Author Jonathan E. Palmer
Consulting Editor Mary Rose Paradis

HIGH-RISK PREGNANCY

BASICS

DEFINITION

A pregnancy that by virtue of maternal, fetal, and/or placental abnormalities in structure or function is prone to premature termination, delivery of a compromised foal, and/or prolongation.

PATHOPHYSIOLOGY

Maternal systemic disease, fetal abnormalities, and/or placental infection, insufficiency, separation, or other abnormalities resulting in maternal and/or fetal death, premature initiation of the labor, or prolonged gestation

SYSTEMS AFFECTED

- Reproductive
- Other organ systems, depending on the nature of the maternal, systemic disease and occurrence of complications—dystocia; RFM

GENETICS

N/A

INCIDENCE/PREVALENCE

Sporadic

SIGNALMENT

- May be nonspecific.
- Thoroughbred, Standardbreds, or draft mares and related breeds (for twinning)
- Mares of >15 years
- American Miniature Horse mares

SIGNS

Historical Findings

- Maternal disease during gestation—colic, hyperlipemia, prepubic tendon rupture, uterine torsion, and so on
- Previous examination or problem pregnancy indicating placentitis or fetal compromise
- Mucoid, hemorrhagic, serosanguinous, or purulent vulvar discharge
- Premature udder development and dripping of milk
- History of abortion, high-risk pregnancy, or dystocia
- History of delivering a small, dysmature, septicemic, and/or congenitally malformed foal
- Pre-existing maternal disease at conception—laminitis, equine Cushing's-like disease, endometrial inflammation and/or fibrosis, and so on

Physical Examination Findings

- Anorexia, fever, or other signs of concurrent, systemic disease
- Abdominal discomfort
- Mucoid, hemorrhagic, serosanguinous, or purulent vulvar discharge
- Premature udder development and dripping of milk
- Evidence of fetal distress, delayed development, or other abnormalities by transrectal or transabdominal ultrasonography
- Placentitis, placental separation, or hydrops of fetal membranes by transrectal or transabdominal ultrasonography
- Excessive swelling along the ventral midline and evidence of ventral body wall weakening by palpation or transabdominal ultrasonography; excessive abdominal distention

CAUSES AND RISK FACTORS

- Pre-existing maternal disease—Cushing's-like disease; chronic, moderate to severe endometrial inflammation and/or fibrosis; laminitis
- Gestational maternal conditions—malnutrition, colic, endotoxemia, hyperlipemia, prepubic tendon rupture, uterine torsion, ovarian granulosa cell tumor, laminitis, musculoskeletal disease, equine fescue toxicosis, and xenobiotics
- Fetal conditions—twins, fetal abnormalities (e.g., hydrocephalus), delayed fetal development (e.g., small for gestational age, growth retardation), and fetal trauma
- Placental conditions—placentitis, placental insufficiency, placental separation, and hydrops of fetal membranes

DIAGNOSIS

DIFFERENTIAL DIAGNOSIS

- Normal, uncomplicated pregnancy—see sections for specific maternal, fetal, and placental abnormalities.
- Other organ system involvement depends on the presence of placentitis, stage of gestation, and the presence of maternal disease, infection, and/or toxemia.
- Hyperlipemia is of special concern in American Miniature Horses, ponies, and donkeys.

CBC/BIOCHEMISTRY/URINALYSIS

CBC and serum biochemistry profile may be indicated based on physical examination findings to determine the presence of an inflammatory, stress, or left shift (e.g., degenerative, regenerative) leukocyte response or other organ system involvement.

OTHER LABORATORY TESTS

Maternal Progesterone

- May be indicated with a history of abortion or high-risk pregnancy, an old mare with endometrial inflammation and fibrosis in a biopsy specimen before breeding, and cases of suspected maternal, fetal, or placental disease.
- ELISA or RIA for progesterone before 80 days of gestation—acceptable levels vary from >1 to >4 ng/mL, depending on the reference.
- After 100 days of gestation, RIA for progesterone detects both progesterone (may be very low after 150 days) and cross-reacting 5α-pregnanes of uterofetoplacental origin (maternal levels decrease with equine fescue toxicosis).
- Acceptable levels of 5α-pregnanes vary by stage of gestation and laboratory.

Maternal Estrogens

- Reflection fetal estrogen production and viability, especially conjugated estrogens—estrone sulfate
- Normal values vary by laboratory.

Maternal Relaxin

- Decreases with placental abnormalities.
- Assay not yet commercially available

Maternal T_3/T_4

- Anecdotal reports of lower levels in mares with history of conception failure, EED, or abortion.
- Significance of low T_4 levels not clear at present

Maternal Xenobiotics

- Assays may be indicated in cases of specific intoxications.
- Samples to submit—whole blood, plasma, or urine

Allantoic/Amniotic Fluid

- Potential method to assess fetal karyotype and pulmonary maturity, to measure fetal proteins, and to detect bacteria, meconium, or inflammatory cells
- Equine sampling technique is a higher-risk procedure than in humans.
- Utility has not yet been established.

Feed

Analysis may be indicated for specific xenobiotics (e.g., ergopeptine alkaloids, phytoestrogens, heavy metals) or endophyte (*Neotyphodium coenophialum*).

IMAGING

General Comments

Transrectal and transabdominal ultrasonography are used to confirm pregnancy, diagnose twins, evaluate fetal viability and development, assess placental health, and diagnose other gestational abnormalities—hydrops of fetal membranes.

Confirm Pregnancy and Diagnose Twins

- Performed whenever serious disease occurs or when considering surgical intervention in a mare bred within the last 11 months.
- Twin pregnancy is confirmed by the presence of two fetuses (easier at <90 days of gestation by transrectal ultrasonography) or is ruled out by presence of a nonpregnant uterine horn (by transabdominal ultrasonography during late gestation).

Fetal Viability and Development

- Best determined by transabdominal ultrasonography during late gestation.
- View the fetus in both active and resting states, and record both fetal presentation and position.

Fetal Activity and Normal Muscle Tone

- Before 330 days of gestation—normal FHR is $\leq$100 bpm after activity and $\geq$60 bpm resting.
- After 330 days of gestation—normal FHR is $\geq$50 bpm resting and $\leq$40 bpm between resting and active rates.

Normal Fetal Heart Rhythm

Assessed by echocardiography.

Normal Fetal Breathing Movements

Appropriately Sized Fetus for Gestational Stage

- Fetal aortic diameter of $\cong$2.1 cm at 300 days and 2.7 cm at 330 days of gestation
- Record length and width of fetal eye.

Normal Quantities of Fetal Fluids

- Normal range for maximal allantoic fluid depth is 4.7–22.1 cm.
- Normal range for maximal amniotic fluid depth is 0.8–14.9 cm.

Placental Health

- Normal uteroplacental thickness as assessed by transabdominal ultrasonography is 7–20 mm.
- Normal uteroplacental thickness as assessed by transrectal ultrasonography—271–300 days of gestation, $\leq$8 mm; 300–330 days, $\leq$10 mm; >330 days, $\leq$12 mm
- Look for evidence of absent or very small areas of uteroplacental discontinuity.

DIAGNOSTIC PROCEDURES

- Pre-breeding reproductive evaluation is indicated in individuals predisposed to problem pregnancies—barren, old mares; mares with history of abortion
- Fetal ECG—to detect twins; to assess fetal viability and distress; now largely replaced by transabdominal ultrasonography.

PATHOLOGIC FINDINGS

Endometrial biopsy—moderate to severe, chronic endometritis and/or fibrosis

TREATMENT

GENERAL COMMENTS

- With a history of abortion or evidence of moderate to severe endometritis and/or fibrosis, evaluate and treat the mare before breeding.
- Consider progestin supplementation during gestation, especially *if* clinical diagnosis was for luteal insufficiency (anecdotal), premature CL regression was thought to be implicated in early pregnancy loss, or the mare has a history of abortion.
- Progestin supplementation may be indicated in placentitis and instances of maternal endotoxemia.
- ET may be the best way to continue breeding mares considered to be at high risk during pregnancy.
- Fescue toxicosis and prolonged gestation can be treated with D_2-dopamine-receptor antagonists.
- Induction of parturition and/or cesarean section may be indicated in specific instances of maternal disease, fetal stress/distress/viability, and/or placental separation.
- Closely supervise parturition in high-risk pregnancies; the neonatal foal may need treatment as well.

APPROPRIATE HEALTH CARE

- When detected early, high-risk pregnancies may be treated on an ambulatory basis.
- Closely supervise foaling in all cases; foaling may be done best at a facility equipped to handle high-risk pregnancies.

NURSING CARE

Depending on nature of the maternal disease, presence of fetal distress, and necessity of surgical intervention, intensive nursing care may be required for the mare and/or neonatal foal.

ACTIVITY

- In most cases, exercise will be somewhat limited and supervised.
- Cases of prepubic tendon rupture, laminitis, and hydrops of fetal membranes may necessitate complete restriction of exercise.

DIET

- Feed the mare an adequate, late-gestational diet with proper levels of energy, protein, vitamins, and minerals, unless contraindicated by concurrent maternal disease.

CLIENT EDUCATION

- Owners of pregnant mares with maternal disease should be made aware of the added risks and poorer prognosis for reaching term and that the neonate may need extended intensive care and a nurse mare.

SURGICAL CONSIDERATIONS

Cesarean section may be indicated if vaginal delivery is not possible or in cases of dystocia that cannot be corrected by manipulation alone.

HIGH-RISK PREGNANCY

MEDICATIONS

DRUGS OF CHOICE

• See specific conditions for drug recommendations.
• For endotoxic/Gram-negative septicemic mares <80 days of gestation—altrenogest (0.088 mg/kg PO SID initially, 0.044 mg/kg SID thereafter, continue until at least day 100, then taper administration dose over 14 days at the end of the treatment period)
• For endometritis/previous-abortion mares (i.e., no active infectious component) and/or mares with fibrosis—altrenogest (0.044–0.088 mg/kg PO SID commencing 2–3 days after ovulation or on diagnosis of pregnancy, continue to at least day 100 of gestation, then taper dose over 14 days at the end of the treatment period)
• Altrenogest may be started later, continued longer, or used for only short periods depending on serum progesterone levels during the first 80 days of gestation (>1 to >4 ng/mL), clinical circumstances, risk factors, and clinician preference.
• If used near term, altrenogest frequently is discontinued 7–14 days before the expected foaling date, depending on the case, unless otherwise indicated by assessment of fetal maturity/viability or by questions regarding accuracy of the gestational age.
• Domperidone (1.1 mg/kg PO SID), beginning when fescue toxicosis is diagnosed or in cases of prolonged gestation. Continue until parturition with normal mammary development and lactation occurs

CONTRAINDICATIONS

Altrenogest:
• Only use to prevent abortion when a fetus has been demonstrated.
• Not recommended to prevent spontaneous, infectious abortion other than those caused by placentitis and endotoxemia

PRECAUTIONS

• Initially, monitor fetal viability at least weekly.
• Retention of mummified fetuses has been described with use of supplemental progestins.
• Altrenogest is absorbed through the skin, so those handling it should wear gloves and wash their hands.
• Successful reports of supplemental progestins for pregnancy maintenance are mainly anecdotal.
• Depending on the cause of the risk to pregnancy, progestin supplementation may be unsuccessful.

ALTERNATIVE DRUGS

• Injectable progesterone (150–500 mg IM SID, oil base) can be administered instead of altrenogest.
• Flunixin meglumine (0.25 mg/kg IM or IV SID–QID)—may be prophylactic for endotoxemia if endotoxin release is anticipated; higher doses may be used for analgesia and anti-inflammatory effect; also may help to decrease premature uterine contractions.
• Thyroxine supplementation has had some anecdotal success in treating subfertile mares, but its use remains controversial and is considered deleterious by some clinicians.

FOLLOW-UP

PATIENT MONITORING

• Anticipate frequent monitoring until completion of pregnancy.
• Vaginal speculum examination and uterine cytology and culture may be indicated 7–10 days postpartum.
• Postpartum endometrial biopsy may help in making decisions regarding the problem mare's reproductive future and making appropriate treatment decisions.

PREVENTION/AVOIDANCE

• Early recognition of high-risk pregnancies
• Correction of poor perineal conformation, especially in mares with a history of placentitis
• Complete breeding records—double ovulations
• Early diagnosis of twins
• Selective embryonic or fetal reduction
• Resolution of endometritis before breeding
• Removing mares from fescue pasture a minimum of 30 days prepartum
• Removing problem mares from the brood population
• ET
• Prudent use of medications in pregnant mares
• Avoid exposure to known toxicants.

POSSIBLE COMPLICATIONS

• Abortion, dystocia, RFM, metritis, laminitis, septicemia, endometritis, reproductive tract trauma, and impaired fertility affect the well-being and reproductive value of the mare.
• Neonatal foals from high-risk pregnancies are more likely to be dysmature, septicemic, and subject to angular limb deformities than foals from normal pregnancies.

EXPECTED COURSE AND PROGNOSIS

• Resolution or progression of maternal systemic, fetal, or placental disease determines outcome of the pregnancy.
• Generally a guarded prognosis for maintenance of high-risk pregnancies
• Guarded to poor prognosis for maintenance of pregnancy in mares with a history of abortion or pre-existing, moderate to severe chronic endometritis and/or fibrosis

HIGH-RISK PREGNANCY

MISCELLANEOUS

ASSOCIATED CONDITIONS
- Dystocia
- Endometritis
- Fetal distress/stress/viability
- Hydrops allantois and amnion
- Metritis, postpartum
- Prepubic tendon rupture
- Placental insufficiency
- Placentitis
- Premature placental separation
- RFM

AGE-RELATED FACTORS
- Chronic endometritis and endometrial fibrosis in old mares
- Old mares generally have more chronic health problems.

ZOONOTIC POTENTIAL
N/A

PREGNANCY
By definition, the condition is associated with pregnancy.

SYNONYMS
N/A

SEE ALSO
- Dystocia
- Endometrial biopsy
- Endometritis
- ET
- Fetal stress/distress/viability
- Hydrops amnion/allantois
- Metritis
- Placental insufficiency
- Placentitis
- Premature placental separation
- Prepubic tendon rupture
- RFM
- Twin pregnancy

ABBREVIATIONS
- CL = corpus luteum
- EED = early embryonic death
- ELISA = enzyme linked immunoadsorbent assay
- ET = embryo transfer
- FHR = fetal heart rate
- RFM = retained fetal membranes/placenta
- RIA = radioimmunoassay
- T_3 = triiodothyronine
- T_4 = thyroxine

Suggested Reading

Brendemuehl JP. Reproductive aspects of fescue toxicosis. In: Robinson NE, ed. Current therapy in equine medicine 4. Philadelphia: WB Saunders, 1997:571–573.

McGladdery A. Fetal ultrasonography. In: Rantanen NW, McKinnon AO, eds. Equine diagnostic ultrasonography. Baltimore: Williams & Wilkins, 1998:171–180.

Santschi EM. Prepartum conditions. In: Robinson NE, ed. Current therapy in equine medicine 4. Philadelphia: WB Saunders, 1997:541–546.

Troedsson MHT. Transrectal ultrasonography of the placenta in normal mares and mares with pending abortion: a field study. Proc Am Assoc Equine Pract 1997:256–258.

Vaala WE, Sertich PL. Management strategies for mares at risk for periparturient complications. Vet Clin North Am Equine Pract 1994;10:237–265.

Author Tim J. Evans

Consulting Editor Carla L. Carleton

HYDROCEPHALUS

BASICS

DEFINITION
Hydrocephalus is associated with increased CSF volume within the ventricular system (i.e., internal hydrocephalus) or subarachnoid space (i.e., external hydrocephalus) of the cranium.

PATHOPHYSIOLOGY
Internal (within the ventricular system), external (within the subarachnoid space), hypertensive, or normotensive

Normotensive Hydrocephalus
- Usually incidental to hypoplasia with passive filling of space unoccupied by brain tissue.
- The result, not the cause, of CNS disease
- Can be present after cerebral destruction subsequent to viral encephalitis, head trauma, and neonatal maladjustment syndrome.

Hypertensive Hydrocephalus
- Often contributes to signs of disease by damaging surrounding tissues.
- Most often associated with obstruction of the mesencephalic aqueduct and lateral apertures between the choroid plexus (production) in the third and lateral ventricles and the arachnoid villi (absorption) in the subarachnoid space.
- Associated with aplasia to hypoplasia of a conducting or absorbing portion of the CSF circulation. These abnormalities can be congenital or associated with traumatic or infectious inflammation or space-occupying lesions—abscess; neoplasia

SYSTEM AFFECTED
CNS

SIGNALMENT
- Acquired disease is evident at any stage.
- Congenital disease often manifests slowly.

SIGNS

Historical Findings
History of CNS disease and/or trauma sometimes can be seen with acquired disease.

Physical Examination Findings
- CNS disease often is referable to the cerebral cortical white matter, with evident compression.
- Congenital hypertensive disease may be associated with an enlarged calvarium, allowed by open cranial sutures in neonates.
- Lack of affinity for the dam and reduced or absent desire or ability to suckle are common.
- Lack of menace response, blindness, and depression may occur.
- Animals that can survive often are mentally deficient (i.e., dummies) and unthrifty.

CAUSES
See *Pathophysiology*.

RISK FACTORS
- Acquired —similar to those of the primary CNS disease processes that may be associated
- Congenital—possible genetic relationship

DIAGNOSIS

DIFFERENTIAL DIAGNOSIS
Any inflammatory or metabolic disease that can induce stupor or seizures

CBC/BIOCHEMISTRY/URINALYSIS
No pathognomonic abnormalities

OTHER LABORATORY TESTS
N/A

IMAGING
Classically, plain-film, lateral radiographs show a homogeneous, ground-glass appearance of the cranial cavity.

DIAGNOSTIC PROCEDURES
Lateral ventricular centesis may be performed.

PATHOLOGIC FINDINGS
See *Pathophysiology*.

HYDROCEPHALUS

TREATMENT

Consider euthanasia.

MEDICATIONS

DRUGS OF CHOICE

N/A

CONTRAINDICATIONS

N/A

PRECAUTIONS

N/A

POSSIBLE INTERACTIONS

N/A

ALTERNATIVE DRUGS

N/A

FOLLOW-UP

PATIENT MONITORING

N/A

POSSIBLE COMPLICATIONS

N/A

MISCELLANEOUS

ASSOCIATED CONDITIONS

Any inflammatory, traumatic, or space-occupying CNS disorder

AGE-RELATED FACTORS

- Acquired—can occur at any age.
- Congenital—often manifests at birth.

ZOONOTIC POTENTIAL

N/A

PRENANCY

N/A

SYNONYMS

N/A

SEE ALSO

Viral, bacterial, and traumatic encephalitis

ABBREVIATIONS

CSF = cerebrospinal fluid

Suggested Reading

Bester RC, et al. Hydrocephalus in an 18-month-old colt. J Am Vet Med Assoc 1976;168:1041–1042.

Foreman JH, et al. Congenital internal hydrocephalus in a Quarter Horse foal. J Equine Vet Sci 1983;3:154–164.

Ojala M, Huikku I. Inheritance of hydrocephalus in horses, Equine Vet J 1992;24:140–143.

Author Joseph J. Bertone

Consulting Editor Joseph J. Bertone

HYDROPS ALLANTOIS/AMNION

BASICS

DEFINITION

• Excessive fluid accumulation in either the allantoic or amniotic cavities of the pregnant uterus.
• Hydrops allantois relates primarily to placental dysfunction/insufficiency.
• The fetus of a hydrops amnion contributes directly to fluid accumulation by virtue of congenital anomalies (i.e. segmental aplasias) that preclude swallowing and processing/recycling of amniotic fluid.
• The fetus may be delivered alive but is nonviable.

PATHOPHYSIOLOGY

• Dysfunction of either the placenta or fetus results in accumulation of excessive allantoic or amniotic fluid, to the point that the dam's health is undermined by excessive weight of the modest to rapid rate of fluid accumulation, by dehydration, and compromised GI function and respiration.
• Clinical management for both conditions is the same—induction of parturition to save the dam's life and to prevent rupture of the ventral abdominal wall and/or the uterus.

SYSTEM AFFECTED

Reproductive—dam and fetus

GENETICS

Possible hereditary role in development of hydropic conditions

INCIDENCE/PREVALENCE

Rare

SIGNALMENT

• No breed or age predisposition, but more cases have been reported in draft mares.
• Abnormal accumulation of fluid ($\leq$100 L) in the allantoic cavity; abdominal size is abnormally large for stage of gestation.
• Commonly occurs from 6–10 months of gestation.
• Frequently has a rapid onset—over a few days to a few weeks.
• Most mares have a tremendous amount of ventral abdominal edema, and abdominal/uterine rupture can result from excessive weight of the fetal fluid.

SIGNS

• Modest to rapid accumulation of fluid within the uterus—allantoic or amniotic.
• Rapid increase in abdominal size/shape.
• Abdominal pain (moderate to severe), severe ventral edema, elevated pulse, labored respiration from pressure on the diaphragm, difficulty walking, and recumbency as the condition progresses.
• Transrectal palpation reveals abnormal fluid accumulation, with the fetus either difficult or impossible to detect.

CAUSES

N/A

RISK FACTORS

Draft mares

DIAGNOSIS

DIFFERENTIAL DIAGNOSIS

• Twin pregnancy—mid-to late gestation
• Prepubic tendon rupture
• Ventral abdominal wall herniation or rupture
• Possibly uterine torsion

CBC/BIOCHEMISTRY/URINALYSIS

• Possible increase or decrease in PCV secondary to hypovolemia or dehydration, respectively
• Possible increase in BUN and creatinine secondary to dehydration

OTHER LABORATORY TESTS

N/A

IMAGING

Ultrasonography:
• Fluid compartments are grossly enlarged—allantoic or amniotic
• Hydramnios fetus may scan as a grossly widened diameter because of ascites.

DIAGNOSTIC PROCEDURES

• Ultrasonography and transrectal palpation
• Abdominocentesis, ultrasonographically guided, may be helpful in detecting abnormal free fluid in the abdomen and in cases of uterine rupture.

PATHOLOGIC FINDINGS

• Placental insufficiency secondary to placentitis
• Hydrops amnion—swallowing defects (i.e., segmental aplasias) preventing the swallowing and processing of amniotic fluid, which leads to its accumulation in excessive amounts
• Fetal defects (e.g., growth retardation, hydrocephalus) as well as brachygnathia
• Torsion of the umbilical and amnion

TREATMENT

APPROPRIATE HEALTH CARE

• Manual dilation of the cervix, completed gradually over 10–20 minutes.
• Measured drainage of allantoic/amniotic fluid via aseptic insertion of a sterile drain tube through the cervix and fetal membranes.
• Slow removal of fluid to prevent possible shock in the mare because of sudden loss of pressure on the abdominal vessels (i.e., vascular pooling) as the uterus is drained.
• For the dam—IV fluids (i.e., balanced electrolyte solutions) and corticosteroids (e.g., Solu-Delta Cortef, 0.5–1 g IV; dexamethasone, 0.5–1 mg/kg or 20–40 mg per 500-kg mare) to decrease likelihood of hypovolemic shock.
• Once sufficient fluid has been removed, rupture the CA membrane, and remove the fetus by forced extraction. (NOTE: in some cases, the CA membrane may be thickened and difficult to rupture, in which case it should be pulled into the anterior vagina to facilitate easier opening of the membrane and fetal extraction.)

NURSING CARE

Close monitoring of the mare for signs of shock and/or infection after removal of fluids and the fetus.

ACTIVITY

Limited by inability of dam to move.

DIET

N/A

HYDROPS ALLANTOIS/AMNION

CLIENT EDUCATION
Mares that appear excessively large for stage of gestation should be evaluated, particularly if signs of systemic disease or disability develop.

SURGICAL CONSIDERATIONS
- Induction of parturition.
- Cesarean section, but fetal survival is unlikely.

MEDICATIONS

DRUGS OF CHOICE
- Because most mares with hydrops spontaneously abort, direct treatment at terminating the pregnancy.
- Oxytocin usually is not effective, because most affected mares have uterine inertia (i.e., atony) because of uterine musculature stretching.

CONTRAINDICATIONS
N/A

PRECAUTIONS
N/A

POSSIBLE INTERACTIONS
N/A

ALTERNATIVE DRUGS
N/A

FOLLOW-UP

PATIENT MONITORING
- Once a diagnosis is made, termination of pregnancy is the appropriate follow-up.
- Monitor for respiratory distress and stability of the dam's vital signs.

PREVENTION/AVOIDANCE
Hydrops amnion—breed to a different sire once the mare recovers from cesarean section.

POSSIBLE COMPLICATIONS
- Loss of pregnancy
- Prepubic tendon rupture
- Ventral belly wall rupture
- Maternal death

EXPECTED COURSE AND PROGNOSIS
- Prognosis for fetal survival is poor.
- Prognosis for dam survival is guarded if parturition is induced before more serious damage occurs.
- Prognosis for future reproduction is guarded for mare with hydrops allantois or hydrops amnion mare, with the recommendation that the mare be bred to a different stallion.

MISCELLANEOUS

ASSOCIATED CONDITIONS
- Placentitis
- Adventitious placentation has been reported in cattle.

AGE-RELATED FACTORS
Older, multiparous mares, but has been reported in all ages.

ZOONOTIC POTENTIAL
N/A

PREGNANCY
By definition, a pregnancy-related condition

SYNONYMS
N/A

SEE ALSO
- Dystocia
- Placentitis

ABBREVIATIONS
- CA = chorioallantoic
- GI = gastrointestinal

Suggested Reading

Honnas CH, et al. Hydramnios causing uterine rupture in a mare. J Am Vet Med Assoc 1988;193:332–336.

Immegart HM, Threlfall WR. In: Reed SM, Bayly WM, eds. Equine internal medicine. Philadelphia: WB Saunders, 1998:763–766.

Löfstedt RM. Miscellaneous diseases of pregnancy and parturition. In: McKinnon AO, Voss JL, eds. Equine reproduction. Philadelphia: Lea & Febiger, 1993:596–597.

Reimer JM. Use of transcutaneous ultrasonography in complicated latter-middle to late gestation pregnancies in the mare: 122 cases. Proc Am Assoc Equine Pract 1997:259–261.

Vandeplassche M, et al. Dropsy of the fetal sacs in the mare: induced and spontaneous abortion. Vet Rec 1976;99:67–69.

Author E. Ricardo Bridges

Consulting Editor Carla L. Carleton

HYPERFIBRINOGENEMIA

BASICS

OVERVIEW

• Increased plasma fibrinogen concentration above the normal reference range (i.e., >400 mg/dL)
• Most commonly results from increased hepatic synthesis of fibrinogen in response to acute inflammatory conditions in virtually any organ system.
• Fibrinogen normally functions in blood clotting and inflammation through its conversion to fibrin, giving support to proliferating fibroblasts during tissue healing.
• Tissue products of inflammation activate the mononuclear phagocyte system, resulting in synthesis of cytokines (e.g., interleukins 1 and 6) and tumor necrosis factor, which induce hepatic synthesis of acute-phase proteins, including fibrinogen.
• Plasma fibrinogen concentration peaks at 5–7 days and can exceed 1000 mg/dL; normal half-life for plasma fibrinogen is ≅3 days.
• Plasma fibrinogen concentrations may be decreased with severe hepatic disease because of decreased production or with disseminated intravascular coagulation because of increased utilization.

SIGNALMENT

N/A

SIGNS

• No clinical signs specifically referable to hyperfibrinogenemia; usually relate to the underlying disease process (e.g., dyspnea with respiratory tract disease, colic with GI tract disease) or nonspecific indicators of inflammation (e.g., fever)
• History varies with the underlying primary disease or may nonspecifically reflect inflammation (e.g., fever, inappetance, weight loss).

CAUSES AND RISK FACTORS

• Any infectious, inflammatory, or neoplastic disorder may stimulate hyperfibrinogenemia.
• Gastrointestinal—large colon torsion, ruptured esophagus, intussusception, mesenteric abscessation, peritonitis, tooth root abscess, right dorsal colitis, parasitism, gastric squamous cell carcinoma, lymphosarcoma, other neoplasia, salmonellosis, enteritis, and surgery
• Respiratory—aspiration pneumonia, guttural pouch infections, sinusitis, neoplasia, bronchopneumonia, pyothorax, pleuropneumonia, and lung abscessation (*Rhodococcus equi*)
• Hemic/lymphatic/immune—septicemia, thrombophlebitis, bacterial endocarditis, urachal and umbilical remnant disease (omphalophlebitis), lymph node abscessation (*Streptococcus equi, Corynebacterium pseudotuberculosis*), and immune-mediated vasculitis
• Renal/urologic—cystitis, urinary calculi, glomerulonephritis, neoplasia, and pyelonephritis
• Reproductive—placentitis, endometritis, and orchitis
• Musculoskeletal—wound infection, fracture, exertional rhabdomyolysis, abscess, septic arthritis, bacterial osteomyelitis, cellulitis, and fistulous withers
• Nervous—bacterial meningitis and abscess
• Skin—pemphigus foliaceus, dermatophilosis, and chronic dermatitis

DIAGNOSIS

DIFFERENTIAL DIAGNOSIS

• Hyperfibrinogenemia should prompt a thorough, systematic physical examination and perhaps further diagnostic testing to establish the origin of the inflammatory stimulus.
• Historical or physical examination findings—colic, abdominal mass, diarrhea, or weight loss should prompt closer investigation of the GI tract; tachycardia, dyspnea, abnormal nasal discharge, or malodorous breath should prompt closer investigation of the respiratory tract; weight loss and lymph node enlargement might indicate lymphosarcoma, other neoplasia, or *S. equi* or *C. pseudotuberculosis* infection.
• Any area of heat, pain, or swelling is a likely source of the inflammatory stimulus for increased fibrinogen production.

CBC/BIOCHEMISTRY/URINALYSIS

• Leukocyte count and number of band (i.e., immature) neutrophils frequently increased
• Changes in biochemistry profile may reflect specific organ system involvement; lipemia and dehydration may result in falsely increased plasma fibrinogen concentrations.
• Urinalysis may reveal urinary system involvement.

OTHER LABORATORY TESTS

N/A

IMAGING

Radiography, ultrasound, or nuclear scintigraphy can be helpful in further localizing and possibly quantitating involvement of a specific organ system.

OTHER DIAGNOSTIC PROCEDURES

Ancillary diagnostic tests (e.g., specific organ biopsies, abdominocentesis, thoracocentesis, endoscopy, exploratory laparoscopy) can be helpful adjuncts in confirming organ involvement.

HYPERFIBRINOGENEMIA

TREATMENT

Degree of hyperfibrinogenemia may roughly indicate severity of the disease process and can be used with other clinical findings in determining the level of care required to appropriately treat the primary disease process.

MEDICATIONS

DRUGS

Therapeutic choices should be based on a tentative or definitive diagnosis of the primary underlying disease process; broad-spectrum bactericidal antimicrobial or anti-inflammatory agents often are indicated.

CONTRAINDICATIONS/POSSIBLE INTERACTIONS

N/A

FOLLOW-UP

PATIENT MONITORING

- Treatment efficacy monitored by serial evaluation of CBC and plasma fibrinogen concentrations at 2–3-day intervals
- Improvement indicated by decreasing fibrinogen concentrations and normalization of total leukocyte and neutrophil counts

POSSIBLE COMPLICATIONS

Increasing plasma fibrinogen concentrations positively correlate with mortality from the associated disease process.

MISCELLANEOUS

ASSOCIATED CONDITIONS

N/A

AGE-RELATED FACTORS

N/A

ZOONOTIC POTENTIAL

N/A

PREGNANCY

N/A

SEE ALSO

Specific disease processes

ABBREVIATION

- GI = gastrointestinal

Suggested Reading

Meyer, Coles, Rich. In: Veterinary laboratory medicine: interpretation and diagnosis. Philadelphia: WB Saunders, 1992:41.

Schalm OW. Equine hematology. Part 3. Significance of plasma fibrinogen concentration in clinical disorders in horses. Equine Pract 1979;1:4,22,24–29.

Schalm OW. Significance of plasma fibrinogen in clinical disorders in the horse. Proc First Int Symp Equine Hematol. In, AAEP. 1977:159–167.

Author Rodney Belgrave
Consulting Editor Debra C. Sellon

HYPERLIPIDEMIA

BASICS

DEFINITION

• Higher-than-normal blood concentrations of circulating lipids (primarily triglyceride)
• May be mild and quickly resolve with early detection and treatment, or may be severe and life-threatening.
• All cases involve elevated serum TG, with serum or plasma becoming milky in appearance at higher concentrations.
• In some texts, *hyperlipidemia* is used to describe mild disease (serum TG concentration <500 mg/dL) and *hyperlipemia* to describe the severe condition.

PATHOPHYSIOLOGY

• Negative energy balance or stress stimulates lipolysis within adipose tissues and mobilizes FFAs.
• Lipolysis is mediated by hormone-sensitive lipase under the influence of several hormones—glucagon, insulin, and glucocorticoids
• Most circulating FFAs are removed from the blood by the liver, in which FFAs either serve as substrates for energy production and ketogenesis or are esterified to TG. In turn, TG is stored within hepatocytes or packaged into VLDLs and exported to other tissues via the blood, and TG within VLDLs is utilized by peripheral tissues under the action of LpL, an enzyme on endothelial surfaces.
• FFAs are generated from TG hydrolysis and used as a source of energy.
• If a high rate of lipolysis within adipose tissue persists, blood FFA concentrations rise, and hepatic uptake of FFAs accelerates. Rates of TG-rich VLDL synthesis and export substantially increase, and accumulation of TG-rich VLDL within the blood (i.e., hyperlipidemia) develops as hepatic production exceeds the maximal clearance rate of particles by LpL.
• In severe cases, accumulation of TG within the liver results in hepatic lipidosis and TG deposits in other tissues, causing fatty infiltration followed by organ dysfunction. A vicious cycle then develops as elevated serum TG concentrations further suppress appetite.
• Generally, the degree of tissue sensitivity to insulin varies between equine subspecies, with ponies being more insulin resistant.
• Obesity further exacerbates the insulin resistance.
• Reduced inhibition of hormone-sensitive lipase by insulin is thought to predispose patients to exaggerated activation of lipolysis.

SYSTEMS AFFECTED

• Endocrine/metabolic
• Hemic/lymphatic/immune
• Hepatobiliary

GENETICS

No studies support a familial association, but several authors have suspected certain families of ponies to show a higher incidence of the disease.

INCIDENCE/PREVALENCE

• Incidence generally is considered to be low.
• No geographic variations in incidence are reported.

SIGNALMENT

• Ponies, donkeys, and miniature horses are more susceptible and are considered "high-risk" subspecies.
• All ages, including foals
• Mares are more susceptible during pregnancy and lactation.

SIGNS

• Early signs are nonspecific—lethargy, inappetence, and depression
• As the disease progresses, patients cease eating and drinking and develop clinical signs associated with organ dysfunction. Fetid, mucus-covered feces are produced (eventually in the form of diarrhea), and neurologic signs consistent with hepatic encephalopathy develop—severe depression, head pressing, ataxia, and sham drinking
• Pregnant mares may abort.
• Severely affected patients show progressive deterioration in neurologic status and require euthanasia.

CAUSES

• Most often develops in animals with a negative energy balance or that have recently been stressed.
• May be the primary disease or arise as a secondary complication in patients suffering from other diseases—enterocolitis, parasitism, dental problems, dysphagia, and esophageal obstruction
• Endotoxemia directly stimulates adipose mobilization.
• The additional strain of pregnancy and lactation on energy metabolism predispose to hyperlipidemia.
• Old patients with equine Cushing's disease also are more likely to develop hyperlipidemia.

RISK FACTORS

• Subspecies—ponies, donkeys, and miniature horses
• Breed—Shetland ponies are most commonly affected
• Stress
• Concurrent disease
• Endotoxemia
• Parasitism
• Pregnancy
• Lactation
• Both obesity and emaciation, secondary to malnutrition and/or parasitism, have been associated.

HYPERLIPIDEMIA

DIAGNOSIS

DIFFERENTIAL DIAGNOSIS

- Acute infectious diseases with nonspecific signs of depression and inappetence
- Liver disease
- Neurologic disease
- GI disease

CBC/BIOCHEMISTRY/URINALYSIS

NOTE: Markedly elevated blood lipid concentrations may interfere with analyzer functions, particularly biochemical analysis.

- A simple diagnostic test can be performed by standing the blood sample (collected in EDTA) upright and examining the plasma once the RBC mass has settled. Lipemic (i.e., visible lipid) plasma usually is detected with a blood TG concentration >500 mg/dL (Normal range in our laboratory, 11–65 mg/dL).
- Hypoglycemia
- Abnormalities associated with hepatic dysfunction/damage—elevated concentrations of total bilirubin, GGT, ALP, and SDH
- Abnormalities associated with renal dysfunction—elevated BUN and azotemia with normal urinalysis. Assessment of BUN should account for the adequacy of hepatic function at the time.

OTHER LABORATORY TESTS

- Blood gas analysis—consistent with metabolic acidosis (i.e., unmeasured acid accumulation)
- Elevated blood ammonia concentration.
- Prolonged coagulation profile—advanced liver failure
- Diagnostic evaluation for equine Cushing's disease

IMAGING

Ultrasonography—liver enlargement and alterations in echogenicity are associated with hepatic lipidosis.

DIAGNOSTIC PROCEDURES

Liver biopsy to confirm hepatic lipidosis

PATHOLOGIC FINDINGS

- Findings are consistent with fatty infiltration of tissues.
- Liver and kidneys may be pale and swollen, with a greasy, cut surface.
- Capsular rupture and hemorrhage in severe cases
- Additional sites of fatty infiltration—skeletal muscle, myocardium, and adrenal glands
- Pancreatitis may be evident
- Nonspecific gross findings—sites of hemorrhage, venous thrombosis, and ischemia
- Histopathologic findings indicate the degree of fatty infiltration of tissues.
- Glomerulonephritis, hyaline degeneration of skeletal muscle, and atrophy of the exocrine pancreas also have been reported.

TREATMENT

APPROPRIATE HEALTH CARE

- In mild cases detected early, appropriate care can be provided on the farm.
- Patient assessment is based on serum TG concentrations, duration of inappetence, and seriousness of concurrent disease conditions.
- Regardless of the initial presentation, monitor patients closely, and provide treatment early in the course of disease.
- Hospitalize severely affected patients immediately.

NURSING CARE

The primary goal of these recommendations is to reverse the patient's negative energy balance.

Increase Feed Intake

- Mildly affected patients improve as their feed intake increases.
- Provide a large variety of feedstuffs or treats until a preferred diet is identified.
- If a preferred feed is identified, provide fresh samples frequently to maintain interest.
- Allow patients access to better pasture or grassy areas to improve appetite and consumption.
- In more depressed patients, hand feeding may be necessary.
- For patients that maintain a poor appetite, clients can administer an oral solution of dextrose powder (50–100 g) in 500 mL (one pint) of warm water or of 50% corn syrup in a warm-water solution.
- Administration of dextrose solution or feed via nasogastric intubation is recommended.

IV Fluid Support

- Severely affected patients require an IV catheter and a nasogastric or indwelling esophageal feeding tube.
- IV fluid therapy should consist of a 5–10% dextrose solution prepared with polyionic fluids (e.g., lactated Ringer's solution) and delivered as a continuous infusion. An initial rate of 20–40 mL/kg per day is recommended.
- Ideally, blood glucose measurements and urine dipstick testing should be used to establish a rate that minimizes renal overflow of glucose into urine.
- An additional fluid line for polyionic fluids may be required to maintain hydration status (dextrose administration may result in diuresis), to address renal compromise, or to provide sodium bicarbonate solution if metabolic acidosis is severe.

HYPERLIPIDEMIA

Enteral and Parenteral Feeding

- With low oral feed intake, enteral feeding via a nasogastric or indwelling nasoesophageal feeding tube is recommended.
- Commercial enteral diets such as Nutrifoal HN (Osmolite HN) and Nutriprime (ProMod) are ideal for smaller patients.
- If a larger-diameter nasogastric tube can be passed, liquid preparations of alfalfa meal or soaked, pelleted feedstuffs with added dextrose can be carefully pumped into the stomach. Administer small quantities frequently (as often as q4h).
- For patients that cannot tolerate enteral feeding or to minimize stress, TPN can be administered. A solution primarily consisting of dextrose and amino acids (8.5% Travasol with electrolytes) should be prepared.
- Addition of lipid to TPN solutions for hyperlipidemic patients is controversial.

ACTIVITY

No specific restrictions, but minimize stress.

DIET

- Once a preferred diet is identified, provide it ad libitum until a positive energy balance is established, after which gradual substitution of alternate feedstuffs may be started.
- See *Nursing Care*.

CLIENT EDUCATION

- Inform clients who keep high-risk breeds (e.g., Shetland ponies, donkeys, miniature horses) about hyperlipidemia and to seek advice if patients exhibit inappetence.
- Clients should recognize obesity as a serious predisposing factor, particularly in pregnant animals.

SURGICAL CONSIDERATIONS

N/A

MEDICATIONS

DRUGS OF CHOICE

Insulin

- Increases cellular uptake of glucose, and inhibits hormone-sensitive lipase.
- Reduction of lipolysis and promotion of TG synthesis within adipose tissue reduces the rate of FFA production; however, the extent to which exogenous insulin can overcome insulin resistance at times of high glucagon (i.e., fasting) or glucocorticoid (i.e., stress) activity is questionable.
- Dosage in hyperlipidemic patients has not been established. (Previously reported doses were for protamine zinc insulin, which as of this writing is no longer available.)
- Regular insulin, because of its short half-life, is best administered within IV fluids.
- Use of ultralente insulin (2 IU SC q24h) has been reported in an American miniature horse.

Heparin Sulfate

- Potentiates LpL activity, resulting in increased VLDL clearance from the blood; if LpL activity is already maximized, as several reports suggest, administration of heparin would be ineffective.
- Can be administered at a dose of 20–40 IU/kg IM or IV twice a day.

Other Drugs

- Consider medications administered in cases of liver failure and hepatic encephalopathy for severely hyperlipidemic patients.
- Anthelmintics should be administered to remove intestinal parasites.

CONTRAINDICATIONS

- Insulin administration in hypoglycemic patients
- Use heparin sulfate with caution in hyperlipidemic patients exhibiting liver failure—reduced coagulation factors

PRECAUTIONS

Monitor blood glucose concentrations.

POSSIBLE INTERACTIONS

N/A

ALTERNATIVE DRUGS

N/A

FOLLOW-UP

PATIENT MONITORING

Repeated measurement of serum TG concentration

PREVENTION/AVOIDANCE

- Maintain appropriate body condition, and avoid obesity.
- Minimize stressful conditions for high-risk breeds, particularly when metabolic demands are high—pregnancy or lactation
- Awareness of the disease, and early intervention when feed intake is reduced.

POSSIBLE COMPLICATIONS

- Liver and renal failure
- Neurologic deficits
- Death
- Colic and laminitis may result from dietary changes.

EXPECTED COURSE AND PROGNOSIS

- The course of this disease is rapid.
- Mildly affected patients can recover quickly if the disease is detected early and the negative energy balance is reversed.
- Severely affected patients with signs of organ failure or neurologic deficits have a poor prognosis; mortality rates of 57–85% have been reported.

MISCELLANEOUS

ASSOCIATED CONDITIONS

- Hepatic lipidosis and subsequent liver failure
- Hepatic encephalopathy
- Renal failure

AGE-RELATED CONDITIONS

N/A

ZOONOTIC POTENTIAL

N/A

PREGNANCY

In pregnant animals, organ failure, metabolic acidosis, and stress may compromise the fetus, resulting in abortion.

SYNONYMS

- Hyperlipemia
- Hyperlipoproteinemia
- Hypertriglyceridemia

SEE ALSO

- Equine Cushing's disease
- Hepatic encephalopathy
- Liver disease

ABBREVIATIONS

- ALP = alkaline phosphatase
- FFA = free fatty acid
- GGT = γ-glutamyltransferase
- GI = gastrointestinal
- LpL = lipoprotein lipase
- SDH = sorbitol dehydrogenase
- TG = triglyceride
- VLDL = very low-density lipoprotein

Suggested Reading

Golenz MR, Knight DA, Yvorchuk-St. Jean KE. Use of a human enteral feeding preparation for the treatment of hyperlipemia and nutritional support during healing of an esophageal laceration in a miniature horse. J Am Vet Med Assoc 1992;7:951–953.

Mogg TD, Palmer JE. Hyperlipidemia, hyperlipemia, and hepatic lipidosis in American miniature horses: 23 cases (1990–1994). J Am Vet Med Assoc 1995;5:604–607.

Rush Moore B, Abood SK, Hinchcliff KW. Hyperlipemia in 9 miniature horses and miniature donkeys. J Vet Intern Med 1994;8:376–381.

Watson TDG, Love S. Equine hyperlipidemia. Compend Contin Educ Pract 1994;16:89–98.

Watson TDG, Murphy D, Love S. Equine hyperlipaemia in the United Kingdom: clinical and blood biochemistry of 18 cases. Vet Rec 1992;131:48–51.

Author Nicholas Frank

Consulting Editor Michel Levy

HYPERTHERMIA AND HEAT STROKE

BASICS

DEFINITION

- An abnormally high body temperature in which the hypothalamic temperature set-point is not altered but the heat-dissipating mechanisms fail
- As opposed to a fever, in which the body temperature is elevated because of upward resetting of the set-point with the heat-dissipating mechanisms remaining intact
- Heat stroke occurs when hyperthermia is combined with dehydration and electrolyte derangement.
- Critical temperature above which the CNS becomes impaired—106° F (41° C)

PATHOPHYSIOLOGY

- The normal physiologic body temperature is set by the hypothalamic thermoregulatory center at 99.5°–101.5° F (37.5–38.5° C).
- With fever, the set-point is altered upward by the pyrogenic effects of mediators (e.g., IL-1) released during disease states.
- With hyperthermia, the mechanisms of heat dissipation are overwhelmed or inadequate.
- Body heat is generated by muscles working and solar radiation.
- Heat is dissipated by conduction, convection, radiation, and evaporation.
- Evaporative loss is through sweating and breathing.
- Dilation of surface vasculature allows heat to be lost by convection.
- Heat from the body core is dissipated to the cooler surface tissues by the circulation of blood (i.e., conduction).
- Heat is lost from the body surface to cooler ambient air by radiation.
- A body temperature >103° F (39.5° C) can be considered hyperthermia.
- Heat denaturation of cellular proteins results in organ dysfunction, failure, and death. The central nervous system is most sensitive to hyperthermic damage. As the temperature continues to increase and/or persist, other systems also become affected.

SYSTEMS AFFECTED

All systems are susceptible to damage by hyperthermia.

GENETICS

Genetic predisposition to hyperthermia during anesthesia (i.e., MH) and rhabdomyolysis

INCIDENCE/PREVALENCE

Greater in hot, humid climates

SIGNALMENT

Breeds with a massive body size:skin ratio have increased heat production with a relatively smaller surface area for heat dissipation.

SIGNS

Historical Findings

- Prolonged muscular exertion
- Weakness
- Stilted gait
- Fatigue
- Depression
- Impaired performance
- Respiratory distress
- Seizures
- Anesthesia
- Transport

Physical Examination Findings

- Elevated temperature associated with panting, tachypnea, tachyarrhythmia, and tachycardia
- Excessive, patchy, or lack of sweating associated with dehydration
- Weakness with ataxia, collapse, muscle rigidity, and SDF
- Decreased anal tone
- Prolapsed penis
- Colic
- Ileus
- Diarrhea
- Seizures
- Dark urine
- Dilated cutaneous vasculature

CAUSES

- Excessive muscular activity—prolonged work; seizures
- Drugs—erythromycin, halothane anesthesia (i.e., MH), phenothiazine tranquilizers, and endophyte-infested tall fescue
- Anhidrosis
- Confinement in closed trailers or buildings during hot weather

RISK FACTORS

- Poor physical condition, insufficient conditioning, and lack of acclimatization
- High ambient temperature and relative humidity
- No air movement and high solar radiation
- Large body mass relative to body surface area and prolonged work
- Long hair coat (i.e., equine Cushing's syndrome), anhidrosis, and obesity
- Dehydration—no access to drinking water during work
- Possible risk of hyperthermia during anesthesia of horses with HPP.

DIAGNOSIS

DIFFERENTIAL DIAGNOSIS

- Fever from disease does not usually exceed 106° F.
- Rule out COPD, anhidrosis, exertional rhabdomyolysis, and equine Cushing's syndrome.

CBC/BIOCHEMISTRY/URINALYSIS

- CBC—stress; hemoconcentration
- Biochemistry—elevated muscle enzymes (i.e., CK and AST) with exertional rhabdomyolysis; electrolyte depletion (i.e., Ca^{++}, K^{+}, Mg^{++}); azotemia with dehydration; elevated renal and hepatic enzymes with organ damage; elevated K^{+} with HPP
- Urinalysis—concentrated urine; myoglobinuria

OTHER LABORATORY TESTS

- Intradermal epinephrine/terbutaline test for decreased sweating—anhidrosis
- Genetic-marker blood test for HPP
- Blood gas disorders—possible alkalosis or acidosis
- Clotting profile—development of DIC, liver failure, thrombocytopenia, prolonged clotting time, and elevated FDPs
- Halothane—caffeine contracture test to identify individuals with MH

IMAGING

N/A

DIAGNOSTIC PROCEDURES

N/A

PATHOLOGIC FINDINGS

N/A

HYPERTHERMIA AND HEAT STROKE

TREATMENT

- Enhance cooling mechanism by providing air movement—fans
- Provide misting fans
- Repeatedly applying cold water can be used to provide rapid cooling; this does not lessen heat loss.
- Correct dehydration by providing drinking water if patient is not critical and IV fluids if heat stroke has occurred.
- Identify and correct electrolyte and acid–base derangements.
- Recovery from anesthesia, if used
- Clip long hair coat.
- Identify and treat accordingly other conditions—rhabdomyolysis; renal failure
- Monitor rectal temperature and continue cooling until $<104°$ F (40° C) for 15–30 minutes.
- SDF—administer 300 mL of 20% calcium borogluconate in a 1:4 ratio with saline or 5% dextrose.
- Cerebral edema—dilute DMSO solution IV; furosemide; glucocorticoids

MEDICATIONS

DRUGS OF CHOICE

- Oral and IV sources of K^+, Na^+, Cl^-, Ca^{++}, Mg^{++} as indicated
- IV saline, lactated Ringer's solution to restore blood volume and renal function
- Appropriate adjunctive therapy with rhabdomyolysis—muscle relaxants; anti-inflammatories
- Antipyretic drugs usually are not indicated for nonpyrogenic hyperthermia but may be useful for their anti-inflammatory properties.
- Dantrolene sodium—MH

CONTRAINDICATIONS

Supplemental K^+ in cases of HPP

PRECAUTIONS

Use NSAIDs cautiously in cases of renal compromise or dehydration.

POSSIBLE INTERACTIONS

N/A

ALTERNATIVE DRUGS

N/A

FOLLOW-UP

PATIENT MONITORING

- Monitoring body temperature frequently
- Assess for renal compromise and urination
- Assess hydration, PCV, and total solids
- Assess response of electrolyte and blood gas adjustments

PREVENTION/AVOIDANCE

N/A

POSSIBLE COMPLICATIONS

- CNS failure—seizures; coma; death
- Renal and hepatic failure
- DIC
- Laminitis
- Pulmonary edema
- May be more prone to subsequent hyperthermia.

EXPECTED COURSE AND PROGNOSIS

Favorable to grave, depending on early detection and reversal of hyperthermia

MISCELLANEOUS

ASSOCIATED CONDITIONS

N/A

AGE-RELATED FACTORS

N/A

ZOONOTIC POTENTIAL

N/A

PREGNANCY

N/A

SYNONYMS

- Heat exhaustion
- Heat stress
- Heat stroke

SEE ALSO

- Exertional Rhabdomyolysis
- Fever
- MH

ABBREVIATIONS

- AST = aspartate aminotransferase
- CK = creatinine phosphokinase
- CNS = central nervous system
- DIC = disseminated intravascular coagulation
- DMSO = dimethyl sulfoxide
- FDPs = fibrinogen degradation products
- HPP = hyperkalemic periodic paralysis
- IL-1 = interleukin 1
- MH = malignant hyperthermia
- PCV = packed cell volume
- SDF = synchronous diaphragmatic flutter

Suggested Reading

Cohn CW, Hinchcliff KW, McKeever KH. Evaluation of washing with cold water to facilitate heat dissipation in horses exercised in hot, humid conditions. Am J Vet Res 1999;60:299–305.

Geor RJ, McCutcheon LJ. Thermoregulation and clinical disorders associated with exercise and heat stress. Compend Cont Educ Pract Vet 1996;18:436–444.

White SL. Alterations in body temperature. In: Smith BP, ed. Large animal internal medicine. 2nd ed. St. Louis: Mosby, 1996:35–45.

Williamson LH. Heat-related illness and fluid deficits in eventing horses. Compend Cont Educ Pract Vet 1996;18:937–941.

Author Wendy Duckett
Consulting Editor Michel Levy

HYPERTHYROIDISM

BASICS

OVERVIEW

• A multisystemic disease caused by increased amounts of the hormones (i.e., T_3, T_4) produced by the thyroid gland.
• Either iatrogenic, caused by the overdose of replacement supplements, or naturally occurring, caused by the increased production of the thyroid gland.
• Only one case report of naturally occurring hyperthyroidism in horses.
• Iatrogenic hyperthyroidism, though not well documented in the literature, may occur in overmedicated horses.
• Primary organ systems—endocrine, musculoskeletal, and nervous; the nervous system is included because of behavioral changes observed in hyperthyroid horses.

SIGNALMENT

• The one horse described with naturally occurring hyperthyroidism was 21 years of age.
• Thyroid tumors generally occur in old horses, so it is reasonable to expect other animals with this disease to be old as well.
• Horses with iatrogenic hyperthyroidism tend to be young race or show horses.
• No known breed or sex predilections.

SIGNS

• Weight loss
• Nervousness
• Cold intolerance
• Behavioral disturbances—pacing and difficulty when being handled
• Tachypnea and tachycardia also may be present.

CAUSES AND RISK FACTORS

• Naturally occurring hyperthyroidism is caused by an active thyroid adenocarcinoma.
• Iatrogenic hyperthyroidism is caused by giving more than the recommended amount of exogenous T_4.

DIAGNOSIS

DIFFERENTIAL DIAGNOSIS

• The diagnosis is established based on a combination of physical signs and history. It should be suspected in an old horses with an enlarged thyroid gland, unexplained weight loss, and change in behavior, and in young horses on thyroid supplements if they exhibit change in behavior and display increased aggressiveness or nervousness.
• The primary differential in old horses is a nonactive thyroid tumor, leading to an enlarged thyroid gland without increased circulating hormone levels.
• Other reasons for weight loss and nervousness primarily result from management and/or training; rule out by a careful history and observation of the amount and type of feed being offered.

CBC/BIOCHEMISTRY/URINALYSIS

These tests were normal in the one report of naturally occurring hyperthyroidism.

OTHER LABORATORY TESTS

• In the horse described in the one case report, free T_4 concentrations were quite elevated above the normal range, but total T_4 levels were not.
• Iatrogenic hyperthyroidism—both free and total T_4 are elevated.
• Free T_4 concentrations must be determined by the equilibrium dialysis method, not by RIA, to be diagnostically beneficial.

IMAGING

• A thyroid tumor may be imaged via ultrasonography as a nodule in the thyroid gland.
• A thyroid tumor large enough to enlarge the entire gland may be seen on radiographs of the cervical region as a soft-tissue density.

DIAGNOSTIC PROCEDURES

• Serum free and total T_4 levels consistently above reference ranges are diagnostic.
• A fine-needle aspiration or biopsy of the thyroid gland may be useful in diagnosing a thyroid tumor.

PATHOLOGIC FINDINGS

A thyroid adenocarcinoma was responsible for the one reported case of naturally occurring hyperthyroidism.

TREATMENT

- Thyroid tumor—surgical removal of the affected thyroid lobe is curative, unless metastatic disease has occurred.
- Suspected iatrogenic hyperthyroidism—removal of exogenous hormone or decreasing the dosage of T_4 to recommended levels (20 μg/kg) is curative.

MEDICATIONS

DRUGS

- Use of antithyroid drugs to treat thyroid tumors has not been reported in horses, possibly because surgical removal is curative unless metastatic spreading of the tumor has occurred.
- Thyroid tumors in horses very rarely metastasize.

CONTRAINDICATIONS/POSSIBLE INTERACTIONS

N/A

FOLLOW-UP

- Anesthetic complications have been reported after removal of thyroid tumors; thus, perform surgery in a controlled setting where monitoring equipment and emergency treatments are available.
- After tumor removal, the horse should gradually regain its weight and former temperament.
- Horses with iatrogenic hyperthyroidism slowly regain their former temperament after discontinuing the supplement.
- All clinical signs should be resolved within 6 months of appropriate actions and return to the euthyroid state.

MISCELLANEOUS

ASSOCIATED CONDITIONS

N/A

AGE-RELATED FACTORS

Horses with thyroid tumors tend to be old (>10 years).

ZOONOTIC POTENTIAL

N/A

PREGNANCY

N/A

SEE ALSO

Thyroid tumors

ABBREVIATIONS

- RIA = radioimmunoassay
- T_3 = triiodothyronine
- T_4 = thyroxine

Suggested Reading

Ramirez S, McClure JJ, Moore RM, et al. Hyperthyroidism associated with a thyroid adenocarcinoma in a 21-year-old gelding. J Vet Intern Med 1998;12:475–477.

Author Janice Sojka

Consulting Editor Michel Levy

HYPOCALCEMIA

BASICS

OVERVIEW

• A fall below the normal reference range for serum calcium, which leads to increased membrane excitability, particularly in skeletal and cardiac muscle
• In cases of profound hypocalcemia. muscle contractility is reduced, which may lead to flaccid paralysis.
• Clinical signs occur at serum calcium concentrations > those leading to clinical signs in lactating cattle.
• The most prominent clinical signs involve the respiratory/cardiovascular and musculoskeletal systems.
• The two major syndromes seen are tetany and SDF.

SIGNALMENT

• Any age, sex, or breed
• Lactation tetany is seen in lactating or recently weaned mares.

SIGNS

• Tetanic animals have a stiff gait and may be hypermetric.
• Muscle twitches and fasciculations may be seen, together with dysphagia and sweating.
• Horses with SDF have heart and respiratory rates that may be equal and synchronous; for every beat of the heart, a simultaneous and synchronous contraction of the diaphragm occurs.

CAUSES AND RISK FACTORS

• Lactation—particularly in stressed or heavily worked mares
• Endurance competition—loss of water and electrolytes in sweat can lead to marked electrolyte and acid–base abnormalities.
• Long-distance transportation—transit tetany
• Colitis
• Colic
• Blister beetle toxicity

DIAGNOSIS

DIFFERENTIAL DIAGNOSIS

• Tetanic conditions may be confused with a variety of others, depending on the severity of clinical signs.
• Classical tetanus caused by the toxins of *Clostridium tetani* is a progressive and often very pronounced tetanic condition, though in the early stages, it is very similar to hypocalcemic tetany. Serum electrolyte determinations assist in differentiation.
• SDF may be differentiated from acute respiratory conditions by the unique synchrony of the heart and respiratory rates and the lack of any abnormal respiratory sounds on thoracic auscultation.

CBC/BICHEMISTRY/URINALYSIS

• Possible concurrent hyponatremia, hypochloremia, and metabolic alkalosis.
• Some of the total serum calcium is bound to serum albumin. In hypoalbuminemic animals, total serum calcium may be marginally low. This is not usually associated with clinical signs, however, and should be remembered when assessing laboratory data in horses showing signs consistent with hypocalcemia.
• Ideally, the ionized calcium concentration allows for a more accurate assessment of severity, but this is not usually available in most practice settings.
• CBC—usually normal, although a stress leukogram may be present.

OTHER LABORATORY TESTS

N/A

IMAGING

N/A

DIAGNOSTIC PROCEDURES

N/A

TREATMENT

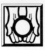

• Reduce stress, and avoid exercise.
• If poor nutrition may have played a role in the cause, make appropriate dietary adjustments.
• Manage animals with acute colitis or colic appropriately.

MEDICATIONS

DRUGS

• Other than medications for specific diseases (e.g., colitis, colic), treatment of all horse with clinical signs from hypocalcemia is similar.
• Calcium borogluconate solutions are the most likely to be available to most practitioners, but calcium chloride solutions may be more appropriate.
• Horses seem more sensitive than cattle to the effects of IV calcium solutions, and they must not be given at the same rate or concentration as used when treating "milk fever" in cows. Dilute the stock calcium solution with at least an equal volume (preferably threefold the volume) of polyionic sterile fluid before administration. Administer the diluted solution slowly to effect, and monitor the heart rate constantly.
• Because the exact deficit in serum calcium is not usually known, the amount of calcium solution needed cannot be determined; resolution of clinical signs often is the only guide.

CONTRAINDICATIONS/POSSIBLE INTERACTIONS

Do not mix calcium solutions with fluids containing bicarbonate, because calcium carbonate precipitate then forms.

HYPOCALCEMIA

FOLLOW-UP

PATIENT MONITORING

- Depending on the cause, follow-up care varies, but even if clinical signs resolve after treatment with IV calcium solutions, recheck serum calcium concentrations 24 hours after treatment. In many cases the levels will have increased but may still be well below the reference ranges.
- Most animals will not need additional therapy if they are eating and drinking well, but some will decline. Clinical signs may recur; if so, additional therapy is needed.
- The specific conditions that caused the hypocalcemia may require specific follow-up actions.

PREVENTION/AVOIDANCE

- Although hypocalcemia is associated with many clinical conditions, the specific causative mechanisms are not always clear. Thus, preventative actions are difficult to recommend.
- Provide endurance horses with adequate and frequent access to water and electrolytes during competition, and monitor these animals carefully at each checkpoint.
- Lactating mares should not be stressed or worked hard.

POSSIBLE COMPLICATIONS

N/A

EXPECTED COURSE AND PROGNOSIS

- Once the underlying problem is resolved, hypocalcemia usually does not recur.
- Prognosis depends mostly on the primary disease.

MISCELLANEOUS

ASSOCIATED CONDITIONS

See *Causes and Risk Factors.*

AGE RELATED FACTORS

N/A

ZOONOTIC POTENTIAL

N/A

PREGNANCY

Lactating mares are prone to lactation tetany.

SEE ALSO

- Colic
- Colitis
- SDF

ABBREVIATIONS

SDF = synchronous diaphragmatic flutter

Suggested Reading

Kaneps AJ, Knight AP, Bennett DG. Synchronous diaphragmatic flutter associated with electrolyte imbalances in a mare with colic. Equine Pract 1980;2:18–24.

Author Christopher M. Brown
Consulting Editor Michel Levy

HYPOTHYROIDISM

BASICS

DEFINITION

Production of hormones produced by the thyroid gland (i.e., T_3 and T_4) insufficient to support normal metabolic functions in the body

PATHPHYSIOLOGY

- Can result from disruption of any portion of the thyroid-pituitary-hypothalamus axis.
- When the hypothalamus senses low thyroid hormone levels, it produces the peptide hormone TRH. This travels to the pituitary gland and stimulates release of TSH, which causes the thyroid gland to release T_4 into the circulation. In turn, T_4 is deiodinated to T_3 at the peripheral tissues, and T_3 diffuses into cells and up- or down-regulates many of the genes in the cell, particularly those affecting the basal metabolic rate and energy metabolism.
- The net effect of hypothyroidism is decreased basal metabolic rate and decreased ability to respond appropriately to increased metabolic demands—the need to increase heat production in cold weather.
- In utero, thyroid hormones are necessary for proper bone, pulmonary, and nervous system development. Thus, foals born with congenital hypothyroidism often have angular limb deformities (caused by incomplete development of the carpal and tarsal bones) and other skeletal deformities, and they often are weak and dysmature.

SYSTEMS AFFECTED

Endocrine/Metabolic

- The endocrine system primarily is affected; however, because thyroid hormones have such widespread effects, many other body systems are affected as well.
- Energy metabolism is altered.
- Affected horses secrete less-than-normal amounts of insulin and have increased serum cholesterol levels.

Musculoskeletal

- In foals with congenital hypothyroidism, the musculoskeletal system is most dramatically affected. These foals are born with underdeveloped tarsal and carpal bones, prognathism, ruptured common digital extensor tendons, and forelimb contracture.
- Foals often are weak and need assistance to stand.
- Adults have an increased incidence of myositis and muscle abnormalities.

Behavioral

Behavior may be altered; both increased aggression and lethargy have been attributed to hypothyroidism.

Cardiovascular

- Thyroidectomized horses have decreased cardiac output compared with normal horses; this results in exercise intolerance.
- Immature respiratory tract and inadequate ability to ventilate in hypothyroid foals.

GENETICS

Congenital hypothryoidism is the best characterized form, but it is thought to result from ingested excess or deficient iodine or other goitrogens by the dam and is not genetic.

INCIDENCE/PREVALENCE

- Poorly characterized in adults, but has a sporadic incidence and low prevalence.
- Two recognized forms of congenital hypothyroidism—idiopathic and congenital
- Idiopathic hypothryoidism primarily occurs in the northwestern portion of North America. Some farms have a very high incidence, with most of the foal crop affected.
- Congenital hypothyroidism can occur on any farm if pregnant mares receive increased amounts of dietary iodine; levels of 35–40 mg/day have led to outbreaks of congenital goiters and hypothyroidism. This occurs sporadically, but the percentage of affected foals is high on such farms.

SIGNALMENT

- Any sex or breed
- Can occur at any age and exist in utero, with the foal showing characteristic signs at birth.

SIGNS

- Common signs in foals with congenital hypothyroidism—prognathism, ruptured common digital extensor tendon, forelimb contracture, retarded ossification and crushing of the carpal and tarsal bones, weakness, and poor suckle reflex
- Less common signs in foals with congenital hypothyroidism—goiters, angular limb deformities, respiratory distress, abdominal hernia, poor muscle development, and osteoporosis
- Adults—hypothermia, bradycardia, myositis, anhydrosis, laminitis, infertility, agalactia, poor hair coat, and poor growth
- Experimentally induced hypothyroidism—edema of the distal limbs and coarsened features

CAUSES

- In most adult cases, the cause is not known.
- Iodine deficiency can cause hypothyroidism, but this occurs extremely rarely.
- Iodine deficiency or excess in the diets of broodmares can cause hypothyroidism in their foals. Ingestion of endophyte-infected fescue also can result in congenital hypothyroidism.
- The cause for the outbreaks among foals in the northwestern portions of North America is not known, but a toxic plant is suspected.
- Rarely, thyroid tumors cause hypothyroidism in adults. In most instances, they are clinically silent.

RISK FACTORS

- Primarily dietary—intake of excess or inadequate iodine or ingestion of other goitrogen
- In old horses, thyroid tumor is a risk factor.

DIAGNOSIS

DIFFERENTIAL DIAGNOSIS

- The primary differential diagnosis in adults suspected of hypothyroidism is a pituitary hyperplasia or adenoma (i.e., equine Cushing's disease). Most of the clinical signs ascribed to hypothyroidism (e.g., laminitis, abnormal fat distribution) actually result from Cushing's disease, which should be ruled out before pursuing a diagnosis of thyroid problems.
- Differentials in foals with congenital hypothyroidism—fescue toxicosis, prematurity, angular limb deformities, dysmaturity, and sepsis

CBC/BIOCHEMISTRY/URINALYSIS

Hypothyroid horses may exhibit anemia, leukopenia, and hypercholesterolemia.

OTHER LABORATORY TESTS

- Low serum T_3 and T_4 provide the diagnostic criteria for hypothyroidism. Both T_3 and T_4 exist in two forms in the blood: total and free. The free hormone is biologically active, so low serum free T_3 and T_4 is more likely associated with hypothyroidism than low total values.Total T_3 and T_4 would be low if serum proteins, particularly albumin, were low or other substances were in the blood that compete with thyroid hormone for protein-binding sites.
- Measurement of serum thyroid hormone levels alone can not be relied on to establish a definitive diagnosis of hypothyroidism.

IMAGING

- Rarely useful
- An enlarged thyroid gland resulting from a tumor or goiter can be seen via ultrasonography or radiography.

DIAGNOSTIC PROCEDURES

- Provocative testing of the thyroid gland is the most definitive way to diagnose hypothyroidism. A test dose of either TSH or TRH is given, and serum thyroid hormone levels are determined before administration and at 2 and 4 hours later.
- In normal horses, T_3 is twice baseline at 2 hours, and T_4 is twice baseline at four hours.
- If resting thyroid hormone levels are low and fail to increase after administration of TSH or TRH, the diagnosis of hypothyroidism can be confidently made.

HYPOTHYROIDISM

PATHOLOGIC FINDINGS
Foals with congenital hypothyroidism often have pathologic changes in their thyroid glands, including large or irregular follicles with no resorption vesicles.

TREATMENT

APPROPRIATE HEALTH CARE
Foals with congenital hypothyroidism may require inpatient treatment if the disease is severe; all other horses can be treated as outpatients.

NURSING CARE
- Foals may need assistance standing as well as milk administered via nasogastric tube if they are too weak to suckle.
- Mechanical ventilation may be required if the affected horse cannot breathe on its own.
- Animals with poor hair coat may need to be kept warm with blankets; cold temperatures should be avoided.

ACTIVITY
Limit in foals with musculoskeletal deformities—incomplete ossification of the carpal or tarsal bones

DIET
- Examine the diet of any affected horse and of dams with affected foals to ensure the proper amount of iodine is given.
- Pregnant mares should not receive endophyte-infected fescue hay, particularly during their last months of gestation.

CLIENT EDUCATION
- The prognosis for soundness is poor with most foals suffering from congenital hypothyroidism; thus, discuss this with owners before beginning expensive treatments.
- Adults respond well to exogenous replacement hormone, and their prognosis generally is good.

SURGICAL CONSIDERATIONS
If the cause is a tumor of the thyroid gland, surgical removal of the affected lobe should be curative.

MEDICATIONS

DRUG OF CHOICE
Replacement therapy with T_4—20 μg/kg maintains T_4 and T_3 levels in the normal range for 24 hours; this constitutes a dose of 10 mg in a 1000-pound horse.

CONTRAINDICATIONS
In horses with low resting T_3 and T_4 values because of some other severe disease (e.g., euthyroid sick syndrome), thyroid replacement therapies may cause further deterioration; thus, perform provocative testing to diagnose hypothyroidism in any horse that is debilitated or exhibits signs of any other systemic disease.

PRECAUTIONS
Exogenous thyroid hormone causes down-regulation and potential thyroid gland atrophy; thus, when a supplement is discontinued, do so gradually (over several weeks).

POSSIBLE INTERACTIONS
N/A

ALTERNATIVE DRUGS
- If there is a reason not to use synthetic T_4, other sources of thyroid hormone replacement may be used.
- Iodinated casein (5.0 g/day) and concentrated bovine thyroid extract (10 g/day) also may be used.

FOLLOW-UP

PATIENT MONITORING
- Monitor horses on thyroid supplement by retesting serum T_4 and T_3 levels every 30–60 days. If serum levels are low, increase the dosage until levels are in the normal range. If the serum levels are too high or in the higher end of the normal range, decrease the dosage, and retest the horse in 30–60 days.
- Reconsider the original diagnosis of hypothyroidism if the patient fails to respond clinically after 6 weeks of therapy.

PREVENTION/AVOIDANCE
- Iatrogenic hypothyroidism can be avoided by feeding the NRC recommended amount of iodine in the diet—1–2 mg/horse per day.
- Never feed high-iodine feedstuffs to broodmares.
- Feed broodmares forage that does not contain endophyte-infested fescue.

POSSIBLE COMPLICATIONS
- The most severe complications occur in foals.
- Musculoskeletal abnormalities, particularly ruptured tendons and incomplete ossification of the carpal or tarsal bones, may lead to permanent angular limb deformities and lameness.
- Weakness and failure to suckle may lead to failure of passive transfer and subsequent sepsis in foals.
- Adults may have reduced fertility and be prone to myositis and agalactia.

EXPECTED COURSE AND PROGNOSIS
- Once on a thyroid supplement, the horse should experience no further problems, and its course is expected to go well.
- The prognosis for foals with congenital hypothyroidism is poor because of the severe lameness that usually accompanies this disease.

MISCELLANEOUS

ASSOCIATED CONDITIONS
- Angular limb deformities, hypognathism, weakness, and respiratory distress often are associated with congenital hypothyroidism.
- Infertility and myositis have been associated with hypothyroidism in adults.

AGE-RELATED FACTORS
The congenital form is only observed in newborn foals.

ZOONOTIC POTENTIAL
N/A

PREGNANCY
Pregnant animals are at risk of bearing affected foals if they are on unbalanced diets of iodine or ingest fescue forage in the later part of gestation.

SYNONYMS
N/A

SEE ALSO
- Goiter
- Thyroid tumors
- TRH and TSH stimulation tests
- T_4 and T_3 determination

ABBREVIATIONS
- NRC = National Research Council
- TRH = thyroid-releasing hormone
- TSH = thyroid-stimulating hormone
- T_4 = thyroxine
- T_3 = triiodothyronine

Suggested Reading

Allen AL, Doige CE, Fretz PB, et al. Congenital hypothyroidism, dysmaturity, and musculoskeletal lesions in Western Canadian foals. Proc AAEP 1993;39:207–208.

Harris P, Marlin D, Grey J. Equine thyroid function tests: a preliminary investigation. Br Vet J 1992;148:71–80.

Messer NT. Clinical and diagnostic features of thyroid disease in horses. Proc Am Coll Vet Intern Med 1993;11:649–651.

Sojka JE. Hypothyroidism in horses. Compend Contin Educ Pract Vet 1995;17:845–852.

Author Janice Sojka

Consulting Editor Michel Levy

HYPOXEMIA

BASICS

DEFINITION

- A decreased amount of oxygen carried in the arterial blood
- Can be measured indirectly as a PaO_2 of <80 mm Hg or as arterial hemoglobin saturation levels <95%.
- Cellular function is adversely affected at a PaO_2 of <60 mm Hg.
- Venous oxygen levels of <40 mm Hg are highly suggestive of arterial hypoxemia.

PATHOPHYSIOLOGY

- Can develop by several mechanisms—hypoventilation; diffusion impairment from interstitial exudate, edema, or fibrosis; right-to-left cardiac or intrapulmonary shunt; and V/Q mismatch.
- Low levels of inspired oxygen as seen at high altitudes result in hypoxemia.
- Abnormalities of hemoglobin structure or function (e.g., methemoglobinemia) decrease the oxygen-carrying capacity of hemoglobin (SaO_2); however, PaO_2 may be normal.
- More than one mechanism often is present in many patients.
- V/Q mismatch is the most frequent and significant cause in anesthetized or recumbent patients, because many factors contribute to this phenomenon—any alteration of pulmonary blood flow or ventilation as well as the matching of these two components can limit the amount of oxygen transferred.

SYSTEMS AFFECTED

- Cardiovascular
- Nervous
- Respiratory

SIGNALMENT

- Any horse
- Most anesthetized horses maintained on room air develop hypoxemia from V/Q mismatch, which develops from atelectasis and variations in pulmonary blood flow, which develop with recumbency.

SIGNS

Historical Findings

Owners may report signs of exercise intolerance, respiratory difficulty, coughing, lethargy, and other signs referable to the primary problem.

Physical Examination Findings

- Tachypnea and tachycardia usually are present.
- Cyanosis does not develop until PO_2 is <40 mm Hg.
- Mucous membranes may be pale, hyperemic, or muddy with endotoxemia or cardiovascular disease/compromise.
- Other clinical signs relative to primary disease states may be present—nasal discharge, coughing, and abnormal lung sounds with respiratory disease; jugular vein distention, murmurs, arrhythmias, and ventral edema with cardiac failure or congenital defects.

CAUSES

- Hypoventilation has many causes (see *Respiratory Acidosis*) but rarely is the sole factor responsible for hypoxemia, because a PaO_2 of <60 mm Hg stimulates respiration and increases minute ventilation. This may correct hypercapnia but often does not improve oxygen levels. Oxygen does not diffuse as quickly as CO_2 and is more dependent on the matching of blood flow to ventilation to obtain normal levels.
- Diffusion impairment results from respiratory diseases such as viral, bacterial, or interstitial pneumonia; allergic small airway disease; COPD; and inhalation of toxic substances (e.g., smoke). Pulmonary edema is uncommon in horses but may occur with anaphylaxis, airway obstruction, hypoxemia, chordae tendinea rupture, or cardiac failure.
- V/Q inequality develops with changes in pulmonary blood flow locally, as with pulmonary hypertension, or systemically, as with hypotension. Atelectasis and other causes of hypoventilation also contribute to V/Q mismatch.
- General anesthesia is a major cause of both atelectasis and alterations of pulmonary blood flow; V/Q mismatch generally is always present in anesthetized horses and can be severe enough to result in hypoxemia even when the FiO_2 is 100%.
- Right-to-left cardiac shunts (e.g., tetralogy of Fallot, truncus arteriosus, tricuspid atresia) produce hypoxemia, because pulmonary blood flow is greatly diminished. Persistent fetal circulation produces hypoxemia via right-to-left shunting through the foramen ovale and ductus arteriosus and pulmonary hypertension.
- Cardiac failure is uncommon in horses but results in hypoxemia via pulmonary edema and pulmonary hypertension and, sometimes, hypoventilation if pleural or peritoneal effusion is significant.
- Endotoxic shock produces hypoxemia via several mechanisms—pulmonary hypertension, endothelial cell damage, decreased cardiac contractility, systemic hypotension, and so on

RISK FACTORS

- All horses are susceptible to hypoxemia during general anesthesia, especially if oxygen supplementation is not utilized.
- Premature foals or term neonates born to mares with systemic illness during pregnancy or that experience dystocia or asphyxia during parturition are predisposed.
- Horses with allergic airway diseases may develop hypoxemia with acute attacks or with progression of the disease.
- Acidotic patients and those with cardio-vascular compromise are more likely to develop hypoxemia.

DIAGNOSIS

DIFFERENTIAL DIAGNOSIS

Diseases that present with tachypnea, dyspnea, or cyanosis

HYPOXEMIA

LABORATORY FINDINGS

Drugs That May Alter Lab Results

N/A

Disorders That May Alter Lab Results

- With poor peripheral perfusion or cardiovascular shunt, results of blood gas analysis on samples taken from peripheral arteries may differ from those taken elsewhere or may not reflect the patient's overall systemic condition.
- Exposure to room air via air bubbles in the sample may change the PO_2 level, because the sample equilibrates with the air.

Valid If Run in Human Lab?

Yes, if properly submitted

CBC/BIOCHEMISTRY/URINALYSIS

N/A

OTHER LABORATORY TESTS

- Arterial blood gas analysis is the definitive method for documenting hypoxemia.
- Take a heparinized blood sample anaerobically, cap with a rubber stopper, and analyze within 15–20 minutes.
- If the sample is stored on ice, results are valid for up to 3–4 hours if analysis must be delayed.
- Handheld analyzers are available for use with equine patients, or the sample may be sent to a commercial laboratory or hospital.

IMAGING

Radiography or ultrasound (with or without contrast enhancement) is very helpful in evaluating cardiac and pulmonary disease.

DIAGNOSTIC PROCEDURES

- Pulse oximetry can be used to measure and monitor hemoglobin saturation.
- The oximeter calculates the amount of oxygenated versus deoxygenated hemoglobin in blood based on light absorption.
- Inaccurate readings can be seen with decreased blood flow in the area where the probe is attached because of hypotension, vasoconstriction, or local or systemic hypothermia.
- Probes designed for the tongue or earlobe of other species can be used on the tongue of anesthetized horses.
- Conscious patients require use of a nasal probe.

TREATMENT

Resolution of the primary cause of hypoxemia is the most effective therapy.

OXYGEN THERAPY

- Oxygen therapy via nasal insufflation can be quite effective in elevating the PaO_2. Inspired concentrations are limited to 30%–45% with nasal insufflation. Higher levels may be obtained via insufflation directly into the trachea.
- Inspired gases must be humidified to avoid damage to mucous membranes from desiccation. This is readily accomplished by use of a humidifier or passing the oxygen through a bottle of sterile water before exposure to the airway. The bottle must be secured in an upright position to prevent inspiration of fluid.
- To avoid oxygen toxicity, maintain the FiO_2 at the lowest level that produces a PO_2 of >80 mm Hg. If insufflation eliminates hypoxemia, PCO_2 levels may increase if the low PO_2 was the primary stimulus of respiratory drive.
- Begin insufflation at 3–5 L/min in foals and 5–10 L/min in adults.

POSTURAL THERAPY AND THORACIC PERCUSSION

- Helpful to improve ventilation and drainage of secretions, especially in foals.
- Maintenance in sternal recumbency is best; turning every few hours is necessary for those in lateral recumbency.

MECHANICAL VENTILATION

- Necessary in patients with severe hypoventilation (PCO_2 persistently >65 mm Hg) and hypoxemia, and feasible in foals and anesthetized adults.
- Conscious foals can be intubated nasotracheally and connected to the rebreathing circuit of a small-animal anesthesia machine.
- Two flowmeters (or one that allows mixing of O_2 and room air) are necessary, as is a monitor that can measure FiO_2 level.
- Assisted rather than controlled ventilation usually is better, because most foals are more comfortable and respiratory drive is not eliminated, making weaning somewhat easier.
- Sedation may be necessary in some patients, but many relax once ventilation improves.
- Periodic suctioning of the nasotracheal tube is necessary to prevent obstruction from accumulated secretions.
- After weaning from mechanical ventilation, temporary nasal insufflation of oxygen is recommended in foals, because their functional residual capacity will decrease and hypoxemia may reoccur.

SUPPLEMENTAL OXYGEN

- Should improve PaO_2 levels with all causes of hypoxemia, except right-to-left cardiac shunts, persistent fetal circulation, and severe V/Q mismatch, which is essentially an intrapulmonary physiologic shunt.

MEDICATIONS

DRUGS OF CHOICE

- Supportive therapy aimed at improvement in any factors contributing to hypoxemia is useful.
- Hypovolemic or hypotensive patients benefit from fluid therapy and inotropes—dobutamine or dopamine
- Endotoxemic patients may improve with anti-inflammatory therapy.
- Bronchodilation may help in some respiratory conditions, especially small airway diseases.
- Methylxanthines or β_2-agonists (e.g., clenbuterol, albuterol) PO or via aerosol therapy may improve gas exchange in some cases if bronchospasm exists.
- Infusions of doxapram or methylxanthines (e.g., aminophylline, caffeine) may improve respiratory function in neonates.

HYPOXEMIA

CONTRAINDICATIONS

• Do not use doxapram to improve respiratory function in healthy anesthetized patients, especially during weaning. Its effects are temporaty, and if the patient's CO_2 levels are still low or the patient remains depressed once it wears off, apnea may occur.
• Mechanical ventilation for meconium aspiration because of the risk of air-trapping behind obstructed bronchioles and subsequent alveolar damage.

PRECAUTIONS

• Do not allow combustible materials or smoking in the vicinity of the patient or the tanks.
• Securely attach tanks to a wall or other immovable structure, because they can rupture or explode violently if knocked over.
• Wear safety glasses, and the operator should keep his or her face out of range of the valves during setup and disconnection.
• Use aseptic technique in handling endotracheal tubes to prevent secondary pneumonia.
• Side effects of methylxanthines and β_2-agonists are not uncommon; therapeutic doses are close to toxic doses. Monitor patients for restlessness, sweating, tachycardia, and arrhythmia.
• Use fluid therapy carefully in neonates and cardiac patients to avoid volume overload.
• Arrhythmias are not uncommon with inotrope therapy; monitor cardiac rhythm closely.
• Oxygen toxicity can occur with administration of $>50\%$ O_2 or maintenance of a PaO_2 >100 mm Hg for long periods.

POSSIBLE INTERACTIONS

• Cimetidine, erythromycin, and other inhibitors of hepatic microsomal activity may decrease clearance and increase serum levels of methylxanthines.
• Rifampin, chloramphenicol, and other inducers of hepatic metabolism decrease serum levels of xanthine derivatives by increasing clearance.

ALTERNATIVE DRUGS

N/A

FOLLOW-UP

PATIENT MONITORING

• Serial evaluation of arterial PO_2.
• Pulse oximetry can be used to monitor hemoglobin saturation. However, measure blood gases intermittently, because the hemoglobin-O_2 cannot be $>100\%$ even when the FiO_2 may be much higher.
• As the PaO_2 improves, provide decreasing levels of FiO_2. Eventually, periodic trials on room air can be attempted.
• Evaluate patient demeanor and degree or quality of respiratory effort as blood gas levels. When the patient can maintain a PO_2 of >70 mm Hg (>60 mm Hg in premature neonates) on room air, oxygen therapy may be discontinued.

HYPOXEMIA

POSSIBLE COMPLICATIONS

• Damage to nervous tissue from prolonged periods of hypoxemia may result in brain damage as exhibited by altered consciousness, blindness, seizures, and so on.
• Cardiac arrhythmias may be caused by hypoxemic damage to the myocardium.

MISCELLANEOUS

ASSOCIATED CONDITIONS

Metabolic acidosis caused by accumulation of lactic acid from anaerobic glycolysis may develop with prolonged hypoxemia, especially if hypotension exists.

AGE-RELATED FACTORS

Premature neonates are highly predisposed to hypoxemia.

ZOONOTIC POTENTIAL

N/A

PREGNANCY

• Heavily pregnant mares are at greater risk of hypoxemia under general anesthesia.
• Prolonged hypoxemia during gestation may result in fetal growth retardation and hypoxic-ischemic syndrome at parturition.

SYNONYMS

N/A

SEE ALSO

N/A

ABBREVIATIONS

• COPD = chronic obstructive pulmonary disease
• V/Q = ventilation-perfusion
• FiO_2 = fractional percent inspired oxygen concentration
• PaO_2 = partial pressure of arterial oxygen tension, mmHg
• $PaCO_2$ = partial pressure of arterial carbon dioxide tension, mmHg
• SaO_2 = arterial oxygen saturation—the % of hemoglobin sites that are bound to oxygen
• HbO_2 = hemoglobin saturation

Suggested Reading

Coons TJ, Kosch PC, Cudd TA. Respiratory care. In: Koterba AM, et al., eds. Equine clinical neonatology. Philadelphia: Lea & Febiger, 1990:200–239.

Hartsfield SM. Airway management and ventilation. In: Thurmon JC, et al., eds. Lumb & Jones' veterinary anesthesia. 3rd ed. Baltimore: Williams & Wilkins, 1996:515–556.

Haskins S. Monitoring the anesthetized patient. In: Thurmon JC, et al., eds. Lumb & Jones' veterinary anesthesia. 3rd ed. Baltimore: Williams & Wilkins, 1996:409–425.

McDonell W. Respiratory system. In: Thurmon JC, et al., eds. Lumb & Jones' veterinary anesthesia. 3rd ed. Baltimore: Williams & Wilkins, 1996:115–147.

Palmer J. Ventilatory support of the neonatal foal. Vet Clin North Am Equine Pract 1994;10:167–186.

Soma LR. Equine anesthesia: causes of reduced oxygen tension and increased carbon dioxide tensions. Compend Contin Educ Pract Vet 1980:2:S57–S63.

West JB. Respiratory physiology: the essentials. 5th ed. Baltimore: Williams & Wilkins, 1995.

Author Jennifer G. Adams
Consulting Editor Claire B. Andreasen

ICTERUS (PREHEPATIC, HEPATIC, AND POSTHEPATIC)

BASICS

DEFINITION

Hyperbilirubinemia with subsequent bilirubin deposition in tissues causes icterus, which is characterized by yellow discoloration of the sclerae, nonpigmented skin, and mucous membranes.

PATHOPHYSIOLOGY

- Bilirubin, the chief bile pigment, derives primarily from the breakdown of heme, which first is converted to biliverdin and then to unconjugated bilirubin. In turn, this is bound to albumin in plasma for transfer to the liver. It is water insoluble and is not removed by the kidneys.
- Unconjugated bilirubin is taken into the hepatocyte and conjugated, primarily to glucose but also to glucuronide.
- Some conjugated bilirubin, which is water soluble, enters the general circulation; if the concentration is high enough, it is filtered by the kidneys.
- Conjugated bilirubin is secreted into the bile and then enters the intestine, where most of it is converted by anaerobic bacteria to urobilinogen.
- Hyperbilirubinemia can result from increased bilirubin production, impaired hepatic uptake or conjugation of bilirubin, or impaired bilirubin excretion.

SYSTEMS AFFECTED

- Skin/exocrine—bilirubin has an affinity for elastic tissues; therefore, icterus is most evident in the sclera and vulva.
- Hepatobiliary—accumulated bilirubin may contribute to hepatocellular injury and cholestasis.
- Renal—bile casts may cause tubular injury.
- Nervous—bilirubin accumulation may cause degenerative lesions (i.e., kernicterus, a rare condition reported in neonates).

GENETICS

N/A

INCIDENCE/PREVALENCE

N/A

SIGNALMENT

All ages and breeds.

SIGNS

Historical Findings

- Icterus
- Dermatitis—photodermatitis from accumulation of phylloerythrin in skin
- Pruritus (uncommon)—from accumulation of bile salts in skin
- Severely altered mentation—HE attributed to hypoglycemia, hyperammonemia, decreased BCAA:AAA ratio, increased concentrations of mercaptans, sulfur-containing amino acids, and short-chain fatty acids in plasma
- Weight loss—anorexia and failure of hepatic metabolic functions (e.g., chronic liver disease)
- Diarrhea (uncommon)—altered intestinal microflora, portal hypertension, and bile acid deficiency (e.g., chronic liver disease)
- Acute or recurrent subacute abdominal pain—acute hepatocellular disease and biliary obstruction (i.e., cholelithiasis)
- Polydipsia and polyuria—sodium retention from increased blood aldosterone concentration and reduced medullary interstitial urea

Physical Examination Findings

- Fever—accompanies hepatic abscesses, acute hepatitis, chronic active hepatitis, obstructive cholelithiasis, or neoplasia
- Pain on palpation over right caudal rib area—swollen and painful liver
- Pale mucous membranes—icterus caused by hemolysis or intracorporeal blood loss
- Bleeding diathesis—inadequate hepatic synthesis of clotting factors
- Pigmenturia—hemolytic crisis in terminal liver failure or other causes of intravascular hemolysis
- Dependent edema (rare)—hypoalbuminemia or vascular thrombosis in ponies with lipemia

CAUSES

Prehepatic (Hemolytic) Icterus

- Intravascular hemolysis and/or extravascular hemolysis or with massive intracorporeal hemorrhage
- Oxidative injury—red maple-leaf (*Acer rubrum*) toxicosis, wild onion (*Allium* sp.) toxicosis, phenothiazine toxicosis, and nitrate poisoning
- Immune mediated—neonatal isoerythrolysis, IMHA (secondary to *Clostridium perfringens* septicemia, purpura hemorrhagica, lymphosarcoma, penicillin administration, etc.), AIHA, DIC (i.e., microangiopathic hemolytic anemia)
- Infectious—EIA, equine piroplasmosis, equine granulocytic ehrlichiosis, leptospirosis
- Iatrogenic—concentrated DMSO (>10%) IV and hypotonic or hypertonic fluids
- Miscellaneous—snake venoms (e.g., rattle snake, copper head, water moccasin) and terminal hepatic failure

Hepatic (Retention) Icterus

Impaired uptake and/or conjugation of bilirubin

Hepatic Causes of Hepatic Icterus

Acute hepatic diseases (adult horses):

- Idiopathic—Theiler's disease (i.e., serum hepatitis)
- Bacterial—secondary bacterial cholangiohepatitis (sequela to bile stasis), bacterial endotoxemia, primary bacterial cholangiohepatitis (e.g., *Salmonella* sp., *Escherichia coli*, other enteric bacteria), and infectious necrotic hepatitis (i.e., *Clostridium novyi* type B)
- Viral—EIA and EVA
- Parasitic—migration of *Strongylus equinus* and *S. edentatus* or thromboembolic disease from *S. equinus*
- Toxic—arsenic, carbon tetrachloride, chlorinated hydrocarbons, monensin, pentachlorophenols, phenol, phosphorus, paraquat, afflatoxin, and rubratoxin
- Drugs—anabolic steroids and erythromycin

Acute hepatic diseases (foals):

ICTERUS (PREHEPATIC, HEPATIC, AND POSTHEPATIC)

- Bacterial—Tyzzer's disease (i.e., *Bacillus piliformis*), bacterial septicemia, and bacterial endotoxemia
- Viral—EHV-1
- Parasitic—*Parascaris equorum* and strongyli
- Toxic—iron toxicity (i.e., ferrous fumarate) and toxins listed for adults

Chronic hepatic diseases (adults):

- Idiopathic—chronic active hepatitis
- Bacterial—hepatic abscessation (*Streptococcus equi*)
- Metabolic—hyperlipemia and hepatic lipidosis
- Neoplastic—primary (e.g., cholangiocarcinoma, hepatocellular carcinoma) and secondary (e.g., lymphosarcoma)
- Immunologic—amyloidosis
- Toxic—chronic megalocytic hepatopathy (e.g., *Senecio* sp., *Crotolaria* sp., *Heliotropium* sp.).

Chronic hepatic diseases (foals):

- Bacterial—hepatic abscessation (secondary to septicemia or ascending from omphalophlebitis)
- Neoplastic—mixed hamartoma

Extrahepatic Causes of Hepatic Icterus

- Anorexia
- Heparin administration
- Prematurity
- Congenital deficiencies of hepatocellular binding proteins or conjugating enzymes—Criggler-Najjar–like syndrome

Posthepatic (Obstructive) Icterus

- Partial or complete obstruction of the biliary tree that inhibits biliary excretion of conjugated bilirubin.
- Usually accompanied by bilirubinuria
- Adults—cholelithiasis, large colon displacement, cholangitis, neoplastic infiltration, fibrosis or hyperplasia of the biliary tract, and hepatitis
- Foals—acquired biliary obstruction (i.e., healing duodenal ulcer adjacent to hepatopancreatic ampulla) or congenital biliary atresia

RISK FACTORS

- Previous administration of equine-origin biologic (i.e., tetanus antitoxin)—Theiler's disease
- Septicemia or omphalophlebitis in foals—hepatic abscessation
- Duodenal ulceration—neonatal acquired biliary obstruction
- Poor parasite control—hepatic ascarid and strongyli migration
- Inadequate vaccination—EHV-1 in foals and EVA in adults
- Exposure to toxic plants and environmental toxins—hepatocellular damage or hemolysis
- Use of certain drugs—macrolides, anabolic steroids, and heparin
- Biliary stasis (secondary cholangitis)—cholelithiasis, hepatic neoplasia, pancreatitis, enterocolitis, intestinal parasitism, intestinal obstruction
- Obese pony or miniature horse with anorexia—hyperlipemia

DIAGNOSIS

DIFFERENTIAL DIAGNOSIS

- Prehepatic icterus generally is characterized by abrupt onset of exercise intolerance, weakness, fever, tachypnea and dyspnea, tachycardia, mucous membrane pallor, mild jaundice, and in some cases, pigmenturia.
- History and clinical signs for hepatic and posthepatic icterus are quite similar but differ from those of prehepatic icterus.
- Signs generally not reported in horses with prehepatic icterus—photodermatitis, pruritus, severely altered mentation, chronic weight loss, diarrhea, and abdominal pain.
- The hemolytic crisis that occurs in some horses with terminal liver failure could lead to a misdiagnosis of prehepatic icterus.
- Icterus generally is more pronounced in posthepatic than hepatic icterus, because conjugated bilirubin causes more pronounced icterus than similar amounts of unconjugated bilirubin.
- Recurrent abdominal pain is a frequent feature of posthepatic icterus, as is pyrexia caused by secondary bacterial cholangitis.

CBC/BIOCEHEMISTRY/URINALYSIS

Prehepatic Icterus

- Severe anemia (usually regenerative), Heinz bodies, and spherocytes
- Marked increase in unconjugated bilirubin (80 mg/dL), with some increase in conjugated bilirubin
- Mildly increased ALP and SDH
- Normal to low glucose
- Normal to high BUN
- Normal albumin
- Bilirubinuria

Hepatic Icterus

- Mild, nonregenerative anemia
- Moderate increase in unconjugated bilirubin (rarely >25 mg/dL), and mild to moderate increase in conjugated bilirubin (up to 25% of total bilirubin)
- Mild to moderate increases in GGT, AST, and SDH; mild increase in ALP
- Normal to low glucose
- Normal to low BUN
- Normal to low albumin
- Normal to slight increase in urinary bilirubin
- Normal to low urinary urobilinogen

Posthepatic Icterus

- Mild, nonregenerative anemia
- Normal to mild increase in unconjugated bilirubin; marked increase in conjugated bilirubin (>25–50% of total bilirubin)
- Normal to mild increase in AST and SDH; moderate to marked increase in GGT; and marked increase in ALP

ICTERUS (PREHEPATIC, HEPATIC, AND POSTHEPATIC)

- Albumin, glucose, and BUN often are normal
- Marked bilirubinuria
- Urinary urobilinogen (absent) with complete bile duct obstruction.

OTHER LABORATORY TESTS

Prehepatic Icterus

- Giemsa or NMB stain for intraerythrocytic parasites
- Saline agglutination test
- Direct antiglobulin (Coombs') test
- Osmotic fragility test

Hepatic and Posthepatic Icterus

- Serum bile acids—highest in obstructive liver disease, but not discriminating
- Blood ammonia concentration not correlated with severity of hepatic encephalopathy and not discriminating
- Serum prothrombin time may be prolonged, but not discriminating
- Serology for infectious diseases (e.g., EIA, EVA, leptospirosis) in patients with hepatic icterus
- Serum triglycerides—marked increased in hyperlipemia
- Clearance of foreign dyes (BSP) is not discriminating.

IMAGING

Utrasonography for:

- Determining general liver size
- Demonstrating changes in hepatic parenchyma—abscesses, cysts, and neoplastic masses
- Detecting dilated bile ducts or obstructions with choleliths
- Demonstrating (sometimes) abnormal intra- or extrahepatic blood flow
- Guiding biopsy

DIAGNOSTIC PROCEDURES

Liver biopsy:

- Yields diagnostic, prognostic, and therapeutic information.
- Samples—obtained using blind or ultrasound-guided percutaneous techniques; in formalin for histopathologic evaluation and transport media for microbiologic culture
- Complications—hemorrhage, pneumothorax, spread of infectious hepatitis, and peritonitis (i.e., contamination with bile or colonic ingesta)
- Complications minimized by performing hemostasis profile and using ultrasound guidance.

TREATMENT

APPROPRIATE HEALTH CARE

Varies, depending on the underlying cause.

NURSING CARE

- In the first 24 hours, use IV fluid therapy (5% dextrose at 2 mL/kg per hour) for hypoglycemic patients with signs of HE.
- After 24 hours, substitute 2.5–5% dextrose in lactated Ringer solution (60 mL/kg per day).
- In anorexic patients, add potassium chloride (20–40 mEq/L) to fluids.
- Treatment can best be accomplished in a hospital environment.

ACTIVITY

Restrict activity, and avoid sunlight.

DIET

For patients with hepatic and posthepatic icterus, a diet that provides 40–50 kcal/kg in the form of low-protein, high-energy feeds rich in BCAAs (e.g., milo, sorghum, beet pulp) is recommended.

CLIENT EDUCATION

Foals nursing from hyperlipemic ponies should be weaned.

SURGICAL CONSIDERATIONS

Surgery may be required in foals with acquired bile duct obstruction or horses with colonic displacement causing acute bile duct obstruction.

MEDICATIONS

DRUGS OF CHOICE

Prehepatic Icterus

- Treatment of IMHA with parenteral corticosteroids.
- Whole-blood transfusion is indicated in patients with PCV <10–12% and/or exhibiting signs of hypoxia.
- Fluid therapy (lactated Ringer's solution [60 mL/kg per day]) to promote diuresis.

Hepatic and Posthepatic Icterus

- Manage clinical signs of HE with sedation (e.g., xylazine [0.5–1.0 mg/kg], diazepam [0.05–0.4 mg/kg]) if the patient is convulsing, and decrease production and absorption of toxic metabolites (mineral oil via nasogastric tube: lactulose [0.3 ml/kg PO q6h] or neomycin [10–100 mg/kg PO q6h]). Oral BCAA concentrates can be formulated, and IV preparations are available.
- Weekly supplementation with vitamin K_1 (40–50 mg/450 kg SQ) as well as vitamin B_1 and folic acid when cholestasis is present.
- Antimicrobial therapy is based on results of culture and sensitivity. Empiric therapy for suppurative cholangitis includes trimethoprim-sulfamethoxazole or a β-lactam and an aminoglycoside. Use metronidazole if an anaerobic infection is suspected.

ICTERUS (PREHEPATIC, HEPATIC, AND POSTHEPATIC)

• Chronic active hepatitis is treated with corticosteroids—dexamethasone (0.05–0.1 mg/kg per day for 4–7 days, then gradually tapering the dose over 2–3 weeks), followed by prednisolone (1 mg/kg for several weeks).

CONTRAINDICATIONS

• Hepatotoxic drugs—anticonvulsants, anabolic steroids, phenothiazines, and macrolides (e.g., erythromycin).
• Tetracyclines, which suppress hepatic protein synthesis.
• Drugs eliminated primarily by the liver—analgesics, anesthetics, barbiturates, and chloramphenicol

PRECAUTIONS

• Avoid use of the antimicrobials listed above.
• Use sedatives (e.g., xylazine, diazepam) at reduced dosages, because they are metabolized by the liver.
• Use corticosteroids cautiously, because they may exacerbate intercurrent infections.

POSSIBLE INTERACTIONS

For many drugs, duration and intensity of action may be increased in patients with hepatobiliary disease.

FOLLOW-UP

PATIENT MONITORING

Prehepatic Icterus

• Recheck PCV as needed.
• Repeat transfusions may be required.

Hepatic and Posthepatic Icterus

• Monitor liver enzyme activities and bilirubin concentration as dictated by the disease.
• Repeat liver biopsies may be indicated to monitor disease progression.

PREVENTION/AVOIDANCE

N/A

POSSIBLE COMPLICATIONS

Horses that are icteric because of anorexia or cholestatic drugs (e.g., heparin) do not suffer long-term complications.

EXPECTED COURSE AND PROGNOSIS

N/A

MISCELLANEOUS

ASSOCIATED CONDITIONS

Prehepatic Icterus

• Hemoglobinemic nephrosis
• Hemic murmur

Hepatic Icterus

• Hepatoencephalopathy
• Photodermatitis
• Pruritus
• Diarrhea
• Colic
• Coagulopathy
• Terminal hemolytic crisis
• See *Signs.*

AGE RELATED FACTORS

• Foals—biliary atresia, Tyzzer's disease, EHV-1 hepatitis, and neonatal isoerythrolysis commonly cause icterus.
• Adults—cholelithiasis, Theiler's disease, and megalocytic hepatopathy commonly cause icterus
• See *Differential Diagnosis.*

ZOONOTIC POTENTIAL

Leptospirosis may affect humans.

PREGNANCY

Pregnant and lactating, obese ponies and miniature horses susceptible to hyperlipemia.

SYNONYMS

• Hyperbilirubinemia
• Jaundice

SEE ALSO

• Hemolytic anemia
• Liver disease topics

ABBREVIATIONS

• AAA = aromatic amino acids
• AIHA = autoimmune-mediated hemolytic anemia
• ALP = alkaline phosphatase
• AST = aspartate aminotransferase
• BCAA = branched-chain amino acid
• BSP = bromosulphothalein
• DIC = disseminated intravascular coagulation
• DMSO = dimethyl sulfoxide
• EIA = equine infectious anemia
• EHV-1 = equine herpes virus 1
• EVA = equine viral arteritis
• GGT = γ-glutamyltransferase
• HE = hepatoencephalopathy
• IMHA = immune-mediated hemolytic anemia
• NMB = new methylene blue
• PCV = packed cell volume
• SDH = sorbitol dehydrogenase

Suggested Reading

Barton MH, Morris DD. Diseases of the liver. In: Reed SM, Bayly WM, eds. Equine internal medicine. Philadelphia: WB Saunders, 1998.

Engelking LR, Paradis MR. Evaluation of hepatobiliary diseases in horses. Vet Clin North Am Equine Pract 1987;3:563–583.

Meyer DJ, Coles EH, Rich LJ. Hepatic test abnormalities. In: Meyer DJ, Coles EH, Rich LJ, eds. Veterinary laboratory medicine: interpretation and diagnosis. Philadelphia: WB Saunders, 1992.

Author Jeanne Lofstedt
Consulting Editor Michel Levy

IDIOPATHIC COLITIS

BASICS

DEFINITION
An inflammatory condition involving the large colon resulting in a variety of clinical signs, the most prominent of which is diarrhea. The cause is unknown, and it was formerly referred to as *colitis X.*

PATHOPHYSIOLOGY
In the adult horse, diarrhea represents a disturbance of the normal balance in fluid and electrolyte secretion and absorption in the large intestine. Due to the variety of possible causes, the exact pathophysiology in cases of idiopathic colitis cannot be determined.

SYSTEMS AFFECTED
Gastrointestinal

The main clinical sign in idiopathic colitis is diarrhea. Signs of colic varying from mild to severe may be present.

Cardiovascular

Varying degrees of dehydration and cardiovascular shock may be present. Venous thrombosis of injection or catheter sites can occur, mainly due to the presence of endotoxemia.

Musculoskeletal

Laminitis is a serious secondary problem that may develop in affected animals. Peripheral edema commonly occurs due to hypoproteinemia.

Respiratory

Septic emboli leading to pulmonary abscess formation may be observed in the lungs.

GENETICS
There is no known genetic basis for idiopathic colitis.

INCIDENCE/PREVALENCE
Idiopathic colitis is a sporadic condition.

SIGNALMENT
There are no reported breed, age, or sex predilections. Foals as young as 24 hr of age may be affected.

SIGNS
Historical Findings

Occasionally, animals may be presented before the development of diarrhea with depression, anorexia, and pyrexia. When present, diarrhea can range from cow-pie consistency to profuse and watery, and may be hemorrhagic. There may be a history of recent antibiotic use. Feeding, deworming, transport, and other management changes (stressors) may have occurred.

Physical Examination Findings

Diarrhea is present in most cases. Dehydration may be present and can be detected by the presence of decreased skin turgor, tacky oral mucous membranes, and increased capillary refill time. Rectal temperature is increased in many cases of colitis, although it may also be normal or subnormal. Tachycardia is often present. Gastrointestinal sounds have a fluid nature, and may be hypermotile or hypomotile. Characteristic sounds may be detected on auscultation of the ventral abdomen in colitis secondary to chronic sand impaction. Signs of endotoxemia such as hyperemic mucous membranes may be present. Marked intestinal distension may be present, especially in peracute, severe cases, and may cause colic. Peripheral edema may be present secondary to hypoproteinemia or vasculitis.

CAUSES
It is likely that there are a variety of enteric pathogens that are involved in a significant percentage of cases of idiopathic colitis, but are not recognized. Pathogens currently recognized as causing colitis in horses include *Salmonella* spp., *Clostridium difficile, C. perfringens, Ehrlichia risticii,* and cyathostomes. Other possible causes include NSAIDs, cantharadins, and chronic sand impaction. Toxins (e.g., heavy metals, mycotoxins) may be involved in some cases.

RISK FACTORS
Many are postulated, including transportation, dietary changes, surgery, and other gastrointestinal disorders (e.g., impactions). Antibiotic use is a well-documented risk factor and is presumed to be a significant one in the horse.

DIAGNOSIS

DIFFERENTIAL DIAGNOSES
- Salmonellosis
- *Clostridium difficile* enterocolitis
- Potomac horse fever
- *Clostridium perfringens* enterocolitis
- Cyathostomiasis
- NSAID-induced colitis
- Cantharidin toxicosis
- Chronic sand impaction

CBC/BIOCHEMISTRY/URINALYSIS
CBC

The packed cell volume is often elevated, indicative of hemoconcentration from dehydration. In some cases serum total protein levels are increased, reflecting hemoconcentration. In other cases they are decreased despite hemoconcentration, as there is protein loss into the gastrointestinal tract. Leukopenia with neutropenia is often present early, frequently with a left shift, depending on the severity and stage of disease. Toxic changes may be present in neutrophils. At later stages of disease or in milder cases, a leukocytosis and neutrophilia may be present.

Biochemistry

Serum sodium and chloride levels are typically decreased. Potassium levels may be increased in animals with a metabolic acidosis, or decreased concurrently with sodium and chloride, especially in anorexic animals. Hypocalcemia and hypoalbuminemia are also common. These losses are likely due to secretion of electrolyte- and protein-rich fluid into the intestinal lumen. A prerenal azotemia is common in dehydrated animals. These are usually only mild elevations and return to normal after rehydration. If more significant elevations are present, urea and creatinine levels plus urinalysis should be monitored.

Urinalysis

An increase in urine specific gravity is frequently present as a response to dehydration.

OTHER LABORATORY TESTS

- Acid–base assessment: In severe cases a marked metabolic acidosis develops, and the extent of negative base–excess has been used as a prognostic indicator for survival.
- As idiopathic colitis is a diagnosis of exclusion, appropriate samples should be submitted to rule out the common infectious causes of colitis. In endemic areas, hay should be inspected for the presence of *Epicauta* beetles.

IMAGING

Abdominal Ultrasonography

The large colon may appear fluid filled and excess motility may be observed. Edematous large colon may be identified.

DIAGNOSTIC PROCEDURES

Rectal palpation should be performed to ensure that other problems, such as a surgical lesion, are not present. This should be performed with caution, as the rectal mucosa may be friable.

PATHOLOGIC FINDINGS

Gross pathologic findings are variable. The only abnormality visible may be fluid intestinal contents. More severe cases may have marked intestinal edema and hemorrhage, with petechiae and ecchymoses. Histologically, evidence of mild inflammation to severe hemorrhagic necrotizing enterocolitis may be present.

TREATMENT

APPROPRIATE HEALTH CARE

This condition is best managed with intensive inpatient care. If the diarrhea is not very severe and adequate hydration can be maintained, treatment on the farm could be attempted. If this treatment option is chosen, close monitoring is required because affected animals may deteriorate quickly.

NURSING CARE

Intravenous fluid therapy is the most important factor in treatment using a balanced electrolyte solution (e.g., lactated Ringer's solution). The rate of fluid administration depends on the degree of dehydration and the amount and fluid content of the diarrhea. In severely dehydrated animals, intravenous administration of up to 1 L/min for the first 30 min can greatly improve hydration status. This can be accomplished with a fluid pump system. The use of two large-bore catheters in separate veins can also deliver a large volume of fluid without the need for a pump system. The remaining fluid deficit should be corrected over 12–24 hr. After correction of dehydration, intravenous administration of maintenance fluids (50–100 mL/kg/day) plus the estimated fluid loss through diarrhea should be continued. Once the diarrhea begins to resolve, the fluid rate can be decreased. Hydration status should be assessed frequently because affected animals may become dehydrated even in the presence of fluid therapy. Mild to moderate cases of metabolic acidosis typically resolve with fluid therapy. Sodium bicarbonate may be required in certain cases to correct a severe metabolic acidosis. In severely hypokalemic horses, 20–40 mEq/L of potassium chloride can be added to lactated Ringer's solution or saline. Intravenous administration of KCl should not exceed 0.5 mEq/kg/hr.

An oral electrolyte solution containing 35 g KCl and 70 g NaCl in 10 L of water should be provided, along with clean, fresh drinking water.

Intravenous administration of hypertonic saline (4–6 mL/kg of 5–7.5% NaCl) may be indicated in severely dehydrated animals. It is essential that isotonic fluid therapy follow the use of hypertonic saline.

Due to the high incidence of venous thrombosis in colitis, the catheter site should be monitored frequently.

If distal limb edema develops due to hypoproteinemia, leg wraps should be applied and changed daily.

Deep bedding should be provided if there are any signs of laminitis.

ACTIVITY

Due to the need for continuous intravenous fluid therapy in most cases, stall confinement is required. Diarrhetic horses should be considered infectious and managed appropriately.

DIET

Affected horses should be provided with free-choice hay. It is recommended to feed hay in a hay-net because hypoproteinemic horses eating off the ground may develop severe facial edema. Higher-energy feeds can also be provided, but should be introduced slowly. Large amounts of grain should be avoided. Anorexic animals may benefit from forced enteral feeding. Partial or total parenteral nutrition may be indicated, but is expensive.

CLIENT EDUCATION

Clients should be made aware that colitis is a potentially life-threatening condition, with the potential for the development of secondary problems, such as laminitis and jugular vein thrombosis. In multi-horse environments, it is important to explain the risk of infection to other animals and be made aware that salmonellosis and possibly *C. difficile* colitis are zoonotic.

SURGICAL CONSIDERATION

N/A

IDIOPATHIC COLITIS

MEDICATIONS

DRUG(S) OF CHOICE

Antimicrobial Agents

The use of these drugs in idiopathic colitis is controversial. In a noncontrolled clinical trial, metronidazole (15–25 mg/kg q6–8hr) has been reported to be useful in the treatment of idiopathic colitis. Zinc bacitracin (50 g of feed additive containing 110 g active zinc bacitracin/kg cereal base carrier q24 hr until diarrhea has resolved) has been used by some clinicians successfully in the treatment of idiopathic colitis, although controlled clinical trials supporting this treatment are lacking. Broad-spectrum antibiotic therapy may be indicated in animals that are severely leukopenic or exhibiting signs of endotoxemia. Ceftiofur sodium (2 mg/kg IV or IM q12 h) may be used; however, this drug has been implicated anecdotally as a cause of clostridial colitis. Trimethoprim–sulfamethoxazole (24 mg/kg IV q12hr) also provides broad-spectrum antibiotic coverage.

Flunixin Meglumine

A dose of 0.25 mg/kg q8hr can be used for its purported anti-endotoxic effects. A dose of 1.1 mg/kg can be used for analgesia in horses displaying signs of colic.

Fresh-frozen plasma is beneficial in severely hypoproteinemic animals (<40 g/L); 3–10 L of plasma can be given intravenously, with close attention paid to the recipient for signs of transfusion reaction.

Hyperimmune Serum

Some clinicians believe that the use of serum from horses hyperimmunized to *E. coli* J5 strain helps moderate the effects of endotoxemia.

Lamitinis Treatment

See Laminitis.

CONTRAINDICATIONS

Metronidazole may be teratogenic, and is therefore contraindicated in pregnant mares.

PRECAUTIONS

The 1.1 mg/kg dose of flunixin meglumine may be nephrotoxic in dehydrated animals. Bacitracin and metronidazole should not be used concurrently; combined effects of these two antibiotics on the intestinal microflora are unknown.

POSSIBLE INTERACTIONS

Cimetidine should not be used concurrently with metronidazole because there is interaction through hepatic inhibition.

ALTERNATIVE DRUGS

N/A

FOLLOW-UP

PATIENT MONITORING

Patients should be monitored frequently. Initially, packed cell volume and total protein levels should be evaluated at least daily. If azotemia was present on presentation, this should be re-evaluated after rehydration to ensure it was pre-renal and not due to renal failure. Serum or plasma electrolytes should be monitored to determine whether supplementation, especially with potassium and calcium, is required. The intravenous catheter site should be monitored frequently. The feet should be checked frequently for increased digital pulses or hoof wall temperature, indicative of laminitis.

PREVENTION/AVOIDANCE

Antibiotics should be used judiciously to decrease the risk of disruption of the gastrointestinal microflora.

POSSIBLE COMPLICATIONS

- Endotoxemia
- Laminitis
- Jugular vein thrombosis
- Renal failure

IDIOPATHIC COLITIS

EXPECTED COURSE AND PROGNOSIS

There is a wide variety in the severity of idiopathic colitis. Overall mortality rates for colitis in animals presented to referral centers has been reported to range from 10% to 40%.

MISCELLANEOUS

ASSOCIATED CONDITIONS

- Laminitis
- Venous thrombosis

AGE-RELATED FACTORS

None

ZOONOTIC POTENTIAL

All affected horses should be treated as zoonotic until shown to be negative for *Salmonella* spp. and *C. difficile.*

PREGNANCY

Metronidazole should not be administered to pregnant mares. An increased risk of abortion may be present due to endotoxemia and hypovolemic shock.

SYNONYMS

Colitis X

SEE ALSO

- Laminitis
- Salmonellosis
- *Clostridium difficile* enterocolitis
- Potomac horse fever
- Sand impaction
- Cantharidin toxicosis
- Endotoxemia

ABBREVIATIONS

N/A

Suggested Reading

Cohen ND, Divers TJ. Acute colitis in horses. Part 1. Assessment. Comp Contin Educ Pract Vet. 1998;20:92-98.

Cohen ND, Divers TJ. Acute colitis in horses. Part II. Initial management. Comp Contin Educ Pract Vet. 1998;20:228-233.

McGorum BC, Dixon PM, Smith DG. Use of metronidazole in equine acute idiopathic toxaemic colitis. Vet Rec. 1998;142:635-638.

Staempfli HR, Prescott JF, Carman RJ, McCutcheon LJ. Use of bacitracin in the prevention and treatment of experimentally-induced idiopathic colitis in horses. Can J Vet Res. 1992;56:233-236.

Staempfli HR, Townsend HGG, Prescott JF. Prognostic features and clincial presentation of acute idiopathic enterocolitis in horses. Can Vet J. 1991;32:232-237.

Author J. Scott Weese

Consulting Editor Henri Stämpfli

IDIOPATHIC TRANSIENT SPINAL ATAXIA IN LATE WEANLINGS

BASICS

DEFINITION
Transient cervical spinal cord ataxia of late weanlings

PATHOPHYSIOLOGY
Unknown

SYSTEM AFFECTED
CNS

SIGNALMENT
- Late weanlings of either sex can be affected.
- No breed predilection has been identified.
- The author has seen this condition in Thoroughbreds, Quarter Horses, Arabian breeds, and mixed-breed horses.

SIGNS

Historical Findings

Foals apparently are neurologically normal until late in the first year of life.

Physical Examination Findings

Symmetric cervical spinal ataxia in otherwise normal foals

CAUSES
Unknown

RISK FACTORS
Unknown

DIAGNOSIS
Foals with no cerebral spinal fluid, radiographic, or other abnormalities

DIFFERENTIAL DIAGNOSIS
- Cervical vertebral malformation
- Transient cerebellar disease

CBC/BIOCHEMISTRY/URINALYSIS
No specific abnormalities

OTHER LABORATORY TESTS
N/A

IMAGING
Radiographic findings are within normal limits.

DIAGNOSTIC PROCEDURES
N/A

PATHOLOGIC FINDINGS
Foals recover, so no pathologic features are known.

TREATMENT
- No treatment is indicated.
- Foals recover after a few months, usually by the following spring.

MEDICATIONS

DRUGS OF CHOICE
N/A

CONTRAINDICATIONS
N/A

PRECAUTIONS
N/A

POSSIBLE INTERACTIONS
N/A

ALTERNATIVE DRUGS
N/A

IDIOPATHIC TRANSIENT SPINAL ATAXIA IN LATE WEANLINGS

FOLLOW-UP

PATIENT MONITORING
N/A

POSSIBLE COMPLICATIONS
N/A

PROGNOSIS
Good

MISCELLANEOUS

ASSOCIATED CONDITIONS
N/A

AGE-RELATED FACTORS
Seen in late weanling foals, often in the fall of the year.

ZOONOTIC POTENTIAL
N/A

PREGNANCY
N/A

SYNONYMS
N/A

SEE ALSO
N/A

Suggested Reading

N/A

Author Joseph J. Bertone
Consulting Editor Joseph J. Bertone

ILEAL HYPERTROPHY

BASICS

OVERVIEW

Ileal hypertrophy is hypertrophy of the muscular layers of the ileum and results in a decrease in the luminal diameter. It is either a primary idiopathic condition or secondary to an aboral stenosis. Suggested etiologies for the primary idiopathic hypertrophy include inflammation of the ileal mucosa, including mucosal edema; an imbalance in the autonomic nervous system; and dysfunction of the ileocecal valve. Ileocecal intussusception is a cause of distal stenosis that can in turn cause a compensatory muscular hypertrophy of the ileum. Parasitic damage may be associated with mucosal irritation. There is an increased risk of ileal impaction in horses with tapeworm burdens, and the same may be true of ileal hypertrophy. Hemomelasma ilei is a common finding in horses with ileal hypertrophy. Failure of normal cecal motility has also been proposed as an etiologic factor.

SIGNALMENT

Occurs in adult horses of all ages, but tends to be more frequent in mature horses. There is no sex or breed predilection.

SIGNS

Clinical signs are dependent on the degree of luminal obstruction. Horses with partial obstruction have intermittent pain of mild to moderate severity. The small intestine is often hypermotile. Colic episodes are worse after eating; horses can become anorectic and exhibit weight loss if the condition is chronic. If complete obstruction occurs, horses develop a more severe, continuous colic with ileus and nasogastric reflux.

CAUSES AND RISK FACTORS

Risk factors for idiopathic hypertrophy are unknown, although poor parasite control and poor-quality roughage may be contributory factors. With compensatory ileal hypertrophy, risk factors also include parasitism and poor-quality roughage, as well as intestinal neoplasia, lipoma formation, and previous abdominal surgeries (adhesions).

DIAGNOSIS

DIFFERENTIAL DIAGNOSIS

Ileal impactions and ileocecal intussusception may be associated with ileal muscular hypertrophy, and the treatments are similar. Conservative therapy is attempted, but progression of clinical signs, and in particular increasing small intestinal distension are indicators for surgical intervention. One study found a relationship between duration of colic signs prior to surgery and rate of survival for ileal impaction; however, successful medical treatment has also been reported.

There is little evidence that these conditions can be differentiated by examination per rectum; however, ileocecal intussusception has a characteristic ultrasonographic "target" image. Adhesions may be detected per rectum, and may be suspected following previous abdominal surgery.

Small intestinal displacement (epiploic foramen) and strangulating lipomas can be difficult to diagnose, but the acute onset and severe colic signs differentiate them from ileal hypertrophy, and further diagnosis is often made via exploratory celiotomy. The diagnosis of small intestinal inguinal herniation is made via scrotal palpation.

CBC/BIOCHEMISTRY/URINALYSIS

There are no specific laboratory tests for ileal hypertrophy.

OTHER LABORATORY TESTS

Abdominocentesis is useful, but there are no abnormalities specific to ileal hypertrophy. Biopsy of the ileum at the time of exploratory celiotomy may be used to confirm the diagnosis.

IMAGING

Ultrasound images of the ileum may detect ileal hypertrophy and are likely to detect the presence of small intestinal distension orally and small intestinal hypermotility. The hypertrophied wall of the ileum is usually between 15- and 25-mm thick, becoming less thick orally. Narrowing of the ileal lumen may also be discernible. Ultrasonography of the ileum is usually performed from the right dorsal paralumbar fossa, but transrectal ultrasound may be beneficial, particularly when the thickened ileum is palpable.

DIAGNOSTIC PROCEDURES

Rectal examination findings may include a thickened ileum palpable in the right dorsal quadrant and loops of distended small intestine. Not all cases have these findings, and the diagnosis may only be revealed after evaluation of a biopsy of the ileum taken at the time of exploratory celiotomy. Passage of a nasogastric tube is mandatory to test for the presence of reflux.

ILEAL HYPERTROPHY

PATHOLOGIC FINDINGS

There is muscular hypertrophy of both circular and longitudinal smooth muscle layers for variable lengths along the ileum, and possibly also the jejunum. Individual muscle cells are enlarged, with elongated vesicular nuclei. Mucosal diverticula through the muscularis layer were found in approximately half of the specimens from one study. Fibrosis of the mucosa is often present, and may indicate parasitic damage or damage from a resolved intussusception.

TREATMENT

Surgical treatments include ileal myotomy, ileocecal bypass, and jejunocecostomy. Ileal myotomy consists of longitudinal incisions made through the serosa and muscularis to allow expansion of the submucosa and relief of the ileal obstruction. This technique is not considered the treatment of choice, particularly if there are abnormalities in ileal motility, or if there is a dysfunction of the ileocecal valve. Ileocecal bypass has been used, but ingesta may still pass through the ileum, causing pain. In addition, complications associated with this anastomosis are more likely if the ileum is markedly thickened at the anastomosis. A jejunocecostomy with blind stumping of the ileum distally and removal of the proximal ileum may be the treatment of choice.

A laxative diet may be palliative in horses in which surgery is not an option.

MEDICATIONS

DRUG(S) OF CHOICE

Medical therapy for colic and ileus is mentioned elsewhere. There is no specific medication for ileal hypertrophy.

CONTRAINDICATIONS/POSSIBLE INTERACTIONS

Prokinetics may exacerbate colic pain severity if there is a partial or complete intestinal obstruction. Similarly, gastrointestinal osmotic cathartics, such as Epsom salts, may increase proximal small intestinal distension.

FOLLOW-UP

Routine post-surgical monitoring for colic cases is required. Prognosis after surgical correction is considered good, provided that the hypertrophy is focal (i.e., the proximal small intestine is normal).

MISCELLANEOUS

ASSOCIATED CONDITIONS

See Differential Diagnosis.

AGE-RELATED FACTORS

There are little data on age related factors, but whereas compensatory ileal hypertrophy may occur in horses of any age, idiopathic muscular hypertrophy appears to be more common in mature horses. In one study of 11 cases of idiopathic ileal muscular hypertrophy, the age range was 5–18 yr with a median age of 10 yr.

Suggested Reading

Chaffin MK, Carmen Fuenteabla I, Schumacher J, et al. Idiopathic muscular hypertrophy of the equine small intestine: 11 cases (1980–1991). Equine Vet J 1992;24:372-378.

Author Simon G. Pearce
Consulting Editor Henry Stämpfli

ILEUS

BASICS

DEFINITION

A loss or reduction of intestinal motility that results in impaired aboral transit of ingesta. Ileus can be further classified as paralytic (adynamic) ileus to differentiate it from obstructive causes of impaired intestinal transit. Obstructive intestinal diseases are sometimes referred to as *obstructive ileus.*

PATHOPHYSIOLOGY

The enteric nervous system is well developed and is primarily under control from the autonomic nervous system. Gastrointestinal motility is stimulated by parasympathetic activity (acetylcholine), whereas sympathetic stimulation (norepinephrine) has an inhibitory effect. Other neurotransmitters such as serotonin and dopamine also play a role in regulating gastrointestinal activity. Many reflexes are present that are essential to proper functioning of intestinal motility, some of which occur locally within the enteric nervous system and are responsible for peristalsis and mixing contractions. Other reflexes travel to sympathetic ganglia, the spinal cord, or the brain stem to coordinate more complex activities, such as the gastrocolic reflex, in which signals from the stomach cause evacuation of the colon, and pain reflexes, which cause generalized inhibition of the gastrointestinal tract. Knowledge of normal control mechanisms of intestinal motility allows for insight into some of the causes of ileus. For example, intestinal distension can cause pain, which reflexively causes ileus. Pain can also cause a systemic release of epinephrine from the adrenal medullae, which decreases intestinal motility. Knowledge of motility regulating mechanisms has also helped in the development of treatments for this condition. Adynamic ileus most commonly affects the small intestine and can occur as a sequel to numerous diseases that affect the gastrointestinal tract. It is a frequent sequel to gastrointestinal surgery. Other factors that potentiate ileus include pain, endotoxemia, electrolyte imbalances, and certain drugs. Cecal impaction is a common manifestation of ileus of the large intestine. The pathogenesis of cecal impaction is poorly understood; however, there appears to be a correlation between its development and painful musculoskeletal injuries or orthopedic surgery.

SYSTEMS AFFECTED

Gastrointestinal

Cardiovascular

Hypovolemia due to fluid sequestration in the intestinal tract can result in depressed cardiovascular function. Endotoxemia can further contribute to depressed cardiac function.

SIGNALMENT

No age, breed, or sex predilections.

SIGNS

Historical Findings

Depression, mild to moderate signs of abdominal pain, anorexia and decreased fecal output. Adynamic ileus can occur secondary to many diseases (see Causes). Historical findings that are consistent with a primary disease may also be present.

Physical Examination Findings

Heart rate and respiratory rate are often elevated due to abdominal discomfort, and the horse usually exhibits mild to severe signs of colic. Signs associated with hypovolemia are often present due to intestinal sequestration of fluids. Abdominal auscultation usually reveals an absence or reduction of borborygmi (although some intestinal sounds may be present due to non-peristaltic motility). On palpation per rectum, small intestinal loops may be present if small intestinal distension is pronounced. In cases of cecal impaction, the impaction may be palpable or tension on the base of the cecum may be identified due to the weight of the impaction. Passage of a nasogastric tube is a vital diagnostic and therapeutic tool. Build-up of fluid in the stomach occurs because of a lack of progressive motility. Decompression with a nasogastric tube not only prevents gastric rupture and provides pain relief, but it also allows for the volume of fluid to be quantified for intravenous replacement fluid therapy, thereby providing a rough estimate of the severity of disease.

CAUSES

Adynamic ileus can be induced by virtually any intestinal insult. Causes of ileus include intestinal distension or impaction, enteritis/colitis, and serosal irritation from abdominal surgery or peritonitis. Ileus can also be caused by vascular or obstructive intestinal injuries, endotoxemia, or pain.

RISK FACTORS

Any factor that predisposes the development of a previously mentioned cause of ileus can be considered a risk factor. Electrolyte imbalances (hypokalemia or hypocalcemia) can alter intestinal smooth muscle function and have a deleterious effect on motility. Certain drugs (alpha-2 agonists or opioid analgesics) also inhibit intestinal motility.

DIAGNOSIS

DIFFERENTIAL DIAGNOSIS

Adynamic ileus should be differentiated from obstructive diseases that require surgical intervention.

CBC/BIOCHEMISTRY/URINALYSIS

- Increase in PCV due to dehydration and/or splenic contraction. Azotemia may also be present.
- Hypo- or hyper-proteinemia, depending on the underlying cause of ileus and degree of dehydration. Colitis or enteritis can cause a loss of protein-rich fluid into the intestines, which results in hypoproteinemia. If an inflammatory response is present, hyperproteinemia can result.
- Leukopenia may be present if ileus is associated with an acute inflammatory response. A long-standing inflammatory response can cause a leukocytosis.
- Hypokalemia, hypocalcemia, hypochloremia, and hyponatremia may be present due to sequestration of fluid in the intestines.

OTHER LABORATORY TESTS

Abdominal Paracentesis

Adynamic ileus usually results in no detectable abnormalities except in cases of duodenitis/proximal jejunitis. In these cases, an elevation of abdominal protein is usually present. In cases of ileus secondary to peritonitis, a marked increase in white blood cells and protein is usually present. If an obstructive ileus is present, the peritoneal fluid can be serosanguinous due to intestinal compromise and the cellular and protein levels are often high.

IMAGING

Ultrasonography

Ultrasonography allows for evaluation of the quantity of abdominal fluid and can also be helpful in identifying a site for paracentesis. Small intestinal distension or mural thickening (edema) can also be assessed.

TREATMENT

Feed and water should be withheld. Gastric decompression via a nasogastric tube should be performed to relieve discomfort and to prevent gastric rupture.

Parenteral fluid therapy is vital due to the inability to administer oral fluids. Fluid rates should be calculated based on deficit + maintenance + ongoing loss. The fluid deficit can be calculated as percent dehydration × body weight (kg) = fluid deficit (liters).

ILEUS

Maintenance fluid requirements for adult horses are 40–50 mL/kg/day. Ongoing losses can be determined by quantifying the amount of fluid lost as reflux. Horses suffering from hypovolemic or endotoxemic shock may benefit from hypertonic saline administration to rapidly expand the vascular fluid volume. Hypertonic saline (5–7%) can be administered at a dose of 4 mL/kg as a rapid bolus, followed by isotonic fluids because the volume expansion by hypertonic fluids is short-lived (<30 min). Horses with severe hyponatremia (<120 mmol/L) should not be given hypertonic saline due to the potential for cerebral edema to develop. Electrolyte imbalances should be addressed due to the negative effect of hypokalemia and hypocalcemia on motility. KCl may be added to parenteral fluids. The rate of potassium administration should not exceed 0.5 mEq/kg/hr due to the potential for cardiac effects. When treating an adult horse, a potassium concentration of 20 mEq/L in parenteral fluids results in a rate of administration <0.5 mEq/kg/hr, even at fast fluid rates. To correct hypocalcemia, 200–500 mL of 23% calcium borogluconate can be administered slowly (diluted in lactated Ringer's solution).

If ileus persists, an exploratory laparotomy for surgical decompression can be performed to relieve discomfort. If the horse appears to deteriorate clinically with medical management, then surgery is indicated due to the potential for an obstructive/ischemic lesion.

MEDICATIONS

DRUG(S) OF CHOICE

Analgesics

Pain relief is important when correcting ileus. Non-steroidal anti-inflammatory drugs are a good choice for analgesia because they do not inhibit motility. If additional analgesia is needed, then alpha-2 agonists can be given alone or in conjunction with butorphanol (opioid). Alpha-2 agonists appear to function synergistically with butorphanol; however, these drugs can inhibit motility for <2 hr and should be used judiciously.

- Non-steroidal anti-inflammatory drugs (NSAIDs)—flunixin meglumine (0.5–1.1 mg/kg IV q8–12hr), phenylbutazone (2.2–4.4 mg/kg IV q12–24hr).
- Alpha-2 agonists—xylazine (0.25–0.5 mg/kg IV or IM), detomidine (5–10 μg/kg IV or IM), romifidine (0.02–0.05 mg/kg IV or IM)
- Opioids—butorphanol (0.02–0.04 mg/kg IV)

Prokinetic Agents

- Cisapride—Improves motility of the entire gastrointestinal tract by increasing acetylcholine release from enteric nerves and may directly improve intestinal smooth muscle contractility by increasing calcium influx. Can be administered orally (0.1–0.6 mg/kg orally q8hr); however, unlike other species, rectal administration is not efficacious in horses.
- Erythromycin lactobionate—Improves small and large intestinal motility by stimulating endogenous motilin release via cholinergic and seratoninergic mechanisms. May also cause direct stimulation of intestinal motilin receptors (1 g IV in 1 L saline over 60 min q6hr).
- Metoclopramide—Improves gastric and proximal small intestinal motility by increasing acetylcholine release from intestinal neurons and by dopamine antagonism (0.1 mg/kg/hr in a constant drip infusion).

Laxatives

- Large intestinal motility can be enhanced by increasing the water content of the ingesta. Lubrication of ingesta has less of an effect on transit time but can ease transport. In addition to the direct effect on ingesta, enhanced motility may result when laxatives are administered by nasogastric tube via the gastrocolic reflex.
- Mineral oil—10 mL/kg via nasogastric tube
- Osmotic laxative—sodium sulfate (0.5g/kg) or magnesium sulfate (0.5–1 g/kg) in 4 L of warm water via nasogastric tube.
- Dioctyl sodium succinate (DSS) via nasogastric tube (10–30 mg/kg of a 10% solution)

CONTRAINDICATIONS

Oral drug administration is contraindicated in horses with ileus of the small intestine (nasogastric reflux or with distended small intestine on rectal palpation).

PRECAUTIONS

Metoclopramide crosses the blood–brain barrier and can cause signs associated with central dopamine antagonism (muscle tremors, excitement, aggression).

FOLLOW-UP

PATIENT MONITORING

The patient should be monitored closely to ensure that intravenous fluid therapy is appropriate and that decompression of gastric and small intestinal distension is adequate.

POSSIBLE COMPLICATIONS

- Circulatory shock
- Gastrointestinal rupture

ASSOCIATED CONDITIONS

N/A

AGE-RELATED FACTORS

N/A

ZOONOTIC POTENTIAL

N/A

SYNONYMS

N/A

ABBREVIATIONS

N/A

Suggested Reading

White NA. Treatment to alter intestinal motility. In: White NA. The equine acute abdomen. Philadelphia: Lea & Febiger 1990:178-184.

White NA, Byars TD. Analgesia. In: White NA. The equine acute abdomen. Philadelphia: Lea & Febiger 1990:154-159.

Guyton AC, Hall JE. General principles of gastrointestinal function—Motility, nervous control, and blood circulation. In: Textbook of medical physiology, 9th ed. Philadelphia: WB Saunders Co. 1996:793-802.

Authors Christopher P. Boutros and Nathalie Coté

Consulting Editor Henry Stämpfli

IMPACTION

BASICS

DEFINITION

An impaction is obstruction of the alimentary tract, and depending on the portion affected, may result in a variety of clinical signs. The obstruction may consist of feed material, fecal material, or foreign matter that slows or stops the movement of ingesta. This may result in distension of a viscus, causing abdominal pain. Impactions may be primary or secondary, and may cause partial to complete obstructions.

PATHOPHYSIOLOGY

Any disease that causes decreased gastric or intestinal motility may cause an impaction (see Ileus). There are feed-associated factors (coarse, high-fiber feed), and insufficient water intake, poor dentition, or a change in diet that may affect the breakdown of feed material resulting in delayed passage. Factors such as dehydration, change in exercise, and transport are thought to be important in initiating an obstruction. In addition, general anesthesia and surgical manipulations may affect the gastrointestinal motility; therefore, post-anesthetic impactions are not uncommon. Portions of the bowel where the intestinal lumen size narrows are common areas for impactions. These include the stomach, distal small intestine, cecum, pelvic flexure, right dorsal colon, transverse colon, and small colon. Impactions may also occur in areas where pacemakers controlling motility are located (cecum, pelvic flexure). In some cases, the cause of impactions may not be delineated.

SYSTEMS AFFECTED

Gastrointestinal

- Decreased appetite
- Decreased fecal output
- Increased or decreased borborygmi
- Abdominal distension
- Colic
- Other signs caused by primary disease

Behavioral

Behavioral changes range from vague changes in demeanor to severe signs of colic and toxemia.

Cardiovascular

- Normal to increased heart rate and capillary refill time
- Tacky mucus
- Greater signs of cardiovascular compromise as severity increases

Renal/Urologic

Changes associated with hypovolemia.

Reproductive

Cecal impaction following parturition.

Respiratory

- Mild tachypnea
- Shallow respiration due to pain and abdominal distension

Skin/Exocrine

Sweating

SIGNALMENT

Any age, breed, or sex.
- Ascarid impactions—occurs in foals, weanlings, and yearlings
- Small colon impactions—may be more common in ponies and American Miniature Horses
- Cecal impaction—more common in post-parturient mares and in horses following general anesthesia

SIGNS

- Abdominal distension
- Anorexia (partial to complete)
- Decreased fecal output
- Diarrhea—sand impaction, although may occur in course of treatment of other impactions
- Feces—firm/hard, dry, mucus covered
- Flank watching
- Frequent attempts to defecate
- Increased or decreased borborygmi
- Lethargy
- Nasogastric reflux
- Pawing
- Rectal prolapse
- Recumbency
- Rolling
- Straining to defecate
- Tail swishing

CAUSES

Gastric Impaction

Abrupt increase in amount of concentrates fed, especially those that swell; outflow obstructions due to pyloric dysfunction or small intestinal ileus or other disease that decreases small intestinal motility.

Small Intestine Impaction

Associated with coarse feed, such as Coastal Bermuda grass, or with mesenteric vascular disease; ascarid impactions in young horses are usually associated with anthelmintic treatment with a paralytic medication, such as ivermectin, piperazine, or organophosphates.

Cecal Impaction

Multifactorial problem that occurs in the adult horse and is rare in foals. May occur as a primary problem due to an abrupt change in feed or may be secondary to altered motility due to general anesthesia, surgery, parturition, or sand ingestion. Parasitic or vascular damage affecting the cecal pacemaker may alter cecal motility.

Large Colon Impaction

- Decreased water intake
- Diet alteration
- Poor dentition
- Decreased exercise
- Sand ingestion
- Enteric parasitism

Small Colon Impaction

Similar to causes of large colon impaction.

IMPACTION

DIAGNOSIS

DIFFERENTIAL DIAGNOSIS

Determination of the cause of colic should include a thorough collection of historical information (including management, exercise, and prior treatments), physical examination, abdominal palpation per rectum, and passage of a nasogastric tube.

Gastric Impaction

Rule out many other causes of colic, including causes of small intestinal/gastric reflux.

Small Intestine Impaction

Ileal hypertrophy, ileum-associated mass, small intestinal or ileal–cecal intussusception. Other causes of small intestinal distension include proximal duodenitis/jejunitis, small intestinal volvulus, and strangulating lipoma.

Cecal Impaction

Differentials for cecal distension include cecocecal intussusception and cecocolic intussusception. For a "simple" cecal impaction, a cecum that is distended with ingesta should be palpable in the upper right abdominal quadrant. A medial and ventral band may be palpated. The cecum should be palpated to course cranioventral as palpate from the base toward the apex. An apical impaction, early in the disease process, may not be palpable.

Large Colon Impaction

Displacements, early large colon/cecal torsions. Impaction of the left large colons should be palpable per rectum. The impacted pelvic flexure is usually located within the pelvic inlet and is positioned with the dorsal and ventral colon in a horizontal plain. A nephrosplenic entrapment (NSE) may closely resemble a simple impaction of the left colons. With an NSE, the position of the left colons is often reversed (ventral colon located in a dorsal position), and the colon and associated bands may be palpated from the pelvic brim to the nephrosplenic space. Ultrasound exam is very helpful in making the diagnosis. Palpation of impactions of the right dorsal or transverse colon is not possible, and diagnosis would require a celiotomy or necropsy.

Small Colon Impaction

Major differential is impaction of the small intestine. Differentiation requires the detection of the large antimesenteric band on the small colon. Multiple loops of impacted small colon are usually palpable.

CBC/BIOCHEMISTRY/URINALYSIS

Usually normal; abnormalities may occur with progressive disease due to hypovolemia and debilitation of the bowel.

Abdominal Fluid Analysis

Abdominal fluid should be collected judiciously if an impaction is suspected because enterocentesis may cause rupture of a distended viscus. Consider identifying fluid pocket with ultrasound prior to centesis and using a blunt tipped cannula such as a 4-in. teat cannula. The fluid should be normal in appearance and have normal cytologic parameters. Abnormal cell count, cell differential, protein level, presence of bacteria or foreign material consistent with compromised bowel or another problem.

IMAGING

Radiographs

Radographs are helpful in assessing foal abdomens or searching for foreign bodies, enteroliths, or sand in adult horses.

Ultrasound

Ultrasound is a useful tool in evaluating foal and adult abdomens. Can be used transcutaneously or per rectum to assess intestinal distension, intestinal wall thickness, and intestinal motility. Possible to detect intussusceptions and masses. Select areas can be evaluated in adult horses, but there are limitations due to size of adult abdomen and inability to penetrate through cecum or colon. Hyperechoic fluid may have high cell count, protein level, or feed/fecal material. Can also assess presence of fibrin deposition and peripheral abscess formation.

TREATMENT

Gastrointestinal Impactions

Resolve primary problem (feed, dentition, hydration, exercise). Medical therapy should include withholding feed; however, small amounts of feed may help maintain gastrointestinal motility and may be considered in impactions of the large or small colon. Grass or grass hay should be considered. Further medical therapy may include intravenous crystalloid fluids given at a high rate to increase the fluid content in the bowel to break down impaction. If tolerated, fluids may be given via an indwelling nasogastric tube at rates up to 6 L/hr in a 400-kg horse. Medications may be given orally to soften the feces and analgesics may be administered as needed. Exploratory surgery may be required depending on the type of disease and its severity, duration, and progression. Factors that should be considered include deteriorating signs of pain, increasing heart rate, retrieving gastric reflux, increased abdominal distension, increased distension of viscera on rectal examination, lack of fecal production, and indications of loss of visceral integrity, such as increased nucleated cells, protein level, presence of bacteria, or presence of feed material in peritoneal fluid.

Gastric

Medical therapy should include withholding feed and maintenance of the hydration status. The stomach may be lavaged through a nasogastric tube; however, caution must be used to prevent further gastric distension and rupture.

IMPACTION

MEDICATIONS

Laxatives

- Mineral oil—2–4 L/450-kg horse, q12hr via nasogastric tube
- Dioctyl sodium sulfosuccinate—120–240 mL/450-kg horse of 4% DSS with water
- Psyllium hydrophilic muciloid—0.25–0.5 kg/450-kg horse

Cathartics

- Magnesium sulfate (Epsom salts)—0.5–1.0 kg q24hr
- Sodium sulfate (Glauber's salts)—0.25–0.5 kg q24hr

DRUGS OF CHOICE

NSAIDs

- Flunixin meglumine—0.5–1.1 mg/kg IV q24hr/12hr/8hr.
- Ketoprofen—2.2 mg/kg IV q24hr/12hr/8hr
- Phenylbutazone—2.2–4.4 mg/kg IV q24hr/12hr

Analgesia and Sedation

- Xylazine—use α_2 adrenergic agonist sparingly due to decreased motility
- Romifidine—40–80 μg/kg IM, IV
- Detomidine—10–30 μg/kg IM, IV
- Butorphanol—0.01–0.05 mg/kg (some horses may need prior or concurrent α adrenergic agonist treatment to prevent tremors)

CONTRAINDICATIONS

NSAIDs

NSAIDs may cause renal papillary necrosis or gastrointestinal ulceration; side effects may be worse in a dehydrated animal. Decreasing order of toxicity: ketoprofen, flunixin, phenylbutazone.

α Adrenergic Agonists

Side effects include transient hypertension followed by longer-lasting hypotension, bradycardia, 2° AV blockade, decreased gastrointestinal motility, sweating, and diuresis.

Salt Cathartics

Animal must be well hydrated; may cause distension and more severe colic. Toxic to enterocytes with repeated administration.

POSSIBLE DRUG INTERACTIONS

N/A

ALTERNATIVE DRUGS

N/A

SURGERY

Consider abdominal surgery for unmanageable pain, displacement of intestine, abnormal peritoneal fluid, or deterioration in condition.

PROGNOSIS

- Good for cecal impaction if primary and detected and treated early in disease
- Guarded for cecal impaction if it persists for >24–48 hr
- Very good for pelvic flexure impaction
- Guarded for ileal and small colon impactions

FOLLOW-UP

PATIENT MONITORING

N/A

POSSIBLE COMPLICATIONS

Magnesium sulfate therapy can lead to hypermagnesemia, especially if there is deficiency in renal function, hypocalcemia, or compromised vascular integrity.

MISCELLANEOUS

ASSOCIATED CONDITIONS

N/A

AGE-RELATED FACTORS

N/A

ZOONOTIC POTENTIAL

N/A

PREGNANCY

N/A

SYNONYMS

N/A

SEE ALSO

Colic

ABBREVIATIONS

N/A

Suggested Reading

White NA, Dabareiner RM. Treatment of impaction colics. Vet Clin North Am [Equine Prac] 1997;13:243-259.

Hanson RR, et al. Medical treatment of horses with ileal impactions: 10 cases (1990–1994). J Am Vet Med Assoc 1996;208:898-900.

Dart AJ, et al. Abnormal conditions of the equine descending (small) colon: 102 cases (1979–1989). J Am Vet Med Assoc 1992;200:971-978.

Snyder JR, Spier SJ. Disorders of the small intestine associated with acute abdominal pain. In: Smith BP, ed: Large animal internal medicine, 2nd ed. St. Louis, Mosby 1996;755-783.

Author Daniel G. Kenney

Consulting Editor Henry Stämpfli

INDUCTION OF PARTURITION

BASICS

DEFINITION

• Elective and attended termination of pregnancy in a mare at term, in order to assist in parturition of the mare. The procedure is not without some inherent risk to the mare and more significant risk to the foal, if parameters assessing both the dam's and foal's readiness for birth are not met. • Gestation length for a particular mare tends to be similar year to year. The variability between two individual mares can be extreme; thus, it is imperative that induction be done only once the fetus is determined to be mature and its viability will not be compromised by the procedure.

PATHOPHYSIOLOGY

The intent with induction is to use drugs/procedures that most closely mimic the normal parturition sequence.

SYSTEM AFFECTED

Reproductive

SIGNALMENT

General Comments

Induction of parturition ensures that adequate and appropriate obstetric assistance is available, if needed. Specific factors and criteria must be taken into consideration before the decision is made to induce parturition. It is essential that these criteria and their limitations be understood by the farm owner/manager.

Clinical indications for induction include:

• Delayed parturition due to uterine atony, most commonly seen in older, multiparous mares. They are typically at term and exhibit all the signs of being ready to foal. • Prolonged gestation (>365 days) may be complicated by the fetus becoming so large that there is a danger to the mare and fetus at parturition. • Mare has experienced a pelvic fracture or other injury to the genital tract/birth canal, such that the size of the canal is reduced. • Mare is developing excessive amounts of ventral edema or hydrops of the amnion such that rupture of the prepubic tendon appears imminent. • Mare with a history of premature placental separation and delivery of hypoxic foals. • Mare is an embryo-transfer (ET) recipient of a very expensive embryo and an attended parturition is essential and may be required by an insurance company. • Other indications for induction include mares with a history of producing a foal that develops neonatal isoerythrolysis (NI), imminent death of the mare due to systemic disease, or preparturient colic. • Mare is leaking colostrum and there is no other source of colostrum available.

SIGNS

The stages of parturition are altered little by standard induction regimens. The biggest difference is in the duration of stage I, which is reduced significantly when induction is achieved with the administration of oxytocin.

RISK FACTORS

• Fetal prematurity, immaturity, or dysmaturity • Dystocia • Premature placental separation

DIAGNOSIS

DIFFERENTIAL DIAGNOSIS

N/A

CBC/BIOCHEMISTRY/URINALYSIS

N/A unless the mare is under care for other conditions/systemic illness.

OTHER LABORATORY TESTS

Evaluation of mammary secretions for calcium, sodium, potassium, magnesium.

DIAGNOSTIC PROCEDURES

Determining Readiness for Birth

Criteria to determine the mare's readiness:

• Gestation length of at least 330 days. Requires accurate breeding records, including ultrasound dates and vesicle sizes. Successful inductions have been performed as early as 320 days, but it appears that the best results are obtained at 330 days. • Mammary development and the presence of colostrum. Udder development can vary tremendously depending on parity, age, size, and breed of the mare. Major changes in udder development occur within the 2 weeks prepartum, however, colostrum may be present for only hours or days. Must assess udder secretions on a daily basis or instruct owner to do so as the mare approaches term. Several weeks before term, udder secretions are commonly straw-colored, are initially watery changing to viscous. Closer to term they change to a smokey gray, and finally to the opaque-white color of colostrum within a few days or hours of foaling. If the mare has no colostrum in the gland, she is likely not close enough to term to safely induce and have a viable foal. Mares with a history of poor lactation may require the farm to procure an alternate source; this requires planning ahead. • Relaxation of the perineum and sacrosciatic ligaments. Due to the difficulty in detecting subtle changes in the ligament in some mares, it should not be used to any great extent in the decision-making process. Other criteria serve as more accurate parameters for determining readiness for birth. • Cervical relaxation: the degree of relaxation is one of the most important criteria to be evaluated. The findings can be quite variable with regard to prepartum relaxation. The cervix of some mares may remain closed and capped until the end of stage I labor, whereas the cervix of other mares may relax several days or more before term. It is therefore imperative to evaluate critically the degree of cervical relaxation in any mare that may be a candidate for induction. Many practitioners anticipate cervical softening and dilation of 3–4 cm must be present before deciding to induce. This degree of relaxation would easily allow insertion of 1–2 fingers into the cervix. Proper obstetric technique must be used when examining the mare. The tail should be wrapped and the perineal area cleansed with a mild, non-residual soap. The degree of cervical softening and dilation can best be evaluated digitally, using a sterile, single-use sleeve and sterile lubricant.

Mammary Secretions

There are several commercial test kits that can quantitate calcium concentrations in the mare's mammary secretions. The Predict-a-Foal Test (Animal Healthcare Products, Chino, CA) is one of several that are available to measure calcium levels in the secretions. There are also kits used to measure water hardness that may be used to measure calcium. Most of these kits provide a scale or guide by which the color changes reveal the adequacy of milk calcium in the prepartum period.

Fetus

Fetal maturity and survivability cannot always be correlated with gestational age. The most reliable way to determine the maturity and readiness for induction is the use of electrolyte concentrations in the prepartum mammary secretions. The electrolyte changes have been positively associated with fetal maturity and should be used in conjunction with the other criteria.

The concentrations of calcium, sodium, and potassium in prepartum mammary secretions undergo distinct changes associated with maturity of the fetus/readiness for birth. Calcium concentrations >40 mg/dL are associated with a mature fetus. Values of 12 mg/dL are associated with fetal immaturity and reduced viability. Sodium concentrations in the mammary secretions are usually higher than potassium, but as the mare gets closer to term an inversion occurs, and potassium concentrations become higher than sodium concentrations. Anticipate sodium value of ~30 mEq/L with potassium of ~35 mEq/L.

TREATMENT

APPROPRIATE HEALTH CARE

• Prior to the administration of the induction agent, the perineum of the mare should be washed thoroughly and the tail should be

wrapped. The mare should be placed in a quiet, clean, and dry stall away from the usual activities of the barn. • After oxytocin is administered, the mare demonstrates normal signs of stage I labor. She becomes restless and exhibits colicy signs, such as lying down and getting up frequently, posturing as if to urinate, and beginning to sweat along the neck, flank, and behind the elbows. These signs occur within 20 min of the first injection.
• Rupture of the chorioallantoic (CA) membrane signals the onset of stage II labor, along with the beginning of the abdominal press. These events begin within 20–30 min of administration of oxytocin. In the majority of mares, foaling should be completed within 60 min of oxytocin. Expulsion of the fetal membranes should occur within 3 hr of foaling. If they are not, treatment for rupture of fetal membranes (RFM) should be instituted.
• If 20–30 min have elapsed and the mare's straining has not caused the CA membrane to rupture, it is imperative that a manual vaginal examination using aseptic technique be performed. This exam allows an assessment of progress of parturition and aids in the early diagnosis of possible complications.

NURSING CARE
Because the foaling is attended, it provides an opportunity to ensure that the mare accepts and cares for the newborn. Observations should be made of the neonate for normal activities within normal time ranges (e.g., suckling reflex, attempts to stand, nursing, ingestion of colostrum within the first 1–2 hr of life).

ACTIVITY
Unless the newborn is ill, a dummy, or exhibits a congenital abnormality that affects its ability to follow the mare, normal activity can be permitted.

CLIENT EDUCATION
Elective induction is not to be used simply as a convenient method to terminate pregnancy. It is imperative to communicate to the client all of the potential risks to both the mare and fetus during induction. These risks must be outlined in a concise manner such that the client has a thorough understanding and accepts responsibility for the decision to induce when there is no medically justified reason.

MEDICATIONS

DRUG(S) OF CHOICE
Oxytocin is the drug most often used for induction. It is administered in doses ranging from 2.5–10 IU to 40–60 IU IV, IM. When oxytocin is administered at a dose of 40–60 IU as an IV bolus, assuming all criteria and parameters for maternal and fetal readiness are in place, foaling can be expected to occur within 60–90 min. When low doses are administered intravenously, less discomfort is exhibited by the mare and there is a shorter delivery time than is seen with the higher doses. Administration of low doses intravenously results in an initiation of foaling in 15–30 min with foaling completed within the hour. A common effective low-dose regimen uses 2.5–10 IU in 30–60 mL saline administered via an IV catheter. This regimen can be repeated every 20 min or as a single 20 IU bolus.

PRECAUTIONS
Lutalyse[or] (Upjohn, Kalamazoo, MI), $PGF_2\alpha$, the natural prostaglandin, should never be used to induce a mare. Because of the strong uterine contractions associated with its use, premature placental separation occurs and it has been associated with ~90% fetal death due to hypoxia and other parturient complications.

POSSIBLE INTERACTIONS
N/A

ALTERNATIVE DRUGS
Prostalene or fenprostalene, synthetic prostaglandins, are less commonly used for induction at doses of 4 mg SQ and 0.5 mg SQ, respectively, at 2-hr intervals. Both of these drugs were used in mares that had electrolyte concentrations in mammary secretions that coincided with the foals' readiness for birth. The results from studies using both of these synthetic prostaglandins for induction indicate that viable foals can be delivered within a mean of approximately 4 hr after administration.

FOLLOW-UP

PATIENT MONITORING
Serial manual vaginal examinations allow assessment of presentation, position, and posture of the fetus. If any malpresentation exists, it can be corrected early in the process, before uterine contractions and abdominal straining move the fetus up into the birth canal (known as *becoming engaged in the pelvis*), making these manipulations more difficult.

POSSIBLE COMPLICATIONS
• The two most common complications associated with induction include premature separation of the fetal membranes and fetal malpresentation with dystocia. • Premature separation of the placental membranes can commonly occur as two scenarios. In the first situation, the red velvet–like bag of the CA membrane may be seen protruding from the vulvar lips. If this should occur, the CA membrane should be opened as quickly as possible and the foal delivered to prevent death by anoxia. In the second scenario, the placental membranes may separate from the uterus, and on vaginal examination the CA is found lying free within the uterus. The membrane should be incised and the foal delivered as quickly as possible. Other complications associated with induction include prolonged fetal membrane retention (not with oxytocin) and the associated systemic illnesses (metritis, laminitis) and delivery of premature or dysmature foals.

EXPECTED COURSE AND PROGNOSIS
• If the process proceeds in an unremarkable manner, the foal should be delivered within 45–60 min after administration of oxytocin.
• The foal should be standing and nursing within 1–2 hr post-delivery. • The mare should pass the fetal membranes within 1–3 hr after delivering the foal.

MISCELLANEOUS

PREGNANCY
This procedure should be used only at term gestation and when justified to protect the mare's health or to guarantee that assistance is available at the time of parturition of a high-risk or valuable offspring. If properly carried out, the procedure should not compromise the survival of the fetus.

SYNONYMS
Elective parturition

SEE ALSO
• Parturition • Dystocia • Premature placental separation • Retained fetal membranes

ABBREVIATIONS
• CA = chorioallantois • ET = embryo transfer • NI = neonatal isoerythrolysis
• RFM = retained fetal membranes/placenta

Suggested Reading

Carleton CL and Threlfall WR. Induction of parturition in the mare. In: Current therapy in large animal theriogenology, 2nd ed. Morrow DA, ed. Toronto, WB Saunders 1986;689-692.
LeBlanc MM. Induction of parturition. In: Equine reproduction. McKinnon AO and Voss JL, eds. Philadelphia, Lea & Febiger 1993;574-577.

Author E. Ricardo Bridges
Consulting Editor Carla L. Carleton

INFECTIOUS ANEMIA (EIA)

BASICS

DEFINITION

• An infectious disease caused by EIAV, a lentivirus of the family Retroviridae.
• EIAV is closely related to HIV-1, the cause of AIDS in humans.

PATHOPHYSIOLOGY

• EIAV is transmitted primarily by blood-feeding insects, especially tabanids (i.e., horseflies and deerflies); iatrogenic transmission can occur via contaminated needles, syringes, and surgical instruments as well as through transfusion of contaminated blood.
• Once infected, a horse remains so for life.
• EIAV infects cells of the monocyte/macrophage lineage and can be detected in the cytoplasm of this cell type in the liver, spleen, lymph nodes, lung, bone marrow, and circulation.
• EIA can be characterized by three clinical syndromes—acute, chronic, and inapparent carrier; not all horses progress through all three syndromes.
• Acute disease—usually occurs 1–4 weeks after infection; is associated with high levels of viremia; can be characterized by fever, anorexia, lethargy, ventral edema, thrombocytopenia, anemia, and occasionally, epistaxis and death; and is usually <1 week in duration and sometimes mild enough to go completely unnoticed.
• Chronic disease—associated with recurrent episodes of viral replication, causing repeated bouts of clinical signs; classic signs of anemia, ventral edema, and weight loss occur during this phase.
• With time, episodes of clinical disease decrease in duration and severity, and most horses control the infection within 1 year, becoming inapparent carriers.
• Inapparent carriers show no clinical signs, are seropositive, and are reservoirs of infection, capable of transmitting the virus to uninfected horses.

SYSTEMS AFFECTED

• Hemic/lymphatic/immune—anemia caused by immune-mediated intravascular and extravascular hemolysis as well as bone marrow suppression. Likewise, thrombocytopenia is caused by both bone marrow suppression and enhanced platelet destruction; severe thrombocytopenia can lead to mucous membrane petechia and epistaxis.
• Cardiovascular—immune-mediated vasculitis leads to hemorrhage, thrombosis, and edema.
• Hepatobiliary—accumulations of lymphocytes and macrophages in the liver can result in hepatomegaly, fatty degeneration, and hepatic cell necrosis.
• Renal/urologic—immune complex deposition can result in glomerulonephritis.
• Neurologic—vasculitis and lymphocyte accumulation in meninges occasionally result in ataxia.

GENETICS

N/A

INCIDENCE/PREVALENCE

• Worldwide distribution
• In the United States, the true incidence is unknown, because only $\cong$10–20% of the total U.S. horse population is routinely tested. Of those horses tested, <0.5% are infected. The incidence is higher in the Gulf Coast states, because the climate is favorable for virus transmission.

SIGNALMENT

• Horses, ponies, mules, and donkeys are susceptible; however, donkeys and mules appear to be less severely affected.
• No breed, age, or sex predilections

SIGNS

General Comments

• Clinical signs—vary, depending on the stage of disease.
• Inapparent carriers—clinically normal.
• Chronic stage—affected animals may show no signs between clinical episodes.

Historical Findings

• Signs can go unnoticed.
• May be a history of inappetence, lethargy, and fever.
• Severely affected horses may have a history of high fever (105–106° F), depression, ventral edema, weight loss, ataxia, and epistaxis.

Physical Examination Findings

Normal, or could include poor body condition, lethargy, fever, mucosal petechiation, ventral edema, pale mucous membranes, epistaxis, and ataxia

CAUSES

Infection with EIAV

RISK FACTORS

Contact with other equids during warm weather, when tabanids are abundant

DIAGNOSIS

DIFFERENTIAL DIAGNOSIS

• List of differential diagnoses depends on the predominant clinical signs.
• Horses affected with these other diseases are seronegative for EIAV and easily differentiated from those infected with EIAV.
• Anemia/thrombocytopenia—blood loss, anemia of chronic disease, red-maple intoxication, immune-mediated thrombocytopenia/hemolytic anemia, and neoplasia
• Fever—other viral/bacterial/inflammatory diseases and neoplasia
• Weight loss—inadequate feed intake, dental abnormalities, parasitism, other chronic diseases, and neoplasia
• Ventral edema—hypoalbuminemia, pleuropneumonia, vasculitis, neoplasia, protein-losing enteropathy, and peritonitis
• Ataxia—cervical stenotic myelopathy, EHV-1 myeloencephalitis, and equine protozoal myeloencephalitis

CBC/BIOCHEMISTRY/URINALYSIS

• Thrombocytopenia—the first laboratory abnormality detected in acutely infected horses, occurs coincident with fever, resolves along with resolution of the clinical disease, but recurs with subsequent disease cycles
• Decreases in PCV and RBCs can occur shortly after infection but generally are more severe during the chronic stage; leukopenia, lymphocytosis, and monocytosis are observed in many infected horses.
• Hypergammaglobulinemia may be present.
• Increases in liver enzyme activities may occur.

OTHER LABORATORY TESTS

• Diagnosis confirmed by serologic testing—AGID (Coggins test) and C-ELISA are approved by the USDA and detect serum antibody to the EIAV group–specific core protein, p26.
• Acute infection produces detectable antibody within 45 days.
• Coggins test—the most widely used and 95% accurate in diagnosing EIAV infection; occasional false-negative results may occur.
• C-ELISA may be more sensitive than AGID, leading to possible false-positive results.
• All horses testing positive with either test should be retested for confirmation.

IMAGING
N/A

DIAGNOSTIC PROCEDURES
N/A

PATHOLOGIC FINDINGS
- In horses that die or are euthanized during a febrile episode, lesions include splenomegaly, hepatomegaly, accentuated hepatic lobular structure, lymphadenopathy, mucosal and visceral hemorrhages, ventral subcutaneous edema, and vessel thrombosis.
- Accumulations of lymphocytes and macrophages in the periportal regions of the liver and in the spleen, lymph nodes, adrenal gland, lung, and meninges
- Lymphoproliferative lesions are thought to result from the spread of virus-reactive T lymphocytes to control infection.
- Fatty degeneration of the liver and hepatic cell necrosis
- Glomerulitis can be present.
- Necropsy of inapparent carriers—unremarkable

TREATMENT

APPROPRIATE HEALTH CARE
- No effective treatment
- Immediately isolate seropositive horses from other equidae.

NURSING CARE
- Provide general supportive care during clinical episodes; the nature of this care varies, depending on the types and severity of signs.
- Whole-blood transfusions may benefit horses with severe anemia or thrombocytopenia.
- Standing leg wraps may benefit horses with ventral pitting edema.
- Cold-water hosing may decrease the temperature in horses with high fever that is nonresponsive to NSAIDs.

ACTIVITY
N/A

DIET
N/A

CLIENT EDUCATION
- A reportable disease in the United States
- Federal law prohibits interstate travel of infected animals, except for slaughter, return to place of origin, or transport to a recognized research facility or diagnostic laboratory.
- Individual states regulate intrastate travel, and most control measures include the following options for seropositive horses—euthanasia, permanent identification and life-long quarantine, or transport to a recognized research facility.

SURGICAL CONSIDERATIONS
N/A

MEDICATIONS

DRUGS OF CHOICE
- Because no treatment for EIAV is effective and infected horses remain so for life, only rarely is treatment attempted.
- NSAIDs may be administered for control of fever and inflammation during viremic, febrile episodes—flunixin meglumine (1.1 mg/kg IV q12h)

CONTRAINDICATIONS
N/A

PRECAUTIONS
N/A

POSSIBLE INTERACTIONS
N/A

ALTERNATIVE DRUGS
N/A

FOLLOW-UP

PATIENT MONITORING
N/A

PREVENTION/AVOIDANCE
- Federal and state control measures have lowered the U.S. incidence of EIA, but outbreaks still occur.
- Veterinarians, horse owners, and others in the equine industry can reduce the chance of exposure by requiring an EIA test as part of every prepurchase examination; a recent, negative EIA test before admitting any new horse to a farm; recent, negative EIA tests for horses entering shows, sales, race tracks, and other events; annual testing of all horses for EIA exposure; never injecting different horses with a common needle or syringe; thoroughly disinfecting instruments that come into contact with blood; and practicing rigorous fly control.

POSSIBLE COMPLICATIONS
N/A

EXPECTED COURSE AND PROGNOSIS
- Occasionally, horses may die of EIA, but most eventually control the infection and become life-long, inapparent carriers.
- Inapparent carriers are clinically normal but remain reservoirs of infection.

MISCELLANEOUS

ASSOCIATED CONDITIONS
N/A

AGE-RELATED FACTORS
N/A

ZOONOTIC POTENTIAL
N/A

PREGNANCY
- EIAV can be transmitted transplacentally in pregnant mares and may cause abortion.
- EIAV also may be transmitted via colostrum or milk.

SYNONYMS
Swamp fever

SEE ALSO
- Immune-mediated hemolytic anemia
- Thrombocytopenia

ABBREVIATIONS
- AGID = agar gel immunodiffusion
- AIDS = acquired immunodeficiency syndrome
- C-ELISA = competitive enzyme-linked immunoadsorbent assay
- EHV = equine herpes virus
- EIAV = equine infectious anemia virus
- HIV = human immunodeficiency virus
- PCV = packed cell volume
- USDA = United States Department of Agriculture

Suggested Reading

Cheevers WP, McGuire TC. Equine infectious anemia virus: immunopathogenesis and persistence. Rev Infect Dis 1985;7:83–88.

Clabough DL. Equine infectious anemia: clinical signs, transmission, and diagnostic procedures. Vet Med 1990;85:1007–1019.

Clabough DL. The immunopathogenesis and control of equine infectious anemia. Vet Med 1990;85:1020–1028.

Montelaro RC, Ball JM, Rushlow KE. Equine retroviruses. In: Levy JA, ed. The retroviridae. New York: Plenum Press, 1993:257–360.

Sellon DC, Fuller FJ, McGuire TC. The immunopathogenesis of equine infectious anemia virus. Virus Res 1994;32:111–138.

Author Robert H. Mealey
Consulting Editor Debra C. Sellon

INFLAMMATORY LOWER AIRWAY DISEASE IN YOUNG PERFORMING HORSES

BASICS

DEFINITION

- A recurrent, reversible allergic airway obstruction caused by accumulation of inflammatory cells leading to excess mucus production and airway hyperresponsiveness.
- Shares some features with heaves. The signs are less severe, however, and it affects young horses.
- If no action is taken, may progress to clinical signs of heaves over several years.

PATHOPHYSIOLOGY

Horses develop an increased sensitivity to dust, molds, pollens, and other irritants, causing mast cells, neutrophils, eosinophils, lymphocytes, and alveolar macrophages to release potent mediators.

SYSTEM AFFECTED

- Strictly limited to the respiratory system.
- Pathologic changes occur in the small airways (i.e., bronchioles), but the alveoli are not affected.

INCIDENCE/PREVALENCE

- Widespread in the northern hemisphere, where horses are stabled or trained in enclosed environments.
- In warmer climates, where horses are pastured year-round, the disease is recognized but rare.

SIGNALMENT

- Any breed
- May be recognized in horses <1 year.
- Seems to progress to a chronic form with age.

SIGNS

Historical Findings

- In athletic horses, reduced exercise tolerance or poor performance, with a prolonged recovery period after exercise, is the most commonly reported clinical sign.
- Other observations—intermittent to frequent coughing while the horse is eating or early in exercise, nasal discharge, and occasionally, increased respiratory rate (>18–20 breaths/min).

Physical Examination Findings

- The cardinal signs are within the normal range, except on occasion, when the resting respiratory rate may exceed 18 breaths/min or when a prolonged return to normal respiratory rate after exercise is observed.
- Nasal discharge—rare, but occasionally, a serous to mucopurulent discharge may be observed.
- Significant increase in bronchial sounds over both lung fields.
- With a rebreathing bag, wheezes frequently are detected over the dorsal area of the lung fields, and coughing may be elicited.
- Lung-field percussion may identify dorsal and caudal areas of hyperresonance, detectable beyond the sixteenth rib.
- A keen observer may notice a slight abdominal lift on expiration.

CAUSES

Airborne environmental allergens are beleived to be the primary causative agents—mold and dust from hay and bedding.

RISK FACTORS

Predisposing and exacerbating factors include respiratory viral infections (e.g., equine herpes virus and influenza virus) or hot days with high humidity.

DIAGNOSIS

DIFFERENTIAL DIAGNOSIS

- Respiratory viral infections (e.g., equine herpes virus and influenza virus) generally affect several horses in the same stable within a defined period of time, whereas inflammatory lower airway disease affects and persists on one to two horses and worsens over time.
- If not treated appropriately, often misdiagnosed as chronic persistent viral infection.
- Bacterial tracheitis and bronchitis, usually secondary to respiratory viral infection, normally are responsive to a 5–7-day course of broad-spectrum antibiotic.
- Any persistence of respiratory clinical signs without elevated body temperature suggests inflammatory lower airway disease.
- Localized pulmonary abscess may present a similar history, but clinical signs indicate fever, inappetence, and pain on chest percussion over the anteroventral area of the lung fields.

CBC/BIOCHEMISTRY/URINALYSIS

Normal

OTHER LABORATORY TESTS

- Total count and differential of cells harvested from bronchoalveolar lavage fluid. These cells are analyzed quantitatively and qualitatively to determine major changes in the inflammatory cell population—neutrophils, mast cells, eosinophils, lymphocytes, and exfoliated epithelial cells
- Lung biopsies permit histologic examination of the small airways and provide information on severity and prognosis but are not routinely done.
- Histamine provocation is a specific test that determines the degree of airway hyperresponsiveness, which manifests as increased sensitivity to a wide variety of allergic and nonallergic agents resulting from the underlying airway inflammation.

IMAGING

Thoracic radiography has little value except to demonstrate small, 2–4-mm diameter, donut-shaped lesions representing accumulation of inflammatory cells in the periphery of bronchioles.

DIAGNOSTIC PROCEDURES

- Bronchoscopy and bronchoalveolar lavage to retrieve cells of the lower airways and alveoli.
- Lung biopsy to assess alveoli and small airway pathology
- Histamine provocation to assess airway hyperresponsiveness

PATHOLOGIC FINDINGS

- Lesions are restricted to the small airways (<5 mm).
- Accumulation of inflammatory cells in the airways and mucus plugging of the airways caused by goblet cell hyperplasia are early changes.
- Smooth muscle hyperplasia from frequent constriction or spasm of the airways

INFLAMMATORY LOWER AIRWAY DISEASE IN YOUNG PERFORMING HORSES

TREATMENT

APPROPRIATE HEALTH CARE
N/A

NURSING CARE
N/A

ACTIVITY
No limitations with a proper therapeutic plan

CLIENT EDUCATION
The disease is not curable and will remain active for the horse's life, but it can be controlled.

SURGICAL CONSIDERATIONS
N/A

MEDICATIONS

DRUGS OF CHOICE

Corticosteroids (Mature Horses)

• Oral—prednisone (300 mg BID for 7–10 days, then 300 mg once a day for 7–10 days, and a maintenance dose of 200–300 mg once a day on alternate days for as long as needed)
• Metered dose inhalers with special delivery devices—beclomethasone dipropionate (250 μg/puff; 12 puffs BID for 2 weeks, then on alternate days for as long as needed) or fluticasone proprionate (250 μg/puff; eight puffs BID for 2 weeks, then on alternate days for as long as needed)

Mast Cell Stabilizer

Nedocromil sodium (2 mg/puff; 12 puffs BID for 2 weeks, then on alternate days for as long as needed)

Bronchodilators

• Clenbuterol (see the label recommendation; dosage varies from country to country)
• Ipatropium bromide (20 μg/puff; five to six puffs given 10–15 minutes before exercise)
• Salbutamol/albuterol (100 μg/puff; 5–10 puffs given 10-15 minutes before exercise)

CONTRAINDICATIONS
Do not use corticosteroids in cases with suspected concomitant viral or bacterial infection, or with of active laminitis.

PRECAUTIONS
• Oral corticosteroids are not recommended in mares while in late gestation; however, inhaled corticosteroids appear safe because of their very low systemic effect.
• Verify medication regulations for withdrawal times before racing and or competition.

POSSIBLE INTERACTIONS
N/A

ALTERNATIVE DRUGS
Herbal therapy and allergen desensitization have not been shown to control the airway inflammatory process.

FOLLOW-UP

PATIENT MONITORING
N/A

PREVENTION/AVOIDANCE
• Avoid moldy hay and straw.
• Maximize fresh-air periods, and reduce stabling time.
• Change diet—haylage, complete feed, or hay cubes with low-dust content

POSSIBLE COMPLICATIONS
Acute exacerbations may lead to heaves if the horse is exposed to an environment rich in mold and dust.

EXPECTED COURSE AND PROGNOSIS
The disease is a lifelong condition, and prognosis largely depends on early diagnosis and owner compliance with maintaining a low-allergen environment and a therapeutic corticosteroid regimen.

MISCELLANEOUS

ASSOCIATED CONDITIONS
N/A

AGE-RELATED FACTORS
The condition tends to progress with age.

ZOONOTIC POTENTIAL
N/A

PREGNANCY
See *Medications* and *Precautions.*

SYNONYMS
• Allergic lower airway disease
• Inflammatory airway disease

SEE ALSO
Heaves

Suggested Reading

Viel L. Lower airway inflammation in young horses. In: Robinson NE, ed. Current Therapy in Equine Medecine, 4th ed. Philadelphia:WB Saunders, 1997.

Author Laurent Viel
Consulting Editor Jean-Pierre Lavoie

INFLUENZA

BASICS

DEFINITION

Equine influenza is a highly contagious viral disease of horses. It is the single most important equine respiratory disease in many countries.

PATHOPHYSIOLOGY

Equine influenza viruses belong to the orthomyxovirus family. There are two subtypes: influenza A/equine/1 and influenza A/equine/2. These subtypes are classified on the basis of the antigenic characteristics of their surface glycoproteins, the hemagglutinin (HA) and the neuraminidase (NA). A/equine/1 viruses carry an H7HA and an N7NA; A/equine/2 viruses carry an H3HA and an N8NA.

An important characteristic of influenza viruses is their ability to undergo antigenic drift, which decreases the degree and duration of protection conferred by previous infection or vaccination because cross-reacting antibody is less efficient and durable than homologous antibody in neutralizing virus. It allows the virus to avoid neutralization by antibody present in the equine population, and thus it can continue to infect seropositive animals. This is caused by mutations, especially mutations that occur in the genes coding for the HA and NA, resulting in changes in the antigenic character of the surface glycoproteins. A/equine/1 viruses undergo less antigenic drift, so are more antigenically stable and less pathogenic than A/equine/2 viruses, which undergo extensive antigenic drift. Strains of A/equine/2 viruses have been responsible for all known outbreaks of the disease since 1980.

SYSTEMS AFFECTED

Respiratory System

Influenza is contracted by inhalation and is extremely contagious. The virus infects the epithelial cells lining the upper and lower airways. The hemagglutinin spike is a key component of the virus, as this enables the virus particle to attach to the epithelium and gain entry to the cell. Infection of ciliated epithelium causes loss of cilia within 3–4 days of infection, which compromises the mucociliary clearance mechanism. This predisposes the compromised airways to secondary bacterial infection.

Musculoskeletal

Myalgia

Cardiovascular

Vasculitis and occasionally myocarditis

GENETICS

N/A

INCIDENCE/PREVALENCE

Worldwide distribution except for Australia and New Zealand, where equine influenza has not yet been reported. Equine influenza is endemic in North America and Europe.

SIGNALMENT

Effects horses, donkeys, mules, and zebras. No known breed or sex predilections for the disease. Usually affects animals between 1 and 3 years old, but can affect animals of any age.

SIGNS

General Comments

Sudden onset disease with short incubation period of 1–3 days. Horses remain infective for 3–6 days after the last signs of disease. Spread is very rapid, with morbidity reaching 100% in immunologically naive populations. Mortality rate is usually low in uncomplicated cases, with the exception of foals. Foals lacking maternal antibody show very severe clinical signs of viral pneumonia, which may lead to death within 48 hr.

Historical Findings

- Cough
- Nasal discharge
- Fever
- Depression
- Lethargy
- Inappetance
- Stiffness
- Lower limb swelling

Physical Examination Findings

In unprimed animals, the clinical signs are very characteristic. Pyrexia may reach 41° C/106 °F, is acute in onset and often biphasic, and usually persists for 7–10 days. There is a dry, hacking cough that may persist for 2–3 weeks. Serous nasal discharge may become mucopurulent, especially if secondary bacterial infection occurs. Other symptoms include dullness, depression, inappetance, submandibular lymph node enlargement, muscular soreness, distal limb edema, and cardiac arrythmias secondary to a viral myocarditis.

In animals that have been previously infected or are vaccinated, clinical signs are modified, thus making it impossible to distinguish between influenza and other respiratory pathogens. These individuals may develop no more than transient mild pyrexia and an occasional cough.

CAUSES

N/A

RISK FACTORS

Rapid national and international transportation of horses incubating the infection or asymptomatically infected with influenza virus without adequate quarantining facilitates widespread distribution of the disease. Although subclinically infected animals are not recognizable as a source of infection, it is likely that they play an important role in the maintenance and spread of the disease because there is no evidence of a carrier state. Epizootics frequently start at large congregations of immunologically naive horses, such as at racetracks, shows, and sales. Viral antigenic drift and failure to vaccinate horses regularly lead to outbreaks in partially immune populations. Infection can occur year round, but outbreaks are more frequent in the winter and spring because the low ambient temperature and humidity enhance virus survival.

DIAGNOSIS

DIFFERENTIAL DIAGNOSIS

Equine rhinovirus has a very similar clinical presentation, but this disease is less contagious than influenza and affected animals usually do not have a cough. Equine herpesvirus types 1 and 4 (EHV-1/EHV-4) respiratory infection is indistinguishable from influenza on clinical signs alone. Equine viral arteritis (EVA) may present with ocular signs (e.g., conjunctivitis, corneal edema) and signs related to vasculitis (e.g., sheath, scrotal, limb, eyelid, and ventral midline edema). *Streptococcus equi* (strangles) presents with characteristic submandibular and retropharyngeal lymph node enlargement and abscessation.

CBC/BIOCHEMISTRY/URINALYSIS

Horses may initially exhibit a lymphopenia followed by a monocytosis.

OTHER LABORATORY TESTS

Definitive diagnosis can be made by isolating virus from nasopharyngeal swabs collected during the acute stages of the infection (i.e., first 24 hr). A retrospective diagnosis can be made by detection of a four-fold or greater rise in antibody titer in paired serum samples, collected 10–14 days apart (both an acute and a convalescent serum sample are necessary to establish a definitive diagnosis). Enzyme-linked immunosorbent assay (ELISA) kit for detection of influenza antigen in nasal secretions is available, simple to use, and useful for making a rapid tentative diagnosis (although diagnosis should still be confirmed with more conventional methods).

IMAGING

Thoracic radiographs may reveal a mixed bronchoalveolar pattern with increased interstitial markings.

DIAGNOSTIC PROCEDURES

Endoscopy of the pharynx, larynx, and trachea may reveal evidence of inflammation. Transtracheal wash samples can be submitted for culture and cytology, particularly if secondary bacterial infection is suspected.

PATHOLOGIC FINDINGS

Pharyngitis, laryngitis, and tracheitis are evident in the upper airways. In the lower airways, bronchitis and bronchiolitis, interstitial pneumonia, congestion, edema, and neutrophil infiltration are present.

TREATMENT

APPROPRIATE HEALTH CARE

Immediate isolation of affected animals to decrease the level of virus in the environment. Outpatient medical management is appropriate.

NURSING CARE

Treatment is symptomatic and supportive. Infected horses should not be subjected to undue stresses.

ACTIVITY

Horses must be rested completely. Rest decreases the severity of the clinical signs, minimizes the viral shedding, and shortens the recovery period. One week of rest for each febrile day is recommended, with a gradual return to work. Horses that suffer severe infections may be unfit for competition for 50–100 days after infection.

DIET

Inappetant, sick horses may need to be encouraged to eat. A variety of good-quality, palatable feed should be offered to ensure adequate nutritional intake.

CLIENT EDUCATION

All new arrivals on a premises or horses suspected of being infected should be promptly isolated to minimize spread of the disease. Secondary complications and sequelae to equine influenza are common in stressed or neglected animals, so it is vital to emphasize the importance of supportive care and adequate rest.

SURGICAL CONSIDERATIONS

N/A

MEDICATIONS

DRUG(S) OF CHOICE

Non-steroidal anti-inflammatory drugs (NSAIDs) may be indicated to decrease fever, eliminate myalgia, and improve appetite (e.g., flunixin meglumine, 1 mg/kg BID IV, IM, or PO). Antibiotic choice to treat secondary bacterial infection should be based on trans-tracheal wash culture results.

CONTRAINDICATIONS

Corticosteroids should not be used due to the risk of secondary bacterial infection of the compromised airways.

PRECAUTIONS

NSAID toxicity results in ulceration of the mucosa, particularly the oral, gastric, and right dorsal colon mucosa.

POSSIBLE INTERACTIONS

N/A

ALTERNATIVE DRUGS

N/A

INFLUENZA

FOLLOW-UP

PATIENT MONITORING

Monitor temperature daily and watch for resolution of cough and nasal discharge. During infection, frequent examination of the respiratory tract is indicated to detect development of secondary complications (e.g., bacterial pneumonia or pleuropneumonia).

PREVENTION/AVOIDANCE

Vaccination against equine influenza can effectively reduce the severity of the disease and decrease spread of infection, but at the present time vaccination rarely prevents infection. All current vaccines are administered by intramuscular injection and contain formalin-inactivated antigens of both types of influenza virus. The immunity stimulated by these vaccines lasts for only 2–3 months due to the fact that they are inactivated and do not contain the most relevant recent field isolates of the influenza virus. As the virus is so inherently mutable, the development of a safe live vaccine is difficult. Following natural infection, immunity lasts for approximately 12 months. Vaccine manufacturers recommend a primary course of two doses of vaccine 4–6 weeks apart, followed by a booster dose 6 months later. In high-risk situations, it may be beneficial to give a third dose of vaccine before 6 months. Ideally, horses should be monitored serologically to ensure that they have responded well to the vaccination and that their antibody titers are at a protective level. Serologic screens also identify poor responders that would require additional boosters. Young horses should be vaccinated every 6 months and if they are competing regularly, vaccination at intervals of 3–4 months is recommended to provide optimal protection. Older horses can be vaccinated every 9–12 months, especially if they seldom attend horses shows and competitions. On stud farms it is important to ensure a good supply of colostral antibody to protect the foals. Pregnant mares should be vaccinated during late gestation. Foals should not begin vaccination until they are weaned. Maternal antibody interferes with the vaccine, and may even inhibit the response to subsequent doses of vaccine administered after colostral antibodies have declined to a level that would not be expected to block the response to vaccination. In foals with no maternal immunity, vaccination can be started as early as 1 month of age. Side effects of the influenza vaccine include fever, depression, muscle stiffness, and pain and swelling around the vaccination site. These signs should resolve within 1–2 days, but it is not recommended to vaccinate horses for influenza within 7–10 days of an athletic event. Prompt isolation of any new arrivals or suspects is very important in limiting spread of the disease. Horses sharing the same airspace can be infected within hours of the introduction of an infected horse. The persistent dry cough that affected horses develop releases large quantities of aerosolized virus particles into the atmosphere. The virus can also be carried on the wind and infect horses on neighboring premises. Transmission of virus can occur from contact with contaminated personnel, housing, and vehicles. Housing and transport vehicles should be thoroughly disinfected before reuse by uninfected animals. Personnel should not move between infected and uninfected premises. The virus is very susceptible to sunlight and disinfectants such as chlorine bleach, which is inexpensive and highly effective. The virus does not persist in the environment for long periods unless protected by proteinaceous solutions (e.g., nasal discharge).

POSSIBLE COMPLICATIONS

Secondary bacterial pneumonia or pleuropneumonia and the development of bronchitis resulting in long-term coughing are potential complications that may follow viral respiratory disease in horses that have not been adequately rested before returning to training, or before undergoing stressful events (e.g., long trailer rides). Another possible complication following a viral infection is myocarditis, resulting in cardiac arrhythmias.

EXPECTED COURSE AND PROGNOSIS

Prognosis for recovery and return to athletic function for an uncomplicated case of equine influenza is good, as long as appropriate treatment is given and adequate rest is allowed. Secondary bacterial pneumonia and pleuropneumonia worsen the prognosis for return to athletic function and significantly prolong the recovery period.

MISCELLANEOUS

ASSOCIATED CONDITIONS

N/A

AGE-RELATED FACTORS

Foals lacking maternal antibody show very severe clinical signs of viral pneumonia. These animals require emergency inpatient intensive care, and the prognosis for their recovery is very guarded.

ZOONOTIC POTENTIAL

N/A

PREGNANCY

NSAIDs are particularly indicated in the treatment of febrile pregnant mares to decrease the risk of abortion. Corticosteroids, which are contraindicated in the treatment of this disease, are always contraindicated in pregnant mares due to the risk of inducing abortion.

SYNONYMS

N/A

SEE ALSO

N/A

ABBREVIATIONS

- ELISA = Enzyme-linked immunosorbent assay
- EHV-1 = Equine herpesvirus type 1
- EHV-4 = Equine herpesvirus type 4
- EVA = Equine viral arteritis
- HA = Hemagglutinin
- NA = Neuraminidase

Suggested Reading

Reed SM, Bayly WM. Equine internal medicine. Philadelphia: WB Saunders, 1998:267-270.

Robinson NE. Current therapy in equine medicine 4. Philadelphia: WB Saunders, 1997:443-448.

Smith BP. Large animal internal medicine, second edition. Mosby, 1996:584-588; 1636-1638.

Timoney RJ. Equine influenza. Comparative immunology, microbiology & infectious diseases. 1996;19(3):205-211.

Author Nuala Summerfield, BVM&S, MRCVS

Consulting Editor Corinne R. Sweeney

INSECT HYPERSENSITIVITY

DEFINITION

- Most common cause of equine pruritus
- Generally seasonal, highly pruritic, and can involve urticaria
- Some species (e.g. C. variipennis) transmit the filarid parasite, Onchocerca cervicalis hich in itself may result in similar clinical signs with ventral crusting/pruritus

PATHOPHYSIOLOGY

- Culicoides hypersensitivity immediate and/or delayed hypersensitivity reactions to salivary components, causing pruritus and self-trauma.
- Whole body extracts of Culicoides used in intradermal testing of affected horses are capable of inducing skin test reactions.
- Tendency to develop the disease is multifactorial (familial; therefore genetic tendency ??; associated with the major histocompatibility complex; geographic)
- The bite itself is painful, due to the chewing mouth parts of these flies.

SIGNALMENT

- No sex, or breed predilections
- Age of onset is typically between 2 and 4 years of age

SIGNS

- Pruritus with varying degrees of severity followed by papules or wheals
- Secondarily, alopecia, crusting, excoriations, hypopigmentation, & lichenification occur
- Distribution pattern is determined by the species of Culicoides (ventral only, mane and tail, dorsal, all of the aforementioned).
- Severe pruritus, sometimes to the point of being steroid non-responsive.
- Secondary Staphylococcus infections are common and may exacerbate the pruritus.
- Seasonal to non-seasonal

CAUSES

- Hypersensitivity to salivary antigens of biting insects or inhalation of desicated insects
- *Culicoides* spp., black flies, horn flies and stable flies most commonly
- Occasionally mosquitoes, deer flies, and horse flies

RISK FACTORS

- Flies feed at dawn and dusk, and require standing water in which to breed

DIFFERENTIAL DIAGNOSES

- Atopy/Food allergy
- Onchocerciasis, especially if not on an ivermectin deworming protocol
- Other ectoparasites (pediculosis, fleas, ticks, chorioptic and psoroptic acariasis)
- Oxyuris equi
- Besnoitiosis, dermatophytosis, dermatophilosis
- Mane & tail dystrophy
- Cutaneous drug reaction

DIAGNOSIS

- History, Physical examination concentrating on the distribution pattern
- Seasonality (for example spring—C. niger and alachua; summer—C. stellifer; fall—C. insignis; depending on the region)
- Evidence of breeding grounds for insects (forrested area, ponds/still water within a mile)
- Response to stringent insect control

DIAGNOSTIC PROCEDURES

- Intradermal skin testing is being used extensively as a diagnostic tool (Greer Labs, Lenoir, NC) using Culicoides variipennis which cross-reacts with other species of Culicoides and possibly other insects (1:5000 w/v)
- Other insects based on regional distribution
- In vitro testing is not reliable for insect hypsersensitivities

PATHOLOGIC FINDINGS

- Dermatopathology is supportive but not conclusive of insect hypersensitivity
- Mild to severe perivascular eosinophilic/lymphocytic dermatitis and folliculitis
- Areas of epidermal damage as a result of the bite
- Eosinophilic vasculitis and dermal fibrosis may be seen depending on lesion chronicity

TREATMENT

APPROPRIATE HEALTH CARE

Non-pharmacologic treatment methods are paramount to help minimize the need for pharmacologic therapy and to provide a successful outcome treatment of insect hypersensitivity.

NURSING CARE

- Fly control is mandatory (late afternoon) with a 2% permethrin-based product (Flypel by Allerderm) or Avon's Skin-So-Soft (50:50 with water) daily in the late afternoon
- Frequent bathing using cool water (tar, sulfur/salicylic acid, anitmicrobial shampoos such as EquiTar (DVM) or Equine Medicated Shampoo (Vet Solutions) +/− colloidal oatmeal rinses with Pramoxine HCl such as Relief Crème Rinse (DVM) or Resiprox (Allerderm)).

ACTIVITY

- Change the environment
  - —move away from standing water
  - —stable before dusk to after dawn
  - —+/−32 × 32 per 2.5 cm grid meshing painted with permethrins regularly
  - —fans within the stall blowing over the patient's affected area(s)
  - —timed-release insecticide sprays

DIET

N/A

CLIENT EDUCATION

A concerted effort and consistency are required to achieve success. Seasonal aggressiveness is regionally dependent. Serious consideration to moving the patient to an area that is less favorable for insect proliferation may be required if little success is obtained from medicinal therapy.

Due to the potential hereditary factor, owners should be encouraged to remove the affected individuals from their breeding program.

SURGICAL CONSIDERATIONS

N/A

MEDICATIONS

DRUGS OF CHOICE

- Antihistamines—blocks the action of histamines at receptor sites
  - —antipruritic, reduce urticarial reactions
  - —stabilizing mast cells and having anti-serotonin properties
  - —exact dosing and pharmacokinetics are lacking in the horse
  - —typically have fewer side effects than corticosteroids but not as effective
  - —pyrilamine maleate 1 mg/kg
  - —hydroxyzine hydrochloride 1–1.5 mg/kg TID (urticaria $\gg$ pruritus)
  - —diphenhydramine 0.75–1 mg/kg BID
  - —doxepin hydrochloride 0.5–0.75 mg/kg BID
  - —chlorpheniramine 0.25 mg/kg BID

- Corticosteroids—often required in many of our allergic skin disorders
  - —judicious use, appropriate amounts and intervals, individual treatment are key
  - —prednisone and prednisolone
    - —prednisone is converted to prednisolone
    - —0.5–1.5 mg/kg/day 7–14 days (induction), then taper to 0.2–0. 5 mg/kg every 48h over 2–5 weeks
  - —dexamethasone
    - —initial loading/pulse dose is needed at 0.02–0.1 mg/kg
    - —oral maintenance dosage of 0.01–0.02 mg/kg every 48–72h
    - —this regime is particularly helpful in more refractory cases

CONTRAINDICATIONS/PRECAUTIONS

Due to the side effects of antihistamines including light sedation and occasional personality changes, judicious use is recommended in working horses. As well, most Horse Associations recommends withdrawal periods from both these medications before any show/competition.

Pregnant mares, horses with prior history of laminitis, and any patient experiencing internal organ complications should be omitted from a treatment regimen that includes steroids.

ALTERNATIVE DRUGS

- Essential Fatty Acid (EFA) supplementation—has had increased use in the horse
  - —modifies the arachidonic acid cascade
  - —recent study in 14 horses with seasonal *Culicoides* hypersensitivity demonstrated that 20 g daily of evening primrose and cold water marine fish oil (80:20) resulted in 4 horses that were no better, 5 horses were better and 5 horses were much improved.
  - —a University of Florida study of 17 horses fed 200 ml of linseed per day for a 6 week period, showed no significant change in pruritus or lesional surface areas (time frame too short??)
  - —response has been variable
  - —DVM's Derm Caps or 3VCaps Liquid Econo @ double the dose
  - —Allerderm's EFA Caps HP @ double the dose
  - —Vet Solutions EFA @ 2 2/3 pumps per 500kg
  - —use these fatty acids as adjunctive therapy
- Hyposensitization—approximately 50% of the horses have good to excellent responses
  - —hyposensitization based on IDAT provides optimal responses
  - —after an induction period, injections are given every 7–28 days
  - —response seems faster than in dogs and humans
  - —response is variable. Dr. Gail Anderson demonstrated benefit of a mycobacterial cell wall adjuvant based Culicoides extract with 80–90% response
- Methylsulfonylmethane (MSM, Vita-Flex Nutrition Co.)
  - —initially at 2 heaping tsp (around 10–12 gm) BID, then taper to SID dose

FOLLOW-UP

PATIENT MONITORING

Follow-up visits and recheck calls should be pursued a minimum of every 4 weeks to ensure owner compliance and to make any adjustments for any seasonal changes.

PREVENTION/AVOIDANCE

Indeed avoidance is the key to therapy. Starting fly control early in the season and consistency will prevent any further recurrence. Modifying the environment by means of an enclosed stall or a change in the environment are essential to minimize clinical signs.

POSSIBLE COMPLICATIONS

The major complication involves the development of secondary bacterial infections and longterm scarring.

EXPECTED COURSE AND PROGNOSIS

Seasonal recurrence is expected unless the patient is moved to a more desirable location. Potential desensitization may occur in a minority of cases; most require on-going longterm therapy.

MISCELLANEOUS

ASSOCIATED CONDITIONS

- Atopy
- Food allergy
- Combined allergies are common

AGE-RELATED FACTORS

- Not typically seen in horses less than 1 year of age
- Age of onset may be greater than 4 years if the patient has recently moved from a low to a high allergen load region

ZOONOTIC POTENTIAL

N/A

PREGNANCY

N/A

SYNONYMS

Queensland itch
Sweet itch
No-See-Um hypersensitivity

ABBREVIATIONS

N/A

Suggested Reading

Pascoe RRR, Knottenbelt DC. Manual of Equine Dermatology. WB Saunders, London, England, 1999.

Perris EE. Parasitic dermatoses that cause pruritus in horses. In: Fadok VA, ed. VCNA; equine practice: dermatology. WB Saunders, Philadelphia, 1995; vol. 11(1): pp. 11–28.

Stannard AA. Immunologic Diseases. Vet Derm 2000 Vol 11(3):166–168.

Author Anthony A. Yu

INSPIRATORY DYSPNEA

BASICS

DEFINITION

- *Dyspnea* is a term that describes the sensation of difficult breathing.
- In animals, dyspnea is used to describe the clinical signs associated with respiratory distress, which can be present throughout the respiratory cycle or primarily be associated with either inhalation (i.e., inspiratory dyspnea) or exhalation (i.e., expiratory dyspnea).

PATHOPHYSIOLOGY

- Generally a sign of impaired gas exchange, with the increased effort to inhale being associated with an increased need to ventilate the lung
- Primary causes—failure of delivery of air into the lung (i.e., alveolar hypoventilation) and of exchange between the lung and blood (i.e., an exchange problem). The former can result from airway obstruction, pleural disease, chest wall or diaphragmatic injury, pneumothorax, encroachment of the abdomen on the thorax (e.g., advanced pregnancy), or CNS disease. Relevant exchange problems primarily are those causing alveolar disease (e.g., pneumonia, pulmonary edema).
- Can also be a sign of decreased oxygen delivery to the tissues (e.g., cardiovascular disease, anemia) and of the need to eliminate more carbon dioxide to correct a metabolic acidosis.
- The most severe cases usually result from obstruction of the extrathoracic airway, because the negative pressure generated in the airways during inhalation tends to collapse these structures. Thus, cases originating in the extrathoracic airway often become worse during exercise.

SYSTEMS AFFECTED

- Respiratory
- Cardiovascular
- Hemic/lymphatic/immune
- Endocrine/metabolic—response to metabolic acidosis
- Nervous

SIGNALMENT

Depends on the underlying cause—foals with guttural pouch tympani, young mature horses with pleuritis, and old animals with neoplasia encroaching on the airway

SIGNS

General Comments

Inspiratory dyspnea is a sign, but associated signs can indicate the source of the dyspnea.

Historical Findings

- Sudden onset of inspiratory dyspnea can indicate acute inflammatory disease of the lung or pleural space; trauma to the chest wall, diaphragm, or extrathoracic airway; or acute blood loss.
- Dyspnea of slower onset may result from a space-occupying mass encroaching on the respiratory system.
- Inappetence indicates inflammatory disease or inability to eat resulting from the severity of the dyspnea.
- Cough indicates inflammation of the tracheobronchial tree and can be a sign of pneumonia.
- Bilateral mucopurulent nasal discharge usually originates distal to the larynx and indicates inflammation of the lower airway.
- Unilateral nasal discharge, either purulent or hemorrhagic, suggests nasopharyngeal (including the sinuses and guttural pouches) disease.
- Noisy breathing indicates obstruction of the extrathoracic airway.

Physical Examination Findings

- Flared nostrils, increased excursions of the thorax during breathing, and retractions (i.e., "sinking in") of the intercostal spaces, particularly if the horse is laboring against a severe upper airway obstruction.
- Prolonged inhalation
- Exaggerated excursions of the diaphragm are indicated by increased movement of the anal sphincter.
- Nasal obstruction—unilateral nasal discharge, foul breath, or noisy breathing
- Strangles—fever, mucopurulent nasal discharge, swollen, or draining lymph nodes
- Guttural pouch tympani—fluctuant, air-filled swelling of the parotid region (usually bilateral)
- Pharyngeal or laryngeal paralysis—if severe or bilateral, severe inspiratory dyspnea and inspiratory noise
- Laryngeal hemiplegia does not produce signs in resting animals, but reduced exercise tolerance is associated with inspiratory noise (i.e., "roaring") during strenuous exercise.
- Pneumonia—fever, tracheal sensitivity, or increased breath sounds audible by stethoscope over the affected region (can be silent if consolidation is extensive or there is overlying pleural fluid)
- Pulmonary edema—fine, inspiratory crackles
- Pneumothorax—lack of breath sounds, possible resonance on percussion, and little air movement despite large effort
- Pleural effusion/pleuritis—lack of lung sounds ventrally, harsh sounds dorsally, can be friction rubs, abducted elbows indicating pain, fever, or depression
- Fractured ribs—signs of trauma, sounds of air entering and leaving wound, or signs of pain
- Diaphragmatic hernia—reduction in lung sounds, signs of colic, or borborygmi audible in chest

(**NOTE:** Borborygmi usually are heard in the ventral thorax, adjacent to the heart)

- Anemia—pallor
- Cardiac disease—murmurs, thrills, or arrhythmias

CAUSES

Respiratory causes

Extrathoracic Airway:

- Paresis of the external nares
- Severe atheroma
- Congestion of the nasal mucosa—Horner's syndrome; inflammatory disease
- Deviation of the nasal septum
- Space-occupying lesion affecting the nasal cavity—foreign body, intraluminal mass, ethmoid hematoma, or extraluminal mass or swelling
- Congenital pharyngeal cysts
- Pharyngeal or laryngeal paresis
- Space-occupying masses encroaching on the pharynx—enlarged lymph nodes; guttural pouch enlargement (usually by tympanites)
- Trauma to the hyoid bone or larynx—edema; chondritis
- Laryngeal or pharyngeal paresis—degenerative nerve disease, lead poisoning, or trauma to left recurrent laryngeal nerves by jugular perivascular injection
- Tracheal foreign body or collapse—Shetland ponies; miniature horses

Lower Respiratory Tract:

- Severe bronchiolitis or heaves—accompanied by expiratory dyspnea, which is more pronounced
- Pulmonary edema—cardiogenic or noncardiogenic
- Pneumonia—bacterial, viral, or fungal
- Pleuritis/pleuropneumonia
- Accumulation of pleural fluid
- Pneumothorax
- Diaphragmatic hernia
- Fractured ribs
- Flail chest
- Mediastinal masses

Nonrespiratory Causes

- Cardiovascular—congenital cardiac defect with right-to-left shunt, right-sided failure, or pulmonary embolus
- Hemic—anemia, methemoglobinemia, or carbon monoxide or cyanide poisoning
- Endocrine/metabolic—metabolic acidosis; hyperthermia
- Nervous—trauma to recurrent laryngeal nerves or pharyngeal plexus, lead poisoning, phrenic nerve injury, or diaphragmatic paralysis
- Reproductive—advanced pregnancy; hydrops amnion

RISK FACTORS

See the individual conditions causing inspiratory dyspnea.

DIAGNOSIS

DIFFERENTIAL DIAGNOSIS

Differentiating Similar Signs

- Expiratory dyspnea is characterized by an enhanced abdominal component to exhalation, with a tucking up of the abdomen toward the end of exhalation.
- Tachypnea, a rapid breathing in response to severe heat stress, is not accompanied by prolonged inhalation.
- Deep breathing with a marked inspiratory effort also follows strenuous exercise.

Differentiating Causes

- Upper airway obstructions can produce severe respiratory distress and are accompanied by inspiratory noise.
- Lung and pleural disease often is inflammatory and, therefore, accompanied by fever, malaise, and inappetence.
- Damage to the respiratory pump (i.e., chest and diaphragm) may result in strenuous efforts to breathe, with little movement of air.
- Cardiac disease usually is accompanied by other signs—murmurs, thrills, and irregularities of rate and rhythm.
- Metabolic acidosis is accompanied by signs of disease of the kidneys, gastrointestinal, or endocrine systems.

CBC/BIOCHEMISTRY/URINALYSIS

A hemogram identifies anemia and inflammatory disease.

OTHER LABORATORY TESTS

- Arterial blood gas analysis identifies hypoventilation (i.e., increased Pa_{CO_2}) and hypoxemia (i.e., low Pa_{O_2}).
- Elevated Pa_{CO_2} (>45 torr) accompanied by hypoxemia (Pa_{O_2} <85 torr) indicates severe upper airway obstruction, damage to the respiratory pump, or severe lung disease.
- Low Pa_{CO_2} (<40 torr) accompanied by decreased pH and elevated Pa_{O_2} (>100 torr) indicates metabolic acidosis; low Pa_{CO_2} accompanied by hypoxemia indicates pulmonary disease.

IMAGING

Radiography

- Skull—nasal obstructions; sinus disease
- Throat—guttural pouch tympani and empyema, hyoid bone injury, or laryngeal injury
- Neck—tracheal damage, foreign bodies, or tracheal collapse
- Thorax—pleuritis, pleural fluid, pneumonia, pulmonary edema, pneumothorax, cardiac enlargement, fractured ribs, or diaphragmatic hernia

INSPIRATORY DYSPNEA

Ultrasonography

- Very useful for identifying pleural fluid or focal loculated regions of pleural effusion
- Also may identify masses in the lung—abscesses; neoplasia
- Echocardiography can identify chamber enlargement, congenital defects, and valvular disease.
- Doppler flow can determine the severity of regurgitant blood flow.

Endoscopy

- Essential for diagnosing space-occupying lesions of the extrathoracic airway
- Videoendoscopy during exercise may be necessary to determine the significance of pharyngeal or laryngeal collapse.
- Endoscopy also can assess for mucopurulent exudate in the trachea, which is a sign of inflammation of the lower airways and lung.

OTHER DIAGNOSTIC PROCEDURES

- Cytology of lower airways, preferably with bronchoalveolar lavage, can determine the presence of lower airway inflammation.
- Bronchoalveolar lavage may overlook a focal lesion if the lavage tube is not lodged specifically in the affected region.
- Bacterial culture of tracheal mucus or tracheal lavage revealing a relatively pure culture of a known pathogen is significant.
- Pleurocentesis determines the presence and nature of pleural fluid.

TREATMENT

RELIEVING UPPER AIRWAY OBSTRUCTION

- Relieve upper airway obstruction sufficient to cause panic or life-threatening hypoxemia (indicated by cyanosis) by tracheotomy.
- Nasotracheal intubation can be used to bypass the obstruction, especially if that obstruction will be corrected surgically within a short time.
- **NOTE:** Tracheotomy is not useful for relief of dyspnea originating in the lower airway, lungs, or thorax.

SUPPORTIVE VENTILATION

- Animals with hypoventilation resulting from thoracic damage may need positive-pressure ventilation, which can be accomplished via a nasotracheal tube until the horse is anesthetized for correction of the injury.
- Ventilation to maintain gas exchange in an animal with pulmonary disease is difficult.

OXYGEN THERAPY

- Supplemental oxygenation via a nasotracheal or nasopharyngeal catheter relieves hypoxemia and accompanying distress when dyspnea results from lung disease.
- In cases of upper airway obstruction or thoracic trauma, oxygen can be life-saving until the problem is surgically corrected.
- Anemia (PCV <10 L/L) sufficient to cause dyspnea requires administration of blood to restore the PCV; without hemoglobin, blood cannot carry oxygen.

CHEST TAP

- Can be both diagnostic and therapeutic.
- Drainage of pleural fluid allows lung expansion.
- Removal of air in cases of pneumothorax restores the negative pressure necessary for breathing.

MEDICATIONS

DRUGS OF CHOICE

Depend on cause of the dyspnea.

CONTRAINDICATIONS

N/A

PRECAUTIONS

N/A

POSSIBLE INTERACTIONS

N/A

ALTERNATIVE DRUGS

N/A

FOLLOW UP

PATIENT MONITORING

- After surgery for upper airway obstruction, monitor patients carefully for signs of further obstruction caused by postoperative swelling.
- Tracheotomy tubes need to be removed and cleaned regularly to prevent occlusion by mucus and exudates.
- Once tracheotomy tubes are removed, stricture at the site of tracheotomy may lead to further inspiratory dyspnea.
- Carefully monitor for redevelopment of pleural effusion and recurrence of pneumothorax.

POSSIBLE COMPLICATIONS

N/A

MISCELLANEOUS

ASSOCIATED CONDITIONS

N/A

AGE-RELATED FACTORS

N/A

ZOONOTIC POTENTIAL

N/A

PREGNANCY

Fetal growth retardation and death may occur in mares with severely compromised respiratory function.

SYNONYMS

N/A

SEE ALSO

- Acute epiglottiditis
- Arytenoid chondritis
- Aspiration pneumonia
- Atheroma of the false nostril
- Diaphragmatic hernia
- Expiratory dyspnea
- Guttural pouch tympany
- Pleuropneumonia
- Pneumothorax
- Respiratory distress syndrome
- Thoracic trauma

ABBREVIATION

PCV = packed cell volume

Suggested Reading

Ames TR, Hmidouch A. Pathophysiology and diagnosis of respiratory disease. In: Kobluk CN, Ames TR, Geor RJ, eds. The horse: diseases and clinical management. Philadelphia: WB Saunders, 1995:199–212.

Hannas CM, Derksen FJ. Principles of emergency respiratory therapy. In: Colahan PT, Mayhew IG, Merritt AM, Moore JM, eds. Equine medicine and surgery. 4th ed. Goleta: American Veterinary Publications, 1991;1:372–374.

Laverty S. Thoracic trauma. In: Robinson NE, ed. Current therapy in equine medicine. 4th ed. Philadelphia: WB Saunders, 1997:463–465.

Parente EJ. Diagnostic techniques for upper airway obstruction. In: Robinson NE, ed. Current therapy in equine medicine. 4th ed. Philadelphia: WB Saunders, 1997:401–403.

Author N. Edward Robinson

Consulting Editor Jean-Pierre Lavoie

Inspiratory dyspnea: Robinson Page 7

INSULIN LEVELS/INSULIN TOLERANCE TEST

BASICS

DEFINITION

• Serum insulin concentrations may be measured to evaluate a horse's ability to regulate its blood glucose appropriately.
• In normal horses, insulin secretion is closely tied to blood glucose concentrations. Insulin concentrations are quite low when the horse is fasting but increase rapidly when the horse receives glucose or eats a meal high in soluble carbohydrates.
• Blood insulin concentrations are consistently elevated in horses with pars intermedia tumors.
• Because insulin concentrations are so labile, insulin response or tolerance tests may give a better picture of the horse's endocrine status.
• Insulin tolerance test—give crystalline insulin (0.05 U/kg IV) or regular insulin (0.4–8 IU/kg IV), and determine blood glucose at baseline and then every 15 minutes for 3 hours. In normal horses, expect to see a decrease $\geq 50\%$ in blood glucose at 30 minutes.
• Serum insulin response also can be measured after administering dextrose (0.5 g/kg IV). Insulin should be low when starting, increase within 5 minutes of the dextrose load, and decrease rapidly once blood glucose levels begin to drop. Serum glucose should normalize within 3 hours after dextrose.
• The most common pathologic process leading to abnormal results is insulin resistance in horses with pars intermedia tumors—equine Cushing's syndrome.

PATHOPHYSIOLOGY

• Inappropriately low insulin levels—pancreatitis, leading to destruction of beta cells and development of type 1 diabetes mellitus
• Increased insulin levels in hypoglycemic horse—insulin-secreting tumor (i.e., insulinoma) or iatrogenic insulin administration
• Increased serum insulin levels in euglycemic or hyperglycemic horses—peripheral insulin resistance caused by type II diabetes mellitus or an insulin antagonist (e.g., cortisol).
• Increased blood cortisol—equine Cushing's syndrome, stress, or glucocorticoid therapy
• Horses with hyperlipemia also exhibit insulin resistance.

SYSTEM AFFECTED

The endocrine system is primarily affected by abnormal blood insulin and insulin response tests—decreased insulin is diagnostic of diabetes mellitus; increased insulin most commonly is associated with insulin antagonists.

SIGNALMENT

• Ponies tend to have higher blood insulin levels than horses and are more prone to hyperlipemia.
• No sex difference
• Obese animals, particularly ponies, are more insulin resistant than thinner animals.
• Cushing's syndrome tends to occur in old horses (>10 years).

SIGNS

• The most common signs in horses with an abnormal insulin response test are those of equine Cushing's syndrome—hirsutism and failure to shed a winter coat; abnormal fat distribution, pendulous abdomen, weight loss, polyuria and polydipsia, laminitis, and tendency to suffer chronic infections also are common.
• The eyelids can look swollen, and the supraorbital fat pad may look bulged.
• Owners may report the horse is dull or depressed.
• Similar clinical signs, but without hirsutism or an abnormal hair coat, are seen in horses with type II diabetes mellitus.
• Clinical signs in horses with Type I diabetes mellitus—weight loss, polyuria and polydipsia, lethargy, or depression
• Signs of excess insulin caused by exogenous overdose or insulinoma are those of hypoglycemia—muscle trembling, ataxia, nystagmus, depression, and facial twitching, leading to convulsions, coma, and death
• Signs of hyperlipemia—include depression, anorexia, and icterus

CAUSES

• The primary cause of increased serum insulin, abnormal response to an insulin response test, or increased insulin after IV glucose is the presence of insulin antagonists. Exogenous or endogenous corticosteroids are the most common, insulin antagonists, but other hormones (e.g., growth hormone, epinephrine) also have this effect.
• When insulin resistance occurs without a predisposing cause, type II diabetes mellitus is diagnosed.
• The most common reason for increased blood insulin without insulin resistance is an insulin-secreting tumor.
• The most common reason for type I diabetes mellitus is pancreatic damage secondary to parasite migration.

RISK FACTORS

• Pituitary tumor is the most common risk factor for development of abnormal insulin secretion.
• Glucocorticoid administration or increased cortisol from a stress response also lead to insulin resistance and hyperglycemia.
• Obesity, particularly in ponies, is associated with insulin resistance, as is hyperlipidemia.

DIAGNOSIS

DIFFERENTIAL DIAGNOSIS

• Polyuria, polydipsia, and glucosuria in horses with suspected endocrine disorders should alert the practitioner to a disorder in glucose homeostasis and, thus, in insulin levels.
• Hypoglycemia from excess insulin—myositis, neurologic disease, and colic
• Determination of abnormally low blood glucose should cause the practitioner to suspect inappropriate insulin levels.

LABORATORY FINDINGS

Drugs that May Alter Lab Results

N/A

Disorders that May Alter Lab Results

Delayed separation of serum from cells falsely lowers blood glucose values, making interpretation of insulin levels more difficult.

Valid If Run in Human Lab?

Yes

CBC/BIOCHEMISTRY/URINALYSIS

• Horses with abnormal insulin levels caused by Cushing's syndrome exhibit stress response with mature neutrophilia, lymphopenia, and eosinopenia. They may also have increased blood glucose and glucosuria.
• Horses with type I or II diabetes mellitus have hyperglycemia.
• Horses with insulinoma or exogenous insulin overdose have hypoglycemia.
• Horses with hyperlipemia have high serum bilirubin and lipid levels.

OTHER LABORATORY TESTS

• Pituitary function—endogenous ACTH determination and dexamethasone suppression test.
• If these results are consistent with equine Cushing's syndrome, this supports that diagnosis; if they do not indicate Cushing's syndrome, suspect stress response or type II diabetes mellitus.

IMAGING

Increased pituitary gland size may be depicted with specialized modalities—CT or venous contrast

DIAGNOSTIC PROCEDURES

Exploratory laparotomy or abdominocentesis may reveal a damaged pancreas but should be considered extremely low yield procedures, because the pancreas normally is difficult to visualize and pancreatic tumors often are microscopic.

INSULIN LEVELS/INSULIN TOLERANCE TEST

TREATMENT

APPROPRIATE HEALTH CARE

- Horses with hypoglycemia require inpatient medical management if the disease is severe and IV dextrose to maintain blood glucose at adequate levels.
- Horses with hyperlipemia also require inpatient medical management that includes IV dextrose, balanced electrolyte solutions, caloric replacement, heparin, and exogenous insulin.
- All other horses with abnormal insulin levels may be treated as outpatients.

NURSING CARE

- Carefully monitor hypoglycemic animals to prevent them from collapsing and injuring themselves.
- Horses with laminitis need corrective hoof trimming and shoeing.

ACTIVITY

- Limit the activity of horses with laminitis.
- Increase the activity of sound, obese horses in an effort to lose weight.

DIET

- Horses with laminitis generally benefit from a low-carbohydrate, high-fiber diet—grass hay
- Keep any horse with insulin resistance on a low-carbohydrate diet.
- Restrict or increase caloric intake until a condition score of 4–6 out of 10 is achieved.

CLIENT EDUCATION

- Horses with Cushing's syndrome may be managed with medication and nursing care, but their prognosis is quite variable. Some do well for several years; others are refractory to treatment. Owners need to understand that treatment of Cushing's syndrome is palliative and is required for life.
- Encourage clients to maintain their horses at condition scores of 4–6 out of 10 and to prevent obesity from developing.

SURGICAL CONSIDERATIONS

N/A

MEDICATIONS

DRUGS OF CHOICE

- The two agents most commonly used to alter the symptoms of Cushing's syndrome are cyproheptadine (0.25–1.2 mg/kg PO SID) and pergolide (0.5–2 mg/day). These two drugs also have been used in horses with suspected type II diabetes with some success.
- Insulin-deficient horses (i.e., type I diabetes mellitus) require insulin supplementation, with the dose being changed in response to the blood glucose level. Protamine zinc insulin (0.5 IU IM BID) normalized blood glucose in a case report of a pony with insulin deficiency.
- Exogenous insulin for the treatment of hyperlipemia—protamine zinc insulin (0.075–0.4 IU/kg SQ or IM BID or SID). Regular insulin (0.4 IU/kg) also has been recommended.

CONTRAINDICATIONS

N/A

PRECAUTIONS

- Dextrose for injection should always be available when administering insulin to any horse. If signs of hypoglycemia occur, treat immediately with IV dextrose.
- Horses that receive an overdose of cyproheptadine or pergolide may exhibit lethargy and ataxia.

POSSIBLE INTERACTIONS

N/A

ALTERNATIVE DRUGS

N/A

FOLLOW-UP

PATIENT MONITORING

- Retest horses with Cushing's syndrome every 6–12 weeks with endogenous ACTH determination or dexamethasone response testing. Abnormal results indicate the need for an increased dose or a change in medication.
- Check the glucose level of horses with diabetes mellitus receiving insulin therapy twice a day. Insulin doses should be increased or decreased in response to blood glucose values outside the normal range.

POSSIBLE COMPLICATIONS

N/A

MISCELLANEOUS

ASSOCIATED CONDITIONS

- Hirsutism, chronic infections, and laminitis are commonly associated with equine Cushing's syndrome.
- Obesity and hyperlipemia are commonly associated with insulin resistance.

AGE-RELATED FACTORS

N/A

ZOONOTIC POTENTIAL

N/A

PREGNANCY

Pregnant mares tend to have higher blood insulin levels than nonpregnant horses. This tendency is most profound early during gestation, and blood glucose levels remain normal.

SYNONYMS

N/A

SEE ALSO

- ACTH
- Pituitary tumors

Suggested Reading

Beech J. Endocrine system. In: Colahan PT, Mayhew IG, Merritt AM, Moore JN, eds. Equine medicine and surgery. 5th ed. St. Louis: Mosby, 1999:1947–1968.

Beech J, Garcia M. Hormonal response to thyrotropin-releasing hormone in healthy horses and in horses with pituitary adenoma. Am J Vet Res 1985;46:1941–1943.

Coffman JR, Colles CM. Insulin tolerance in laminitic ponies. Can J Comp Med 1983;47:347–351.

Riggs WL. Diabetes mellitus secondary to necrotizing pancreatitis in a pony. Southwest Vet 1972;25:149–152.

Ruoff WW, Baker DC, Morgan SJ, et al. Type II diabetes mellitus in a horse. Equine Vet J 1986;18:143–144.

Author Janice Sojka

Consulting Editor Michel Levy

INTERNAL ABDOMINAL ABSCESSES

BASICS

DEFINITION

Internal abdominal abscesses can be defined as an insidious clinical disease characterized by internal sepsis in different localizations presenting in two typical distinct clinical presentations, characterized by weight loss or prolonged colic.

PATHOPHYSIOLOGY

The pathogenesis of mesenteric abscesses has not been elucidated; however, it has been proposed that the development of the internal infection is associated with the inability of the animal to develop adequate immune response to the microorganism involved, thereby allowing systemic spread of the infection. It is thought by some authors that given the high frequency of these abscesses being caused by *Streptococcus equi,* treatment with penicillin prior to abscess maturation and drainage in strangles results in more frequent occurrence of metastatic abscesses. Other authors have pointed out that withholding therapy to allow maturation of the abscess does not help in preventing hematogenous spread of the organisms.

Once the internal abdominal abscess has developed, it can remain dormant as an abscess or peritonitis may develop. This seems to be responsible for the different clinical presentations. Colic events seem to be due to prolonged tension on the mesentery or from adhesions or scarring of the small intestine with acute or chronic obstruction.

SYSTEMS AFFECTED

The internal abdominal abscesses usually involve the mesentery, but can also occur in liver, spleen, kidneys, and uterus.

INCIDENCE AND PREVALENCE

There is no information regarding incidence or prevalence.

SIGNALMENT

Internal abscessation may affect any domestic species. In the equine, all individuals at any age or either sex are at risk. In a study of 25 cases, it was observed that horses <5 yr of age were more commonly affected.

SIGNS

Usually, horses with internal abdominal abscesses present with one of two chief complaints. The first is a history of intermittent or prolonged colic. However, there are cases with history of colic of sudden onset. These animals show depression, congested mucous membranes, increased rectal temperature (> 38.6°C), increased and shallow respiratory rate, groaning on expiration, partial or complete anorexia, constipation, decreased peristaltic sounds, and dehydration. Dysuria can be noticed in some cases.

In the second form of presentation of internal abdominal abscesses, the chief complaint is chronic ongoing weight loss. The body condition in these animals ranges from the cachectic horse to the thin horse that is unable to gain weight. Some animals are depressed, inconsistently anorexic, and have poor shaggy haircoats. The rectal temperature and heart and respiratory rates may be elevated. Abdominal peristaltic sounds are usually normal.

Combinations of the two forms can occur.

In some cases there is evidence of diarrhea, and this seems to be more commonly associated with abscesses caused by *Rhodococcus* infection in foals and growing horses.

CAUSES

The agents more commonly involved are *Streptococcus equi, Streptococcus zooepidemicus, Corynebacterium pseudotuberculosis, Salmonella* spp., *E. coli,* and *R. equi* in foals.

RISK FACTORS

There have no been epidemiologic studies that have determined specific risk factors. However, it has been indicated that heavily parasitized animals are more prone to internal abdominal abscessation. In a review of clinical cases it was noted that many affected animals had a previous history of respiratory disease or lymphadenitis. The problem is more likely to occur on farms where infections with *S. equi* and *R. equi* are common.

DIAGNOSIS

DIFFERENTIAL DIAGNOSIS

Internal abdominal abscessation must be differentiated from the different cases of chronic weight loss, such as pleuropneumonia, neoplasia, chronic hepatic disease, chronic intestinal malabsorption disease, chronic renal failure, severe parasitism, and dental problems. In the colic presentation, it must be differentiated from peritonitis of different origin or surgical or medical colics.

CBC/BIOCHEMISTRY/URINALYSIS

The CBC may indicate a slight to moderate anemia of chronic inflammation. The PCV can be <0.3 L/L (30%). The WBC shows a leukocytosis with neutrophilia and a left shift evident in most horses. Plasma fibrinogen concentration is frequently increased, with values close to 1000 mg/dL (10 g/L). Plasma proteins are increased, usually due to increased globulin fractions; albumin may be below normal levels. The albumin to globulin (A/G) ratio is below normal, ranging from 0.17 to 0.63 (normal 0.65–1.46).

OTHER LABORATORY TESTS

Peritoneal fluid is usually determined to be an exudate based on a specific gravity (>1.017), protein level (>2.5 g/dL [25 g/L]), and WBC count (>10000 cells/μL [> 10^9 cells/L]). The protein levels, WBC, and fibrinogen can be as high as 8.5 g/dL (85 g/L), 365,000 cells/μL (365×10^9 cells/L), and 500 mg/dL (5 g/L), respectively. Intracellular bacteria (both cocci and bacilli) can be observed, but only on rare occasions are free bacteria observed.

IMAGING

Ultrasonography, conducted transrectally or percutaneously, can be useful in diagnosing these abscesses when they can be located during rectal examination.

DIAGNOSTIC PROCEDURES

Rectal palpation may be limited by the fact that some animals during the colic episodes often show severe abdominal straining and rectal expulsive efforts. In both clinical presentations, detailed rectal examination may allow the detection of an abdominal mass.

Abdominal laparoscopy could well be indicated in these instances and may allow visualization of the mass. Fine-needle aspirate of the abscess could be done percutaneously with ultrasound guidance or by laparoscopy.

A Gram stain and culture of the peritoneal fluid should be carried out. The clinician should request anaerobic and aerobic methods for bacterial isolation from the cultures submitted. In some instances, exploratory laparotomy might be indicated.

PATHOLOGIC FINDINGS

Abdominal abscessation can involve the mesentery or several internal organs, such as intestines, spleen, liver, or kidneys. When localized in the mesentery, adhesions to various organs might be present.

TREATMENT

APPROPRIATE HEALTH CARE

Most cases can be managed in a farm setting.

ACTIVITY

Animals with internal abdominal abscesses should have stall or pasture rest until the problem has resolved.

DIET

Normal diet

CLIENT EDUCATION

Cases that are managed with long-term antibiotic therapy can be treated by the owner. If owners are unfamiliar with the administration of medication to horses, they must be trained to do this. Compliance can be a problem, particularly with parenteral therapy, as many horses rapidly become intolerant of twice-daily intramuscular injections.

SURGICAL CONSIDERATIONS

In cases in which colic presentation is the chief complaint, the severity of the colic may warrant intensive care management and even surgical management in some cases.

Surgical treatment could be attempted in cases with a grave prognosis, but it is complicated by the need to drain the abscess without contaminating the abdominal cavity. It is usually very difficult to excise the abscess. In cases of abdominal obstruction, it may be necessary to bypass the abscess. Abdominal lavage is indicated in cases when rupture of the abscess occurs. This procedure is not without constraints and difficulties.

MEDICATIONS

DRUG(S) OF CHOICE

Medical treatment of abdominal internal abscesses is usually preferred. For the most part it is empirical, as the causative organism(s) is not usually positively identified. Farm history and clinical findings are the basis for antibiotic selection. Antibiotic therapy should last for a minimum of 30 days and may extend up to 90 days in some cases, depending on the response to therapy. Procaine penicillin (40,000–100,000 UI/kg divided in two doses daily has been recommended. It may be combined with trimethoprim–sulfadiazine (16–30 mg/kg BW). It may be very efficacious to use a combination of rifampin (10 mg/kg BW BID) and erythromycin estolate (15 mg/kg two to three times daily) or trimethoprim–sulfadiazine. Metronidazole (20–25 mg/kg TID) could be added in the case of a suspected or isolated anaerobic pathogen.

FOLLOW-UP

PATIENT MONITORING

In order to follow-up the patient evolution, repeated rectal examinations, abdominocentesis, and ultrasound examinations are necessary.

PREVENTION/AVOIDANCE

On problem farms, careful monitoring of all horses may lead to early detection of the problem. If *S. equi* is the etiologic agent, then consideration should be give to a vaccination program.

POSSIBLE COMPLICATIONS

- Peritonitis
- Purpura hemorrhagica

EXPECTED COURSE AND PROGNOSIS

The prognosis is usually guarded to good when there has been good response within 2 weeks of treatment. The prognosis becomes grave if there is either intestinal obstruction or internal rupture of the abscess, lack of response to the treatment, and evidence of intestinal adhesions.

Suggested Reading

Byars, DT. Miscellaneous acute abdominal diseases. In: NA White (ed.), The equine acute abdomen. Philadelphia: Lea & Febiger 1990;403-404.

Golland LC, Hodgson DR, Hodgson JL, Brownlow MA, Hutchins DR, Rawlinson RJ, Collins MB, McClintock SA, Riasis AL. Peritonitis associated with *Actinobacillus equuli* in horses: 15 cases. J Am Vet Med Assoc. 1994;205:340-343.

Hawkins JF, Bowman KF, Roberts MC, Cowe P. Peritonitis in horses: 67 cases. J Am Vet Med Assoc 1993;203:284-288.

Rumbaugh GE, Smith BF, Carlson GP. Internal abdominal abscesses in the horse: a study of 25 cases. J Am Vet Med Assoc. 1978;172:304-308.

Author Oliver Olimpo

Consulting Editor Henry R Stämpfli

INTESTINAL AGANGLIONOSIS

BASICS

OVERVIEW

• An autosomal recessive defect in foals from two phenotypically overo paint parents characterized by an unpigmented haircoat, light blue irises, and the absence of myenteric ganglia in the terminal portions of the ileum, cecum, and colon
• A polymorphism in the *EDNRB* gene is associated with the defect.
• EDNRB plays a role in regulating the neural crest cells in the fetus that become the enteric ganglia and melanocytes.
• Carriers of this allele have been reported in some Tobiano and solid-colored horses as well.
• Also known as lethal white syndrome

SIGNALMENT

No sex predilections in affected foals

SIGNS

• Foals are born with a white coat color, light blue irises, and pigmented retinas.
• Foals may appear normal at birth, stand, and nurse.
• Colic is the primary problem that develops within the first 24 hours of life. Abdomens become progressively distended, and affected foals do not pass meconium.

CAUSES AND RISK FACTORS

• Genetic disease.
• Breeding of two overo paint horses with each other or an overo paint to a nonovero paint horse that has overo breeding in its pedigree
• If two heterozygotes for the mutant lethal white gene are bred, there is a 25% chance of getting a lethal white, a 50% chance of getting an overo-colored, and a 25% chance of a solid-colored offspring.

DIAGNOSIS

DIFFERENTIAL DIAGNOSIS

• White haircoat and parentage—fairly strong indicators that signs of colic may be due to intestinal aganglionosis
• Other problems that may present with similar colic signs—meconium retention and intestinal atresia
• Unlikely that foals with these differentials would be unpigmented

CBC/BIOCHEMISTRY/URINALYSIS

N/A

OTHER LABORATORY TESTS

• Recently, an allele-specific PCR test has been developed to identify the mutation site of the DNA sequence responsible for the lethal white overo foal. This test can be performed on either whole blood or hair samples with roots and used to detect carriers, noncarriers, and affected animals.
• Laboratories currently performing this test include the veterinary schools at the University of California–Davis and the University of Minnesota.

IMAGING

Abdominal radiography—intestinal distention with gas may be seen on plain radiographs.

DIAGNOSTIC PROCEDURES

N/A

PATHOLOGIC FINDINGS

Gross Pathology

• Milk in the stomach
• Meconium in the colons
• Gas distention of the ileum and the large and small colon
• Occasionally, the small colon may be contracted.
• No atresia of the colon

Histopathology

Myenteric ganglia—absent in the terminal ileum, cecum, and colon; present in the stomach and small intestine

TREATMENT

• No treatment for this genetic disease
• Euthanasia is recommended.

INTESTINAL AGANGLIONOSIS

MEDICATIONS

DRUGS
N/A

CONTRAINDICATIONS/POSSIBLE INTERACTIONS
N/A

FOLLOW-UP

PREVENTION/AVOIDANCE
- Because of the genetic implications, breeding an overo mare with an overo stallion without genetic testing is unwise.
- The problem has also occurred between an overo and nonovero mating in which the nonovero parent had overo coloring in its pedigree.

EXPECTED COURSE AND PROGNOSIS
- Grave prognosis
- Foals generally begin showing signs of colic within the first 24 hours of life and, if not euthanized, naturally die within 2–3 days.

MISCELLANEOUS

ASSOCIATED CONDITIONS
N/A

AGE-RELATED FACTORS
The problem is evident at or soon after birth in all cases.

ZOONOTIC POTENTIAL
N/A

PREGNANCY
N/A

SEE ALSO
Meconium impaction

ABBREVIATIONS
- ENDRB = endothelial receptor B
- PCR = polymerase chain reaction

Suggested Readings

Hultgren BD. Ileocolonic aganglionosis in white progeny of overo spotted horses. J Am Vet Med Assoc 1982;180:289–292.

Metallinos DL, Bowling AT, Rine J. A missense mutation in the endothelial-B receptor gene associated with white foal syndrome: an equine version of Hirschsprung disease. Mamm Genome 1998;9:426–431.

Santschi EM, Purdy AK, Valberg SJ, Vrotsos PD, Kaese H, Mickelson JR. Endothelial receptor B polymorphism associated with lethal white foal syndrome in horses. Mamm Genome 1998;9:306–309.

Schneider JE, Leipold HW. Recessive lethal white in two foals. J Equine Med Surg 1978;2:479–482.

Author Mary Rose Paradis
Consulting Editor Mary Rose Paradis

INTRA-ABDOMINAL HEMORRHAGE

BASICS

DEFINITION

Loss of blood into the abdominal cavity

PATHOPHYSIOLOGY

Rate of blood loss determines the pathophysiologic responses.

Acute Abdominal Hemorrhage

- Acute, massive blood loss ≥30% of total blood volume results in hypovolemic shock.
- Loss of blood initially results in decreased venous pressure and venous return to the heart; consequently, cardiac output and arterial pressure decrease.
- Physiologic compensation for hypovolemic shock includes redistribution of interstitial fluid from tissue spaces into capillaries to expand circulating fluid volume and increased sympathetic activity. Tachycardia and peripheral vasoconstriction to increase cardiac output result from this physiologic compensation, and splenic contraction subsequent to the increased sympathetic activity occurs. In turn, this results in initial maintenance of PCV concentrations.
- As hemorrhage progresses, more vital organs (e.g., kidneys and pancreas, followed by intestines and liver) undergo vasoconstriction, and the oncotic pressure and oxygen-carrying capacity of the blood decrease. Because of this lack of oxygen, cells revert to anaerobic metabolism, which causes production of organic acids (e.g., lactic acid).
- Blood flow to the most vital organs (e.g., brain, heart) is maintained for the longest period.

Chronic Abdominal Hemorrhage

- At least 30% of total blood volume must be lost with chromic or slow hemorrhage before clinical signs become evident.
- This compensation can be attributed to an immediate release of erythrocytes via splenic contracture, redistribution of interstitial fluid intravascularly during a 12- to 24-hour period, and enhanced erythropoiesis within 1 week.

SYSTEMS AFFECTED

- Cardiovascular—because abdominal hemorrhage may result in hypovolemic shock, the cardiovascular system is the most affected.
- Urinary—during acute hemorrhage, urine output decreases, because the vascular supply to kidneys undergoes vasoconstriction.

SIGNALMENT

Breed

N/A

Sex/Age

- Blood loss from the reproductive tract occurs in broodmares.
- Multiparous mares >11 years are the prime candidates.

SIGNS

General Comments

Clinical manifestations frequently are nonspecific and can be easily misinterpreted.

Historical Findings

Initial clinical signs include depression, lethargy, partial or complete anorexia, and colic.

Physical Examination Findings

- As anemia and hypovolemia intensify, tachycardia, tachypnea, weak peripheral pulses, pale mucous membranes, and holosystolic murmur develop.
- Ileus and abdominal distention may be observed if a large volume of blood accumulates.

CAUSES

Hemorrhage from the Reproductive Tract

- The ovaries, uterus, or utero-ovarian blood vessels are the most common locations from which intra-abdominal bleedings occur in females.
- Ovarian hemorrhage can originate from capsular rupture of granulosa cell tumors and from ovarian follicular hematomas.
- Uterine bleeding can be associated with birth-related trauma to the uterine vessels or with uterine neoplasia—leiomyomas or leiomyosarcoma

Hemorrhage from the GI Tract and Related Structures

- Rupture of the mesenteric arteries secondary to *Strongylus vulgaris* larval migration is less frequent since the introduction of ivermectin dewormers.
- Splenic rupture secondary to blunt trauma to the left caudal abdomen or to splenic neoplasia—hemangiosarcoma
- Entrapment of the small intestine within the epiploic foramen—distention of the bowel incarcerated within the foramen or surgical manipulation may rarely result in rupture of the caudal vena cava.
- GI vascular leakage secondary to neoplasia or abscessation, coagulopathies, or surgery
- Renal trauma
- Hepatic rupture

RISK FACTORS

Age

- Periparturient hemorrhage associated with rupture of the uterine or ovarian arteries is most frequently observed in older broodmares.
- An age-related degeneration within the arterial walls leads to the formation of aneurysms, and arterial rupture at the aneurysm site occurs subsequent to uterine contractions and fetal movement during late gestation and parturition.
- Rupture of the caudal vena cava, particularly in old horses with epiploic foramen entrapment

Pregnancy

Peripartum hemorrhage can occur before, during, or after foaling.

Blunt External Trauma

Splenic, renal, or hepatic rupture

Parasitism

- Infestation by *S. vulgaris*

Ingestion of Anticoagulants

Warfarin and related compounds

DIAGNOSIS

DIFFERENTIAL DIAGNOSIS

- All equine disorders resulting in abdominal pain should be included.
- In broodmares, consider peripartum conditions—uterine torsion, uterine rupture, and dystocia; rectal palpation and ultrasonography help to differentiate these disorders.
- Consider any condition causing mild to moderate abdominal distension—intestinal obstruction, ascites, and pregnancy.
- Consider other causes of hypovolemia and blood loss—intrathoracic hemorrhage, internal carotid artery rupture in the guttural pouch, or chronic GI or genitourinary hemorrhage.
- Many of these causes will be obvious based on history and physical examination findings.

CBC/BIOCHEMISTRY/URINALYSIS

- Hematologic abnormalities associated with acute blood loss are seen after the initial 24-hours period and include anemia (e.g., decreased PCV, erythrocyte count, and hemoglobin concentration) and decreased total plasma protein.
- These changes are observed when intercompartmental fluid shifts or IV fluid replacement occurs.
- Hypoproteinemia usually is noted before the decline in hematocrit.
- Anemic horses show no evidence of a regenerative response in the peripheral blood—no reticulocytosis
- Sequential PCV measurements help to determine if the blood loss and resulting anemia are progressive or controlled.
- Coagulation profile reveals thrombocytopenia in conjunction with a normal activated partial thromboplastin time and prothrombin time.
- Thrombocytopenia is secondary to blood loss.

OTHER LABORATORY TESTS

Abdominocentesis

- Hemoperitoneum is definitively diagnosed on the basis of abdominal paracentesis. The fluid collected has an elevated erythrocyte count, which during the early stages generally is less than or equal to the erythrocyte count in the peripheral blood. At cytology, platelets typically are not present, unless the hemorrhage is peracute. However, blood may be introduced into the peritoneal fluid during sampling by aspiration of splenic blood or laceration of a subcutaneous vessel. Cytologic evidence of erythrophagocytosis suggests the hemorrhage occurred before paracentesis, unless the fluid is not analyzed promptly.
- Normally, splenic blood clots readily because of the increased fibrinogen concentration.
- In chronic intra-abdominal hemorrhage, the erythrocyte count usually is equal to or greater than the erythrocyte count in peripheral blood, and the protein content is less because of resorption. At cytology, hypersegmented pyknotic neutrophils and hemosiderophages are observed.

Blood Gas Analyses

- Measurement of arterial or venous PCO_2, PO_2, pH, and HCO_3^- provide useful information in hypovolemic shock states.
- Lactic acidosis, resulting from anaerobic metabolism, causes a nonrespiratory acidosis (i.e., decreased pH and HCO_3^- concentration) with respiratory compensation (i.e., decreased PCO_2).

IMAGING

Abdominal ultrasonography, either transabdominal or transrectal, permits assessment of fluid distribution; occasionally, particularly when neoplasia is present, the origin of the hemorrhage can be identified.

OTHER DIAGNOSTIC PROCEDURES

Rectal palpation—fluid accumulation within the abdomen, abnormal (i.e., neoplastic) masses, abnormalities within the reproductive tract, rupture of the left kidney, or gas-distended intestines may be noted.

TREATMENT

Initial treatment of abdominal blood loss is directed at controlling hemorrhage and restoring normal intravascular volume.

Fluid Therapy

- Hypovolemic shock is addressed by prompt IV therapy with isotonic crystalloid solutions (lactated Ringer solution [20–40 mL/kg per hour) to increase vascular volume. Replacement fluid volume necessary to maintain perfusion in hemorrhagic shock usually is two- to sevenfold the actual blood loss, because redistribution within the entire extracellular space occurs. Monitor the clinical response to fluid replacement—improved jugular distensibility and capillary refill time, increased pulse strength, and decreased heart rate indicate improved cardiovascular status.
- Replacement of intravascular volume also may be accomplished with hypertonic saline (7.5% NaCl [4 mL/kg]), which expands vascular volume, enhances vascular tone, and restores intravascular pressure. When blood loss is not controlled, however, hypertonic saline increases bleeding from the mesenteric vasculature and decreases mean arterial pressure.

Blood Transfusion

- Usually, crystalloid solutions only are used to treat acute abdominal hemorrhage, but when the PCV is decreasing toward 15% (0.15 L/L), whole-blood transfusion is required to increase oncotic pressure and oxygen-carrying capacity.
- The rate at which the PCV falls determines the urgency and need for transfusion.
- The volume of blood transfused depends on the rate and quantity of blood loss.
- Administer whole blood at 15–25 mL/kg, and repeat if necessary. Administer balanced crystalloid solutions concurrently to maintain perfusion.
- Transfused RBCs survive only 4–6 days in horses, so the increase in PCV is transient.

Surgery

An attempt to stop hemorrhage arising from tumors, rupture of a viscus, or leaking GI vessels may be undertaken at surgery.

MEDICATION

DRUGS OF CHOICE

- Opioid antagonist—naloxone (one treatment of 8 mg IV)
- Buffered neutral formalin (10–30 mL of 10% solution added to 500 mL of 0.09% NaCl) administered through an IV catheter placed in the jugular vein. The rational for its use is unclear, but many anecdotal reports testify to its efficacy.

CONTRAINDICATIONS

Phenothiazine tranquilizers (e.g., acepromazine) are contraindicated in horses with hemorrhagic shock, because these drugs have a direct vasodilatory effect on blood vessels and decrease systemic arterial blood pressure.

PRECAUTION

Use α_2-Agonists(e.g., xylazine, detomidine) with extreme caution in horses with intra-abdominal hemorrhage, because these drugs decrease cardiac output.

POSSIBLE INTERACTIONS

N/A

ALTERNATIVE DRUGS

N/A

FOLLOW-UP

PATIENT MONITORING

Assess cardiovascular status by monitoring heart rate, pulse strength, capillary refill time, and jugular vein distensibility from every 5 minutes to a few times a day, depending whether hemorrhage is controlled.

POSSIBLE COMPLICATIONS

- Cardiovascular collapse and death
- In postparturient broodmares with rupture of the utero-ovarian artery, two clinical outcomes are possible, depending whether hemorrhage is contained in the uterine broad ligament. If it is, a large hematoma develops in the broad ligament, and the mare survives. If it is not, death can occur within minutes to days after parturition.

MISCELLANEOUS

ASSOCIATED CONDITIONS

N/A

AGE-RELATED FACTORS

N/A

ZOONOTIC POTENTIAL

N/A

PREGNANCY

N/A

SYNONYMS

N/A

SEE ALSO

N/A

ABBREVIATIONS

- GI = gastrointestinal
- PCV = packed cell volume

Suggested Reading

Edens LM. Intra-abdominal hemorrhage in horses. Proc12th ACVIM Forum 1994:607–609.

Author Ludovic Boure

Consulting Editor Henry R. Stämpfli

INTRACAROTID INJECTION

BASICS

DEFINITION
Accidental injection of drugs into the carotid artery associated with acute neurologic signs

PATHOPHYSIOLOGY
• Drugs that are accidentally injected into the carotid artery
• The proximity of the common carotid artery to the jugular vein and patient movement make this condition a real hazard.
• Injected material often travels via the carotid artery, distributes to the ipsilateral forebrain, and is associated with acute and, possibly, severe cerebral disturbances.
• Marked cardiovascular changes (e.g., bradycardia, arrhythmias, blood pressure fluctuations) may accompany CNS signs.
• Local cerebral histopathologic and clinical signs depend on the drug's potential to induce tissue abnormalities and both the rate and quantity of the injection (see *Expected Course and Prognosis).*

SYSTEMS AFFECTED
• CNS
• Cardiovascular—bradycardia, ectopia, and hypotension

SIGNALMENT
No specific signalment

SIGNS

Historical Findings
Very recent history of parenteral drug administration

Physical Examination Findings
• A violent reaction typically occurs within 5–30 seconds of initiating the injection.
• Signs range from apprehension, facial twitching, head-shaking, kicking, and propulsive circling to recumbency, loss of consciousness, and seizure-like activity.
• Episodes can be variable in length, and on occasion, death occurs.

CAUSES
See *Pathophysiology.*

RISK FACTORS
Fractious animals and attempts at IV injection

DIAGNOSIS
Established by history and onset of clinical signs.

DIFFERENTIAL DIAGNOSIS
N/A

CBC/BIOCHEMISTRY/URINALYSIS
No specific abnormalities

OTHER LABORATORY TESTS
No specific abnormalities

IMAGING
N/A

DIAGNOSTIC PROCEDURES
N/A

PATHOLOGIC FINDINGS
• Unusual for affected horses not to recover, because xylazine is the most common drug administered in these situations.
• In horses that do not survive, diffuse perivascular necrosis with marked edema, vascular endothelial damage, hemorrhage, and neuronal degeneration are evident.

TREATMENT
• Largely supportive and symptomatic
• Padding and sedation for thrashing, delirious horses
• Hypertonic (7%) saline solution may useful.

MEDICATIONS

DRUGS OF CHOICE
Dexamethasone (0.1–0.25 mg/kg IV), DMSO (1 g/kg IV diluted 1:6 in physiologic saline), and anticonvulsant therapy may be useful.

CONTRAINDICATIONS
Mannitol may be contraindicated because of cerebral hemorrhage.

INTRACAROTID INJECTION

PRECAUTIONS
- The techniques used to avoid intra-arterial injection are controversial.
- All IV techniques of drug administration can be argued to have disadvantages.

POSSIBLE INTERACTIONS
N/A

ALTERNATIVE DRUGS
N/A

FOLLOW-UP

PATIENT MONITORING
N/A

POSSIBLE COMPLICATIONS
Complications often arise from self-induced trauma during the early seizure-like response.

EXPECTED COURSE AND PROGNOSIS

Water-Soluble Drugs
- Injection of water-soluble drugs (e.g., xylazine, butorphanol, acetylpromazine) usually is associated with complete recovery within hours, though some horses may require as long as 7 days and, on rare occasions, may die.
- Common signs during recovery—facial hypalgesia, blindness, and deficient menace response contralateral to the side of injection.

Other Drugs
- Intracarotid injection of procaine penicillin, phenylbutazone, and oil-based or poorly water-soluble drugs are associated with a poorer prognosis.
- Intracarotid injection of such drugs often is associated with prolonged and intractable seizures, coma, or stupor.

MISCELLANEOUS

ASSOCIATED CONDITIONS
N/A

AGE-RELATED FACTORS
N/A

ZOONOTIC POTENTIAL
N/A

PREGNANCY
N/A

SYNONYMS
N/A

SEE ALSO
N/A

ABBREVIATIONS
DMSO = dimethyl sulfoxide

Suggested Reading

Hahn CN, Mayhew IG, Mackay RJ. Intracarotid injection. In: Colohan PT, Mayhew IG, Merritt AM, Moore JN, eds. Equine medicine and surgery. 5th ed. St. Louis: Mosby, 1999:907.

Author Joseph J. Bertone
Consulting Editor Joseph J. Bertone

IONOPHORE TOXICOSIS

BASICS

DEFINITION

• Several polyether ionophorous drugs (i.e., ionophores) are approved for use as coccidiostats or growth promoters—laidlomycin propionate (Cattlyst), lasalocid (Avatec, Bovatec), maduramycin (Cygro), monensin (Coban, Rumensin), narasin (Maxiban, Monteban), and salinomycin (Biocox, Coxistat, Saccox).
• Ingestion of toxic amounts of ionophores results in a physicochemical or pathologic disruption of the cardiac muscle, skeletal muscle, nerves, liver, and kidney.
• Clinical signs usually develop within 24 hours of ingesting a toxic dose but can be delayed for several days.
• Animals that survive acute episodes can have permanent damage.
• Some ionophores have not been evaluated in horses, but all should be considered toxic, with similar adverse effects.
• Reported median lethal doses in horses—lasalocid, 21.5 mg/kg; monensin, 2–3 mg/kg; salinomycin, 0.6 mg/kg; laidlomycin propionate, >2 mg/kg per day

PATHOPHYSIOLOGY

• Ionophorous compounds embed in the biologic membranes of cells and subcellular organelles and transport ions across membranes down concentration gradients. This results in loss of ionic gradients across the membranes of excitable cells (i.e., muscle, nerve) and across mitochondrial membranes.
• Ion gradient loss across mitochondrial membranes prevents oxidative metabolism, results in mitochondrial swelling and rupture, and is the ultimate cause of cell death.

SYSTEMS AFFECTED

Cardiovascular

• Mitochondrial damage results in loss of aerobic ATP production and myocardial cell necrosis.
• Loss of ion gradients alters the polarity of cardiac myofibers.
• Cardiac function, including conductance, is altered.
• In animals surviving acute toxicosis, connective tissue fills the voids left by myocardial necrosis, which can result in permanent myocardial dysfunction.

Musculoskeletal

• Effects on skeletal muscle are similar to those on myocardial muscles; however, skeletal muscle damage is less severe.
• Muscular scarring can occur in animals surviving acute intoxication.

Neuromuscular

Ionophores can alter nerve conduction through muscle fibers, which results in altered reflexes and muscle co-ordination.

Renal/Urologic

• Renal tubular damage can occur, which generally is associated with myoglobin casts.
• Urinary bladder distention may be seen.

Hepatobiliary

Hepatocellular necrosis and decreased function can occur.

GENETICS

N/A

INCIDENCE/PREVALENCE

Though not uncommon, equine cases of ionophore poisoning are not as common today as when ionophores were first introduced because of recognition regarding the sensitivity of horses and warnings on ionophore products.

SIGNALMENT

• Poisoning can occur at all ages.
• Male and female horses are equally susceptible.

SIGNS

Acute Poisoning

• Feed refusal/anorexia
• Weakness
• Ataxia/inco-ordination
• Stumbling
• Exaggerated stepping
• Sweating
• Tremors
• Tachycardia
• Hesitance to move or turn
• Congested mucous membranes
• Dyspnea
• Hyperpnea
• Hypotension
• Recumbency
• Prolonged capillary refill
• Jugular pulse
• Increased or decreased borborygmus
• Arrhythmias
• Bladder distention
• Pitting edema
• Death

Long-Term Effects

Horses surviving acute intoxication can experience numerous long-term effects caused by initial myocardial damage—unthriftiness, poor performance, poor exercise tolerance, arrhythmias, pitting edema, hyperpnea, and death, both with or without observed clinical signs

CAUSES

Ionophore toxicoses primarily result from feeding horses medicated feed prepared for another species or contaminated feeds.

RISK FACTORS

Vitamin E or selenium deficiency may predispose to more severe tissue damage, but adequate concentrations do not prevent toxicosis.

DIAGNOSIS

DIFFERENTIAL DIAGNOSES

• Vitamin E/selenium deficiency—low serum, whole-blood, or liver selenium concentrations
• White snakeroot (*Eupatorium rugosum*) poisoning—evidence of plant consumption

CBC/BIOCHEMISTRY/URINALYSIS

Incidences of the following abnormalities can be quite variable and are not good indications for the severity of intoxication:
• CBC—increased hematocrit
• Biochemistry—increased LDH, CPK, bilirubin, AST, ALP, creatinine, BUN, phosphate, glucose, and serum osmolarity; hypocalcemia; hypokalemia
• Urinalysis—hypo-osmolar urine

OTHER LABORATORY TESTS

• Analyze feed or stomach contents for ionophores to verify exposure.
• Tissue analysis can be performed, but if death is >1–2 days after exposure, the ionophore may not be detected.

IMAGING

Echocardiography—not useful in acute cases, but can help in determining the amount of myocardial damage in surviving horses; absence of identifiable scarring, however, does not rule out small or microscopic lesions.

DIAGNOSTIC PROCEDURES

• ECG abnormalities have been identified in both acute poisonings and in animals that survive; however, horses with myocardial lesions have had normal ECGs.
• ECG changes occasionally are identified but are quite variable and are not reliable indices for the severity of intoxication.
• Abnormalities include prolonged atrial and ventricular depolarization, AV block, increased S-wave amplitude, absent P wave, increased T-wave amplitude, depressed ST segment, atrial fibrillation, ventricular tachycardia, ventricular extrasystole, ventricular fibrillation, and intermittent and premature ventricular contractions.

PATHOLOGIC FINDINGS

Gross Findings

- Lesions generally are associated, either directly or indirectly, with myocardial damage, but renal lesions occasionally are identified.
- Some horses have no gross lesions.
- Lesions include pale streaks in the ventricular myocardium, increased myocardial friability, epicardial or endocardial hemorrhage, pericardial effusion, ascites, pulmonary congestion and edema, pleural effusion, systemic congestion, subcutaneous edema, hyperemic kidneys, accentuated hepatic lobular pattern, pale skeletal musculature, and urinary bladder distension.

Histopathologic Findings

- Generally some degree of myocardial damage, but renal, hepatic, and skeletal muscle lesions also may occur.
- Lesions in acute cases include myocardial necrosis; swollen myocardial fibers with loss of striations; intracytoplasmic myocardial vacuolization; hemorrhage and edema of myocardial or skeletal muscles; skeletal muscle necrosis; pulmonary congestion and edema; renal tubular vacuolization, necrosis, myoglobin casts, and congestion; hepatocellular vacuolization; mild bile duct proliferation; acute toxic hepatitis; and adrenal vacuolization.
- Fibrous connective tissue replacement of myocardial cells and hepatic congestion with centrilobular degeneration are seen in individuals surviving ≥1 week.

TREATMENT

APPROPRIATE HEALTH CARE

- Inpatient management generally is not necessary, because severely affected horses rarely survive.
- No effective medical management has been identified; therefore, outpatient management generally is recommended—preventing further exposure, GI decontamination, and general supportive care
- GI decontamination may decrease the duration and severity of signs; if exposure is recognized early, decontamination can prevent absorption and toxicosis.
- AC may bind ionophores, and cathartics (e.g., mineral oil, magnesium sulfate [Epsom salt]) can decrease GI transit time, thus minimizing absorption.

NURSING CARE

IV normal saline if dehydrated (see *Contraindications*)

ACTIVITY

Give horses exposed to ionophores complete rest.

DIET

N/A

CLIENT EDUCATION

- Horses surviving acute intoxication may have residual heart damage.
- Sudden death can occur unexpectedly or after excitement or exercise.
- Recovered horses may be used for breeding, but the stress of breeding or foaling may cause death, which makes these animals potentially dangerous.

SURGICAL CONSIDERATIONS

N/A

MEDICATIONS

DRUGS OF CHOICE

- AC (2–5 g/kg PO in a water slurry [1 g of AC in 5 mL of water])
- One dose of cathartic PO with AC if no diarrhea or ileus—70% sorbitol (3 ml/kg) or sodium or magnesium sulfate (250–500 mg/kg as a 20% solution).

CONTRAINDICATIONS

- Do not give AC with mineral oil, because the oil prevents binding of compounds to the AC.
- Do not give IV fluids if cardiac function is compromised, because this may increase systemic congestion and edema.

PRECAUTIONS

N/A

POSSIBLE INTERACTIONS

N/A

ALTERNATIVE DRUGS

N/A

FOLLOW-UP

PATIENT MONITORING

- Serum chemistries, ECGs, and echocardiography can be used to monitor progress; however, these are not good prognostic indicators.
- Severe abnormalities can indicate that severe damage has occurred and death is likely.
- A complete lack of serum chemistry abnormalities, monitored daily for 2 weeks, plus an absence of ECG and echocardiographic changes may indicate a lack of or minimal exposure, but this does not rule out tissue effects by the ionophores.

PREVENTION/AVOIDANCE

- Purchase feed from a manufacturer with a good quality-control program.
- Never use feeds prepared for another species.

POSSIBLE COMPLICATIONS

Myocardial damage can result in long-term effects that cannot be corrected (see *Client Education*).

EXPECTED COURSE AND PROGNOSIS

- Clinical signs can occur as early as a few hours to days or weeks after exposure.
- Death can occur as long as several months after intoxication.
- Horses exhibiting moderate to severe clinical signs within the first few days likely will die or suffer permanent myocardial damage; however, mildly affected horses also may suffer long-term effects.

MISCELLANEOUS

ASSOCIATED CONDITIONS

N/A

AGE-RELATED FACTORS

N/A

ZOONOTIC POTENTIAL

N/A

PREGNANCY

Ionophores do not cause birth defects or impair fertility; however, stress or poor cardiac function associated with acute intoxication can result in loss of the fetus.

SYNONYMS

N/A

SEE ALSO

N/A

ABBREVIATIONS

- AC = activated charcoal
- ALP = alkaline phosphatase
- AST = aspartate aminotransferase
- CPK = creatine phosphokinase
- GI = gastrointestinal
- LDH = lactate dehydrogenase

Suggested Reading

Novilla MN. The veterinary importance of the toxic syndrome induced by ionophores. Vet Hum Toxicol 1992;34:66–70.

Author Jeffery O. Hall

Consulting Editor Robert H. Poppenga

IRIS PROLAPSE IN THE HORSE

BASICS

OVERVIEW

• Most frequently follows acute ocular trauma (i.e., TIP), particularly sharp, perforating corneal injuries or blunt injuries causing rupture of the cornea, limbus, or sclera.
• Corneal perforation also occurs secondary to rapid, enzymatic degradation of stromal collagen and ground substance due to infectious and noninfectious ulcerative keratitis (i.e., UIP).

SIGNALMENT

All ages and breeds in all types of environments are at risk.

SIGNS

• Cloudy, red, and painful eye
• Blepharospasm and tearing
• Slight droopiness of the upper eyelid lashes may be a subtle sign of corneal ulceration.
• Corneal edema—focal or generalized
• Brown to red structure protruding through a corneal or scleral laceration is diagnostic.
• Anterior chamber—shallow or collapsed from loss of aqueous humor

CAUSES AND RISK FACTORS

Corneal perforation with iris prolapse may be a sequel to traumatic insult to the globe or orbit, or to ulcerative infectious and noninfectious corneal ulcerations.

DIAGNOSIS

DIFFERENTIAL DIAGNOSIS

Ocular pain may be found with corneal ulcers, uveitis, conjunctivitis, glaucoma, blepharitis, and dacryocystitis.

CBC/BIOCHEMISTRY/URINALYSIS

N/A

OTHER LABORATORY TESTS

N/A

IMAGING

N/A

DIAGNOSTIC PROCEDURES

Fluorescein dye indicates the site of a corneal perforation; the dye may leak into the anterior chamber, or the dye will change color when exposed to leaking aqueous.

TREATMENT

• Clinical and surgical guidelines based on the possibility of useful vision and ocular survival assist in choosing therapy.
• Perforating lacerations confined to the cornea and ≤15 mm in length tend to have favorable visual outcome after surgical repair. Iridectomy generally does not exacerbate postoperative uveitis or adversely affect visual outcome and may facilitate postoperative mydriasis and prevent septic endophthalmitis.
• Perforating corneal lacerations >15 mm and extending to, along, or beyond the limbus tend to have poor visual outcome and to require enucleation. Chances of retaining vision also may be substantially reduced in perforating corneal wounds accompanied by hyphema, even when comprising only 10–50% of the anterior chamber. Enucleation should be more seriously considered in cases with these clinical and surgical findings.
• Intensive postoperative medical therapy, especially use of systemic NSAIDs, is critical for successful management of profound iridocyclitis and endophthalmitis. By inhibiting the cyclo-oxygenase inflammatory pathway, flunixin meglumine reduces uveal prostaglandin synthesis and, subsequently, vasodilation and permeability of the uveal vasculature.

MEDICATIONS

DRUGS

• Topically applied antibiotics (chloramphenicol, bacitracin-neomycin-polymyxin B, gentamicin; QID), atropine (1%; QID), and serum (QID) are recommended.
• Systemic NSAIDs (phenylbutazone, 2 mg/kg PO BID; flunixin meglumine, 1 mg/kg PO, IM, or IV BID), and broad-spectrum parenteral antibiotics also are indicated.

CONTRAINDICATIONS/POSSIBLE INTERACTIONS

N/A

IRIS PROLAPSE IN THE HORSE

FOLLOW-UP

PATIENT MONITORING

- Horses with iris prolapse and secondary uveitis should be stall-rested till healed; intraocular hemorrhage and increased severity of uveitis are sequela to overexertion.
- Protect the horse from self-trauma with hard or soft cup hoods.
- Monitor for signs of eye pain and colic; the ocular pain should gradually diminish after surgical repair.
- Diet should be consistent with the training level of the horse.

PREVENTION/AVOIDANCE

N/A

POSSIBLE COMPLICATIONS

Infectious endophthalmitis and blindness that require enucleation

EXPECTED COURSE AND PROGNOSIS

- Prognosis of perforating corneal lacerations generally is guarded, depending on the size, location, and mechanism of injury. Perforating lacerations caused by sharp injuries generally have a better prognosis than those caused by blunt or missile injuries. High-energy blunt ocular trauma may result in hyphema or globe rupture, most often occurring at the limbus or equator, where the sclera is thinnest.
- If uncontrolled, iridocyclitis may predispose to fibropupillary membrane formation, with subsequent posterior synechiae and cataract development.
- Prognosis of corneal lacerations and mild hyphema is slightly more favorable, albeit guarded, compared to corneal lacerations and total hyphema. TIP and hyphema comprising more than an estimated 10% of the AC often result in blindness, phthisis bulbi, or enucleation.
- With TIP, corneal wounds ≤ 15 mm may have a positive visual outcome.
- Wound lengths >15 mm result in either blindness, phthisis bulbi, or enucleation.
- Prolonged ulcerative keratitis before UIP relates directly to poor visual outcome. Perforating corneal ulcers due to ulcerative keratitis of $>$2-weeks duration, and melting ulcers or ulcers with concomitant fungal and bacterial infections tend to produce a poor visual outcome or to result in enucleation due to endophthalmitis in most cases.

MISCELLANEOUS

ASSOCIATED CONDITIONS

- Ulcerative keratitis frequently incites severe anterior uveitis mediated by reflex axonal pathways.
- Infection.

AGE-RELATED FACTORS

N/A

ZOONOTIC POTENTIAL

N/A

PREGNANCY

N/A

SEE ALSO

N/A

ABBREVIATIONS

- AC =
- TIP = traumatic iris prolapse
- UIP = ulcerative iris prolapse

Suggested Reading

Brooks DE. Equine ophthalmology. In: Gelatt KN, ed. Veterinary ophthalmology. 3rd ed. Philadelphia: Lippincott Williams & Wilkins, 1999.

Chmielewski NT, Brooks DE, Smith PJ, et al. Visual outcome and ocular survival following iris prolapse in the horse: a review of 32 cases. Equine Vet J 1997;29:31–39.

Author Dennis E. Brooks

Consulting Editor Dennis E. Brooks

IRON TOXICOSIS

BASICS

OVERVIEW

• Iron is an essential mineral required for a variety of physiologic functions involving oxidation–reduction reactions.
• Horses often are supplemented with iron, either in their feed or via parenteral administration.
• Oral forms include ferrous fumarate, ferrous sulfate, ferrous gluconate, ferrous carbonate, and ferric phosphate.
• Injectable forms include ferric ammonium citrate and iron–dextran complexes.
• Iron toxicosis in horses most often is associated with oral exposure to iron-containing supplements, with most documented cases occurring in neonates <3 days of age from oral administration of a digestive inoculant containing ferrous fumarate.
• Toxicity of iron salts depends on the amount of elemental iron present—ferrous sulfate is 20% elemental iron; ferrous gluconate is 12% elemental iron.
• Iron toxicosis is associated with both local and systemic effects.
• Ingestion of iron salts causes corrosive damage to the GI mucosa, resulting in edema, ulceration, and hemorrhage.
• After absorption, ferrous iron (Fe^{+2}) is converted to ferric iron (Fe^{+3}), releasing an unbuffered hydrogen ion and causing metabolic acidosis.
• Intracellularly, iron disrupts oxidative phosphorylation and causes free-radical formation and lipid peroxidation, resulting in cell death.
• Periportal hepatocytes are especially vulnerable to damage and necrosis.
• Iron also can result in a coagulopathy from inhibition of thrombin.
• Iron is cardiotoxic, resulting in decreased cardiac output.
• Hypovolemia from GI fluid loss and decreased cardiac output contribute to circulatory shock.

SIGNALMENT

• Most reported cases involve neonates.
• The sensitivity of neonates is believed to result from their lower capacity to bind iron to transferrin and their increased absorption of orally administered iron.
• The toxicity of elemental iron to horses has not been firmly established, but toxic doses for neonates are estimated to be 25-fold less than those for adults.

SIGNS

• Early signs associated with oral ingestion of iron salts include colic, diarrhea, and melena.
• Intoxicated horses often present with anorexia, lethargy, and icterus.
• Signs of hepatoencephalopathy (e.g., ataxia, head pressing, coma) may be seen.

CAUSES AND RISK FACTORS

Iron is more toxic in selenium- or vitamin E–deficient individuals.

DIAGNOSIS

DIFFERENTIAL DIAGNOSIS

Adult Horses

• Other hepatotoxicants—aflatoxins (detection in feed, histopathologic lesions), blue-green algae toxins (presence of algal bloom, detection of toxins, histopathologic lesions), PAs (evidence of PA-containing plant consumption, histopathologic lesions)
• Theiler's disease—history of equine immune serum administration
• Causes of hemolytic anemia—red-maple ingestion (evidence of plant consumption, Heinz bodies, methemoglobinemia); equine infectious anemia (positive Coggins test)
• Immune-mediated thrombocytopenia—positive Coombs' test
• DIC—detection of underlying disease, thrombocytopenia, moderately prolonged PT and APTT, and increased serum FDPs
• Bacterial cholangiohepatitis—liver biopsy
• Lymphosarcoma—evaluation of blood smears, cytologic evaluation of bone marrow, and enlarged lymph nodes or tumor masses

Foals

• Septicemia—fever; neutrophilia
• Neonatal isoerythrolysis—low PCV; positive Coombs' test
• Tyzzer's disease—histopathologic examination
• Equine herpes virus—histopathologic lesions

CBC/BIOCHEMISTRY/URINALYSIS

• Thrombocytopenia, lymphopenia, and prolonged PT and APTT
• Increased serum GGT, ALP, total and conjugated bilirubin, bile acids, fibrinogen, FDP, and ammonia
• Anion gap metabolic acidosis

OTHER LABORATORY TESTS

• High serum iron concentration, high saturation of iron binding, and high free iron in tissues
• Postmortem interpretation of high liver iron concentrations is difficult in the absence of compatible histopathologic lesions.

IMAGING

N/A

DIAGNOSTIC PROCEDURES

N/A

PATHOLOGIC FINDINGS

Gross Findings

Lesions include icterus, small livers with dark red areas or tan discoloration and uneven surfaces, GI hemorrhages, and thymic atrophy in foals.

Histopathologic Findings

• Lesions include hepatocellular necrosis that may be primarily periportal or panlobular, varying degrees of bile duct proliferation, fibrous connective tissue proliferation, mixed inflammatory cell infiltration, and cholestasis.
• There may be multifocal to locally extensive areas of necrosis and hemorrhage in the gastric glandular mucosa and areas of necrosis in the lamina propria of the small intestine.
• Mild to severe lymphoid lesions, including thymic lymphoid necrosis and necrosis in splenic lymphoid follicles

IRON TOXICOSIS

TREATMENT

- Stabilize the patient, paying particular attention to cardiovascular support and acid–base status.
- GI decontamination is unlikely to be beneficial after oral ingestion of iron because of the delay in presentation and inability of AC to bind iron.
- Use of the specific iron-chelator deferoxamine mesylate is possible. Appropriate dosage regimens have not been determined, however, and efficacy and safety studies in horses are lacking.

MEDICATIONS

DRUGS

- Chelator of choice—deferoxamine mesylate, which forms a stable, water-soluble compound readily excreted by the kidneys; veterinary experience is limited.
- For mild intoxications, chelation therapy probably offers little advantage compared with supportive care.
- A suggested deferoxamine dosage based on experience in humans and dogs is 15 mg/kg per hour IV; if used, therapy probably should be limited to 24 hours

CONTRAINDICATIONS/POSSIBLE INTERACTIONS

- Do not give deferoxamine to patients with renal impairment.
- Rapid administration of deferoxamine can cause cardiac dysrhythmias and exacerbate existing hypotension.
- Do not give deferoxamine to pregnant animals because of possible fetal skeletal abnormalities.
- Do not give corticosteroids to iron-intoxicated patients because of possible increased serum free-iron concentrations.

FOLLOW-UP

PATIENT MONITORING

Monitor serum iron concentrations, liver function, and cardiovascular status.

PREVENTION/AVOIDANCE

- Do not oversupplement iron in individuals without confirmed iron deficiency.
- A normal dietary requirement of iron in adult horses is 40 ppm.

POSSIBLE COMPLICATIONS

N/A

EXPECTED COURSE AND PROGNOSIS

- Individuals with mild liver pathology have a good prognosis with good supportive care.
- Individuals with severe liver pathology or hepatoencephalopathy have a guarded prognosis.

MISCELLANEOUS

ASSOCIATED CONDITIONS

N/A

AGE-RELATED FACTORS

N/A

ZOONOTIC POTENTIAL

N/A

PREGNANCY

N/A

SEE ALSO

N/A

ABBREVIATIONS

- AC = activated charcoal
- ALP = alkaline phosphatase
- APTT = activated partial thromboplastin time
- DIC = disseminated intravascular coagulation
- FDP = fibrin degradation product
- GGT = γ-glutamyltransferase
- GI = gastrointestinal
- PA = pyrrolizidine alkaloid
- PCV = packed cell volume
- PT = prothrombin time

Suggested Reading

Acland HM, Mann PC, Robertson JL, et al. Toxic hepatopathy in neonatal foals. Vet Pathol 1984;21:3–9.

Divers TJ, Warner A, Vaala WE, et al. Toxic hepatic failure in newborn foals. J Am Vet Med Assoc 1983:1407–1413.

Edens LM, Robertson JL, Feldman BF. Cholestatic hepatopathy, thrombocytopenia and lymphopenia associated with iron toxicity in a Thoroughbred gelding. Equine Vet J 1993;25:81–84.

Mullaney TP, Brown CM. Iron toxicity in neonatal foals. Equine Vet J 1988;20:119–124.

Author Robert H. Poppenga

Consulting Editor Robert H. Poppenga

ISCHEMIC OPTIC NEUROPATHY

BASICS

OVERVIEW

• Optic nerve atrophy as a sequel to infarction or injury to the vascular supply of the optic nerve.
• After a sudden loss of blood supply, the optic disc at first appears slightly pale.
• Within 3–5 days, a papilledema due to ischemia and infarction of the optic nerve is seen, which may progress to white, raised lesions overlying the optic nerve and its margins.
• After several weeks, ophthalmoscopic signs of optic nerve atrophy, with pallor and vascular attenuation of the optic disc
• Peripapillary retinal ischemia results in microinfarcts of the nerve fiber layer, which appear clinically as whitish, indistinct spots; these are areas of thickened nerve fiber layer consisting of aggregates of ruptured and swollen axons.
• With time, increasing signs of retinal atrophy
• Organ system—ophthalmic

SIGNALMENT

N/A

SIGNS

• Rapidly developing blindness
• Dilated pupil
• Absent PLR
• No signs of pain

CAUSES AND RISK FACTORS

• Head trauma
• Severe systemic hemorrhage
• Septic embolism
• Optic neuritis
• Surgical ligation of the carotid artery for treatment of epistaxis caused by guttural pouch mycosis

DIAGNOSIS

DIFFERENTIAL DIAGNOSIS

• Traumatic neuropathy
• Exudative optic neuritis
• Retinal detachment
• ERU

CBC/BIOCHEMISTRY/URINALYSIS

N/A

OTHER LABORATORY TESTS

N/A

IMAGING

N/A

DIAGNOSTIC PROCEDURES

ERG

ISCHEMIC OPTIC NEUROPATHY

TREATMENT

Symptomatic

MEDICATIONS

DRUG(S)

Choice of drug depends on the cause and whether any specific etiologic agent has been determined.

CONTRAINDICATIONS/POSSIBLE INTERACTIONS

N/A

FOLLOW-UP

EXPECTED COURSE AND PROGNOSIS

Poor prognosis for return of vision

MISCELLANEOUS

ASSOCIATED CONDITIONS

N/A

AGE-RELATED FACTORS

N/A

ZOONOTIC POTENTIAL

N/A

PREGNANCY

N/A

SEE ALSO

- ERU
- Exudative optic neuritis
- Retinal detachment
- Traumatic neuritis

ABBREVIATIONS

- ERG = electroretinogram
- ERU = equine recurrent uveitis
- PLR = pupillary light reflex.

Suggested Reading

Brooks DE. Equine ophthalmology. In: Gelatt KN, ed. Veterinary ophthalmology. 3rd ed. Philadelphia: Lippincot Williams & Wilkins, 1999.

Author Maria Källberg
Consulting Editor Dennis E. Brooks

ISOCOMA WRIGHTII (RAYLESS GOLDENROD) TOXICOSIS

BASICS

OVERVIEW

- In the past, *Isocoma wrightii* (rayless goldenrod) has been known as *Haplopappus heterophyllus.*
- The plant is an erect, bushy, unbranching perennial shrub that grows 2–4 feet in height.
- The leaves are alternate, linear, and generally have a smooth margin but can be toothed; the leaves also may have a sticky feel to them.
- The flowers are yellow, tubular, terminal, and number 7–15 per head.
- The plant prefers the arid Southwest and is found in dry rangelands of southern Colorado, through New Mexico and Arizona, western Texas, and into northern Mexico.
- The plant grows well in river valleys, along drainage areas, and is abundant along the Pecos River.
- Tremetone, a ketone, is reportedly the toxic agent.

SIGNALMENT

N/A

SIGNS

- No cases of *I. wrightii* intoxication have been documented in horses.
- The toxin is the same as that found in *Eupatorium rugosum* (white snakeroot), and presumptive evidence exists that the same clinical signs could be expected—heart muscle degeneration, muscle tremors, ataxia, reluctance to walk, heavy sweating, myoglobinuria, and depression.
- Horses that eat *E. rugosum* have an onset of clinical signs within 2–3 weeks after ingestion; generally, 2–3 days of ingestion is required.
- Affected horses stand with their legs wide apart and develop swelling near the thoracic inlet and along the ventral neck.
- There may be a jugular pulse and associated tachycardia.
- ECG changes—increased heat rate, ST elevation, and variable QRS complexes
- Cardiac arrhythmias often are present and detectable on auscultation.

CAUSES AND RISK FACTORS

- Environmental conditions such as drought result in less desirable forages or weeds being consumed.
- Hungry or thirsty horses that are unfamiliar with a given area are more likely to consume *I. wrightii.*

DIAGNOSIS

DIFFERENTIAL DIAGNOSIS

- Evidence of consumption and compatible clinical signs remain the best way of diagnosing intoxication.
- Examination of the pasture may reveal that the plant has been browsed.
- Selenium/vitamin E deficiency (white muscle disease)—measurement of selenium and vitamin E in whole blood, serum, or liver
- Ionophore intoxication—detection of ionophore in feed or GI contents.

CBC/BIOCHEMISTRY/URINALYSIS

- Horses intoxicated with *E. rugosum* have elevated serum CK, AST, and AP activities.
- Presumably, horses consuming *I. wrightii* have similar abnormalities.

OTHER LABORATORY TESTS

- ECG changes may be noted as described above.
- Detection of toxin may be possible.

IMAGING

N/A

DIAGNOSTIC PROCEDURES

N/A

PATHOLOGIC FINDINGS

- Horses ingesting *E. rugosum* have nonspecific histopathologic lesions.
- Lesions associated with suspected *I. wrightii* intoxication—myocardial degeneration, necrosis, and fibrosis.
- The pericardial sac may contain straw-colored fluid, and the subendocardium may have extensive pale areas.

TREATMENT

- Decontamination with AC and a saline cathartic may be helpful.
- Monitor ECG, and treat arrhythmias accordingly.
- Animals that survive may be left with a severely scarred heart and circulatory dysfunction; therefore, symptomatic and supportive care is always appropriate.

ISOCOMA WRIGHTII (RAYLESS GOLDENROD) TOXICOSIS

MEDICATIONS

DRUGS

- AC (2–5 g/kg PO in a water slurry [1 g of AC per 5 mL of water)].
- Sodium or magnesium sulfate (250 mg/kg PO as a 20% solution)

CONTRAINDICATIONS/POSSIBLE INTERACTIONS

N/A

FOLLOW-UP

PATIENT MONITORING

N/A

PREVENTION/AVOIDANCE

- Preventing access to the plant is the best solution for avoiding intoxication.
- Herbicides can be used to control plant growth.

POSSIBLE COMPLICATIONS

N/A

EXPECTED COURSE AND PROGNOSIS

N/A

MISCELLANEOUS

ASSOCIATED CONDITIONS

N/A

AGE-RELATED FACTORS

N/A

ZOONOTIC POTENTIAL

N/A

PREGNANCY

N/A

SEE ALSO

E. rugosum (white snakeroot)

ABBREVIATIONS

- AC = activated charcoal
- AST = aspartate aminotransferase
- AP = alkaline phosphatase
- CK = creatine kinase

Suggested Reading

Olson CT, Keller WC, Gerken Reed SM. Suspected tremetol poisoning in horses. J Am Vet Med Assoc 1984;185:1001–1003.

Sanders M. White snakeroot poisoning in a foal: a case report. Equine Vet Sci 1983;3:128–131.

Author Tam Garland

Consulting Editor Robert H. Poppenga

ISOERYTHROLYSIS, NEONATAL (NI)

BASICS

DEFINITION

Immune-mediated destruction of a neonate's RBCs, triggered by maternal antibodies ingested in colostrum

PATHOPHYSIOLOGY

- Several independent events contribute to development of the condition.
- First, a mare, which lacks a particular inherited antigenic RBC factor, is exposed to that blood factor via transfusion of incompatible RBCs or exposure to fetal RBCs containing the factor. This exposure may occur at parturition or because of placentitis. As a result, the mare produces antibody directed against the factor. These antibodies do no harm to the mare.
- Second, the mare conceives a foal, sired by a stallion with that particular antigenic RBC factor, and the resulting foal inherits the factor from the sire.
- Third, at birth, the foal ingests and absorbs colostrum containing maternal antibodies, including the anti-RBC factor antibodies from the mare.
- Fourth, the antibodies attach to the foal's RBCs and result in lysis or premature removal of the cells by the reticuloendothelial system, leading to anemia.

SYSTEMS AFFECTED

- Hemic/lymphatic/immune—intravascular or extravascular hemolysis leads to anemia, hemoglobinemia, and icterus
- Renal/urologic—hemoglobinuria; pigment nephrosis that may lead to renal failure
- Cardiovascular—tachycardia; shock may result from the anemia
- Nervous—anoxia because of anemia leads to weakness and convulsions

GENETICS

- The underlying pathogenesis is based on a genetic difference between the dam and the foal and sire, in that the dam lacks the gene producing an inherited RBC factor and both the sire and foal have that gene.
- Many antigenic RBC factors are inherited, any one of which theoretically could be involved, but two factors, Aa in the A system and Qa in the Q system, are involved in nearly all equine cases.
- In mules, "donkey factor," an RBC factor found in virtually all donkeys but not in horses, is involved.
- Presence or absence of antigenic factors is determined by blood typing.

INCIDENCE/PREVALENCE

- In Standardbred and Thoroughbred foals, the prevalence is 1–2%.
- In mule foals, the prevalence is estimated to be as high as 10–25%.
- Prevalence varies somewhat among breeds and is influenced primarily by the frequency with which genes for the various blood group factors are found in each breed.
- Gene frequency can be used to estimate how many mares are "at risk" because they lack a factor and how many stallions are "incompatible" with these mares because they have the factor.
- Virtually all mares bred to jacks are at risk.

SIGNALMENT

Species

- Horses and mules
- Similar conditions occur in cattle, cats, and humans; however, the antigenic factors involved in each species are different.

Breed Predilections

- The antigenic factors involved are not specific for, or limited to, any single breed of horse.
- Virtually all mule pregnancies are incompatible regarding the blood group factor donkey factor, which donkeys have and horses do not.

Mean Age and Range

0–8 days

SIGNS

General Comments

Severity of clinical signs depends on the rate of hemolysis.

Historical Findings

- Foals are healthy at birth and nurse normally.
- Lethargy and other signs develop within hours to days after colostral ingestion.
- Icterus or pallor may be present.
- Mares may have a history of producing foals with jaundice or known NI.

Physical Examination Findings

- Lethargy
- Tachypnea; tachycardia
- Pallor (acutely) or icterus (subacutely)
- Hemoglobinuria
- Recumbency
- Mild fever occasionally is present.
- Anoxia may lead to colic, melena, and convulsions.

ISOERYTHROLYSIS, NEONATAL (NI)

CAUSES

Sensitization of the dam to produce antibody results from exposure to incompatible fetal RBCs because of placentitis, at parturition, or via incompatible blood transfusion.

RISK FACTORS

• Mares lacking RBC factors Aa and/or Qa are at higher risk to produce antibodies to these antigens if exposed than are mares with incompatibilities involving other blood group factors.
• All mares bred to donkeys are at risk for production of antibody to donkey factor.

DIAGNOSIS

DIFFERENTIAL DIAGNOSIS

• The differential diagnosis includes septicemia, hepatopathy, and hypoxic ischemic encephalopathy (i.e., neonatal maladjustment syndrome); anemia and hemoglobinuria distinguish NI from these.
• Consider neonatal piroplasmosis if in an endemic area.

CBC/BIOCHEMISTRY/URINALYSIS

• Anemia—decreased PCV, decreased hemoglobin, and decreased RBC count
• Hemoglobinemia
• Hyperbilirubinemia
• Hemoglobinuria
• Azotemia
• Mild leukocytosis
• Hypoglycemia

OTHER LABORATORY TESTS

Coomb's Test (Direct Antiglobulin Test)

• Detects immunoglobulin-coated RBCs. This test may remain positive for several weeks, until the maternal antibody is metabolized.
• Detects anti-RBC factor antibody in mare serum or colostrum. A sample of the mare's fluids is preferable to foal serum, because colostral antibody ingested by the foal may be adsorbed to RBCs and not be free in sera.

JFA Test

Useful for screening colostrum before the foal nurses

Saline Agglutination or Complement-Mediated Hemolytic Tests

Must be performed by blood-typing laboratories, but can determine the presence and specificity of antibody—against which factor the antibody is directed

IMAGING

N/A

DIAGNOSTIC PROCEDURES

N/A

PATHOLOGIC FINDINGS

• Pallor if the animal dies acutely, or icterus, often marked, if the animal survives long enough to convert hemoglobin to bilirubin
• Splenic enlargement; dark, pigment-stained kidneys secondary to hemoglobin nephrosis, and bloody, dark intestinal contents may be found.
• Hypoplastic bone marrow

TREATMENT

APPROPRIATE HEALTH CARE

Peracute Cases

• Emergencies requiring rapid and aggressive treatment, including provision of RBCS without the factor (i.e., antigen) against which the maternal antibody is directed.
• Affected foals can die within hours, often leaving little time for diagnosis and treatment.

Acute Cases

Emergencies requiring prompt, aggressive therapy in the form of IV fluids, nursing care, and perhaps, RBC replacement.

Subacute Cases

Generally require little more than stall confinement and enforced rest.

NURSING CARE

Nutritional Support

Mare's milk or supplements provided via nasogastric tube to recumbent foals or those not nursing may be required.

IV Balanced Polyionic Crystalloid Solutions

• Promote diuresis in cases with pigment nephropathy.
• Glucose-containing fluids in cases with hypoglycemia

ISOERYTHROLYSIS, NEONATAL (NI)

Intranasal Oxygen

May be useful to ensure maximal oxygen transport for the existing volume of RBCs.

RBC Transfusion

• Consider if PCV is 15–18% and dropping. Transfusion may not be necessary until the PCV reaches 12–14%, but because of the time required to obtain suitable RBCs, the need should be anticipated before the PCV reaches this level.
• Providing RBCs that do not react with the maternal anti-RBC antibody is the goal of transfusion. This excludes the sire as a donor. A suitable compatible donor is unlikely to be chosen by random selection, regardless of sex or relation to the patient, because of the frequencies of offending antigens in equine populations. Perform cross-matching, if possible.
• Administer RBCs as whole blood (if donor plasma is free of anti-RBC antibody) or as washed RBCs (if from the dam or a donor with compatible RBCs but with anti-RBC antibody in the plasma). Washed RBC from the dam are ideal in the absence of cross-matching.
• Always use a blood administration set with a filter for transfusion of blood or blood components.

ACTIVITY

Confine the mare and foal to restrict exercise until the foal's PCV returns to the normal range.

DIET

• Withhold colostrum until the anti-RBC antibody titer has declined or the foal's gut has "closed" to further absorption.
• Colostral titers, as measured by JFA test, decrease rapidly (often within 6–8 hours), and after 12–24 hours of life, further absorption of ingested antibody is unlikely from the GI tract.

CLIENT EDUCATION

If the mare has produced a previous foal with NI, she is at higher risk for a second affected foal.

SURGICAL CONSIDERATIONS

N/A

MEDICATIONS

DRUGS OF CHOICE

N/A

CONTRAINDICATIONS

N/A

PRECAUTIONS

Avoid administration of nephrotoxic medications (e.g., aminoglycoside antibiotics) because of pigment nephropathy.

POSSIBLE INTERACTIONS

N/A

ALTERNATIVE DRUGS

N/A

FOLLOW-UP

PATIENT MONITORING

• CBC and PCV to monitor anemia; frequency depends on the severity and rapidity of decline in PCV. In acute cases, monitoring may be necessary every 4–8 hours to evaluate the progress of and need for transfusion.
• BUN and creatinine levels to monitor pigment nephropathy; perform daily for the first several days.
• Evaluate glucose multiple times a day if the foal is depressed, recumbent, or being maintained on IV glucose.

ISOERYTHROLYSIS, NEONATAL (NI)

PREVENTION/AVOIDANCE

- Prebreeding—select a compatible stallion (e.g., one lacking the factor to which the mare is producing antibody) based on blood typing.
- Postbreeding—evaluate the mare's serum during the last month of gestation for anti-RBC antibody; if detected, withhold the dam's colostrum and provide an alternative, safe source of colostrum or serum for the foal.
- Test colostrum at birth against the foal's RBCs using the JFA test before allowing the foal to nurse, and provide an alternative source of colostrum or other immunoglobulins if a reaction is detected.

POSSIBLE COMPLICATIONS

At risk mares may have recurrence on subsequent pregnancies, depending on the genetics of the stallion and the foal.

EXPECTED COURSE AND PROGNOSIS

- Peracute cases—prognosis is poor, because rapidity and severity of onset often compound recognition and treatment.
- Acute cases—prognosis depends on rapidity of onset and aggressiveness of treatment; the more rapid the onset, the more aggressive the therapy needs to be for survival.
- Subacute cases—prognosis is excellent, even without treatment, and a full recovery is expected.

MISCELLANEOUS

ASSOCIATED CONDITIONS

Neonatal alloimmune thrombocytopenia

AGE-RELATED FACTORS

- Because foals obtain essentially all the maternal antibody they will ever obtain within approximately the first 12 hours of life, the severity and, to some extent, duration of NI usually are determined by the time of diagnosis.
- Foals >8 days that continue to show persistent, progressive anemia long after colostral immunoglobulin has declined and absorption by the gut has ceased may suffer from some other mechanism of immune-mediated hemolysis—IgA-mediated or production of antibody by maternally derived cells absorbed via the GI tract

ZOONOTIC POTENTIAL

N/A

PREGNANCY

Immunoglobulins do not normally cross the equine placenta; thus, the fetus is protected from the disease and from the ingestion and absorption of maternal immunoglobulins until after birth.

SYNONYMS

- Hemolytic disease of the newborn
- Jaundiced foal syndrome

SEE ALSO

N/A

ABBREVIATIONS

- GI = gastrointestinal
- JFA = jaundiced foal agglutination test
- PCV = packed cell volume

Suggested Reading

Bailey E. Prevalence of anti-red blood cell antibodies in the serum and colostrum of mares and its relationship to neonatal isoerythrolysis. Am J Vet Res 1982;43:1917–1921.

Bailey E, Conboy S, McCarthy PF. Neonatal isoerythrolysis of foals: an update on testing. Proc Am Assoc Equine Pract 1987,00:341–353.

McClure JJ. Strategies for prevention of neonatal isoerythrolysis in horses and mules. Equine Vet Educ 1997;9:118–122.

Stormont C. Neonatal isoerythrolysis in domestic animals: a comparative review. Adv Vet Sci Comp Med 1975;19:23–45.

Swiderski CE, McClure JJ. Immunodiagnostic assays. Vet Clin North Am Equine Pract 1995;11:455–489.

Author Jill Johnson McClure

Consulting Editor Mary Rose Paradis

JUGLANS NIGRA (BLACK WALNUT) TOXICOSIS

BASICS

OVERVIEW

• *Juglans nigra* (black walnut) is a large tree native to the eastern U.S.; its wood is prized for furniture and gun stocks.
• When fresh black walnut shavings are used as bedding, horses can develop laminitis and pyrexia within 12–24 hours.
• The condition usually presents as a stable-wide outbreak, but not all horses in contact with black walnut–contaminated bedding develop problems.

SIGNALMENT

No breed, age, or sex predilections

SIGNS

• Laminitis—can be severe
• Pyrexia
• Depression
• Limb edema
• Colic

CAUSES AND RISK FACTORS

• An unknown compound in fresh, black walnut shavings.
• Toxicity decreases with exposure of shavings to light and air.
• Problems can occur when as little as 5–20% of bedding is black walnut.

DIAGNOSIS

DIFFERENTIAL DIAGNOSIS

• Other causes of laminitis
• *Berteroa incana* ingestion
• History will indicate several to many of the horses bedded with black walnut shavings develop laminitis during a relatively short period.

CBC/BIOCHEMISTRY/URINALYSIS

N/A

OTHER LABORATORY TESTS

• Black walnut shavings can be identified by their dark brown color (with a hint of purple).
• Samples can be submitted to diagnostic laboratories or forestry departments for positive identification.

IMAGING

N/A

DIAGNOSTIC PROCEDURES

N/A

PATHOLOGIC FINDINGS

Laminitis

TREATMENT

• Remove all animals from suspect bedding.
• Wash legs with mild soap and water.
• Treat for laminitis.

JUGLANS NIGRA (BLACK WALNUT) TOXICOSIS

MEDICATIONS

DRUGS

- If black walnut is ingested, AC (2–5 g/kg PO in a water slurry)
- Treat for laminitis.

CONTRAINDICATIONS/POSSIBLE INTERACTIONS

N/A

FOLLOW-UP

PATIENT MONITORING

N/A

PREVENTION/AVOIDANCE

Inspect bedding deliveries for black walnut contamination.

POSSIBLE COMPLICATIONS

Ventral rotation of the third phalanx

EXPECTED COURSE AND PROGNOSIS

Good with no complications

MISCELLANEOUS

ASSOCIATED CONDITIONS

N/A

AGE-RELATED FACTORS

N/A

ZOONOTIC POTENTIAL

N/A

PREGNANCY

N/A

SEE ALSO

Laminitis

ABBREVIATIONS

AC = activated charcoal

Suggested Reading

Uhlinger C. Black walnut toxicosis in 10 horses. J Am Vet Med Assoc 1989,195:343–344.

Author Larry J. Thompson
Consulting Editor Robert H. Poppenga

LAMINITIS

BASICS

DEFINITION

• Strictly speaking, inflammation of the laminae of the foot.
• More broadly, the pathology and pathophysiology of the condition, namely a degeneration and then failure of the attachments between P3 and the inner hoof wall.
• Acute and chronic forms, with the chronic form loosely defined as more than 2 days' duration or as clear failure of the attachment between the hoof wall and P3.

PATHOPHYSIOLOGY

• Mechanisms that lead to failure of attachment between the hoof wall and P3 are not clearly defined.
• Much research has focused on the hemodynamic changes and tissue fluid shifts that occur in the foot during the onset of laminitis. Recent reports suggest that these changes more likely result from failure of the P3–hoof wall bond rather than cause it.
• During normal hoof wall growth, attachments between epidermal lamellae and basement membrane (firmly attached to P3) are constantly being broken down and reformed. It is proposed that the cell–cell, and cell–basement membrane, attachments are released under the influence of MMPs.
• MMPs have been demonstrated in normal lamellar tissue and at increased quantities in lamellar tissues from horses with both experimentally induced and spontaneous laminitis.
• Electron microscopy has shown that early and severe changes occur in the basement membranes in the lamellae of affected horses. In some areas, the membrane disappears; in others, connections between the basal cells and basement membranes break down. Thus, the P3–hoof wall bond is broken, which sets the scene in the foot for the serious changes that follow.
• The substance or substances that induce MMPs in spontaneous and experimentally induced laminitis have not been identified.
• Associated with a wide range of diseases, many of which are severe and multisystemic (see *Causes*) and many of which probably are associated with release or production of cytokines (i.e., tumor necrosis factor, interleukin-1, and transforming growth factor). These substances increase MMP production in other species.
• By the time the horse shows clinical signs, major and potentially irreversible changes have already occurred in the digit. This emphasizes the need for early and aggressive preventative and therapeutic actions.

SYSTEM AFFECTED

Musculoskeletal

• Primarily a disease of the foot, leading to varying degrees of lameness.
• Depending on the inciting cause, all four feet, only one foot, or only the front feet may be involved.

Other Systems

See *Causes*.

GENETICS

N/A

INCIDENCE/PREVALENCE

N/A

SIGNALMENT

• No consistent associations between age, breed, sex, or weight for acute laminitis, but this form rarely is seen in foals and weanlings.
• Horses with chronic laminitis tend to be old, and more females than males tend to be affected.

SIGNS

General Comments

Clinical signs of the primary problem may overshadow those of laminitis during the early stages of the acute phase.

Historical Findings

• The horse is reluctant to move, particularly when made to turn or to walk on hard surfaces.
• At rest, the animal may constantly shift weight from one leg to another.
• The front feet often are more frequently or severely affected than the hind feet, so the horse may attempt to place more of its weight on the hind limbs by drawing them forward under the belly and extending the fore limbs out in front.
• Horses with severe pain may become recumbent.

LAMINITIS

Physical Findings

Acute Laminitis:

• Affected feet may be warm to the touch, and digital arteries may have an increased pulse.
• Degree of pain may be reflected by tachycardia, muscle tremors, and sweating.
• Examination with a hoof tester will reveal pain over the sole, particularly at the toe, and tapping on the hoof wall may cause pain.
• In severe cases, the horse will not allow the feet to be picked up.

Chronic Laminitis:

• Passage from acute to chronic laminitis is marked by pain that persists for 2 days, by displacement of P3, or both.
• Displacement can be a rotation of P3, with a marked separation of the parallel alignment between the hoof wall and the dorsal surface of P3, or palmar displacement, in which P3 migrates toward the sole but remains parallel to the hoof wall. The latter situation, which sometimes is called "sinking" of P3, may involve a palpable depression at the coronary band and also serum oozing from the coronary band.
• Examination of the sole may reveal a separation just dorsal to the apex of the frog, which indicates the tip of P3 is close to penetrating the sole. This is a very grave sign.
• If the problem persists for a few weeks, then there is abnormal growth of the hoof wall, with irregular rings that are close together at the toe and more widely spaced at the heels.
• The sole may be flatter than normal, and the white line may be much wider, particularly at the toe.
• The material of the white line often is soft and granular, and it often is referred to as "seedy toe." This softer material may allow foreign material to penetrate the white line, and infection may ensue.

CAUSES

• Agents responsible for failure of the bond between P3 and the hoof laminae have not been identified, but they appear to be released or induced in a wide variety of circumstances.
• Acute colitis—salmonellosis, Potomac horse fever, and grain overload
• Acute metritis—retention of fetal membranes
• Acute septic peritonitis
• Acute pleuropneumonia
• Ingestion of lush pasture, particularly in overweight horses
• Concussion; working unfit horses on hard surfaces
• Cushing's syndrome
• Increased weight bearing—laminitis may develop in the contralateral limb in a horse with a severe leg injury (e.g., a fracture).
• Black walnut toxicity
• Possible associations include ingestion of large amounts of cold water and administration of corticosteroids.

RISK FACTORS

See *Causes.*

DIAGNOSIS

DIFFERENTIAL DIAGNOSIS

• Any severely painful condition, particularly of the limbs, should be considered in horses with clinical signs of laminitis. Absence of digital pulses and the localization of pain to a specific site will allow differentiation.
• In horses with laminitis in only one foot, all acute and chronic conditions of the foot should be considered, including subsolar abscesses and fractures of P3.
• Acute myopathies may mimic laminitis, because the horse may be reluctant or unable to move. Such horses do not have the characteristic digital pulses associated with acute laminitis, and serum enzymes associated with myopathies usually are markedly elevated.

CBC/BIOCHEMISTRY/URINALYSIS

• No specific laboratory findings
• Marked abnormalities resulting from the inciting cause or causes

OTHER LABORATORY TESTS

N/A

IMAGING

• Lateromedial radiography of the foot to assess the relationship of soft tissues to P3 and to monitor progress of the condition.
• Severity of the changes, including the degree of rotation, can be used to provide a prognosis.

DIAGNOSTIC PROCEDURES

Perineural anesthesia is not usually indicated for diagnostic purposes but may have benefit therapeutically.

PATHOLOGIC FINDINGS

Consistent with the clinical and radiographic findings

TREATMENT

APPROPRIATE HEALTH CARE

Acute Laminitis

• Much of the treatment is aimed at the primary disease inducing the laminogenic agents.
• Pending or established acute laminitis is an emergency and should be treated as such.
• Most acute cases can be managed on the farm, but the underlying problem may warrant referral to a hospital.

LAMINITIS

Chronic Laminitis

Can be managed on the farm.

NURSING CARE

Acute Laminitis

- Bed affected horses on deep sand or other soft bedding. This helps to spread the weight across the sole, unloading the hoof wall, and reduces the tension on the laminae.
- Frog support bandages or shoes have a similar effect.
- The agents inducting MMPs are thought to be carried to the digit via the bloodstream, so reducing blood flow to the digit has been suggested as being indicated in horses at high risk of laminitis. This can be achieved by surrounding the feet with crushed ice or ice water.

Chronic Laminitis

- Depending on the displacement of P3, secondary effects of infection, and abnormal hoof growth, affected horses may require extensive, long-term, and expensive foot care.
- Requires good client cooperation as well as an experienced farrier.

ACTIVITY

Acute Laminitis

- Some argue that limited forced exercise is beneficial, because it promotes digital blood flow. Equally, however, if the laminar degeneration is ongoing due to continued release of mediators, increased blood flow could be detrimental.
- Exercise, particularly on hard ground, will increase the tension on the laminae.
- Generally, encourage horses to lie down to unload the laminae.

Chronic Laminitis

- Activity may be restricted in some cases, particularly those undergoing extensive trimming and shoeing.
- Footing should be soft and severe exertion avoided.

DIET

Acute Laminitis

- A low-carbohydrate, grain-free diet is indicated.
- Grass hay is suitable.

Chronic Laminitis

- Grass hay and low carbohydrates are preferred.
- Keep the horse on the lean side to maintain the load on affected feet as low as possible.

CLIENT EDUCATION

Acute Laminitis

Advise clients of the potentially catastrophic nature of the disease and the long-term problems that may ensue.

Chronic Laminitis

- Instruct clients on the severity of the problem and the long-term management issues they face.
- Inform clients they may never have a sound riding horse.

SURGICAL CONSIDERATIONS

Acute Laminitis

N/A

Chronic Laminitis

Tenotomy of the deep digital flexor tendon has been advocated for horses with rotation of P3 $>10–15°$.

MEDICATIONS

DRUGS OF CHOICE

- NSAIDs are the cornerstone of most therapeutic regimens.
- Phenylbutazone (4.4 mg/kg BID) or flunixin meglumine (1.1 mg/kg BID) frequently are used, occasionally at initially higher doses, with the objective of reducing the dosage as soon as possible to the level that maintains adequate pain control.
- Other medications have been used to promote increased blood flow to the foot, including acepromazine (0.02–0.04 mg/kg IM QID). No data, however, support the value of these and other medications.
- In one study, topical application of glyceryl trinitrate to the pasterns of affected horses reduced the strength of the digital pulse, and lameness was improved.

CONTRAINDICATIONS

N/A

PRECAUTIONS

N/A

POSSIBLE INTERACTIONS

N/A

ALTERNATIVE DRUGS

N/A

FOLLOW-UP

PATIENT MONITORING

- Monitor acute cases frequently, at least daily (and probably more).
- Usually, the underlying inciting condition requires frequent monitoring.
- Chronic cases require periodic monitoring, depending on severity of the problem. This may include repeated radiography to assess status of the foot components.

PREVENTION/AVOIDANCE

Laminitis usually is secondary to other diseases, so direction actions to reduce the development or recurrence of the problem at the primary causes.

POSSIBLE COMPLICATIONS

- In acute cases, the most serious complication is total separation of the epidermal and bony structures, with subsequent sloughing of the hoof.
- In chronic cases, recurrent infections, often associated with penetration of P3 through the sole, are the most serious complication.

EXPECTED COURSE AND PROGNOSIS

- Vary with the severity of the initial problem, inciting cause, and response to treatment.
- The more severe the disruption of the P3–hoof wall bond, the worse the prognosis.
- With massive and rapid loss of the bond, affected feet may deteriorate in a matter of 2–3 days to a point beyond salvage.
- Other, more chronic cases may have problems for weeks to months, and some may never have normal feet.
- The rotation of P3 seen on lateral radiographs has been suggested as a reasonable prognostic indicator, with horses having 10–15° of rotation carrying a poor prognosis.

MISCELLANEOUS

ASSOCIATED CONDITIONS

See *Causes.*

AGE-RELATED FACTORS

N/A

ZOONOTIC POTENTIAL

N/A

PREGNANCY

N/A

SYNONYMS

Founder

SEE ALSO

See *Causes.*

ABBREVIATIONS

- MMPs = metalloproteinases
- P3 = third phalanx

Suggested Reading

Pollitt CC. Equine laminitis: a revised pathophysiology. Proc 45th Annu Conv Am Ass Equine Pract, Albuquerque, New Mexico, Dec 6–8, 1999:188–192.

Slater MR, Hood DM, Carter GK. Descriptive epidemiological study of equine laminitis. Equine Vet J 1995;27:364–367.

Stashak TS. Laminitis. In: Stashak TD, ed. Adams' lameness in horses. 4th ed. Baltimore: Williams & Wilkins, 1987:486–499.

Author Christopher M. Brown

Consulting Editor Christopher M. Brown

LANTANA CAMARA (LANTANA) TOXICOSIS

BASICS

OVERVIEW

- *Lantana camara* (lantana or red sage) is an herbaceous perennial, ornamental shrub.
- It is erect or sprawling, clumped, stout, hairy, and grows to 210 cm tall, with several stems arising out of the base.
- It has square twigs or stems that have small, scattered spines.
- The leaves are simple, opposite or whorled, and are oval shaped, with a petiole up to 1.5 cm long.
- The net-veined leaf blade is aromatic when crushed; the blades are broadly lanceolate and between 5–11 cm long and 2.5–6 cm wide, with a wedge-shaped base and regularly spaced, toothed margins.
- The flowers most often consist of two colors, ranging from white, yellow or orange, red, blue, or even dark violet; the flowers are small and tubular, in flat-topped clusters.
- A green, immature, berry-like fruit also is found, with hard seeds that turn blue to black at maturity.
- The plant is regarded as ornamental, but some varieties have escaped cultivation. These most often are found in fence lines and around old houses or fields over most of the U.S.
- This plant is known to grow in southern Florida and into the northern U.S. and Canada and as far west as California.
- The green berry apparently is the most toxic, although the entire plant is toxic.
- The toxins are polycyclic triterpenoids—lantadene A and lantadene B
- Lantana toxins cause intrahepatic cholestasis, characterized by inhibition of bile secretion without extensive hepatocyte necrosis.
- The plant has been extensively studied in ruminants and produces secondary or hepatogenous photosensitization secondary to hepatobiliary damage.
- Horses are suspected of developing liver disease, but not photosensitization, after ingestion.

SIGNALMENT

N/A

SIGNS

- Anecdotally, horses may develop some liver and renal dysfunction after ingestion that may be evident on clinicopathologic tests, although somewhat nonspecific, and at necropsy.
- Horses are not believed to develop photosensitization, but one report of ingestion by horses described associated crusty, contact-type lesions around the muzzles and light-skinned areas.
- Some owners report icterus of the sclera and mucus membranes after ingestion.

CAUSES AND RISK FACTORS

- Plants accessible to animals are subject to being consumed, and animals that are hungry or unfamiliar with the plants are more likely to consume *L. camara.*
- Hepatic metabolism differences between species may account for differences in susceptibility to lantana toxins.
- Injury to the liver cells could result from the action of metabolite rather than the parent compound.

DIAGNOSIS

DIFFERENTIAL DIAGNOSIS

- Consider other hepatotoxins—aflatoxin (detection in feed and histopathology), PAs (ingestion of alkaloid-containing plants and histopathology), and iron toxicosis (tissue iron concentrations and histopathology).
- In addition to PA-containing plants, consider exposure to other hepatotoxic plants—*Nolina texana, Agave lecheguilla, Panicum* spp., and *Trifolium hybridum.*
- A nontoxic differential includes Theiler's disease (history, histopathology).

CBC/BIOCHEMISTRY/URINALYSIS

Hyperbilirubinemia (conjugated) is the most consistent finding.

OTHER LABORATORY TESTS

- Lantadenes may be detected in stomach contents if death occurs close to the time of consumption. Portions of the plant may be identified in the stomach contents by a competent microscopist.
- The most valuable tool is a good history.

IMAGING

N/A

DIAGNOSTIC PROCEDURES

N/A

LANTANA CAMARA (LANTANA) TOXICOSIS

PATHOLOGIC FINDINGS
- Liver lesions—cholestasis, pigmentation and degeneration of hepatocytes, and fibrosis
- Kidney lesions—vacuolation and degeneration of convoluted tubule epithelium and presence of various casts. Occasionally, multifocal, interstitial, mononuclear cell infiltration and fibrosis may be evident.

TREATMENT
- No specific treatment
- Consider GI decontamination.
- Symptomatic and supportive care

MEDICATIONS

DRUGS
AC (2–5 g/kg in a water slurry [1 g of AC per 5 mL of water])

CONTRAINDICATIONS/POSSIBLE INTERACTIONS
N/A

FOLLOW-UP

PATIENT MONITORING
Monitor hepatic function.

PREVENTION/AVOIDANCE
- Preventing access to the plant is the best solution for avoiding toxicities.
- Herbicides can be used to control the plant.

POSSIBLE COMPLICATIONS
N/A

EXPECTED COURSE AND PROGNOSIS
N/A

MISCELLANEOUS

ASSOCIATED CONDITIONS
N/A

AGE-RELATED FACTORS
N/A

ZOONOTIC POTENTIAL
N/A

PREGNANCY
N/A

SEE ALSO
N/A

ABBREVIATIONS
- AC = activated charcoal
- GI = gastrointestinal
- PA = pyrrolizidine alkaloid

Suggested Reading

Pass MA. Poisoning of livestock by lantana plants. In: Keeler RF, Tu AT, eds. Toxicology of plant and fungal compounds: handbook of natural toxins. New York: Marcel Dekker, 1991;6:297–311.

Author Tam Garland
Consulting Editor Robert H. Poppenga

LARGE COLON TORSION

BASICS

DEFINITION

- A displacement characterized by rotation of the large colon about the mesocolic axis in a dorsomedial or dorsolateral direction.
- Most commonly originates at the cecocolic fold, where the right ventral colon and cecum attach to the body wall.
- Less commonly occurs at any level of the large colon aboral to the cecocolic fold.
- The transverse colon or cecum may be involved.
- Most torsions are in a dorsomedial direction.
- A rotation $<180^\circ$ is within normal physiologic limits.
- A rotation between 180° and $<360^\circ$ often results in nonstrangulating obstruction of the large colon, with mild vascular compromise; a rotation $\geq 360^\circ$ results in strangulating obstruction of the large colon, which manifests as severe, acute abdominal crisis.

PATHOPHYSIOLOGY

- The large colon consists of left and right, dorsal and ventral colons.
- The dorsal and ventral portions of the large colon are joined by the ascending mesocolon, which originates from the root of the mesentery.
- The only attachment of the large colon to the body wall is by the right ventral colon, at the level of the cecocolic fold.
- Because of its lack of anchoring attachments, the left colon is mobile, predisposing it to displacement.
- Torsion causes varying degrees of mechanical bowel obstruction, which decreases normal colonic absorption and results in electrolyte imbalances and hypomotility, which in turn may contribute to displacement and torsion.
- Blood supply to the colon is via the colic arteries, which enter the colon at the level of the cecocolic fold. A torsion $>180^\circ$ may cause venous obstruction, resulting in congestion and edema of the large colon; a torsion $>270^\circ$ may cause both arterial and venous obstruction, resulting in colonic ischemia.
- With venous obstruction, blood accumulates in the veins and, eventually, extravasates into the submucosa and colonic lumen. This extravasation disrupts the colonic epithelium that sloughs into the lumen, and these phenomena produce increased gas and fluid accumulation within the colonic lumen. The accumulation of gas results in painful distension of the colon.
- Vascular damage results in degeneration of blood vessels and intraluminal hemorrhage.
- With damage to the bowel wall, bacteria and endotoxins, as well as fluid and protein, leak into the peritoneal cavity, which results in endotoxemia, hypovolemia, and hypoproteinemia. Within 4–5 hours, the colonic mucosa undergoes complete necrosis.
- Severe systemic shock leads to cardiovascular collapse and death.
- With complete arterial and venous obstruction, tissue perfusion decreases, with resultant hypoxia and ischemia that cause reduced absorption and hypomotility. Prolonged ischemia causes bowel necrosis, with leakage of bacteria and endotoxins into the peritoneal cavity.
- Endotoxemia and hypovolemia result in severe systemic shock, cardiovascular collapse, and death.

SYSTEMS AFFECTED

- GI
- Cardiovascular

GENETICS

No known genetic basis

INCIDENCE/PREVALENCE

The reported incidence ranges between 11–26% of horses undergoing surgical treatment of colic.

SIGNALMENT

Old horses and broodmares, especially during the postparturient period, appear to be more commonly affected.

SIGNS

Historical Findings

Owners typically report a sudden onset of severe abdominal pain.

Physical Examination Findings

- With strangulating large colon torsion, horses usually present with acute, severe abdominal pain that is nonresponsive to analgesia.
- With progression of clinical signs, horses may become depressed.
- Horses typically have tachycardia and tachypnea, though some have normal heart and respiratory rates.
- As the condition progresses, abdominal distension is evident.
- Borborygmi are reduced to absent in all GI quadrants.
- Mucous membranes may be normal initially, with progression to pallor or congestion.

CAUSES

- The exact cause is unknown, but hypomotility and increased intraluminal gas accumulation are theorized to initiate a dorsomedial or dorsolateral rotation of the left or right ventral colon. Nonstrangulating obstructions may progress to strangulating obstructions by this mechanism as well.

• Horses undergoing a sudden dietary change may be predisposed to increased gas production and altered GI motility. Similarly, horses fed lush pasture or large volumes of grain have significant fermentation processes within the ventral colon, producing excessive amounts of gas that may initiate torsion.
• Postparturient broodmares are thought to be predisposed because of increased space within the abdomen.

RISK FACTORS

A diet high in grain, rich grass, or a sudden change in feed may predispose because of increased fermentation, subsequent gas production, and hypomotility.

DIAGNOSIS

DIFFERENTIAL DIAGNOSIS

• Nonstrangulating obstruction—torsion $<360^\circ$
• Right dorsal colon displacement
• Left dorsal colon displacement
• Large colon impaction
• Enterolithiasis
• Adhesions
• Colonic or cecal tympany
• Strangulating obstruction—torsion $\geq 360^\circ$
• Large intestinal intussusception
• Incarceration of the large intestine through the epiploic foramen, gastrosplenic space, or mesenteric rents
• Colonic or cecal tympany
• A definitive preoperative diagnosis may be difficult to establish, because significant gas distension within the large colon may preclude thorough rectal examination. However, the severe, unrelenting abdominal pain, tachycardia, and abnormal rectal findings allow recognition of need for surgical intervention, and a definitive diagnosis may be established at the time of exploratory surgery.

CBC/BIOCHEMISTRY/URINALYSIS

• CBC and biochemistry may be normal or show evidence of hemoconcentration (i.e., elevated PCV and serum proteins) and prerenal or renal azotemia.
• With endotoxemia, a leukopenia characterized by neutropenia, with or without a left shift, may be evident.
• Nonstrangulating obstruction may cause mild metabolic alkalosis, whereas strangulating obstruction may cause severe metabolic acidosis.
• Other changes are nonspecific.
• In chronic, nonstrangulating obstruction or strangulating obstruction, hypovolemia and shock, if they ensue, may cause prerenal or renal azotemia, which can result in isosthenuria, glucosuria, proteinuria, and casts or RBCs at urinalysis.

OTHER LABORATORY TESTS

• Attempt abdominocentesis with caution, because distended large intestines increase the risk of enterocentesis.
• Peritoneal fluid may be normal or reveal elevated protein concentration and RBC count.

IMAGING

Nonspecific, but may be used for differentiation from other causes of nonstrangulating obstructions—enterolithiasis (i.e., abdominal radiography) and left dorsal colon displacement (i.e., abdominal ultrasonography).

DIAGNOSTIC PROCEDURES

• Nasogastric intubation and rectal examination
• Nasogastric reflux has been reported in as much as 35% of cases because of tension on the duodenocolic fold.
• Findings at rectal examination may be normal early during the course of the disease. With progression, increasing gaseous distension of the large colon is found, and tight colonic bands may be palpable.
• With careful palpation, sacculations of the ventral colon may be palpable dorsally, indicating colon torsion.
• Colonic edema may be palpable as thickening of the colonic wall.
• In some cases, gas distension is so severe that it fills the abdomen, preventing a complete rectal examination.

PATHOLOGIC FINDINGS

• The torsion, its origin, and its direction are determined at postmortem examination.
• Varying degrees of large colon and cecal necrosis or rupture may be present, depending on the level, degree, and duration of the torsion.

LARGE COLON TORSION

TREATMENT

APPROPRIATE HEALTH CARE

- Successful treatment of colonic torsion is reported only after surgery.
- Initial evaluation—physical examination, nasogastric intubation, and rectal examination.
- Nonstrangulating torsion often results in progression to strangulation and worsening clinical signs with time, requiring emergency surgical intervention.
- Strangulating torsion is a rapidly progressive condition and represents a surgical emergency; early recognition and prompt surgery are paramount for patient survival.

NURSING CARE

Refer affected horses to a surgical facility immediately after initial diagnosis.

ACTIVITY

- Limit activity to stall rest with handwalking.
- Stall rest with handwalking is recommended for the first 4 weeks after surgery.
- Full return to exercise or breeding is not recommended for at least 6 months.

DIET

- Discontinue oral intake until the postoperative period.
- Gradually reintroduce feed postoperatively.

CLIENT EDUCATION

- Inform clients that prompt diagnosis and surgical intervention maximize the outcome for survival.
- Varying degrees of endotoxemia, hypovolemia, and abdominal distension pose added risks for general anesthesia.
- Many potential postoperative complications may worsen the prognosis—laminitis and colitis
- Inform clients of the 5–8% recurrence rate.
- Advise owners of pregnant mares regarding the risk of fetal compromise.

SURGICAL CONSIDERATIONS

Surgical correction is performed via exploratory laparotomy.

MEDICATIONS

DRUGS OF CHOICE

- Administer a single dose of flunixin meglumine or similar NSAID.
- Further analgesics may be administered based on severity of the clinical signs.

CONTRAINDICATIONS

As described for other causes of colic.

PRECAUTIONS

- Worsening of symptoms may be masked by repeated administration of analgesics.
- Avoid repeated dosing of drugs because of the potential for toxicity.

POSSIBLE INTERACTIONS

N/A

ALTERNATIVE DRUGS

N/A

FOLLOW-UP

PATIENT MONITORING

- Perform routine postoperative monitoring for alterations in attitude or appetite, recurrence of colic, and laminitis.
- Initially (1–2 weeks after surgery) monitor rectal temperature daily; fever may be an early indication of impending colitis, pleuropneumonia, thrombophlebitis, incisional infection, or peritonitis.

PREVENTION/AVOIDANCE

- Employ careful feeding practices that avoid large quantities of lush pasture and large amounts of grain wherever possible.
- Make all dietary changes gradually over a period of several days.

LARGE COLON TORSION

POSSIBLE COMPLICATIONS

• Because of the rapid progression of colonic torsion, bowel necrosis and rupture may occur before surgical intervention, resulting in death. Similarly, severe endotoxic and hypovolemic shock may ensue before treatment, resulting in cardiovascular collapse and death.
• Postoperative complications—recurrence of colic, laminitis, thrombophlebitis, pleuropneumonia, incisional infections or herniation, colitis, and peritonitis

EXPECTED COURSE AND PROGNOSIS

• Prognosis for survival after conservative, medical management is poor.
• Historically, the prognosis has been poor despite surgical intervention, with a short-term survival rate of 21–42%. A 1996 study, however, reported that early diagnosis, rapid referral, and prompt surgery improves short-term survival rate to 83%.
• No data have been reported regarding long-term survival rates for horses undergoing surgical treatment.

MISCELLANEOUS

ASSOCIATED CONDITIONS

Endotoxemia

AGE-RELATED FACTORS

N/A

ZOONOTIC POTENTIAL

N/A

PREGNANCY

• Broodmares appear to be predisposed, especially during the postparturient period.
• In affected pregnant mares, severe systemic deterioration and the added stress of general anesthesia and surgery pose a significant risk to the fetus.

SYNONYMS

Large colon volvulus

SEE ALSO

• Acute abdomen
• Dorsal colon displacements
• Endotoxemia

ABBREVIATIONS

• GI = gastrointestinal
• PCV = packed cell volume

Suggested Reading

Embertson RM, Cook G, Hance SR, et al. Large colon volvulus: surgical treatment of 204 cases (1986–1995). Proc AAEP 1996;42:254–255.

Fischer AT, Meagher DM. Strangulating torsions of the equine large colon. Compend Contin Educ 1986;8:S25–S30.

Harrison IW. Equine large intestinal volvulus: a review of 124 cases. Vet Surg 1988;17:77–81.

Hughes FE, Slone DE. Large colon resection. Vet Clin North Am Equine Pract 1997;13:341–349.

Johnston JK, Freeman DE. Diseases and surgery of the large colon. Vet Clin North Am Equine Pract 1997;13:317–339.

Author Mollie C.M. Ferris
Consulting Editor Henry R. Stämpfli

LARGE OVARY SYNDROME

BASICS

DEFINITION

The term includes a number of conditions, both normal and abnormal, that result in one or both ovaries achieving a size that is significantly larger than normal as detected by transrectal palpation and/or ultrasonography.

PATHOPHYSIOLOGY

- Equids are long-day breeders—estrous cycles and ovulatory period normally occur during spring and summer months.
- Light is the predominant influence on ovarian activity and estrous cycles.
- Outside the optimal season for breeding activity, the gonads are waxing or waning relative to follicular activity and occurrence of ovulation.
- Persistent follicles in vernal (spring) transition—those present late in transition either regress after persisting for a month or more or eventually ovulate (of their own accord if time is not an issue, or ovulation may be stimulated by the administration of hCG).
- Autumnal (fall) transition follicles—early in transition, some can be stimulated to ovulate, especially those identified during the first half of autumnal transition and of $\geq$35 mm; all eventually regress (i.e., decrease in size) as daylight wanes and endogenous GnRH, LH, and FSH decrease and the mare slips into winter anestrus (i.e., bilateral, small, inactive ovaries).

SYSTEM AFFECTED

Reproductive

GENETICS

N/A

INCIDENCE/PREVALENCE

Persistent Follicles

- Potentially $\geq$80% of reproductively normal mares.
- $\cong$20% of northern hemisphere mares continue to experience estrous cycle activity year-round, albeit with some variation in length from the "standard" of 21 days.

Hematoma

Uncommon, but a few cases are recognized each year within a normal population of mares during the breeding season.

Tumors

- GCT/GTCT is the most common ovarian tumor, but its occurrence is rare.
- All other tumors occur even less often.

SIGNALMENT

- Females of breeding age—postpubertal and preovarian senescence.
- All breeds.

SIGNS

- Seasonal component—typically during one of the two transition periods.
- Usually tease in/positive response to a stallion for extended periods of time ($\geq$1 month).
- Estrous behavior persists longer than during a normal estrous cycle (>12–14 days in the spring)
- Transrectal palpation and ultrasonography reveal the presence of follicles that may be multiple and of varying size; however, their appearance remains that of follicles—they do not take on the irregular appearance of the multilocular spaces, characteristic of a granulosa cell tumor.
- May increase in size/diameter with time, but the increase is slower than that observed with dominant follicles (5–6 mm/day) during the ovulatory period.

CAUSES

Normal Ovary, Persistent Follicles

- Most common cause.
- May be single or multiple, present on one or both ovaries, the presence/characteristics of which primarily result from the season (late spring/early fall) and the increasing or decreasing duration of light.
- Such follicles do not indicate ovarian disease—normal structures that will resolve if left alone.

Normal Ovary, Hematoma

- Second most common cause.
- Enlargement resolves without assistance over time, unless treated with prostaglandin to stimulate earlier initiation of estrous cyclic activity.
- Only considered pathologic if the hematoma causes destruction of ovarian tissue sufficient to preclude future normal activity.

Tumors and Other Causes

Based on hormone treatments (hCG or $PGF_2\alpha$) failing to elicit a desirable response, transrectal palpation, radiography, ultrasonography, systemic illness of the mare, and type of cell identified at histopathologic examination.

RISK FACTORS

N/A

DIAGNOSIS

DIFFERENTIAL DIAGNOSIS

Ovaries During Pregnancy (>37–40 Days of Gestation)

- With formation of endometrial cups and eCG production, secondary follicles luteinize to become secondary CL. The ovaries of the pregnant mare become bilaterally enlarged.
- Mare's behavior may mimic the aggression of some mares with GCT/GTCT. This most likely relates to increased circulating testosterone stemming from fetal gonads, which may be >100 pg/mL by 60–90 days of gestation, peaks at $\cong$200 days, and declines to basal levels by foaling.

Ovarian Hematoma

- Follows estrus and ovulation.
- The CH increases to a size substantially larger than the follicle preceding it.
- At diagnosis, the mare's behavior is that of a diestrous mare—normal (i.e., teases out/rejects the stallion)
- The initial rise of progesterone may be delayed slightly compared with a normal CH, but blood progesterone will rise (>1 ng/mL) by 5–6 days after ovulation, indicating that ovulation has occurred.
- Contralateral ovary is normal; ultrasonographic appearance is similar to a CH, albeit a large one.
- The rapid size increase of the hematoma stretches the tunic surrounding the ovary. The mare may exhibit pain/colic in the short term.
- Resolution—time or prostaglandin.

GCT/GTCT

- Transrectal palpation—characterized by a unilateral gonad enlargement (rate of tumor growth varies significantly by case); surface of tumor remains smooth but may have gentle lobulations; ovulation fossa disappears (i.e., fills in) early in development of tumor.
- Over time, contralateral ovary shows evidence of suppression. Initially, the number/size of follicles decreases, then the total volume/size of parenchyma decreases.
- Chronic GCT/GTCTs are coupled with a contralateral ovary that may become so small it is difficult for the novice to detect. Rarely, the contralateral ovary will continue to experience follicular activity and ovulations.
- Mares exhibit one of three primary behaviors—chronic anestrus (80%), stallion-like (increased aggression, 15%), or persistent estrus (nymphomanic, 5%).
- Because of the slower rate of increase stretching the ovarian tunic, the mare rarely exhibits acute (Colicky) pain because of that (contrast with rapid formation of a hematoma). The mare may, however, exhibit discomfort at the trot or refuse to go over jumps—weight of the enlarging ovary coupled with impact bounces the ovary, which is felt as a sharp, painful stretching of the mesovarium.

Teratoma/Dysgerminoma

- Rare; not hormonally active.
- Transrectal palpation—contralateral ovary is normal; teratoma surface may exhibit some sharper protuberances, reflecting its potential for eclectic contents.
- No impact on behavior or estrous cycle activity.
- Teratoma is benign; dysgerminoma can be highly malignant.

Cystadenoma

- Unilateral; no effect on contralateral ovary.
- No effect on behavior.
- Large, cystic structures that may be confused early on with persistent follicles.
- Remains nonresponsive to hCG.
- Rare hormonal impact—elevated testosterone.

Ovarian Abscess

- Rare
- Early reports may have been associated with attempts to reduce the size and number of persistent follicles via a flank-approach aspiration.
- Contralateral ovary is normal.
- No effect on behavior or estrous cycle activity

CBC/BIOCHEMISTRY/URINALYSIS

N/A

OTHER LABORATORY TESTS

GCT/GTCT

- Elevation of circulating inhibin levels (>0.7 ng/mL) in 90%.
- Elevation of testosterone (>50–100 pg/mL) in 50%–60%.
- Progesterone levels usually are <1 ng/mL.

Ovarian Hematoma

Blood progesterone will increase by 5–7 days of formation of the enlarged ovary.

Dysgerminoma

- Two reports of hypertrophic pulmonary osteoarthropathy developing secondary to metastatic dysgerminoma.
- Initial presentation was for intermittent, chronic colic; weight loss; and stiff extremities.
- Radiography and biopsies for metastasis.

IMAGING

Ultrasonography:

- Persistent follicle—appearance, but for size, is similar to that of a normal follicle.
- Hematoma—early, fluid-filled space (black); 2–10 days, hyperechoic areas began to show as blood clotting and clot contraction occur; eventually, takes on the uniform hyperechoic appearance of a large CH.
- GCT/GTCT—multicystic, the spaces of which can appear quite irregular; at detection, most are <30 cm in diameter.
- Teratoma—echogenicity can be quite variable, reflecting the nature of its contents (i.e. soft tissue, fluid, hair, bone, teeth).

DIAGNOSTIC PROCEDURES

Serial palpation and ultrasonography; blood hormone evaluations:

Hormone	Normal Range GCT/GTCT
Progesterone, estrus	<1 ng/mL
Progesterone, diestrus	>1 ng/mL
Progesterone, GCT/GTCT	<1 ng/mL
Testosterone	>50–100 pg/mL
Inhibin 0.1–0.7 ng/mL	>0.7 ng/mL

PATHOLOGIC FINDINGS

- Persistent Follicles—N/A
- Hematoma—N/A
- Neoplasms—can potentially arise from any tissue type in the ovary; classification based on their origin in surface epithelium, sex cord–stromal tissue, germ cell, or mesenchymal tissue
- GCT/GTCT—sex cord–stromal tumor; endocrine effects; specific in mare: inhibin production by thecal cells (i.e., GTCT).
- Teratoma—many tissue types, as well as germ cells, within the mass; including hair, skin, respiratory epithelium, tooth, and bone; high metastatic potential in mice and humans, but not a routine concern in mares; immature teratomas consist of tissue resembling embryonic origins; mature teratomas also are known as dermoid cysts.
- Cystadenoma—from epithelium; forms cystic neoplastic masses.
- Dysgerminoma—from germ cells; analogous to seminoma of the testis; cells are arranged in sheets and cords, with a dense population of large, pleomorphic cells; all are malignant.

LARGE OVARY SYNDROME

TREATMENT

APPROPRIATE HEALTH CARE
N/A

NURSING CARE
N/A

ACTIVITY
N/A

DIET
N/A

CLIENT EDUCATION
- Serial examinations are important for establishing an accurate diagnosis and avoiding unnecessary ovariectomy.
- Most cases result from persistent follicles and hematoma.
- GCT/GTCT is the most common tumor causing ovarian enlargement, but it is still uncommon.

SURGICAL CONSIDERATIONS
- Ovariectomy.
- See rule-outs in *Expected Course and Prognosis.*

MEDICATIONS

DRUGS OF CHOICE

Hematoma
- No treatment, wait for ovary to regress in size and other follicular activity to develop
- Alternatively, administer $PGF_2\alpha$ (10 mg IM; Lutalyse, Upjohn, Kalamazoo, MI) when hematoma has developed >7–10 days after ovulation.
- May be unresponsive to treatment within first 2+ weeks.
- Successful treatment is noted by the mare returning to estrus within 2–5 days after treatment.

Persistent Follicles
- Time (no treatment); wait for estrous activity to begin (vernal transition) or cease (autumnal transition).
- Alternatively, to shorten the extended duration of teasing in vernal transition, administer Regumate, but do not institute treatment before significant follicular activity is present (multiple 15–20 mm follicles present on Mare's Ovaries). This is behavioral, not physiologic, estrus (see estrus, abnormal intervals).
- hCG (2500–3000 IU IV) to induce ovulation *late* in vernal transition (see estrus, abnormal intervals).

CONTRAINDICATIONS
N/A

PRECAUTIONS
- Some behavioral changes can be dramatic. Use caution around mares showing aggressive behavior; such mares may need an individual paddock, distant from other mares in estrus, and separation from foals and stallions.
- Large ovarian tumors can develop extensive blood supplies. Intraoperative time can be significantly lengthened because of the time required to properly ligate vessels supplying the tumor, resulting in greater risk from surgery.

POSSIBLE INTERACTIONS
N/A

ALTERNATIVE DRUGS
N/A

FOLLOW-UP

PATIENT MONITORING
Routine postoperative care for ovariectomy.

PREVENTION/AVOIDANCE
N/A

POSSIBLE COMPLICATIONS

Surgery
Any operative procedure/anesthesia holds a potential risk for death.

GCT/GTCT
- Time from ovariectomy to resumption of estrous cycle activity is influenced by the months/years of suppression.
- Usually <1–3 years, rare cases of suppression being permanent.
- Rare case of remaining ovary also developing into a GCT/GTCT.
- A few mares with this tumor continue to develop follicles and ovulate on the contralateral ovary.

EXPECTED COURSE AND PROGNOSIS

Poor Prognosis
Dysgerminoma—potential for metastasis; usually advanced by the time diagnosis is made.

Good Prognosis for Future Reproduction
- Hematoma—large size returns nearly to normal over 1–6 months; rarely, will destroy remaining ovarian tissue.
- Persistent follicles—100% resolve with time and season.

Good Prognosis for Life
- GCT/GTCT
- Abscess
- Cystadenoma
- Teratoma

Recommendation for Ovariectomy
- GCT/GTCT—for reproductive function of affected (smaller) gonad to return, prognosis is fair to good depending on size of tumor, surgical route, and duration of suppression of contralateral ovary.
- Cystadenoma—rare; reported testosterone production.
- Abscess; teratoma—dysfunctional ovary.

LARGE OVARY SYNDROME

MISCELLANEOUS

ASSOCIATED CONDITIONS

- Dysgerminoma—hypertrophic pulmonary osteoarthropathy developing secondary to metastatic dysgerminoma; initial presentation was for intermittent chronic colic, weight loss, and stiff extremities.
- Behavior modification with GCT/GTCT.

AGE-RELATED FACTORS

- Hematoma; persistent follicles—of breeding age (i.e., capable of estrous activity).
- Tumors—no age limitation.

ZOONOTIC POTENTIAL

N/A

PREGNANCY

N/A

SYNONYMS

N/A

SEE ALSO

- Abnormal estrus intervals
- Anestrus
- Ovulation failure
- Pregnancy
- Prolonged diestrus

ABBREVIATIONS

- CH = corpus hemorrhagicum
- CL = corpus luteum
- eCG = equine chorionic gonadotropin
- FSH = follicle stimulating hormone
- GCT = granulosa cell tumor
- GnRH = gonadotropin releasing hormone
- GTCT = granulosa theca cell tumor
- hCG = human chorionic gonadotropin
- LH = luteinizing hormone

Suggested Reading

Carleton CL. Atypical, asymmetrical, but abnormal? Large ovary syndrome. In: Proceedings of Mare Reproduction Symposium, American College of Theriogenologists/Society for Theriogenology 1996:27–39.

Foley GL. Proceedings of Reproductive Pathology Symposium, American College of Theriogenologists/Society for Theriogenology 1997:60–65.

McCue PM. Review of ovarian abnormalities in the mare. Proc Am Assoc Equine Pract 1998:125–133.

Schlafer DH. Non-neoplastic lesions of the ovaries of the mare. In: Proceedings of Reproductive Pathology Symposium, American College of Theriogenologists/Society for Theriogenology 1997:69–72.

Stangroom JE, Weevers RG. Anticoagulant activity of equine follicular fluid. J Reprod Fertil 1962;3:269–282.

Author Carla L. Carleton

Consulting Editor Carla L. Carleton

LARGE STRONGYLE INFESTATION

BASICS

OVERVIEW

• In the past, infections with the large strongyles (i.e., *Strongylus vulgaris, S. edentatus,* and *S. equinus*) were considered to be the most common and important equine intestinal parasites.
• Their perceived importance has decreased, however, and that of the small strongyles (i.e., cyathastomes) has increased, from widespread application of preventative and control programs and from reported experimental and clinical findings.
• The worms can cause significant damage and, in combination with cyathastomes, probably are responsible for many cases of equine colic.
• Eggs are passed in the feces of infected horses.
• The rate of strongyle development depends on climatic conditions and is favored by warm, moist conditions.
• Development of the infective L3 larvae occurs after larval growth and a molt. The L3 are ensheathed and, under moist conditions, migrate up to the tips of grass blades, increasing the likelihood of ingestion by a grazing horse.
• Dry, hot conditions lead to rapid desiccation of larvae.
• The larvae exsheath in the intestine and penetrate the walls of the small intestine, cecum, and colons.
• In $\cong$8–11 days, L4 larvae are produced, inducing a marked inflammatory response in the bowel wall. The larvae then begin to migrate, the pattern of which varies with each species.
• *S. vulgaris* larvae penetrate the intima of the arterioles and migrate within the vessel wall to the cranial mesenteric artery, arriving there $\cong$14 days after infection. Severe arteritis, with fibrosis and thrombus formation, is noted. Rarely, an aneurysm occurs. At $\cong$45 days postinfection, larvae migrate back to the subserosa of the large intestine, where they encyst for $\cong$45 more days and develop into L5 larvae. These larvae enter the lumen of the gut and mature, with egg production starting $\cong$6–7 months postinfection.
• *S. edentatus* larvae penetrate the cecal mucosa, enter the hepatic portal system, and then enter the liver. Here, they molt to L4 larvae, which by the tenth-week postinfection may have migrated to various sites, such as the body wall, where they cause nodules, and L5 larvae develop. They then migrate back to the cecum and colon and mature. Egg production starts $\cong$11 months postinfection, although it can be as short as 6 months.
• *S. equinus* larvae follow a similar path to those of *S. edentatus,* but the migration of L4 larvae is more likely to involve the pancreas and peritoneal cavity. The prepatent period of this latter parasite is $\cong$9 months.
• Clinical signs caused by larval migration are thought to result from direct damage to the tissues through which the larvae migrate, release of various inflammatory mediators, and potential impacts on blood flow to the bowel. This latter aspect is thought to be particularly important with *S. vulgaris* infection, in which reduced blood flow is speculated to arise due to vasoconstriction and thromboembolism, which then leads to ischemia, altered motility and colic. This hypothesis, however, has not been totally supported by experimental findings.
• Adult worms attach to the mucosa and feed on mucosal cells, blood, and tissue fluids.

SIGNALMENT

• All ages, breeds, and genders
• Young animals, particularly those with little previous exposure to enteric parasites, are more susceptible than old horses.

SIGNS

• Infections often are mixed, with both large and small strongyles, so clinical signs cannot be attributed to a specific infestation with one species.
• In experimental infections with infective larvae of one species, specific clinical signs have been observed.
• With *S. vulgaris,* an acute syndrome has been described, characterized by colic, fever, and diarrhea, that may coincide with the initial invasion of the intestinal mucosa by the infective larvae.
• With *S. equinus,* experimental heavy infections caused colic, anorexia, and depression, and a similar infection with *S. edentatus* larvae caused peritonitis, jaundice, and fever. These latter three syndromes often are not recognized in the clinical setting. More typically there are signs of colic, which can be severe and acute or, more commonly, recurrent and moderate. In addition, signs of ill thrift and, sometimes, occasional diarrhea may be noted. These nonspecific signs may be the result of the mixed infection.
• Rarely, aberrant larval migration and clinical signs may ensue—into the central nervous system, renal artery, or iliac artery

CAUSES AND RISK FACTORS

• Grazing pasture with infective larvae is the primary risk factor.
• Lack of a co-ordinated parasite monitoring and control program on a particular farm is likely to sustain pastures as high risk.

LARGE STRONGYLE INFESTATION

DIAGNOSIS

DIFFERENTIAL DIAGNOSIS

- Many conditions can cause signs of colic—impactions, ileus, bowel displacements and strangulations, incarcerated hernias, enteroliths, severe enteritis, and peritonitis
- Strongyle infestations may play a significant role in development of some of these conditions, but not others.
- Detailed evaluation of the GI system helps to determine the most likely cause of the problem.
- Vague signs of ill thrift and weight loss also can have a wide range of causes and be differentiated based on physical and laboratory findings.

CBC/BIOCHEMISTRY/URINALYSIS

Possible neutrophilia during the early stages and an eosinophilia later

OTHER LABORATORY TESTS

- Serum β- and α-globulins may be elevated later during the disease, but not consistently.
- Fecal analysis may reveal eggs in patent infections. This may have little diagnostic value, however, because most damage occurs during the prepatent period.

IMAGING

N/A

DIAGNOSTIC PROCEDURES

N/A

TREATMENT

- Pasture management may help to reduce exposure to infective larvae.
- Regular manure removal (e.g., every 2 days) significantly reduces the numbers of infective larvae on the pasture.
- Mixed grazing, using cattle or sheep, also may help to reduce the pasture load.

MEDICATIONS

DRUGS

- A cornerstone of treating strongyle infections is an appropriate anthelmintic regimen both with respect to drug selection and frequency of use.
- The efficacy of drugs against larvae dictates their frequency of use—pyrantel (6.6 mg/kg) every 4 weeks, ivermectin (0.2 mg/kg) every 8 weeks, or moxidectan (0.4 mg/kg) every 12 weeks.
- Timing also may be influenced by local climatic conditions and be focused on the times of highest risk (see *Overview*).

FOLLOW-UP

- Develop a parasite monitoring and management plan for all horses on a farm; this should include regular fecal analysis for eggs as well as a co-ordinated use of appropriate anthelmintics.
- Prognosis for individual horses with large strongyles infections varies, depending on the extent and severity of the damage caused by migrating larvae. Those with massive bowel infarcts and ischemia may die, but most do not and, with appropriate immediate care and follow-up, they recover.

MISCELLANEOUS

ASSOCIATED CONDITIONS

Usually a mixed infection with cyathastomes

AGE-RELATED FACTORS

N/A

ZOONOTIC POTENTIAL

N/A

PREGNANCY

N/A

SEE ALSO

N/A

ABBREVIATIONS

GI = gastrointestinal

Suggested Reading

Uhlinger CA. Equine strongyle disease. In: Smith BP, ed. Large animal internal medicine. 2nd ed. Philadelphia: Mosby, 1996:1689–1693.

Author Christopher M. Brown
Consulting Editor Henry Staempfli

LARYNGEAL HEMIPARESIS/HEMIPLEGIA

BASICS

DEFINITION

• Failure of an anatomically normal left (rarely right) arytenoid cartilage to abduct fully during forced inspiration, which results in inspiratory respiratory obstruction.
• The cause generally is unknown; therefore, the disease is referred to as idiopathic laryngeal hemiparesis/hemiplegia.
• The condition is graded from I–IV, with IV being the most severe.

PATHOPHYSIOLOGY

• Trauma to the left recurrent laryngeal nerve can produce the condition, but in most cases, the underlying pathologic basis is peripheral neuropathy characterized by distal loss of large myelinated fibers (i.e., distal axonopathy). This neuropathy affects long nerves of large-statured horses.
• Because the left recurrent laryngeal nerve is the longest equine nerve, it is the most severely affected, resulting in clinical signs of left-sided laryngeal hemiparesis/hemiplegia. Interestingly, the right recurrent laryngeal nerve and long nerves in the limbs also are affected histologically. Lesions in these latter nerves are far less severe, however, and clinical signs rarely, if ever, are associated with these abnormalities.
• The peripheral neuropathy is progressive and accompanied by attempts at axonal regeneration such that both axonal degeneration and regeneration are observed histologically.
• Distal axonopathy of the left recurrent laryngeal nerve leads to neurogenic atrophy of the intrinsic laryngeal muscles supplied by this nerve.
• The loss of abductory function associated with neurogenic atrophy of the CAD muscle causes the clinical signs. Impaired CAD function leads to inability of the left arytenoid cartilage to abduct and to resist pressure swings in the upper airway during exercise. As a result, negative pressure during inspiration leads to adduction of the left arytenoid cartilage, and positive pressure during expiration leads to abduction of the left arytenoid cartilage. The paradoxic adduction during inspiration obstructs the airway, leading to inspiratory stridor and diminished airflow during inspiration, which in turn results in decreased ventilation and, therefore, hypoxemia, hypercarbia, and consequent impaired athletic performance.
• Horses respond to inspiratory obstruction by modifying their breathing strategies during exercise to restore minute volume. Strategies include more negative inspiratory (i.e., driving) pressure, increased inspiratory time, and increased tidal volume.

SYSTEM AFFECTED

Respiratory—upper respiratory tract

GENETICS

Evidence beyond the tendency to have tall offspring suggests this is an inheritable defect.

INCIDENCE/PREVALENCE

Worldwide

SIGNALMENT

• Males are more commonly affected.
• Horses of large height, particularly Thoroughbreds, Warmbloods, and draft horses, are predisposed.
• Approximately 5% of Thoroughbreds and draft breeds are affected (range, 1.8–9.5%); the condition is far less common in Standardbreds and almost nonexistent in ponies.
• In Thoroughbreds, the incidence is reported to increase from 6.5% in 2-year-old horses to 9.5% in 6-year-olds.

SIGNS

• Horses are presented for upper respiratory noise, exercise intolerance, or both.
• Laryngeal hemiplegia significantly interferes with ventilation in horses that perform at high speed. The longer the high-intensity exercise, the more severe the hypoventilation; therefore, the horse does not finish or close well.
• In show horses, loss of points during competition because of upper respiratory noise is the main owner concern. Upper airway noise at low airflow or speeds is best described as a soft whistle that increases in intensity as airway pressures become more negative during high-intensity exercise.

CAUSES

• Most commonly idiopathic on the left
• Genetic predisposition.
• Any abnormality affecting the left or right recurrent laryngeal nerve can result in laryngeal hemiparesis/hemiplegia—perivenous jugular vein injection, jugular thrombophlebitis, common carotid artery puncture, cervical trauma, esophageal rupture and subsequent cellulitis, and any surgical procedure in the vicinity of the recurrent laryngeal nerve.
• Viral neuritis
• Neurologic diseases (e.g., equine lower motor neuron disease) that may affect neurons of the nucleus ambiguous
• Intoxications (e.g., organophosphate, lead) may cause bilateral paresis of the laryngeal nerves.

RISK FACTORS

• Perivenous injection—look for damage to vagosympathetic trunk (e.g., Horner's syndrome).
• Cervical trauma
• Surgical procedures near the left recurrent nerve

DIAGNOSIS

DIFFERENTIAL DIAGNOSIS

• Unlike horses with arytenoid chondritis, horses with laryngeal hemiparesis/hemiplegia have a normally shaped arytenoid cartilage.
• Right-sided hemiplegia is rare, so careful examination of the arytenoid cartilage shape is necessary to identify horses with arytenoid chondritis. In addition, be suspicious for congenital malformation of the muscular process of the arytenoid cartilage or of the thyroid lamina in right-sided paresis/paralysis.
• Other causes of upper respiratory obstruction
• Other causes of diminished athletic performance

CBC/BIOCHEMISTRY/URINALYSIS

Of no value

OTHER LABORATORY TESTS

Arterial blood gases during exercise, with which hypoventilation can be evaluated—in affected horses at maximal exercise, $PaCO_2$ can be >55 torr and PaO_2 can be <65 torr.

IMAGING

Radiography

Lateral radiographs of the larynx in old (>8 years) horses may reveal ossification of the laryngeal cartilage, which may interfere with placement of laryngeal prosthesis sutures or degree of abduction obtained with surgery.

Videoendoscopy at Rest

• Diagnosis of complete laryngeal hemiplegia (i.e., grade IV) is confirmed by videoendoscopy at rest. Marked laryngeal asymmetry is observed with the left arytenoid cartilage in the midline or paramidline position. No substantial movement of the left arytenoid cartilage is observed during any phase of respiration.
• Diagnosis of laryngeal hemiparesis (i.e., grade III) also is obtained by videoendoscopy at rest. These horses have asynchronous movement (e.g., hesitation, flutter, adductor weakness, etc.) of the left arytenoid cartilage during inspiration or expiration, and they cannot achieve and maintain full abduction of the left arytenoid cartilage by swallowing or nasal occlusion.
• Horses with laryngeal grade I and II are normal.
• Grade II—asynchronous movement (e.g., hesitation, flutter, adductor weakness, etc.) of the left arytenoid cartilage during inspiration or expiration; full abduction of the left arytenoid cartilage (compared with the right) inducible by swallowing or nasal occlusion.
• Grade I—synchronous, full abduction and adduction of the left and right arytenoid cartilages.

• Videoendoscopy during high-speed treadmill exercise, if available, is indicated in horses with resting laryngeal grade III to determine if full abduction of the left hemilarynx is maintained during exercise. Note that 20—25% of these horses can still have normal arytenoid abduction during exercise.

OTHER DIAGNOSTIC PROCEDURES

• Respiratory mechanics—during exercise, affected horses have more negative inspiratory tracheal pressures than normal horses as well as loss of the linear relationship between tracheal and pharyngeal pressures during inspiration and increased translaryngeal pressures during inspiration.
• On external palpation, the left CAD muscle may be atrophied compared to the right.
• "Slap" test—normally, reflex adduction of the contralateral arytenoid cartilage occurs when the withers are slapped with the hand; loss of this reflex suggests recurrent laryngeal nerve dysfunction.

PATHOLOGICAL FINDINGS

Gross Findings

• Atrophy of all intrinsic laryngeal muscles innervated by the left recurrent laryngeal nerve—lateral cricoarytenoideus, dorsal cricoarytenoideus, vocalis, and ventricularis muscles
• Atrophy of the left lateral cricoarytenoideus dorsalis usually is most severe.
• Atrophy of the dorsal cricoarytenoid dorsalis muscle is most obvious clinically and can be estimated by manual palpation of the dorsal aspect of the cricoid and muscular process of the arytenoid cartilage.

Histopathologic Findings

• Distal loss of large, myelinated fibers in the left recurrent laryngeal nerve
• Left intrinsic laryngeal muscles exhibit angular fiber atrophy and fiber-type grouping.

TREATMENT

APPROPRIATE HEALTH CARE

N/A

NURSING CARE

N/A

ACTIVITY

N/A

DIET

N/A

CLIENT EDUCATION

Inform clients regarding the possible genetic basis for this disease and that breeding to affected horses may not be indicated.

SURGICAL CONSIDERATIONS

• Treatment is not necessary if exercise intolerance is not present and owners are willing to tolerate the upper respiratory noise.
• Placement of laryngeal prosthesis that fixes the left arytenoid cartilage in near-maximal abduction coupled with cordectomy or ventriculocordectomy is the treatment of choice in horses used for strenuous athletic activities. Chronic coughing during eating is seen in as many as 20% of horses after this surgery.
• Cordectomy or ventriculocordectomy can successfully decrease respiratory noise and restore exercise tolerance in selected horses with laryngeal grade III, in which arytenoid abduction is adequate yet vocal cord collapse is present.
• Laryngeal reinnervation of the CAD muscle in yearlings

MEDICATIONS

DRUGS OF CHOICE

None, other than routine, perioperative antimicrobial and anti-inflammatory agents.

CONTRAINDICATIONS

N/A

PRECAUTIONS

N/A

POSSIBLE INTERACTIONS

N/A

ALTERNATIVE DRUGS

N/A

FOLLOW-UP

PATIENT MONITORING

• Upper airway endoscopy is required 6 weeks after surgery to monitor response to surgery.
• Determining final response to treatment or monitoring of affected horses is made on the basis of evaluating exercise tolerance and upper respiratory noise.

PREVENTION/AVOIDANCE

N/A

POSSIBLE COMPLICATIONS

Horses undergoing laryngeal prosthesis may experience chronic coughing and, rarely, aspiration pneumonia.

EXPECTED COURSE AND PROGNOSIS

• Laryngeal hemiplegia—horses with grade IV will not exhibit any further deterioration of athletic activity or upper respiratory noise.
• Laryngeal hemiparesis—horses with grade III may exhibit further deterioration of athletic activity or upper respiratory noise.

MISCELLANEOUS

ASSOCIATED CONDITIONS

Untreated horses may be predisposed to EIPH if submitted to strenuous exercise.

AGE-RELATED FACTORS

N/A

ZOONOTIC POTENTIAL

N/A

PREGNANCY

N/A

SYNONYMS

N/A

SEE ALSO

• Dynamic collapse of the upper airway
• EIPH

ABBREVIATIONS

• CAD = dorsal cricoarytenoid muscle
• EIPH = exercise-induced pulmonary hemorrhage

Suggested Reading

Duncan ID, Griffith IR. A light and electron microscopic study of the neuropathy of equine idiopathic laryngeal hemiplegia. Acta Neuropath 1978;4:483–501.

Greet TR, Jeffcott LB, Whitwell KE, Cook WR. The slap test for laryngeal adductory function in horses with suspected cervical spinal cord damage. Equine Vet J 1980;12:127–131.

Parente EJ, Martin BB, Tulleners EP, Ross MW. Upper respiratory dysfunctions in horses during high-speed exercise. Proc Am Assoc Equine Pract 1994;40:81–82.

Rakestraw PC, Hackett RP, Ducharme NG, Nielan GJ, Erb HN. Arytenoid cartilage movement in resting and exercising horses. Vet Surg 1991;20:122–127.

Shappel KK, Derksen FJ, Stick JA, Robinson NE. Effects of ventriculectomy, prosthetic laryngoplasty, and exercise on upper airway function in horses with induced left laryngeal hemiplegia. Am J Vet Res 1988;49:1760–1766.

Authors Norm G. Ducharme and Richard P. Hackett

Consulting Editor Jean-Pierre Lavoie

LENS OPACITIES/CATARACTS (MINI)

BASICS

OVERVIEW

Cataracts are opacities of the lens. Very small incipient lens opacities are common and not associated with blindness. As cataracts develop or mature, they become more opaque, and blindness develops. The basic mechanism of cataract formation is a decrease in soluble lens proteins, failure of the lens epithelial cell sodium pump, a decrease in lens glutathione, and lens fiber swelling and fiber membrane rupture.

SIGNALMENT

All ages and breeds of horses are at risk for cataract development. Cataracts are a frequent congenital ocular defect in foals.

SIGNS

- Horses manifest varying degrees of blindness as cataracts mature. The tapetal reflection is seen with incipient and immature cataracts, but is not seen in mature cataracts. In most instances, the rate of cataract progression and development of blindness cannot be predicted.
- Due to associated uveitis, blepharospasm and lacrimation may accompany cataracts in horses.
- Assessment of visual function can be made by distant observation of the horse walking, feeding, and interacting with other horses. Visually impaired horses may demonstrate a reluctance to run or even walk, although some horses with bilateral cataracts appear to do quite well in a familiar environment. Differences in head posture may be associated with cataracts, as a unilaterally blind horse may attempt to keep its sighted eye towards activity in its environment.

CAUSES AND RISK FACTORS

- Heritable, traumatic, nutritional, and postinflammatory etiologies have been proposed.
- Cataracts may be associated with microphthalmos.
- Cataracts secondary to equine recurrent uveitis (ERU) or trauma are frequently seen, whereas juvenile onset cataracts are uncommon in horses. True senile cataracts that interfere with vision are found in horses older than 20 years.
- Dominant inheritance has been reported for cataracts in Belgian and Thoroughbred horses. Morgan horses have nonprogressive, nuclear, bilaterally symmetrical cataracts that generally do not interfere with vision.

DIAGNOSIS

DIFFERENTIAL DIAGNOSIS

Increased cloudiness of the lens occurs with age and is called nuclear or lenticular sclerosis. It is common in older horses, but vision is clinically normal as nuclear sclerosis does not cause vision loss.
Blindness in horses is also due to ERU, glaucoma, or retinal disease.

CBC/BIOCHEMISTRY/URINALYSIS

N/A

OTHER LABORATORY TESTS

N/A

IMAGING

B-scan ultrasound is beneficial in assessing the anatomic status of the retina if a cataract is present.

DIAGNOSTIC PROCEDURES

Electroretinography is beneficial in assessing the functional status of the retina if a cataract is present.

PATHOLOGIC FINDINGS

Lens fiber swelling, epithelial cell metaplasia, liquefaction of lens material, and lens fiber swelling are noticed.

TREATMENT

Most veterinary ophthalmologists recommend surgical removal of cataracts in foals less than 6 months of age if the foal is healthy, no uveitis or other ocular problems are present, and the foal's personality tolerates aggressive topical therapy, but adults with visual impairment due to cataracts are also candidates for cataract surgery. Therapy for cataracts is necessarily surgical, although some degree of spontaneous cataract resorption may occur with hypermature cataracts. Horses considered for lens extraction should be in good physical condition.
Complete ophthalmic and general physical examinations should be performed.
Preoperative complete blood counts and serum chemistries are important for evaluating systemic organ function. A complete ophthalmic examination is necessary.
Slow or absent pupillary light reflexes (PLRs) may indicate active iridocyclitis with or without posterior synechiation, retinal disease, optic nerve disease, or iris sphincter muscle atrophy.
Afferent pupillary defects in a cataractous eye cannot be attributed to the cataract alone, as well as the fact that normal PLRs do not exclude some degree of retinal or optic nerve disease.
Any signs of anterior uveitis should delay cataract surgery until the cause of the inflammation is diagnosed and has been treated successfully. Cataract surgery should also be delayed in the presence of active eyelid, conjunctival, or corneal disease.
Examination of the fundus may be difficult due to the cataract. Preoperative electroretinography and b-scan ultrasonography are beneficial to evaluate outer retinal function and the integrity of intraocular structures, respectively.
Phacoemulsification cataract surgery is most useful for equine cataract surgery as it involves a small corneal incision of 3.2 mm. Immature, mature, and hypermature cataracts have been removed successfully in horses with this technique.
Intraocular lenses of 25 Diopters have been used in horses following cataract surgery.

MEDICATIONS

DRUG(S)

Topically applied antibiotics, such as chloramphenicol, gentamicin, ciprofloxacin, or tobramycin ophthalmic solutions, may be used pre- and postoperatively. Frequency of medication varies from q2h to q8h.
Topically applied 1 to 2% atropine is effective in stabilizing the blood–aqueous barrier, minimizing pain from ciliary muscle spasm, and causes pupillary dilatation. Atropine may be used as often as q4h, with the frequency of administration reduced as soon as the pupil dilates.
Topically applied corticosteroids, such as prednisolone acetate (1%), are beneficial to suppress pre- and postoperative inflammation.
Systemically administered NSAIDs, such as phenylbutazone (2 mg/kg BID PO) or flunixin meglumine (1 mg/kg BID, IV, IM, or PO), can be used orally or parenterally, and are effective in reducing anterior uveitis in horses with cataracts.
Topically administered NSAIDs, such as flurbiprofen and suprofen, can be used TID to QID to suppress signs of anterior uveitis.

LENS OPACITIES/CATARACTS (MINI)

CONTRAINDICATIONS/POSSIBLE INTERACTIONS

Infectious endophthalmitis is a devastating complication.
General anesthesia with its attendant risks is required for cataract surgery.

FOLLOW-UP

PATIENT MONITORING

Horses with cataracts should be monitored for blepharospasm and lacrimation, as cataracts can cause uveitis.
Blind horses should be monitored in their environment.
Horses who have had cataract surgery should be monitored for signs of eye pain, self-trauma, a reoccurrence of blindness, and colic.

PREVENTION/AVOIDANCE

Breeding of horses with cataracts is to be avoided.

POSSIBLE COMPLICATIONS

Postoperative complications include persistent iridocyclitis and plasmoid aqueous, fibropupillary membranes, synechiae, iris bombè, corneal ulceration, corneal edema, corneal fibrovascular infiltrates, posterior capsular opacification, retained lens cortex, wound leakage, vitreous presentation into anterior chamber, retinal degeneration, retinal detachment, and infectious endophthalmitis.

EXPECTED COURSE AND PROGNOSIS

Foals are easiest to operate on because the globe size is small enough that the standard cataract surgical equipment is of satisfactory size, general anesthesia is of less risk in foals, and foals heal very quickly following cataract surgery. Early return of vision is paramount in foals for development of the higher visual centers. Slight corneal edema is usually present from 24 to 72 hours postoperatively. One week following surgery, the pupil should be functional, any fibrin in the anterior chamber resorbing, and the fundus visible. Three weeks following surgery the eye should be nonpainful, the patient visual, pupillary movement normal, and the ocular media clear. Most reliable reports of vision in successful cataract surgery in horses indicate vision is functionally normal postoperatively. From an optical standpoint, the aphakic eye should be quite far-sighted or hyperopic postoperatively, and was +9.94D in one study. Images close to the eye would be blurry and appear magnified.

MISCELLANEOUS

ASSOCIATED CONDITIONS

Retinal detachment and ERU

AGE-RELATED FACTORS

N/A

ZOONOTIC POTENTIAL

N/A

PREGNANCY

N/A

SYNONYMS

N/A

SEE ALSO

N/A

ABBREVIATIONS

- D = Diopters
- ERU = equine recurrent uveitis
- NSAID = nonsteroidal anti-inflammatory drug
- PLR = pupillary light reflex

Suggested Reading

Brooks DE: Equine ophthalmology. In Gelatt KN, Veterinary ophthalmology. 3rd ed. Chapter 30. 1999. Philadelphia: Lippincott Williams & Wilkins, 1999.

Author Dennis E. Brooks, DVM, PhD
Consulting Editor Dennis E. Brooks, DVM, PhD

LEPTOSPIROSIS

BASICS

DEFINITION

Leptospirosis is a bacterial disease caused by pathogenic serovars of *Leptospira interrogans.* It affects wildlife and domestic animals and has a zoonotic potential. Serologic surveys show that equine exposure to leptospires is common but clinical disease is uncommon. Clinical leptospirosis is primarily associated with recurrent uveitis, abortions, stillbirths, and neonatal infections. Hepatic and renal disease is sporadic.

PATHOPHYSIOLOGY

Leptospires are spirochetes that are both host-adapted and non-host adapted. Infection by host-adapted serovars results in an increase in endemic disease or clinical disease in immunologically naïve animals. Infection by non-host-adapted serovars results in sporadic infections or disease outbreaks. If the serovar is host adapted, then infection is often for life; if the serovar is non-host-adapted, then infection and shedding are usually brief. *Leptospira bratislava* is the presumed host-adapted serovar of horses. Leptospires penetrate mucosal and skin surfaces and result in a bacteremia and an invasion of internal organs 4–10 days later. Outcome of infection depends on the horse's humoral response and the pathogenicity of the serovar. Organisms multiply in organs and release metabolites that, combined with immune-mediated damage, cause the clinical signs associated with the disease. Leptospires evade the immune system in the proximal renal tubules, genital tract, central nervous system, and eyes. Leptospira are shed into the environment in high concentrations in the urine, although all body secretions may contain leptospires during the bacteremic phase.

SYSTEMS AFFECTED

Ophthalmic

Recurrent uveitis

Reproductive

Abortion, stillbirth

Renal/Urologic

Renal disease and pyuria

Neonatal Disease

Hepatic and renal disease, weakness, pulmonary hemorrhage

Hepatobiliary

Liver disease and jaundice

GENETICS

N/A

INCIDENCE/PREVELENCE

Serologic surveys have identified worldwide exposure to leptospires. Predominant serovars vary with geographic area and leptospire antigens used in the surveys. *L. bratislava* seroprevalence of 40–70% has been reported in North America, Australia, and the United Kingdom. Serology has been used as the main method of diagnosing leptospirosis due to the difficulties with culturing leptospires and lack of adequate diagnostic tests. However, it is hoped that improved diagnostic tests and increased awareness of the disease will increase its reported occurrence.

SIGNALMENT

Nonspecific

SIGNS

General Comments

Signs associated with the bacteremia include pyrexia, depression, lethargy, and anorexia. Signs associated with organ invasion are indicative of the specific organ involved. Subclinical infections and carrier states are asymptomatic. Chronic disease is associated with recurrent uveitis and abortions.

Physical Examination Findings

• Ophthalmic—initially, blepharospasm, excessive tearing, photophobia, chemosis, miosis, aqueous flare, hypopyon, and corneal edema. Chronic sequelae include synechia formation, retinal detachment, chorioretinitis, cataracts, atrophy of corpora nigra, and phthisis bulbi.
• Reproductive—abortion (usually late gestation), stillbirth, or premature birth or neonatal disease depending on stage of gestation and infection.
• Renal/urologic—azotemia, polyuria/polydipsia, pyuria, hematuria, pyrexia.
• Neonatal disease—weakness, icterus. One outbreak also reported respiratory distress, pyrexia, depression.
• Hepatobiliary—jaundice, pyrexia, lethargy.

CAUSES

Pathogenic serovars of *L. interrogans.* Serovars reported in serologic surveys in horses are *L. arboreae, L. bratislava, L. canicola, L. grippotyphosa, L. hardjo, L. icterohaemorrhagiae, L. lora, L. muenchen,* and *L. pomona.*

RISK FACTORS

• Direct transmission—Host to-host contact via infected urine, exposure to postabortion discharge, and aborted fetuses.
• Indirect transmission—Contaminated environment from exposure to shedding animals. Swine, cattle, and sheep are the definitive hosts for *L. hardjo;* deer, raccoon, and swine for *L. pomona;* dogs for *L. canicola;* badgers and rats for *L. icterohaemorrhagiae;* and raccoons for *L. grippotyphosa.*
• Environmental factors—Warm, moist environment; neutral to slightly alkaline soil pH; and a high density of carrier and susceptible animals.

DIAGNOSIS

DIFFERENTIAL DIAGNOSIS

Clinical signs associated with the bacteremic phase can be attributed to a variety of infectious disease processes.

Recurrent Uveitis

Toxoplasma spp., *Onchocerca cervicalis, Streptococcus* spp., viral agents, ocular trauma. *Onchocerca* microfilariae and viral inclusion bodies are found in conjunctival scraping and biopsy. Rising serum titers are associated with *Toxoplasma* spp.

Abortion

• Infectious causes—EHV-1 is differentiated by a lack of maternal parturition signs and a well-preserved fetus with focal necrosis of the lung, liver, adrenal cortex, and lymphoid tissue with intranuclear eosinophilic inclusion bodies. Placentitis (bacterial and fungal) is differentiated by gross evidence of placentitis, isolation of organisms from the placenta and fetal organs, especially the stomach. EIA is associated with high a EIA titer in the mare. EVA is differentiated by viral isolation from placental and fetal tissues. *Ehrlichia risticci* is differentiated by histopathology of the fetus and isolation of the organism from the fetus.
• Noninfectious causes—Placental abnormalities, twinning, and maternal systemic disease.
• Renal/Urologic—Bacterial pyelonephritis is identified by pyuria and the presence of bacteria in the urine. Hemodynamic renal dysfunction is differentiated by other physical examination findings. Nephrotoxicity is identified by exposure to a source.
• Neonatal disease—NI is associated with hemolytic anemia. Tyzzer's disease is usually seen in older foals; organisms are seen in the liver with Warthin–Starry stain.
• EHV-1—See above; also, severe leukopenia.
• *Actinobacillus equuli*—The organism is isolated from blood culture and postmortem specimens, especially the kidney.
• Septicemia
• Hepatobiliary—Hemolytic anemia, fasting, and cholelithiasis, often seen with ultrasonographic examination.

CBC/BIOCHEMISTRY/URINALYSIS

Serum biochemistry profile reflects specific organ involvement; leukocytosis, hyperfibrinogenemia. Urinalysis (if renal involvement) shows red and white blood cells and casts.

OTHER LABORATORY TESTS

• Culture of *Leptospira* is difficult. Antemortem body fluids (urine, blood, aqueous humor) or postmortem tissues (kidney, liver, fetus, placenta) must be placed in 1% BSA at 1:10 dilution. The collection of midstream urine samples from second urination after furosemide administration enhances isolation, and repeat sampling increases the chances of isolation. Dark-phase microscopy can also be used, although it is less reliable. Leptospires need not be viable for fluorescent antibody test (FAT) of urinary sediment because urine on ice can be sent overnight to the lab. Blood culture is performed during bacteremia.

• Serology—MAT and ELISA (more sensitive). MAT titer > 1:100 is an indication of exposure; however, paired samples 1 month apart showing a four-fold increase are more definitive. Compare with other farm individuals to assist with interpretation. Aqueous humor titers are greater than serum titers. FAT of placenta, uterine fluid, fetal aqueous humor, liver, lung, kidney, and stomach contents can be performed.

IMAGING

Ultrasonography may assist in the evaluation of hepatic and renal disease.

PATHOLOGY FINDINGS

Fetus and Neonates

Most common findings are icterus and interstitial nephritis and nephrosis. Warthin–Starry stain of tissue samples.

TREATMENT

APPROPRIATE HEALTH AND NURSING CARE

Ophthalmic

Uveitis is immune mediated; therefore, specific antibiotic therapy is unlikely to be effective. Therapy is aimed at reducing immune-mediated inflammation and providing mydriasis and analgesia.

Reproductive

Aborting mares should be isolated and the areas they inhabited should be disinfected.

Renal/Urologic

Appropriate antimicrobials and supportive intravenous isotonic polyionic fluids should be administered.

Neonatal Disease

Appropriate antimicrobials and supportive care should be administered.

Hepatobiliary

Appropriate antimicrobials and supportive care should be administered.

ACTIVITY

Acivity should be restricted to decrease environmental contamination.

CLIENT EDUCATION

The client should be informed as to the zoonotic potential from infected urine and body fluids of affected horses.

SURGICAL CONSIDERATIONS

N/A

MEDICATIONS

DRUG(S) OF CHOICE

(Recommendations for antimicrobial therapy have been extrapolated from other species.) Oxytetracycline (5–10 mg/kg), streptomycin (10 mg/kg IM q12h), penicillin (10,000–15,000 IU/kg q12h) for 1 week. Potassium penicillin G (20,000 IU/kg IV q6h) used in pregnant mares with rising titers, and acute leptospirosis.

CONTRAINDICATIONS

N/A

PRECAUTIONS

Avoid use of potentially nephrotoxic drugs if renal disease is suspected. Colitis may occur secondary to tetracycline therapy.

POSSIBLE DRUG INTERACTIONS

N/A

ALTERNATIVE DRUGS

Synthetic penicillins (ampicillin, amoxicillin) and combinations (ticarcillin/clavulonic acid), cefotaxime, erythromycin may be used.

FOLLOW-UP

PATIENT MONITORING

Ophthalmic

Recurrent episodes of uveitis.

Reproductive

Therapy should be instituted if fetal membranes are retained or if signs of systemic illness become evident. Monitor other mares in contact for signs of pyrexia, anorexia, and lethargy. Monitor serum titer levels and consider antibiotic therapy of in-contact pregnant mares.

Renal/Urologic, Neonatal Disease, and Hepatobiliary

Monitor hepatic and renal function.

PREVENTION/AVOIDANCE

Approved vaccinations are not available for use in horses. Isolate affected animals, and consider antibiotic therapy for in-contact pregnant mares. Limit access to wet environments, and avoid contamination with other domestic animals and wildlife.

POSSIBLE COMPLICATIONS

Ophthalmic

Blindness associated with recurrent uveitis.

Reproductive

Abortion outbreak.

Neonatal Disease

Foals from infected dams may be born diseased.

EXPECTED COURSE AND PROGNOSIS

Ophthalmic

Alternating periods of acute and quiescent disease.

Reproductive

Uneventful recovery of mare.

Neonatal Disease, Renal/Urologic, and Hepatobiliary

Prognosis is guarded in severe acute disease and depends on the extent of organ invasion and the severity of tissue injury.

MISCELLANEOUS

ASSOCIATED CONDITIONS

N/A

ZOONOTIC POTENTIAL

Leptospira spp. are reported to cause Weil's disease, flu-like symptoms, meningitis, and hepatorenal failure in humans. Prophylatic antibiotic therapy may be indicated if humans or animals are exposed to urine or body fluids from an infected horse.

PREGNANCY

Abortion, stillbirths, and neonatal disease can be sequellae, depending on the stages of infection and gestation.

SYNONYMS

N/A

SEE ALSO

N/A

ABBREVIATIONS

• EHV-1 = equine herpesvirus 1
• EIA = enzyme immunoassay
• ELISA = enzyme-linked immunosorbent assay
• EVA = equine viral arteritis
• FAT = fluorescent antibody test
• MAT = mixed agglutination test

Suggested Reading

Bernard, WV. Leptospirosis. Vet Clin North Am Eq Pract 1993;9:435-444.

Heath SE, Johnson R. Leptospirosis. JAVMA 1994;205:1518-1523.

Author Jane E. Axon

Consulting Editor Corinne R. Sweeney

LEUKOENCEPHALOMALACIA (ELEM)

BASICS

DEFINITION
A generally fatal, rapidly progressing neurologic disease caused by ingestion of the mycotoxin fumonisin and characterized by liquefactive necrosis of subcortical white matter of the cerebral hemispheres

PATHOPHYSIOLOGY
Fumonisin mycotoxins interfere with sphingolipid metabolism, resulting in damage to the vascular endothelium of the brain and, with some animals, in hepatocellular necrosis and vacuolization.

SYSTEMS AFFECTED
- CNS—damage to vascular endothelium
- Hepatobiliary—pathogenesis not definitively known

GENETICS
N/A

INCIDENCE/PREVALENCE
- Sporadic incidence, yet one of the most common equine toxicoses
- Worldwide, but most often in temperate, humid climates after a dry summer and a wet harvest season.
- Outbreaks often are seasonal, with most occurring from fall through early spring.
- Although quite variable, 15–25% or more of horses in a group can be affected.

SIGNALMENT
- Only affects horses and other equine species.
- Mature horses appear most susceptible.

SIGNS
Neurologic Syndrome
- Anorexia
- Depression, with little response to stimuli, although some horses may become hyperexcitable
- Progressive ataxia and proprioceptive defects
- Delirium
- Blindness
- Aimless wandering
- Eventual recumbency
- Coma
- Body temperature generally normal
- Death from 12 hours to as long as 1 week after onset of signs

Hepatotoxic Syndrome
- Occurs occasionally and perhaps concurrently with the neurologic syndrome.
- Severe icterus
- Swelling of the lips and nose
- Petechiae in mucous membranes
- Lowered head
- Reluctance to move
- Abdominal breathing
- Cyanosis
- Hemoglobinuria
- Death within hours to a few days.

CAUSES
Ingestion of corn products contaminated with fumonisin mycotoxins, especially fumonisin B_1, which are produced by *Fusarium moniliforme* and *F. proliferatum* molds growing on corn.

RISK FACTORS
- The causative fusarium molds invade corn during the stress of hot, dry weather at the time of pollination, and they continue to increase when temperature and moisture remain high into harvest.
- Fumonisins are produced in corn under these conditions before harvest, then contaminate corn products used for horse feed. Corn screenings present a special risk, because they contain small, shrunken, and broken kernels often heavily contaminated with fumonisin.
- Development of disease depends on fumonisin concentration in the feed and the duration of exposure. As little as 10 ppm for 30 days can cause death.
- Onset of clinical disease generally occurs 2–9 weeks after the start of continuous consumption of fumonisin-containing feeds but may vary from 1–21 weeks.

DIAGNOSIS

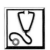

DIFFERENTIAL DIAGNOSIS
- Rabies
- Equine encephalomyelitis
- Equine herpesvirus myeloencephalopathy
- Botulism
- Hepatoencephalopathy
- Head trauma
- Bacterial meningoencephalitis
- Tick paralysis
- Pyrrolizidine alkaloid hepatotoxicosis
- Aflatoxicosis

CBC/BIOCHEMISTRY/URINALYSIS
- Most parameters are inconsistent between affected horses.
- Anemia may occur
- WBC counts are variable.
- Total bilirubin often is elevated with hepatotoxicosis, especially with icterus.
- Elevations of GGT and AST vary with the amount of liver damage
- CSF may be normal but often shows elevated total protein and neutrophils.

OTHER LABORATORY TESTS
- Analysis of feeds for fumonisin (especially B_1)—more than 5 ppm is significant; many contaminated feeds contain 40–100 ppm.
- Alteration of the sphinganine:sphingosine ratio in serum or tissues is consistent with fumonisin ingestion.

IMAGING
N/A

DIAGNOSTIC PROCEDURES
N/A

PATHOLOGIC FINDINGS
- Primary lesion—necrosis of internal white matter of the cerebral hemispheres, although the brain surface often is normal in appearance.
- Massive softening of the interior of the hemispheres may create large cavitations of liquefactive necrosis or discrete focal areas of necrosis and hemorrhage.
- Microscopically, liquefaction and proliferation of macrophages in response to the necrosis are seen.

TREATMENT

APPROPRIATE HEALTH CARE
- Horses showing neurologic signs usually die or are euthanized.
- By the time clinical signs appear, significant and irreversible cerebral necrosis usually is present; however, therapy may be an option in selected clinical cases.

LEUKOENCEPHALOMALACIA (ELEM)

NURSING CARE
• Supportive therapy as needed, including PO and IV fluids for rehydration and tube feeding.
• Sedate excited horses to prevent injury to themselves and caregivers.
• Oral administration of AC with a saline cathartic may help to eliminate toxin already in the GI tract.

ACTIVITY
N/A

DIET
Immediately eliminate feeds suspected of contamination with fumonisin.

CLIENT EDUCATION
• Inform clients about the risk of using corn-based feeds, especially those containing corn screenings or that appear moldy.
• Inform clients of the added risk in years with drought stress during the growing season and periods of high moisture during harvest.

SURGICAL CONSIDERATIONS
N/A

MEDICATIONS

DRUGS OF CHOICE
No specific antidote for the toxin.

CONTRAINDICATIONS
N/A

PRECAUTIONS
N/A

POSSIBLE INTERACTIONS
N/A

ALTERNATIVE DRUGS
N/A

FOLLOW-UP

PATIENT MONITORING
• Continue supportive care.
• Monitor for progression or remission of neurologic signs.

PREVENTION/AVOIDANCE
• Do not use feed with >5 ppm fumonisin.
• Do not use corn screenings.

POSSIBLE COMPLICATIONS
Neurologic deficits may remain in the few horses that recover.

EXPECTED COURSE AND PROGNOSIS
• Treatment of horses with significant neurologic signs rarely is successful; death generally occurs from 12 hours to 1 week after onset of signs, regardless of treatment.
• Euthanasia of advanced cases and confirmation of the diagnosis often are advised.

MISCELLANEOUS

ASSOCIATED CONDITIONS
Corn and other grains infected with *Fusarium* spp. molds also may contain DON, but feeds with $\leq$14 ppm have no effect on horses.

AGE-RELATED FACTORS
N/A

ZOONOTIC POTENTIAL
N/A

PREGNANCY
N/A

SYNONYMS
• Corn stalk poisoning
• Fumonisin toxicosis
• Moldy corn poisoning

SEE ALSO
N/A

ABBREVIATIONS
• AC = activated charcoal
• AST = aspartate transaminase
• CSF = cerebrospinal fluid
• DON = deoxynivalenol, vomitoxin
• GGT = γ-glutamyltransferase
• GI = gastrointestinal

Suggested Reading

Lewis LD. Feed-related poisonings of horses. In: Equine clinical nutrition. Baltimore: Williams & Wilkins, 1995.
McCue PM. Equine leukoencephalomalacia. Compend Contin Educ Pract Vet 1989;11:646.
Uhlinger C. Leuko encephalomalacia. Vet Clin North Am Equine Pract 1997;13:13.
Wang E, Ross PF, Wilson TM, et al. Increases in serum sphingosine and sphingamine and decreases in complex sphingolipids in ponies given feed containing fumonisins, mycotoxins produced by *Fusarium moniliforme.* J Nutr 1992;122:1706.

Author Thomas L. Carson
Consulting Editor Robert H. Poppenga

LEUKOENCEPHALOMALACIA (MOLDY CORN POISONING)

BASICS

OVERVIEW

- A sporadic disease of horses, ponies, donkeys, and mules caused by the mycotoxin fumonisin B1, a metabolite of *Fusarium monoliforme.*
- Worldwide distribution, with seasonal outbreaks occurring from late fall through early spring.
- Most outbreaks have been associated with a dry growing period followed by a wet period.
- Two clinical syndromes, neurotoxicosis and hepatotoxicosis, result from *F. monoliforme* toxicosis.
- Typical cross lesions include liquefactive necrosis and degeneration of the subcortical white matter of the cerebral hemispheres.
- Progression of clinical signs is rapid, with most severely affected horses succumbing in 2–3 days.

SIGNALMENT

- Horses, ponies, donkeys, and mules
- Old animals appear to be more susceptible than young animals.
- Moldy corn fed to nonequine species (e.g., goats, pigs, monkeys, hamsters, rats, mice, rabbits, and chickens) did not result in illness or death.

SIGNS

- Two clinical syndromes are associated with *F. moniliforme* toxicosis. The neurotoxic syndrome is the most common, but hepatotoxicosis occurs in some horses.
- Initial signs occur 3–4 weeks after daily ingestion of the toxin.

Neurologic Syndrome

- Characterized by intermittent anorexia, lethargy, and depression, followed by progressive ataxia, blindness, circling, head-pressing, agitation, hyperexcitability, and delirium.
- Death usually occurs in 2–3 days.
- Before death, animals may become recumbent and show clonic–tetanic convulsions.
- Many of these horses are found dead, without observation of any clinical signs.

Hepatotoxic Syndrome

- Clinical signs include swelling of the lips, severe depression, severe icterus, petechiae of mucous membranes, and cyanosis.
- Death usually occurs within a few hours to days.

CAUSES AND RISK FACTORS

- The association between acute, fatal neurologic disorders in horses and ingestion of moldy feed has been recognized since the nineteenth century.
- Caused by the mycotoxin fumonisin B1, a metabolite of *F. moniliforme.*
- Both the neurologic and hepatotoxic syndromes have been experimentally reproduced by PO and IV administration of fumonisin B1.
- Ingestion of smaller quantities of infected material over an extended period of time are suggested to result in the neurologic disease, whereas ingestion of larger amounts of the toxin may result in fatal hepatotoxicosis.

DIAGNOSIS

DIFFERENTIAL DIAGNOSIS

- Include, but is not limited to, EHV-1 myeloencephalopathy, EEE, rabies, botulism, and Theiler's disease.
- Horses affected with EHV-1 myeloencephalopathy usually show signs of rapid progression of ataxia (most severe in the hindlimbs) for 24–48 hours, after which clinical signs usually subside.
- CSF analysis of EHV-1 infection is characterized by xanthochromia and elevated protein with a normal nucleated cell count.
- Horses with EEE are febrile, with signs primarily occurring during summer months.
- Horses infected with rabies have behavioral changes occurring at any time of year.
- Clinical signs of botulism are characterized by flaccid paralysis and weakness, with dysphagia and decreasing tongue and tail tone.
- In addition to CNS signs, horses affected by Theiler's disease may have areas of photosensitization, hemorrhage, and icterus.

CBC/BIOCHEMISTRY/URINALYSIS

- Abnormal biochemistry results are nonspecific but usually indicate some degree of liver dysfunction.
- Increased serum concentrations of bilirubin, GGT, SDH, and AST have been observed.
- Urinalysis usually is normal.

OTHER LABORATORY TESTS

Serologic tests for infectious agents are inconclusive.

LEUKOENCEPHALOMALACIA (MOLDY CORN POISONING)

IMAGING
N/A

DIAGNOSTIC PROCEDURES
- CSF abnormalities include elevated protein and elevated nucleated cell count.
- Feed (i.e., corn) may be cultured for *F. moniliforme*. More specifically, fumonisin B1 may be assayed in feed materials by various analytic methods. Feed-containing >10 ppm fumonisin B1 can be lethal to horses and, therefore, is not safe to use. An appropriate feed sample should be submitted, because feed currently being used may not contain the toxin. This most likely is because horses usually require a fairly long exposure to the toxin for clinical signs to occur.
- Definitive diagnosis can be established only by necropsy.
- Typical gross lesions include liquefactive necrosis and degeneration of the cerebral hemispheres.
- Gross liver changes are not pronounced, but the liver may be discolored and swollen.

TREATMENT
- No definitive treatment or antidote for horses with clinical signs.
- Laxatives and activated charcoal may be given to eliminate toxins in the digestive tract, but if clinical signs are observed, significant necrosis of the cerebrum usually has occurred.
- Sedate extremely agitated horses to prevent injury to themselves and their handlers.
- Remove any contaminated feed to decrease further exposure.

MEDICATIONS

DRUGS
N/A

CONTRAINDICATIONS/POSSIBLE INTERACTIONS
N/A

FOLLOW-UP
N/A

MISCELLANEOUS

ASSOCIATED CONDITIONS
N/A

AGE-RELATED FACTORS
N/A

ZOONOTIC POTENTIAL
N/A

PREGNANCY
N/A

SEE ALSO
N/A

ABBREVIATIONS
- AST = aspartate aminotransferase
- CSF = cerebrospinal fluid
- EEE = eastern equine encephalomyelitis
- EHV = equine herpes virus
- GGT = γ-glutamyltransferase
- SDH = sorbitol dehydrogenase

Suggested Reading

McCue PM. Equine leukoencephalomalacia. Compend Contin Educ Pract Vet 1989;11:646–651.

Uhlinger C. Clinical and epidemiological features of an epizootic of equine leukoencephalomalacia. J Am Vet Med Assoc 1991;198:126–128.

Wilson BJ, Maronpot RR, Hildebrandt PK. Equine leukoencephalomalacia. J Am Vet Med Assoc 1973;163:1293–1294.

Wilkins PA, Zivotofsky WD, Twitchell E. A herd outbreak of equine leukoencephalomalacia. Cornell Vet 1994;84:53–59.

Author Steven T. Grubbs
Consulting Editor Joseph J. Bertone

LIMBAL KERATOPATHY

BASICS

OVERVIEW
• Ulceration of the perilimbal cornea
• Organ system—ophthalmic

SIGNALMENT
All ages and breeds

SIGNS
Peripheral, superficial to midstromal, deep, sterile ulcers involving the perilimbal region and that can enlarge centripetally and circumferentially

CAUSES AND RISK FACTORS
• Immune-mediated
• The limbus is a very active region of immune activity because of its vasculature.

DIAGNOSIS

DIFFERENTIAL DIAGNOSIS
• Lid abnormalities—distichiasis, trichiasis, and entropion
• Neuroparalytic and neurotrophic keratitis
• Keratoconjunctivitis sicca
• Corneal dystrophies and foreign bodies
• Inappropriate topical corticosteroid therapy causing delayed corneal healing
• Chronic epithelial erosion—indolent ulceration

CBC/BIOCHEMISTRY/URINALYSIS
N/A

OTHER LABORATORY TESTS
• Rule out infectious causes (bacterial or fungal) with corneal scrapings for cytology and culture.
• Biopsy can support the diagnosis.

IMAGING
N/A

DIAGNOSTIC PROCEDURES
N/A

PATHOLOGIC FINDINGS
Conjunctiva adjacent to ulcer contains lymphocytes, plasma cells, and eosinophils.

TREATMENT
• Superficial grid keratotomy for debridement of ulcers
• Postoperatively, temporary partial tarsorrhaphy prevents trauma to ulcers from blepharospasm.

LIMBAL KERATOPATHY

MEDICATIONS

DRUGS

Topical corticosteroid therapy—1% prednisolone acetate or 0.1% dexamethasone four to six times per day; limbal keratopathy is the only type of equine ulcer for which topical corticosteroid therapy is indicated.

CONTRAINDICATIONS/POSSIBLE INTERACTIONS

Evaluate evidence of infectious organisms by cytology and culture before instituting topical corticosteroid treatment.

FOLLOW-UP

Ulcers heal rapidly once topical corticosteroid medication is applied; if the ulcer does not heal rapidly, re-evaluate whether topical corticosteroids are indicated.

MISCELLANEOUS

ASSOCIATED CONDITIONS

- Infection
- Uveitis

SEE ALSO

- Burdock pappus bristle keratopathy
- Calcific band keratopathy
- Corneal laceration
- Corneal stromal abscessation
- Corneal ulceration
- Eosinophilic keratitis
- Glaucoma
- Herpes keratitis
- Keratomycosis
- Nonulcerative keratouveitis
- Recurrent uveitis
- Superficial corneal erosions with anterior stromal sequestration

Suggested Reading

Brooks DE. Equine ophthalmology. In: Gelatt KN, ed. Veterinary ophthalmology. 3rd ed. Philadelphia: Lippincott Williams & Wilkins, 1999.

Author Andras M. Komaromy
Consulting Editor Dennis E. Brooks

LIPIDS, HYPERLIPIDEMIA/HYPERLIPEMIA

BASICS

DEFINITIONS

- Hyperlipidemia—concentration of lipid (i.e., cholesterol, triglyceride) in the blood exceeding the upper range of normal
- Lipemia—excess concentration of triglycerides in serum or plasma sufficient (≅500 mg/dL or greater) to impart a milky appearance (i.e., lactescence)
- Hyperlipemia—disturbance in metabolism causing lipemia
- Equine hyperlipidemia/hyperlipemia—disorder of lipid metabolism seen primarily in ponies, donkeys, and miniature horses; characterized by hypertriglyceridemia; may be called equine hyperlipemia when severe enough for lipemia to be present.

PATHOPHYSIOLOGY

- In equids, various disorders causing anorexia result in mobilization of body fat stores to satisfy energy demands. This leads to hypertriglyceridemia, which often is severe enough to cause lipemia. Fatty degeneration of the liver, kidney, and possibly, other organs then ensues.
- Insulin resistance may be a predisposing factor.
- Ponies are insulin insensitive relative to horses, and obesity accentuates this insensitivity.
- Insulin resistance increases during gestation.

SYSTEMS AFFECTED

- Endocrine/metabolic
- Hepatobiliary
- Renal/urologic

SIGNALMENT

- Primarily ponies (especially Shetlands), donkeys, and miniature horses
- Occasionally seen in full-size horses
- Most common in mares, especially those >4 years

SIGNS

Historical Findings

- Inappetence progresses to anorexia, often with lethargy, incoordination, and weakness.
- Diarrhea is common.
- May progress to severe nervous dysfunction with ataxia, dysphagia, head pressing, and circling, followed by recumbency.
- Agonal events may include paddling convulsions, champing, nystagmus, and mania.

Physical Examination Findings

- Variable
- May include fever, increased heart and respiratory rates, congested mucous membranes, icterus, halitosis, and ventral subcutaneous edema.

CAUSES

- Anorexia/negative energy balance (often from an underlying disease or metabolic disturbance) is the most common cause of equine hyperlipidemia.
- Many cases are associated with metabolic stresses of late pregnancy or lactation.

RISK FACTORS

- Obesity
- Stress
- Feed restriction
- Lactation
- Late pregnancy
- Diseases causing anorexia

DIAGNOSIS

DIFFERENTIAL DIAGNOSIS

- Starvation may cause mild hyperlipidemia without evidence of hepatic disease.
- Equine Cushing's-like disease (e.g., pituitary pars intermedia dysfunction, adenoma) may cause lipemia but is characterized by hirsutism, abnormal shedding patterns, polyuria, polydipsia, and hyperhydrosis.

LABORATORY FINDINGS

Sample Handling

- Submit serum.
- Lipemia can cause hemolysis, which may become more severe if separation of the serum from the clot is delayed.
- Do not clear lipemia from serum to be submitted for cholesterol and triglyceride determinations.

Drugs That May Alter Lab Results

- Corticosteroids
- Thiazides
- Phenothiazines

Disorders That May Alter Lab Results

- Lipemia, hemolysis, and icterus are likely to adversely affect several parameters on a general chemistry panel.
- Effects depend on the specific laboratory methodology used and the lab's success in clearing lipemia before chemical analysis of the specimen; check with the lab regarding possible artifactual results.

Valid if Run in Human Lab?

Yes

CBC/BIOCHEMISTRY/URINALYSIS

- Serum/plasma is lipemic, except in some mild or early cases.
- Serum TG >400 mg/dL in early or mild cases, and possibly >6500 mg/dL in severe cases.
- Cholesterol may be elevated.
- Glucose may be low.
- Ketonemia/ketonuria is absent.
- Metabolic acidosis usually is present—decreased total CO_2
- Fatty infiltration of the liver generally causes increased GTT, ALP, LDH, and SDH.
- Total bilirubin may be increased.
- Urea and creatinine increase during later stages.
- Lipemia may interfere with some laboratory tests and give misleading results; check with the lab. (**NOTE**: Healthy ponies generally have higher TG levels than horses. Healthy donkeys may have TG levels as high as 290 mg/dL, and pregnant ponies may have levels as high as 250 mg/dL by the end of gestation.)

LIPIDS, HYPERLIPIDEMIA/HYPERLIPEMIA

OTHER LABORATORY TESTS
- Phospholipids and free fatty acids may be elevated.
- Serum bile acids may be increased.
- Coagulation abnormalities may be present—prolonged prothrombin and partial thromboplastin times

IMAGING
N/A

DIAGNOSTIC PROCEDURES
- Postmortem findings/histopathology—excess lipid may be present in many tissues, with the liver and kidneys most severely affected.
- Other possible findings—pancreatitis, focal hemorrhages, pulmonary edema, left ventricular infarcts, renal infarcts, venous thrombosis, proliferative glomerulitis, skeletal muscle degeneration, pancreatic atrophy, and lymphoid depletion of the spleen and lymph nodes

TREATMENT
- Directed at any underlying disease; beyond that, provide nutritional support and correct fluid/electrolyte imbalances.
- IV fluid (acetated Ringer's solution with 5 g of dextrose per 100 mL and 20–40 mEq KCl/L) for rehydration and maintenance
- Restrict administration of sodium bicarbonate to those patients with established acidosis; the dose should not exceed 2 L of 5% sodium bicarbonate.
- Offer fresh, highly palatable foodstuffs.
- If food intake is inadequate, provide nutritional support.
- Enteral feeding (e.g., oral drenches or nasogastric tube feeding of commercial glucose and electrolyte solutions or slurries made of alfalfa hay or feed pellets 4–8 times daily) can be used if no GI abnormalities (e.g., diarrhea, ileus) are present. The volume of each feeding should not exceed 3 L for miniature horses, 5 L for ponies, and 7 L for larger ponies and horses.
- Parenteral nutrition may be attempted in valuable horses that are completely off feed. An appropriate solution can be made by mixing 50% dextrose and an amino acid solution formulated for patients with hepatic failure. The final solution should be 20% dextrose with 4–5% amino acid and can be given at a rate of 2 mL/kg per hour if serum glucose is not >180 mg/dL during treatment.

MEDICATIONS

DRUGS OF CHOICE
- Exogenous insulin (30 IU per 200 kg of protamine zinc insulin IM BID in combination with PO or IV glucose) may help to decrease plasma lipid levels.
- Flunixin meglumine (0.25 mg/kg TID) may improve attitude and appetite.

CONTRAINDICATIONS
Glucocorticoids, which may exacerbate hyperlipidemia

PRECAUTIONS
- Neutralize metabolic acidosis slowly to prevent exacerbation of hepatic encephalopathy.
- Overdosing with bicarbonate can lead to persistent alkalosis and respiratory depression and cause hypokalemia in anorexic animals.
- Overdosing with glucose can cause diuresis, dehydration, hyponatremia, and worsen metabolic acidosis.

POSSIBLE INTERACTIONS
N/A

ALTERNATIVE DRUGS
Heparin (100 U/kg IV q12h) may be used to decrease hyperlipemia. The efficacy of this is questionable, however, and heparin may increase the risk of hemorrhage.

FOLLOW-UP

PATIENT MONITORING
- Monitor serum chemistry to establish the presence and severity of organ failure.
- Monitor blood glucose, acid–base status, and hepatic and renal function to determine response to therapy and assess prognosis.

POSSIBLE COMPLICATIONS
- Multiple organ failure may develop.
- The mortality rate is 60–80%.

MISCELLANEOUS

ASSOCIATED CONDITIONS
- Often secondary to a disorder causing anorexia
- May lead to multiple organ failure.

AGE-RELATED FACTORS
Most common in horses >4 years

ZOONOTIC POTENTIAL
N/A

PREGNANCY
Pregnancy is a risk factor.

SYNONYMS
N/A

SEE ALSO
Equine Cushing's-like disease

ABBREVIATIONS
- ALP = alkaline phosphatase
- GI = gastrointestinal
- GTT = gamma glutamyl transferase
- LDH = lactate dehydrogenase
- SDH = sorbitol dehydrogenase
- TG = triglycerides

Suggested Reading

Divers TJ. Hepatic disorders. In: Robinson NE, ed. Current veterinary therapy in equine medicine 4. Philadelphia: WB Saunders, 1997:214–222.

Mogg TD, Palmer JE. Hyperlipidemia, hyperlipemia, and hepatic lipidosis in American Miniature Horses: 23 cases. J Am Vet Med Assoc 1995;207:604–607.

Pearson EG, Maas J. Hepatic lipidosis. In: Smith BP, ed. Large animal internal medicine. 2nd ed. St. Louis: Mosby, 1996:937–944.

Watson TDG, Love S. Equine hyperlipidemia. Compend Contin Educ Pract Vet 1994;16:89–98.

Author Marlyn S. Whitney
Consulting Editor Claire B. Andreasen

LOCOMOTOR STEREOTYPIC BEHAVIORS

BASICS

DEFINITION

• A stereotypy is as an invariant, repetitive pattern of movement with no apparent purpose.
• The basic pattern arises from a normal maintenance behavior (e.g., walking), but the behavior is performed excessively and out of context, to the exclusion of normal behaviors.
• Performance of the stereotypy usually interferes with the animal's well-being.
• Equine locomotor stereotypies include head shaking, swinging, or bobbing; stall walking; weaving; fence running; and stall kicking.

PATHOPHYSIOLOGY

• Unclear
• Several mechanisms have been postulated implicating serotonergic and dopaminergic dysfunction, but the exact contribution of each system is undetermined.
• Endogenous endorphin concentrations are suspected to be aberrant among horses engaging in stereotypic behaviors with a self-injurious component—self-mutilation or wall kicking

SYSTEMS AFFECTED

• Behavioral—may interfere with expression of normal maintenance behaviors or affect performance of learned responses.
• CNS—proposed causes involve serotonergic, dopaminergic, or endogenous opioid system abnormalities at the gross anatomic or molecular level.
• Musculoskeletal—uneven hoof wear or muscle development, or decreased performance if the behavior is performed to the point of fatigue or self-injury.

SIGNALMENT

• No breed, age, or sex predilection
• Onset may be more common at the time of social maturity (≅ 4–5 years) but may occur earlier or later.

SIGNS

General Comments

• The amount of time spent performing the behavior varies with the severity of the problem.
• Performance of the behaviors usually is elicited by increased emotional arousal—when being fed, led to and from barns or pastures, or led toward or away from herdmates; or in anticipation of pleasurable experiences (e.g., feeding time).
• When the behavior is performed during a large proportion of the horse's waking hours, the intensity of the stereotypy may be exaggerated during situations of increased emotional arousal.
• Head shaking, swinging, or bobbing—side to side, circular, or up and down motions of the head, neck, or both when the horse is at rest, moving at liberty, or under saddle.
• Stall walking—circular pacing when confined to a stall. The horse may circle in one or both directions; when severe, the behavior may be exhibited as fence walking or running when the horse is turned out.
• Weaving—rhythmic stepping in place with the front limbs, alternating from one foot to the other and usually accompanied by a side to side swaying of the head and neck. In some cases, the hindlimbs also march, in which case the overall foot placing corresponds to a trotting pattern but without any moment of suspension (unlike a true trot.)
• Fence running—the horse walks, trots, or canters in a repetitive pattern along a fence line or before a gate, with the distance traveled and the location and features of the turns being invariant.
• Stall kicking—the horse repetitively strikes the wall of its stall, typically with one or both hindlegs. It also may strike the wall with the hoof, the plantar aspect of the metatarsus, or the tarsometatarsal joint.

Historical Findings

• Owners may report a gradual onset or an incitatory event after which the behavior was seen or became more noticeable.
• Information on related horses (e.g., sire, dam, full- or half-siblings) sometimes may reveal other affected individuals.

Physical Examination Findings

Unremarkable, except for lesions resulting from self-injurious behavior or uneven shoe or hoof wear or muscle development secondary to increased ambulation.

CAUSES

• One of the suspected causes is dysregulation of neurotransmitter systems and function.
• Environments or management practices that inhibit expression of normal behaviors are believed to increase anxiety and can precipitate or exacerbate expression of stereotypic behaviors.

RISK FACTORS

Offspring of affected horses may be at a higher risk—a genetic component is suspected, but the precise contribution of inheritance has not been determined.

LOCOMOTOR STEREOTYPIC BEHAVIORS

DIAGNOSIS

DIFFERENTIAL DIAGNOSIS

• Stall kicking—any painful medical condition (e.g., colic) may cause a horse to strike with or toward the affected area.
• Do not confuse anxiety specific to separation from herdmates with a locomotor stereotypy, unless the signs fit the diagnostic criteria.
• Headshaking—rule out trigeminal neuritis, photophobia, orodental disease, auricular disease, guttural pouch disease, tracheopharyngeal disease, poor horsemanship (if the behavior occurs while under saddle), and response to an airborne allergen.
• The behavior can be a learned response, and undesirable behaviors can be repeated to obtain a reward (e.g., a horse bangs the stall door at feeding time and is fed first by the caretaker; thus, the horse only bangs the door at feeding time to be fed first).

CBC/BIOCHEMISTRY/URINALYSIS

Ancillary tests to rule out medical problems; results should be unremarkable if no underlying disease is present.

OTHER LABORATORY TESTS

Aggression associated with equine hypothyroidism has been reported; perform thyroid function testing in cases of self-injurious stereotypic behavior if other clinical signs suggest the possibility of hypothyroidism.

IMAGING

Only necessary to rule out lameness as a contributing factor or for treatment of injuries secondary to performance of the stereotypy.

DIAGNOSTIC PROCEDURES

Endoscopy of the oropharynx, larynx, and related structures may be indicated to rule out medical problems in headshaking horses.

TREATMENT

• A number of past devices and management measures focused on preventing performance of the behavior without addressing the psychologic well-being of the horse. Antiweaving stall doors prevent the neck from swaying, but the horse will continue to march with its feet. Even in a straight stall, a horse can still weave. Chains attached to the horse's pasterns may temporarily decrease kicking, but the anxiety level resulting from frustration and the inability to kick may express itself in a different way. Horses have been known to rearrange obstacles placed on the stall floor, such as tires, in order to continue stall walking. An ethologically based approach is indicated.
• The most feasible treatment plan focuses on management practices that allow the horse to express a wider range of normal behaviors while decreasing confinement, isolation, and emotional arousal.
• Horses with locomotor stereotypies are managed as outpatients.
• Recommended modifications in management practices—increased turnout time, preferably with a compatible companion; increased grazing time; increased opportunities for social contact within the confines of the stall; increased aerobic exercise; increased roughage:concentrate ratio in feed; and replacement of sweet feed (or other highly palatable grain) with a complete pelleted or extruded feed.
• Stall floors and walls can be fitted with heavy rubber mats or padding to decrease wear and tear on the stall and the horse's feet and extremities. Stall toys can be useful with young horses, who may still be actively exploring their environment. Stall toys that dispense small amounts of food when moved about by the horse can help to direct locomotive patterns into an activity that resembles the walk-and-nibble sequence of a grazing horse. Food dispensed this way gets mixed with the bedding; in addition, picking and cleaning the stall likely requires more time. Both these inconveniences can be overcome by using the feeding device in a small, dirt-floored paddock if available.
• Another way to simulate grazing within a stall or paddock is to place hay in nested haybags, but before pulling the drawstring tight, a second and a third bag are placed inside the first, always with some hay between the added haybags. Two or three of these nested bags can be hung at a safe height in different corners of the stall. Some horses walk from bag to bag but stop at these, because the nesting of hay layers makes the horse work harder to get the hay.
• Caution owners against reinforcing undesirable, repetitive behaviors. Reinforcing a stereotypic behavior is unlikely to be the single underlying inciting factor, but externally provided rewards could promote the behavior.

LOCOMOTOR STEREOTYPIC BEHAVIORS

MEDICATIONS

DRUGS OF CHOICE

- Use of medications is limited by drug's cost and or its frequency and route of administration.
- Opioid antagonists may have a role in treatment of self-injurious stereotypies (e.g., self-mutilation) and may help in cases of stall kicking—naltrexone (0.4 mg/kg IV) and naloxone (0.2 mg/kg IV), but their short half-life (these drugs must be given q4–6h), cost, and route of administration make currently available forms impractical for the long-term treatment.
- Tricyclic antidepressants and serotonin-specific reuptake inhibitors have been used to treat obsessive-compulsive disorders in humans and small animals and may have a place in treatment of locomotor stereotypies in horses—amitriptyline (0.5–1.0 mg/kg PO q12–24h), clomipramine (1–2 mg/kg PO q12–24h), and fluoxetine (1 mg/kg PO q24h). These dosages are extrapolated from human and companion animal use; few (if any) studies of these drugs in horses exist.
- Other anxiolytics (e.g., benzodiazepines) may help, but their use in treatment of stereotypies is underexplored—buspirone (0.5–1 mg/kg PO q8–12h).
- Individual response to drugs from different classes, and even between drugs from the same group, varies greatly. Base drug selection on possible contraindications, cost, and ease of administration.

CONTRAINDICATIONS

Tricyclics have anticholinergic and antihistaminic properties; in humans, their use is contraindicated in patients receiving thyroxine supplementation or in cases of cardiac conduction abnormalities, glaucoma, seizures, and urinary and fecal retention. Horses with a history of recurrent ileus may be at higher risk of an adverse reaction. Concurrent hepatic or renal disease warrant adjustment of starting dosages and careful monitoring of serum chemistry values and clinical signs.

PRECAUTIONS

- Owners should be aware that use of psychotropic medication constitutes experimental and off-label use; owners should sign an informed consent form and receive an explanation (preferably in writing) of the medication selection rationale, expected benefits, and possible side effects.
- Before use of medication, perform a CBC and serum chemistry panel.
- ECG—suggested before administration of tricyclics, which are arrhythmogenic in humans and companion animals and may be so in horses.
- Ancillary tests— can be repeated 6 weeks after start of medication or whenever clinical signs warrant.

POSSIBLE INTERACTIONS

- Phenothiazines may potentiate the effect of buspirone through inhibition of dopaminergic function.
- Combinations of tricyclics and serotonin-reuptake inhibitors may be synergistic, so initial dosages should be lowered if the two drug classes are used together.

ALTERNATIVE DRUGS

N/A

FOLLOW-UP

PATIENT MONITORING

- Drug dosages may need adjustment, so weekly follow-up is recommended.
- If long term use of medication is intended, annual to biannual monitoring of CBC and serum chemistry is recommended.
- Perform an ECG if tricyclics are used.
- Monitor owner compliance with recommendations; the time period for follow-up varies depending on the severity of the problem.

LOCOMOTOR STEREOTYPIC BEHAVIORS

POSSIBLE COMPLICATIONS

- Very little is known about the actual neurochemical basis of stereotypic disorders in horses. Treatment is aimed at minimizing the display of the behaviors, but owners must be cautioned that complete elimination cannot be guaranteed.
- Situations likely to increase stress and anxiety (e.g., rigorous training program, extensive travel schedule, or other disruptions in the environment or routine) may increase the incidence of the behaviors.

MISCELLANEOUS

ASSOCIATED CONDITIONS

If stereotypies are performed to the exclusion of normal maintenance behaviors, unthriftiness and poor performance could be secondary problems.

AGE RELATED FACTORS

N/A

ZOONOTIC POTENTIAL

N/A

PREGNANCY

- Avoid the mentioned drugs during pregnancy, because their use has not been studied in such animals.
- Use of tricyclics is contraindicated in pregnant individuals.

SYNONYMS

- Compulsive disorders
- Obsessive-compulsive disorders
- Stable vices
- Stereotypies

SEE ALSO

- Oral stereotypic behaviors
- Self-mutilation

Suggested Readings

Dodman NH, et al. Equine self-mutilation syndrome. J Am Vet Med Assoc 1994;204:1219–1223.

Dodman NH, Shuster L, eds. Psychopharmacology of animal behavior disorders. Malden, MA: Blackwell Science, 1998.

Houpt KA. New perspective on equine stereotypic behaviour. Equine Vet J 1995;27:82–83.

Houpt KA, McDonnell SM. Equine stereotypies. Comp Contin Ed Pract Vet 1993;15:1265–1272.

Author Soraya V. Juarbe-Díaz

Consulting Editor Daniel Q. Estep

LYME DISEASE

BASICS

DEFINITION

Lyme disease is caused by the spirochete *Borrelia burgdorferi*. It is the most frequent tick-borne disease of humans in the United States and has been reported in cats, dogs, cattle, and horses. Serologic surveys indicate the disease is endemic in various regions of the United States and United Kingdom; however, only isolated clinical cases of Lyme disease in horses have been documented.

Definitive diagnosis in horses is difficult and clinical diagnosis is usually presumptive, based on clinical signs, a history of tick exposure in an endemic region, supportive serology, and response to treatment.

Shifting lameness is the most common presenting complaint. Associated clinical signs include polyarthritis, limb edema, stiffness, lethargy, unwillingness to work, and low-grade fever. Uveitis and neurologic disease have been described, and there is a possibility that multi-organ involvement and transplacental transmission may occur.

PATHOPHYSIOLOGY

• The pathogenesis is not known. The disease has not been reproduced experimentally. The incubation period is unknown. Infection has resulted in shedding of the spirochete in the urine and seroconversion 3–8 weeks later.
• There has been seroconversion of in-contact research animals, but no seroconversion has been reported in horses. • *Borrelia* organisms are transmitted by an *Ixodes* tick. The ticks become infected with their first blood meal from an infected host. The spirochete penetrates the gut epithelium and invades the salivary gland. The *Borrelia* cause a localized skin infection after the tick has been feeding for 24 hr. The *Borrelia* multiplies at the site of the tick bite. A bacteremia follows, disseminating the spirochete. • It is currently unknown whether the arthritis is caused by deposition of immune complexes or due to joint sepsis.
• Because *Borrelia* is a gram-negative organism, the release of endotoxin may be involved as a mediator of clinical signs.

SYSTEMS AFFECTED

• Musculoskeletal—polyarthritis, stiffness, lameness • Hemic/lymphatic/immune—distal limb edema • Ophthalmic—uveitis
• Nervous—encephalitis, meningitis

INCIDENCE/PREVALENCE

Borrelia burgdorferi has a worldwide distribution in humans, with reports of disease in horses limited to the United States and the United Kingdom. Seroprevalence from horses in the United States has ranged from <1% in nonendemic areas to 68% in endemic areas. Seroprevalence in horses in the United Kingdom is increased in areas that have a high incidence of human and canine Lyme disease.

SIGNALMENT

Non-specific

SIGNS

• Suspected clinical cases of Lyme disease have been reported only from endemic areas. The common reported clinical findings are arthritis, polyarthritis, shifting lameness, distal limb edema, low-grade fever, and lethargy. Lameness usually shifts in location. The lameness can be associated with joint or periarticular pain without swelling, lasting hours to a few days in each location; or it can be overt arthritis, with swelling of one or more joints, lasting days to a few weeks and often reoccurring. Reoccurring episodes can lead to chronic inflammatory arthritis. • Behavior changes may be seen with reluctance to work and lethargy.
• Anterior uveitis with the clinical signs of blepharospasm, photophobia, aqueous flare, hypopyon, and miosis have been reported to occur but are rare. This may reoccur, resulting in chronic sequelae associated with recurrent uveitis. • Neurologic diseases with clinical signs relating to meningitis and encephalitis have been reported, but are rare. Multiple organ system involvement with clinical signs relating to the organ systems involved has been reported, but is rare. *Borrelia burgdorferi* have been isolated from the kidney, liver, and brain of two foals and a yearling in which transplacental transmission was suspected to have occured; the clinical significance is questionable.

CAUSES

The usual life cycle for *B. burgdorferi* involves an *Ixodes* tick as the vector and a small mammal as the intermediate host for the larval and nymph stage, with a deer or small mammal as the final host for the adult. *Ixodes pacificus* (western black-legged tick) and *I. scapularis* [black-legged tick, now including the reclassified *I. dammini* (deer tick)] are the principal vectors for *B. burgdorferi* in the United States. *Ixodes rinicus* (sheep tick) is the main vector in the United Kingdom. *Ixodes* ticks have a 2-year life cycle. Larvae hatch in the spring and become infected by feeding on the infected intermediate host. The following spring, the larvae molt into nymphs and stay infected; those not infected become infected by feeding on the intermediate host. In fall of the second year, the nymphs molt into adults. After mating, the adult female ticks become engorged with blood from deer or other mammals, fall off, and remain dormant until the following spring, when they lay eggs. Transmission of *B. burgdorferi* usually occurs after 24 hr of feeding by the nymphal-stage or adult female. *Borrelia burgdorferi* have also been found in other arthropods, but none have a proven role in transmission.

RISK FACTORS

Contact with *Ixodes* ticks in Lyme endemic areas. Contact transmission has not been reported between horses.

DIAGNOSIS

DIFFERENTIAL DIAGNOSIS

• Lyme arthritis should be differentiated from infectious causes of arthritis by synovial fluid cytology and culture. Traumatic causes of arthritis can be differentiated by history, radiographic findings, and lack of response to antibiotic therapy. Immune-mediated causes of arthritis can be differentiated on the presence of other systemic clinical signs, synovial fluid cytology, synovial biopsy, and laboratory data, including antinuclear antibodies, lupus erythematosus preparations, and rheumatoid arthritis factor. • Distal limb edema due to Lyme disease should be differentiated from cellulitis, vasculitis (purpura hemorrhagica, EVA, EIA, equine erlichiosis), stocking up from inactivity, and systemic diseases that are immune-mediated or associated with hypoproteinemia. The presence of other physical examination findings, laboratory data, and serologic tests assist in differentiation.
• Cervical vertebral malformation, the encephalitides, rabies, equine protozoal myeloencephalitis, cauda equina syndrome, spinal nematodiasis, space-occupying lesion, and equine herpes-virus-1 should differentiated from the neurologic manifestation of Lyme disease by radiographs, serology, and cerebrospinal fluid analysis. • Causes of uveitis, including ocular trauma and infectious agents such as *Toxoplasma, Onchocerca cervicalis, Leptospira* spp., *Streptococcus,* and viral agents should be investigated. *Onchocerca* microfilariae and viral inclusion bodies can be found in conjunctival scraping and biopsy. Rising serum titers may be associated with *Leptospira* spp. and *Toxoplasma.*

CBC/BIOCHEMISTRY/URINALYSIS

Hematologic and biochemical analysis of blood is usually unremarkable. Serum biochemistry profile may reflect specific organ involvement.

OTHER LABORATORY TESTS

• Culture and isolation of *B. burgdorferi* is difficult and requires special media (Barbour-Stoenner-Kelly). It may be possible from blood, urine, and CSF. • Immunofluorescence assay (IFA), enzyme-linked immunosorbent assay (ELISA), and Western immunoblot have been used to detect *B. burgdorferi* antibodies in serum, CSF, synovial fluid, and aqueous humor. ELISA is reportedly more sensitive and specific than IFA. The Western immunoblot is recommended if false positives are suspected. • Positive serologic results indicate exposure to *B. burgdorferi* but do not indicate clinical disease. Four-fold rising titers from samples 2 weeks apart support recent exposure to *Borrelia*. False-negative results with ELISA can occur in first few weeks of infection prior to seroconversion and with concurrent use of antibiotics. False-positive results may occur due to cross-reactivity with other *Borrelia* spp. More recently, polymerase chain reaction (PCR) testing has been described that will further assist in the diagnosis of the clinical disease.

IMAGING

Radiographs are useful in assisting with the differential diagnosis of lameness and neurologic dysfunction, as well as in evaluating chronic Lyme arthritis.

DIAGNOSTIC PROCEDURES

• Synovial fluid analyses—may have a neutrophilic inflammation, 10,000–25,000 neutrophils. • Synovial biopsy—histopathology, IFA, PCR. • CSF analysis—higher titer of IgG antibody to *B. burgdorferi* in CSF compared to serum suggests an active intrathecal infection.

PATHOLOGIC FINDINGS

Gross findings in cases with suspected Lyme disease in horses relate to the organ system involved. Joints from Lyme arthritis and polyarthritis may have a congested hyperplastic synovial membrane, with a small number of small pale nodules. Histopathology of affected tissues may show a lymphoplasmacytic infiltrate. Immunohistochemical staining and PCR may detect *B. burgdorferi* in affected tissues.

TREATMENT

APPROPRIATE HEALTH CARE

Horses with Lyme disease can be treated as outpatients.

NURSING CARE

Polyarthritis and distal limb edema—cold hosing, supportive standing wraps.

ACTIVITY

Reduced activity until clinical signs have resolved.

DIET

No diet change necessary.

CLIENT EDUCATION

Examine horse after riding through bush and remove ticks with tweezers or gloves.

SURGICAL CONSIDERATIONS

Synovial biopsy via arthroscopic guidance for assistance in diagnosis.

MEDICATIONS

DRUG(S) OF CHOICE

The recommended antibiotics for treatment are procaine penicillin G (20,000–40,000 IU/kg q12h IM), oxytetracycline (6.6–11 mg/kg q12h IV), and ampicillin (10–15 mg/kg q6h IV). Duration of antibiotic therapy is guided by clinical response. Early infections are generally treated for 2–3 weeks. If CNS involvement is present, penicillin G (20,000–40,000 IU/kg q6h IV) or a third-generation cephalosporin with the ability to penetrate the blood–brain barrier, such as ceftriaxone (20–50 mg/kg q12h IV) is recommended. Anti-inflammatory therapy may be used with antibiotic therapy, but can make monitoring response to treatment difficult by masking clinical signs. Therapy for uveitis is aimed at reducing inflammation and providing mydriasis and analgesia.

PRECAUTIONS

Colitis may occur secondary to antimicrobial therapy.

POSSIBLE INTERACTIONS

Jarisch–Herxheimer reactions have been reported in humans during the treatment of spirochetal disease. This reaction involves the exacerbation of clinical signs with antibiotic therapy. It is believed to be an immune-associated reaction caused by the release of endotoxin protein and products of lysed spirochetes. Pyrexia associated with the initiation of tetracycline therapy has been documented in one equine case.

ALTERNATIVE DRUGS

Corticosteroid therapy remains controversial. Corticosteroids administered intra-articularly have been used occasionally in human patients. If some manifestations of Lyme disease are immune-mediated, response to antibiotics may be slow or absent, and corticosteroid therapy may be useful.

FOLLOW-UP

PATIENT MONITORING

A marked improvement in clinical signs should be seen after the commencement of antibiotic therapy.

PREVENTION/AVOIDANCE

No vaccine is currently available for horses. Avoid tick-infested areas endemic for Lyme disease. The horse should be carefully groomed daily to remove ticks. Use appropriate insecticide sprays approved for horses for tick removal (not amitraz). Isolation of horses suspected of having Lyme disease is not necessary.

POSSIBLE COMPLICATIONS

• Chronic inflammatory arthritis • Recurrent episodes of uveitis • Irreversible CNS damage

EXPECTED COURSE AND PROGNOSIS

Recovery should be expected within a week of commencement of antibiotic therapy. The reported cases with multi-organ involvement did not survive. Horses with neurologic dysfunction or arthritis may survive, but be unable to return to previous athletic performance.

MISCELLANEOUS

AGE-RELATED FACTORS

No reported age predisposition.

ZOONOTIC POTENTIAL

No zoonotic potential. Humans in contact with infected horses may have increased risk of infection due to increased exposure from animals bringing ticks into their environment.

PREGNANCY

Evidence of intrauterine infection of foals has been reported with *B. burgdorferi* isolated from the kidney and brain of one foal with positive serum titers and from the kidney from another foal without serum titers. The significance of the isolated organisms is questionable.

SYNONYMS

• Borreliosis • Lyme arthritis • Lyme borreliosis

ABBREVIATIONS

• EIA = Enzyme immunoassay • ELISA = Enzyme-linked immunosorbent assay
• EVA = Equine viral arteritis • IFA = Immunofluorescence assay • PCR = polymerase chain reaction

Suggested Reading

Madigan JE. Lyme disease (Lyme borreliosis) in horses. Vet Clin North Am Eq Pract 19XX;9:429-434.

Cohen ND. Borreliosis (Lyme disease) in horses. Eq Vet Ed 1996;8:213-215.

Manion TB, Bushmich SL, Mittel L, et al. Lyme disease in horses: serological and antigen testing differences. AAEP Proc 1998;44:144-145.

Cohen ND, Cohen D. Borreliosis in horses: a comparative review. Comp Cont Ed 1990;44:1449-1457.

Author Jane E. Axon
Consulting Editor Corinne R. Sweeney

LYME DISEASE, BORRELIOSIS

BASICS

DEFINITION
An immune-mediated disorder associated with a tick-borne spirochete, *Borrelia burgdorferi*

PATHOPHYSIOLOGY
See *Lyme Disease.*

SYSTEMS AFFECTED
Multisystem disease

SIGNALMENT
Nonspecific

SIGNS
Historical Findings
- Chronic, nonresponsive disease often is present.
- Findings can include chronic weight loss, lameness, laminitis, chronic fever, enlarged and distended joints, myalgia, anterior uveitis, and less frequently, generalized neurologic disease.

Physical Examination Findings
- Neurological disease often manifests peracutely.
- Early signs can vary from subtle clumsiness and/or stiffness to dog-sitting and to recumbency.
- Severe trunkal and limb paresis and ataxia occurs in 24–72 hours.
- A distended, paralytic bladder, with urinary incontinence, often is present.
- Reduced tail muscle tone with perineal hypalgesia can be seen.
- Brain-stem deficits rarely are seen.
- Affected horses most often have normal mentation, but depression can occur.
- Clinical signs often stabilize and improve a few days after onset but, occasionally, can worsen.
- Initially, neurologic deficits can be symmetric or asymmetric in one or more limbs.
- Thoracolumbar lesions seem to occur most commonly.
- Pelvic limb signs tend to be most severe.

CAUSES
Tick-borne spirochete, *B. burgdorferi*

RISK FACTORS
Horses maintained in high-risk regions

DIAGNOSIS

DIFFERENTIAL DIAGNOSIS
- Equine herpes virus-1
- Trauma
- Equine protozoal myeloencephalitis

CBC/BIOCHEMISTRY/URINALYSIS
No consistent abnormalities

OTHER LABORATORY TESTS
No consistent abnormalities

IMAGING
N/A

DIAGNOSTIC PROCEDURES
- Positive serology with suspect clinical signs must be interpreted with caution.
- Positive PCR from synovial fluid or CSF samples should be considered confirmatory.

LYME DISEASE, BORRELIOSIS

TREATMENT

Supportive management

MEDICATIONS

DRUGS OF CHOICE

- Oxytetracycline (1mg/kg IV q24h)
- Cephalosporins may be used if neural disease associated with *B. burgdorferi* is suspected.

CONTRAINDICATIONS

N/A

PRECAUTIONS

N/A

POSSIBLE INTERACTIONS

N/A

ALTERNATIVE DRUGS

N/A

FOLLOW-UP

PATIENT MONITORING

Prognosis is fair for complete recovery.

POSSIBLE COMPLICATIONS

- Trauma associated with weakness and attempts at rising
- Decubital sores
- Paralytic bladder with secondary urinary tract infection

MISCELLANEOUS

ASSOCIATED CONDITIONS

Secondary urinary tract infection

AGE-RELATED FACTORS

N/A

ZOONOTIC POTENTIAL

N/A

PREGNANCY

Abortion may occur before, during, or after development of neurologic signs.

SYNONYMS

N/A

SEE ALSO

N/A

ABBREVIATIONS

- CSF = cerebrospinal fluid
- PCR = polymerase chain reaction

Suggested Reading

Hahn CN, et al. A possible case of lyme borreliosis in a horse in the UK. Equine Vet 1996;28:84–88.

Parker JL, White KW. Lyme borreliosis in cattle and horses: a review of the literature. Cornell Vet 1992;82:253–274.

Author Joseph J Bertone

Consulting Editor Joseph J Bertone

LYMPHADENOPATHY

BASICS

DEFINITION

A local, regional, or generalized enlargement of lymph nodes

PATHOPHYSIOLOGY

- Depends on the underlying disease process. Lymph nodes may be enlarged locally from regional drainage of pathologic processes; lymph nodes enlarge due to inflammation (i.e., acute or chronic lymphadenitis) and neoplasia.
- Lymph nodes in acute lymphadenitis frequently are soft, hyperemic, and may be necrotic. Lymph nodes in chronic lymphadenitis are hard and somewhat indurated. A classification of benign or malignant hyperplasia is based on histologic evaluation.
- Benign enlargement is characterized by variably sized lymphocytes with mixed populations of plasma cells, neutrophils, and macrophages. Neoplastic processes have a monomorphic population of cells that may obliterate the normal node architecture. Generalized enlargement of lymph nodes throughout the body usually reflects a neoplastic process or systemic infection.

SYSTEM AFFECTED

- Depends on underlying cause
- Hemic/lymphatic/immune—most common
- Thoracic and abdominal lymphadenopathy—may have primary respiratory or abdominal signs

SIGNALMENT

N/A

SIGNS

General Comments

History and clinical signs depend on underlying cause and location of enlarged lymph nodes.

Physical Examination Findings

- Palpable enlargement of regional or all lymph nodes depending on cause; may be warm, painful swellings or draining, purulent material.
- Submandibular and retropharyngeal lymphadenopathy may cause anorexia and dysphagia.
- Anorectal lymphadenopathy may cause dyschezia and abdominal pain.
- Nonspecific signs—pale mucous membranes, depression, anorexia, weight loss, tachypnea, tachycardia, respiratory distress, elevated rectal temperature, ventral edema, edema of the peripheral limbs, ascites, pleural effusion, or other signs associated with the underlying disease

CAUSES

Infectious

Multiple viral, bacterial, fungal, and protozoal infections, including *Streptococcus equi, Corynebacterium pseudotuberculosis, Mycobacterium avium-intracellulare,* nonspecific blood-borne infections, strongylus infection, echinococcosis, and trypanosomiasis

Neoplastic

Lymphoma, melanoma, and leukemia

Toxic

Silicosis

Idiopathic

Anorectal lymphadenopathy

RISK FACTORS

Recent respiratory infections in stablemates

DIAGNOSIS

DIFFERENTIAL DIAGNOSIS

- Primary thoracic lesion—complete work-up for upper or lower respiratory insufficiency indicated, including endoscopy of upper and lower airways and radiography/ultrasound of throat and thorax
- Primary intestinal lesion–complete work-up for abdominal pain indicated, including abdominal auscultation, rectal examination, nasogastric intubation, abdominocentesis, and exploratory celiotomy
- Abdominal abscess–CBC for increased WBC, fibrinogen, and total protein; abdominocentesis for high WBC count and elevated protein; cytology for inflammation; culture for bacteria; rectal examination for abdominal mass
- Abdominal neoplasia–sonography of all abdominal organs; work-up similar to abdominal abscess

CBC/BIOCHEMISTRY/URINALYSIS

Highly variable—anemia, thrombocytopenia, leukopenia or leukocytosis, neutropenia or neutrophilia, lymphopenia or lymphocytosis, hyperproteinemia or hypoproteinemia, and hyperfibrinogenemia

OTHER LABORATORY TESTS

Bone marrow aspirate and biopsy, abdominocentesis, serology for infectious agents, and blood culture

LYMPHADENOPATHY

IMAGING

- Ultrasonography of local and regional drainage areas (thorax or abdomen) to assess size, detect extent of multiple lymph node involvement, detect infiltrative disease, and allow for guided biopsy
- Thoracic radiography for pulmonary lymphadenopathy

DIAGNOSTIC PROCEDURES

- Rectal palpation
- Lymph node aspiration
- Lymph node biopsy and culture

TREATMENT

Aimed at the underlying disease—antimicrobials, antiparasitics, anti-inflammatories, antineoplastics, surgical drainage or removal, and supportive care

MEDICATIONS

Vary with the underlying cause

DRUGS OF CHOICE

N/A

CONTRAINDICATIONS

N/A

PRECAUTIONS

N/A

POSSIBLE INTERACTIONS

N/A

ALTERNATIVE DRUGS

N/A

FOLLOW-UP

PATIENT MONITORING

N/A

POSSIBLE COMPLICATIONS

N/A

MISCELLANEOUS

ASSOCIATED CONDITIONS

Lymphadenopathy usually is representative of another underlying disease process; a complete diagnostic work-up is warranted to evaluate the extent of disease.

AGE-RELATED FACTORS

N/A

ZOONOTIC POTENTIAL

N/A

PREGNANCY

N/A

SYNONYMS

N/A

SEE ALSO

- *Streptococcus equi* (strangles)
- *Corynebacterium pseudotuberculosis*
- Neoplasia
- Lymphosarcoma

Suggested Reading

Jubb RVFK, Kennedy PC, Palmer N, eds. Pathology of domestic animals. 4th ed. San Diego: Academic Press, 1998.

Author Maureen T. Long
Consulting Editor Debra C. Sellon

LYMPHOCYTIC–PLASMACYTIC ENTERITIS

BASICS

OVERVIEW

Lymphocytic–plasmacytic enteritis (LPE) is a pathologic description of a type of infiltrative intestinal disease within the complex of idiopathic inflammatory bowel disease in the horse. Malabsorption and protein-losing enteropathy results due to the diffuse infiltration of well-differentiated lymphocytes and plasma cells into the lamina propria, between crypts, and sometimes in the submucosa of the small intestine and to a lesser extent the large intestine. Normal fecal consistency indicates that the majority of the large intestine is functional.

SIGNALMENT

Median age 13 yr ($n = 10$)

SIGNS

- Chronic weight loss
- Thin to emaciated
- Generalized weakness
- Depression (mild)
- Poor appetite
- Normal feces consistency
- Normal vital signs
- Intermittent colic
- Per rectal examination—Firm mass in craniodorsal abdomen suggestive of enlargement of the lymph nodes in the region of the cranial mesenteric artery

CAUSES AND RISK FACTORS

Exact cause unknown, although there is a strong probability that LPE is an immune-mediated disorder.

DIAGNOSIS

DIFFERENTIAL DIAGNOSIS

- Malnutrition
- Internal parasitism
- Granulomatous enteritis
- Alimentary lymphosarcoma
- Eosinophilic enteritis
- Multisystemic eosinphilic epitheliotropic complex
- Tuberculosis
- Histoplasmosis
- Basophilic enterocolitis

CBC/BIOCHEMISTRY/URINALYSIS

- Hypoproteinemia
- Marked hypoalbuminemia
- Marked hyperglobulinemia
- Normal urinalysis

OTHER LABORATORY TESTS

- D-xylose absorption test/oral glucose absorption test: abnormal
- Serum protein electrophoresis abnormal

IMAGING

N/A

DIAGNOSTIC PROCEDURES

- Rectal biopsy—Moderate to large numbers of lymphocytes and plasma cells seen in the lamina propria.
- Definitive diagnosis by small intestine biopsy—Standing flank or laparosopy; infiltration with lymphocytes and plasma cells

LYMPHOCYTIC-PLASMACYTIC ENTERITIS

TREATMENT

Poor prognosis

MEDICATIONS

DRUG(S) OF CHOICE

Corticosteroids (e.g., prednisolone at 2.2 mm/kg SID IM. Anecdotal reports of some response in some cases when given for several weeks.

CONTRAINDICATIONS/POSSIBLE INTERACTIONS

Corticosteroids at this dosage are immunosuppressive and also may have significant metabolic side effects. Therapy should be withdrawn gradually.

FOLLOW-UP

N/A

MISCELLEANEOUS

ABBREVIATION

- LPE = lymphocytic–plasmacytic enteritis

Suggested Reading

Clark ES, Morris DD, Allen D, Tyler DE. Lymphocytic enteritis in a filly. J Am Vet Med Assoc 1988;193:1281-1283.

Kemper DL, Perkins GA, Schumacher, Edwards JF, Valentine BA, Divers T J, Cohen ND. Equine lymphocytic–plasmacytic enterocolitis: 10 cases. Proc 6th Equine Colic Res Sympos 1998;20.

MacAllister CG, Mosier D, Qualls CW Jr, Cowell RL. Lymphocytic-plasmacytic enteritis in two horses. J Am Vet Med Assoc 1990;196:1995-1998.

Author John D. Baird

Consulting Editor Henry Stämpfli

LYMPHOCYTOSIS

BASICS

DEFINITION
• An absolute number of circulating lymphocytes greater than the reference interval, or $>5.1 \times 10^3$ cells/μL
• Absolute lymphocyte counts may be greater in young horses.

PATHOPHYSIOLOGY
• Lymphocytes originate from lymphoid stem cells in the bone marrow and are necessary for both acquired and innate immunity to pathogens.
• B lymphocytes derive from the bone marrow and are responsible for antibody production and antigen presentation.
• T cells mature in the thymus, regulate the immune response, and provide cell-mediated immunity.
• Both B and T cells are found in peripheral blood, but T cells greatly predominate.
• T cells recirculate from blood to the lymphoid tissues.
• Antigenic stimulation can cause memory T and B cells, and then clonal proliferation of these cells.
• In general, B and T cells cannot be differentiated on a peripheral blood smear.
• Antigenically stimulated lymphocytes are called reactive lymphocytes or immunocytes. These are large cells with deeply basophilic cytoplasm and large nuclei with rather coarse chromatin.
• NK cells are present in the peripheral blood of horses but constitute a very small percentage of the lymphoid population. They contain few numbers of small, azurophilic cytoplasmic granules and are important to the innate immune response.

SYSTEM AFFECTED
Hemic/Lymph/Immune:
• Spleen and liver affected as a result of hyperplasia or neoplasia
• Bone marrow affected as a result of neoplasia
• Lymphosarcoma can present as multicentric, alimentary, cutaneous, or mediastinal forms.

SIGNALMENT
All horses

SIGNS
• With a physiologic cause, an excited horse exhibiting increased heart rate and blood pressure is presented.
• With antigenic stimulation, look for signs of infectious process—respiratory disease
• Mediastinal or visceral lymphosarcoma can result in thoracic or abdominal effusion containing neoplastic cells. Affected horses may present with weight loss, diarrhea, depression, fever, lymphadenopathy, anorexia, venous distention, subcutaneous edema, and anemia.

CAUSES

Physiologic
• Physiologic lymphocytosis associated with excitement or exercise commonly occurs in horses < 2 years of age.
• Lymphocyte counts are 6000–15,000 cells/μL.
• Epinephrine is released in response to fear, excitement, or vigorous exercise. Epinephrine may block receptors on endothelial cells of postcapillary venules in lymph nodes, prevent lymphocytes from re-entering lymphoid tissue, or increase capillary blood flow with release of marginated cells.
• Lymphocytes also may be released into the general circulation from other sources.
• The lymphocytosis develops in minutes and lasts 20–30 minutes.

Antigenic Stimulation
• Occasionally causes lymphocytosis.
• Chronic inflammation—severe bacterial infection or viral infection; often see reactive lymphocytes on peripheral blood smears.
• Vaccination—reactive lymphocytes on peripheral blood smears

Lymphosarcoma or Lymphoid Leukemia
• Lymphosarcoma affects horses of all ages but is most common in adults.
• Lymphocytosis or neoplastic cells are uncommon in the peripheral blood of horses with lymphosarcoma.
• Lymphoid leukemia is uncommon in horses.

RISK FACTORS
N/A

DIAGNOSIS

DIFFERENTIAL DIAGNOSIS
Thin horses with depression, fever, and lymphadenopathy—consider lymphosarcoma or chronic inflammatory diseases.

LABORATORY FINDINGS

Drugs That May Alter Lab Results
• Epinephrine and other β-adrenergic agonists
• Corticosteroids
• Methimazole

Disorders That May Alter Lab Results
• Must be able to differentiate lymphoblasts (i.e., neoplastic cells) from reactive lymphocytes.
• Incorrect identification of nucleated RBC or monocytes as lymphocytes.

Valid If Run in Human Lab?
Human labs often do not review equine blood smears; such smears must be reviewed by veterinary-trained technologists.

LYMPHOCYTOSIS

CBC/BIOCHEMISTRY/URINALYSIS

- Mature neutrophilia (WBC count, 12,000–25,000 cells/μL)—consider physiologic response and antigenic stimulation.
- Lymphocytosis of > 20,000 cells/μL—consider lymphoid leukemia.
- Immature, bizarre lymphocytes in circulation—consider acute lymphoid leukemia (rare); rule out reactive lymphocytosis.
- Nonregenerative anemia, leukopenia, and thrombocytopenia—consider myelophthisic disease (i.e., lymphosarcoma/lymphoid leukemia).
- Hypercalcemia—consider lymphosarcoma.

OTHER LABORATORY TESTS

Protein electrophoresis may detect polyclonal or, rarely, monoclonal gammopathy with lymphosarcoma.

IMAGING

Hepatosplenomegaly, mediastinal mass—consider lymphosarcoma.

DIAGNOSTIC PROCEDURES

Aspiration cytology of pleural fluid, liver, or mass or biopsy of tumor mass may establish the diagnosis of lymphosarcoma.

TREATMENT

Directed toward the primary disease causing lymphocytosis.

MEDICATIONS

DRUGS OF CHOICE

Lymphosarcoma—chemotherapy (see appropriate topics)

CONTRAINDICATIONS

N/A

PRECAUTIONS

N/A

POSSIBLE INTERACTIONS

Levamisole can act as an immunomodulator to increase lymphocyte function.

ALTERNATIVE DRUGS

N/A

FOLLOW-UP

PATIENT MONITORING

N/A

POSSIBLE COMPLICATIONS

N/A

MISCELLANEOUS

ASSOCIATED CONDITIONS

N/A

AGE-RELATED FACTORS

Physiologic lymphocytosis commonly occurs in horses < 2 years of age.

ZOONOTIC POTENTIAL

N/A

PREGNANCY

N/A

SYNONYMS

N/A

SEE ALSO

- Leukemia, lymphoid
- Lymphosarcoma

ABBREVIATION

NK = natural killer

Suggested Reading

Duncan JR, Prasse KW, Mahaffey EA. Veterinary laboratory medicine: clinical pathology. Ames: Iowa State University Press, 1994.

Eades SC, Bounous DI. Laboratory profiles of equine diseases. St. Louis: Mosby–Year Book, 1997.

Author Denise I. Bounous

Consulting Auther Claire B. Andreasen

LYMPHOSARCOMA

BASICS

DEFINITION
A malignant, neoplastic disorder of lymphoid tissue

PATHOPHYSIOLOGY
- Classification of equine lymphoid tumors by cell type is still being determined. Neoplastic cells may be either B cells (most common), T cells, or non-B, non-T cells; other cell types generally are present within the tumor as well.
- Clinical signs may result from several mechanisms—infiltration of tissues by neoplastic lymphocytes leading to loss of normal function, physical obstruction by tumor masses, or activity of tumor cytokines
- Compromised humoral or cellular immunity has been identified in some cases and may contribute to secondary infections.
- Occasionally associated with immune-mediated hemolytic disease or thrombocytopenia, possibly due to antibody production by neoplastic B cells

SYSTEMS AFFECTED
- Hemic/lymphatic/immune—a neoplastic condition of lymphoid tissue.
- Four major anatomic forms based on the site of tumor involvement—multicentric, alimentary, mediastinal, and cutaneous.
- A leukemic form characterized by peripheral lymphocytosis with circulating atypical lymphocytes or lymphoblasts is uncommonly encountered.
- Considerable overlap between forms
- Almost any tissue may be affected—most common: lymph nodes, liver, spleen, GI tract, kidneys, and lungs; occasional involvement: nervous, ophthalmic, and reproductive systems

GENETICS
N/A

INCIDENCE/PREVALENCE
- Most common neoplasm of the equine hemolymphatic system
- Prevalence estimated at 2–5%

SIGNALMENT
- Age of onset typically 5–10 years (range, birth to 25 years; also identified in an aborted fetus).
- No breed or sex predilections

SIGNS

General Comments
- Clinical signs vary depending on the lesion location and duration and often are vague, making diagnosis difficult.
- Tends to be slowly progressive, although the onset may appear to be acute.

Historical Findings
- Client complaints vary depending on the systems involved.
- Weight loss, depression, or decreased performance frequently are reported.

Physical Examination Findings
- Most common—depression and weight loss
- Fever
- Lymphadenopathy—usually regional (e.g., intra-abdominal); only occasionally peripheral lymphadenopathy
- Ventral edema
- Thoracic involvement may result in dyspnea, cough, or pleural effusion.
- GI involvement may result in colic, diarrhea, or weight loss.
- Variable neurologic signs depending on location of the lesion
- Rectal palpation may reveal splenic enlargement, internal lymphadenopathy, or abdominal mass
- Cutaneous—multiple dermal or subcutaneous nodules, 1–20 cm, regional or generalized; seldom associated with internal organ involvement

CAUSES
- Undetermined
- No documented viral cause

RISK FACTORS
N/A

DIAGNOSIS

DIFFERENTIAL DIAGNOSIS
- Chronic inflammatory disease—particularly internal abscessation
- Infectious diseases associated with anemia, fever, and weight loss (e.g., EIA and babesiosis). Appropriate diagnostic tests to rule out specific infectious agents may be indicated when considering lymphosarcoma.
- Immune-mediated hemolytic disease from other causes
- Plasma cell myeloma—characterized by proliferation of neoplastic plasma cells.
- Diagnosis supported by monoclonal gammopathy, light-chain proteinuria, and plasmacytosis in bone marrow or soft tissues

CBC/BIOCHEMISTRY/URINALYSIS
- Laboratory findings—variable and nonspecific
- Most common findings—nonspecific changes consistent with chronic inflammatory disease (i.e., anemia, hyperglobulinemia, and a mild neutrophilic leukocytosis with hyperfibrinogenemia).
- In addition to suppression of erythropoiesis from chronic disease, possible causes of anemia in these cases include bone marrow infiltration, immune-mediated hemolytic disease, and blood loss.
- Hyperglobulinemia—most often due to a polyclonal gammopathy; however, monoclonal gammopathy has been described.
- Total plasma protein varies, but the albumin:globulin ratio often is decreased. Total protein may be markedly decreased in cases with alimentary involvement.
- Lymphocytic leukemia characterized by peripheral lymphocytosis and large numbers of circulating neoplastic lymphocytes—rare and typically associated with bone marrow involvement.
- Atypical lymphocytes—occasionally seen in the circulation, even in cases with normal or decreased total lymphocytes.
- Chemistry—variable, depending on the location and severity of internal organ involvement
- Hypercalcemia associated with pseudohyperparathyroidism of malignancy has been reported.

OTHER LABORATORY TESTS
- Bone marrow examination may reveal neoplastic lymphocytes.
- Oral glucose or xylose absorption test may be abnormal in cases with intestinal involvement.
- Coombs' test—positive in cases with associated immune-mediated hemolytic disease
- Low serum IgM concentration reported in some cases, but this is an inconsistent and nonspecific finding.

IMAGING

Ultrasound and radiography may be useful in demonstrating internal organ involvement and in guiding biopsies.

DIAGNOSTIC PROCEDURES

- Definitive diagnosis depends on demonstration of neoplastic lymphocytes. In some cases, differentiating neoplastic lymphocytes from reactive lymphocytes or mesothelial cells is difficult.
- Histologic examination of a biopsy specimen from affected tissue is most reliable; an excisional biopsy is preferred. Without lymphadenopathy or the presence of masses, the diagnosis often is difficult to make.
- Cytologic evaluation of pleural or peritoneal fluid, tissue aspirates, and rarely, peripheral blood smears.
- Laparoscopy or exploratory laparotomy may be helpful, but in some cases, definitive diagnosis can be made only at postmortem examination.

PATHOLOGIC FINDINGS

- Gross lesions may include lymphadenopathy, solitary or multiple masses, splenomegaly, or diffuse infiltration of tissues.
- Neoplastic lymphocytes have variable morphology and may be poorly to well differentiated; disruption of normal tissue architecture aids in diagnosing neoplasia.
- Characteristics of neoplastic lymphocytes—large lymphoid cells with a variable nuclear:cytoplasmic ratio, multiple nucleoli, nuclear chromatin clumping, cytoplasmic basophilia, vacuolation, mitotic figures, and binucleate cells

TREATMENT

APPROPRIATE HEALTH CARE

Inpatient or outpatient, depending on the location and extent of disease

NURSING CARE

N/A

ACTIVITY

Depends on the extent of disease

DIET

N/A

CLIENT EDUCATION

N/A

SURGICAL CONSIDERATIONS

Limited studies in horses with alimentary lymphosarcoma suggest that surgical resection of the mass and associated intestine may prolong survival in cases without evidence of metastasis.

MEDICATIONS

DRUGS OF CHOICE

- Generalized forms—still uncommon. Corticosteroids have been used as symptomatic treatment or to control paraneoplastic disorders (e.g., hemolytic anemia). Combination chemotherapy protocols similar to those for small animals and radiation therapy have caused remission, but the response usually is transient.
- Cutaneous—some cases spontaneously regress, with or without recurrence; may respond to corticosteroids.

CONTRAINDICATIONS

N/A

PRECAUTIONS

N/A

POSSIBLE INTERACTIONS

N/A

ALTERNATIVE DRUGS

N/A

FOLLOW-UP

PATIENT MONITORING

Reduced lymphadenopathy or mass size, weight gain, and improvement in attitude or clinical signs (e.g., colic) can be used to monitor the efficacy of therapy.

PREVENTION/AVOIDANCE

N/A

POSSIBLE COMPLICATIONS

N/A

EXPECTED COURSE AND PROGNOSIS

Grave for most forms, with most horses succumbing within 6 months of the onset of clinical signs.

MISCELLANEOUS

ASSOCIATED CONDITIONS

- Immune-mediated hemolytic disease and thrombocytopenia
- Immunosuppression

AGE-RELATED FACTORS

N/A

ZOONOTIC POTENTIAL

N/A

PREGNANCY

Chemotherapy and radiation therapy pose potential risk to the fetus; however, chemotherapy has successfully maintained two pregnant mares with lymphoproliferative disease until foaling, with the result of viable foals.

SYNONYMS

- Malignant lymphoma
- Lymphoma

SEE ALSO

Selective IgM deficiency

ABBREVIATIONS

- EIA = equine infectious anemia
- GI = gastrointestinal

Suggested Reading

Byrne BA, Yvorchuk-St. Jean K, Couto CG, Kohn CW. Successful management of lymphoproliferative disease in two pregnant mares. Proc Vet Cancer Soc 1991:8–9.

Carlson GP. Lymphosarcoma in horses. In: Smith BP, ed. Large animal internal medicine. 2nd ed. St. Louis: Mosby–Year Book, 1996:1242–1243.

Dabreiner RM, Sullins KE, Goodrich LR. Large colon resection for treatment of lymphosarcoma in two horses. J Am Vet Med Assoc 1996;208:895–897.

Rebhun WC, Bertone A. Equine lymphosarcoma. J Am Vet Med Assoc 1984;184:720–721.

Author Melissa T. Hines

Consulting Editor Debra C. Sellon

MAGNESIUM, HYPOMAGNESEMIA

BASICS

DEFINITION

- Serum magnesium $<$ the reference interval (e.g., <1.1 mg/dL or <0.45 mM/L)
- Published reports list 1.82 ± 0.73 mg/dL as normal, but most laboratories list a higher interval.

PATHOPHYSIOLOGY

- Magnesium is the second most abundant intracellular cation (after potassium) in the horse.
- The equine body contains $\cong 0.05\%$ magnesium by weight, 60% of which is in the bones.
- Because $<1\%$ of magnesium is in the serum, serum concentrations may not be a good indicator of total-body magnesium.
- Digestive secretions contain considerable magnesium (0.5–5.1 mg/kg per day), so continual losses occur in the feces. If absorption by the distal small intestine does not keep up with this loss, magnesium levels decrease.
- Magnesium is excreted by the kidneys, which play a major role in regulating magnesium balance by controlling tubular reabsorption.
- Magnesium also is secreted into the milk of lactating mares.
- Magnesium has numerous physiologic functions, especially with enzyme activity, but its importance in muscle contraction and neurotransmission accounts for most of the clinical signs when concentrations are inappropriate.
- Magnesium is antagonistic to the actions of calcium.
- Low magnesium levels increase the release of acetylcholine at nerve endings, which can induce tetany.

SYSTEMS AFFECTED

- Neuromuscular
- Nervous
- Endocrine/metabolic
- Cardiovascular

SIGNALMENT

- Lactating mares
- Hard-working draft horses

SIGNS

- Muscle fibrillation
- Weakness
- Hyperreflexia
- Arrhythmias
- Hyperpnea
- Tetany

CAUSES

- Insufficient intake because of poor diet, severe anorexia, or small intestinal disease prevents adequate absorption of magnesium to replace the endogenous loss by intestinal secretions, which continues even without dietary consumption.
- Green forage supplies adequate magnesium, because it is present in chlorophyll. High levels of potassium or nitrogen, however, reduce magnesium absorption.
- The most common causes of low serum magnesium include lack of food intake, diets low in available magnesium, gastrointestinal disturbances, increased lactation, exhaustion, hyperaldosteronism, and hyperthyroidism.

RISK FACTORS

- Anorexia
- Transport
- Surgery
- Lactation
- Diuretics

DIAGNOSIS

DIFFERENTIAL DIAGNOSIS

- The signs of hypomagnesemia vary, so any condition manifesting neuromuscular abnormalities must be considered.
- Other conditions that must be investigated and may have a greater prevalence than hypomagnesemia—eclampsia, botulism, equine lower motor neuron disease, and other less common neuromuscular conditions

LABORATORY FINDINGS

Drugs That May Alter Lab Results

N/A

Disorders That May Alter Lab Results

Hemolysis may increase serum magnesium concentrations.

Valid If Run in Human Lab?

Yes

CBC/BIOCHEMISTRY/URINALYSIS

- Calcium—may be low and accentuate signs.
- Elevated BUN or creatinine, or inability to concentrate urine, could indicate a renal cause.
- Decreased fractional excretion of magnesium indicates inadequate intake.
- Inappropriate, high fractional excretion of magnesium indicates renal disease.
- Other electrolytes may be abnormal—sodium; potassium

OTHER LABORATORY TESTS

Fractional excretion of magnesium, as determined by comparing urinary magnesium and creatinine to serum magnesium and creatinine, helps to differentiate renal from dietary causes.

IMAGING

N/A

DIAGNOSTIC PROCEDURES

- An accurate history of food intake and recent activity is more useful than other invasive tests.
- An electromyogram may reveal the effect, but not the cause, of hypomagnesemia on the muscles.

TREATMENT

- Initiate treatment of the underlying cause, or the condition will persist.
- Increase dietary intake of magnesium, because total body stores may be depleted and, thus, the condition will reoccur.

MEDICATIONS

DRUGS OF CHOICE

If the serum magnesium concentration is low enough to cause clinical signs, administer 20% $MgSO_4$ in water or glucose at 1 mEq/kg IV or to effect; a 10% solution of $MgCl_2$ also can be used.

CONTRAINDICATIONS

Magnesium may potentiate the toxic effect of aminoglycosides.

PRECAUTIONS

- Administer solutions slowly if given IV.
- Use diuretics with caution—excessive doses may lead to hypermagnesemia and CNS depression or potentiation of CNS-depressant drugs.

POSSIBLE INTERACTIONS

- Magnesium sulfate is incompatible with sodium bicarbonate and hydrocortisone.
- Calcium-containing compounds lower serum magnesium concentrations.

ALTERNATIVE DRUGS

N/A

FOLLOW-UP

PATIENT MONITORING

- Determine serum magnesium and calcium concentrations once or twice a day to detect overdosage or recurrence.
- ECG is helpful if arrhythmias are detected.
- Monitor TPR and presenting physical signs both during and after treatment.

POSSIBLE COMPLICATIONS

- Severe hypomagnesemia can lead to tetany, coma, and death.
- Cardiac arrhythmias may develop.

MISCELLANEOUS

ASSOCIATED CONDITIONS

- Hypocalcemia
- Hyponatremia
- Hypokalemia

AGE-RELATED FACTORS

Adult horse, especially lactating mares, and nursing foals are more susceptible.

ZOONOTIC POTENTIAL

N/A

PREGNANCY

Effect on the fetus is the same as that on the dam.

SYNONYMS

Transport tetany

ABBREVIATION

- TPR = temperature, pulse, and respiration

Suggested Reading

Holley DC, Evans JW. Determination of total and ultrafilterable calcium and magnesium in normal equine serum. Am J Vet Res 1977;38:259–262.

Magneson GR, Puvathingal JM, Ray WJ. The concentrations of free Mg^{2+} and free Zn^{2+} in equine blood plasma. J Biol Chem 1987;262:11140–11148.

Rosol TJ, Capen CC. Calcium and magnesium. In: Kaneko JJ, Harvey JW, Bruss ML, eds. Clinical biochemistry of domestic animals. 5th ed. San Diego: Academic Press, 1997:674–687.

Author Erwin G. Pearson

Consulting Editor Claire B. Andreasen

MALABSORPTION

BASICS

DEFINITION

Malabsorption or malassimilation from the intestine occurs when there is diffuse or localized intestinal disease that inhibits the transference of nutrients from the intestinal lumen to the vasculature. Transient malabsorption occurs with enteritis caused by viral and bacterial agents. Chronic malabsorption is caused by parasitism, infiltrative bowel diseases, amyloidosis, and neoplasia. Besides parasitism, the causes of chronic inflammatory bowel disease are uncommon. The small intestine is usually affected in the chronic diseases; however, the large intestine may also be involved.

PATHOPHYSIOLOGY

Malabsorption is caused by loss of the intestinal absorptive area (villus atrophy), loss of absorptive villus epithelial cells, and enlargement of junctional areas between epithelial cells. Thickening of the intestinal wall with edema, inflammatory cells, or fibrous tissue inhibits the absorptive capacity. Blockage of normal lymphatic drainage (lymphangiectasia) and decreased intestinal blood flow due to verminous arteritis may be involved. Horses that have had extensive small intestinal resection may also suffer from malabsorption.

Viral and bacterial infections of the bowel wall can result in the temporary loss of the absorptive capacity of the small intestine.

Chronic malabsorption is caused by uncontrolled immune reactions (infiltrative bowel diseases, such as lymphocytic/plasmacytic enteritis, granulomatous enteritis, or eosinophilic granulomatous enteritis). The initiating factors in this group of diseases are unknown; however, allergens or infectious agents may be stimuli. Chronic diseases include infections with *Mycobacterium avium, Mycobacterium paratuberculosis,* and fungi (*Aspergillus* spp., *Histoplasma* spp.). Alimentary neoplasia may also cause similar signs.

Transient malabsorption may result in short-term weight loss, delayed growth, and diarrhea. These problems should resolve once the infection and immune reaction subside and the intestines achieve normal structure and function. The signs of chronic malabsorption persist; however, the progression and severity may vary. A hallmark of chronic disease is hypoproteinemia resulting from decreased protein intake (due to inappetance), malabsorption of nutrients, and protein loss into the bowel. Decreased albumin production may occur due to negative feedback mechanisms in response to elevated globulin levels, thus maintaining plasma oncotic pressure.

Other disease entities cause protein-losing enteropathy than malabsorptive diseases.

SYSTEMS AFFECTED

Gastrointestinal

Normal feces or diarrhea if diffuse colonic involvement with weight loss

Endocrine/Metabolic

Altered protein levels and ratios

Hemic/Lymphatic/Immune

Lymphadenopathy with neoplasia or granulomatous disease

Hepatobiliary

Decreased feed intake may cause mild increase in bilirubin; eosinophilic epitheliotropic disease may affect many organs, including the liver.

Musculoskeletal

- Weight loss
- Muscle atrophy

Skin/Exocrine

Due to malnutrition, vasculitis, or inflammatory cell infiltration

Behavioral

Mild depressed demeanor

SIGNALMENT

Any breed or sex; younger horses usually involved (1–6 yr)

SIGNS

- Colic
- Cutaneous lesions—alopecia; rough, dry haircoat
- Dermatitis
- Coronitis
- Depressed demeanor
- Diarrhea or normal feces
- Edema
- Lethargy
- Lymphadenopathy
- Pyrexia
- Weakness
- Weight loss

CAUSES

Parasitic damage due to *Strongylus* spp. or cyathostomes. *Parascaris equorum* may cause disease in young horses. Infiltrative diseases may be due to an allergic response or uncontrolled response to infectious agent. Familial occurrence has been reported. The causes of alimentary neoplasia, such as lymphosarcoma, are unknown.

DIAGNOSIS

DIFFERENTIAL DIAGNOSIS

A detailed history and physical examination are required. Initially, common causes of weight loss should be considered, such as inadequate nutritional intake for metabolic demands (poor feed quality, bad dentition, competition for food). Many other diseases should be considered using a systematic approach.

Differential diagnosis for hypoproteinemia include decreased protein absorption (inadequate intake, gastroenteric disease), decreased production (liver failure), sequestration into third spaces (pleural cavity, peritoneal cavity, abscesses), or loss (alimentary or renal). Protein-losing enteropathy may be caused by acute/subacute colitis, parasitism, non-steroidal anti-inflammatory drug use, gastrointestinal neoplasia (lymphosarcoma, adenocarcinoma), infiltrative bowel disease, tuberculosis, or congestive heart failure.

Chronic inflammatory bowel disease is caused by lymphocytic/plasmacytic enteritis, eosinophilic granulomatous enteritis, and granulomatous enteritis.

CBC/BIOCHEMISTRY/URINALYSIS

CBC

Common findings include neutrophilia, anemia (due to chronic inflammatory disease or blood loss from ulcerations), and hypoproteinemia. The neutrophil level can be normal or low.

Biochemistry

- Hypoalbuminemia
- Globulin level—low, normal, or elevated
- Fibrinogen—mild elevation
- Hypocalcemia (due to loss of protein-bound calcium)
- Elevations of hepatobiliary parameters:
  - γ-glutamyl transferase
  - Aspartate amino transferase
  - Alkaline phosphatase
  - Bilirubin (conjugated)
  - Lactate dehydrogenase, glutamate dehydrogenase, iditol deydrogenase (sorbitol dehydrogenase)
  - Bile acids

Urinalysis

Normal

Abdominal Fluid Analysis

Normal

Fecal Examination

Identification of large or small strongyles; if present, strongyles do not pinpoint parasites as the cause of malabsorption.

Ultrasound Imaging

Determine thickness of wall of small intestine and the presence of masses

Carbohydrate Absorption Tests

Horse should be fasted for at least 12 hr but not >24 hr. A blood sample should be collected before the administration of the sugar, then at 30-min intervals for up to 4 hr. Water intake should be restricted for the initial 2 hr of the test period. Low or no absorption levels are consistent with delayed gastric emptying, enteric disease, or delayed intestinal transit. In addition to absorption, distribution, metabolism, and excretion are important factors to consider.

D-Xylose Absorption Test

Give 0.5 g/kg as a 10% solution via nasogastric tube. Samples may be collected into heparinized tubes. A peak is expected at approximately 60 min.

Glucose Absorption Test

Give 1 g/kg as a 20% solution via nasogastric tube. Collect blood samples into tubes containing sodium fluoride to prevent cellular metabolism of glucose. Heparinized samples can be used if the glucose level is determined immediately after collection. Normal absorption is a two-fold increase in the baseline glucose level within 90–120 min. Low levels may occur if there is metabolism of the glucose in the lumen. Levels also reflect the metabolic/endocrinologic status of the animal.

Rectal Mucosal Biopsy

Use uterine biopsy forceps or other instrument (bottlecap, syringe-case cap); collect mucosal sample from dorsal or lateral rectal wall in region of retroperitoneal space (30-cm orad to anus). Samples with infiltration of lymphocytes, plasmacytes, eosinophils, and/or histocytes represent diffuse disease. Negative sample is non-diagnostic, necessitating intestinal biopsy.

Small Intestinal Biopsy

Requires general anesthesia, celiotomy, and wedge biopsies. Risks of anesthesia, surgery, and poor wound healing due to catabolic state with hypoalbuminemia.

TREATMENT

Symptomatic care or specific treatment for transient diseases.

DIET

Consider feeding highly digestible feed; high-quality fiber should be fed for colonic digestion. Multiple small feedings should be given. Intestinal resection for localized small intestinal disease.

MEDICATION

Anthelmintics

Treatment should be aimed for appropriate worm; repeat treatment may be required for encysted stages of nematode.

- Ivermectin—0.2 mg/kg PO
- Moxidectin—0.4 mg/kg
- Fenbendazole—10 mg/kg PO once daily for 5 days. Consider prior treatment with dexamethasone if treating for encysted cyathostomes.
- Pyrantel tartrate—2.2 mg/kg/day. Used as a preventative; other anthelmintics should be used to kill adult worms

Corticosteroids

- Infiltrative bowel disease
- Prednisone—1–2 mg/kg, PO, IM BID
- Dexamethasone—0.1–0.2 mg/kg PO SID or by parenteral administration

Antibiotics

Trimethoprim–sulfonamide 30 mg/kg PO or IV, sulfasalazine

CONTRAINDICATIONS

Corticosteroids have been associated with laminitis.

POSSIBLE DRUG INTERACTIONS

N/A

ALTERNATIVE DRUGS

N/A

PROGNOSIS

- Parasitism—poor to good
- Infiltrative bowel disease—poor
- Neoplasia—poor

FOLLOW-UP

PATIENT MONITORING

- Appetite
- Demeanor
- Feces
- Body condition

POSSIBLE COMPLICATIONS

Drug associated (immunosuppression; laminitis; Cushing's or Addison's disease)

MISCELLANEOUS

ASSOCIATED CONDITIONS

N/A

AGE-RELATED FACTORS

N/A

ZOONOTIC POTENTIAL

May be possible if shedding Mycobacterial organisms or *Salmonella* spp.

PREGNANCY

Debilitation may lead to infertility, early embryonic death, or abortion.

SYNONYMS

- Chronic inflammatory bowel disease
- Granulomatous bowel disease
- Infiltrative bowel disease

SEE ALSO

Colic

ABBREVIATIONS

N/A

Suggested Reading

Brown CM. The diagnostic value of the D-xylose absorption test in horses with unexplained chronic weight loss. Br Vet J 1992:148:41-44.

Lindberg R, Nygren A, Persson SG. Rectal biopsy diagnosis in horses with clinical signs of intestinal disorders: a retrospective study of 116 cases. Equine Vet J 1996; 28:275-284.

MacAllister CG, et al. Lymphocytic–plasmacytic enteritis in two horses. J Am Vet Med Assoc 1990;196:1995-1998.

Schumacher J, et al. Effect of intestinal resection on two juvenile horses with granulomatous enteritis. J Vet Int Med 1990;4:153-156.

Sweeney RW. Laboratory evaluation of malassimilation in horses. Vet Clin North Am [Equine Pract] 1987;3:507-515.

Author Daniel G. Kenney

Consulting Editor Henry Stämpfli

MALICIOUS INTOXICATION

BASICS

OVERVIEW

- Determining underlying causes for sudden or unexplained equine deaths has significant medicolegal importance. Potentially all horses are at risk, but there likely is more incentive to kill those that are insured or involved in some form of competition.
- Determining the cause and manner of death is critical to substantiating claims and the ultimate liability of insurers.
- A systematic and thorough postmortem examination is essential to confirm death caused by toxicant exposure. Documentation of proper sample collection, storage, and laboratory submission is crucial.
- It is important to keep an open mind when investigating the death of any animal and not to be misled by allegations of malicious intent.

SIGNALMENT

N/A

SIGNS

- Signs vary considerably depending on the specific toxicant used; however, most malicious intoxications are associated with administration of highly toxic drugs or chemicals intended to kill quickly.
- An ideal toxicant used maliciously would cause rapid death, not result in specific postmortem lesions, and be difficult to detect in postmortem tissue or fluid samples. Fortunately, the list of toxicants meeting all three criteria is rather limited.
- Most toxicants that result in sudden death impair the central or peripheral nervous systems, cardiovascular system, or respiratory system. Thus, if signs are noted before death, they generally relate to failure of one or more of these systems.
- Depending on the toxicant used, there may be evidence of struggle before death, as might occur following CNS stimulation or respiratory impairment. Alternatively, some toxicant-induced deaths are associated with no struggle before death, as might occur after administration of a barbiturate or other CNS depressant.
- Most malicious deaths follow administration of a single dose of a highly toxic compound, but repeated administration of a less toxic or cumulative drug or chemical also occurs.

CAUSES AND RISK FACTORS

- Exclusive of plants for which ingestion is associated with sudden death, potential toxicants include strychnine, phosphides, cholinesterase-inhibiting insecticides (e.g., OPs, carbamates), nicotine, metaldehyde, cyanide, fluoroacetate, illicit drugs (e.g., amphetamines, cocaine, heroin, morphine), metals (e.g., mercury, arsenic, lead, selenium, iron), drugs (e.g., insulin, barbiturates, reserpine, succinylcholine), electrolytes (e.g., potassium, calcium) and vitamins A, D, and E.
- Ingestion of toxic plants is a less common cause but still a possibility. Exposure to extremely toxic plants (e.g., *Taxus* spp. [yew], *Conium maculatum* [poison hemlock], *Cicuta* spp. [water hemlock]) should be considered, as should zootoxins (e.g., cantharidin).

DIAGNOSIS

DIFFERENTIAL DIAGNOSIS

- There are many causes of sudden or unexplained death other than toxicants.
- Physical causes—trauma, electrocution, lightning strike, suffocation, heat stroke, and gunshot
- Natural or genetic causes—hyperkalemic periodic paralysis, cardiac conductive disturbances, acute myocardial necrosis, cerebral thromboembolism, aortic aneurysm or other vessel rupture, and neoplasia
- Infectious or parasitic causes—acute clostridial diseases, salmonellosis, Tyzzer's disease, anthrax, equine monocytic ehrlichiosis, foal actinobacillosis, babesiosis, and verminous arteritis
- Metabolic and nutritional causes—hypoglycemia, hypocalcemia, hypomagnesemia, and selenium or vitamin E deficiencies

CBC/BIOCHEMISTRY/URINALYSIS

- When possible, collect whole blood, serum, plasma, and urine before death for routine clinicopathologic tests; this helps to delineate pathophysiologic processes, which aids in refining an initial differential list.
- If these samples can be obtained, collect additional quantities beyond those needed for clinicopathologic testing for possible toxicologic analysis.

OTHER LABORATORY TESTS

- In addition to samples collected for clinicopathologic testing, other samples for toxicologic analysis include stomach contents, urine, liver, kidney, brain, eyeball, and heart blood.
- With any suspicion of an injection site, obtain tissue from around that site.
- Collect representative feed and water samples.
- Because of medicolegal considerations, handle all samples under chain-of-custody procedures. These records specifically identify each specimen, document their condition and container in which they are packaged, time and date of both transfer and receipt of samples, and all individuals involved in their handling, transfer, or receipt.

IMAGING

N/A

DIAGNOSTIC PROCEDURES

N/A

PATHOLOGIC FINDINGS

- Conduct a complete and thorough postmortem examination.
- Consider transporting the animal to a veterinary diagnostic facility as soon as possible. If this is not an option, conduct a thorough field postmortem examination, and record any actual or suspected abnormalities.
- Carefully examine stomach and GI tract contents for evidence of toxic plant fragments or unexpected grain or forage ingestion.
- Collect formalin-fixed samples from all major organ systems and any gross lesions, and submit these samples to a veterinary pathologist for histopathologic examination.
- Pathologic findings in suspected intoxication often are nonspecific in nature; however, lesions may suggest specific target organs and help to narrow the list of differentials.

TREATMENT

- In many situations, treatment is not possible; however, if the animal is alive, direct treatment toward stabilization of vital organ systems—establish and maintain an open airway, control seizures, correct life-threatening cardiac dysrhythmias, and begin fluid administration.
- Once the animal is stabilized, initiate oral and dermal decontamination procedures if there is any suspicion of exposure via one of these routes; this includes administration of AC and a cathartic or washing of the skin.
- Antidotes are not available for many toxicants, but fortunately, many animals survive with timely decontamination and appropriate symptomatic and supportive care.

MEDICATIONS

DRUGS

- AC (2–5 g/kg PO in water slurry [1 g of AC in 5 mL of water])
- One dose of cathartic PO with AC if no diarrhea or ileus—70% sorbitol (3 mL/kg) or sodium or magnesium sulfate (250–500 mg/kg)
- Administration of other drugs depending on the individual situation

CONTRAINDICATIONS/POSSIBLE INTERACTIONS

N/A

FOLLOW-UP

PATIENT MONITORING

- Appropriate follow-up depends on the specific toxicant under suspicion or analytically confirmed.
- Residual neurologic or cardiac damage may result.
- Monitoring of vital functions is critical.

PREVENTION/AVOIDANCE

N/A

POSSIBLE COMPLICATIONS

Potential complications depend on the specific toxicant involved.

EXPECTED COURSE AND PROGNOSIS

Depend on the specific toxicant involved.

MISCELLANEOUS

ASSOCIATED CONDITIONS

N/A

AGE-RELATED FACTORS

N/A

ZOONOTIC POTENTIAL

N/A

PREGNANCY

N/A

SEE ALSO

N/A

ABBREVIATIONS

- AC = activated charcoal
- GI = gastrointestinal
- OP = organophosphate insecticide

Suggested Reading

Brown CM, Mullaney TP. Sudden and unexpected death in adult horses and ponies. In Pract 1991;13:121–125.

Haliburton JC, Edwards WC. Medicolegal investigation of the sudden or unexpected equine death: toxicologic implications. In: Robinson, NE, ed. Current therapy in equine medicine 4. Philadelphia: WB Saunders, 1997:657–659.

Author Robert H. Poppenga

Consulting Editor Robert H. Poppenga

MASTITIS

BASICS

DEFINITION
Inflammation of the mammary gland, most commonly caused by bacterial colonization within the gland, other causes being nematode migration, mycotic infection, and neoplasia.

PATHOPHYSIOLOGY
Pathophysiology of mastitis depends on pathogen and route of infection. Initial infection occurs via three possible routes, hematogenous, adjacent dermatologic inflammation, or, most commonly, ascending via the teat canal. Bacterial colonization of the teat cistern does not automatically lead to mastitis. This suggests that failure of the immune system either locally at the teat canal or systemically as seen with endotoxemia is necessary for mastitis to occur. The equine mammary gland consists of two glands separated by a fascial septum. Each gland is divided into two or three lobes by fibroelastic capsules, with one teat cistern emptying each lobe. Inflammation may involve one or several lobes of one or both glands. In the case of ascending infection via the canal a cycle is created, with cellular debris clogging the teat canal and leading to an increase in pressure and no effective drainage of the infected material, thus encouraging it to spread into surrounding tissues.

SYSTEM AFFECTED
Mammary, however, other systems may be affected if primary mammary gland infection leads to systemic endotoxemia or if the mastitis is secondary to infection in other systems.

GENETICS
No genetic predisposition has been documented.

INCIDENCE/PREVALENCE
The incidence of infectious mastitis in the mare is quite low, and several factors may play a role in this, such as frequent nursing by the foal, which keeps the mammary gland empty. Also, the mare's lactation period is often less than 6 months, and mares have small teats, which are concealed and less likely to be traumatized. In addition, mares experience less human manipulation of teats than other species, such as cattle, in which mastitis is more common.

SIGNALMENT
Most clinical cases are in lactating mares, but it has been documented in nonlactating mares and has also been observed in foals.

SIGNS

Historical Findings
Owners report reluctance to allow the foal to nurse the lactating mare; may also report depression, anorexia, and severe adverse behavior when udder is palpated.

Physical Examination Findings
- Abnormal size or swelling of the mammary gland
- Heat or pain associated with palpation
- Abnormal mammary secretions, serous, purulent, or bloody in nature
- Fever
- Ventral edema
- Hindlimb lameness or circumduction of the ipsilateral limb if one gland is affected or bilateral if both glands are affected
- Signs associated with concurrent disease

Note: Not all signs are seen in every animal; any combination may occur.

CAUSES

Infectious
Agents that cause infectious mastitis are most often bacterial. The most common isolate is *Streptococcus zooepidemicus*. Other isolates are *Staphylococcus, Actinobacillus, Pseudomonas, Klebsiella,* and *Escherichia coli*. Fungi documented to cause mastitis are *Aspergillus* spp. and *Coccidioides immitis*. Aberrant parasitic migration.

Noninfectious
Neoplasia, the most common being primary mammary adenocarcinoma.

RISK FACTORS
- Primary infection of the mammary gland occurs most commonly via the teat canal. Lactation, trauma to the teats, or insects feeding on the teats allow for colonization through this route.
- Hematogenous spread due to other disease process within the body.
- Dermatologic route via cellulitis, wounds on the abdomen, culicoides hypersensitivity.
- Recent surgical incision.
- Lactation does not appear to be a significant predisposing factor; mastitis can occur in any female horse of any age or breed.

DIAGNOSIS

DIFFERENTIAL DIAGNOSIS

Other Causes of Mammary Heat, Pain, or Abnormal Secretions
Mammary abscess is differentiated from diffuse mastitis by palpation of the udder, which indicates a focal site of inflammation. Mares may show signs of pain on palpation of the udder if their foal has suddenly stopped nursing and the udder is transiently distended. These signs of discomfort should resolve completely with stripping of the udder.

Other Causes of Abnormal Udder Development
Placentitis in the pregnant mare that is differentiated by history; reproductive examination findings indicative of placentitis. Impending parturition or abortion is differentiated by history and response to treatment. Hyperplasia of the mammary gland.

CBC/BIOCHEMISTRY
All laboratory data may be normal or there may be a leukocytosis with neutrophilia and hyperfibrinogenemia. Other abnormalities such as azotemia, leukopenia, increased non-segmented white cell count, or toxic changes in neutrophils may be seen if systemic endotoxemia, bacteremia, or concurrent disease is present. Anemia of chronic disease may also be present.

IMAGING
Sonographic imaging of the mammary gland may be useful in the following cases to identify and document a mammary abscess and its subsequent response to treatment.

OTHER DIAGNOSTIC PROCEDURES
Culture and cytology of mammary secretions and/or milk is necessary for a definitive diagnosis. Samples from each teat cistern should be collected, with attention paid to aseptic technique. Each sample should be submitted for cytologic examination and culture. Cytology is important because culture results may be negative with clinical mastitis. Cytologic examination of milk from normal mares is often acellular or with rare neutrophils present. During the drying-off period, normal mammary secretions contain macrophages with vacuoles present, often called *foam cells,* and lymphocytes. Smears of milk or mammary secretions from mares with signs of mastitis show numerous intact and degenerated neutrophils and cellular debris, and may show large numbers of bacteria or fungal hyphae if a mycotic infection is present. Gram-stain preparations of mammary secretions or milk may guide initial treatment until culture results are available. Aerobic culture and sensitivity is recommended. Anaerobes are not considered significant bacterial pathogens in equine mastitis, so anaerobic culture is not necessary.

Mammary gland biopsy may be indicated if clinical signs are not responsive to initial treatment for bacterial infection, or if cytologic examination of mammary secretions is not suggestive of infectious mastitis. Biopsy may show other causes of mastitis, such as parasitic migration, mycotic infections, or neoplasia.

MASTITIS

TREATMENT

• Most important therapy is local treatment, consisting of frequent stripping out of the affected lobes to remove pathogens and inflammatory cells
• Hot packing
• Hydrotherapy
• Mild exercise, consisting of hand walking, to decrease edema formation
• Surgery may be indicated if sonographic examination reveals a mammary abscess requiring drainage, or if neoplasia is the causative agent and removal of the neoplasm is attempted

MEDICATIONS

DRUG(S) OF CHOICE

Local antimicrobial therapy with lactating cow intramammary treatments. Choice of antimicrobial agent is dictated by culture and sensitivity results. Prior to local infusions, the teat orifice must be cleaned and disinfected with iodine solution or chlorhexadine solution. Intramammary infusions of 0.1% gentamicin solutions made from 100 mg gentamicin added to 100 mL of sterile saline have been used. Caution is needed when administering intramammary treatments because the equine teat canal is smaller and shorter than the bovine, for which the teat cannulae are designed. Systemic antimicrobial therapy may not be necessary in every case. Trimethoprim sulfadiazine (15 mg/kg q12h) pending culture and sensitivity results. Penicillin alone is not effective, but if used in combination with an aminoglycoside, it is very effective. Procaine penicillin 30,000 units/kg IM q12h. Gentamicin 8 mg/kg IM q24h.

ALTERNATIVE MEDICATIONS

Antiflammatory treatment flunixin meglumine 1.1mg/kg IV or PO q24h or phenylbutazone 1–2mg/lb IV or PO q12 or 24h.

FOLLOW-UP

PATIENT MONITORING

Initial treatment should be aimed at bacterial infection unless another etiology is suggested. Only after the patient does not respond to treatment should other causes of mastitis be considered and further diagnostic tests, as outlined above, be performed. The udder should be palpated manually daily. Response to treatment should be seen within 3 days. Resolution of signs should be seen within 5–7 days. Treatment should be continued until 24 hr after signs have resolved or for 5–7 days. If abnormalities in the peripheral blood were noted, follow-up CBC or fibrinogen should be checked within 1 week of discontinuing treatment. If long-term systemic aminoglycoside or non-steroidal anti-inflammatory administration is indicated to monitor renal function, serum creatinine should be monitored. Rectal temperature should be evaluated at least once a day for 14 days if the mare was febrile prior to treatment.

POSSIBLE COMPLICATIONS

Possible complications include sepsis, bacteremia, endotoxemia, laminitis, colitis, lymphadenopathy, lymphangitis, and fibrosis of the affected mammary glands with subsequent decreased milk production.

MISCELLANEOUS

ASSOCIATED CONDITIONS

There is one reported case of acute mastitis that was followed by abortion; however, no association was found.

AGE-RELATED FACTORS

No age predilection has been documented.

ZOONOTIC POTENTIAL

N/A

PREGNANCY

N/A

SYNONYMS

N/A

SEE ALSO

N/A

ABBREVIATIONS

N/A

Suggested Reading

McCue PM, Wilson WD. Equine mastitis—a review of 28 cases. Eq Vet J 1989;2:351-353.
Perkins N, Threlfall WR. Mastitis. In: Reed S, ed. Equine Internal Medicine. Philadelphia: WB Saunders, 1998:804-806.

Author Brett Dolente
Editor Corinne R. Sweeney

MATERNAL FOAL REJECTIONS

BASICS

DEFINITION

• Two major forms—rejection of the foal's attempts to suckle, and overt aggression toward the foal.
• Because a mare's identification of a foal as her own largely depends on smell, iatrogenic foal rejection can occur if the foal's odor changes because of extensive clinical treatments.

PATHOPHYSIOLOGY

Not a pathologic condition per se and can occur without any physical pathology; however, any painful condition (e.g., mastitis) may cause this behavior.

SYSTEMS AFFECTED

• Behavioral—inadequate maternal behavior and increased aggressiveness
• CNS—mechanism unknown

SIGNALMENT

• More common in primiparous and Arabian mares but can occur in any breed at any age.
• Most common immediately postpartum but can occur hours or days after initial acceptance.

SIGNS

• Rejection of attempts to suckle—squealing and signs of fear and avoidance, including repeatedly moving the hindquarters away from the foal or walking away from the foal, especially when the foal moves its head toward the teats
• Aggressive rejection—squealing, head-threat (i.e., ears laid back against the neck), threatening to bite, biting, threatening to kick, kicking, threatening to strike, and striking

CAUSES

• Genetics may be a contributing factor; the problem has been identified as being more common in a specific breed and in certain pedigrees.
• Turgid udders and lack of experience in primiparous mares probably are the most relevant factors in failure to allow suckling with a first birth; the mare has not yet learned that allowing the foal to suckle relieves her discomfort.

RISK FACTORS

• First birth
• Arabians, especially if relatives have exhibited this behavior
• Previous foal rejection, especially with a second or later birth
• A highly disrupted environment or unusual circumstances at the time of birth

DIAGNOSIS

DIFFERENTIAL DIAGNOSIS

Any pathologic condition that might cause pain or discomfort (e.g., mastitis or musculoskeletal disease)

CBC/BIOCHEMISTRY/URINALYSIS

• Should be normal if the problem is purely behavioral.
• Abnormalities supporting the diagnosis of a physical pathology suggest that rejecting behavior is secondary to pain.

OTHER LABORATORY TESTS

N/A

IMAGING

N/A

DIAGNOSTIC PROCEDURES

N/A

TREATMENT

PRIMIPAROUS MARES

• Restraint until the foal can suckle allows the mare to learn that suckling relieves the discomfort in her udder and familiarizes her with the process of standing for nursing.
• Punishment of the mare is contraindicated, because she already is fearful and may associate the presence of the foal with the physical punishment.

AGGRESSIVE MARES

• Restraint so that the mare cannot injure the foal is necessary—cross-tying may be sufficient but still allows the mare to kick; a pole or partition the foal can reach under to suckle while the mare is held in place provides greater protection.
• Provide close supervision for at least the first 24 hours.
• Restrain the mare during all interactions with the foal for at least 3 days; if the mare's behavior does not improve in 7 days, acceptance of the foal is unlikely.

MATERNAL FOAL REJECTIONS

MEDICATIONS

DRUGS OF CHOICE

- Acepromazine (0.02–0.06 mg/kg IV, IM, or SC q2–4h to effect)
- Butorphanol (0.05 mg/kg IV) to relieve pain from turgid udder; if no complicating painful conditions are present, do not repeat.

CONTRAINDICATIONS

Benzodiazepines (e.g., diazepam) are contraindicated in aggressive animals, because these drugs may disinhibit aggression.

PRECAUTIONS

- Administration of anxiolytics and progestins for foal rejection constitutes extralabel use, and owners should be so informed.
- Review all side effects, and prepare an informed consent form for the owner to sign.

POSSIBLE INTERACTIONS

N/A

ALTERNATIVE DRUGS

- Anxiolytics (e.g., diazepam) may help with fearful mares.
- Progestins may help with aggressive mares.
- Diazepam (10–20 mg q6–8h)
- Altrenogest (1 mL/day for every 50 kg)

FOLLOW-UP

PATIENT MONITORING

Intensive monitoring until the mare consistently allows the foal to suckle and fails to show aggression for several hours.

POSSIBLE COMPLICATIONS

Inadequate supervision and restraint of an aggressive mare may result in injury to or death of the foal.

MISCELLANEOUS

ASSOCIATED CONDITIONS

Mastitis

AGE RELATED FACTORS

Most common in primiparous mares, probably due to lack of experience.

ZOONOTIC POTENTIAL

N/A

PREGNANCY

N/A

SYNONYMS

N/A

SEE ALSO

Aggression

Suggested Reading

Crowell-Davis SL, Houpt KA. Maternal behavior. Vet Clin North Am Equine Pract 1986;2:557–571.

Houpt KA. Foal rejection—a review of 23 cases. Equine Pract 1984;6:38–40.

Houpt KA. Foal rejection and other behavioral problems in the postpartum period. Comp Cont Educ Pract Vet 1984;6:S144–S148.

Houpt KA, Lieb S. A survey of foal rejecting mares. Appl Anim Behav Sci 1994;39:188.

Juarbe-Diaz SV, Houpt KA, Kusunose R. Prevalence and characteristics of foal rejection in Arabian mares. Equine Vet J 1998;30:424–428.

Author Sharon L. Crowell-Davis

Consulting Editor Daniel Q. Estep

MECONIUM RETENTION

BASICS

OVERVIEW

• Meconium, the first fecal material produced by a newborn foal, is composed of cellular debris, amniotic fluid, and intestinal secretions and generally is passed within 30 minutes of first suckling (≅2 hours after birth)
• Total amount voided is a little more than 1% of body weight.
• Meconium generally is dark brown and formed; in meconium retention, fecal consistency is dry and hard.
• Meconium retention occurs when the foal fails to pass the meconium and begins to experience abdominal pain.

SIGNALMENT

• Seen in the first day or two of life
• Affects colts more often than fillies

SIGNS

• Abdominal pain (i.e., colic)—manifested by tail swishing, restlessness, and reluctance to eat; may progress to recumbency and violent rolling.
• Abdominal distention
• Fecal production—scant or absent
• Tenesmus—foals usually stand with their tail lifted and their back "humped up."
• Eversion of the rectal mucosa

CAUSES AND RISK FACTORS

• Often, no direct cause is found.
• Asphyxia at birth has been suggested to affect intestinal motility.
• Hydration status may affect the passage of fecal material.
• Male foals have a narrower pelvis and a convex pubis, which may predispose to impaction.

DIAGNOSIS

DIFFERENTIAL DIAGNOSIS

• Ruptured bladder may result in signs that are mistaken as straining to defecate when they actually signal straining to urinate.
• Atresia coli present with similar signs; the most consistent finding is an absence of meconium staining after repeated enemas.
• Foals with intestinal aganglionosis present with no meconium production and colic; these are white foals of two overo paint parents.

CBC/BIOCHEMISTRY/URINALYSIS

N/A

OTHER LABORATORY TESTS

N/A

IMAGING

Abdominal radiography—meconium may be seen as fecal material in the large colon, small colon, and rectum; gas-distended loops of bowel may be seen proximal to the meconium; and barium enemas may outline the meconium pellets.

DIAGNOSTIC PROCEDURES

Small, hard fecal material may be felt on careful digital rectal examination of the foal.

TREATMENT

MEDICAL

• Enemas are the best treatment.
• Phosphate enemas manufactured for use in humans are effective for mild meconium impactions.
• Enemas of warm soapy water (1-L volume, use a mild hand soap) or 4% *N*-acetylcysteine (add 20 g of $NaHCO_3$ + 8 g of acetylcysteine to 200 mL of water) have effectively relieved more persistent impactions. These enemas may be given via a soft-rubber tube or a 30-Fr Foley catheter, respectively. With the Foley catheter, gradually inflate the balloon, blocking expulsion of the enema for 4–5 minutes.
• Enemas must be done gently to prevent irritation and injury to the delicate rectal mucosa; rectal irritation causes continued straining, even after the meconium has passed.
• If the impaction has not resolved after use of enemas, nasogastric intubation and mineral oil (240 mL for a 40-kg foal) may be indicated; however, do not administer mineral oil before 18 hours of age to allow adequate colostrum absorption.
• IV fluid therapy—beneficial in dehydrated foals

SURGICAL

• Rarely necessary, but may be indicated in foals that do not respond to medical therapy.
• Bowel massage with simultaneous enema or enterotomy may be performed.

MECONIUM RETENTION

MEDICATIONS

DRUGS

• Foals may require analgesics if in discomfort.
• Flunixin meglumine (0.5 mg/kg IV) or butorphanol (0.1mg/kg IV or IM) may be helpful in alleviating pain.

CONTRAINDICATIONS/POSSIBLE INTERACTIONS

Foals are susceptible to gastric ulceration, especially with use of NSAIDs, which should be administered with caution and only in well-hydrated foals.

FOLLOW-UP

PATIENT MONITORING

Observation after treatment for passage of meconium

POSSIBLE COMPLICATIONS

• Rough administration of enemas may injure or even perforate the foal's rectum; depending on the extent of damage, this may result in peritonitis or rectal stricture.
• Surgical complications—peritonitis, adhesion formation, and chronic colic

EXPECTED COURSE AND PROGNOSIS

Most respond well to medical therapy and without complication.

MISCELLANEOUS

ASSOCIATED CONDITIONS

N/A

AGE-RELATED FACTORS

Seen during the first day or two of life.

ZOONOTIC POTENTIAL

N/A

PREGNANCY

N/A

SEE ALSO

• Acute abdominal pain
• Gastric ulcers
• Intestinal aganglionosis
• Ruptured bladder

Suggested Reading

Ganesan S, Bhuvanakumar CK. Weighing meconium—an approach to prevent meconium retention in foals. Centaur Mylapore 1993;10:23–24.

Hughes FE, Moll HD, Slone DE. Outcome of surgical correction of meconium impactions in 8 foals. J Equine Vet Sci 1996;16:172–175.

Kurtz-Filho M, Depra NM, Alda JL, Castro FD, Silva CAM. Physiological and behavioral parameters in the newborn Thoroughbred foal. Braz J Vet Res Anim Sci 1997;34:103–108.

Madigan JE, Goetzman BW. Use of an acetylcysteine solution enema for meconium retention in the neonatal foal. Proc AAEP 1990:117–119.

Author Mary Rose Paradis
Consulting Editor Mary Rose Paradis

MELENA AND HEMATOCHEZIA

BASICS

OVERVIEW

Melena is the presence of digested blood in the feces. It appears as dark, black, or tarry feces. Hematochezia is the presence of blood in the feces. Melena can be present from blood that enters the gastrointestinal tract (GIT) from the mouth to the colons. This would include blood from the respiratory tract that was in turn swallowed. However, microbes in the equine large colon proficiently degrade blood/hemoglobin. Therefore, large quantities of blood must be present for melena to be evident, and fecal occult blood tests are frequently negative despite the loss of blood into the GIT.

SIGNALMENT

There is no age, breed, or sex predisposition for this condition.

SIGNS

Historical Findings

Clients frequently have observed dark or bloody feces.

Physical Examination Findings

Dark or tarry feces or frank blood in feces. Additional signs present depend on underlying cause. If substantial blood loss has occurred, mucous membranes may become pale and capillary refill time extended.

CAUSES AND RISK FACTORS

- Parasitism
- Bacterial enteritis/colitis
- Toxicoses (acorn, aflatoxin, arsenic, cantharidin, *crotolaria* spp., mycotoxin, NSAIDs, oak, organophosphate, warfarin)
- Neoplasia
- Colonic hematomas
- Rectal tears
- Swallowed blood from the respiratory tract
- Gastroduodenal ulcers (rare with this condition)
- Purpura hemorrhagica
- Thrombocytopenia
- Coagulopathies
- Mesenteric arterial aneurysm
- Previous rectal examination or rectal trauma

DIAGNOSIS

DIFFERENTIAL DIAGNOSIS

History of exposure to risk factors is helpful in establishing the diagnosis.

CBC/BIOCHEMISTRY/URINALYSIS

Hemogram may show anemia from blood loss. Leukopenia is present in many bacterial enterocolitis cases. Hypoproteinemia possible from loss of protein into the GIT lumen. Thrombocytopenia if present may result in significant GIT hemorrhage. Electrolyte and acid–base abnormalities with many diarrheas. Mild azotemia may be associated with dehydration. Urine typically concentrated from fluid retention, with the exception of cantharidin toxicosis. With cantharidin toxicosis there is frequently hyposthenuria (SG 1.003–1.006) despite clinical dehydration.

OTHER LABORATORY TESTS

- Fecal examination for parasite ova and bacterial cultures
- Coagulation profile may reveal clotting abnormality

DIAGNOSTIC PROCEDURES

Gastroscopic Examination

Check for the presence of gastric squamous cell carcinoma or bleeding gastric ulcers. Caution! It is not uncommon for mild iatrogenic hemorrhage to occur with gastric ulcers in the stratified squamous mucosa when the stomach is insufflated for gastroscopy. In addition, it is rare to have melena from bleeding gastric ulcers in the horse.

Proctoscopy

Useful in hematochezia, as this is most often due to hemorrhage in the lower GIT.

MELENA AND HEMATOCHEZIA

TREATMENT

Most patients with melena or hematochezia should be hospitalized to determine a cause of the condition and provide supportive care. Fluid electrolyte and acid–base abnormalities should be corrected.

MEDICATIONS

Blood transfusion should be considered if the PCV is <12%; 0.12 L/L or is low and rapidly falling. A 1000-lb (454-kg) horse with a PCV <12% should receive 5–8 L of whole blood.

DRUG(S) OF CHOICE

N/A

CONTRAINDICATIONS

NSAIDs should not be administered to patients with NSAID toxicosis.

PRECAUTIONS

NSAIDs should be used with caution in patients with gastroduodenal ulceration.

POSSIBLE INTERACTIONS

N/A

ALTERNATIVE DRUGS

N/A

FOLLOW-UP

PATIENT MONITORING

PCV should be checked twice daily until stabilized

POSSIBLE COMPLICATIONS

Right dorsal colitis and chronic, low-grade colic with NSAID toxicosis.

MISCELLANEOUS

Administration of bismuth compounds such as bismuth subsalicylate turns the feces black and can be misinterpreted as melena.

ASSOCIATED CONDITIONS

N/A

AGE-RELATED FACTORS

N/A

ZOONOTIC POTENTIAL

The zoonotic potential of *Salmonella* spp. and *Cryptosporidium* (foals) should be considered when treating patients with diarrhea of unknown etiology.

PREGNANCY

Mares receiving blood transfusions develop alloantibody to the transfused RBCs. The alloantibody may be transferred to subsequent foals via the colostrum. If sufficient quantities of the alloantibody are present in the colostrum and the foal's RBCs contain the same antigens as the transfused RBCs, the foal could develop neonatal isoerythrolysis.

SYNONYMS

N/A

SEE ALSO

ABBREVIATIONS

- GIT = gastrointestinal tract
- PCV = packed cell volume

Suggested Reading

Pearson EG, Smith BB, McKim JM. Fecal blood determinations and interpretations. Proc Am Assoc Equine Pract 1987:77-81.

Smith BP. Alterations in alimentary and hepatic function. In: B Smith, ed. Large animal internal medicine. St. Louis: Mosby, 1996;118-141.

Author Charles G. MacAllister

Consulting Editor Henry Stämpfli

MERCURY TOXICOSIS

BASICS

OVERVIEW

- A toxic syndrome involving the GI and renal systems, resulting primarily from the ingestion or dermal absorption of blistering agents containing inorganic mercury salts—mercuric iodide; mercuric chloride
- Toxicosis from ingesting seeds treated with mercury-containing fungicides is unlikely, because such fungicides no longer are available.
- Mercury binds to a variety of sulfhydryl-containing enzymes, resulting in nonspecific cell injury and death.

SIGNALMENT

No breed, age, or sex predilections

SIGNS

- Depression
- Colic
- Diarrhea
- Weakness
- Skin erosions, ulcerations, and crusting
- Dehydration
- Oliguria
- Laminitis

CAUSES AND RISK FACTORS

- Excessive application of blistering agent
- Application of blistering agent to damaged skin
- Failure to prevent the animal from ingesting a dermally applied agent
- Application of blistering agent in combination with DMSO

DIAGNOSIS

DIFFERENTIAL DIAGNOSIS

- Lead toxicosis—likely evidence of neurologic dysfunction; measurement of whole-blood or tissue lead concentrations
- Arsenic toxicosis—measurement of whole-blood, urine, or tissue arsenic concentrations
- NSAIDs toxicosis—history of previous use; measurement in plasma or serum
- Cantharidin toxicosis—evidence of cystitis; detection of cantharidin in stomach contents or urine
- *Quercus* spp. (oak) toxicosis—detection of plant material in the GI tract; evidence of oak consumption
- Salmonellosis—fecal cultures
- Ehrlichial colitis—serology
- Acute cyathastomiasis—fecal egg counts
- Clostridial colitis—isolation of pathogenic clostridia; identification of toxins
- Antimicrobial-induced colitis (e.g., lincomycin, tetracycline)—history of drug use

CBC/BIOCHEMISTRY/URINALYSIS

- Increased PCV
- Hyperfibrinogenemia
- Serum electrolyte changes—hyponatremia, hypochloremia, hyperphosphatemia, and hyperkalemia
- Hyperglycemia
- Azotemia
- Urinalysis—glycosuria, proteinuria, isosthenuria, hematuria, waxy or granular casts
- Occult blood in feces

OTHER LABORATORY TESTS

- Antemortem—measurement of mercury in urine or blood
- Postmortem—measurement of mercury in liver or kidney tissue

IMAGING

N/A

DIAGNOSTIC PROCEDURES

N/A

PATHOLOGIC FINDINGS

Gross Findings

- Watery feces
- Intraluminal hemorrhage
- GI mucosal edema
- Mucosal ulcerations in the oral cavity, stomach, and colon
- Subcutaneous edema
- Pale, soft, and swollen kidneys

Histopathologic Findings

- Acute, severe renal tubulonephrosis
- Severe, extensive ulcerative colitis and enteritis

TREATMENT

- Remove source of mercury.
- Control abdominal pain.
- Treat for dehydration, circulatory shock, and renal failure.
- Enhance mercury elimination with a chelator.
- Provide a bland diet containing reduced amounts of high-quality protein.

MEDICATIONS

DRUGS

- Dimercaprol (British anti-lewisite) is classic mercury chelator—loading dose of 4–5 mg/kg by deep muscular injection followed by 2–3 mg/kg q4h for 24 hours and then 1 mg/kg q4h for 2 days; adverse reactions include tremors, convulsions, and coma.
- DMSA is a less toxic chelator—dose not established for horses, but 10 mg/kg PO q8h is suggested.
- Appropriate fluid therapy
- Flunixin meglumine (1.1 mg/kg IV q12–24h) or butorphanol tartrate (0.1 mg/kg IV q3–4h up to 48 h)
- Xylazine hydrochloride (1.1 mg/kg IV) may be used in conjunction with butorphanol (0.01–0.02 mg/kg IV).
- Demulcents—mineral oil; kaolin-pectin

CONTRAINDICATIONS/POSSIBLE INTERACTIONS

Use NSAIDs cautiously because of possible adverse GI and renal effects.

FOLLOW-UP

PATIENT MONITORING

Monitor renal function.

PREVENTION/AVOIDANCE

- Identify and properly dispose of the source of exposure.
- Avoid use of mercury-containing blisters.

POSSIBLE COMPLICATIONS

N/A

EXPECTED COURSE AND PROGNOSIS

- Dependent on the severity of clinical signs.
- Renal impairment suggests a poor prognosis.
- One equine case report described brain neuronal degeneration.
- Long-term neurologic deficits are possible after recovery.

MISCELLANEOUS

ASSOCIATED CONDITIONS

N/A

AGE-RELATED FACTORS

N/A

ZOONOTIC POTENTIAL

N/A

PREGNANCY

- Most forms of mercury can cross the placenta.
- The significance of fetal exposure after use of mercury salts on pregnant mares is unknown.

SEE ALSO

N/A

ABBREVIATIONS

- DMSA = 2,3-dimercaptosuccinic acid, succimer
- DMSO = dimethyl sulfoxide
- GI = gastrointestinal
- PCV = packed cell volume

Suggested Reading

Guglick MA, MacAllister CG, Sundeep Chandra AM, Edwards WC, Qualls CW, Stephens DH. Mercury toxicosis caused by the ingestion of a blistering compound in a horse. J Am Vet Med Assoc 1995;206:210–213.

Author Robert H. Poppenga
Consulting Editor Robert H. Poppenga

METHEMOGLOBINEMIA

BASICS

DEFINITION

• Methemoglobin is an oxidized form of hemoglobin that cannot bind oxygen reversibly and contains an oxidized ferric (+3) ion with five electron pairs but lacks the electron pair required for oxygen binding.
• Methemoglobinemia results when formation of methemoglobin exceeds the ability of RBCs to reduce it back to the native ferrous (+2) state found in hemoglobin and the methemoglobin content of blood exceeds 3%.

PATHOPHYSIOLOGY

• Normally, a small amount of methemoglobin is produced in the blood.
• Methemoglobin is continuously reduced back to hemoglobin by several mechanisms—NADH-dependent methemoglobin reductase, which is the principal conversion mechanism under physiologic conditions, or the NADPH-diaphorase and NADPH-methemoglobin reductase systems; these two enzymatic systems gain importance in the presence of dyes (e.g., methylene blue) used to treat severe cases.
• Nonenzymatic mechanisms of methemoglobin reduction—ascorbic acid and reduced glutathione.
• Methemoglobin can form during the physiologic process of oxygen binding to hemoglobin, after exposure to oxidants (e.g., superoxide anion, hydrogen peroxide), or because of decreased red cell glutathione and glutathione reductase content.
• Familial methemoglobinemia and hemolytic anemia associated with glutathione and glutathione reductase deficiency have been reported.

SYSTEMS AFFECTED

• The condition leads to reduced oxygen-carrying capacity of blood, which may be fatal with as little as 22% methemoglobinemia in horses with red-maple (*Acer rubrum*) leaf toxicity.
• Coma and death may result when the methemoglobin content of blood reaches or exceeds 80%.
• Hypoxia resulting from the condition affects the neuromuscular, hepatobiliary, and cardiovascular systems as well as the upper urinary tract. In addition to the ischemic injury to the kidneys resulting from hypoxic injury, nephrotoxicosis may occur from the resulting pigmenturia.

SIGNALMENT

• No breed, age or gender predispositions, given that the condition generally results from oxidant injury caused by ingestion of dried red-maple leaves and, uncommonly, from nitrate poisoning.
• Rarely, familial methemoglobinemia and hemolytic anemia have been reported in association with decreased erythrocytic glutathione and glutathione reductase.

SIGNS

• Vary with the severity and organ systems involved.
• Muddy-brown cyanotic mucous membranes may be noted in addition to brownish discoloration of the blood (methemoglobin content of blood >10%) and urine.
• Additional signs—weakness, lethargy, ataxia, anorexia, tachycardia, tachypnea, exercise intolerance, icterus, or scleral petechiation.
• With nitrate poisoning, salivation, diarrhea, colic, or increased urination may be noted.

CAUSES

• Red-maple (*A. rubrum*) toxicity, which also can cause Heinz-body hemolytic anemia.
• Nitrite poisoning (uncommon in horses)
• Rarely, glutathione and glutathione reductase deficiencies

RISK FACTORS

Access to dry red-maple leaves or nitrates

DIAGNOSIS

DIFFERENTIAL DIAGNOSIS

• Cyanosis and dark-colored blood can result from hypoxemia as well as methemoglobinemia.
• In hypoxemia, arterial PO_2 is low; in methemoglobinemia, PO_2 is normal or high.

LABORATORY FINDINGS

Drugs That May Alter Test Results

N/A

Disorders That May Alter Laboratory Results

Sample hemolysis may falsely raise the methemoglobin value.

Valid If Run in Human Lab?

Valid, unless saponin is used as the red cell–lysing agent in the methemoglobin assay.

CBC/BIOCHEMISTRY/URINALYSIS

• CBC may reveal anemia and concurrent Heinz-body formation in red-maple leaf toxicity.
• Depending on severity, clinical chemistry panel can reveal evidence of injury to various organ systems—high BUN, creatinine, liver enzymes, or bilirubin
• Urinalysis may reveal hemoglobinuria, bilirubinuria, and proteinuria.

METHEMOGLOBINEMIA

OTHER LABORATORY TESTS

- Determination of methemoglobin content requires rapid submission to an appropriate laboratory, because levels fall quickly in vitro even in cold storage.
- The spot test consists of comparing the patient's whole blood with a normal control sample. A drop of patient blood is placed on absorbent paper and compared with a normal control. Methemoglobin content >10% results in a brown discoloration of patient blood compared with the frank red color of control blood.
- The brown discoloration of blood combined with the high PO_2 content of arterial blood aids in establishing the diagnosis by distinguishing methemoglobinemia from hypoxemia.

IMAGING

N/A

OTHER DIAGNOSTIC PROCEDURES

Examine a new methylene blue–stained blood smear for Heinz bodies, which indicate concurrent hemolytic anemia.

TREATMENT

- Eliminate access to source of the toxin—red-maple leaves or other oxidant
- Treatment required in moderate or marked cases.
- As little as 22% methemoglobin content of blood may be fatal in horses with red maple leaf poisoning, which may result from the concurrent Heinz-body hemolytic anemia that frequently occurs.
- Supportive therapy—whole-blood transfusion if severe anemia develops, oxygen therapy, and laxatives (e.g., mineral oil)
- IV fluid therapy for dehydration, and IV hemolysis to limit hemoglobin-induced nephrotoxicosis
- Correction of electrolyte or acid–base disturbance may be required with evidence of renal injury or shock.

MEDICATIONS

DRUGS OF CHOICE

In nitrate poisoning, methylene blue (4.4 mg/kg) may be administered slowly IV as a 1–2% solution in isotonic saline, and repeated if necessary after 30 minutes.

CONTRAINDICATIONS

N/A

PRECAUTIONS

Methylene blue administration can cause or exacerbate concurrent Heinz-body hemolytic anemia.

POSSIBLE INTERACTIONS

N/A

ALTERNATIVE DRUGS

N/A

FOLLOW-UP

PATIENT MONITORING

- Cyanosis should resolve if methemoglobin content of blood falls below critical levels, and blood should again become red (i.e., spot test) if the content falls below 10%.
- If methylene blue is administered, carefully monitor PCV over 3 days to ensure severe anemia does not develop because of Heinz-body formation.

POSSIBLE COMPLICATIONS

Coma and death if methemoglobin content of blood exceeds 80%.

MISCELLANEOUS

ASSOCIATED CONDITIONS

Heinz-body hemolytic anemia.

AGE-RELATED FACTORS

N/A

ZOONOTIC POTENTIAL

N/A

PREGNANCY

N/A

SYNONYMS

N/A

SEE ALSO

- Anemia
- Heinz body

ABBREVIATION

- PCV = packed cell volume

Suggested Reading

George LW, Divers TJ, Mahaffey EA, Suarez JH. Heinz body anemia and methemoglobinemia in ponies given red maple (*Acer rubrum*) leaves. Vet Pathol 1982;19:521–533.

Jain NC. Hemolytic anemias of noninfectious origin. In: Essentials of veterinary hematology. Philadelphia: Lea & Febiger, 1991.

Schmitz DG. Toxicologic problems. In: Reed SM, Bayly WM, eds. Equine internal medicine. Philadelphia: WB Saunders, 1998.

Tennant B, Glickman LT, Mirro EJ, et al. Acute hemolytic anemia, methemoglobinemia and Heinz body formation associated with ingestion of red maple leaves by horses. J Am Vet Med Assoc 1981;179:143–150.

Author Anne Lanevschi

Consulting Editor Claire B. Andreasen

METHYLXANTHINE TOXICOSIS

BASICS

OVERVIEW

• Methylxanthines include theobromine, caffeine, and theophylline.
• Generally, they cause release of catecholamines (i.e., epinephrine, norepinephrine), increased muscular contractility, and stimulation of the CNS.
• Only theobromine (from cocoa bean hulls) has been associated with clinical intoxication and death in horses. Use and detection in race horses is of concern; the diagnosis is established based on a history of ingestion and determination of theobromine in serum, plasma, urine, or stomach contents.

SIGNALMENT

All Equidae are susceptible to theobromine intoxication, but the few reported cases of theobromine poisoning in horses do not allow for determination of breed or sex predilections.

SIGNS

• One case of theobromine ingestion by horses has been reported, with "violent excitement" as the outstanding clinical sign.
• The sole other case in the literature reported only sudden death.
• Clinical signs of toxicosis reported in other species (primarily dogs)—hyperactivity, diarrhea, diuresis, muscle tremors, ataxia, cardiac arrhythmias, and death

CAUSES AND RISK FACTORS

• Theobromine is found in cocoa bean hulls, chocolate, chocolate-containing bakery waste, and formerly, in some diuretics.
• Toxicoses and deaths have been reported through ingestion of cocoa bean hulls used as bedding or in feed.
• Roughly, a dose of 100 mg/kg of theobromine given over 4 days as cocoa bean hulls in feed has been reported to cause death; the possibility of toxicosis at lower doses has not been investigated.
• Cocoa bean hulls are reported to contain as much as 0.5% theobromine by weight.
• Theobromine and caffeine have been detected in the urine of race horses fed small amounts of chocolate candy or incorporated into feed.

DIAGNOSIS

DIFFERENTIAL DIAGNOSIS

Other causes of rapid/sudden death in horses from cardiac arrhythmias include accidental ingestion of ionophore feed supplements (test for ionophores in the feed), ingestion of *Eupatorium rugosum* or white snakeroot (history; evidence of ingestion and myocardial necrosis), or ingestion of bark and leaves of *Robinia pseudoacacia* or black locust (history; evidence of ingestion).

CBC/BIOCHEMISTRY/URINALYSIS

No abnormalities have been reported with theobromine toxicoses.

OTHER LABORATORY TESTS

N/A

IMAGING

N/A

DIAGNOSTIC PROCEDURES

• The diagnosis of theobromine toxicosis is established based on clinical history, evidence of ingestion, and presence of theobromine in serum, plasma, urine, or stomach contents.
• ECG to monitor for possible cardiac arrhythmias.

TREATMENT

• Eliminate exposure.
• Restrict activity because of possible cardiac arrhythmias.

MEDICATIONS

DRUGS

• Administer AC unless contraindicated (2–5 g/kg in a water slurry).
• Because of the limited number of reported cases, pharmacological intervention in equine theobromine toxicosis has not been evaluated.

CONTRAINDICATIONS/POSSIBLE INTERACTIONS

N/A

METHYLXANTHINE TOXICOSIS

FOLLOW-UP

PATIENT MONITORING
Monitor ECG to evaluate cardiac status.

PREVENTION/AVOIDANCE
Do not allow horses to eat cocoa bean hulls or chocolate products.

POSSIBLE COMPLICATIONS
N/A

EXPECTED COURSE AND PROGNOSIS
The rarity of theobromine toxicosis precludes generalization to all prospective equine cases; however, when less-than-toxic amounts are ingested and ECG abnormalities are not present, the prognosis is excellent.

MISCELLANEOUS

ASSOCIATED CONDITIONS
N/A

AGE-RELATED FACTORS
N/A

ZOONOTIC POTENTIAL
N/A

PREGNANCY
N/A

SEE ALSO
N/A

ABBREVIATION
AC = activated charcoal

Suggested Reading

Blakemore F, Shearer GD. The poisoning of livestock by cacao products. Vet Rec 1943;55:165.

Harkins JD, Rees WA, Mundy GD, Stanley SD, Tobin T. An overview of the methylxanthines and their regulation in the horse. Equine Pract 1998;20:10–16.

Author Stephen B. Hooser

Consulting Editor Robert H. Poppenga

MITRAL REGURGITATION

BASICS

DEFINITION
• Occurs when the mitral valve becomes insufficient, allowing blood to leak backward into the left atrium during systole and creating a systolic murmur with its PMI in the mitral to aortic valve area.
• The murmur radiates toward the left base or dorsally and caudally.

PATHOPHYSIOLOGY
• The mitral leaflets do not form a complete seal between the left atrium and ventricle.
• During systole, blood regurgitates into the left atrium, causing increased left atrial pressure and a left atrial and ventricular volume overload.
• As the regurgitation becomes more severe, further increases in left atrial pressure produce increased pulmonary venous pressure, increased pulmonary capillary pressure, pulmonary edema, pulmonary hypertension, and clinical signs of left-sided congestive heart failure.
• As the pulmonary hypertension becomes more severe, clinical signs of right-sided congestive heart failure appear.

SYSTEMS AFFECTED
Cardiovascular

GENETICS
N/A

INCIDENCE/PREVALENCE
N/A

SIGNALMENT
N/A

SIGNS
General Comments
Usually an incidental finding during routine auscultation

Historical Findings
• Poor performance
• Sometimes congestive heart failure

Physical Examination Findings
• Grade 2–6/6, band-shaped, crescendo or musical holosystolic or pansystolic murmur with PMI in the mitral to aortic valve area and radiating dorsally to the left heart base
• Other, less common findings—atrial premature beats, atrial fibrillation, accentuated third heart sounds, tachypnea, cough, and congestive heart failure

CAUSES
• Degenerative changes of the mitral leaflets
• Nonvegetative valvulitis
• Ruptured chordae tendineae
• Bacterial endocarditis
• Congenital malformation

RISK FACTORS
N/A

DIAGNOSIS

DIFFERENTIAL DIAGNOSIS
Aortic stenosis—rare; murmur radiates up the carotid arteries and to the right side; weak arterial pulses; differentiate echocardiographically.

CBC/BIOCHEMISTRY/URINALYSIS
May have neutrophilic leukocytosis and hyperfibrinogenemia with bacterial endocarditis.

OTHER LABORATORY TESTS
• Elevated cardiac isoenzymes may be present (e.g., cardiac troponin I, CK-MB, HBDH, LDH 1 and 2) with concurrent myocardial disease.
• Positive blood culture may be obtained from horses with bacterial endocarditis.

IMAGING
Electrocardiography
• Atrial premature depolarizations may be present in horses with acute onset of severe regurgitation and left atrial enlargement.
• Atrial fibrillation often is present in affected horses with significant left atrial enlargement.
• Ventricular premature depolarizations may be present in affected horses with diffuse myocardial disease.

Echocardiography
• Most affected horses have thickened mitral valve leaflets. Diffuse thickening of the leaflet free edge is more common than nodular thickening.
• Prolapse of a mitral leaflet (usually an accessory leaflet) into the left atrium is frequently detected.
• A ruptured chorda tendineae, flail mitral leaflet, or bacterial endocarditis infrequently are detected.
• Left atrium—enlarged and dilated, with a rounded appearance
• Left ventricle—enlarged and dilated, with a rounded apex
• Thinning of the left ventricular free wall and interventricular septum
• Pattern of left ventricular volume overload
• Normal or decreased fractional shortening in a horse with left ventricular enlargement is consistent with myocardial dysfunction.
• Dilatation of the pulmonary veins and, later, the pulmonary artery in severely affected horses
• Pulsed-wave or color-flow Doppler reveals a jet or jets of regurgitation in the left atrium. Size and extent of the regurgitation jet is a good method of semiquantitating severity, as is the strength of the regurgitation signal.

Thoracic Radiography
• Left-sided cardiac enlargement may be detected.
• Pulmonary edema may be detected in horses with left sided congestive heart failure.

DIAGNOSTIC PROCEDURES
Cardiac Catheterization
• Right sided catheterization can be performed to directly measure pulmonary arterial and pulmonary capillary wedge pressures.
• Severely affected horses should have elevated pulmonary capillary wedge pressures and pulmonary arterial pressures, with normal oxygen saturation.
• Right atrial and ventricular pressures also may be elevated with right-sided heart failure.

Continuous 24-Hour Holter Monitoring
Useful in the diagnosis of horses with suspected atrial or ventricular premature depolarizations

PATHOLOGIC FINDINGS
• Focal or diffuse thickening or distortion of one or more mitral leaflets may be present.
• Ruptured chordae tendineae, flail mitral leaflets, bacterial endocarditis, or congenital malformations of the mitral valve infrequently are detected.
• Jet lesions usually are detected in the left atrium.
• With significant regurgitation, left atrial enlargement and atrial myocardial thinning, as well as left ventricular enlargement and thinning of the left ventricular free wall and interventricular septum
• Dilatation of the pulmonary veins in severely affected horses
• Dilatation of the pulmonary artery in affected horses with pulmonary hypertension
• Pale areas may be seen in the atrial myocardium, with areas of atrial fibrosis detected histopathologically.
• Inflammatory cell infiltrate has been documented in affected horses with myocarditis.
• Myocardial necrosis occasionally is detected in affected horses with primary myocardial disease.

TREATMENT

APPROPRIATE HEALTH CARE
• Most affected horses require no treatment and can be monitored on an outpatient basis.
• Horses with moderate to severe regurgitation may benefit from long-term vasodilator therapy, particularly with ACE inhibitors.
• Treat horses with severe regurgitation and congestive heart failure for the congestive heart failure with positive inotropic drugs, vasodilators, and diuretics on an inpatient basis, if possible, and monitor response to therapy.

MITRAL REGURGITATION

NURSING CARE
N/A

ACTIVITY
- Affected horses are safe to continue in full athletic work until the regurgitation becomes severe or ventricular arrhythmias develop.
- Monitor horses with moderate to severe regurgitation by ECG during high-intensity exercise to ensure they are safe to compete. These horses can be used for lower-level athletic competitions until they begin to develop congestive heart failure.
- Horses with significant ventricular arrhythmias or pulmonary artery dilatation are no longer safe to ride.

DIET
N/A

CLIENT EDUCATION
- Regularly monitor the cardiac rhythm; any irregularities other than second-degree AV block should prompt ECG.
- Carefully monitor for exercise intolerance, respiratory distress, prolonged recovery after exercise, increased resting respiratory or heart rate, or cough; if detected, seek a cardiac re-examination.

SURGICAL CONSIDERATIONS
N/A

MEDICATIONS

DRUGS OF CHOICE
- Severe regurgitation—enalapril (0.25–0.5 mg/kg PO SID or BID) or another ACE inhibitor
- ACE inhibitors prolong the time to valve replacement in humans with moderate to severe regurgitation.
- Affected horses in heart failure—treat with digoxin, furosemide, and vasodilators.

CONTRAINDICATIONS
ACE inhibitors in horses actively competing in types of athletic work that involve drug testing; these drugs must be withdrawn before competition to comply with the medication rules of the various governing bodies of equine sports.

PRECAUTIONS
ACE inhibitors can cause hypotension; thus, do not give a large dose without time to accommodate to this treatment.

POSSIBLE INTERACTIONS
N/A

ALTERNATIVE DRUGS
Most other vasodilatory drugs should have some beneficial effect in horses with moderate to severe regurgitation but may be less effective than ACE inhibitors.

FOLLOW UP

PATIENT MONITORING
- Frequently monitor cardiac rhythm and respiratory system.
- Horses with mild to moderate regurgitation should be re-examined echocardiographically every year.
- Horses with severe regurgitation should be re-examined echocardiographically every 3–6 months, depending on severity of the regurgitation and its probable speed of progression, to ensure the horse continues to be safe to ride.

PREVENTION/AVOIDANCE
N/A

POSSIBLE COMPLICATIONS
Chronic regurgitation—atrial fibrillation; congestive heart failure

EXPECTED COURSE AND PROGNOSIS
- Many affected horses have a normal performance life and life expectancy.
- Prognosis for horses with mitral valve prolapse and mild regurgitation is excellent; in many, the amount of regurgitation remains unchanged for years.
- Progression of regurgitation associated with degenerative valve disease usually is slow; if the regurgitation is mild, these horses also have a good prognosis.
- Horses with ruptured chordae tendineae, flail mitral valve leaflets, or bacterial endocarditis have a more guarded prognosis, because regurgitation usually becomes more severe and results in shortened performance life and life expectancy.
- Affected horses with congestive heart failure usually have severe underlying valvular heart and myocardial disease and a guarded to grave prognosis for life.
- Most affected horses being treated for congestive heart failure respond to supportive therapy and improve. This improvement usually is short lived, however, and most are euthanized within 2–6 months of initiating treatment.

MISCELLANEOUS

ASSOCIATED CONDITIONS
N/A

AGE-RELATED FACTORS
Old horses are more likely to be affected.

ZOONOTIC POTENTIAL
N/A

PREGNANCY
- Affected mares should not experience any problems with pregnancy unless the regurgitation is moderate to severe.
- The volume expansion of late pregnancy places an additional load on the already volume-loaded heart and may precipitate the onset of congestive heart failure in mares with severe regurgitation.
- Pregnant affected mares with congestive heart failure should be treated for the underlying cardiac disease with positive inotropic drugs and diuretics; ACE inhibitors are contraindicated because of potential adverse effects on the fetus.

SYNONYMS
Mitral insufficiency

SEE ALSO

- Atrial fibrillation
- Bacterial endocarditis
- Congestive heart failure—left sided
- Congestive heart failure—right sided
- Systolic murmurs

ABBREVIATIONS
- ACE = angiotensin-converting enzyme
- AV = atrioventricular
- CK-MB = MB isoenzyme of creatine kinase
- HBDH = α-hydroxybutyrate dehydrogenase
- LDH = lactate dehydrogenase
- PMI = point of maximal intensity

Suggested Reading

Else RW, Holmes JR. Cardiac pathology in the horse. I. Gross pathology. Equine Vet J 1972;4:1–8.

Reef VB. Cardiovascular ultrasonography. In: Reef VB, ed. Equine diagnostic ultrasound. Philadelphia: WB Saunders, 1998:215–272.

Reef VB. Heart murmurs in horses: determining their significance with echocardiography. Equine Vet J 1995;19(Suppl):71–80.

Reef VB. Mitral valvular insufficiency associated with ruptured chordae tendineae in three foals. J Am Vet Med Assoc 1987;191:329–331.

Reef VB, Bain FT, Spencer PA. Severe mitral regurgitation in horses: clinical, echocardiographic, and pathologic findings. Equine Vet J 1998;30:18–27.

Author Virginia B. Reef

Consulting Editor N/A

MONOCYTOSIS

BASICS

DEFINITION

An absolute number of circulating monocytes > the reference interval for the laboratory performing the determination (i.e., >1.0 × 10^9 cells/L or >1000 cell/μL [mm^3]).

PATHOPHYSIOLOGY

• No available information specifically regarding equine monopoiesis; the following description is based on the assumption that equine kinetics and proliferation are similar to those of other species.
• Monocytes originate in the bone marrow; the hematopoietic progenitor that precedes recognizable monocyte precursors is the CFU-GM.
• Monocytes apparently have a considerably shorter marrow generation time than granulocytes. Their generation involves at least three mitotic divisions during maturation from monoblasts (or myeloblasts) through promonocytes to monocytes.
• Monocytes are released to the peripheral blood shortly after their last division, without storage or further maturation. Thus, they are still relatively immature compared to granulocytes.
• Monocytes have a half-life in the blood of ≅3 days.
• Some early investigations suggested a marginated pool, but kinetic studies have not supported this.
• In other species, monopoiesis is regulated by a variety of mediators, including colony-stimulating factor, PGE_2, and various interleukins, but no specific information is available for horses.
• On exiting the blood to tissues, monocytes continue differentiation into a variety of macrophages, which are named for the tissues in which they occur—Kupffer cells in the liver, alveolar macrophages in the lungs, osteoclasts in bone, and microglial cells in the CNS.
• Macrophages are found in almost every tissue, but they do not acquire specialized names in all.
• Tissues with a significant macrophage component include the pleural and peritoneal cavities, lymph nodes, bone marrow, and spleen.
• Macrophages may fuse to form multinucleated giant cells, often in response to fungi, mycobacterium, syncytial virus, and foreign material.
• Monocytes accumulate in areas of acute or chronic inflammation in response to chemotactic factors, some of which also attract neutrophils. Most macrophages in inflammatory foci derive from circulating monocytes, but under special circumstances, they can be locally produced.
• Monocytes/macrophages have numerous functions—phagocytosis, microbiocidal activity, tumor cytolysis, regulation of the immune system, coagulation, fibrinolysis, and bone repair
• Monocytes/macrophages are very important in the body's response to many infectious agents, especially intracellular bacteria (e.g., *Mycobacterium, Listeria,* and *Brucella* sp.), mycotic agents, protozoa, and viruses.

SYSTEMS AFFECTED

• Any system can be affected by an underlying infectious disease that has caused monocytosis.
• In monocytic myeloproliferative disease, the bone marrow, lymph nodes, spleen, and liver commonly are infiltrated by neoplastic cells.

SIGNALMENT

N/A

SIGNS

Referable to primary cause of the monocytosis

CAUSES

• Any inflammatory process that stimulates neutrophilia, because monocytes and neutrophils share a common progenitor, CFU-GM. In fact, monocytosis without neutrophilia may not occur in horses.
• Causes of monocytosis and neutrophilia include hemorrhage, hemolysis, necrosis, suppurative inflammation, and pyogranulomatous inflammation.
• Glucocorticoids do not stimulate any consistent monocyte changes in equine blood.
• Without a marginated pool, epinephrine-induced monocytosis cannot occur.
• Monocytic and myelomonocytic leukemia (i.e., the neoplastic proliferation of the monocyte cell line or the combined myeloid and monocyte cell lines, respectively) are rare but can produce monocytosis. Only the acute forms of these diseases have been reported, and affected animals are presented with leukocytosis caused by immature, bizarre-appearing monocytoid cells.

RISK FACTORS

• Failure of passive transfer
• Combined immunodeficiency

MONOCYTOSIS

DIAGNOSIS

DIFFERENTIAL DIAGNOSIS

• If accompanied by neutrophilia, consider the caused listed above.
• If not accompanied by neutrophilia and splenomegaly or lymphadenopathy are noted, consider leukemia.

LABORATORY FINDINGS

Drugs That May Alter Lab Results
N/A

Disorders That May Alter Lab Results
N/A

Valid If Run in Human Lab?
Metamyelocytes and other immature neutrophils, especially if toxic, can be confused with monocytes; thus, an erroneous monocytosis may be reported.

CBC/BIOCHEMISTRY/URINALYSIS

• Severe monocytosis (i.e., >10,000 monocytes/μL), with normal or low neutrophils—consider leukemia; immature or bizarre cells in the circulation support this conclusion.
• Neutrophilia—consider inflammatory diseases.
• Anemia—consider hemolysis or hemorrhage.

OTHER LABORATORY TESTS

N/A

IMAGING

N/A

DIAGNOSTIC PROCEDURES

N/A

TREATMENT

Directed at the underlying cause of the monocytosis or neutrophilia.

MEDICATIONS

DRUGS OF CHOICE

N/A

CONTRAINDICATIONS

N/A

PRECAUTIONS

N/A

POSSIBLE INTERACTIONS

Levamisole increases migration rate of monocytes, enhances chemotaxis, and increases phagocytosis.

ALTERNATIVE DRUGS

N/A

FOLLOW-UP

PATIENT MONITORING

N/A

POSSIBLE COMPLICATIONS

N/A

MISCELLANEOUS

ASSOCIATED CONDITIONS

N/A

AGE-RELATED FACTORS

N/A

ZOONOTIC POTENTIAL

N/A

PREGNANCY

N/A

SYNONYMS

N/A

SEE ALSO

N/A

ABBREVIATIONS

CFU-GM = colony-forming unit–granulocyte monocyte

Suggested Reading

Burkhardt E, Saldern FV, Huskamp B. Monocytic leukemia in a horse. Vet Pathol 1984;21:394–398.
Lassen DE, Swardson CJ. Hematology and hemostasis in the horse: normal functions and common abnormalities. Vet Clin North Am Equine Pract 1995:351–389.
Monteith CN, Cole D. Monocytic leukemia in a horse. Can Vet J 1995;36:765–766.

Author G. Daniel Boon
Consulting Editor Claire B. Andreasen

MORBILLIVIRUS

BASICS

OVERVIEW

Equine morbillivirus (EMV) is an acute and rapidly fatal viral pneumonia in horses. An outbreak of EMV pneumonia (EMP) was reported in Queensland, Australia; two horses in a separate occurrence, remote from the outbreak, were diagnosed retrospectively. Both have been associated with human fatalities and illness. EMV is a member of the Paramyxoviridae family and is distantly related to the morbilliviruses rinderpest, measles, and canine distemper. Pylogenetic analysis suggests that the virus emerged from its natural host and is not a mutation. The natural host has not been identified; however, serum neutralization antibodies to EMV in *Pteropus* bats (flying foxes) have been found, the significance of which is unknown. Cats and guinea pigs are susceptible to experimental infection via parenteral and non-parenteral routes; rabbits and mice are not.

SIGNALMENT

Horses described in the outbreaks were racing thoroughbreds, pregnant mares, and a stallion.

SIGNS

The incubation period is up to 10 days. Clinical course is very acute, with death occurring 1–3 days after onset of clinical signs. Initial signs include anorexia, depression, fever (up to 41°C), sweating, edema around the lips and head, cyanosis, and slightly jaundiced mucous membranes. Clinical signs indicative of severe respiratory difficulty include shallow, rapid respiration; and nasal discharge that varies from clear to serosanginous. Terminal signs include headpressing, dependent edema, ataxia, and copious frothy nasal discharge. Two of the recovered horses showed mild transient neurologic signs of myoclonic twitches. All seropositive horses were euthanized.

CAUSES AND RISK FACTORS

No outbreaks of EMV have been identified in countries other than Australia. EMV is not endemic in the Queensland horse population. Very close contact appears necessary for disease transmission via infected aerosols, nasal secretions, or blood from infected horses or from contaminated tack or handlers.

DIAGNOSIS

DIFFERENTIAL DIAGNOSIS

African horse sickness is differentiated by serology, virus isolation, histopathology, and immunofluorescence. Equine influenza has a lower mortality and coughing is a more common clinical sign, and is differentiated by virus culture from acute phase collection of nasal secretions, ELISA antigen detection, or immunofluorescence. Equine viral arteritis differentiated by virus isolation from nasal or conjunctival swabs, heparinized blood, and virus neutralization on serum. Clinical signs are not as severe for the encephalitides and relate to the nervous system, as do postmortem findings and serology. Anthrax is differentiated by postmortem findings, black tarry exudates, and organisms in blood smears. Hantavirus infection is differentiated by serology. Toxins—paraquat, monensin, heavy metals, mycotoxins—are differentiated by a history of exposure; presence of the toxin in the stomach, urine, or feed; lack of supportive serology; and postmortem findings.

MORBILLIVIRUS

CBC/BIOCHEMISTRY/URINALYSIS
No characteristic abnormalities were detected from a few affected horses.

OTHER LABORATORY TESTS
- Serum neutralization test and indirect fluorescent antibody test should be performed for serologic diagnosis and to confirm the identity of the virus. Death may occur prior to seroconversion.
- Virus isolation from fresh specimens of the lung, liver, spleen, and kidney. Duplicate tissues in 10% formal saline for histopathology.

IMAGING
N/A

DIAGNOSTIC PROCEDURES
N/A

PATHOLOGIC FINDINGS
Most changes are restricted to the lower respiratory tract. There is marked subpleural edema, severe pulmonary edema and congestion, and airways filled with blood-stained stable froth. Histologically, the main lesion is an acute interstitial pneumonia. Syncytial giant cells, which are typical of a morbillivirus infection, are found in the endothelium of lung capillaries and arterioles.

TREATMENT
No known treatment. Persons in close contact with affected animals should wear protective facemasks, goggles, and gloves.

MEDICATIONS
There is no medication for EMV.

CONTRAINDICATIONS/POSSIBLE INTERACTIONS
N/A

FOLLOW-UP
Control of outbreak by quarantine, containment, early identification of the causal agent, and disinfection of the area.

MISCELLANEOUS

ZOONOTIC POTENTIAL
Two fatalities and one illness have been associated with EMV outbreaks. Influenza-like illness caused the fatality of the trainer and illness of a stablehand in one outbreak. The other fatality was from acute progressive encephalitis in a farmer assisting with necropsies of two affected horses.

ABBREVIATIONS
- EMV = equine morbillivirus
- EMP = equine morbillivirus pneumonia

Suggested Reading

Hodgson DR, Hodgson JL. Acute Equine Respiratory Syndrome. In: Robinson NE, ed. Current Therapy in Equine Medicine,Vol 4. Philadelphia: WB Saunders, 1997:459-460.

Author Jane E. Axon
Consulting Editor Corinne R. Sweeney

MOTOR NEURON DISEASE (MND)

BASICS

DEFINITION

An acquired, neurodegenerative disease primarily affecting somatic motor neurons

PATHOPHYSIOLOGY

- The cause is unproven, but EMND is strongly associated with vitamin E deficiency.
- Ventral horn motor neuron cells become dysfunctional or die, presumably from oxidative damage that likely results from an imbalance in pro- and anti-oxidants.
- Excessive pro-oxidants axe unproven, but excessive copper or iron would be the most likely.
- Early dysfunctional changes in the motor neuron cells likely are associated with mitochondrial damage, followed by disintegration of the nucleus and nucleolus and neurofibrillary accumulation.
- Dead motor neurons eventually may be removed by glial cells.
- Clinical signs become apparent only when $\cong$30% of the motor neurons become dysfunctional, some of which may be dead but others only diseased.
- Ventral horn motor neurons that supply the postural muscles (i.e., predominantly type 1) are preferentially affected. This is believed to occur because of the higher oxidative activity of predominant type I muscle and its corresponding parent motor neuron.
- The oxidative disease causes lipopigment (i.e., ceroid) accumulation in the endothelium of spinal cord capillaries, neurons, and RPE. The RPE ceroid generally can be seen at fundoscopy as brown streaks.
- Excessive lipopigment may, on occasion, be found in livers of affected horses.

SYSTEMS AFFECTED

- Neuromuscular—motor neuron cell dysfunction causing neurogenic muscular atrophy and weakness
- Ocular—lipopigment accumulation in RPE causes electroretinographic abnormalities and, undoubtedly, affects vision, even though owners rarely report this.
- GI—a functional abnormality in carbohydrate absorption occurs in severely affected horses and may relate to mitochondrial dysfunction in the enterocyte; rarely, abnormal light microscopy changes are seen; hepatic lipofuscinosis occurs in a few cases.

GENETICS

- No known genetic basis
- Superoxide dismutase activity is abnormally low in red cells and nervous tissue. This is believed to result from excessive oxidative stress, however, because no abnormal polymorphism is seen in the SOD gene of affected horses versus controls.

INCIDENCE/PREVALENCE

- Affected $\cong$1 horse per 10,000 per year in the northeastern United States from 1990–1996
- Worldwide distribution, but most commonly seen in those areas less likely to have alfalfa hay (e.g., the northeastern United States and Canada) and lack of pasture (e.g., urban areas).
- Clusters may occur on certain premises.

SIGNALMENT

Environment

Adult horses kept without pasture and leafy green hay for at least 1 year

Breed Predilection

- Quarter Horses are more commonly affected, because they are more likely (in the United States) to be on farms with conducive environmental conditions.
- All breeds of horses and ponies may be affected.

Mean Age and Range

- Mean age—12 years
- Range—2–25 years

Predominant Sex

N/A

SIGNS

- Clinical signs vary depending on the stage/duration of the disorder.
- Signs are best summarized into subacute and chronic forms.

Subacute Form

- Acute onset of trembling, fasciculations, lying down more often than normal, frequent shifting of weight in the rear legs, and abnormal sweating
- Head carriage may be abnormally low.
- Appetite and gait usually are not noticeably affected.
- Owners may mention the horse had been losing weight (i.e., loss of muscle mass) for 1 month before the trembling.

Chronic Form

- Trembling and fasciculations subside, and the horse stabilizes, but with varying degrees of muscle atrophy.
- In some cases, atrophy is so severe that the horse looks emaciated. In others, noticeable improvement in muscle mass and/or fat deposition is seen.
- The tail head frequently is in an abnormally high resting position.

CAUSES

- Dysfunction and death of motor neurons is an oxidative disorder that, presumably, results from low concentrations of vitamin E and inability to protect against oxidative (i.e., pro-oxidant) stress.
- Clinical signs occur when $\cong$30% of motor neurons are affected. Some of these neurons may only be diseased, however, and may regain function.

DIAGNOSIS

DIFFERENTIAL DIAGNOSIS

- Colic, because of the propensity to stand for only brief periods during the subacute form. Normal appetite and fecal production should rule out an abdominal disorder.
- Laminitis, because of the almost-constant shifting of weight in the subacute form. The ease of motion and even the desire to walk (as seen in EMND) is contradictory to this diagnosis.
- Other neuromuscular disorders (e.g., botulism), myositis/myopathy, and EPM may have similarities to EMND. Normal appetite, elevated tail head, and lack of cranial nerve dysfunction should separate EMND from botulism. Chronic myopathies (e.g., PSSM) may appear very similar to EMND, and consideration of breed (for PSSM) and muscle biopsy may be required to delineate the two. EMND causes symmetric muscle weakness and atrophy without ataxia and elevation of muscle enzymes (in subacute cases), as opposed to EPM.
- The severe muscle wasting with normal appetite in the chronic form may look similar to intestinal malabsorption syndrome. Plasma albumin is low in most infiltrative bowel syndromes but is normal in EMND.

CBC/BIOCHEMISTRY/URINALYSIS

- CBC generally is within the nornal range.
- The most common abnormal biochemical finding is a moderate elevation in muscle enzymes in subacute case.
- A few affected horses may have elevated liver enzymes.
- Urinalysis is normal in most cases, but some may have myoglobinuria.
- CBC, biochemistry, and urinalysis are all normal in chronic cases.

OTHER LABORATORY TESTS

- Subacute cases—plasma or serum vitamin E (i.e., α-tocopherol) is abnormally low (mean, 0.56 μg/mL); serum ferritin often is abnormally high.
- Chronic cases—α-tocopherol values may have returned to normal.

IMAGING

N/A

MOTOR NEURON DISEASE (MND)

DIAGNOSTIC PROCEDURES

- Biopsy of the sacrocaudalis dorsalis medialis muscle (i.e., tail-head muscle) or ventral branch of the spinal accessory nerve biopsy are reliable diagnostic tests.
- Fundoscopy frequently reveals brown streaking of the retina, which is specific for vitamin E deficiency and only supportive for EMND.
- Glucose malabsorption generally is present in subacute cases but is only supportive for EMND.

PATHOLOGIC FINDINGS

Gross Findings

- Few or no gross lesions
- An abnormal paleness of some muscles (e.g., vastus intermedius) containing most type I fibers may be observed.
- Body fat stores are variable.

Histopathologic Findings

- CNS lesions are confined to the spinal cord ventral horn cells and nuclei of cranial nerves V, VII, VIII, IX, X, XI, and XII. Demyelination of corresponding motor nerves and neurogenic muscle atrophy are found.
- Lipofuscinosis of the RPE layer and spinal cord endothelium in all cases and of the liver in a few.
- No light microscopic lesions in the intestine in 90% of cases, but ultrastructural changes may be seen.

TREATMENT

APPROPRIATE HEALTH CARE

- Affected horses can be treated either on the farm or in the hospital.
- Trailering can worsen the clinical signs.

NURSING CARE

N/A

ACTIVITY

Affected horses should not have free movement restricted but should not be exercised or ridden.

DIET

Provide leafy green hay or grass with additional vitamin E—2000–7000 U/day

CLIENT EDUCATION

N/A

SURGICAL CONSIDERATIONS

N/A

MEDICATIONS

DRUGS OF CHOICE

- The only recommended treatment is a diet high in vitamin E (natural and/or supplemental).
- Feeding small amounts of corn oil may enhance absorption of vitamin E.
- Corticosteroids have been used in hopes of decreasing hypersensitivity (seen in a small percentage of cases) and neuronal oxidative damage (unproven effect).
- Lazaroids, vitamin therapy, neurotrophic growth factors, and glutamate inhibitors have been used in humans with motor neuron disease.

CONTRAINDICATIONS

No proven contraindications to vitamin E therapy.

PRECAUTIONS

N/A

POSSIBLE INTERACTIONS

N/A

ALTERNATIVE DRUGS

N/A

FOLLOW-UP

PATIENT MONITORING

- Subacute cases—improvement in clinical signs often corresponds to return of serum muscle enzymes to normal values.
- Monitor vitamin E concentrations to determine that levels return to normal.

PREVENTION/AVOIDANCE

Supplement all other horses kept under similar conditions with vitamin E.

POSSIBLE COMPLICATIONS

N/A

EXPECTED COURSE AND PROGNOSIS

- Of horses subacutely affected, ≅40% will stabilize within 3–8 weeks and regain some of the lost muscle mass. Other horses will have progressive deterioration in clinical signs or no improvement despite vitamin E treatment. This might reflect the number of motor neurons that have died (as opposed to being temporarily dysfunctional), reinnervation, or a continued imbalance between pro- and anti-oxidants.
- Horses with the chronic and more stabilized form may have several years of quality life, but not performance. Their life expectancy would be shorter than normal, and another acute onset of clinical signs may occur years later (similar to the human postpolio paresis). Horses diagnosed with EMND should not be ridden, because they can be unsafe and because moderate to severe exercise likely will shorten their life expectancy.

MISCELLANEOUS

ASSOCIATED CONDITIONS

N/A

AGE-RELATED FACTORS

N/A

ZOONOTIC POTENTIAL

N/A

PREGNANCY

N/A

SYNONYMS

N/A

SEE ALSO

N/A

ABBREVIATIONS

- EPM = equine protozoal myelitis
- GI = gastrointestinal
- PSSM = polysaccharide storage myopathy
- RPE = retinal pigment epithelium
- SOD = superoxide dismutase

Suggested Reading

Cummings JF, de Lahunta A, George C, et al. Equine motor neuron disease: a preliminary report. Cornell Vet 1990;80:357–379.

Divers TJ, et al. Simple and practical muscle biopsy test for equine motor neuron disease. AAEP Proc 1996;42:180–181.

Divers TJ, Mohammed HO, Cummings JF, et al. Equine motor neuron disease: findings in 28 horses and proposal of a pathophysiological mechanism for the disease. Equine Vet J 1994;24:409–415.

Jackson CA, de Lahunta A, Cummings JF, et al. Spinal accessory nerve biopsy as an antemortem diagnostic test for equine motor neuron disease. Equine Vet J 1996;28:215–219.

de la Rua-Domenech R, Mohammed HO, Cummings JF, et al. Association between plasma vitamin E concentration and the risk of equine motor neuron disease. Vet J 1997;154:203–213.

Author Thomas J. Divers

Consulting Editor Joseph J. Bertone

MULTIPLE MYELOMA

BASICS

OVERVIEW

- An uncommon malignant neoplasm of plasma cells characterized by multifocal or diffuse bone marrow involvement.
- The abnormal plasma cells produce paraprotein, a homogenous immunoglobulin or immunoglobulin fragment.

SIGNALMENT

- Most reported cases are light-breed horses.
- Affected ages range from 3 months to 22 years.
- No sex predilection
- A genetic link has not been documented in horses, but familial cases and chromosomal abnormalities have been detected in humans.

SIGNS

- Nonspecific clinical signs, but most commonly progressive weight loss, anorexia, fever, and limb edema
- Pneumonia, recurrent local infections, ataxia, epistaxis, petechiae, bleeding, lymphadenopathy, and bone pain (lameness) also reported
- Other signs may develop relative to specific tissue invasion

CAUSES AND RISK FACTORS

The disease is uncommon and sporadic, with no known risk factors or predisposing causes in horses; however, in humans, radiation exposure and chronic antigenic stimulation may predispose.

DIAGNOSIS

DIFFERENTIAL DIAGNOSIS

- Lymphosarcoma is differentiated by cytology of tissue or bone marrow or immunofluorescent or immunohistochemical staining to differentiate plasma cells.
- Chronic infection (i.e., abscess, pulmonary or peritoneal), chronic liver failure, other neoplasms, and immune-mediated disorders are differentiated by the presence of polyclonal gammopathy and the absence of atypical plasma cell populations.
- Benign, transient monoclonal gammopathy is differentiated by the absence of homogeneity (morphologic or immunohistochemical) of plasma cell populations.

CBC/BIOCHEMISTRY/URINALYSIS

- Hyperproteinemia characterized by hyperglobulinemia with hypoalbuminemia
- Anemia, sometimes macrocytic
- Thrombocytopenia
- Leukopenia, characterized by neutropenia
- Plasma cell leukemia may be present.
- Hyponatremia
- Rare azotemia
- Variable proteinuria

OTHER LABORATORY TESTS

- Serum or urine electrophoresis, immunoelectrophoresis, or immunodiffusion indicate the presence of monoclonal gammopathy, typically subclasses of IgG, and decreased concentrations of other polyclonal immunoglobulins.
- Bence-Jones proteinuria may be present.
- Hyperviscosity

IMAGING

Radiography—focal, punctate bone lysis; adjacent periosteal reaction and sclerosis; and diffuse osteoporosis

OTHER DIAGNOSTIC PROCEDURES

- Cytologic evidence of bone marrow plasmacytosis (>10% plasma cells) or presence of atypical plasma cells confirms the diagnosis; however, bone marrow cytology may be normal.
- Cytologic evidence of extramedullary plasmacytosis in conjunction with serum or urine monoclonal gammopathy or osteolytic lesions
- Immunofluorescent or immunohistochemical labeling of cytoplasmic or surface immunoglobulins, antigens, or neoplastic markers have been used in humans to distinguish benign from malignant monoclonal gammopathy.

PATHOLOGIC FINDINGS

- Multifocal or diffuse bone marrow involvement with associated bone destruction and normal to increased numbers of plasma or atypical plasma cells
- Extraosseous accumulation of plasma cells in essentially any tissue, but most commonly in the lymph nodes, spleen, liver, kidney, and lung
- Immunohistochemical staining of tissues may be helpful.

TREATMENT

No successful long-term treatment regimens have been reported; if attempted, initial therapy may be best managed under hospitalized conditions.

MEDICATIONS

DRUGS

- Melphalan (7 mg/m^2 PO q24h for 5 days every 3 weeks) stabilized one horse's condition for 1 year.
- Unreported doses of melphalan, prednisolone, and cyclophosphamide were used in an 18-year-old, pregnant Quarter Horse mare that survived an additional 7 months.
- Plasmapheresis
- Treatment of acquired secondary infections

CONTRAINDICATIONS/POSSIBLE INTERACTIONS

Bone marrow suppression, gastrointestinal upset, and laminitis are possible side effects of therapy.

FOLLOW-UP

- Average life expectancy after diagnosis is 4 months, but one horse reportedly survived 2 additional years.
- Even with extensive chemotherapy, cure is exceedingly uncommon in humans.

MISCELLANEOUS

ASSOCIATED CONDITIONS

N/A

AGE-RELATED FACTORS

N/A

ZOONOTIC POTENTIAL

N/A

PREGNANCY

N/A

SEE ALSO

Lymphosarcoma

Suggested Reading

Edwards DF, Parker JW, Wilkinson JE, Helman RG. Plasma cell myeloma in the horse. A case report and literature review. J Vet Intern Med 1993;7:169–176.

Author Michelle Henry Barton
Consulting Editor Debra C. Sellon

MULTIPLE PREGNANCIES

BASICS

DEFINITION
Simultaneous intrauterine production of two or more embryos/fetuses

PATHOPHYSIOLOGY
- Most multiple pregnancies are twins, and most twins are dizygotic and result from double ovulations. Early twin vesicles behave similarly to a singleton conceptus. The vesicles traverse the full extent of the uterine lumen until 15 days of gestation, when they "fix" in one or both uterine horns around 16–17 days; ≅75% of twin vesicles fix in the same horn—unicornual
- Of unicornual pregnancies, ≅75% undergo natural reduction to one embryo before 40 days, and the remaining embryo develops normally to term as a singleton. If natural reduction does not occur in unicornual twins by 40 days of gestation, there is a strong probability that the twins will continue to develop only to abort later in gestation.
- Bicornual twins do not undergo natural reduction. Instead, they usually develop through the last trimester of gestation, when abortion is common.

SYSTEM AFFECTED
Reproductive

GENETICS
N/A

INCIDENCE/PREVALENCE
- Incidence of twin pregnancy relates to age, breed, and reproductive status.
- Twin pregnancy occurs more frequently in old mares, barren mares, Thoroughbreds, and draft breeds.
- Arabians, Quarter Horses, ponies, and primitive breeds have a lower incidence of twin pregnancy.

SIGNALMENT
Mares that develop twin pregnancies tend to have twins in subsequent pregnancies.

SIGNS
N/A

CAUSES
- Ovulation and fertilization of multiple ova, in most cases
- Rare incidence of monozygotic multiple pregnancies

RISK FACTORS
- Breed
- Age
- Reproductive status

DIAGNOSIS

DIFFERENTIAL DIAGNOSIS
Differentiating Similar Signs:
- Uterine cysts can be confused with developing embryonic vesicles, causing an improper diagnosis of twin pregnancy.
- Differentiation of uterine cysts from embryonic vesicles may be simplified by recording the location, size, and shape of uterine cysts before pregnancy.
- Embryonic vesicles also may be differentiated from uterine cysts by observation of an embryonic heartbeat at ≥24 days of gestation.

CBC/BIOCHEMISTRY/URINALYSIS
N/A

OTHER LABORATORY TESTS
N/A

IMAGING
Transrectal Ultrasonography
- Ultrasonography of the reproductive tract early in gestation allows for prompt diagnosis and treatment of twin pregnancies.
- Pregnancies may be detected as early as 9 days of gestation; however, twin pregnancies may differ in age by as much as 2 days.
- Because of possible differences in the age and size of twin pregnancies, ultrasonographic diagnosis is recommended between 13 and 15 days of gestation. At this time, the embryonic vesicle is an anechoic, spheric yolk sac averaging 12–20 mm in height.
- Twin vesicles are highly mobile for the first 15–16 days and can be located adjacent to one another or in different locations within the uterus.
- To properly determine if twin vesicles are present, scan both uterine horns and the uterine body to the cervix, sequentially.

Transabdominal Ultrasonography
- Useful for diagnosing twin pregnancies at >75–100 days of gestation
- Diagnosis generally is established by identifying two fetal heartbeats.

DIAGNOSTIC PROCEDURES
Transrectal palpation of the reproductive tract:
- Pregnancy diagnosis based on transrectal palpation at 25–30 days of gestation is characterized by distinct uterine tone and a narrow, elongated cervix.
- A bulge the size of a small hen's egg can be appreciated at the caudoventral aspect of a uterine horn, adjacent to the uterine bifurcation.
- If twin vesicles are bicornual, it may be possible to diagnose twin pregnancies at this time.
- If vesicles are located within the same uterine horn, it is impossible to diagnose twin pregnancies using transrectal palpation alone.

PATHOLOGIC FINDINGS
N/A

TREATMENT

APPROPRIATE HEALTH CARE
Twins Before 40 Days of Gestation
- Twin pregnancies detected during the mobility phase of the conceptus (9–15 days) are best managed by crushing one embryonic vesicle.
- One vesicle is manipulated, transrectally, to the tip of a uterine horn. Pressure then is placed on the vesicle, and it is crushed.
- The remaining vesicle survives in ≅90% of the cases.
- The crush technique is useful for twins in the mobility phase and bilateral twins before 30 days of gestation. After 30 days of gestation, fluid released from the crushed vesicle tends to disrupt the remaining pregnancy.
- Unicornual twins usually are both destroyed when crushing of one vesicle is attempted.

Twins After 40 Days of Gestation
- Management of twin pregnancies in the fetal period (>40 days) is further complicated by the formation of endometrial cups.
- Pregnancy loss in the presence of endometrial cups causes irregular estrous cycles and/or delayed return to fertile cycles.
- Maintenance of a singleton pregnancy from twin pregnancies is critical to the reproductive success of the mare after 40 days.

MULTIPLE PREGNANCIES

Potassium Chloride
• Using transcutaneous ultrasonography, one fetal heart is located, and fetal death is caused by intracardiac injection of potassium chloride.
• The technique has been successful in ≅50% of cases.
• Most useful from 115–130 days of gestation.

NURSING CARE
N/A

ACTIVITY
N/A

DIET
In one study, mares with twin pregnancies (diagnosed by transrectal palpation) were limited to poor-quality grass hay early during gestation (21–49 days); one viable foal was delivered in 56% (23/41) of the cases examined.

CLIENT EDUCATION
N/A

SURGICAL CONSIDERATIONS
Surgical Removal of One Twin
• Surgical removal of one twin has been attempted in seven unicornual and eight bicornual twins at 41–62 days of gestation.
• No unicornual twins have survived.
• Five of the eight bicornual twin pregnancies were successfully reduced to a singleton.

Transvaginal Allantocentesis
• Has been used to aid in identifying the allantoic sac in one twin fetus, to pass a needle into the allantois, and to aspirate the allantoic fluid.
• Fluid aspiration collapses the vesicle and causes fetal death.
• To date, this technique has been successful in ≅30% of cases.
• Most applicable for bicornual twins.

MEDICATIONS

DRUGS OF CHOICE
• Flunixin meglumine (1 mg/kg IV) often is administered during attempted twin reduction to prevent prostaglandin release from the uterus and subsequent lysis of the corpus luteum.
• Exogenous progestins (e.g., altrenogest [0.044–0.088 mg/kg PO SID]) at double the recommended dose may be administered when attempting twin reduction to maintain uterine tone after uterine manipulation and to counter the effects of possible fetal fluid release into the uterine lumen.

CONTRAINDICATIONS
N/A

PRECAUTIONS
N/A

POSSIBLE INTERACTIONS
N/A

ALTERNATIVE DRUGS
N/A

FOLLOW-UP

PATIENT MONITORING
• After any method of twin reduction is performed, monitor the progress and viability of the remaining embryo/fetus using ultrasonography.
• Critical to monitor the mare for embryo/fetal death if being treated with exogenous progestins
• Weekly ultrasonography is warranted for the first 3 weeks after the procedure. After the initial examinations, a monthly schedule is useful to monitor fetal progress.
• Monitor the mare for signs of abortion—mammary development, vulvar discharge, or fetal expulsion

PREVENTION/AVOIDANCE
• Serial, complete transrectal palpations and maintenance of individual records for broodmares
• Record sizes for all follicles >30 mm on both ovaries during estrus (average growth, 5–6 mm/day) to account for whether they ovulate or regress. Double ovulation is the earliest indicator for mares at higher risk for twinning.
• Early diagnosis of pregnancy in mares from families with a history of twinning or with an individual history of or twinning in previous pregnancies
• Earlier reduction is associated with greater success in achieving a singleton pregnancy.

POSSIBLE COMPLICATIONS
• Embryonic or fetal loss
• Abortion
• Dystocia

EXPECTED COURSE AND PROGNOSIS
Reduction Technique:
• 90% success with early crush of a bicornual twin
• 50% success with potassium chloride (intracardiac injection) between days 115–130
• 20%–30% success with transvaginal aspiration of allantoic fluid from one bicornual twin

MISCELLANEOUS

ASSOCIATED CONDITIONS
N/A

AGE-RELATED FACTORS
N/A

ZOONOTIC POTENTIAL
N/A

PREGNANCY
N/A

SYNONYMS
N/A

SEE ALSO
• Abortion
• Early embryonic death
• Dystocia and parturient complications
• Placenta
• Placentitis

Suggested Reading
Ginther OJ. Reproductive biology of the mare. 2nd ed. Cross Plains: Equiservices, 1992.
Ginther OJ. Ultrasonic imaging and reproductive events in the mare. Cross Plains: Equiservices, 1986.
Author Margo L. Macpherson
Contributing Editor Carla L. Carleton

MYELOPROLIFERATIVE DISEASES

BASICS

DEFINITION

Abnormal, unregulated proliferation of myeloid hematopoietic cells; differentiated from lymphoproliferative diseases (e.g., lymphoma, lymphocytic leukemia, and plasma cell myeloma)

PATHOPHYSIOLOGY

- Proliferation of cells occurs within the medullary cavity but also can occur outside the marrow.
- Myelomonocytic leukemia is the most commonly reported myeloproliferative disease. Single cell-line leukemias in horses include monocytic, histiocytic (malignant histiocytosis), neutrophilic, and eosinophilic; primary erythrocytosis has been suspected. Basophilic leukemia and absolute thrombocythemia have not been reported.
- A specific inciting factor has not been described, but the disturbance is believed to occur between the pluripotential and committed stem cell level. Unregulated proliferation of cells within the medullary cavity results in "overcrowding" of healthy precursor cells and destruction of the marrow architecture.

SYSTEMS AFFECTED

- Hemic/lymphatic/immune
- Most cases have a tendency to anemia, neutropenia, and thrombocytopenia; this secondary effect is responsible for many of the reported clinical signs.
- Subsequent immune suppression leads to secondary infections; bacterial or fungal pneumonia has been reported and contributes to fever.

GENETICS

Genetic predisposition suggested in humans; no evidence in horses.

INCIDENCE/PREVALENCE

Rare (<1% of all reported neoplasms)

SIGNALMENT

Most common in young adult animals but also reported in horses from 10 months to 16 years of age.

SIGNS

Historical Findings

Most horses have a short history (days to weeks) of weight loss, depression, exercise intolerance, and fever.

Physical Examination Findings

- Prevalent—fever, ventral and peripheral edema, mucosal petechiation, and lymphadenopathy
- Less common—hemorrhagic diathesis (e.g., epistaxis), oral ulceration, pneumonia, and abdominal pain

CAUSES

- None known
- Retroviruses implicated in other species; exposure to certain chemicals or ionizing radiation may produce disease in humans.

RISK FACTORS

N/A

DIAGNOSIS

DIFFERENTIAL DIAGNOSIS

- History and clinical signs—nonspecific and can be indicative of bacterial infection, including pneumonia, pleuritis, peritonitis, or abdominal abscessation; these conditions are ruled out by thoracic auscultation and percussion, rectal palpation, CBC, and peripheral blood smear.
- Cytology and culture of peritoneal or tracheal fluid aspirates may be indicated, but affected animals are at risk for secondary bacterial or fungal infections.
- Horses with acute lymphoproliferative disease often share signalment, history, and physical examination findings similar to those of animals with myeloproliferative disease. The abnormal circulating lymphocytes in primary or late secondary lymphoid leukemias are differentiated from myeloid dysplasia based on morphology and histochemical staining.
- Differentiate eosinophilia from eosinophilic leukemia.
- Consider alternative causes of ventral and peripheral edema, including hypoproteinemia, vasculitis, or impaired lymphatic drainage. Edema due to vasculitis is warm and painful on firm palpation.

CBC/BIOCHEMISTRY/URINALYSIS

- Examine peripheral blood smear for evidence of neoplasia.
- Total WBC counts vary widely depending on whether a leukemic, subleukemic, or aleukemic leukemia is present.
- Pancytopenia may be present due to an overcrowding effect of the proliferating cells on the marrow architecture (myelophthisis).
- Immune-mediated anemia and thrombocytopenia may coexist.
- Anemias—typically nonregenerative
- Gammopathy may be present.

OTHER LABORATORY TESTS

Decreased erythropoietin concentration with normal PaO_2 and elevated hematocrit could be consistent with primary erythrocytosis.

IMAGING

- Hepatomegaly or splenomegaly may be evident at abdominal ultrasound.
- Radiography and ultrasound examination of the thorax may demonstrate pathology in horses with secondary respiratory infection.

MYELOPROLIFERATIVE DISEASES

DIAGNOSTIC PROCEDURES

- Bone marrow aspiration and core biopsy are indicated if abnormal circulating cells or pancytopenia exist. A monomorphic population of neoplastic cells is expected, resulting in an elevated myeloid:erythroid ratio (normal, 0.5–3.75). Megakaryocytes may be absent; morphologic examination may determine the cell type.
- Further characterization by histochemical and immunohistologic methods. Positive cytochemical staining with Sudan black B or PAS suggests myeloid rather than lymphoid origin. Granulocytic cells are differentiated from monocytic and megakaryocytic cells by a nonspecific esterase stain, α-naphthyl-butyrate esterase. The latter can be separated using a megakaryocyte stain (Megacolor®).
- Some poorly or undifferentiated leukemias may be difficult to classify with cytochemical staining; electron microscopy can aid in further differentiation.
- Malignant histiocytosis can be differentiated from acute monocytic leukemia based on histologic features.

PATHOLOGIC FINDINGS

- Gross examination may reveal lymphadenopathy, hepatomegaly, splenomegaly, and discoloration of the marrow cavities.
- Myeloblastic cells are evident histologically in bone marrow and occasionally in lymph nodes, spleen, liver, kidneys, lung, or heart.

TREATMENT

- Invariably fatal—the disease course is unlikely to be affected by housing, activity, or diet.
- Based on the nature of the disease and the poor response to treatment, euthanasia is usually warranted.

MEDICATIONS

DRUGS OF CHOICE

- Generally resistant to common antineoplastic therapy in all species.
- Treatment with cytosine arabinoside (10 mg/m^2 BID for 3 weeks) has been successful (promotes terminal differentiation of the neoplastic cell line and diminishes clonal expression).

CONTRAINDICATIONS

Horses appear to be sensitive to the toxic side effects of most chemotherapeutic agents.

PRECAUTIONS

N/A

POSSIBLE INTERACTIONS

N/A

ALTERNATIVE DRUGS

N/A

FOLLOW-UP

PATIENT MONITORING

N/A

PREVENTION/AVOIDANCE

N/A

POSSIBLE COMPLICATIONS

N/A

EXPECTED COURSE AND PROGNOSIS

Usually rapid deterioration; based on published cases, death can be expected within weeks.

MISCELLANEOUS

ASSOCIATED CONDITIONS

N/A

AGE-RELATED FACTORS

N/A

ZOONOTIC POTENTIAL

N/A

PREGNANCY

N/A

SYNONYMS

N/A

SEE ALSO

- Anemia
- Anemia, aplastic
- Lymphosarcoma
- Multiple myeloma
- Pancytopenia
- Thrombocytopenia

ABBREVIATIONS

N/A

Suggested Reading

Savage CJ. Lymphoproliferative and myeloproliferative disorders. Vet Clin North Am Equine Pract 1998;14:563–578.

Author Guy D. Lester
Consulting Editor Debra C. Sellon

NARCOLEPSY AND CATAPLEXY

BASICS

DEFINITION

Cerebral cortical and voluntary muscle disassociation

PATHOPHYSIOLOGY

- Both narcolepsy and cataplexy are pathologic syndromes and, therefore, different forms of sleep deprivation.
- In my opinion, sleep deprivation is far more common in horses with a history of sudden, episodic collapse than narcolepsy or cataplexy, which are rare.
- Narcolepsy is a neurologic disorder characterized by excessive daytime sleepiness and pathologic manifestations of REM sleep.
- Cataplexy is characterized by episodes of muscle weakness with full consciousness—cerebral cortical and voluntary muscle disassociation

SYSTEM AFFECTED

CNS

SIGNALMENT

- Two clinically distinct syndromes of narcolepsy and cataplexy
- The more common form is transient and affects foals through yearlings.
- The rare form is persistent and seen in some light breeds, ponies, Suffolk horses, and miniature horses.

SIGNS

Historical Findings

Most commonly, these signs are present from early in life but, occasionally, seem to be acquired.

Physical Examination Findings

- Horses are normal between attacks.
- Severity of episodes can vary.
- Mild signs include drowsiness, head droop, and knee and fetlock buckling.
- More severe episodes are characterized by sudden, complete collapse.
- Frequency of episodes can vary from rare to several per day.
- When forced to walk, horses are ataxic and difficult to arouse, which contrasts with sleep deprivation, in which horses are easily awakened.
- The narcoleptic and cataplectic state is similar to REM sleep with atonia and areflexia, with some maintenance of facial responses.
- No spinal reflexes can be elicited from horses that are recumbent in association with a cataplectic state. Again, this contrasts with sleep deprivation, in which horses often will not lie down.
- Attacks often are preceded by an external stimulus, such as grooming, feeding, and leading the horse out of a stall, which also contrasts with sleep deprivation. The precipitating stimulus is consistent in an individual with narcolepsy and cataplexy.
- Narcoleptic attacks while horses are under saddle have been reported; hence, these horses present a safety risk. This sharply contrasts with sleep deprivation.
- Narcolepsy and cataplexy usually do not worsen.
- A self-limited disease occurs in newborn foals of many breeds. Affected foals may have one or multiple episodes, which usually resolve with age.

CAUSES

No specific cause has been identified.

RISK FACTORS

None identified.

DIAGNOSIS

DIFFERENTIAL DIAGNOSIS

- Sleep deprivation
- Cardiac arrhythmias
- Seizure syndrome

CBC/BIOCHEMISTRY/URINALYSIS

No specific abnormalities

OTHER LABORATORY TESTS

N/A

IMAGING

N/A

DIAGNOSTIC PROCEDURES

- Clinical signs are diagnostic, however, when warranted, physostigmine provocation can be attempted.
- In this test, physostigmine (0.06–0.08 mg/kg IV) is administered, and an attack is induced within minutes.
- Unfortunately, a lack of positive response does not rule out the diagnosis of narcolepsy, and adverse effects (i.e., diarrhea and colic) can accompany this test.

PATHOLOGIC FINDINGS

No associated findings

NARCOLEPSY AND CATAPLEXY

TREATMENT

See *Drugs of Choice.*

MEDICATIONS

DRUGS OF CHOICE

- Atropine (0.08 mg/kg IV) can resolve signs for as long as 30 hours after administration.
- Imipramine (1–2 mg/kg IM or IV q6–12h), a tricyclic antidepressant, may be useful. Signs seem to be relieved for 5–10 hours, but oral absorption is poor and variable.

CONTRAINDICATIONS

N/A

PRECAUTIONS

N/A

POSSIBLE INTERACTIONS

N/A

ALTERNATIVE DRUGS

N/A

FOLLOW-UP

PATIENT MONITORING

N/A

POSSIBLE COMPLICATIONS

N/A

EXPECTED COURSE AND PROGNOSIS

- Poor prognosis with the persistent form
- Excellent prognosis with the neonatal form

MISCELLANEOUS

ASSOCIATED CONDITIONS

N/A

AGE-RELATED FACTORS

N/A

ZOONOTIC POTENTIAL

N/A

PREGNANCY

N/A

SYNONYMS

N/A

SEE ALSO

N/A

ABBREVIATIONS

REM = rapid eye movement

Suggested Reading

Guilleminault C, Anagnos A. Narcolepsy. In: Kryger M, Roth T, Dement W, eds. Principle and practices of sleep medicine. 3rd ed. Philadelphia: WB Saunders, Philadelphia, 2000:676–686.

Hines MT, et al. Adult-onset narcolepsy in the horse. Proc 39th Annu Conv AAEP 1993:289–296.

Lunn DP, et al. Familial occurrence of narcolepsy in miniature horses. Equine Vet J 1993;25:483–487.

Mignot EM, Dement WC. Narcolepsy in animals and man. Equine Vet J 1993;25:476–477.

Sweeney CR, et al. Narcolepsy in a horse. J Am Vet Med Assoc 1983;183:126–128.

Author Joseph J. Bertone

Consulting Editor Joseph J. Bertone

NASAL REGURGITATION OF MILK

BASICS

DEFINITION

Abnormal flow of milk from the nares of foals after nursing

PATHOPHYSIOLOGY

- Appearance of milk at the nares of newborn foals after nursing usually indicates an abnormality in swallowing, which may result from a physical deformity in the structures forming the pharyngeal/laryngeal area or a muscular/neurologic dysfunction of these structures.
- In normal nursing, a foal creates negative pressure in the oral cavity as it wraps its tongue around the mare's teat and presses it against the hard palate. Milk flows into the oral cavity, moving back to the oral pharynx. The milk bolus is directed up both sides of the larynx, and the soft palate creates a seal on the dorsal pharyngeal wall, preventing milk from entering the nasal passages. The vocal cords close, the epiglottis moves over the glottis, and the upper esophageal sphincter relaxes, allowing the bolus to enter the esophagus. These events are co-ordinated by the swallowing center in the medullary portion of the brainstem and by the trigeminal, glossopharyngeal, vagus, and hypoglossal nerves.
- Muscles involved in the swallowing reflex include those of the tongue and jaw, pharyngeal constrictors, and pharyngoesophageal sphincters. Disruption of any of these structures can result in lack of laryngeal closure, esophageal relaxation and constriction, and sealing off of the proximal pharynx.
- Upper airway obstruction may result in stridor and respiratory distress as well as dysphagia.

SYSTEMS AFFECTED

- Respiratory—foals with laryngeal/pharyngeal dysfunction likely have milk in their nares after suckling; this dysfunction also may result in respiratory stridor and aspiration of milk into the lungs.
- Gastrointestinal—decreased milk generally is ingested.
- Immune—foals with severe dysphagia may not ingest adequate colostrum from their dam, which can result in failure of passive transfer.

SIGNALMENT

Usually seen soon after birth.

SIGNS

Historical Findings

- Owners usually report milk dripping from the foal's nares soon after nursing.
- Owners sometimes report respiratory stridor.

Physical Examination Findings

- Milk reflux from the nares after suckling
- Increased respiratory rate and effort
- Crackles and wheezes heard on auscultation of the lung fields
- Respiratory stridor, leading to distress

CAUSES

- Numerous
- Congenital defects of the oral cavity such as cleft palate are the most obvious, but subepiglottic or pharyngeal cysts, dorsal displacement of the soft palate, and rostral displacement of the palatopharyngeal arch also are congenital causes.
- Laryngeal paralysis, either uni- or bilateral, has been implicated.
- Muscular, neuromuscular, and neurologic problems may affect the function of swallowing in foals. Vitamin E/selenium deficiency, prematurity, dysmaturity, pharyngeal paralysis, hydrocephalus, arytenoiditis, myotonia congenita, and hypoxic ischemic encephalopathy fall in this category.

RISK FACTORS

Any condition causing depression and weakness in foals

DIAGNOSIS

DIFFERENTIAL DIAGNOSIS

Other causes of respiratory distress—meconium aspiration, septic pneumonia, respiratory distress syndrome secondary to lack of surfactant, and pulmonary hypertension

CBC/BIOCHEMISTRY/URINALYSIS

- An inflammatory or stress leukogram may be seen in cases that develop aspiration pneumonia.
- No consistent changes in biochemistry or urinalysis

OTHER LABORATORY TESTS

- Hypoxemia may be found at arterial blood gas analysis in foals experiencing significant aspiration pneumonia or upper airway obstruction from laryngeal paralysis or pharyngeal cyst formation.
- Serum IgG levels <800 mg/dL may be seen in cases with severe dysphagia

IMAGING

- Thoracic radiography—in the cases with aspiration pneumonia, a heavy interstitial or alveolar lung pattern may be noted in the caudal ventral region of the lung field.
- Pharyngeal/laryngeal radiography—dorsal displacement of the soft palate, guttural pouch tympany, and subepiglottic/pharyngeal cysts may be visualized; administration of PO liquid contrast agents may assist in establishing the diagnosis.

DIAGNOSTIC PROCEDURES

Upper Airway Endoscopy

- Important in identifying laryngeal or pharyngeal abnormalities.
- Cleft palate can be visualized as a failure of the median line of the palate to close; if the defect is significant, one may visualize the tongue ventrally.
- Pharyngeal paralysis presents as a collapsing of the pharyngeal walls on inspiration and may be severe enough to obstruct the larynx.
- Dorsal displacement of the soft palate can be diagnosed if the caudal edge of the soft palate is seen but the epiglottis is hidden.
- Pharyngeal cysts are fluid-filled structures that form from the dorsal wall of the pharynx, whereas subepiglottic cysts develop under the epiglottis, pushing it upward.
- Bi- or unilateral laryngeal paralysis, arytenoiditis, and rostral displacement of the palatopharyngeal arch also can be diagnosed.

Laryngoscopy

The oral cavity and oral pharyngeal region can be visualized with a long-bladed laryngoscope.

NASAL REGURGITATION OF MILK

TREATMENT

• Because of the high risk of aspiration pneumonia, do not initially allow an affected foal to suckle from the mare, and place an indwelling nasogastric tube for feeding. Later, if no aspiration is noted or has cleared and the foal continues to be affected, train the foal to drink from a bucket. This decreases negative pressure in the oral pharynx and lowers the foal's head to provide postural drainage.
• Provide nutrition to the foal at 10–20% of body weight, divided over 24 hours and administered every 1–2 hours for the first week of life.
• With suspected failure of passive transfer, tube feed high-quality colostrum before the foal is 12 hours of age. In old foals, plasma transfusion is recommended.
• With severe respiratory stridor, emergency tracheotomy may be necessary.
• Cleft palate repair has been attempted, but the complications are many and the prognosis poor.
• Surgical drainage and removal of cysts can be performed with laser, electrocautery through an endoscope, or laryngotomy.

MEDICATIONS

DRUGS OF CHOICE

• In cases with aspiration pneumonia, a broad-spectrum antibiotic plan is necessary—amikacin (20 mg/kg SID) combined with ampicillin (20 mg/kg q6–8h) usually is effective.
• Some clinicians feel that cases of soft palate displacement and pharyngeal paralysis are secondary to vitamin E and selenium deficiency; supplementation may be indicated.

CONTRAINDICATIONS

N/A

PRECAUTIONS

Foal should be well hydrated before initiation of aminoglycoside antibiotics because of their potential nephrotoxicity.

POSSIBLE INTERACTIONS

N/A

ALTERNATIVE DRUGS

N/A

FOLLOW-UP

PATIENT MONITORING

• Some causes resolve with supportive care and time. Check patients daily or every other day to evaluate progression of the original problem and resolution of aspiration pneumonia, which may involve repeated endoscopy and radiology.
• If a tracheotomy has been performed, remove and clean the tracheotomy tube daily because of the build up of exudate.

POSSIBLE COMPLICATIONS

• Prognosis for resolution depends on the cause and severity of the problem.
• Foals with soft palate displacement and pharyngeal paralysis may resolve in a few days with supportive care.
• Sometimes the original problem does not resolve completely, and these animals may continue to have a chronic, food-stained nasal discharge as adults.
• Foals with bilateral paralysis of the larynx or arytenoiditis have a poor prognosis for survival because of continued respiratory distress.
• Surgical repair of cleft palates is difficult and may result in complications of chronic nasal discharge, dehiscence of the repair, and osteomyelitis of the mandibular symphysis.
• Surgical removal of pharyngeal/laryngeal cysts carries a good prognosis for recovery.

MISCELLANEOUS

ASSOCIATED CONDITIONS

Foals with severe dysphagia may have experienced failure of passive transfer of antibodies from their dam, which increases the risk of septicemia.

AGE-RELATED FACTORS

Milk regurgitation generally is seen soon after the foal begins to nurse; with arytenoiditis, the first signs may occur later.

ZOONOTIC POTENTIAL

N/A

PREGNANCY

N/A

SYNONYMS

N/A

SEE ALSO

• Failure of passive transfer
• Neonatal pneumonia
• Respiratory distress
• Septicemia

Suggested Reading

Altmaier K, Morris EA. Dorsal displacement of the soft palate in neonatal foals. Equine Vet J 1993;329–332.
Barton MH. Nasal regurgitation of milk in foals. Compend Contin Educ Pract Vet 1993;81–90.
Bowman KF, Tate LP, Evans LH, Donawick WJ. Complication of cleft palate repair in large animals. J Am Vet Med Assoc 1982;652–657.
Haynes PF, Qualls CW. Cleft soft palate, nasal septal deviation and epiglottic entrapment in a Thoroughbred filly. J Am Vet Med Assoc 1981;910–913.

Author Mary Rose Paradis
Consulting Editor Mary Rose Paradis

NERIUM OLEANDER (OLEANDER) TOXICOSIS

BASICS

OVERVIEW

• *Nerium oleander* (oleander) is an evergreen shrub (family Apocynaceae) with leathery, dark, gray-green, sharply pointed leaves 4–12-inches long with a prominent midrib and parallel secondary veins.
• The plant is native to Asia but now is a common ornamental in the southern U.S.
• The plant contains several cardiac glycosides, and ingestion can cause severe cardiac abnormalities and sudden death.
• The plant remains toxic when dry.

SIGNALMENT

All animals are susceptible.

SIGNS

• Onset usually several hours after ingestion
• Anorexia
• Colic
• Diarrhea
• Cardiac arrhythmias
• Tremors
• Seizure-like activity
• Coma
• Death

CAUSES AND RISK FACTORS

• Cardiac glycosides—oleandrin, oleandroside, nerioside, digitoxigenin, and others
• Cardiac glycosides inhibit Na/K-ATPase.
• Ingestion of 0.005% body weight may be lethal.

DIAGNOSIS

DIFFERENTIAL DIAGNOSIS

• *Taxus* (yew) toxicosis—evidence of consumption
• Other cardiac glycoside–containing plants—evidence of consumption
• Other causes of sudden death

CBC/BIOCHEMISTRY/URINALYSIS

N/A

OTHER LABORATORY TESTS

• Identification of oleander leaves in ingesta
• Chemical analysis of ingesta for oleandrin

IMAGING

N/A

DIAGNOSTIC PROCEDURES

ECG disturbances are supportive—widening of the QRS wave, ST-segment depression, enlarged P waves, and a variety of ventricular arrhythmias

PATHOLOGIC FINDINGS

• Identification of oleander leaves in ingesta
• Often no lesions in peracute cases
• Endocardial hemorrhages
• Increased pericardial fluid
• Necrosis of the subendocardium, most often involving the left ventricle
• Pulmonary edema or hepatic congestion may be present.

TREATMENT

• Keep the animal quiet.
• Supportive care

MEDICATIONS

DRUGS

• Evaluate cardiac function (i.e., ECG), and treat appropriately.
• AC (2–5 g/kg PO in a water slurry)

CONTRAINDICATIONS/POSSIBLE INTERACTIONS

N/A

NERIUM OLEANDER (OLEANDER) TOXICOSIS

FOLLOW-UP

PATIENT MONITORING
ECG evaluation

PREVENTION/AVOIDANCE
Remove oleander from animal access

POSSIBLE COMPLICATIONS
N/A

EXPECTED COURSE AND PROGNOSIS
N/A

MISCELLANEOUS

ASSOCIATED CONDITIONS
N/A

AGE-RELATED FACTORS
N/A

ZOONOTIC POTENTIAL
N/A

PREGNANCY
N/A

SEE ALSO
N/A

ABBREVIATION
AC = activated charcoal

Suggested Reading

Galey FD, Holstege DM, Plumlee KH, et al. Diagnosis of oleander poisoning in livestock. J Vet Diagn Invest 1996;8:358–364.

Author Larry J. Thompson
Consulting Editor Robert H. Poppenga

NEUTROPENIA

BASICS

DEFINITION

• Neutrophil count < the laboratory reference interval (e.g., <2100 cells/μL)
• Can develop alone or as a component of pancytopenia.
• May be accompanied by left shift and toxic change—cytoplasmic basophilia, cytoplasmic vacuolation, Döhle bodies, and toxic granulation

PATHOPHYSIOLOGY

• Neutrophils are produced in bone marrow, released into the blood, circulate for ≅10 hours, then migrate into tissue spaces and onto epithelial surfaces.
• Senescent neutrophils are lost via mucosal surfaces and destroyed in the spleen, liver, and bone marrow.
• When tissue demand occurs, colony-stimulating factors increase proliferation and maturation of neutrophil progenitor cells in the bone marrow; transit time for bone marrow granulopoiesis is ≅4–6 days.
• The circulation has two pools of neutrophils—the CNP, which is central within the vessel and sampled during phlebotomy; and the MNP, which marginates along the vessel wall; in horses, the ratio of these pools is 1:1.
• With tissue demand > the CNP, initial recruitment of neutrophils from marrow results in the appearance of immature neutrophils in the circulation, which can include band neutrophils, metamyelocytes, and myelocytes. When this supply is depleted or suppressed, or when ineffective myelopoiesis/neutropoiesis occurs, neutropenia develops.
• Circulating neutrophil numbers are affected by the rate of bone marrow production and release, the rate of exchange between CNP and MNP, and the rate of migration into tissue.
• Neutropenia can result from deficient neutrophil production in the bone marrow, cells shifting from the CNP to MNP, and reduced neutrophil survival because of neutrophil destruction—tissue destruction; endotoxin
• An important factor in equine neutropenia is occurrence secondary to disturbances/devitalization of the GI tract, resulting in endotoxemia/septicemia and leading to shifts from CNP to MNP, complement-activated neutrophil aggregation within the microvasculature, and neutrophil egress to affected tissues.

SYSTEMS AFFECTED

Neutropenia predisposes patients to systemic infection by various pathogens, and many body systems can be affected, in any combination, depending on the sites of infection.

SIGNALMENT

• No specific signalment for generalized infection
• Foals with failure of passive transfer are predisposed to sepsis and endotoxemia.

SIGNS

• Signs of localized or systemic infection
• Pyrexia

CAUSES

Inflammation/Tissue Damage

Associated with overwhelming tissue demand.

Bacteria

• Often related to devitalized GI tract, septicemia, or endotoxemia, resulting in shifts from CNP to MNP and reduced neutrophil survival—salmonellosis
• Neonatal septicemia/bacteremia/endotoxemia can result in profound neutropenias.
• Neutrophil left shift and toxic change are common.

Viral

• EIA is reported to cause pancytopenia, primarily anemia and thrombocytopenia.
• EHV-1 in foals—experimental inoculation

Rickettsia

• *Ehrlichia equi*—neutrophilic ehrlichiosis; may see intracytoplasmic inclusions.
• *E. risticii*—monocytic ehrlichiosis; also have associated thrombocytopenia, anemia, and variable neutropenia.

Drugs/Toxins

• Some may affect more cell lines than neutrophils—pancytopenia
• Estrogen
• Chemotherapy/radiation therapy
• Chloramphenicol
• Cephalosporins
• Trimethoprim-sulfadiazine and -sulfamethoxazole

Bone Marrow Diseases

• Marrow necrosis
• Myelofibrosis
• Myelophthisis
• Neoplastic infiltrates—leukemias, lymphoma, and metastatic neoplasia

Hereditary

• Rare
• Myeloid and megakaryocytic hypoplasia with profound neutropenia have been described in related Standardbreds, in some cases with cyclic neutropenia in peripheral blood.
• Suspected bone marrow defect.

Immune-Mediated

• Antibody associated with systemic immune disease
• Primary disease with antibody directed against neutrophils, or caused by hapten reaction associated with drugs

RISK FACTORS

• Foals with failure of passive transfer are predisposed to sepsis and endotoxemia.
• Horses or neonates from mares treated with sulfa drugs, often for EPM, are at risk for bone marrow suppression.

DIAGNOSIS

DIFFERENTIAL DIAGNOSIS

History should include information concerning drugs and toxins.

LABORATORY FINDINGS

Drugs that May Alter Lab Results

N/A

Disorders that May Alter Lab Results

• Failure to properly mix the blood specimen before sampling for CBC (i.e., laboratory error), especially because equine blood sediments so rapidly.
• Obtaining blood specimen from an IV catheter used for fluid administration—diluted specimen
• Partial clotting of the blood specimen, with leukocyte entrapment or aggregation

Valid If Run in Human Lab?

• Neutrophil counts are valid if equine thresholds are used and the smear is examined to correlate the cell count and to identify cells correctly.
• Bands may be overestimated in human hospital laboratories.

CBC/BIOCHEMISTRY/URINALYSIS

• Results depend on the underlying disease.
• Diagnosis of neutropenia is verified by CBC and leukocyte differential counts.

OTHER LABORATORY TESTS

- Blood culture; bacterial culture and sensitivity
- Serologic testing for infectious agents, when appropriate
- Demonstration of antineutrophil antibodies is essential to establish the diagnosis of immune-mediated neutropenia.

IMAGING

Survey radiography and ultrasonography may help to locate sites of infection not apparent during physical examination.

DIAGNOSTIC PROCEDURES

- Examination of bone marrow aspirate and core biopsy specimen is indicated to evaluate unexplained neutropenia and to exclude myelophthisis, myelonecrosis, and myelofibrosis.
- Cytology of preparations can be used to document excess tissue demand for neutrophils; to verify sequestration of neutrophils in body cavities, respiratory tract, or GI tract; to confirm bacterial infection; and to identify sites of insensible or occult loss of neutrophils from mucous membranes or skin lesions.

TREATMENT

Fluid therapy and supportive care, depending on the underlying disease

MEDICATIONS

DRUGS OF CHOICE

- Appropriate antimicrobial therapy
- Aggressive therapy for septicemia/ endotoxemia

CONTRAINDICATIONS

See drugs listed under *Causes.*

PRECAUTIONS

Proper hydration is needed when administering aminoglycoside and sulfa drugs.

POSSIBLE INTERACTIONS

N/A

ALTERNATIVE DRUGS

N/A

FOLLOW-UP

PATIENT MONITORING

- Rising leukocyte and neutrophil counts to normal reference intervals, resolution of left shift, and disappearance of toxic change denote improvement.
- Rebound neutrophilic leukocytosis may occur during recovery from neutropenia.

POSSIBLE COMPLICATIONS

Secondary infections

MISCELLANEOUS

ASSOCIATED CONDITIONS

Secondary infections

AGE RELATED FACTORS

- Repopulation of bone marrow with hematopoietic cells is more difficult in middle-aged and old animals because of age-related reduction in stem cell numbers.
- Foals may be susceptible to septicemia secondary to failure of passive transfer.
- Reference intervals may vary by age and for miniature ponies as well as hot- and cold-blooded horses.

ZOONOTIC POTENTIAL

Salmonellosis

PREGNANCY

N/A

SYNONYMS

N/A

SEE ALSO

- Monocytic ehrlichiosis (*E. risticii*)
- Neutrophilic ehrlichiosis (*E. equi*)
- Salmonellosis
- Septicemia/endotoxemia

ABBREVIATIONS

- CNP = circulating neutrophil pool
- EIA = equine infectious anemia
- EHV = equine herpes virus
- EPM = equine protozoal myeloencephalitis
- GI = gastrointestinal
- MNP = marginating neutrophil pool

Suggested Reading

Latimer KS. Diseases affecting leukocytes. In: Colahan PT, Mayhew IG, Merritt AM, Moore JN, eds. Equine medicine and surgery. 4th ed. American Veterinary Publications, 1991;2:1809–1813.

Latimer KS. Peripheral blood smears. In: Cowell RL, Tyler RD, eds. Cytology and hematology of the horse. 1st ed. American Veterinary Publications, 1992:191–207.

Latimer KS, Andreasen CB. Bone marrow. In: Cowell RL, Tyler RD, eds. Cytology and hematology of the horse. 1st ed. American Veterinary Publications, 1992:209–219.

Kohn CW, Swardson C, Provost P, Gilbert RO, Couto CG. Myeloid and megakaryocytic hypoplasia in related Standardbreds. J Vet Intern Med 1995;9:315–323.

Author Claire B. Andreasen

Consulting Editor Claire B. Andreasen

NEUTROPHILIA

BASICS

DEFINITION

- Absolute numbers of circulating neutrophils > the laboratory reference interval (e.g., >6,700 cells/μL)
- The magnitude of neutrophilia with strong tissue demand usually is not as marked in horses as in dogs and cats.
- Neutrophils are the predominant cell type in horses, so elevated neutrophil counts usually result in leukocytosis.
- A functional neutrophil mass depends on neutrophil numbers mediated by neutrophil kinetics and the ability of neutrophils to migrate and function when they arrive at their tissue target.
- Absolute neutrophil numbers commonly reflect neutrophil kinetics, because tests for neutrophil function are not commonly available.
- A single leukocyte count and differential taken at a single point in time may, or may not, reflect the complete health status of the animal.
- If marrow demand is met and new neutrophils are not recruited into the circulation, there is no neutrophilia.
- A neutrophil count within the reference interval does not exclude the possibility of concurrent inflammation.

PATHOPHYSIOLOGY

- Neutrophils are produced in bone marrow, released into blood, circulate for ≅10 hours, then migrate into tissue spaces and onto epithelial surfaces.
- Senescent neutrophils are lost via mucosal surfaces and destroyed in the spleen, liver, and bone marrow.
- With tissue demand, colony-stimulating factors increase the proliferation and maturation of neutrophil progenitor cells in the bone marrow; transit time for bone marrow granulopoiesis is ≅4–6 days.
- Mediators of inflammation stimulate bone marrow release and promote margination and adhesion of neutrophils to vascular endothelium.
- Species differences exist in the ability to recruit neutrophils during infection and inflammation.
- The circulation has two pools of neutrophils—the CNP, which is central within the vessel and sampled during phlebotomy; and the MNP, which marginates along the vessel wall. In horses, the ratio of these pools is 1:1.
- Shifts from the MNP to CNP may occur because of cortisol or epinephrine release.
- With tissue demand > the CNP, recruitment of neutrophils from the marrow results in the appearance of immature neutrophils in circulation.
- With intense inflammation, the shift of neutrophils can result in circulating band neutrophils and, possibly, metamyelocytes and myelocytes.
- Numbers of circulating neutrophils are affected by the rate of bone marrow production and release, the rate of exchange between CNP and MNP, and the rate of migration into tissue.
- Neutrophilia results when one or more of the following occur—the rate of marrow production and release increases, neutrophils demarginate from the MNP to the CNP, tissue demand for neutrophils increases, neutrophils cannot exit the vasculature, or neoplasia of granulopoiesis develops.

SYSTEM AFFECTED

Hemic/lymph/immune

SIGNALMENT

N/A

SIGNS

Vary with the cause.

CAUSES

Physiologic Neutrophilia

- An increase in mature neutrophils, but the effects usually are transient.
- Fear, excitement, and vigorous exercise cause epinephrine release (i.e., "fight or flight" reaction), producing increased blood flow, increased neutrophils going into the circulating pool, and decreased margination. This effect can be pronounced in young foals.
- Splenic contraction can affect neutrophil numbers because of the large amount of blood in horses compared with other species.

Corticosteroid- or Stress-Induced Neutrophilia

- Stress response caused by endogenous or exogenous cortisol results in decreased neutrophil margination and ability to emigrate into tissues because of down-regulation of neutrophil adherence molecules and increased marrow release of neutrophils.
- Typical "stress leukogram" consists of neutrophilia, lymphopenia, and variable or no changes in eosinophil and monocyte counts.
- Endogenous hypercortisolemia, secondary to pituitary adenomas, results in a stress leukogram and, sometimes, hypersegmented neutrophils because of prolonged circulation time.

Neutrophilia of Tissue Necrosis/Inflammation

- Inflammation, sepsis, necrosis, and immune-mediated diseases (see below) cause increased tissue demand and increased bone marrow release of segmented and band neutrophils.
- Numerous conditions may produce inflammation—endocarditis or other thromboembolic diseases that may lead to thrombi/infarction of tissues; neoplasia caused by direct tissue inflammation or inflammation that may occur after chemotherapy.
- Numerous organ sites can undergo inflammation or necrosis—internal or cutaneous abscesses, metritis, pyelonephritis, pyoderma, peritonitis, pancreatitis, and pleuritis

Neutrophilia Associated with Infectious Agents

- Bacterial—various types
- Viral—also may produce neutropenia.
- Systemic fungal

Neutrophilia Associated with Immune-Mediated Disease

- Systemic lupus erythematosus, pemphigus, and vasculitis caused by antigen and antibody stimulation of phagocytic leukocytes, including neutrophils
- Autoimmune hemolytic anemia or hemolytic anemias caused by several factors—release of irritating free iron from hemolysis, release of RBC membranes that stimulate tissue inflammation and leukocyte phagocytosis, marrow stimulation during regeneration, possible underlying concurrent diseases, and antigen/antibody deposition (i.e., immune-mediated).

Paraneoplastic Syndromes

- Production of GM-CSF or G-CSF by neoplasms, stimulation of marrow by inflammation of neoplasms, or bone marrow metastasis
- Syndrome reported in dogs with renal cysts or carcinomas, carcinomas (including dermal and pulmonary), rectal adenomatous polyp, and various types of neoplasms as described in humans, including mammary carcinomas.

Chronic Granulocytic Leukemia

- Neutrophilic (i.e., granulocytic) leukemia and chronic granulocytic leukemias may appear similar to a left shift.
- Acute leukemias contain blasts in the circulation.
- In left shifts, always rule out inflammation first.

RISK FACTORS

Depend on the underlying disease.

NEUTROPHILIA

DIAGNOSIS

DIFFERENTIAL DIAGNOSIS

• Animals with inflammatory neutrophilia usually have historical or clinical evidence of septic or nonseptic inflammatory disease, with pyrexia, weight loss, loss of appetite, and specific organ system involvement.
• Stress neutrophilia may be concurrent with infectious inflammatory disease or present in noninflammatory disorders.
• Physiologic neutrophilia affects young, healthy animals, especially foals.
• Bone marrow examination is indicated when ancillary testing does not explain neutrophilia.

LABORATORY FINDINGS

Drugs that May Alter Lab Results

• Corticosteroid administration causes stress leukograms.
• Neutrophilia subsides with long-term therapy, but lymphopenia persists.

Disorders that May Alter Lab Results

• Electronic WBC counts can be falsely high because of large platelets, platelet clumps, and Heinz bodies.
• Leukocyte clumping causes a false decrease in WBC counts.

Valid If Run in Human Lab?

• Valid if equine thresholds are used for accurate hematology analysis and blood smear is examined.
• Some human laboratories unfamiliar with animal neutrophils overestimate the number of bands.

CBC/BIOCHEMISTRY/URINALYSIS

• Assessment of sequential leukograms is important, because numbers of segmented and band neutrophils can change dramatically in a few hours.
• Trends that are persistent, increasing, or decreasing are important in establishing the diagnosis and prognosis.
• Toxic neutrophils indicate severe inflammation, endotoxin, or bacterial infections.
• Neutrophil toxic change is characterized by diffuse cytoplasmic basophilia, foamy vacuolated cytoplasm, Döhle bodies, and eosinophilic cytoplasmic granules.
• Cytoplasmic basophilia is normally increased in immature neutrophils—metamyelocytes and myelocytes

OTHER LABORATORY TESTS

• Blood culture
• Bacterial or fungal culture of urine, tissue samples, and body fluids
• Serologic tests for fungal, protozoal, and rickettsial agents
• Coombs' test or antinuclear antibody test with suspected immune-mediated disease

IMAGING

Radiography and ultrasonography of the abdomen, thorax, soft tissue, or skeleton to detect inflammatory or neoplastic lesions—abscesses, granulomatous lesions, effusions, foreign bodies, and organomegaly

DIAGNOSTIC PROCEDURES

N/A

TREATMENT

• Varies with the identity and severity of the underlying cause.
• Animals with acute sepsis or hemolytic anemia require aggressive intervention.
• Animals with chronic granulocytic leukemia require chemotherapy.
• Animals with inflammatory neutrophilia may require surgical intervention to remove or drain sites of infection.

MEDICATIONS

DRUGS OF CHOICE

Appropriate antimicrobial therapy based on results of culture and sensitivity testing

CONTRAINDICATIONS

Avoid corticosteroids in cases with suspected infectious agents.

PRECAUTIONS

N/A

POSSIBLE INTERACTIONS

N/A

ALTERNATIVE DRUGS

N/A

FOLLOW-UP

PATIENT MONITORING

Animals with inflammatory neutrophilia, especially of acute onset, may require daily or twice-daily hematologic assessment.

POSSIBLE COMPLICATIONS

Animals with acute inflammatory neutrophilia may become neutropenic if migration into the inflamed tissue exceeds the rate of bone marrow production; if neutropenia develops, prognosis is grave.

MISCELLANEOUS

ASSOCIATED CONDITIONS

N/A

AGE-RELATED FACTORS

• In healthy foals, neutrophil counts may exceed 6700 cells/μL, with the highest levels from 1–14 days of age.
• Neutrophil:lymphocyte ratios of 2.8:1 at birth drop to 1.1:1 at 51 days of age because of increasing lymphocyte numbers and some decrease in neutrophil numbers.
• Neutrophil reference intervals for miniature horses as well as for hot- and cold-blooded horses differ.

ZOONOTIC POTENTIAL

N/A

PREGNANCY

N/A

SYNONYMS

N/A

SEE ALSO

• Hyperadrenocorticism/pituitary adenoma.
• Infectious Diseases
• Myeloproliferative disorders/leukemia

ABBREVIATIONS

• CNP = circulating neutrophil pool
• G-CSF = granulocyte colony-stimulating factor
• GM-CSF = granulocyte-macrophage colony-stimulating factor
• MNP = marginal neutrophil pool

Suggested Reading

Latimer KS. Diseases affecting leukocytes. In: Colahan PT, Mayhew IG, Merritt AM, Moore JN, eds. Equine medicine and surgery. 4th ed. American Veterinary Publications, 1991;2:1809–1813.

Latimer KS. Peripheral blood smears. In: Cowell RL, Tyler RD, eds. Cytology and hematology of the horse. 1st ed. American Veterinary Publications, 1992:191–207.

Latimer KS, Andreasen CB. Bone marrow. In: Cowell RL, Tyler RD, eds. Cytology and hematology of the horse. 1st ed. American Veterinary Publications, 1992:209–219.

Author Claire B. Andreasen

Consulting Editor Claire B. Andreasen

NITRATE/NITRITE TOXICOSIS

BASICS

OVERVIEW

- Nitrate intoxication primarily is a problem in ruminants because of their efficient reduction of nitrate to nitrite.
- Monogastrics generally tolerate rather high concentrations of nitrate, because it is not rapidly reduced to nitrite in the GI tract.
- Nitrite is ≅3- to 10-fold more toxic than nitrate for ruminants and monogastrics, respectively.
- Nitrate is found in plants, water, fertilizers, and animal wastes.
- Horses are most likely to be intoxicated after exposure to high concentrations of nitrate or nitrite in fertilizers, but no cases of equine nitrate/nitrite intoxication have been documented.
- Nitrite converts Fe^{+2} in hemoglobin to Fe^{+3}, forming methemoglobin, which cannot bind and transport oxygen. In turn, this leads to generalized tissue hypoxia.

SIGNALMENT

- No breed or sex predispositions
- Neonates may be more sensitive because of their more efficient reduction of nitrate to nitrite, but data are lacking.

SIGNS

- Polypnea
- Dyspnea
- Cyanotic or muddy mucous membranes
- Weakness
- Muscle tremors
- Reluctance to move
- Terminal convulsions
- Death

CAUSES AND RISK FACTORS

The most likely cause is acute exposure to a concentrated source of nitrate or nitrite (e.g., fertilizers); a horse is unlikely to be exposed to sufficient nitrate from other sources to cause intoxication.

DIAGNOSIS

DIFFERENTIAL DIAGNOSIS

Other causes of methemoglobin formation such as *Acer rubrum* (red maple) toxicosis (clinical signs of icterus and anemia) or chlorate toxicosis (identified source of exposure to a chlorate salt, e.g., potassium or sodium chlorate).

CBC/BIOCHEMISTRY/URINALYSIS

- Methemoglobin imparts a brown discoloration to blood.
- All routinely measured parameters are normal.

OTHER LABORATORY TESTS

- Significant methemoglobinemia (>30%)
- High plasma, serum, or ocular fluid nitrate or nitrite concentrations—diagnostic concentrations have not been determined for horses.
- Measurement of high nitrate/nitrite in an environmental source associated with a suspected fertilizer spill.

IMAGING

N/A

DIAGNOSTIC PROCEDURES

N/A

PATHOLOGIC FINDINGS

No specific postmortem findings except for a dark red to brown discoloration of the blood and muscle.

NITRATE/NITRITE TOXICOSIS

TREATMENT

- Reduce methemoglobin to hemoglobin
- Treat acidosis and ischemia-induced ECG changes.

MEDICATIONS

DRUGS

- The standard treatment for methemoglobinemia is methylene blue, which is not believed to be efficacious in horses (although this conclusion is based on limited data).
- Ascorbic acid (30 mg/kg BID given in IV fluids) may be beneficial in reducing methemoglobin, but as with methylene blue, studies of clinical efficacy are lacking.

CONTRAINDICATIONS/POSSIBLE INTERACTIONS

N/A

FOLLOW-UP

PATIENT MONITORING

Monitor methemoglobin concentrations, acid–base status, and ECG.

PREVENTION/AVOIDANCE

N/A

POSSIBLE COMPLICATIONS

N/A

EXPECTED COURSE AND PROGNOSIS

Because methylene blue may not be efficacious, prognosis is guarded.

MISCELLANEOUS

ASSOCIATED CONDITIONS

N/A

AGE-RELATED FACTORS

More efficient reduction of nitrate to nitrite might occur in neonates.

ZOONOTIC POTENTIAL

N/A

PREGNANCY

Fetal hypoxia is a concern in pregnant animals.

SEE ALSO

N/A

ABBREVIATION

GI = gastrointestinal

Suggested Reading

Osweiler GD, Carson TL, Buck WB, Van Gelder GA. Clinical and diagnostic veterinary toxicology. 3rd ed. Dubuque: Kendall Hunt Publishing, 1985:460–467.

Author Robert H. Poppenga
Consulting Editor Robert H. Poppenga

NON-STEROIDAL ANTI-INFLAMMATORY DRUG (NSAID) TOXICITY

BASICS

DEFINITION

Non-steroidal anti-inflammatory drug (NSAID) toxicity refers to the adverse effects on several body systems that result from administration of excessive amounts of the NSAID class of drugs.

PATHOPHYSIOLOGY

NSAIDs inhibit the synthesis of prostaglandins by inhibiting cyclo-oxygenase, which converts arachidonic acid into endoperoxide intermediates. Endoperoxides are converted by specific enzymes to metabolically active prostaglandins; prostacyclin (PGI_2), thromboxane A_2 (TXA_2), PGD_2, PGE_1, PGE_2, PGF_{2a}, and other prostaglandins.

Cyclo-oxygenase exists in both constitutive (COX-1) and inducible (COX-2) forms. The COX-1 enzyme exists in practically all body tissues and is responsible for the normal production of prostaglandins that regulate a multitude of physiologic activities. The inducible cyclo-oxygenase is formed in response to inflammatory stimuli, and prostaglandins that are produced through this enzyme system generally augment inflammation. The NSAIDs currently in use in equine veterinary practice inhibit both COX-1 and COX-2 enzyme systems, and thus there is inhibition of both pro-inflammatory prostaglandins and prostaglandins necessary for regulating physiologic activities.

Most of the adverse effects of NSAIDs occur as a result of local irritation, such as in the stomach, or through inhibition of prostaglandins, mainly PGE_1 and PGE_2, that are important in maintaining mucosal blood flow via regulating synthesis of nitric oxide, a potent vasodilator. Inhibition of these prostaglandins interferes with blood flow, which can be reduced to ischemic levels.

The severity of effects seems to be proportional to the type, dose, interval, and duration of NSAID administered. Phenylbutazone can cause severe ulcerative lesions throughout the alimentary tract, extending from the lips and mouth through the rectum. In most cases, lesions are located in the stomach or the large colon, mainly the right dorsal colon.

NSAID-induced gastric lesions occur primarily in the glandular mucosa because this tissue requires prostaglandins (E_1 and E_2) for mucosal protection against hydrochloric acid and pepsin. Lesions can vary from erosions to deep ulcers. Lesions in the gastric squamous mucosa may also occur because prostaglandins have a mild inhibitory effect on gastric acid secretion, and presumably NSAIDs will block this inhibitory effect. NSAID-induced lesions in the large intestine seem to have a predilection for the right dorsal colon, probably because the greatest constitutive prostaglandin synthesis is in this part of the large intestine. Urinary system lesions are usually confined to the kidneys and range from disruption of medullary blood flow to severe renal medullary and papillary necrosis.

SYSTEMS AFFECTED

The clinical effects of NSAID toxicity are manifested principally in the alimentary and urinary systems.

GENETICS

N/A

INCIDENCE/PREVALENCE

N/A

SIGNALMENT

N/A

SIGNS

The clinical signs are usually referable to the gastrointestinal or urinary systems. Gastrointestinal signs may be overt, such as abdominal discomfort or diarrhea, or more subtle, such as poor appetite. With colon involvement there is often weight loss and peripheral edema secondary to hypoproteinemia. With renal involvement there is often polyuria secondary to impaired urine concentration.

CAUSES

NSAID toxicity is caused by administration of excessive NSAIDs—typically, twice the recommended dosage—for 3 or more days. However, cases of right dorsal colitis have been reported in which phenylbutazone was a suspected cause but was administered at an appropriate dose.

Administration of NSAIDs to equids using the label dose is generally safe and without adverse consequence, even when done chronically. Exceptions to this include concurrent water deprivation and dehydration, hepatic insufficiency, and possibly septicemia/endotoxemia. With water deprivation, NSAIDs can accumulate in the kidneys and cause medullary/papillary damage. Because NSAIDs are generally metabolized by the liver, the effective half-life can be extended with hepatic insufficiency. This is a particular concern with phenylbutazone, which the liver metabolizes to an active metabolite, oxyphenbutazone. With hepatic insufficiency, the half-lives of both the parent drug and the active metabolite are prolonged.

Doubling the recommended dose of NSAID for >2–3 days consistently induces adverse effects, whereas administering 1.5 times the recommended dose is inconsistently and unpredictably tolerated. It is important to recognize that administering 2 or more NSAIDs concurrently, even if each is at or below the recommended dose, increases the risk of inducing NSAID toxicity.

NON-STEROIDAL ANTI-INFLAMMATORY DRUG (NSAID) TOXICITY

RISK FACTORS

- The animal's weight is improperly estimated
- An NSAID is improperly administered by a non-veterinarian
- Two or more NSAIDs are combined
- A paste formulation of NSAID is mistakenly administered instead of the intended product
- Administration of an NSAID with inherent risks for toxicity. Examples:
    - Meclofenamic acid has a very long half-life (up to 36 hr), and thus even once daily dosing can lead to accumulation of the drug to toxic levels.
    - Aspirin consistently causes gastric mucosal irritation when administered orally.
    - Order of gastric and colonic lesion severity: phenylbutazone > flunixin > ketoprofen
- Foals may be at greater risk of NSAID toxicity compared to adult horses. In one study, flunixin given at 1.1 mg/kg/day for 30 days induced gastric lesions.
- Pharmacokinetics of NSAIDs may differ in neonatal foals compared to adults, affecting both the dosage (increase) and frequency (decrease) of administration.
- Foals' weights can easily be improperly estimated, and the percentage of error in weight estimation is usually greater for foals than for adult horses.

DIAGNOSIS

DIFFERENTIAL DIAGNOSIS

- Signs of colic may be referable to many other disorders.
- Diarrhea may be referable to many other disorders, particularly salmonellosis and Potomac Horse Fever.
- Peripheral edema may occur secondary to congestive heart failure, vasculitis, other protein-losing enteropathies, and glomerulonephritis.
- Polyuria may occur secondary to hyperadrenocorticism, other renal disorders, or diabetes insipidus.

NSAID toxicity should be strongly suspected in a patient that presents with the following signs and findings concurrently:

- Abdominal discomfort, weight loss, or diarrhea
- Hypoproteinemia
- Azotemia
- Hyposthenuria

CBC/BIOCHEMISTRY/URINALYSIS

CBC

- +/− anemia
- Decreased total solids (<5.0 g/dL;<50gk)
- +/− change in WBC count; often leukopenic with colonic damage
- +/− hyperfibrinogenemia

Serum Chemistries

- Azotemia (creatinine >2.0 mg/dL;>μmol/L)
- Hypoalbuminemia (albumin <2.5 g/dL; <25g/L)
- +/− electrolyte changes if diarrhea present

Urine Analysis

- Hyposthenuria (SG <1.020)
- Hemoglobinuria (if acute)
- Proteinuria (if acute)
- Renal epithelial cells in sediment (if acute)
- Increased RBCs in urine (if acute)

OTHER LABORATORY TESTS

N/A

IMAGING

Transrectal or transabdominal ultrasonography may be used to detect thickening of the large colon that can occur in severe cases of NSAID-induced colitis. Colonic ulceration is difficult to diagnose ante-mortem. A technetium-labeled white blood cell scintigraphic scan may help diagnose right dorsal colitis.

DIAGNOSTIC PROCEDURES

Endoscopy is indicated for diagnosing esophageal and gastric ulceration.

PATHOLOGIC FINDINGS

Erosions and ulcers can occur throughout the alimentary tract, including the oral cavity and tongue. Linear hyperemia and erosions occur in the small intestine, and multifocal to diffuse ulceration occurs in the colon, particularly the right dorsal colon. Perforations of cecal and colonic ulcers have been reported, as has stricture of the right dorsal/transverse colon secondary to severe ulceration. Renal lesions are medullary and papillary necrosis.

TREATMENT

APPROPRIATE HEALTH CARE

N/A

NURSING CARE

Intravenous fluid therapy may be required in acute cases with colitis or renal involvement.

ACTIVITY

N/A

DIET

Dietary management depends on the nature of the disorders. If there are severe oral/lingual lesions, then a palatable, easily consumed mash or gruel should be offered. If there is substantial abdominal discomfort, feed should be withheld. For right dorsal colitis, it has been suggested that there should be only a pelleted feed and no roughage for up to 3 months.

CLIENT EDUCATION

When dispensing an NSAID to a client for a patient, the veterinarian is responsible for the proper administration of the drug and should consider the formulation to be dispensed and the owner/trainer's competence to properly administer the drug.

SURGICAL CONSIDERATION

N/A

NON-STEROIDAL ANTI-INFLAMMATORY DRUG (NSAID) TOXICITY

MEDICATIONS

DRUG(S) OF CHOICE

Treatment of gastric ulceration should include drugs that suppress gastric acidity and agents that enhance mucosal protection and prostaglandin synthesis. Gastric acidity can be reduced using a histamine type-2 receptor antagonist or the proton-pump inhibitor omeprazole.

- Cimetidine (generic), 25 mg/kg PO q8hr
- Ranitidine (generic), 7 mg/kg PO q8hr
- Omeprazole (Gastrogard, Merial Limited, Iselin, NJ), 4 mg/kg PO once daily

Gastric mucosal protection (*glandular mucosa*) can be enhanced using sucralfate (10–20 mg/kg PO q8hr), and possibly misoprostol (1.5–2.5 μg/kg PO q8–12hr). Misoprostol can cause abdominal discomfort and diarrhea, each of which are clinical signs with NSAID toxicity, and a starting dose of 1.5 μg/kg, twice daily is appropriate to determine the animal's tolerance to the drug.

Colonic ulceration is more difficult to treat because drugs with topical effects, such as sucralfate, cannot reach the right dorsal colon at effective levels. Misoprostol may be helpful in some cases of right dorsal colitis at the doses given previously.

If there is acute NSAID-induced renal damage, intravenous fluid diuresis is indicated (4–6 mL/kg/hr). If the renal damage is chronic, fluid diuresis may temporarily improve azotemia, but because the decreased glomerular filtration is a result of tubuloglomerular feedback, fluid therapy will have no permanent effect on renal function.

Plasma therapy may be required if there is severe hypoproteinemia and edema. The amount of plasma given depends on the severity of hypoproteinemia and the response to treatment, but an adult horse with a serum protein <3.5 g/dL, <35g/L may require 5–20 L.

CONTRAINDICATIONS

Many horses with NSAID toxicity have painful conditions, such as laminitis and abdominal discomfort from colitis, that require analgesic administration. Clearly, NSAIDs are contraindicated in such patients and other analgesics should be used. Unfortunately, other analgesics, such as narcotic analgesics, are ineffective for pain from laminitis. If hind limbs are involved, epidural injection of detomidine and morphine can provide analgesia to the pelvic limbs. If an NSAID must be given, one should select an NSAID with minimal adverse effects, use the lowest possible dose, and consider concurrent treatment with misoprostol.

PRECAUTIONS

If glomerular filtration is impaired, administering drugs that depend on renal clearance, particularly aminoglycosides, should be done judiciously. If there is small intestinal involvement, suspected by the presence of hypoproteinemia, orally-administered drugs may have impaired absorption.

POSSIBLE INTERACTIONS

N/A

ALTERNATIVE DRUGS

N/A

FOLLOW-UP

PATIENT MONITORING

- Attitude
- Appetite
- Weight gain
- Serum protein concentration
- Serum creatinine
- Urine specific gravity
- Urine blood, cells

PREVENTION/AVOIDANCE

NSAID toxicity is best prevented by not administering NSAIDs. If NSAIDs are given, use only products licensed for use in horses and follow the recommended dose on the product label.

POSSIBLE COMPLICATIONS

- Chronic, recurrent colic
- Chronic diarrhea
- Chronic poor body condition
- Chronic polyuria, polydipsia

EXPECTED COURSE AND PROGNOSIS

Oral and esophageal ulceration usually heal well, particularly with the influence of growth factors present in saliva. Gastric ulceration usually resolves completely with appropriate treatment. Lesions in the intestine, particularly the right dorsal colon, are more likely to persist as chronic problems and can result in the animal dying or requiring humane destruction.

NON-STEROIDAL ANTI-INFLAMMATORY DRUG (NSAID) TOXICITY

MISCELLANEOUS

ASSOCIATED CONDITIONS
NSAID toxicity is often associated with painful musculoskeletal problems, such as laminitis, or recurrent colic, in which the owner administers repeated and excessive doses of an NSAID.

AGE-RELATED FACTORS
N/A

ZOONOTIC POTENTIAL
N/A

PREGNANCY
An effect of NSAIDs on normal pregnancy or the fetus has not been determined in horses. NSAIDs can cross the placental barrier. Lactating mares pass NSAIDs into their milk, but the concentration is too low to have any adverse consequences.

SYNONYMS
N/A

SEE ALSO
Listed related topics

ABBREVIATIONS
N/A

Suggested Reading

Cohen ND Carter GK Mealey RH, Taylor TS. Medical management of right dorsal colitis in 5 horses: a retrospective study (1987–1993). J Vet Intern Med 1995;9:272-276.

Lees P, Creed RFS, Gerring EEL, et al. Biochemical and hematological effects of phenylbutazone in horses. Equine Vet J 1983;15:158-167.

Murray, MJ. Phenylbutazone toxicity. In: Smith BP, ed. Large animal internal medicine. St. Louis: CV Mosby, 1996.

MacAllister CG, Morgan SJ, Borne AT, Pollet RA. Comparison of adverse effects of phenylbutazone, flunixin meglumine, and ketoprofen in horses. J Am Vet Med Assoc 1993;202:71-77.

Karcher LF, Dill SG, Anderson WI, King JM. Right dorsal colitis. J Vet Intern Med 1990;4:247-253.

Author Michael J. Murray

Consulting Editor Henry Stämpfli

NSAID Toxicosis

BASICS

OVERVIEW
• The mechanism of toxic action by NSAIDs is unknown.
• All NSAIDs are potentially toxic.
• Toxicity generally depends on dose or duration (or both) and probably relates to inhibition of prostaglandin synthesis.
• The role of NSAID metabolites in toxicity is unknown.

SIGNALMENT
No age, breed, or sex predispositions

SIGNS
• Depression
• Anorexia
• Bruxism
• Oral ulceration
• Polyuria
• Diarrhea (occasionally)

CAUSES AND RISK FACTORS
NSAIDs in excessive doses or administered concurrently with other nephrotoxic drugs, concurrent administration of multiple NSAIDs, concurrent administration of highly bound drugs, hypovolemia, dehydration, or pre-existing renal disease predispose to intoxication.

DIAGNOSIS

DIFFERENTIAL DIAGNOSIS
• Nephrotoxicity from other causes (e.g., aminoglycosides, pigment nephropathy, vitamin K_3, heavy metals), acute glomerulopathy, and acute interstitial nephritis
• GI ulceration from other causes, duodenitis/proximal jejunitis, and cantharidin toxicosis
• Protein-losing gastroenteropathies from other causes

CBC/BIOCHEMISTRY/URINALYSIS
• Hypoalbuminemia is the earliest recognized alteration.
• Leukocytosis may develop as injury to tissue continues.
• Polyuria with dilute urine may be evident with cellular injury associated with renal crest necrosis.
• Urinary GGT—elevated

OTHER LABORATORY TESTS
N/A

IMAGING
Nonspecific enlargement of kidneys and perirenal fluid infiltration may be observed on ultrasonography.

DIAGNOSTIC PROCEDURES
TDM is not routinely performed for these drugs, but quantitative assays may reveal abnormal NSAID clearance and accumulation to toxic concentrations.

TREATMENT
• Discontinue NSAID administration.
• Supportive care
• Diuresis with polyionic fluids and urinary alkalization may increase drug clearance.

MEDICATIONS

DRUGS
• Polyionic fluids
• Transfusion with plasma to replace lost proteins
• Alkalinize urine
• Antiulcer medication—H_2-receptor antagonists, sucralfate, antacids, omeprazole or misoprostol

CONTRAINDICATIONS/POSSIBLE INTERACTIONS
See *Causes and Risk Factors.*

NSAID Toxicosis

FOLLOW-UP

PATIENT MONITORING

• Monitor renal function during and after recovery for evidence of residual damage.
• Altered dosage regimen (e.g., lower dose, longer dosage interval) may meet therapeutic needs.

PREVENTION/AVOIDANCE

N/A

POSSIBLE COMPLICATIONS

Laminitis is a commonly reported complication.

EXPECTED COURSE AND PROGNOSIS

Occurrence of severe renal impairment is associated with poor outcome.

MISCELLANEOUS

ASSOCIATED CONDITIONS

N/A

AGE-RELATED FACTORS

N/A

ZOONOTIC POTENTIAL

N/A

PREGNANCY

Do not use misoprostol in pregnant animals.

SEE ALSO

N/A

ABBREVIATIONS

• GGT = γ-glutamyltransaminase
• GI = gastrointestinal
• TDM = therapeutic drug monitoring

Suggested Reading

Mitten LA, Hinchcliff KW. Nonsteroidal anti-inflammatory drugs. In: Robinson NE, ed. Current therapy in equine medicine. Philadelphia: WB Saunders, 1997:724–727.

Author Gordon W. Brumbaugh
Consulting Editor Robert H. Poppenga

NONULCERATIVE KERATOUVEITIS

BASICS

OVERVIEW
• A paralimbal, corneal stromal infiltrate combined with pronounced anterior uveitis
• Organ system—ophthalmic

SIGNALMENT
All ages and breeds

SIGNS
• Nonulcerated, fleshy, stromal infiltrate involving the limbus
• Uveitis, with signs such as miosis, aqueous flare, corneal edema, and blepharospasm

CAUSES AND RISK FACTORS
Immune mediated

DIAGNOSIS

DIFFERENTIAL DIAGNOSIS
• Onchocerciasis
• Stromal abscesses
• Keratomycosis
• β-Radiation keratopathy
• Infiltrating limbal neoplasms
• ERU—keratouveitis does not undergo spontaneous regression.

CBC/BIOCHEMISTRY/URINALYSIS
N/A

OTHER LABORATORY TESTS
Rule out infectious causes (bacterial or fungal) with corneal scrapings for cytology, culture, and possibly, biopsy.

IMAGING
N/A

DIAGNOSTIC PROCEDURES
N/A

PATHOLOGIC FINDINGS
• Corneal epithelial thickening, dermal fibrosis, and mild to moderate suppurative cellular infiltrate
• No evidence of stromal necrosis or infection

TREATMENT
• β-radiation therapy
• Enucleation often results from the inability to control pain.

MEDICATIONS

DRUGS
• Topical corticosteroids (1% prednisolone acetate or 0.1% dexamethasone 4–6 times daily), 2% cyclosporin A (BID), and mydriatics/cycloplegics (1% atropine SID to QID).
• Systemic NSAIDs—flunixin meglumine (0.25–1 mg/kg PO BID) or phenylbutazone (1 mg PO or IV BID)

CONTRAINDICATIONS/POSSIBLE INTERACTIONS
N/A

NONULCERATIVE KERATOUVEITIS

FOLLOW-UP

EXPECTED COURSE AND PROGNOSIS
Persistent, painful uveitis results in enucleation.

MISCELLANEOUS

ASSOCIATED CONDITIONS
Severe iridocyclitis

AGE-RELATED FACTORS
N/A

ZOONOTIC POTENTIAL
N/A

PREGNANCY
N/A

SEE ALSO
- Burdock pappus bristle keratopathy
- Calcific band keratopathy
- Corneal laceration
- Corneal stromal abscessation
- Corneal ulceration
- Eosinophilic keratitis
- ERU
- Glaucoma
- Herpes keratitis
- Keratomycosis
- Limbal keratopathy
- Superficial corneal erosions with anterior stromal sequestration

ABREVIATION
- ERU = equine recurrent uveitis

Suggested Reading

Brooks DE. Equine ophthalmology. In: Gelatt KN, ed. Veterinary ophthalmology. 3rd ed. Philadelphia: Lippincott Williams & Wilkins, 1999.

Author Andras M. Komaromy
Consulting Editor Dennis E. Brooks

NUTRITIONAL SECONDARY HYPERPARATHYROIDISM (NHP)

BASICS

DEFINITION

A skeletal disease that occurs in animals fed a ration with an excess of phosphorus or a deficiency in digestible calcium.

PATHOPHYSIOLOGY

• Three basic mechanisms decrease serum calcium and stimulate secretion of PTH, which may result in NHP. First, sustained consumption of diets containing excess phosphorus (e.g., wheat bran) that binds calcium in the gut, resulting in decreased calcium absorption and subsequent decreased serum calcium concentration. Second, diets high in cereal grain contain excess phosphorus but, more importantly, are calcium deficient. Third, oxalate crystals in certain plants combine with calcium in the gut and cannot be absorbed.
• In all cases, decreased plasma ionic calcium stimulates PTH secretion and inhibits calcitonin secretion, leading to increased calcium and phosphorus mobilization from bone. Also, PTH acts on the renal tubules by increasing calcium reabsorption and inhibiting phosphorus resorption. Intestinal absorption of calcium is increased via PTH stimulation of 1,25-dihydroxycholecalciferol production by the kidney as well.
• The continuous high phosphorous or low calcium intake overwhelms the ability of PTH to eliminate phosphorous and maintain calcium homeostasis. Over time, minerals mobilized from bone are replaced by a larger volume of fibrous connective tissue, leading to fibrous osteodystrophy. The skeleton becomes weakened and more prone to injuries. Bones also may become enlarged from fibrous deposition.
• Clinical manifestations—bilaterally symmetric facial swelling, shifting lameness, and difficulty masticating

SYSTEM AFFECTED

The skeletal system is weakened because of increased bone resorption resulting from elevated PTH production.

GENETICS

N/A

INCIDENCE/PREVALENCE

• Cases resulting from excess phosphorus intake or deficient calcium are rare.
• Commonly occurs in geographic areas with oxalate-containing plants.
• Incidence and severity are highest in horses with high calcium requirements—weanlings, lactating mares, and pregnant mares during the last trimester of gestation
• Prevalence is quite variable but can be up to 100% of herds grazing on these plants.

SIGNALMENT

• Any breed and sex
• Clinical signs are seen in weanlings to old, mature animals.

SIGNS

Historical Findings

May have a history of intermittent or shifting lameness, enlarged jaws, loose teeth, difficult and painful mastication, weight loss, and weakness.

Physical Examination Findings

• Physical manifestations relate to loss of bone minerals and accumulation of soft tissue, particularly at sites of high mechanical stress, that render the skeleton particularly weak.
• Intermittent lameness usually is an early sign and may result from periosteal avulsion, tendon or ligament tear, articular pain, and fractures.
• Swelling of the distal limbs is not uncommon.
• Constant shifting of weight at rest from one side to the other has been described.
• Bilateral facial swelling (i.e., "big head") results from maxillary and mandibular enlargement and represents a classic sign of advanced NHP. The swelling is firm but can be indented by digital pressure without causing pain.
• A "cardboard" sound can be heard on sinus percussion. Extreme deformation of nasal turbinates may impair nasal airflow and result in dyspnea.
• Obstruction of the lacrimal duct results in epiphora.
• Resorption of bone from the laminae durae causes loose teeth and difficulty in chewing; as a result, affected horses tend to lose weight and may become cachectic.
• Severely affected horses may be reluctant to move and have a hopping gait; fit horses may suddenly collapse when ridden.
• The rib cage may appear flat and narrow.

CAUSES

• High phosphorous intake with a diet rich in grain by-products—wheat bran
• Even when calcium was not deficient, rations with a calcium:phosphorus ratio $<1:3$ have caused the disease, but the lower the calcium intake, the more severe the disease.
• A high–cereal grain diet with grass hay usually provides inadequate amounts of calcium compared to phosphorus and may result in the disease.
• Calcium combined with oxalate crystals contained in grass or leaves cannot be absorbed in the gut. Plants more commonly cited are setaria grass, buffel grass, and purple pigeon grass. Plants accumulating larger amounts of oxalate (e.g., halogeton, greasewood, and sorrel) can be found in the US, but they most commonly cause acute oxalate poisoning, which may result in gastroenteritis and renal failure.
• The disease has been described in horses grazing pastures rich in oxalate-containing plants in Australia.

NUTRITIONAL SECONDARY HYPERPARATHYROIDISM (NHP)

• Oxalate-containing plants may cause NHP when the total oxalate concentration exceeds 0.5% of dry matter or when the calcium:total oxalate ratio is <0.5. Grasses with a calcium:total oxalate ratio <0.5 can induce NHP even though total calcium and phosphorous contents are normal.

RISK FACTORS

Diets with deficient calcium or excess phosphorus as well as pastures containing oxalate-rich plants. These plants are usually not appealing to horses, but they may be eaten when no others are available.

DIAGNOSIS

DIFFERENTIAL DIAGNOSIS

• Besides NHP, the major differential diagnosis for fibrous osteodystrophy is primary hyperparathyroidism. In both cases, PTH secretion is increased. However, hypercalcemia is characteristic of primary hyperparathyroidism, whereas serum calcium may be normal or decreased in NHP.
• Chronic renal failure may result in renal secondary hyperparathyroidism in dogs and human beings and lead to signs of fibrous osteodystrophy. Horses in chronic renal failure commonly are hypercalcemic or normocalcemic; therefore, these horses do not develop secondary hyperparathyroidism.

CBC/BIOCHEMISTRY/URINALYSIS

• Serum calcium may be below or in the lower limits of the reference range.
• Serum phosphorus may be within or above the reference range.
• Serum alkaline phosphatase activity usually is normal or slightly elevated.
• The laboratory test of greatest diagnostic value is urinary fractional excretion of phosphorus, which is increased in NHP (reference range, 0–0.5%).
• Excretion of calcium is decreased, but accurate measurement is difficult because of the formation of calcium carbonate crystals in horse urine.

OTHER LABORATORY TESTS

• Analysis of dietary calcium and phosphorus is important to determine the cause and correct any imbalance.
• Calcium content should be $\geq$0.3% of total dietary dry matter for maintenance and up to 0.8% for rapid growth.
• Phosphorus content should be 0.2–0.5% of total dietary dry matter, depending on the requirements.
• Calcium:phosphorus ratio should not be <1:1 or >6:1. If the dietary calcium and phosphorus contents are appropriate in horse exhibiting clinical signs, oxalate-containing plants should be suspected.
• Increased serum PTH with decreased ionized calcium indicates NHP.

IMAGING

• Decreased bone density may be visualized radiographically, however, a minimum decrease of 30% is necessary for detection.
• Loss of laminae durae usually is detected first and is particularly evident on a ventrodorsal view of the rostral end of the mandible.
• Bone loss from mandibles and maxillae may appear as diffuse radiolucency, radiolucent miliary mottling, and subperiosteal resorption.
• Changes in long bones are characterized by endosteal roughening, radiolucent linear striation in the cortex, and coarse trabeculation of the spongious bone of the metaphyseal region.
• Long bone cortical thinning and demineralization are only seen in long-lasting cases.
• Only rarely are two limbs found with the same decrease in bone density.

DIAGNOSTIC PROCEDURES

N/A

PATHOLOGIC FINDINGS

• Bone minerals are replaced by fibrous tissue (i.e., osteodystrophia fibrosa), resulting in increased bone volume but decreased bone density.
• Bone resorption is more pronounced in cancellous bone of the skull, ribs, and metaphyses of long bones.
• Parathyroid gland hypertrophy and hyperplasia are evident in prolonged cases.

TREATMENT

APPROPRIATE HEALTH CARE

Rarely, hospitalization may be necessary in cases of fractured bone or severe lameness, but most cases can be dealt with in the field.

NUTRITIONAL SECONDARY HYPERPARATHYROIDISM (NHP)

NURSING CARE
N/A

ACTIVITY
Confine affected horses for several months, until radiographic evidence indicates bone density normalization.

DIET
- Dietary imbalance can be corrected by increasing calcium or decreasing phosphorus intake. Total dietary calcium and phosphorus intake should be twice the horse's requirement, with a calcium:phosphorus ratio between 1:1 and 3:1 for an initial 2–3-month period. Afterward, feed the horse a normal ration that meets its calcium and phosphorus requirements.
- Legume hay (e.g., alfalfa) is a good source of calcium (0.8–2.0% of total dry matter).
- Mineral supplements (e.g., ground limestone) supply large amounts of digestible calcium (0.38 g calcium/g limestone).
- Treat cases secondary to excess oxalate intake by removing oxalate-containing plants from the horse's diet (this may not be practical) or by supplementing the diet with calcium and phosphorus. A weekly supplementation with 1kg of a mixture containing one part ground limestone for every two parts dicalcium phosphate effectively prevents or treats clinical signs in horses grazing oxalate-rich pastures.

CLIENT EDUCATION
- Emphasize the importance of providing adequate amounts of dietary calcium and phosphorus, with a ratio no less than 1:1.
- Remind owners that wheat bran should be only a small part of the horse's diet.

SURGICAL CONSIDERATIONS
N/A

MEDICATIONS

DRUGS OF CHOICE
N/A

CONTRAINDICATIONS
N/A

PRECAUTIONS
Use NSAIDs with caution, because decreasing pain may result in increased physical activity and skeletal trauma.

POSSIBLE INTERACTIONS
N/A

ALTERNATIVE DRUGS
N/A

FOLLOW-UP

PATIENT MONITORING
Radiography helps to assess return to normal bone density. If care is taken to match for age, gender, and activity, radiographs may be compared with those of nonaffected horses.

PREVENTION/AVOIDANCE
- Avoid large amounts of bran in the diet.
- For horses fed large amounts of grain, supplement the diet with the amount of calcium required to ensure a calcium:phosphorus ratio no less than 1:1.
- Deny horses access to pastures containing oxalate-accumulating plants, or supplement their diets with calcium and phosphorus.

POSSIBLE COMPLICATIONS
In advanced cases, horses may lose teeth or suffer skeletal trauma—fractures of long bones, compression fractures of vertebrae, and periosteal avulsions

EXPECTED COURSE AND PROGNOSIS
- In most cases, lameness disappears after 4–6 weeks on the corrected diet; however, some severely affected horses (or long-lasting cases) may not completely recover.

NUTRITIONAL SECONDARY HYPERPARATHYROIDISM (NHP)

- Lameness and radiographic bone density resolves before bone density actually returns to normal. Full recovery of bone strength may take as long as 9 months to a year.
- In most cases, enlarged skull bones remain deformed or show little regression after the diet is corrected.

MISCELLANEOUS

ASSOCIATED CONDITIONS
N/A

AGE-RELATED FACTORS
N/A

ZOONOTIC POTENTIAL
N/A

PREGNANCY
- Mares are particularly susceptible during the last 3 months of pregnancy and early lactation because of their higher calcium requirements at these times.
- Mares may raise a healthy foal once their diet is corrected.

SYNONYMS
- Big head
- Bran disease.
- Miller's disease

SEE ALSO
N/A

ABBREVIATION
- PTH = parathyroid hormone

Suggested Reading

Joyce JR, Pierce KR, Romane WM, Baker JM. Clinical study of nutritional secondary hyperparathyroidism in horses. J Am Vet Med Assoc 1971,158:2033–2042.

Krook L, Lowe JE. Nutritional secondary hyperparathyroidism in the horse. Pathol Vet J 1964;44–87.

Lewis LD. Minerals for horses. In Lewis LD, ed. Equine clinical nutrition: feeding and care. Baltimore: William & Wilkins, 1995:25–60.

McKenzie RA, Gartner RJW, Blaney BJ, Glanville RJ. Control of nutritional secondary hyperparathyroidism in grazing horses with calcium plus phosphorus supplementation. Aust Vet J 1981;57:554–557.

Author Laurent Couëtil
Consulting Editor Michel Levy

OCULAR/ADNEXAL SQUAMOUS CELL CARCINOMA (SCC)

BASICS

DEFINITION

A malignant, squamous epithelial tumor of the eyelids, nictitans, conjunctiva, cornea, and corneal limbus that is locally invasive but typically slow to metastasize.

PATHOPHYSIOLOGY

- Cause unknown
- Suggested predisposing factors—solar radiation, reduced or absent periocular pigmentation, viral agents, and hormonal, genetic, and immunologic factors
- Most plausible carcinogenic agent—the UV component of solar radiation, because it targets the tumor suppressor gene p53, which is altered in equine SCC.
- Tumors may be preceded by actinic keratosis, solar elastosis, and epithelial dysplasia.

SYSTEMS AFFECTED

- Ophthalmic
- Other systems may be affected by local extension and invasion or by metastasis.

GENETICS

- No proven genetic basis, but apparent breed predispositions suggest possible heritability.
- Reduced or absent periocular pigmentation inherited in certain breeds may predispose to ocular SCC.

INCIDENCE/PREVALENCE

- The most common equine ocular/adnexal tumor, accounting for 40–50% of reported cases
- A national survey of equine ocular/adnexal SCC revealed an increased prevalence with increased longitude, altitude, or mean annual solar radiation.

SIGNALMENT

Species

Reported in horses, cats, cattle, dogs, and sheep

Breed Predilections

- No specific breed predispositions, but increased prevalence is reported in Belgians, Clydesdales, and other draft horses, followed by Appaloosa and Paints, with the least prevalence reported in Arabians, Thoroughbreds, and Quarter Horses.
- White, gray-white, and palomino hair colors predispose, with a lower prevalence occurring with bay, brown, and black hair coats.

Mean Age and Range

- Prevalence increases with age.
- Mean age and range of 11.1 ± 0.39 years in one report.

Predominant Sex

No proven sex predilection, though a recent study found geldings are at higher risk.

SIGNS

Historical Findings

- Excessive tearing or ocular discharge, squinting, redness or cloudiness of the cornea, or redness or ulceration of the eyelid margins or nictitans
- Advanced cases—raised, ulcerated, or pedunculated masses of the eyelids, nictitans, or globe

Physical Examination Findings

- Nonspecific findings—serous to mucopurulent ocular discharge, blepharospasm, nictitans prolapse, and conjunctival hyperemia
- Closer inspection may reveal red to white, plaque-like, proliferative or pedunculated lesions of the eyelids, nictitans, conjunctiva, or corneal limbus. These lesions may be ulcerated or nonulcerated, and infection or hemorrhage may be associated.
- On the eyelids, alopecia and pyoderma may accompany SCC.
- On the cornea, corneal vascularization, cellular infiltration, edema, fibrosis, and occasionally, ulceration may be associated.
- Corneal SCC typically is limited to the superficial cornea, though chronic SCC may invade intraocular structures.
- Chronic SCC of any periocular location may invade the deep tissues of the eyelids and orbit, including the bony orbit.
- Thorough palpation is essential and typically requires topical anesthesia as well as an auriculopalpebral nerve block.

CAUSES

Unknown

RISK FACTORS

- UV radiation
- Lack of periocular pigmentation
- Possible genetic risk factors

DIAGNOSIS

DIFFERENTIAL DIAGNOSIS

- The diagnosis is established based on biopsy results.
- Differentials—other tumors such as papilloma, sarcoid, schwannoma, adenoma, adenocarcinoma, angiosarcoma, mastocytoma, melanocytoma, plasmacytoma, fibroma, and fibrosarcoma; parasites such as *Habronema, Onchocerca,* and *Thelazia* sp.; and inflammatory lesions such as abscesses, granulation tissue, and foreign-body reactions.

CBC/BIOCHEMISTRY/URINALYSIS

Usually normal

OTHER LABORATORY TESTS

Azostix placed over conjunctival, corneal, or nictitans lesions may reveal higher-than-normal tear protein levels and hemorrhage, possibly differentiating active lesions with leaky vessels from inactive scars.

IMAGING

- Skull radiography may be required if orbital or bony involvement is suspected.
- Thoracic radiography if metastasis is suspected.
- Orbital ultrasonography may help in determining extent of orbital invasion.

DIAGNOSTIC PROCEDURES

Cytology of cells obtained by aspiration or scraping, followed by Giemsa or Wright's staining, may reveal abnormal epithelial cells suggestive of SCC.

PATHOLOGIC FINDINGS

Gross Findings

- Appearance varies from erosive to proliferative.
- Proliferative lesions range from small nodules to firm, sessile masses.
- The outer surface may demonstrate inflammation secondary to trauma or bacterial infection, and the mass may be covered by a purulent exudate.
- Possible secondary invasion by *Habronema* sp. or fungal organisms.

Histopathologic Findings

- Nests or cords of epithelial cells, with varying degrees of dermal infiltration
- Mitotic figures are common, and intercellular bridges may be present.
- Well-differentiated tumors form epithelial "pearls"—rings of cells with central areas of keratinization
- Poorly differentiated tumors usually lack epithelial pearls but may exhibit individual cell dyskeratosis.
- Possible inflammatory cells and fibrosis

TREATMENT

APPROPRIATE HEALTH CARE

- Very small, superficial lesions of the eyelids and nictitans may be removed while patient is standing with sedation and local anesthesia.
- Larger, more invasive lesions of the eyelids or nictitans or those involving the conjunctiva or cornea require hospitalization for surgery; alternatively, eyelid lesions may be treated under sedation and local anesthesia using intralesional chemotherapy.

OCULAR/ADNEXAL SQUAMOUS CELL CARCINOMA (SCC)

NURSING CARE
Protect the eye from self-trauma and secondary infection with a soft or hard cup hood.

ACTIVITY
Restrict during the immediate postoperative period.

DIET
N/A

CLIENT EDUCATION
- If postoperative medication is required, the client should wait at least 5 minutes between topical eye medications.
- If intralesional chemotherapy is used, instruct the client to wear gloves when handling the periocular region for several days after injection.
- Inform the client regarding clinical signs that suggest tumor recurrence, metastasis, or development of new lesions on the fellow eye.
- Make the client aware of the possible role of UV radiation in the formation of ocular SCC and of appropriate steps to minimize exposure to solar radiation.

SURGICAL CONSIDERATIONS
- Tumors may be removed by surgical excision alone if adequate margins can be obtained; however, adjunctive therapy often is recommended to improve the chances of a complete cure, especially with large or invasive tumors.
- Adjunctive therapies include cryotherapy, irradiation, radiofrequency hyperthermia, CO_2 laser ablation, and intralesional chemotherapy.
- Reconstructive eyelid surgery may be required when eyelid margins are lost after tumor excision, and conjunctival grafts may be required after keratectomy.
- Cryosurgery with liquid nitrogen or nitrous oxide induces cryonecrosis of malignant cells when temperatures of -20 to -40°C are achieved using a double freeze-thaw technique.
- Radiation therapy with beta irradiation (i.e., ^{90}Sr) is most beneficial in superficial SCC of the cornea and limbus after superficial keratectomy, with reported success rates approaching 70%.
- Brachytherapy using ^{137}Cs, ^{222}Rn, ^{60}Co, or ^{192}Ir may be employed after surgical debulking of invasive eyelid tumors.
- Interstitial radiation therapy provides continuous exposure of the tumor to high levels of radiation over a period of time.
- Small, superficial tumors may be treated with radiofrequency hyperthermia, killing malignant cells with local temperatures of 41–50°C after surgical excision.
- Excision of corneal limbal SCC followed by CO_2 laser ablation also has been advocated.

MEDICATIONS

DRUGS OF CHOICE

Topical and Intralesional Immunotherapy/Chemotherapy
- Immunotherapy with BCG cell-wall extract has been used successfully for large, periocular SCC.
- Chemotherapy of invasive eyelid SCC with intralesional, slow-release cisplatin has been very effective, both with and without surgical debulking. One-year relapse-free rates approach 90%. Four sessions at 2-week intervals using 1 mg/cm^3 tumor are necessary; tumors $\leq$20 cm^3 may be treated using 3.3 mg/mL (10 mg Platinol in 1 ml of water and 2 ml of purified, medical-grade sesame oil).
- Topical 5-FU (1% TID) or mitomycin C (0.02% QID) may be effective for corneal SCC in situ and be beneficial for extensive, periocular SCC.

Antibiotics
- Topical and systemic antibiotics may be required to prevent infection after surgical and adjunctive therapy.
- A broad spectrum ophthalmic antibiotic such as neomycin-polymyxin B-bacitracin (Trioptic P)is an excellent choice for topical prophylactic therapy.
- Broad-spectrum systemic antibiotics such as trimethoprim/sulfamethazone (Tribrissen) are used for more invasive procedures of the eyelids or orbit.

Atropine
Atropine (1%) ophthalmic ointment or solution (q8–24h) may be used to treat "reflex anterior uveitis" after keratectomy for corneal limbal SCC; use with enough frequency to effect mydriasis.

Analgesic/Anti-inflammatory Agents
NSAIDs may be indicated after surgical excision or intralesional chemotherapy—banamine (0.5—1 mg/kg q12–24h PO depending on the degree of intraoperative trauma)

FOLLOW UP

PATIENT MONITORING
- Observed for recurrence of lesions, new lesions, and signs of metastasis.
- Long-term follow-up may be necessary, because tumor recurrence has been reported months to years postoperatively.

PREVENTION/AVOIDANCE
Reduce exposure to solar radiation, either through avoidance of light or protective headgear.

POSSIBLE COMPLICATIONS
- Tumor progression may lead to orbital involvement, with subsequent exophthalmos, necessitating orbital exenteration.
- Limbal SCC may invade intraocular structures, with secondary glaucoma, retinal detachment, uveitis, and globe rupture, necessitating enucleation.
- Chronic ulceration or tissue necrosis may lead to secondary bacterial or fungal infection and possible septicemia.
- Reported metastasis rates range from 0–18.6%, with the regional lymph nodes, parotid salivary glands, and thorax the most frequently affected sites.

EXPECTED COURSE AND PROGNOSIS
- Prognosis is generally good provided that treatment is early in the course of disease and owners are committed to long-term follow-up therapy.
- Factors affecting prognosis—tumor location, degree of invasiveness, presence or absence of metastasis, and number of tumors at diagnosis.
- The initial treatment modality does not appear to affect survival time.
- Recurrence rates range from 25–42%.

MISCELLANEOUS

ASSOCIATED CONDITIONS
Premalignant lesions include actinic keratosis, solar elastosis, and epithelial dysplasia.

AGE-RELATED FACTORS
N/A

ZOONOTIC POTENTIAL
N/A

PREGNANCY
N/A

SYNONYMS
N/A

SEE ALSO
- Equine periocular sarcoid
- Habronemiasis

ABBREVIATIONS
- BCG = bacillus Calmette-Guérin
- 5-FU = 5-fluorouracil

Suggested Reading

Brooks DE. Equine ophthalmology. In Gelatt KN, ed. Veterinary ophthalmology. 3rd ed. Philadelphia: Lippincott Williams & Wilkins, 1999.

Author Dennis Todd Strubbe
Consulting Editor Dennis E. Brooks

OCULAR EXAMINATION

BASICS

OVERVIEW

- Obtaining a thorough history is important before performing the ophthalmic examination.
- If some form of visual disability is suspected, knowledge of how the horse performs under different lighting conditions is valuable.
- A prepurchase ophthalmic examination is designed to detect any ophthalmic disease that may recur or that is associated with decreased vision.
- The purpose for which the horse is to be used determines the emphasis placed on any ocular lesion seen.
- A proper ophthalmic examination requires a good focal light source (e.g., transilluminator and direct ophthalmoscope). In horses, magnification is 7.9 × lateral and 84 × axial with the direct ophthalmoscope and, with a 20-D lens, 0.79 × lateral and 8.4 × axial with the indirect ophthalmoscope.
- Examine the head for symmetry, ocular discharge, and blepharospasm, and note the general appearance of the eyes and adnexa.
- Assess the size, movement, and position of the globe relative to the orbit.
- Examine the angle of the eyelashes on the upper lid to the cornea of the two eyes. Normally, the eyelashes are almost perpendicular to the corneal surface; droopiness may indicate blepharospasm, ptosis, enophthalmos, or exophthalmos. The first sign of a painful eye often is the eyelashes pointing downward.
- Test the palpebral reflex by touching the eyelids and observing for a blink response.
- Test the menace response by making a quick, threatening motion toward the eye to cause a blink response or a movement of the head. Take care not to create air currents toward the eye when performing this test.
- Vision can be further assessed by maze testing, with blinkers alternatively covering each eye. Maze tests should be done under both dim and light conditions.
- Test both direct and indirect PLR. The normal equine pupil responds somewhat sluggishly and incompletely unless the stimulating light is particularly bright.
- IV sedation, a nose or ear twitch, and supraorbital sensory and auriculopalpebral motor nerve blocks may be necessary to facilitate the rest of the examination.
- Examine the margins, outer, and inner surfaces of the upper and lower eyelids and the position and outer surface of the third eyelid with the light source.
- The cornea should be clear, smooth, and shiny. Most have an obvious gray line at the medial and lateral limbus that represents insertion of the pectinate ligaments into the posterior cornea.
- Placing fluorescein dye in the eye to identify corneal ulcers should be a routine part of every examination, because small corneal ulcers that otherwise might be undetected will stain.
- To determine patency of the nasolacrimal system, use irrigation, which is most easily accomplished from the nasal orifice, although fluorescein dye penetration through the nasolacrimal system also may indicate patency.
- The anterior chamber is filled with aqueous humor, should be optically clear, and is best examined with a slit lamp. Any discoloration of the cornea or sign of aqueous flare should be cause for concern.
- Measure IOP with applanation tonometry; normally, IOP is 17–28 mm Hg with a Tonopen applanation tonometer.
- Persistent pupillary membrane remnants are common and have no significance unless they span the pupil or attach to the lens and cornea. Examine the pupillary margin for any posterior synechiae (i.e. adhesions) resulting from uveitis.
- Pupillary dilatation is necessary to examine the whole lens in detail.
- Apply a mydriatic to the eye after the PLR is evaluated. The agent of choice is topical 1% tropicamide, which takes 15–20 minutes to produce mydriasis in normal horses and has an action that persists for ≅ 8–12 hours. Check the lens for position and any opacities or cataract.
- Several lens opacities may be regarded as normal variations—prominent lens sutures, the point of attachment of the hyaloid vessel (i.e., Mittendorf's dot), refractive concentric rings, fine dust-like opacities, and sparse "vacuoles" within the lens substance.
- Normal aging results in cloudiness of the lens nucleus beginning at 7–8 years, but this is not a true cataract. The suture lines and the lens capsule also may become slightly opaque as a normal feature of aging.
- Cataracts are always important. They can be secondary to previous uveitis, congenital, progressive or nonprogressive, and in some breeds, hereditary.
- Adult vitreous should be free of obvious opacities. Vitreal floaters can develop with age or be a sequel to ERU, but they generally are benign in nature.
- Examine the fundus for any signs of ERU (e.g., peripapillary depigmentation). Examine the nontapetal region ventral to the optic disc carefully with a direct ophthalmoscope; this is where focal retinal scars are seen. Retinal detachments may be congenital, traumatic, or secondary to ERU, and they are serious faults because of their association with complete or partial vision loss.
- Optic nerve atrophy can relate to ERU, glaucoma, or trauma and is associated with blindness.
- Proliferative lesions of the optic nerve may be noted in old horses but generally are not sight or life threatening.
- Organ system—ophthalmic

OCULAR EXAMINATION

SIGNALMENT

N/A

SIGNS

N/A

CAUSES AND RISK FACTORS

N/A

DIAGNOSIS

DIFFERENTIAL DIAGNOSIS

N/A

CBC/BIOCHEMISTRY/URINALYSIS

N/A

IMAGING

- ERG
- Ultrasonography (B scan)

DIAGNOSTIC PROCEDURES

- Culture
- Schirmer tear test
- Cytology
- Tonometry
- Ophthalmoscopy

TREATMENT

N/A

MEDICATIONS

DRUGS

- Tropicamide 1% for mydriasis
- Topical local anesthetic for cytology

CONTRAINDICATIONS/POSSIBLE INTERACTIONS

N/A

FOLLOW-UP

N/A

MISCELLANEOUS

ASSOCIATED CONDITIONS

N/A

AGE-RELATED FACTORS

N/A

ZOONOTIC POTENTIAL

N/A

PREGNANCY

N/A

SEE ALSO

All other ocular topics

ABBREVIATIONS

- ERG = electroretinogram
- ERU = equine recurrent uveitis
- IOP = intraocular pressure
- PLR = pupillary light reflex

Suggested Reading

Brooks DE. Equine ophthalmology. In: Gelatt KN, ed. Veterinary ophthalmology. 3rd ed. Philadelphia: Lippincott Williams & Wilkins, 1999.

Author Maria Källberg

Consulting Editor Dennis E. Brooks

OCULAR PROBLEMS IN THE NEONATE (EXPANDED)

BASICS

DEFINITION

- The equine neonatal eye has many features of immaturity that, over time, resolve to yield a healthy, adult eye. Despite normal embryogenesis and a fully developed adnexa and globe, a newborn foal may exhibit lagophthalmos, low tear secretion, round pupil, reduced corneal sensitivity, lack of menace reflex for as long as 2 weeks, hyaloid artery remnants possibly containing blood for hours after birth), prominent lens Y sutures, and a round optic disc with smooth margins.
- Tapetal color relates to coat color and usually is blue-green but may be partially red, orange, or blue. Color-dilute foals have a red fundic reflection from lack of tapetum and consequential exposure of choroidal vessels.
- Knowing the accepted presentation of the neonatal ophthalmic system, as previously mentioned, any further evidence of ocular pathology from abnormal embryogenesis or progression of ocular and periocular inflammation from any cause may define a true neonatal ophthalmic disorder.

PATHOPHYSIOLOGY

- Congenital, inherited, and acquired diseases
- Inactive or dynamic; may or may not have a significant impact on vision.

SYSTEMS AFFECTED

- Ophthalmic
- CNS
- Skin

GENETICS

- Belgian and Thoroughbred horses can get cataracts with a dominant mode of inheritance.
- Congenital stationary night blindness (CSNB) of Appaloosas and Quarter Horses is inherited through a recessive or sex-linked recessive mode of transmission, with the defect on the X chromosome.

INCIDENCE/PREVALENCE

Esotropia (i.e., crossed eyes) has an incidence of 0.5% in mules.

SIGNALMENT

Breed Predilections

- Congenital and dorsomedial strabismus and CSNB in Appaloosas
- Limbal dermoids with iridal hypoplasia and cataracts in Quarter Horses
- Heterochromia iridis, or dual coloration of the iris (usually blue and brown), is common in Appaloosas and in palomino, chestnut, gray, spotted, and white horses; however, it is not considered a true pathologic condition.
- Aniridia (i.e., the complete absence of the iris) is reported in Quarter Horses and Belgians and also is seen with congenital cataracts in Thoroughbreds.
- Morgans have nonprogressive, nuclear, bilaterally symmetric cataracts that do not seriously interfere with vision.
- Superficial, irregular corneal epithelial opacities may be found in one or both eyes in Thoroughbred foals; these do not appear painful and resolve with age.
- Goniodysgenesis and neonatal glaucoma have no breed predilections.

Mean Age and Range

N/A

Predominant Sex

N/A

SIGNS

General Comments

Numerous disease processes exist, each with a specific set of signs; therefore, serious i.e., vision-threatening) and treatable problems in neonatal eyes (i.e., ulcerative keratopathies, iridocyclitis) are emphasized here.

Historical Findings

- The newborn may be suffering from more serious, life-threatening problems and, in addition, develops traumatic or progressive inflammatory ocular or periocular disease.
- The neonate may not be adjusting well to the new environment, gazing off into space with little physical activity, or may be easily startled and running into things with reluctance to move—consider neonatal maladjustment syndrome.
- Occasionally, the owner/trainer may notice an abnormal appearance to one or both eyes, without any visual or behavioral problems.

Physical Examination Findings

- It sometimes helps to sedate a fractious foal for examination with Valium (5–10 mg IV in a 50-kg foal) and to have several people present to handle the mare and to assist in restraining the foal.
- Compare both eyes for symmetry, and note any nystagmus or strabismus.
- The menace reflex is unreliable in neonates, but record PLRs.
- Any painful eye needs a thorough examination of the eyelids, nictitans, conjunctiva, cornea, and anterior chamber. Upper cilia (i.e., eyelashes) tend to point downward in painful eyes. Epiphora, blepharospasm, and photophobia may indicate trauma, foreign body, and possible ocular inflammation and infection.
- Rarely, serious keratitis and blepharitis are noted without any signs of ocular pain.
- Iris prolapse, with or without panophthalmitis, has a poor prognosis and is seen in acute, severe trauma or aggressive infection.
- Congenital and developmental abnormalities have myriad clinical features that may or may not affect vision; each disorder is listed with its possible causes.

CAUSES

Corneal Ulcers

- Fungal or bacterial keratitis—*Pseudomonas, Streptococcus*, and *Aspergillus* sp.
- Entropion
- Lagophthalmos
- Deficient palpebral reflex
- Sicca
- Distichia or ectopic cilia—rare

Iridocyclitis

- Ulcerative keratitis
- Sepsis—immune-mediated causes or from *Rhodococcus equi, Escherichia coli, S. equi, Actinobacillus equuli*, adenovirus, or EVA

OCULAR PROBLEMS IN THE NEONATE (EXPANDED)

Conjunctivitis and Subconjunctival Hemorrhage
- Environmental irritants
- Secondary to pneumonia caused by adenovirus, EHV-1, EVA, influenza virus, *S. equi* subspecies *equi*, or *Rhodococcus* and *Actinobacillus* sp.
- Trauma
- Neonatal maladjustment syndrome

Glaucoma
- Goniodysgenesis
- Trauma

Microphthalmos
Congenital

Strabismus
- Congenital
- Trauma

Blepharitis
- Fly strike
- Dermatophytosis
- *Dermatophilus* sp.
- Staphylococcal folliculitis
- Trauma

Entropion
- Microphthalmia
- Dehydration
- Malnutrition
- Prematurity/dysmaturity
- Eyelid trauma
- Cicatrices

Dermoids
Congenital

Nasolacrimal System Atresia
Congenital

Dacryocystitis
- Systemic illness
- Nasolacrimal system atresia

Heterochromia Iridis
Congenital

Aniridia
Congenital

Iridal Hypoplasia
Congenital

Enlarged Corpora Nigra
Congenital

Iridal Colobomata
Congenital

Persistent Pupillary Membranes
Congenital

Lens Luxation
- Congenital
- Trauma

Cataracts
- Congenital
- Uveitis
- Penetrating trauma/lens rupture or perforation

Retinal Dysplasia
In utero inflammation

Retinal Detachments
- Congenital
- Inflammatory
- Traumatic

Chorioretinitis
Possibly maternal systemic disease late in gestation

Optic Nerve Head Colobomas
Congenital

Optic Nerve Hypoplasia and Optic Nerve Atrophy
- Developmental
- Inflammation in utero

RISK FACTORS
- "Downer" foals are more prone to entropion, blepharitis, conjunctivitis, and infected or persistent corneal ulcers.
- Risk factors in these neonates include malnourishment, sepsis, contact with soiled shavings, and invariable pressure and friction placed on the eyes and eyelids from chronic recumbency.
- Protection of the eyes in these neonates (e.g., padding, eye lubricant) is critical to avoid secondary ophthalmic disorders.

DIAGNOSIS

DIFFERENTIAL DIAGNOSIS
- Distinguish active disease requiring treatment from inactive problems not requiring intervention.
- Consulting with a veterinary ophthalmologist helps to identify treatable eye diseases in the neonate.
- Careful ophthalmic examination is the most important way to localize disease in an eye and to decide on appropriate diagnostic tests and treatment.

CBC/BIOCHEMISTRY/URINALYSIS
Usually normal in pure primary eye disorders

OTHER LABORATORY TESTS
Cytology and microbial (i.e., bacterial, fungal) culture of infected tissue, especially melting corneas, cellular aqueous humor, or purulent ocular or nasolacrimal discharge.

IMAGING
Radiography or dacryocystorhinography to identify nasolacrimal system atresia.

DIAGNOSTIC PROCEDURES
- Sterile corneal scrapings from the edge and base of the ulcer for culture and cytology, Schirmer tear test, and fluorescein stain in painful eyes with suspected ulceration. Apply topical anesthesia before deep scrapings are attempted.
- Aqueocentesis may identify pathogens in cases of severe idiopathic anterior uveitis.
- Complete ophthalmic examination, including IOP as measured with applanation tonometry, slit-lamp biomicroscopy, pupil dilation, and funduscopy. Many suspected congenital abnormalities are confirmed by these special tests.
- Candidates for cataract surgery—ocular ultrasonography and electroretinography.

PATHOLOGIC FINDINGS
- Consistent with the disease process
- Infections—a suppurative inflammation, with or without large numbers of organisms.
- Enucleated eyes that were blind and painful with hypopyon may show panophthalmitis, with or without bacterial sepsis.

OCULAR PROBLEMS IN THE NEONATE (EXPANDED)

TREATMENT

APPROPRIATE HEALTH CARE

- Severe ulcerative keratitis and uveitis need aggressive therapy to preserve vision and eliminate pain. Initially, hourly or bihourly instillation of medication is required to halt a melting ulcer and to prevent corneal perforation. These eyes must be examined several times daily until clinical signs improve. Hospitalization of the foal and mare sometimes is indicated to administer the frequent medication and to enable examinations several times each day.
- Usually, patients can be managed at home when medications are given four times daily or less. Some farms/stables have round-the-clock staff that can give medications in a less stressful environment.
- Deep ulcers must be watched closely; they may progress to descemetoceles and perforate in a matter of hours.
- Glaucoma must be managed on a day-to-day basis until the disease is under control.
- Most other types of neonatal problems, if they need medical therapy, can be managed on an outpatient basis.

NURSING CARE

- "Downer" foals with eye disease not only need correct medical management but also may benefit from a protective eye hood or plenty of padding and supplemental lubrication in the form of artificial tear ophthalmic ointment applied on the eye two to six times daily (depending on other topical medication).
- Monitor all foals in intensive care each day for corneal ulceration.

ACTIVITY

Generally restricted until the eye lesions are healed.

DIET

Good nutrition is essential for neonates to have enough energy not only for growth but for wound healing and recuperation.

CLIENT EDUCATION

- Some diseases threaten vision more than others. Severe inflammatory disease without therapy often results in a phthisical or septic eye that may need removal. Hospitalization may be necessary to initiate aggressive therapy. Treatment can be given over days to weeks for the most severe inflammatory conditions, and surgery may be necessary to preserve vision in cases of deep ulcerations and uncontrolled glaucoma.
- Neonatal anesthesia is a high-risk event and must be weighed heavily against the benefits of surgery, especially if the newborn is debilitated in any way.
- A full workup, including CBC and chest radiography, often is standard, even for elective procedures such as cataract removal.
- Share genetic information with clients as necessary.

SURGICAL CONSIDERATIONS

- Surgery under general anesthesia in neonates is risky and should be done only if the owner concedes to the dangers involved and understands the potential consequences.
- Conjunctival grafting is common to aid in healing of deep corneal ulcers and descemetoceles. Magnification and proper ophthalmic instrumentation are essential to a successful outcome. Corneal scarring is a sequela to surgery but may diminish as the foal matures.
- Entropion in neonates is corrected by placing a temporary suture perpendicular to the eyelid margin in the affected areas (2–3 mm from the eyelid edge) in a vertical mattress pattern. These sutures remain until the cause of the entropion is gone. Do not perform Hotz-Celsus procedures on neonatal eyelids; the foal usually outgrows neonatal entropion but may need temporary tacking in the meantime.
- Cataract surgery is performed in foals as young as 1 week if no other ocular pathology (e.g., retinal detachment or degeneration) is discovered during the diagnostic workup. A veterinary ophthalmologist performs this procedure with phacofragmentation.
- Glaucoma can be surgically treated with valve implants when medical therapy does not control disease progression. This procedure is reserved for veterinary ophthalmologists.
- Eyelid trauma must be corrected with maximal preservation of eyelid tissue. Adequate flushing with a 1:50 povidone-iodine solution, followed by a two-layer closure of skin-orbicularis muscle and tarsal-conjunctival layers, is recommended. Systemic antibiotics are administered.
- Keratectomy or blepharoplasty is indicated in cases of dermoids.
- Restoration of atretic nasal or palpebral puncta is done by flushing and cannulating the duct through one opening and, after creating a new opening at the other end, leaving the polyethylene tubing or silicone in the entire duct for several weeks to allow epithelialization of the new puncta and resolution of any dacryocystitis.
- Anterior lens luxation requires lens removal by a veterinary ophthalmologist to prevent secondary glaucoma. Posterior lens luxation does not necessitate surgical intervention.
- Persistent corneal ulcers in foals may need repeated debridement with topical anesthesia and a dry cotton swab every 3–4 days in addition to medical therapy. If unsuccessful, a grid keratotomy can be carefully made over the ulcer bed with use of topical anesthesia, and a sterile, 20-G needle at a very shallow angle dragged across the ulcer in a grid of linear patterns.

OCULAR PROBLEMS IN THE NEONATE (EXPANDED)

MEDICATIONS

DRUGS OF CHOICE

- Drugs for ulcerative keratitis and iridocyclitis are outlined in the chapters discussing uveitis and corneal ulceration.
- Medical treatment of glaucoma is discussed in the relevant chapter.
- Ranitidine (6.6 mg/kg PO TID) and/or sucralfate (20 mg/kg PO TID or QID) should be given to all hospitalized foals, especially if they are on systemic NSAIDs for iridocyclitis.
- In foals, subconjunctival injections of medications and subpalpebral and nasolacrimal lavage systems effectively deliver drugs without frequent manual manipulation of the eye.

CONTRAINDICATIONS

Do not use topical steroids on eyes with ulcerative keratitis.

PRECAUTIONS

- Watch foals on topical atropine for signs of colic. Persistent dilation of the contralateral pupil indicates systemic absorption of the atropine; when observed, either discontinue or give the atropine frequently until the contralateral pupil function returns to normal.
- Topical ophthalmic gentocin may retard corneal epithelialization.
- Topical ophthalmic medications are not intended for subconjunctival injection and cause a severe inflammatory response if administered under the conjunctiva.
- Use of topical steroids to reduce scarring on a cornea with previous fungal or bacterial ulcerative keratitis is dangerous and may cause a relapse of the infection.

POSSIBLE INTERACTIONS

N/A

ALTERNATIVE DRUGS

N/A

FOLLOW-UP

PATIENT MONITORING

- Not necessary for inactive ophthalmic disorders.
- Rechecks are advised for most inflammatory disorders until the eye shows no sign of active disease. If recurrence of infection or inflammation is apparent, perform a thorough workup to document relapse of microbial infection or other inflammation. A new or nosocomial infection also may be possible.
- Recurrence also may result from failure to correct the underlying cause (e.g., entropion-induced ulcers).

PREVENTION/AVOIDANCE

- A clean, well-ventilated stall in which the neonate can nurse and move about readily helps to prevent infectious and traumatic ocular problems.
- Some congenital lesions (e.g., retinal dysplasia) may be less likely if the mare maintains good health during pregnancy.

POSSIBLE COMPLICATIONS

- Any ocular anomaly or disease, even if successfully treated, can impair vision.
- Modifications to activity and the environment may be necessary when eye disorders are diagnosed.

EXPECTED COURSE AND PROGNOSIS

- With accurate diagnosis and timely treatment, most vision-threatening problems in the neonate can be managed successfully.
- Aphakic foals who had cataracts removed will adjust to their environment but remain permanently hyperopic (i.e., far-sighted).
- Even with complete recovery from an inflammatory disease, the owner must observe for and report any recurrence of ocular pain. The veterinarian should perform a brief ophthalmic examination during routine checkups to assess the eye's health.
- When vision cannot be saved in a neonatal eye, ocular comfort becomes the long-term goal of therapy.

MISCELLANEOUS

ASSOCIATED CONDITIONS

- Sepsis
- Pneumonia

AGE RELATED FACTORS

N/A

ZOONOTIC POTENTIAL

N/A

PREGNANCY

N/A

SYNONYMS

Anterior uveitis = iridocyclitis

SEE ALSO

- Chorioretinitis
- Eyelid diseases
- Glaucoma
- Orbital diseases
- Ulcerative keratitis
- Uveitis

ABBREVIATIONS

- CSNB = Congenital Stationary Night Blindness
- EHV = equine herpesvirus
- EVA = equine viral arteritis
- IOP = intraocular pressure
- PLR = pupillary light reflexes

Suggested Reading

Brooks DE. Equine ophthalmology. In: Gelatt KN, ed. Veterinary ophthalmology. 3rd ed. Philadelphia: Lippincott Williams & Wilkins, 1999.

Brooks DE. Ocular emergencies and trauma. In: Auer JA, ed. Equine surgery. Philadelphia: WB Saunders, 1992:666–672.

Gelatt KN. Congenital and acquired ophthalmic diseases in the foal. Anim Eye Res 1993;1–2:15–27.

Munroe G. Congenital ocular disease. In: Robinson NE, ed. Current therapy in equine medicine 4. Philadelphia: WB Saunders, 1997:355–359.

Author Daniel Biros

Consulting Editor Dennis E. Brooks

OMPHALOPHLEBITIS (NAVEL ILL)

BASICS

OVERVIEW

Bacterial infections of the structures within the internal or external umbilical cord, including the umbilical vein, two umbilical arteries, and urachus

SIGNALMENT

- Most often seen immediately postpartum, but cases have been reported up to 16 months of age.
- Most affected patients are 3–21 days of age.
- No breed or sex predispositions

SIGNS

- Earliest signs often are depression and inappetence.
- Young foals (2–14 days) often present with a separate primary problem (e.g., sepsis) with no external signs of umbilical infection; infected umbilical structures are found at ultrasonography.
- Old foals (14–21 days) usually show signs of external umbilical swelling with associated heat and pain on palpation; purulent umbilical discharge, patent urachus, or both often are seen as well.
- Affected foals may display fever, dysuria, pollakiuria, and tenesmus.
- Untreated cases may progress to show signs consistent with generalized septicemia—septic polyarthritis; bacterial pneumonia

CAUSES AND RISK FACTORS

- Failure of passive transfer
- Umbilical contamination at birth
- Improper care of the umbilical remnant during the postpartum period
- Seeding of bacteria from other sites—intestinal translocation

DIAGNOSIS

DIFFERENTIAL DIAGNOSIS

- Umbilical herniation may cause a similar ventral abdominal swelling, but affected animals are otherwise healthy in uncomplicated cases, with no clinicopathologic abnormalities and a normally involuted umbilical stalk.
- Patent urachus may coexist or present as the primary process; affected animals may be identified by retrograde contrast cystography and observing contrast voiding through the urachus.

CBC/BIOCHEMISTRY/URINALYSIS

- Leukocytosis with neutrophilia, toxic changes within WBCs, and hyperfibrinogenemia
- Possible hypogammaglobulinemia, particularly in cases of generalized septicemia with complete/partial failure of passive transfer
- Protein, WBCs, and bacteria may be present at urinalysis if the urachal remnant is involved.

OTHER LABORATORY TESTS

N/A

IMAGING

Transabdominal ultrasonography—the best method for evaluating internal umbilical structures to determine the severity and extent of infection, which may be detected using this method even before the appearance of external abnormalities.

DIAGNOSTIC PROCEDURES

- Deep aerobic and anaerobic bacterial cultures of the aseptically prepared external umbilical remnant are useful in determining appropriate antibiotic therapy because of the wide variety of organisms that may be involved.
- Blood cultures in neonatal foals because of the association with generalized neonatal septicemia

TREATMENT

- If possible, admit severely ill foals with a primary septicemia to an intensive care facility for supportive care—IV fluids, nutrition, antibiotics, oxygen, etc.
- If failure of passive transfer is a concurrent problem, provide plasma transfusion.
- Surgical intervention with evidence of multisystem involvement or uroperitoneum from urachal rupture or with failure to respond to medical treatment. Surgery should involve resection of the umbilical remnant and all associated infected structures, with ligation of the umbilical vein, both umbilical arteries, and the urachal remnant, followed by primary closure of the abdominal defect.

MEDICATIONS

DRUGS

- Long-term IV antibiotic therapy as dictated by results of bacterial culture and sensitivity. A broad-spectrum combination of antibiotics includes amikacin (20 mg/kg IV SID) and penicillin (22,000 IV/kg IV QID).
- Gastroduodenal ulcer prophylaxis may be helpful—cimetidine (6–20 mg/kg PO TID), ranitidine (6.6 mg/kg PO TID), omeprazole (0.7 mg/kg SID), and sucralfate (1–4 g PO BID–QID).
- Flunixin meglumine (0.25–1.1 mg/kg IV BID for 3–5 days postoperatively) helps to reduce incisional pain and to reduce the risk of adhesion formation.

CONTRAINDICATIONS/POSSIBLE INTERACTIONS

- Use aminoglycoside antibiotics with caution in cases involving dehydration because of their renal toxicity.
- Foals are more susceptible to the ulcerogenic effects of NSAIDs.

FOLLOW-UP

PATIENT MONITORING

- If the primary therapy is medical, serial transabdominal ultrasonography is useful to monitor resolution of infection, which usually is seen after 3–7 days of treatment.
- Medical therapy alone is successful in ≅50% of foals.

PREVENTION/AVOIDANCE

Frequent local disinfection of the external umbilical remnant using 0.5% chlorhexidine or 2% iodine solution after birth and for the first 2 days of life may decrease the risk of infection.

POSSIBLE COMPLICATIONS

- Uroperitoneum is a possible complication of septic omphalophlebitis; infection of the internal umbilical structures may erode through the wall of the urachus, resulting in leakage of urine into the abdomen.
- Surgical treatment carries an excellent prognosis. Complications include recurrence of infection, incisional dehiscence with hernia formation, and intestinal adhesions.

EXPECTED COURSE AND PROGNOSIS

When uncomplicated by sepsis or septic arthritis, the prognosis is good.

MISCELLANEOUS

ASSOCIATED CONDITIONS

- Patent urachus
- Generalized neonatal septicemia
- Septic arthritis

AGE-RELATED FACTORS

N/A

ZOONOTIC POTENTIAL

N/A

PREGNANCY

N/A

SEE ALSO

- Septic arthritis
- Septicemia
- Shock
- Uroperitoneum

Suggested Reading

Adams SB, Fesler JF. Umbilical cord remnant infections in foals: 16 cases (1975–1985). J Am Vet Med Assoc 1987;190:316.

Reimer JM. Ultrasonography of umbilical remnant infections in foals. Proc Annu Meet Am Assoc Equine Pract 1993;39:247–248

Author Enda Currid

Consulting Editor Mary Rose Paradis

OPTIC NERVE ATROPHY

BASICS

OVERVIEW
• Atrophy of the optic nerve due to inflammatory or noninflammatory causes
• During the early stages, the ophthalmoscopic appearance of the optic nerve head may be normal, although the eye is blind.
• With time, the optic disc becomes pale, with profound vascular attenuation and an obvious granularity caused by exposure of the lamina cribrosa.
• Organ system—Ophthalmic

SIGNALMENT
N/A

SIGNS
• Blindness
• Dilated pupil

CAUSES AND RISK FACTORS
• Inflammatory—optic neuritis, ERU, and chorioretinitis
• Noninflammatory—trauma, glaucoma, toxic, neoplasia, and loss of blood

DIAGNOSIS

DIFFERENTIAL DIAGNOSIS
• Optic nerve hypoplasia
• Retinal detachment
• Glaucoma
• Cataract

CBC/BIOCHEMISTRY/URINALYSIS
N/A

OTHER LABORATORY TESTS
N/A

IMAGING
Ultrasonography

DIAGNOSTIC PROCEDURES
ERG

TREATMENT
N/A

OPTIC NERVE ATROPHY

MEDICATIONS

DRUGS
No therapy for this condition

CONTRAINDICATIONS/POSSIBLE INTERACTIONS
N/A

FOLLOW-UP

EXPECTED COURSE AND PROGNOSIS
Poor prognosis.

MISCELLANEOUS

ASSOCIATED CONDITIONS
See *Causes and Risk Factors.*

AGE-RELATED FACTORS
N/A

ZOONOTIC POTENTIAL
N/A

PREGNANCY
N/A

SEE ALSO
Optic nerve hypoplasia

ABBREVIATIONS
- ERG = electroretinogram
- ERU = equine recurrent uveitis

Suggested Reading

Brooks DE. Equine ophthalmology. In: Gelatt KN, ed. Veterinary ophthalmology. 3rd ed. Philadelphia: Lippincott Williams & Wilkins, 1999.

Author Maria Källberg
Consulting Editor Dennis E. Brooks

OPTIC NERVE HYPOPLASIA

BASICS

OVERVIEW
• Congenital lack of retinal ganglion cell development or excessive destruction of embryonic ganglion cells
• Optic discs are small and pale, with retinal vessels absent and a one- to several-diopter, posterior depression of the optic disc.
• Organ system—ophthalmic

SIGNALMENT
• Congenital
• Genetics unknown

SIGNS
• Slight visual impairment to total blindness
• Mydriasis, with slow to absent PLR
• Unilateral or bilateral
• May be associated with microphthalmos, cataracts, and retinal dysplasia.

CAUSES AND RISK FACTORS
See *Pregnancy*.

DIAGNOSIS

DIFFERENTIAL DIAGNOSIS
Optic nerve atrophy

CBC/BIOCHEMISTRY/URINALYSIS
N/A

OTHER LABORATORY TESTS
N/A

IMAGING
N/A

DIAGNOSTIC PROCEDURES
N/A

TREATMENT
N/A

OPTIC NERVE HYPOPLASIA

MEDICATIONS

DRUG(S)

No therapy for this condition

CONTRAINDICATIONS/POSSIBLE INTERACTIONS

N/A

FOLLOW-UP

EXPECTED COURSE AND PROGNOSIS

- Poor prognosis for vision
- Nonprogressive

MISCELLANEOUS

AGE-RELATED FACTORS

Congenital

PREGNANCY

- May relate to uterine infections, liver disease, and exposure to toxic agents by the mare.
- Do not use affected mares for breeding.

SEE ALSO

Optic nerve atrophy

ABBREVIATIONS

PLR = pupillary light reflex

Suggested Reading

Brooks DE. Equine ophthalmology. In: Gelatt KN, ed. Veterinary ophthalmology. 3rd ed. Philadelphia: Lippincott Williams & Wilkins, 1999.

Author Maria Källberg

Consulting Editor Dennis E. Brooks

ORAL NEOPLASIA

BASICS

DEFINITION

Although equine tumors are rather uncommon, a significant proportion occur in the head and neck. Neoplasms of the oral cavity may originate in the mandible, gums, tongue, lips, and oropharynx. However, they may extend to involve surrounding tissues. Oral cavity neoplasia can originate from dental tissue (odontogenic), bone (osteogenic), or soft tissues of the mouth and oropharynx.

Odontogenic

The classification of odontogenic tumors is based on the inductive effect of one dental tissue on another.

- Ameloblastoma (adamantinoma)—Benign but locally invasive. Often interosseus and distorts the mandible.
- Ameloblastic odontoma (odentoameloblastoma)—Benign, slowly expanding, and locally invasive.
- Complex odontoma—Contains all the elements of a normal tooth but structure is disorganized.
- Compound odentoma—Contains all the elements of a normal tooth. Forms a tooth-like structure—denticles. Regarded as a malformation.
- Cementoma—Dense, mineralized structure

Osteogenic

Osteogenic tumors are usually benign and have a predilection for the mandibular symphysis.

- Osteomas
- Osteosarcomas
- Fibro-osteoma
- Ossifying fibromas
- Hemangiosarcoma
- Soft tissue
- Squamous cell carcinoma
- Tongue, gingiva, pharynx, and hard palate
- Lymphosarcoma
- Horse palate
- Fibrosarcoma
- Tongue
- Myosarcoma
- Melanomas
- Adenomas

PATHOPHYSIOLOGY

N/A

SYSTEMS AFFECTED

The neoplasms affect the digestive system but may invade the respiratory tract.

GENETICS

N/A

INCIDENCE

Malignant bone tumors are extremely rare in the horse, but more than 80% of osteosarcomas occur in the head region. Neoplasia of the oral cavity or pharynx is extremely uncommon. In one study of 141 cases with squamous cell carcinomas, only 5% involved the oral or pharyngeal mucosa.

SIGNALMENT

The age of the horse may suggest the type of neoplasm. There is a high incidence of ameloblastic odontomas in young animals (6 weeks to 1 yr of age). Ameloblastomas occur in older horses (5–20 yr of age), whereas osteogenic neoplasms have no age predilection. Horses with osteogenic tumors of the intra-membranous bone of the head are young, 2–14 months of age. Squamous cell carcinoma, which is by far the most common type of soft-tissue tumor, occurs in older horses.
No breed or sex susceptibility has been suggested for any of the neoplasms.

SIGNS

Historical Findings

The clinical signs of oral cavity and oropharyngeal neoplasia are dependent on the location and size of the neoplasm and may include dysphagia, difficulty in prehension or mastication, halitosis, oral discharge, and lymphadenopathy. Nasal discharge may be evident if the tumor has expanded to involve the nasal chamber or paranasal sinuses.
The anatomy of the oral cavity allows for considerable progression and expansion of the lesion before it causes major clinical signs. Therefore, the majority of neoplasms in this region are usually well advanced with extensive local infiltration before clinical signs become apparent.

Physical Examination Findings

Odontogenic neoplasms usually present as slowly developing, firm, immobile swellings of the mandible or maxilla.
The most common presentation of osteogenic tumors is proliferation of bony tissue on the rostral mandible in the young horse. The syndrome has been classified as equine juvenile mandibular ossifying fibroma, and usually presents as a rapidly growing subgingival mass of the rostral mandible or, much less commonly, the premaxilla. The mucosa covering the mass is usually ulcerated. The proliferation can be symmetric or may only involve the rostral aspect of one hemi-mandible. On palpation, the teeth may be loose but the mass is usually non-painful. Prehension and mastication are initially unaltered, but become apparent when the tumor reaches a large size.
The typical appearance of squamous cell carcinoma of the oral cavity is a partially ulcerated multilobular mass projecting from the mucosa. The tumor is usually locally invasive and metastasis can occur. Displacement and loosening of the teeth is present. Horses with squamous cell carcinoma and lymphosarcoma of the hard palate commonly have a foul, fetid odor to their breath.
Although lesions of the rostral mandible are readily identified, those affecting the more caudal part of the oral cavity and pharynx require a more detailed examination. Sedation and the use of a Houssmann gag and headlamp or pen flashlight allow the presence of a tumor to be determined visually or by palpation and a biopsy taken in many cases, but in others general anesthesia is necessary. The regional lymph nodes should be examined.

CAUSES

N/A

RISK FACTORS

N/A

DIAGNOSIS

The definitive diagnosis depends on histologic examination of tissue removed by biopsy or at necropsy.

DIFFERENTIAL DIAGNOSIS

- Swellings of the mandible or maxilla due to underlying dental disease, especially periapical abscessation.
- Foreign bodies in the oropharynx causing dysphagia and halitosis.

CBC/BIOCHEMISTRY

N/A

OTHER LABORATORY TESTS

N/A

IMAGING

Radiography is of considerable value in evaluating the nature and extent of the neoplasm and in differentiating it from a dental problem.
Ameloblastomas appear as a radiolucent multiloculated mass often well marginated by thick, sclerotic bone with cortical expansion on the lingual and buccal surfaces. The tooth roots may appear shortened and lytic with loss of lamina diva and periodontal membrane.
Ameloblastic odontomas appear radiographically as radiopaque masses that may appear to fill the maxillary sinus, obstructing the nasal passage on the affected side. The maxilla and teeth are usually displaced laterally.
Radiographically osteogenic tumors are characterized by a smooth, bony proliferation of the rostral mandible with or without osteolytic change involving the roots of the teeth.
Horses with squamous cell carcinoma of the hard palate show dental displacement and loss of alveolar bone. Extension into the paranasal sinuses results in loss of the normal radiolucent

appearance. Radiography of the pharynx may show its dorsal wall to be deformed and thickened, particularly when affected by lymphosarcoma.
Endoscopy is of value in determining the extent of palatine and nasal involvement. In cases of lymphosarcoma, the pharyngeal wall may be edematous with moderately severe lymphoid hyperplasia and ulceration of the soft palate. Guttural pouch empyema may be noted, particularly if the pharyngeal walls are affected. In some cases an oronasal fistula may be present. Oral endoscopy carried out under general anesthesia allows a thorough examination that may not be possible by other means.

DIAGNOSTIC PROCEDURES

Biopsy

Biopsies of masses involving the mandible or maxilla enable differentiation between odontogenic and osteogenic tumors.
Biopsy of squamous cell carcinoma of the mouth can be obtained without difficulty by breaking off a piece of the proliferative tissue, whereas biopsies of pharyngeal or palatine tissues may be accomplished with a biopsy instrument through an endoscope or using uterine biopsy forceps under general anesthesia.
If lymph node enlargement is present, a fine-needle aspirate or biopsy is necessary to determine if metastasis has occurred.

PATHOLOGIC FINDINGS

Histology

Ameloblastomas contain odontogenic islands set in well-vascularized connective tissue. The periphery of the follicle is composed of a layer of columnar cells with distinct polarization of nuclei away from the basement membrane, resembling ameloblasts. Toward the center of the follicles the cells form a loose network similar to the stellate reticulum of the developing tooth. Differentiation of this tumor from other odontogenic epithelial tumors is based on the degree of stellate reticulum formation without intracellular bridges.
Ameloblastic odontomas differ from amelioblastomas in that the islands of epithelium are smaller, so that the formation of cysts is less frequent and the stellate reticulum is less extensive.
The term *odontoma* implies that there has been induction of both dentine and enamel within the lesion and their presence is evident histologically.
It should be noted, however, that these tumor classifications are subjective, and because of their rarity and difficulties in their histologic recognition, a degree of inconsistency exists with respect to their nomenclature.
Two reports of rostral mandibular enlargement in young horses were described as osteosarcomas, but there were no mitotic cells observed histologically and it is possible that these lesions were related to the equine juvenile ossifying fibroma syndrome.
Histologic diagnosis of oral and pharyngeal neoplasms is much less complicated.

TREATMENT

Whereas neoplasms of the mouth and pharynx, such as squamous cell carcinoma and lymphosarcoma, are usually too advanced when diagnosed to consider anything but euthanasia, there have been several reports of attempted surgical removal of odontogenic and osteogenic tumors of the mandible and maxilla. The ease of surgical debridement is dependent on the size and location of the tumor. Surgical excision and curettage are often followed by recurrence, although this may be delayed for several years. Because the growth of amelobastic odontomas is by expansion rather than infiltration, theoretically they may represent a better prognosis than ameloblastomas. Radical tumor resection in conjunction with partial mandibulectomy and possible stabilization of the resulting defect with internal or external orthopedic devices has met with greater success. Recurrence is more common when the neoplasm is located in the maxilla. Cryosurgery has been used as an adjunct to surgical excision. This has the potential advantage of destroying neoplastic cells at the surgical margins without removing additional bone. The amount of dead space is decreased, and scaffolding is provided for new bone development by creeping substitution.
As previously mentioned, many neoplasms of the oral cavity and oropharynx are advanced before detection; consequently, surgical removal often leads to poor success rates because of difficult access and incomplete removal of the lesion. Confirmation of malignancy by histologic examination in an extensive lesion is an indication for euthanasia.
The use of laser surgery had been advocated for the ablation of certain soft-tissue neoplasms of the oropharynx or nasopharynx, but the success of this therapy is largely dependent on early tumor recognition.

NURSING CARE/ACTIVITY/DIET

Horses that have undergone radical surgical excision, including mandibulectomy, may have difficulty prehending short grass; however, prehending longer grass and mastication have not been complications. Cosmetically the post-operative appearance of the horses is acceptable, even though all horses have some flaccidity of the lower lip. Horses with a mandibulectomy have been able to return to their intended uses, including racing.

MEDICATIONS

CONTRAINDICATIONS

N/A

PRECAUTIONS

N/A

POSSIBLE INTERACTIONS

N/A

ALTERNATIVE DRUGS

N/A

FOLLOW-UP

PATIENT MONITORING

N/A

PREVENTION/AVOIDANCE

N/A

POSSIBLE COMPLICATIONS

N/A

EXPECTED COURSE AND PROGNOSIS

Successful treatment depends on complete removal/destruction of the neoplasm.

MISCELLANEOUS

ASSOCIATED CONDITIONS

N/A

AGE-RELATED FACTORS

N/A

ZOONOTIC POTENTIAL

N/A

PREGNANCY

N/A

SYNONYMS

N/A

Suggested Reading

Hana SR, Bentone AL. Neoplasia. Vet Clin North Am Equine Pract 1993;9(1): 213-234.
Head KW. Tumours of the alimentary tract. In: Moulton JE (Ed.). Tumours in domestic animals, 3rd ed. Los Angeles: University of California Press. 1990:347.
Pirie RC, Tremaine WH. Neoplasia of the mouth and surrounding structure. In: Robinson NE (Ed.). Current therapy in equine medicine, 4th ed. WB Saunders & Co. 199X:153-155.
Richardson DW, Evans LH, Tulleners EP. Rostral mandibulectomy in five horses. J Am Vet Med Assoc 1991;174;734.

Author Garry B. Edwards
Consulting Editor Henry Stämpfli

ORAL STEREOTYPIC BEHAVIORS

BASICS

DEFINITION

- Repetitive, apparently functionless behavior that may be considered to be compulsive
- Two forms—locomotor and oral
- Oral stereotypies—cribbing, tongue flapping, and sucking are common; lip licking, noise making with the head, and tooth grinding are less common.
- Locomotor stereotypies—head bobbing or shaking

PATHOPHYSIOLOGY

- Cribbing is the only stereotypy in which the pathophysiology has been elucidated using endoscopy and fluoroscopy. Air is not swallowed, but a transient dilation of the upper esophagus occurs. The noise is produced when air rushes through the cricopharynx. Contraction of the ventral neck muscles produces negative pressure in the esophagus that allows air to move in; the air then is expelled from the pharynx rostrally, with only a small amount passing into the lower esophagus.
- Endogenous opiates may be involved, because administration of an opiate blocker inhibits cribbing for several hours. Cribbing does not cause release of endogenous opiates, but opiates are necessary for cribbing to occur.

SYSTEMS AFFECTED

- Behavioral—repetitive, apparently functionless behavior involving the head.
- GI—wear of the upper incisors is one definite outcome of cribbing, and a few horses exhibit colic (i.e., "gas colic") afterward. Cribbing may help to maintain GI motility when food is absent.
- Oral problems may cause tongue protrusion.
- Neurologic—these causes of headshaking must be ruled out before the diagnosis of a behavior problem can be established.

SIGNALMENT

Usually an adult horse and one confined in a stall

SIGNS

General Comments

- Cribbing—the horse grasps a horizontal surface with its incisors, flexes its neck, and allows air to pass into the upper esophagus. Tongue movements and tooth grinding may be signs of stereotypic behavior.
- Tongue movements—not as frequent in horses as in cattle, probably because horses do not use their tongues to prehend food as cattle do. Some horses simply protrude their tongue, which probably relates to food-anticipating movements that occur not when horses are free, expecting palatable food, and free-lunged. Other horses move the tongue in and out or flap the tongue.
- Stereotypic behavior that is purposeless must be differentiated from purposeful behavior. Biting the stall wall may be redirected aggression against the horse in the next stall. Tongue movements may have been rewarded by the present or a previous owner. Noise making also may have been rewarded by food (e.g., if a horse happened to be rattling a pail just before feeding time, it would not take many pairings before the horse concluded that rattling led to food). Horses may make noise to increase environmental stimulation, but they more likely do so to attract attention. If the oral behavior occurs mostly at feeding time, consider it anticipatory and not stereotypic behavior. Head bobbing may be stereotypic behavior, but if it occurs or is aggravated by exercise or sunlight, it is not behavioral.

Historical Findings

Stereotypic behavior usually begins with an abrupt change in the environment; taking a horse from pasture and immediately limiting its access to hay can be the initiating factor that leads to cribbing.

Physical Examination Findings

- Cribbing—well developed neck muscles and wear of the upper incisors. Rarely, the horse is very thin, because it spends so much time cribbing that it does not have time to ingest the calories it needs.
- Head bobbing—must be differentiated from head shaking in response to bright light or pain in the nasopharynx. In contrast to stereotypic head bobbing, which is seen in confined horses at rest, head shaking is exacerbated by exercise.

CAUSES

- The cause of stereotypic behavior is unknown.
- Boredom probably is not a cause, because providing stall toys usually does not help.
- The horse is thwarted in some goal, usually grazing, and the frustration leads to repetition of a behavior that is part of the appetitive portion of that behavior (e.g., cribbing as part of biting a mouthful of grass as the first step of ingestion).
- Feeding sweet feed or other highly palatable food stimulates cribbing.

RISK FACTORS

- Genetic predisposition
- Stall confinement with limited (<7 kg) forage, <10 gallons/day of water, bedding other than straw, and minimal visual or tactile contact with other horses
- Race, dressage, and eventing horses are at greater risk than endurance horses.
- No evidence that horses learn to crib by observing other horses; if the environment is conducive to cribbing and the horse has the genetic predisposition, it will crib.

DIAGNOSIS

DIFFERENTIAL DIAGNOSIS

- Differentiate cribbing from wood chewing. The cribbing horse grasps wooden edges but does not ingest them; the wood-chewing horse does. The cribbing horse makes a loud noise; the only sound made by the wood-chewing horse is that of wood being splintered.
- Differentiate head bobbing from a normal, mild threat by a horse or the vertical head shakes of a foal trying to stop its mother to nurse. Also differentiate head bobbing from head shaking, which usually occurs outdoors in response to light, to allergies, or to some other nasopharyngeal irritation.
- Differentiate tongue movements and tooth grinding from oral pathologies. Tooth grinding of sudden onset also can be a sign of pain elsewhere in the body.

CBC/BIOCHEMISTRY/URINALYSIS

Perform a chemistry screen and CBC to determine presence of an underlying disease and to judge whether medication can be administered safely.

OTHER LABORATORY TESTS

N/A

IMAGING

May be necessary to rule out GI tract problems as a cause of cribbing.

DIAGNOSTIC PROCEDURES

Endoscopy of the nasal cavity and pharynx to rule out medical causes of head bobbing

ORAL STEREOTYPIC BEHAVIORS

TREATMENT

• Aimed at creating a normal equine environment, which means the horse has physical contact with other horses and available forage at all times. The cure for stall behavior problems is to remove the horse from the stall and put it in a compatible social group with access to pasture or a hay-free choice. When the use of the horse precludes keeping it in a group with a run-out housing situation, eliminating risk factors (e.g., limited forage, wood shavings as bedding) helps. Stall toys generally are ineffective, except for the food ball (i.e., a barrel that delivers pellets when nudged by the horse), which simulates grazing.
• Punishment—not the preferred method of treatment, but clinicians should be aware of this option. Several types of collars can pinch the horse when it cribs, and a shock collar is available. More humane is a muzzle that prevents the horse from making contact with a horizontal surface.
• Surgery—accessory neurectomy, strap muscle myectomy, or a combination of the two. Reserve these surgical approaches for horses that experience colic when they crib or are emaciated because they crib rather than eat.
• Providing a padded horizontal bar on which the horse can bite without damaging his teeth or the stall fixtures is the best approach, and eliminating grain, molasses, and sugar from the diet also helps.
• Other oral stereotypies—provide oral stimulation in the form of several types of forage, pasture, or a barrel the horse can turn to receive pelleted feed or grain. If the behavior occurs before feeding, the horse probably is frustrated by hunger (i.e., undernourishment); if it occurs after feeding, the horse probably is frustrated from the lack of a specific dietary component (i.e., malnourishment).
• Counter-conditioning—training the horse to do something incompatible with the oral behavior (e.g., teaching horse to hold something in its mouth for a food reward so it does not scrape the teeth on metal or bite and toss the feed bucket)
• Tongue protrusion under saddle is usually treated with a dropped nose band.

MEDICATIONS

DRUGS OF CHOICE

Opiate blockers such as naloxone (0.02–0.04 mg/kg), naltrexone (0.04 mg/kg), or nalmefene (0.08 mg/kg), either IM or IV, inhibit cribbing, but these drugs are too expensive and too short acting to be practical.

CONTRAINDICATIONS

Mares during late pregnancy.

PRECAUTIONS

GI side effects, including diarrhea, inappetence, and behavior indicative of colic, are seen after naloxone administration.

POSSIBLE INTERACTIONS

N/A

ALTERNATIVE DRUGS

• Substitution of fat (e.g., corn oil) for carbohydrates (e.g., molasses and grain)
• Acupuncture

FOLLOW-UP

PATIENT MONITORING

Regular follow-up after 2 weeks of treatment to evaluate the owner's compliance and the success of the treatments given.

POSSIBLE COMPLICATIONS

N/A

MISCELLANEOUS

ASSOCIATED CONDITIONS

N/A

AGE RELATED FACTORS

Usually a disease of mature horses

ZOONOTIC POTENTIAL

N/A

PREGNANCY

N/A

SYNONYMS

• Crib biting
• Wind sucking

SEE ALSO

• Locomotor stereotypic behaviors
• Pica

ABBREVIATIONS

GI = gastrointestinal

Suggested Reading

Dodman NH, Schuster L, Court MH, Dixon R. An investigation into the use of narcotic antagonists in the treatment of a stereotypic behaviour pattern (crib-biting) in the horse. Am J Vet Res 1989;48:311–319.

Gillham SB, Dodman NH, Shuster L, Kream R, Rand W. The effect of diet on cribbing behavior and plasma β-endorphin in horses. Appl Anim Behav Sci 1994;41:147–153.

Houpt KA, McDonnell SM. Equine stereotypies. Compend Cont Educ 1993;15:1265–1272.

Luescher UA, McKeown DB, Halip J. Reviewing the causes of obsessive-compulsive disorders in horses. Vet Med 1991:527–530.

McGreevy PD, Cripps PJ, French NP, Green LE, Nicol CJ. Management factors associated with stereotypic and redirected behaviour in the Thoroughbred horse. Equine Vet J 1995;27:86–91.

McGreevy PD, Richardson JD, Nichol CJ, Lane JG. Radiographic and endoscopic study of horses performing an oral based stereotypy. Equine Vet J 1995;27:92–95.

Ralson SL. Common behavioral problems of horses. Compend Cont Educ 1982;4:S152–S159.

Author Katherine Albro Houpt
Consulting Editor Daniel Q. Estep

ORAL ULCERS

BASICS

DEFINITION

Oral ulcers are disruptions in the integrity of the oral mucosa that may be preceded by lesions such as vesicles, bullae, or crusts.

PATHOPHYSIOLOGY

The pathophysiologic events that lead to oral ulceration are variable and depend on the inciting cause. In the case of vesicular stomatitis, a short incubation period of 24 hr and invasion of oral epithelial cells by the virus occurs. The lesions progress rapidly from blanched macules to vesicles and soon rupture, leaving sloughed epithelium and ulcers.
Phenylbutazone is known to inhibit prostaglandin synthesis by inhibition of cyclooxygenase. This inhibition of prostaglandin synthesis in the gastrointestinal tract results in a depletion of PGE_1 and PGE_2 that is thought to cause vasoconstriction of the microvasculature of the mucosa, leading to ischemia and ulcer formation. The mechanism of action of cantharidin to induce ulcers is not well understood yet, but acantholysis and vesicle formation occur as a result of damage to cell membrane due to interference with oxidative enzymes bound to mitochondria.
The oral ulcers caused by facial paralysis and dental problems are due to impaction of food material between the teeth and the cheek, as well as direct traumatic damage by the teeth.

SYSTEMS AFFECTED

The different systems affected vary depending on the initial cause. When oral ulcers are the result of vesicular stomatitis, the locomotor system is usually affected. The vesicular lesions are present also on the coronary band, and lameness is observed.
In cases of phenylbutazone toxicity, several sections of the gastrointestinal tract are affected, causing gastric and intestinal ulceration and colitis of the right dorsal colon. The kidney is also affected, causing renal medullary crest necrosis. Ventral and peripheral edema is also observed.
Blister beetle toxicosis (Cantharidin toxicosis), besides affecting the mucosal surface, also affects the gastrointestinal tract, causing colic. There is hypocalcemia, hypoproteinemia, and the kidney is slightly affected. Myocardial necrosis is a common finding in affected horses. Some horses show stilted gait, as seen in myositis.
In the uremic syndrome, weight loss is the most common affliction; there is PU/PD due to kidney damage. Gastric ulceration, coagulation disorders, and halitosis (urine odor) have been reported. There is excessive dental tartar, and there is ventral edema because of a decrease in oncotic pressure, increased vascular permeability, and increased hydrostatic pressure. Bone marrow, the endocrine system, and the CNS might be affected.
The other causes of oral ulceration are local phenomena limited to the buccal mucosa.

SIGNALMENT

Oral ulcers can occur at any age, and there is no sex or breed predisposition.

SIGNS

Historical Findings

The history of oral ulceration cases is quite variable and is dependent on the initial cause. In the cases of vesicular stomatitis, it starts as an outbreak. The owner usually reports that the affected animals have excessive salivation, inappetence, and lameness. In the cases where toxicity is involved, there is history of ingestion of toxic material. In the case of phenylbutazone toxicity, the history indicates that an excessive dosage for several days or accidental administration of large amounts has occurred. Facial nerve paralysis is usually preceded by some history of trauma or CNS disease.

Physical Examination Findings

In the majority of the cases of oral ulcers regardless of the cause, there is ptyalism, different degrees of anorexia, and dysphagia due to pain.
Vesicular stomatitis starts with oral vesicles that with time coalesce and turn into ulcers. Lameness of different degrees is observed due to involvement of the coronary band, which has vesicles and is swollen (see Vesicular Stomatitis).
In phenylbutazone toxicity there are signs typical of oral ulcers, but also there may be ventral and peripheral edema, bruxism, diarrhea (see Colitis), melena, ulceration of the digestive tract, and weight loss (see NSAID Toxicity).
In addition to oral ulcers, Cantharidin toxicosis is also manifested by depression, colic, fever, profuse diarrhea, stranguria, synchronous diaphragmatic flutter, and a stiff gait (see Cantharidin Toxicosis). Oral ulcers in uremia are accompanied by all the signs that distinguish the uremic syndrome (see Chronic Renal Failure).

CAUSES

- Vesicular stomatitis
- Phenylbutazone toxicity
- Uremia
- Cantharidin toxicosis
- Chemical stomatitis
- Periodontal disease
- Foxtail and plant thorn stomatitis
- Oral foreign body
- Oral ulcers secondary to yellow bristle grass
- Food impaction between molar teeth and cheek (facial nerve paralysis, dental problems)
- Equine Herpes Virus type II

RISK FACTORS

The risk factors involved in oral ulcers are related to the primary cause (see each clinical entity).

ORAL ULCERS

DIAGNOSIS

DIFFERENTIAL DIAGNOSIS

See Ptyalism

CBC/BIOCHEMISTRY/URINALYSIS

No findings are specific to oral ulceration, but changes may reflect the underlying causes.

IMAGING

Radiographic studies are indicated when there is suspicion of dental problems or trauma has caused facial paralysis.

DIAGNOSTIC PROCEDURES

A thorough physical and oral examination is indicated to rule out the different causes of oral ulceration.

To diagnose vesicular stomatitis, virus isolation from biopsy of the vesicles is done. A complement fixation test and a fluorescent antibody test are used for virus identification. An ELISA is also available.

Cantharidin toxicosis diagnosis is based on detecting cantharidin in stomach contents or in urine or finding blister beetles in the forage.

The diagnosis of phenylbutazone toxicity is suggested by history of inappropriate drug administration and clinical picture compatible with it. Biopsy and histologic examination of lesions may assist in narrowing differential diagnosis and rule out associated neoplastic events.

TREATMENT

Specific therapy for particular conditions may be indicated. The treatment strategies for oral ulcers involves local therapy to relive the pain and irritation, such as mild antiseptic mouthwashes with potassium permanganate (2%), hydrogen peroxide (0.5%), saturated solution of boric acid, or povidone iodine solution (1% v/v). If present, thorns or any foreign body should be extracted. There is also need to remove any chemical irritant that may be causing oral ulceration. This also applies for all toxicoses. When dental problems are the cause, appropriate dental prophylactic measures are indicated.

ZOONOTIC POTENTIAL

Among the causes of oral ulcers, only vesicular stomatis has zoonotic potential.

SYNONYMS

- Vesicles
- Crusts
- Growths

Suggested Reading

Green S. Vesicular stomatitis in the horse. Vet Clin North Am Equine Pract 1993;9:349-353.

Meschter CL, Giñbert M, Krook L, Maylin G, Corradino R. The effects of phenylbutazone on the intestinal mucosa of the horse: A morphological, ultrastructural and biochemical study. Equine Vet J 1990;22:255-263.

Scmitz DG. Cantharidin toxicosis in horses. J Vet Intern Med 1989;3:208-215.

Scrutchfield WL., Schumacher J. Examination of the oral cavity and routine dental care. Vet Clin North Am Equine Pract 1993;9:123-131.

Author Oliver E. Olimpo
Consulting Editor Henry Stämpfli

ORBITAL DISEASE

BASICS

OVERVIEW

- An assortment of diseases and conditions leading to dysfunction of the anatomic orbit, which is composed of a several bones forming a series of canals, fissures, and foramina that communicate with the extraorbital compartments and is a closed, conical cavity with a broad opening anteriorly. Within the orbit are the globe and numerous types of extraocular supportive tissue, including fascia, nerves, blood vessels, muscle, fat, and glands. Pathology of any of these extraocular tissues (including the bony orbit) broadly defines orbital disease.
- Disease progresses as tissue within or adjacent to the orbit loses its ability to function; consequently, vision is endangered.
- Major mechanisms—compression by a space-occupying lesion, anatomic rearrangement by trauma or disease, or invasion of a systemic illness into the orbit.
- Organ systems—ophthalmic, musculoskeletal, vascular, nervous, and upper respiratory, including sinuses

SIGNALMENT

Old horses tend to develop neoplasia; foals and yearlings may be prone to acute trauma.

SIGNS

- Vary depending on the disease process
- Exophthalmos (i.e., anterior displacement of the globe) associated with nictitans protrusion, lagophthalmos, and corneal ulceration
- Enophthalmos (i.e., posterior displacement of the globe) caused by atrophy of tissue behind the globe
- Phthisis bulbi (i.e., globe atrophy)
- Nasal discharge or epistaxis
- Blepharedema, chemosis, or corneal edema
- Epiphora or other ocular discharge
- Strabismus, with associated visual difficulties and abnormal head posture
- Vision loss—usually unilateral
- Orbital asymmetry (OD vs. OS) from fractures, cellulitis, and orbital emphysema
- Fever or pain

CAUSES AND RISK FACTORS

- Trauma causing orbital fractures and proptosis
- Foreign bodies leading to orbital abscesses
- (Pyo)granulomatous diseases
- Guttural pouch disease
- Sinusitis involving the frontal, maxillary, or sphenopalatine sinuses
- Tooth-root abscesses
- Orbital neoplasia—meningioma, neuroendocrine tumor, lipoma, adenocarcinoma, lymphoma, melanoma, sarcoid, squamous cell carcinoma, hemangiosarcoma, multilobular osteoma, medulloepithelioma, schwannoma, and neurofibroma
- Varices (i.e., abnormal distension of venules) causing displacement of normal tissue
- Retro-orbital cysts
- Parasitism—hydatid cysts

DIAGNOSIS

DIFFERENTIAL DIAGNOSIS

- Any cause of ocular pain
- Exophthalmos, a sign of orbital disease, can be confused with buphthalmos, a marked increase in globe diameter associated with advanced glaucoma.
- Primary extraorbital disease close to, but not affecting, the orbit—sinusitis, guttural pouch disorders, and tooth problems

CBC/BIOCHEMISTRY/URINALYSIS

- CBC may show elevated fibrinogen or other nonspecific inflammatory indicators with extensive disease.
- Consider systemic illness.

OTHER LABORATORY TESTS

N/A

IMAGING

- Skull radiography
- Retro-orbital ultrasonography
- CT or MR imaging where available—foals and small ponies primarily

DIAGNOSTIC PROCEDURES

- Digital retropulsion of affected and unaffected eyes helps in confirming retro-orbital masses.
- Fluid aspiration or tissue biopsy
- Cytology, microbial culture and sensitivity, and histopathology
- Orbitotomy can be diagnostic and therapeutic; however, it is difficult surgery that may require orthopedic instruments.
- Trephination into paranasal sinuses may be indicated for microbial culture, irrigation, and drainage.
- Proptosis—careful ophthalmic examination indicates the viability of the eye; miosis with severe hypotony and hyphema indicates severe trauma and poor visual prognosis.

PATHOLOGIC FINDINGS

Vary greatly depending on the particular disease.

TREATMENT

- Orbital diseases, once identified, may be treated medically (e.g., minor trauma) or may need surgical attention (e.g., orbital neoplasia) and short hospital stays until the owner or trainer can monitor and treat the patient at home.
- Activity is based on the degree of vision impairment and comfort of the horse. Some diseases are very painful, especially after invasive surgery. Stall rest may be indicated for the short term.
- No change in diet is necessary unless malnutrition has caused atrophy of the orbital contents.
- Long-term damage may be sustained during orbital trauma, including eyelid paralysis, chronic keratitis, or intermittent nasal or ocular discharge.
- Recurrence of retrobulbar tumors or infections is possible after primary treatment, depending on the definitive diagnosis.

ORBITAL DISEASE

- For primary orbital disease, prognosis for vision is guarded initially. In severe, painful orbital disease with irreversible blindness and orbital neoplasia, the best treatment may be orbital exenteration.
- In a sighted eye, orbitotomy is best for discrete, solitary retrobulbar masses that do not invade the optic nerve.
- Enucleation may be recommended to remove a painful, blind, pathologic eye and its associated conjunctiva and nictitans. An intraorbital prosthesis may replaced the globe if risk of infection or tumor recurrence is low.
- Intrascleral prostheses are an acceptable alternative to enucleation and can be placed in an eviscerated scleral shell if the cornea is not severely diseased and no residual lagophthalmos or exophthalmos is present. Orbital bleeding should be minimized by careful hemostasis.
- Periorbital fractures should be repaired quickly, because fibrous union can occur as soon as 1 week after trauma. Tarsorrhaphies are beneficial to proptosed eyes and should not be removed until most of the periorbital swelling has subsided (usually 5–7 days).

MEDICATIONS

DRUGS

- Systemic antibiotics should be administered in cases of trauma or suspected orbital infection.
- The globe itself may benefit from topical ophthalmic lubricants or antibiotics.
- Periorbital swelling can be alleviated by judicious use of anti-inflammatories.
- Occasionally, uveitis is seen with orbital trauma and should be treated with topical or systemic anti-inflammatories.
- Banamine (1 mg/kg IV, IM, or PO BID) or phenylbutazone (4.4–8.8 mg/kg PO once daily) can be given for pain associated with the orbital disease.
- Intralesional iridium implants or cisplatin chemotherapy into the orbital tumor may be beneficial in some types of neoplasia.

CONTRAINDICATIONS/POSSIBLE INTERACTIONS

- Topical steroids are contraindicated in ulcerative keratitis.
- Long-term use of banamine may cause ulcerative gastroenteritis. Concurrent administration of 60 mL of corn oil PO once daily may lower the risk of ulcers.

FOLLOW-UP

- Recheck visits for more extensive diseases, especially if orbital surgery is performed (e.g., for an aggressive tumor).
- Providing a safe environment with good training may decrease the opportunity for trauma.
- Recurrence of tumor, reinfection of orbit, and persistent pain and swelling can occur during and after the treatment period.
- Blindness and loss of the eye are possible sequela of severe orbital disease.
- Highly variable outcomes depending on correct diagnosis and appropriate treatment. Some orbital diseases (e.g., trauma) are one-time events, with possible long-term side effects. Other diseases (e.g., tumors) can never be cured and only treated palliatively.

MISCELLANEOUS

SEE ALSO

- Intralesional iridium implants or cisplatin chemotherapy into the orbital tumor may be beneficial in some types of neoplasia.
- CNS diseases
- Ocular neoplasia
- Sinus and guttural pouch disorders
- Skull fractures

ABBREVIATIONS

- MR = magnetic resonance
- OD = oculo dextro
- OS = oculo sinistro

Suggested Reading

Brooks DE. Equine ophthalmology. In: Gelatt KN, ed. Veterinary ophthalmology. 3rd ed. Philadelphia: Lippincott Williams & Wilkins, 1999.

Author Daniel Biros

Consulting Editor Dennis E. Brooks

ORGANOPHOSPHORUS (OP) AND CARBAMATE INSECTICIDE TOXICOSIS

BASICS

DEFINITION

- Toxicosis caused by exposure to ACHE-inhibiting OP or carbamate compounds, which are active ingredients in many animal oral and topical parasiticides as well as household and agricultural pesticide products
- More than 50 different, but structurally related, OP and carbamate compounds exist, with hundreds of different formulations containing varying concentrations of AI.
- Toxicity among individual compounds varies tremendously.
- Oral ingestion is the most common form of equine exposure, either from ingesting pasture grass or hay in which pesticide spills or drift have occurred or from overdosing with oral parasiticide products.
- Inhalation exposure is rare but may result from close proximity to aerial applied pesticides.

PATHOPHYSIOLOGY

- Most OP and carbamate pesticides are rapidly absorbed by the respiratory or GI systems and dermally.
- Some are direct-acting compounds; others require metabolic activation by the liver to a toxic metabolite.
- The underlying biochemical lesion responsible for the clinical syndrome is inhibition of ACHE activity in the nervous system, resulting in accumulation of acetylcholine at synapses and myoneural junctions.
- Inhibition of the enzyme by OPs is considered irreversible, particularly once covalent bonding or aging occurs.
- Inhibition of the enzyme by carbamates is reversible.
- To restore ACHE activity after pesticide exposure, the enzyme must be reactivated or resynthesized.

SYSTEMS AFFECTED

- Nervous and musculoskeletal—excess acetylcholine at synapses and myoneural junctions initially excites, then paralyzes, transmission in cholinergic synapses of the CNS and at parasympathetic and a few sympathetic nerve endings (i.e., muscarinic effects) and at somatic nerves and ganglionic synapses of autonomic ganglia (i.e., nicotinic effects).
- Respiratory—buildup of secretions from muscarinic effects can lead to respiratory difficulties, perfusion problems, and secondary bacterial invaders.

GENETICS

N/A

INCIDENCE/PREVALENCE

- Poisonings with these compounds in horses are relatively uncommon.
- Most cases occur during the spring and summer, when agricultural and household pesticide use is highest.
- Poisonings can occur from eating hay that was baled several months previously—any pesticide spilled or drifted onto the hay and then baled has a slower rate of degradation, and some pesticides persist in baled hay for as long as 6 months.
- Most cases occur in agricultural areas.

SIGNALMENT

No breed, age, or sex predilections

SIGNS

General Comments

- Clinical signs vary considerably between different species of animals despite the same mechanism of action.
- In horses, GI signs predominate, and nervous signs may be absent.
- Severity of the clinical syndrome depends on the exposure dose, exposure route, and formulation of the pesticide product.
- Clinical signs can occur immediately, after inhalation or oral exposure, or be delayed by several hours (i.e., oral or dermal route).

Physical Examination Findings

- Abdominal pain accompanied by restlessness, anxiety, and sweating
- Markedly increased intestinal sounds
- Watery diarrhea
- Weakness and depression
- Mild to severe muscle tremors—seizures uncommon
- Tachycardia or bradycardia
- Miosis or mydriasis
- Dyspnea
- Excessive salivation—rare

CAUSES

- Most cases occur via ingestion of pesticide-contaminated grass or hay or from overdosing with oral parasiticide products.
- Horses also can be poisoned by accidental access to spilled or improperly used, stored, or discarded pesticides.

RISK FACTORS

Most OPs are lipophilic and slowly released, so animals with a lean body mass may exhibit more severe symptoms.

DIAGNOSIS

DIFFERENTIAL DIAGNOSIS

- Bacterial or viral gastroenteritis—physical examination; bacteriology; serology
- Intestinal compromise (e.g., twist, torsion, or intussusception)—physical examination
- Peritonitis—physical examination; abdominocentesis
- Inorganic arsenic poisoning—urine, whole-blood, or tissue arsenic determination

CBC/BIOCHEMISTRY/URINALYSIS

N/A

OTHER LABORATORY TESTS

- Inhibition of blood, brain, or retinal ACHE activity suggests exposure, particularly with activity <50% of normal.
- ACHE activity can be assessed up to several days after the suspected exposure.
- Carbamate binding can be reversed during transit to a laboratory facility, so lack of enzyme inhibition does not necessarily rule out carbamate exposure.
- In peracute to acute, high-dose exposures, the animal may die of respiratory compromise before sufficient brain enzyme activity can be inhibited. In addition, some OP and carbamates poorly penetrate the CNS, so lack of brain ACHE inhibition cannot rule out exposure to these compounds.
- Tissue testing (e.g., liver, kidney, stomach contents, skin, fat, urine) for OP or carbamate residues is readily available at most diagnostic facilities and can confirm exposure.

IMAGING

N/A

DIAGNOSTIC PROCEDURES

N/A

PATHOLOGIC FINDINGS

- Visible evidence of insecticide granules in stomach contents
- Most OP and carbamate pesticides have a strong sulfur or "chemical" odor.
- No specific gross or histopathologic lesions—pulmonary edema and effusions sometimes are reported.

ORGANOPHOSPHORUS (OP) AND CARBAMATE INSECTICIDE TOXICOSIS

TREATMENT

APPROPRIATE HEALTH CARE
- Prompt and aggressive treatment is essential to a favorable outcome.
- Save samples of blood, urine, or stomach reflux for toxicologic analysis before initiating any specific treatments.

NURSING CARE
- Administration of IV fluids to correct intestinal fluid and electrolyte losses and to assist in renal excretion of metabolites. Continue fluids until diarrhea and sweating are under control and the horse can eat and drink on its own.
- Decontamination procedures after oral exposures include administration of AC (2–5 g/kg PO in a water slurry [1 g of AC in 5 mL of water]) and a laxative/cathartic via stomach tube. Leave in the stomach for 20–30 minutes, then give a laxative (e.g., mineral oil) to hasten removal of the toxicant. Alternatively, an osmotic cathartic can be given—70% sorbitol (3 ml/kg) or sodium or magnesium sulfate (250–500 mg/kg), the latter two given in a water slurry.
- With significant diarrhea, do not give a laxative/cathartic.
- Use care when administering laxatives to patients that are severely dehydrated because of diarrhea.
- For dermal exposure, bathe the patient with warm, soapy water followed with a thorough rinse.

ACTIVITY
N/A

DIET
N/A

CLIENT EDUCATION
N/A

SURGICAL CONSIDERATIONS
N/A

MEDICATIONS

DRUGS OF CHOICE
- Diazepam (adults: 25–50 mg IV; foals: 0.05–0.4 mg/kg IV) can be used in patients that are overly anxious or restless or have severe muscle tremors or seizures.
- Atropine sulfate (0.22 mg/kg, 25% IV and the remainder SQ or IM, as needed) can be used to control muscarinic signs.
- Xylazine (0.3–1.1 mg/kg IV, repeat as necessary) can be used as a sedative/analgesic to control signs associated with colic, but do not use in conjunction with tranquilizers.
- Butorphanol (0.1 mg/kg IV q3–4h) is an alternative analgesic to relieve pain associated with colic.
- Pralidoxime chloride (20–35 mg/kg slow IV, repeat q4–6h as necessary) reactivates ACHE that has been inactivated by phosphorylation secondary to most OP exposures and is most effective in controlling muscle fasciculations within the first 24 hours of exposure.
- Cost can be an issue in treating adults, but most patients require no more than 1–3 treatments.
- Bronchoconstriction, pulmonary edema, and respiratory muscle weakness may occur. In these cases, a diuretic (e.g., furosemide [0.25–1.0 mg/kg IV]), a bronchodilator (e.g., aminophylline [4–7 mg/kg PO TID]), and mechanical respiratory support may be necessary.

CONTRAINDICATIONS
Phenothiazine tranquilizers may potentiate signs associated with some OP poisonings.

PRECAUTIONS
Avoid overzealous use of atropine and aminophylline.

POSSIBLE INTERACTIONS
Use of OP anthelmintics may potentiate action of succinylcholine chloride for as long as 1 month after administration of the OP.

ALTERNATIVE DRUGS
N/A

FOLLOW-UP

PATIENT MONITORING
Continuously monitor heart rate and rhythm, respiratory system, urination, defecation, and hydration status.

PREVENTION/AVOIDANCE
Take care to read the label carefully on all products containing OPs and carbamates, ensuring they are used, stored, and disposed of appropriately.

POSSIBLE COMPLICATIONS
- Delayed neuropathy may occur after some OP exposures but is uncommon.
- Bilateral laryngeal paralysis has occurred in foals after dosing with an OP anthelmintic.

EXPECTED COURSE AND PROGNOSIS
- Good prognosis in patients that receive prompt and aggressive therapy.
- Most animals recover uneventfully over 24–48 hours.

MISCELLANEOUS

ASSOCIATED CONDITIONS
N/A

AGE-RELATED FACTORS
N/A

ZOONOTIC POTENTIAL
N/A

PREGNANCY
N/A

SYNONYMS
N/A

SEE ALSO
N/A

ABBREVIATIONS
- AC = activated charcoal
- ACHE = acetylcholinesterase
- AI = active ingredient
- GI = gastrointestinal

Suggested Reading

Fikes JD. Organophosphate and carbamate insecticides. Vet Clin North Am Small Anim Pract 1990;20:353–367.

Organophosphorus compounds and carbamates. In: Radostits OM, Blood DC, Gay CC, eds. Veterinary medicine: a textbook of the diseases of cattle, sheep, pigs, goats and horses. Philadelphia: Bailliere Tindall, 1994:1514–1517.

Author Patricia A. Talcott

Consulting Editor Robert H. Poppenga

ORPHAN AND SICK FOAL NUTRITION

BASICS

OVERVIEW

Adequate nutrition must be provided to foals that cannot get sufficient milk from dams to ensure normal growth and health status; starvation and malnutrition are major contributors to stunted growth, morbidity, and mortality.

SIGNALMENT

Foals require adequate feeding of milk or milk replacer until they can be weaned at 2–3 months of age.

SIGNS

- Newborn foals of agalactic or abusive mares may present with depression, hypothermia, and weakness; without intervention, this may progress to stupor and sepsis.
- Older foals whose dams do not produce enough milk to provide adequate nutrition will not achieve the expected daily gains and will be thin.
- Sick foals may not have a good suckle response.

CAUSES AND RISK FACTORS

Death of the mare, agalactia, rejection, or illness

DIAGNOSIS

DIFFERENTIAL DIAGNOSIS

When mares are agalactic or abusive, the depression seen with hypoglycemia must be differentiated from that of septicemia and hypoxic-ischemic encephalopathy.

CBC/BIOCHEMISTRY/URINALYSIS

- If orphaned at birth or born to an agalactic/abusive dam, a foals may present with hypoglycemia.
- If adequate colostrum has not been received, the CBC may be reflective of that seen in septic foals.

OTHER LABORATORY TESTS

Serum IgG concentration—should be measured at 8–12 hours of age and be ≥400 mg/dL (preferably >800 mg/dL)

IMAGING

N/A

DIAGNOSTIC PROCEDURES

N/A

TREATMENT

- Hypoglycemic—IV supplementation is important; a 5–10% dextrose/LRS solution is best.
- Low IgG—in foals younger than 18 hours, administer colostrum either from the mare or from stored colostrum (200 mL q1h by bottle or tube for a total of 800 mL); foals older than 18 hours cannot absorb IgG enterally and should receive fresh or commercially available frozen plasma IV.
- The best option for raising orphan foals is to find a nurse mare or foster mother who will accept the foal. If a nurse mare is not available, hand-rear the foal. For the first few days of hand-rearing, feed by bottle; if the foal is too weak, feed by tube.
- For bottle-feeding, use an infant nipple until the foal is 1-2 weeks old, then use a lamb nipple. Keep the foal's nose below eye level to avoid overextending head and neck, which can increase the risk of aspiration.
- Gradually introduce the foal to bucket-feeding using a shallow bowl or pan. Keep all equipment clean to avoid bacterial contamination.
- Frequency of feeding—during the first week, q2h; after that, a bucket of milk can be left out at all times but changed q12h to avoid spoilage.
- Formula—the first choice is mare's milk; other options include goat's milk, artificial milk replacers, and cow's milk.
- Goat's milk—more concentrated, higher in fat, and lower in lactose than mare's milk, but usually well tolerated (add 30-mL mineral oil daily if constipation is a problem)
- Artificial milk replacers—recommended nutrient levels (on a dry-matter basis) are crude protein, 20–25%; fat, 15–20%; crude fiber, <0.5%; ash, <12%. Artificial milk replacers may cause osmotic diarrhea or constipation; if so, dilute them to 10–15% dry matter to reduce the risk (1.0–1.5 pounds of dry milk replacer/gallon of water, or 110–190 g/L).
- Cow's milk—Use pasteurized skim milk plus dextrose (20 g/L, or 40 ml of 50% dextrose/L). Healthy foals require 120–150 kcal/kg per day; start at 10% of body weight/day, increase to 20–25% of body weight/day for the first 1–4 weeks (for a 50-kg foal, start at 5 L/day and increase to 10–12.5 L/day for the first 1–4 weeks), then provide 17–20% of body weight/day thereafter.

ORPHAN AND SICK FOAL NUTRITION

• Mare's milk provides 0.5–0.6 kcal/mL; most foal and calf milk replacers range from 0.5–0.8 kcal/ml when reconstituted correctly.
• Exact requirements of sick foals are not known but assumed to be similar to healthy foals; however, feeding intolerance often limits the amount that can be fed to sick foals.
• Other feeds—introduce milk pellets at 1 week of age; introduce good-quality hay, creep feed (16% protein), and water at 1 month of age. Weaning can be done at 8 weeks of age, although it is preferable to wait until at least 12 weeks.
• If the foal has no suckle response, an indwelling nasogastric tube may be placed for enteral feedings.
• Total or partial parenteral nutrition may be required in critically ill foals that do not tolerate oral feeding.

MEDICATIONS

DRUGS

• Nutritional problems uncomplicated by sepsis—no drug treatment necessary
• Sepsis secondary to failure of passive transfer—appropriate antibiotic therapy

CONTRAINDICATIONS/POSSIBLE INTERACTIONS

N/A

FOLLOW-UP

PATIENT MONITORING

• The major nutritional concern in hand-reared foals is stunted growth. Micronutrient imbalances also can occur with some milk replacers. Signs of nutritional deficiencies or imbalances include musculoskeletal abnormalities, weakness, and poor haircoat.
• Monitor body weight to assure adequate growth. Foals should gain 1.5 kg/day from 0–4 weeks of age, 1.4 kg/day from 4–8 weeks, and 1.2 kg/day from 8–12 weeks of age.
• Monitor for diarrhea or other abdominal problems (e.g., colic, ileus, bloating, reflux, constipation, or flatulence); if observed, lowering the osmolarity of formula, adding psyllium, or changing to a new diet may help.

MISCELLANEOUS

Orphan foals may develop behavioral problems if they have only human contact; house the foal with other foals or a quiet pony for companionship.

SEE ALSO

• Failure of passive transfer
• Septicemia

ABBREVIATIONS

LRS =

Suggested Reading

Green SL. Feeding the sick or orphaned foal. Equine Vet Educ 1993;5:274–275.
King SS, Nequin LG. An artificial method to produce optimum growth in orphaned foals. Equine Vet Sci 1989;9:319–322.
Lewis LD. Equine clinical nutrition: feeding and care. Baltimore: Williams and Wilkins, 1995:334–349.

Author Lisa M. Freeman
Consulting Editor Mary Rose Paradis

OSMOLALITY, HYPEROSMOLALITY

BASICS

DEFINITION

- Osmolality (mOsm/kg) represents the number of solute particles per kilogram of solvent (e.g., the concentration of a solution expressed as mOsm/kg).
- Osmolality is a thermodynamically more precise term than osmolarity, because it is based on weight, which is temperature independent, versus volume (i.e., osmolarity), which is temperature dependent.
- Osmolarity (mOsm/L) represents the number of solute particles per liter of solvent (e.g., the concentration of a solution expressed as mOsm/L).
- Osmotic pressure governs the movement of water across membranes because of differences in solute content.
- Hyperosmolarity and hyperosmolality are defined in horses as serum concentrations >270–300 mOsm/L or >270–300 mOsm/kg.
- One osmole is the gram molecular weight of a nondissociable substance and contains Avogadro's number of particles.
- A solvent is a liquid holding another substance in solution; for osmolality, this would be water.
- A solute is the dissolved substance in the solution.
- A solution, in this discussion, contains solutes within a solvent.

PATHOPHYSIOLOGY

- In serum/plasma, Na^+ is primarily responsible for osmotically active particles, as well as associated Cl^- and HCO_3^-, with lesser contributions by glucose and urea.
- Anything causing water loss increases the concentrations of solutes in plasma/serum, thereby increasing serum osmolality.
- Dissolved particles that cannot move between adjacent compartments exert osmotic pressure and cause water to move to dilute differences in solute concentrations between compartments.
- Serum osmolality is a measure of ECF osmolality but is not a measure of total body water. The ECF compartment comprises one-third of total body weight, with the remaining two-thirds in the ICF compartment.
- The osmolalities of ICF and ECF are equal, but the ionic compositions differ. ECF is primarily Na^+ and Cl^-, with small concentrations of HCO_3^-, K^+, phosphate, Ca^{2+}, and Mg^{2+}, whereas ICF is high in K^+ and phosphate, with lower concentrations of Na^+, Cl^-, and Ca^{2+}.
- Blood volume, hydration status, and ADH are involved in controlling the ECF volume. Low circulating blood volume stimulates carotid and aortic baroreceptors to respond to changes in blood pressure, causing ADH secretion.
- Hyperosmolality affects osmoreceptors in the hypothalamus and stimulates ADH secretion from the neurohypophysis. The kidney's ability to produce urine of various concentrations maintains body regulation of osmolality. The hypothalamic thirst center also is stimulated and causes an increase in water consumption to counteract serum hyperosmolality. Therefore, regulation is by modifying water loss in urine or water intake
- Rapid increases in serum osmolality cause water movement along its concentration gradient, from ICF to ECF spaces, resulting in neuronal dehydration, cell shrinkage, and cell death.
- Hypo-osmolality is associated with hyponatremia.

SYSTEMS AFFECTED

- Nervous—because of fluid shifts
- Cardiovascular—hypotension and depressed ventricular contractility
- Renal/urologic—low urine output

SIGNALMENT

Any age

SIGNS

General Comments

- Excessive thirst may be the first sign of hyperosmolality.
- Signs are primarily neurologic and behavioral.
- Severity of signs relates more to how quickly hyperosmolality occurs rather than to the absolute magnitude of change.
- Signs are most likely to develop with serum osmolality >350 mOsm/kg, and they usually are severe if >375 mOsm/kg.

Historical Findings

- Anorexia
- Lethargy
- Vomiting
- Weakness
- Disorientation
- Ataxia
- Seizures
- Coma
- Polydipsia, followed by hypodipsia

Physical Examination Findings

- Abnormalities reflect the underlying disease.
- Dehydration, tachycardia, hypotension, weak pulse, and fever may be present.

CAUSES

- Increased solutes—hypernatremia; hyperglycemia; severe azotemia; ethylene glycol toxicosis (potential); propylene glycol toxicosis; salt poisoning; shock; administration of ethanol, mannitol, radiographic contrast solution, and parenteral nutrition solutions; lactate in patients with lactic acidosis; and acetoacetate and β-hydroxybutyrate ketones
- Decreased ECF volume—dehydration (e.g., GI loss, cutaneous loss, third-space loss, low water consumption) and polyuria without adequate compensatory polydipsia

RISK FACTORS

- Predisposing medical conditions—renal failure, diabetes insipidus, diabetes mellitus, hyperadrenocorticism, hyperaldosteronism, and heat stroke
- Therapeutic hyperosmolar solutions—hypertonic saline, sodium bicarbonate, and mannitol
- High environmental temperatures
- Fever
- Limited access to water

DIAGNOSIS

DIFFERENTIAL DIAGNOSIS

- Primary CNS disease from a variety of causes—neoplasia, inflammation, or trauma; serum osmolality usually is normal.
- Assess hydration status, and obtain information regarding previous treatment that may have included sodium-containing fluids or hyperosmolar solutions.

LABORATORY FINDINGS

Drugs that May Alter Lab Results

Excessive administration of sodium-containing fluids or hyperosmolar solutions increases serum osmolality.

OSMOLALITY, HYPEROSMOLALITY

Disorders that May Alter Lab Result
N/A

Valid If Run in Human Lab?
Yes

CBC/BIOCHEMISTRY/URINALYSIS

- High PCV, hemoglobin, and plasma proteins in dehydrated patients; serum electrolytes also may be high
- Hyperosmolality is an indication to evaluate serum sodium, BUN, and glucose concentrations. Estimated serum osmolality can be calculated from serum biochemistries as $2(\text{Na}) + \text{BUN}/2.8 + \text{glucose}/18$. Sodium concentration provides an estimate of the total electrolyte concentrations and, thus, is multiplied by two. The remaining calculation is to convert concentrations into mmol/L; therefore, BUN is divided by 2.8 and glucose by 18.
- Normally, measured osmolality should not exceed the calculated osmolality by more than 10 mOsm/kg. If it does, calculate an osmolar gap (i.e., measured osmolality−calculated osmolality).
- High measured osmolality with a high osmolar gap indicates the presence of unmeasured solutes—not Na^+, K^+, glucose, or BUN.
- High measured osmolality and high calculated osmolality with a normal osmolar gap usually indicate that hyperosmolality results from measured solutes—Na^+, K^+, glucose, or BUN
- Serum sodium may be low in patients with severe hyperglycemia and hyperosmolality.
- Fasting hyperglycemia and glucosuria support a diagnosis of diabetes mellitus.
- Numerous calcium oxalate monohydrate crystals in urine suggest ethylene glycol toxicosis, but this is not well documented in horses.
- High urine specific gravity rules out diabetes insipidus; low urine specific gravity, especially hyposthenuria, suggests diabetes insipidus.

OTHER LABORATORY TESTS

Urine osmolality < serum osmolality suggests diabetes insipidus, whereas concentrated urine rules out diabetes insipidus.

IMAGING

Renal ultrasonography may differentiate renal disease.

DIAGNOSTIC PROCEDURES

N/A

TREATMENT

- Mild hyperosmolality without clinical signs may not warrant specific treatment; however, any underlying diseases should be diagnosed and treated.
- Patients with moderate to high osmolality (>350 mOsm/kg) or exhibiting clinical signs should be hospitalized and their serum osmolality gradually lowered with IV fluid administration while a definitive diagnosis is pursued.
- D_5W or 0.45% saline should be administered slowly IV.
- Initially, 0.9% saline may be used to restore normal hemodynamics and to replace dehydration deficits.

MEDICATIONS

DRUGS OF CHOICE

Seizures can be controlled with appropriate anticonvulsants.

CONTAINDICATIONS

Hypertonic saline and hyperosmolar solutions

PRECAUTIONS

- Normal saline may be used initially, but rapid administration may worsen neurologic signs.
- Rapid administration of hypotonic fluids (e.g., D_5W, 0.45% saline) also may cause cerebral edema and worsen neurologic signs.

POSSIBLE INTERACTIONS

N/A

ALTERNATIVE DRUGS

N/A

FOLLOW-UP

PATIENT MONITORING

- Monitor hydration status; avoid overhydration.
- Monitor urine output and breathing patterns during IV fluid administration.
- Anuria and irregular breathing patterns may be signs of deterioration.
- Monitor mentation and behavior.

POSSIBLE COMPLICATIONS

Altered consciousness and abnormal behavior

MISCELLANEOUS

ASSOCIATED CONDITIONS

- Azotemia
- Hyperglycemia
- Hypernatremia

AGE-RELATED FACTORS

N/A

ZOONOTIC POTENTIAL

N/A

PREGNANCY

N/A

SYNONYMS

Hyperosmolarity

SEE ALSO

- Diabetes mellitus
- Glucose, hyperglycemia
- Sodium, hypernatremia

ABBREVIATIONS

- ADH = antidiurectic hormone
- ECF = extracellular fluid
- GI = gastrointestinal
- ICF = intracellular fluid
- PCV = packed cell volume

Suggested Reading

Carlson GP. Fluid, electrolyte, and acid-balance. In: Kaneko JJ, Harvey JW, Bruss ML, eds. Clinical biochemistry of domestic animals. San Diego: Academic Press, 1997:512–513.

DiBartola SP, Green RA, Autran de Morais HS. Osmolarity and osmolar gap. In: Willard MD, Tvedten H, Turnwald GH, eds. Small animal clinical diagnosis by laboratory methods. 2nd ed. Philadelphia: WB Saunders, 1994:106–107.

Johnson PJ. Physiology of body fluids in the horse. Vet Clin North Am Equine Pract 1998;14:1–22.

Author Claire B. Andreasen
Consulting Editor Claire B. Andreasen

OVULATION FAILURE

BASICS

DEFINITION

• The ovulatory follicle in a mare is generally $\geq$35 mm in diameter.
• Follicles that obtain that size but fail to ovulate are addressed.

PATHOPHYSIOLOGY

• Waves or "clutches" of oocytes are recruited for development into antral follicles.
• Ultimately, one or two follicles become dominant and progress to ovulation, while the remaining follicles undergo atresia. The mechanism for this selection is not well understood.
• Estrogen produced by the dominant follicle stimulates an increase in LH that ultimately induces ovulation. The LH rise in mares is prolonged compared to other species.
• Deficiencies of either follicular estrogen or pituitary gonadotropin can contribute to ovulation failure.

SYSTEM AFFECTED

Reproductive

SIGNALMENT

• Mares of any breed and age.
• Multiple dominant follicle formation is more common in thoroughbred, standardbred, warmblood, and draft mares
• Multiple dominant follicles are most frequently observed from March through May in the northern hemisphere.

SIGNS

Historical Findings

• Mares may exhibit prolonged estrus behavior.
• Discomfort from ovarian enlargement can mimic pain associated with colic or a sore back under saddle.

Physical Examination Findings

• Ovarian palpation: common finding is at least one large ($>$35 mm) fluid-filled structure or simply an enlarged ovary.
• Ovarian ultrasonography: single or multiple follicle(s), polycystic structures typical of neoplasia, a fluid-filled cavity filled with echogenic particles or fibrin-like strands indicative of a hematoma, or, rarely, an ovarian abscess.

CAUSES

Hemorrhagic Anovulatory Follicles

Normal follicular development occurs, but ovulation does not. These follicles can become quite large (60–110 mm diameter), are filled with blood, and may or may not have luteinization of the follicular wall. Such follicles may be estrogen-deficient or result from insufficient GnRH release. Decreased LH secretion/synthesis may be involved in the pathogenesis. The occurrence of hemorrhagic anovulatory follicles is most common during the autumn transition.

Multiple Dominant Follicles

If transrectal palpation is the sole means used to determine follicular growth and ovulation, the presence of two or more adjacent follicles may be interpreted to be one follicle that fails to ovulate.

Persistent Follicles

Most common during late spring or early fall transition. These are not ovarian cysts, which rarely occur in the mare, but are follicles that fail to undergo final maturation and ovulation.

Luteinized Follicles

Described in humans, luteinized follicles may also occur in mares. An association with reproductive senility has been proposed. This form of ovulation failure may occur in the normal mare when secondary corpora lutea form during pregnancy.

Diestrus Follicular Development

Large antral follicles can form during the luteal phase of the estrous cycle and frequently undergo atresia rather than proceed to ovulation.

RISK FACTORS

N/A

DIAGNOSIS

DIFFERENTIAL DIAGNOSIS

Differentiating Similar Signs

• Ovarian neoplasia can mimic persistent follicular development due to similarities of behavior, cycling/teasing, and the presence of fluid-filled cavities (transrectal palpation and ultrasound). See Large Ovary Syndrome.
• Ovarian abscesses have been reported to occur secondary to invasive procedures or as a result of hematogenous infection. It may be confused with a persistent follicle on palpation, but its contents are very echogenic (ultrasound), and the mare may be systemically ill.
• Periovarian cysts can be confused with ovarian follicles if they are in close proximity to the ovary. They can be distinguished from ovarian structures by careful transrectal palpation and ultrasonography.

Differentiating Causes

• Comprehensive history rules out problems that are primarily related to season, sexual behavior, and teasing.
• Transrectal palpation of the reproductive tract at biweekly intervals provides definition to time-related changes: ovarian size, shape, and activity; uterine size and tone; and cervical relaxation are important components of a complete exam.
• Transrectal ultrasonography is important to fully evaluate the abnormal ovary. Normal follicles exhibit increased echogenicity of follicular fluid and change their shape from spherical to pear/triangular shape as ovulation approaches. Persistent follicles appear normal on ultrasound examination. Hematomas may have a distinctly echogenic fluid content with large, criss-crossing fibrin-like strands. The ultrasound appearance of ovarian neoplasia varies depending upon the tumor type. The most common, the GCT/GTCT, frequently appears to be polycystic/multilocular.
• Follicles can develop during diestrus when progesterone concentrations are $>$1 ng/mL.

CBC/BIOCHEMISTRY/URINALYSIS

N/A

OTHER LABORATORY TESTS

• Serum progesterone concentrations: basal levels of $<$1 ng/mL indicate no active/mature CL is present. Mature CL function is associated with levels of $>$4 ng/mL.
• Serum testosterone concentrations: mares typically have values $<$50–60 pg/mL. Values of $>$50–100 pg/mL have been observed in mares with GTCT.
• Serum inhibin concentrations are increased in 90% of mares that have GCT/GTCTs.

IMAGING

N/A

DIAGNOSTIC PROCEDURES

N/A

OVULATION FAILURE

TREATMENT

• If ovulation failure is related to season (transition, anestrus), no treatment is necessary. Transitional follicles eventually regress (may be 30–45 days).
• Tumors or abscess of an ovary—ovariectomy. Luteinized follicles and some hematomas (luteinization may be inadequate, if a recent event) may respond to prostaglandin treatment.
• Ovulation of persistent follicles may be induced using either hCG or deslorelin implants, if they occur late in vernal transition.

MEDICATIONS

DRUG(S) OF CHOICE

• hCG (2500 IU, IV) can be used to induce ovulation.
• Deslorelin (Ovuplant™, 2.1 mg SC implant, Ft. Dodge), a GnRH analog, induces ovulation within 48 hr in mares with a follicle(s) >30 mm in diameter.
• $PGF_2\alpha$ (Lutalyse™, 10 mg, IM, Upjohn) short-cycles a mare that has a functional CL present.
• Progesterone (altrenogest, 0.044 mg/kg SID, P/O, Hoechst) can help shorten the duration of vernal transition, providing the mare has follicles of at least 20 mm in diameter and she is exhibiting estrus. Recommendation: Treat with progesterone for 15 days, give injection of prostaglandin on day 15, and breed on the first estrus post-treatment.

CONTRAINDICATIONS

N/A

PRECAUTIONS

• $PGF_2\alpha$ causes sweating and colic-like symptoms due to its effect on smooth muscle cells. Monitor for 1–2 hr and treat symptomatically, if symptoms persist.
• $PGF_2\alpha$ can cause pregnant mares to abort.
• Progesterone supplementation may cause decreased uterine clearance in mares with a history of uterine infections.
• Antibodies to hCG can develop. Their half-life ranges from 30 days to several months, but not from one breeding season to the next. Administration is thus generally limited to two times during a breeding season.
• As altrenogest can be absorbed across skin, latex gloves should be worn by the individual administering it.
• It is recommended that pregnant women use with caution/limit/avoid contact with prostaglandin and progesterone products.

POSSIBLE INTERACTIONS

N/A

ALTERNATIVE DRUGS

N/A

FOLLOW-UP

PATIENT MONITORING

Serial palpations, as described before.

POSSIBLE COMPLICATIONS

Individual mares may be prone to develop more than one hemorrhagic/anovulatory follicle in a season.

MISCELLANEOUS

ASSOCIATED CONDITIONS

N/A

AGE-RELATED FACTORS

N/A

ZOONOTIC POTENTIAL

N/A

PREGNANCY

Prostaglandin administration can cause pregnant mares to abort. It should not be used until pregnancy has been definitively ruled out.

SYNONYMS

Hemorrhagic anovulatory follicles = autumn follicles

SEE ALSO

• Anestrus
• Large ovary syndrome
• Abnormal estrus intervals

ABBREVIATIONS

• CL = corpus luteum
• GCT/GTCT = granulosa cell tumor/granulosa theca cell tumor
• GnRH = gonadotropin releasing hormone
• hCG = human chorionic gonadotropin
• LH = luteinizing hormone
• $PGF_2\alpha$ = natural prostaglandin

Suggested Reading

Carleton CL. Atypical, asymmetrical, but abnormal? Large ovary syndrome. In: Proceedings of mare reproduction symposium, American College of Theriogenologists and Society for Theriogenology, Hastings, NE, 1996:27-39.
Ginther OJ. Ovaries. In: Ultrasonic imaging and animal reproduction: Horses. Cross Plains, WI. Equiservices 1995;23-42.
Hinrichs K. Irregularities of the estrous cycle and ovulation in mares. In: Current therapy in large animal theriogenology. Youngquist RS, ed. Philadelphia: WB Saunders Co. 1997;166-171.
Pierson RA. Folliculogenesis and ovulation. In: Equine reproduction. McKinnon AO and Voss JL, ed. Philadelphia: Lea & Febiger 1993;161-171.
Sharp DC, Davis SD. Vernal transition. In: Equine reproduction. McKinnon AO and Voss JL, ed. Philadelphia: Lea & Febiger 1993:133-143.

Author Carole C. Miller
Consulting Editor Carla L. Carleton

OXALATE (SOLUBLE) POISONING

BASICS

OVERVIEW

• Disease after ingestion of plants containing oxalic acid or soluble sodium and potassium oxalates
• Oxalate concentration in plant material varies widely with the season, geographic location, and part of the plant.
• Green leaves and fruiting structures tend to contain the highest oxalate concentration.
• *Halogeton* spp. are an exception—oxalate concentration increases as the plant matures and often is highest when the plant is dead and dry.
• Plants containing dangerous amounts of soluble oxalates—*Beta vulgaris, Halogeton glomeratus, Oxalis* spp., *Portulaca oleracea, Amaranthus* spp., *Rheum rhaponticum, Rumex* spp., *Setaria* spp., *Salsola* spp., *Kochia scoparia,* and *Sarcobatus vermiculatus*; most of these plants are considered unpalatable when the oxalate content is high.
• Cases of poisoning are seen in the summer and fall months, when other forage is unavailable and patients eat a large amount of plant material during a short period of time.
• Ingestion of excess soluble oxalates causes GI discomfort along with muscular weakness and paralysis caused by hypocalcemia. Ultimately, this can lead to acute renal damage.
• Nephrosclerosis and osteodystrophia fibrosa have been recorded in horses after chronic ingestion of oxalates but are uncommon.

SIGNALMENT

Equine intoxication is rare; horses appear relatively resistant to acute oxalate-induced nephrosis.

SIGNS

• Acute signs relate predominantly to hypocalcemia.
• Within 2–6 hours of ingestion, signs observed include depression, mild to moderate colic, and muscular weakness.
• Weakness may lead to recumbency, convulsions, unconsciousness, and death.
• Chronic signs may relate to renal disease, including polydipsia, polyuria, and weight loss.

CAUSES AND RISK FACTORS

• Overgrazing areas highly contaminated with oxalate-containing plants
• Not providing adequate supplemental feed.
• Hungry animals are more likely to ingest potentially toxic amounts.
• Low-calcium diets enhance soluble oxalate absorption; calcium binds oxalate in the GI tract to form insoluble calcium oxalate.

DIAGNOSIS

DIFFERENTIAL DIAGNOSIS

• Oxalate-induced hypocalcemic syndrome must be differentiated from hypocalcemia caused by poor diet and starvation, forced exercise, transit tetany (i.e., hypocalcemia during and after transportation), and lactation tetany (occurs 10 days after foaling or 1–2 days after weaning).
• Causes of equine acute renal disease—ischemia, vitamin K_3, NSAIDs, vitamin D, heavy metal (e.g., arsenic, mercury, lead), aminoglycoside, and acorn toxicoses.
• Causes of equine chronic renal failure—proliferative glomerulonephritis, renal glomerular hypoplasia, chronic interstitial nephritis, pyelonephritis, amyloidosis, and neoplasia.
• Known access to oxalate-containing plants is critical in helping to differentiate this disease from all others.

CBC/BIOCHEMISTRY/URINALYSIS

• Hypocalcemia is the most consistent finding.
• Other findings in cattle and sheep—modest elevations in liver enzymes (e.g., AST, ALT), proteinuria, albuminuria, hematuria, hyperglycemia, azotemia, hyperphosphatemia, and hyperkalemia

OTHER LABORATORY TESTS

Oxalate content of suspect plant material can be assayed.

IMAGING

N/A

DIAGNOSTIC PROCEDURES

N/A

PATHOLOGIC FINDINGS

• Erythema and edema of the GI mucosa is most commonly seen.
• Other findings—necrosis of the proximal renal tubules and collecting ducts, with birefringent crystals; crystals also may be seen within vascular spaces.

TREATMENT

• Hospitalize patients for initial medical workup and management.
• Fluid replacement therapy for any volume deficits and correction of any electrolyte and acid–base abnormalities are critical in patients with GI distress or possible renal failure.
• Fluid therapy also tends to slow precipitation of calcium oxalate crystals within the renal tubule lumen.

OXALATE (SOLUBLE) POISONING

MEDICATIONS

DRUGS

• Hypocalcemic patient should receive a slow IV infusion of calcium gluconate (100–500 mL of 23% calcium gluconate diluted in fluids).
• Rare patients exhibiting acute or chronic renal failure should be treated accordingly; treatment options vary depending on whether oliguria or polyuria is present.

CONTRAINDICATIONS/POSSIBLE INTERACTIONS

N/A

FOLLOW-UP

PATIENT MONITORING

• Monitor respiration and cardiac rate and rhythm during administration of calcium gluconate.
• Monitor serum concentrations of sodium, chloride, potassium, bicarbonate, urea nitrogen, creatinine, PCV, total protein, and central venous pressure in patients with severe GI distress or impaired renal function.

PREVENTION/AVOIDANCE

• Prevent access to soluble oxalate–containing plants through pasture management—animal rotation; herbicide treatment
• Do not allow hungry animals access to highly contaminated areas.
• Make adequate supplemental forage available to animals grazing contaminated areas.
• Oral dicalcium phosphate prevents this disease in cattle and sheep.

EXPECTED COURSE AND PROGNOSIS

• Most clinically affected horses do not recover.
• Animals that survive acute intoxication often suffer renal failure, which carries a poor prognosis.
• Horses, being relatively resistant to the renal effects of soluble oxalates, may have a somewhat better prognosis than affected cattle and sheep.

MISCELLANEOUS

ASSOCIATED CONDITIONS

N/A

AGE-RELATED FACTORS

N/A

ZOONOTIC POTENTIAL

N/A

PREGNANCY

N/A

SEE ALSO

N/A

ABBREVIATIONS

• ALT = alanine aminotransferase
• AST = aspartate aminotransferase
• GI = gastrointestinal
• PCV = packed cell volume

Suggested Reading

Divers TJ. Diseases of the renal system. In: Smith BP, ed. Large animal internal medicine. St. Louis: C.V. Mosby, 1990.

Author Patricia A. Talcott
Consulting Editor Robert H. Poppenga

PANCREATIC DISEASE

BASICS

OVERVIEW

Clinical pancreatic disease is rarely recognized in the horse. Acute and chronic pancreatic disease have been reported. Equine pancreatic disorders include inflammatory disease, chronic eosinophilic pancreatitis, endocrine or exocrine insufficiency, and neoplasia. Fibrosis of the pancreas induced by parasitic migration of *Strongylus equinus* is probably the most common cause of pancreatic disease in the horse. Aberrant migration of *S. edentatus, S. vulgaris,* and *Parascaris equorum* may also occur. Pancreatitis has also been reported in horses with cholelithiasis. Diabetes mellitus is rare in the horse, and most cases are secondary to a demonstrable cause of insulin resistance, such as elevated concentrations of hormones, which antagonize the action of insulin. The most common etiology for the secondary diabetes mellitus in the horse is induced by hyperplasia (or adenoma) of the *pars intermedia* of the pituitary gland. Insulin-dependent diabetes mellitus, which is far less common in the horse, has been reported secondary to pancreatic fibrosis. There are a few rare reports of pancreatic neoplasia (adenocarcinoma, adenoma) in the horse. Typically, pancreatic adenocarcinoma occludes the common bile duct and causes cholestasis and severe liver dysfunction. Pancreatic fibrosis is seen in eosinophilic syndrome.

SIGNALMENT

The few published reports of pancreatic neoplasia have been on aged horses and donkeys (>11 yr).

SIGNS

The clinical signs of equine pancreatic disease are not specific. Signs of acute pancreatitis may include:

- Abdominal pain (moderate to severe) due to gastric distension, peritonitis, and hemoabdomen
- Gastric reflux
- Hypovolemic shock
- Signs of cardiovascular compromise (tachycardia, prolonged capillary refill, congested mucous membranes)

Signs of chronic pancreatitis may include:

- Weight loss
- Intermittent colic
- Icterus

Signs of diabetes mellitus may include:

- Polyuria, polydipsia
- Weight loss despite polyphagia
- Rough hair coat

Signs of pancreatic neoplasia may include:

- Pyrexia
- Depression
- Weight loss
- Icterus
- Ascites
- Rectal examination may be able to palpate neoplastic pancreas in the left kidney region

CAUSES AND RISK FACTORS

Causes of pancreatitis that have been documented in the horse include parasitic migration (*Strongylus equinus, S. edentatus, S. vulgaris, Parascaris equorum*); ascending or hematogenous bacterial infections; viral (VEE, EIA) infections; immune-mediated disease; biliary or pancreatic duct inflammation; vitamin E or A deficiency; and selenium, methionine, and vitamin D toxicity. The cause of acute pancreatitis is not known, but the autodigestion of pancreas by activated enzymes has been suggested. Pancreatic neoplasia (e.g., adenocarcinoma, adenoma) is very rare.

DIAGNOSIS

DIFFERENTIAL DIAGNOSIS

- Intra-abdominal abscessation
- Neoplasia

CBC/BIOCHEMISTRY/URINALYSIS

No specific abnormalities associated with pancreatic disease have been documented in the horse.

- Hyperglycemia (persistent)
- Glycosuria (persistent)
- Elevated serum gamma-glutamyl transferase (GGT) when obstruction of the biliary tree
- Elevated serum amylase (normal: 14–35 U/L)
- Elevated lipase activity (normal: 23–87 U/L) (variable)
- Hyperfibrinogenemia (acute pancreatitis)

OTHER LABORATORY TESTS

- Elevated peritoneal fluid amylase concentration (normal: 0–14 U/L) compared to serum amylase concentration (normal 14–35 U/L) in acute pancreatitis
- Dexamethasone suppression test or beta-endorphin assay to rule out a functional pituitary adenoma
- Serum insulin concentration: elevated in insulin resistance and reduced in insulin-dependent diabetes mellitus
- IV glucose tolerance test: 0.5 g/kg glucose administered IV as 50% solution; serum glucose and insulin determined
- Insulin-dependent (type 1) diabetes mellitus: increased blood glucose without accompanying increase in insulin.
- Insulin-resistance (type 2) diabetes mellitus when blood glucose remains elevated for a prolonged period of time after infusion, despite high blood insulin levels. This is the most common type of diabetes mellitus in horses and ponies and is usually associated with pituitary adenoma
- Abdominocentesis—abnormal cells in peritoneal fluid; elevated peritoneal fluid amylase activity (normal 0–14 U/L)

IMAGING

- Abdominal ultrasound has been used to detect pancreatic neoplasia in the horse
- Laparoscopy

OTHER DIAGNOSTIC PROCEDURES

- Elevated peritoneal fluid amylase concentration (normal 0–14 U/L)
- Ultrasound-guided biopsy of pancreas

TREATMENT

- Symptomatic medical management
- Indwelling nasogastric tube to prevent gastric rupture; reflux every 2–4 hr

MEDICATIONS

DRUG(S) AND FLUIDS

Acute pancreatitis:

- Intravenous balanced polyionic electrolyte fluids
- Analgesics (NSAIDs such as flunixin meglumine 1.1 mg/kg q24h) and opiates (e.g., butorphanol 0.02 mg/kg q4h) for abdominal pain
- Broad-spectrum antibiotics to prevent secondary bacterial infection
- Plasma transfusion may be indicated
- Calcium-containing fluids

CONTRAINDICATIONS/POSSIBLE INTERACTIONS

N/A

FOLLOW-UP

- Monitor hydration, serum calcium
- Monitor abdominal pain
- Prognosis poor to grave for acute pancreatitis

MISCELLANEOUS

ABBREVIATIONS

N/A

Suggested Reading

Furr MO, Robertson J. Two cases of equine pancreatic disease and a review of the literature. Equine Vet Educ 1992;4:55-58.

Author John D. Baird
Consulting Editor Henry Stämpfli

PANCYTOPENIA

BASICS

OVERVIEW

• Characterized by a concurrent decrease in circulating red cell mass, leukocytes, and thrombocytes (<90,000 platelets/μL).
• Variety of mechanisms, including decreased production, increased consumption, sequestration, or destruction of RBCs, WBCs, and thrombocytes
• Decreased production—disturbance of pluripotent stem cells within the marrow, infiltration of marrow by neoplastic myeloid or lymphoid cells, and drug-induced suppression of marrow hematopoiesis
• Increased consumption, sequestration, or destruction in excess of production leads to decreases in one or more cell types.
• Can result from malignant histiocytosis via a myelophthisic effect on the marrow and phagocytosis of cells by the malignant monocytes

SIGNALMENT

N/A

SIGNS

Historical Findings

• Onset and duration of clinical signs vary depending on the primary cause.
• History may include lethargy, depression, exercise intolerance, and weight loss.
• Signs of hemorrhagic diathesis, including epistaxis, blood in feces, mucosal bleeding, or prolonged hemorrhage from traumatic wounds, may be observed.
• Fever associated with primary disease process (e.g., myeloproliferative disease) or secondary bacterial infections (due to leukopenia)

Physical Examination Findings

Clinical signs often attributable to the secondary effects of anemia, thrombocytopenia, or leukopenia—pale mucous membranes, lethargy, depression, mucosal petechiation, and fever

CAUSES AND RISK FACTORS

• Idiopathic pancytopenia due to bone marrow hypoplasia (aplastic anemia) or myelofibrosis
• Neoplasia—myeloproliferative (monocytic, myelomonocytic, histiocytic, eosinophilic, or granulocytic cell lines) or lymphoproliferative (plasma cell myeloma or lymphoid leukemia) disease that produces pancytopenia by altering the bone marrow architecture
• Toxic—drugs (trimethoprim, pyrimethamine, phenylbutazone, chloramphenicol, estrogens, and trichloroethylene-extracted soybean meal)
• Infectious—acute infection with *Ehrlichia equi* or EIA virus
• Immune-mediated diseases or disseminated intravascular coagulation may contribute to pancytopenia.

DIAGNOSIS

DIFFERENTIAL DIAGNOSIS

• See **Causes and Risk Factors**.
• Piroplasmosis (babesiosis) also may cause fever, pale mucous membranes, edema, and mucosal hemorrhage.

CBC/BIOCHEMISTRY/URINALYSIS

• Peripheral pancytopenia
• Anemia may occur after neutropenia and thrombocytopenia due to the long erythrocyte life span (≅140 days).
• Examine peripheral smear for evidence of morulae in circulating neutrophils (equine ehrlichiosis), red cell parasites (*Babesia equi* or *B. caballi*), hemosiderophages (EIA), or abnormal leukocytes (leukemic or subleukemic myeloid or lymphoid neoplasia).
• A false diagnosis of lymphoid leukemia can be made, because circulating lymphocytes often are reactive.

OTHER LABORATORY TESTS

Serological tests for EIA, *B. equi* or *caballi*, and *E. equi*

IMAGING

N/A

DIAGNOSTIC PROCEDURES

• Bone marrow examination is important in the evaluation of pancytopenia without obvious cause. Aspirates and core biopsy specimens are best obtained from the sternum of adults or the sternum, ileum, or rib of young horses. Aspiration is indicated in horses with chronic, unresponsive anemia to assess regenerative response. Poorly or nonregenerative anemias result from iron deficiency, anemia of chronic disease, neoplasia, or bone marrow hypoplasia.
• Normal myeloid:erythroid ratio is from 0.5 to 3.75. A ratio <0.5 suggests myeloid suppression or erythroid regeneration.
• Bone marrow evaluation is used in the diagnosis of myeloproliferative or lymphoproliferative diseases. Aspiration may be difficult in animals with hypocellular marrow (aplastic anemia), myelofibrosis, or myelophthisis; antemortem diagnosis is established through core biopsy.

PANCYTOPENIA

TREATMENT

- Remove or treat potential inciting causes (e.g., phenylbutazone or chloramphenicol).
- Supportive treatment—whole-blood or platelet-rich plasma transfusion and broad-spectrum antimicrobial therapy

MEDICATIONS

DRUGS

- Bone marrow hypoplasia—clinical remission was observed in an adult horse after treatment with glucocorticoids, androgens, and broad-spectrum antimicrobials.
- Anabolic steroids enhance erythropoiesis by increasing EPO production and sensitivity of stem cells to EPO.
- Specific therapy for *E. equi* (oxytetracycline, 7 mg/kg IV daily for 7 days) or *Babesia* sp. infection (imidocarb dipropionate) indicated when present.
- No specific therapy for EIA infection
- See appropriate sections for treatment recommendations regarding lymphoproliferative or myeloproliferative diseases.

CONTRAINDICATIONS/POSSIBLE INTERACTIONS

Immune status may be further compromised through use of exogenous glucocorticoids.

FOLLOW-UP

PATIENT MONITORING

- Pancytopenia—weekly monitoring of CBC
- Monitor for signs of fever, lethargy, hemorrhage to indicate worsening leukopenia, anemia, and thrombocytopenia, respectively.

EXPECTED COURSE AND PROGNOSIS

- Myeloproliferative and lymphoproliferative disease—hopeless
- Insufficient number of documented cases of bone marrow hypoplasia to establish a prognosis.

MISCELLANEOUS

ASSOCIATED CONDITIONS

Infection, particularly of the respiratory tract, occurs due to leukopenia.

AGE-RELATED FACTORS

N/A

ZOONOTIC POTENTIAL

N/A

PREGNANCY

N/A

SEE ALSO

- Anemia
- Anemia, aplastic (pure red cell aplasia)
- Ehrlichiosis, equine granulocytic
- EIA
- Lymphosarcoma
- Multiple myeloma
- Myeloproliferative diseases
- Piroplasmosis

ABBREVIATIONS

- EIA = equine infectious anemia
- EPO = erythropoietin

Suggested Reading

Morris DD, Barton MH. Bone marrow aplasia (aplastic anemia). In: Colahan, et al., eds. Equine medicine and surgery, 5th ed. St. Louis: Mosby, 2007–2009.

Author Guy D. Lester
Consulting Editor Debra C. Sellon

PANICUM COLORATUM (KLEINGRASS) TOXICOSIS

BASICS

OVERVIEW

• *Panicum coloratum* (kleingrass, kleingrass 75) is a tufted, perennial grass with stems usually 60–135 cm in height from a firm, knotty base.
• The blades are elongate, 2–8 mm in width, smooth or stiff, with bristly hairs on one or both surfaces.
• Loosely branched, pyramidal flower clusters are mostly 8–25 cm in length, with spikelets on spreading branches; the spikelets are 2.8–3.2 mm in length and smooth.
• The rootstock is hearty and easily develops rhizomes.
• *Panicum* spp. grow in Australia, New Zealand, South Africa, South America, Afghanistan, India, and Texas. In Texas, it reaches from the high plains to the Edward's Plateau and the Trans-Pecos area.
• *Panicum* spp. were introduced into the U.S. during the 1950s; *P. coloratum* was developed by Texas A&M University during the early 1970s and prefers improved pastures.
• Some native species found outside the U.S. generally are not toxic.
• The toxin is a saponin (saponins are sapogenins and a sugar moiety) and probably is the same as that found in *Tribulus, Nolina*, and *Agave* spp.
• Horses have developed liver disease while grazing kleingrass or eating kleingrass hay, but they have not developed photosensitization.

SIGNALMENT

No known breed, sex, or age predispositions

SIGNS

• Horses develop liver disease and become icteric.
• History of anorexia and weight loss
• Horses tend not to develop secondary or hepatogenous photosensitization.

CAUSES AND RISK FACTORS

N/A

DIAGNOSIS

DIFFERENTIAL DIAGNOSIS

• History of grazing kleingrass; compatible clinical signs
• Other hepatotoxins—aflatoxin (detection in feed and histopathology), PAs (ingestion of alkaloid-containing plants and histopathology), and iron toxicosis (tissue iron concentrations and histopathology).
• In addition to PA-containing plants, exposure to other hepatotoxic plants—*Nolina texana, Agave lechuguilla, Panicum* spp., and *Trifolium hybridum.*
• Nontoxic differential—Theiler's disease (history, histopathology).

CBC/BIOCHEMISTRY/URINALYSIS

• Horses on kleingrass have high serum GGT activity, total and direct bilirubin, blood ammonia, and sulfobromophthalein clearance times.
• Serum SDH, AST, and AP activities are variable.

OTHER LABORATORY TESTS

N/A

IMAGING

N/A

DIAGNOSTIC PROCEDURES

N/A

PATHOLOGIC FINDINGS

• Histopathologically, chronic hepatitis with varying degrees of fibrosis, depending on the length of exposure
• Characteristic lesions—bridging hepatic fibrosis, cholangitis, and hepatocellular regeneration

TREATMENT

• Remove animals from the kleingrass pastures or hay.
• Although horses have not shown photosensitization, shade may be helpful.
• Symptomatic and supportive care

MEDICATIONS

DRUGS

No specific therapeutic interventions

PANICUM COLORATUM (KLEINGRASS) TOXICOSIS

CONTRAINDICATIONS/POSSIBLE INTERACTIONS
Impaired hepatic function may prolong clearance of drugs metabolized by the liver.

FOLLOW-UP

PATIENT MONITORING
Monitor hepatic function.

PREVENTION/AVOIDANCE
Do not allow horses to graze *Panicum* spp. or ingest hays containing the grass.

POSSIBLE COMPLICATIONS
Photosensitization

EXPECTED COURSE AND PROGNOSIS
Onset of clinical signs is associated with significant hepatic fibrosis, making the long-term prognosis guarded to poor.

MISCELLANEOUS

ASSOCIATED CONDITIONS
N/A

AGE-RELATED FACTORS
N/A

ZOONOTIC POTENTIAL
N/A

PREGNANCY
N/A

SEE ALSO
N/A

ABBREVIATIONS
- AP = alkaline phosphatase
- AST = aspartate aminotransferase
- GGT = γ-glutamyltransferase
- PA = pyrrolizidine alkaloids
- SDH = sorbitol dehydrogenase

Suggested Reading

Cornick JL, Carter GK, Bridges CH. Kleingrass-associated hepatotoxicosis in horses. J Am Vet Med Assoc 1988;193:932–935.

Author Tam Garland
Consulting Editor Robert H. Poppenga

PARANASAL SINUSITIS

BASICS

OVERVIEW

• Infection of the paranasal sinuses may be primary, following transient, systemic bacterial infection (usually streptococcal); primary mycotic infection of the sinuses is rare.
• Commonly occurs secondary to periradicular infection of a maxillary molar or the caudal portion of the fourth maxillary premolar; the tooth most commonly affected is the first molar.
• Bacterial sinusitis less commonly occurs secondary to facial fracture or tissue necrosis caused by an expanding mass within the sinuses—cyst, neoplasm, osteoma, or progressive ethmoidal hematoma.
• Generally accompanied by empyema that, regardless of its cause, may become inspissated.
• All compartments communicate directly or indirectly with each other, so all may be involved.

SIGNALMENT

Any age, breed, or sex

SIGNS

• The most common clinical sign, regardless of the cause, is persistent unilateral purulent nasal discharge from the affected side.
• Flow of exudate from the naris may increase when the head is lowered.
• Malodorous exudate is characteristic associated tissue necrosis (e.g., sinusitis caused by dental disease) or an expanding mass, whereas odorless exudate is more characteristic of primary sinusitis.
• Other common signs—epiphora, conjunctivitis, and enlargement of the submandibular lymph nodes on the affected side.
• Facial distortion and obstructed airflow are features of horses with expanding masses or accumulation of fluid within the sinuses caused by occlusion of the nasomaxillary opening.

CAUSES AND RISK FACTORS

• Horses 1–5 years old are most susceptible to infection with *Streptococcus equi* var *equi* and, therefore, are most susceptible to primary bacterial sinusitis.
• The incidence of infundibular decay and periodontal disease, both of which are causes of periradicular dental disease, increases with age, as does the incidence of neoplasia.

DIAGNOSIS

DIFFERENTIAL DIAGNOSIS

• Other sources of purulent exudate at the nares—nasal passages, guttural pouches, nasopharynx, and lungs.
• Nasal discharge caused by disease caudal to the caudal edge of the nasal septum usually is bilateral.

CBC/BIOCHEMISTRY/URINALYSIS

Usually normal

OTHER LABORATORY TESTS

N/A

IMAGING

• The different radiodensities of teeth and paranasal sinuses necessitate multiple radiographs with different factors of exposure and positions of the tube head to clearly demonstrate detail of the paranasal sinuses and dental structures. The cassette should be positioned on the affected side of the skull.
• Lateral and dorsoventral radiographs usually show increased opacity of the affected sinuses. On a standing lateral view of the skull, horizontal fluid lines in the sinuses generally are visible. Obtaining radiographs after exudate is lavaged from the sinuses may be necessary to demonstrate masses.
• The VCS is the usual site of inspissated exudate. Identification of a soft-tissue density dorsal to the maxillary molars on a lateral radiograph and medial to those teeth on a dorsoventral radiograph is evidence of a mass in the VCS.
• To examine the maxillary roots, position the cassette on the affected side and the tube dorsally, angled 30° ventrally and centered on the rostral end of the facial crest.
• Periradicular disease of teeth whose roots reside within the paranasal sinuses can be recognized radiographically with confidence in only half of the cases.

PARANASAL SINUSITIS

DIAGNOSTIC PROCEDURES

• Percussion may identify loss of resonance within the sinuses, especially if sinuses are completely filled with fluid or tissue.
• Examine the oral cavity for dental abnormalities.
• Endoscopy of the nasal cavities with sinusitis may reveal exudate discharging from the middle meatus just rostral to the ethmoid labyrinth or distortion of the turbinates caused by an expanding mass within the sinuses.
• The sinuses can be examined endoscopically through trephine holes.
• Cytology and culture of exudate obtained by sinocentesis may help in determining whether sinusitis is caused by primary infection or is secondary to other disease. If infection is caused by periradicular dental disease, plant material sometimes can be identified and multiple bacterial colonies cultured. Sinusitis probably is primary if a single bacterial species is identified during cytology or if a β-hemolytic *Streptococcus* sp. is cultured.

TREATMENT

• Noninspissated empyema of the paranasal sinuses caused by primary bacterial infection—lavage of the sinuses and parenteral administration of an antimicrobial drug.
• Inspissated purulent exudate in the **VCS** should be suspected when primary bacterial sinusitis does not resolve with lavage and parenteral administration of antimicrobial agents; these animals require surgery.
• Primary mycotic paranasal sinusitis—irrigation of the affected sinuses with antifungal agents (e.g., enilconazole, natamycin).
• Sinusitis secondary to other diseases (e.g., periradicular dental disease)—eliminate the cause of the sinusitis, usually by surgical intervention.

MEDICATIONS

DRUGS

• Primary bacterial empyema—parenteral administration of an antimicrobial drug to which streptococci are susceptible, usually a β-lactam antibiotic (e.g., procaine penicillin [20,000–50,000 IU/kg IM q12h) in conjunction with lavage of the sinuses.
• Sinusitis secondary to other disease—antimicrobial drugs, either broad spectrum or based on culture and sensitivity results.

CONTRAINDICATIONS/POSSIBLE INTERACTIONS

N/A

FOLLOW-UP

• Distortion of the turbinates into the nasal passage caused by an expanding mass gradually resolves over several weeks following removal of the mass.
• Increased opacity of the sinuses may be observed radiographically long after the disease has resolved.

MISCELLANEOUS

ASSOCIATED CONDITIONS

Horses affected by primary sinusitis caused by *S. equi* infection also may have additional infection sites, including primary guttural pouch infection.

AGE-RELATED FACTORS

N/A

ZOONOTIC POTENTIAL

N/A

PREGNANCY

N/A

SEE ALSO

• Guttural pouch empyema
• Purulent nasal discharge

ABREVIATION

VCS = ventral conchal sinus

Suggested Reading

Freeman DE. Paranasal sinuses. In: Beech J, ed. Equine respiratory disorders. Philadelphia: Lea & Febiger, 1991.

Author Jim Schumacher
Consulting Editor Jean-Pierre Lavoie

PARAPHIMOSIS

BASICS

DEFINITION

Prolapse of the penis and inner preputial fold with extensive penile and preputial edema and the inability to retract the penis into the prepuce.

PATHOPHYSIOLOGY

- The anatomic location of the penis and prepuce affects how it reacts to injury. The effect of gravity magnifies the inflammatory reaction to an injury with the accumulation of edema, or with the formation of a hematoma or seroma.
- As the penis and prepuce prolapse, further edema accumulates, as vascular and lymphatic drainage are impeded while in the prolapsed state.
- The inelasticity of the preputial ring further promotes fluid retention.
- Chronic prolapse may lead to penile/preputial trauma, balanoposthitis, or penile paralysis.

SYSTEMS AFFECTED

- Reproductive: Prolapse of the penis and prepuce exposes them to trauma. Chronic paraphimosis may result in penile paralysis, fibrosis of the corpus cavernosum, and an inability to achieve an erection.
- Urologic: Urethral obstruction may be the inciting cause of paraphimosis, or it may occur secondary to edema.

SIGNALMENT

- Predominantly stallions, but geldings can also be affected.
- No breed predilection.
- Unlikely to occur in the first month of life, when normal adhesions exist between the free penis and inner lamina of the preputial fold.

SIGNS

Historical Findings

- Acute cases often present as traumatic injury to the penile or preputial area.
- Chronic cases: Delay in presentation for veterinary care may occur if owners believed an injury was minor and attempted care themselves or the injury may only recently have become obvious because of its slow increase in size, e.g., a slow developing enlargement of the penis or preputial area such as is seen with *Habronema* spp. infections or neoplastic growths.

Physical Examination Findings

- Prolapse of the penis and prepuce with severe penile enlargement is readily apparent. Caudoventral displacement of the glans penis is common. A careful visual and digital exam is necessary to properly define the nature of the injury.
- Balanitis (inflammation of the penis), posthitis (inflammation of the prepuce), or balanoposthitis (inflammation of the prepuce and penis) may be present. Serous or hemorrhagic discharges on the surface of the penis and prepuce are common. Lacerations, excoriations, ulcerative lesions, or neoplastic masses may be evident.
- Hematomas, when present, are generally located on the dorsal surface of the penis and usually arise from blood vessels superficial to the tunica albuginea.
- Transrectal palpation may reveal an enlarged urinary bladder indicative of urethral blockage.
- Chronic prolapse may result in penile paralysis.

CAUSES

Noninfectious Causes

- Trauma*—breeding injuries, fighting or kicks, improperly-fitting stallion rings, falls, movement through brush or heavy ground cover, whips, or abuse.
- Priapism, penile paralysis, posthitis, or balanoposthitis.
- Post-surgical complication—castration or cryptorchid surgery.
- Neoplasia of the penis or prepuce—sarcoids, squamous cell carcinoma, melanoma, mastocytoma, hemangioma, or papillomas.
- Debilitation or starvation.
- Spinal injury or myelitis.
- Urolithiasis/urinary tract obstruction.

Infectious Causes

- Bacterial—*Staphylococcus, Streptococcus, Purpura hemorrhagica.*
- Viral—EHV-1 (rhinopneumonitis), EHV-3 (coital exanthema), EIA, EVA.
- Parasitic—*Habronema muscae, Habronema microstoma, Draschia megastoma, Onchocera* spp., *Cochliomyia hominivorax* (screw worm).
- Fungal—phycomycosis due to *Hyphomyces destruens.*
- Protozoal—*Trypanosoma equiperdum* (Dourine).

RISK FACTORS

- Use of phenothiazine tranquilizers in stallions.
- Open-range, not in-hand, stud management.
- More aggressive stallions.
- Poor management, unsanitary conditions, or malnutrition.

DIAGNOSIS

DIFFERENTIAL DIAGNOSIS

- Any injury or condition that leads to chronic protrusion of the penis or prepuce can lead to paraphimosis. The initial cause may be due to injury or disease, but because both accumulate edema and leave the surfaces exposed to further injury, the underlying cause must be determined whenever possible.
- The presence of visible lacerations or hematomas or a history of trauma or surgical intervention is diagnostic.
- The presence of ulcerative or proliferative lesions warrants investigation to determine if the origin of the lesion is neoplastic, parasitic, or infectious.
- Systemic signs indicative of neurologic or systemic disease include ataxia, depression, lymph node enlargement, or increased rectal temperature.

CBC/BIOCHEMISTRY/URINALYSIS

- Generally, there are no abnormal findings unless infectious agents, neoplastic disease, or severe debilitation/starvation are the causative factors.
- Urinalysis may indicate urolithiasis/cystitis.

OTHER LABORATORY TESTS

- Bacterial causes—Cultures of affected tissues.
- EHV-1—Rising antibody titers from paired sera, collected at a 14–21 day interval; virus isolation from nasopharyngeal swabs during the acute stage.
- EHV-3—Rising antibody titer from paired sera, collected at a 14–21 day interval; intranuclear inclusion bodies in cytologic smears; virus isolation from lesions during the acute stage.
- EIA—AGID (Coggins) test.
- EVA—Rising antibody titer from paired sera collected at a 14–21 day interval; virus isolation from nasopharygneal swabs.
- Protozoal—Identification of the causative agent in urethral exudates; serology:CF.

IMAGING

Ultrasound findings are generally unrewarding. In other species, fibrosis of the corpus cavernosum has been visualized in chronic cases.

DIAGNOSTIC PROCEDURES

Cytology or biopsy of masses or lesions may provide a diagnosis in the case of parasitic, neoplastic, or fungal disease.

TREATMENT

- The primary goals: reduce the inflammation and edema and return the penis to the prepuce to improve venous and lymphatic drainage. The initial management of the patient is intensive and may require hospitalization to allow adequate physical restraint and patient access.
- Ensure urethral patency. Catheterize or perform a perineal urethrostomy if necessary.
- Manual reduction of the prolapse:

- Elastic or pneumatic bandaging may reduce edema prior to attempting reduction.
- Preputiotomy if the preputial ring is preventing successful reduction.
- Purse-string suture of umbilical tape around the preputial orifice, tightened to a one-finger opening, to hold the penis within the prepuce; has the additional benefit of maintaining pressure on the penis for sustained reduction of edema.
- Additional support can be gained by putting on a net sling, which covers the cranial aspect of the prepuce but allows urine to drain.

- In cases resistant to manual reduction, support remains of primary importance. Wrap the exposed penis and prepuce to reduce edema. Support in the form of a sling is essential. Nylon slings raise and maintain the penis close to the ventral belly wall. Using netting with small perforations allows urine to drain.
- Hydrotherapy: Cold hydrotherapy for the first 4–7 days until edema and hemorrhage subside, then warm hydrotherapy. Generally applied for 15–30 min BID to QID.
- Massage the penis and prepuce BID to QID to reduce edema.
- Topical emollient ointment application: A&D ointment, lanolin, petroleum jelly, nitrofurazone.
- Exercise: Confinement and limited activity until after active hemorrhage and edema subside, then slowly increase; aids in resolution of dependent edema.
- No sexual stimulation in the early stages of therapy. It may be necessary to prevent exposure to mares for up to 4–8 weeks.
- Local surgical resection, cryosurgery, or radiation therapy of neoplastic or granulomatous lesions, once the edema is resolved.
- Chronic refractory paraphimosis may require surgical intervention, including circumcision (reefing or posthioplasty), penile retraction (Bolz technique), or penile amputation (phallectomy).

MEDICATIONS

DRUG(S) OF CHOICE

- NSAIDs including phenylbutazone (2–4 g/450 kg/day PO) or flunixine meglumine (1 mg/kg/day IV, IM, or PO) for symptomatic relief and to reduce inflammation.
- Systemic or local antibiotics as indicated to treat local infection and prevent septicemia.
- Diuretics—Furosemide (1 mg/kg IV, SID, or BID) if indicated in the acute phase for reduction of edema.
- Specific topical or systemic treatments for parasitic, fungal, or neoplastic conditions as indicated by results of diagnostic testing.

CONTRAINDICATIONS

- Tranquilizers, particularly the phenothiazine tranquilizers, should be avoided in males to avoid drug-induced priapism.
- Avoid sexual stimulation in the early stages and usually for 4–8 weeks after treatment for paraphimosis has begun.

PRECAUTIONS

Diuretics are contraindicated if urinary obstruction is present. Their effectiveness in treating localized edema is in doubt.

POSSIBLE INTERACTIONS

N/A

ALTERNATIVE DRUGS

Dimethyl sulfoxide (DMSO) has been used topically (50/50 mixture by volume with nitrofurazone ointment) or systemically (1 gm/kg IV as a 10% solution in saline BID to TID for 3–5 days) to reduce inflammation and edema. Note that the parenteral administration of DMSO is not approved and is considered an extra-label use.

FOLLOW-UP

PATIENT MONITORING

Initial management is intensive. Frequent evaluation is essential. Reduction of edema, coupled with the horse's ability to retain his penis in the prepuce, are good prognostic indicators.

POSSIBLE COMPLICATIONS

- Excoriations/ulcerations or further trauma of exposed skin surfaces.
- Fibrosis of tissues leading to the inability to achieve erection or urethral obstruction.
- Chronic paraphimosis.
- Continued hematoma enlargement indicates that a rent may be present in the tunica albuginea. The hematoma should be surgically explored.
- Penile paralysis.
- Frostbite due to exposure.
- Myiasis.
- Infertility.

MISCELLANEOUS

ASSOCIATED CONDITIONS

N/A

AGE-RELATED FACTORS

N/A

ZOONOTIC POTENTIAL

N/A

PREGNANCY

N/A

SYNONYMS

N/A

SEE ALSO

- Viral diseases, infectious
- Penile lacerations
- Penile paralysis
- Penile vesicles/erosions
- Priapism
- Venereal diseases

ABBREVIATIONS

- AGID = agar gel immunodiffusion
- CF = complement fixation
- EHV-1 = equine rhinopneumonitis
- EHV-3 = equine coital exanthema
- EIA = equine infectious anemia, swamp fever
- EVA/EAV = equine viral arteritis, equine arteritis virus

Suggested Reading

Clem MF, DeBowes RM. Paraphimosis in horses. Part I. Compend Contin Educ 1989;11:72-75.

Clem MF, DeBowes RM. Paraphimosis in horses. Part II. Compend Contin Educ 1989;11:184-187.

De Vries PJ. Diseases of the testes, penis, and related structures. In: Equine reproduction. McKinnon AO and Voss JL, ed. Philadelphia: Lea & Febiger, 1993;878-884.

Vaughan JT. Surgery of the penis and prepuce. In: Bovine and equine urogenital surgery. Walker DF and Vaughan JT, eds. Philadelphia: Lea & Febiger 1980;125-144.

Vaughan JT. Penis and prepuce. In: Equine reproduction. McKinnon AO and Voss JL, ed. Philadelphia: Lea & Febiger 1993;885-894.

Author Carole C. Miller

Consulting Editor Carla L. Carleton

PARTURITION

BASICS

DEFINITION

• Normal parturition is a relatively rapid process culminating in a series of tightly orchestrated physical and physiologic events between the mare and fetus, ending with passage of the fetus through the birth canal and delivery.
• Most foal between 11 PM and 3 AM.

PATHOPHYSIOLOGY

• *General Comments* Duration of gestation is variable (average, 335–342 days).
• The equine fetus cannot survive if delivered before 300 days of gestation.
• Delivery of foals at 300–320 days generally results in prematurity and reduced survivability.
• Prolonged gestation (>365–480 days) has resulted in spontaneous delivery of normal foals.
• Mares foaling in the winter and early spring months commonly have gestational periods that may be 10 days longer than summer-foaling mares.
• Mares carrying male fetuses tend to have gestations 2–3 days longer than when carrying female fetuses.
• Three stages—(I) preparatory; (II) fetal passage; (III) passage of fetal membranes and involution of the uterus.

Stage I

• Duration 1–4 hr
• Patchy sweating behind the elbows, in the flanks, and along the neck; increased restlessness expressed by pacing/circling in the stall, lying down and rising frequently, and tail switching; posturing as if to urinate; looking at flanks; frequent passage of small amounts of feces; some mares yawn—these signs are a manifestation of abdominal pain (i.e., colic) experienced by the mare and result from the increased myometrial contractions taking place.
• Maternal estrogens increase late in gestation. Threshold sensitivity to oxytocin is greatly diminished in the presence of estrogen. These factors, coupled with point pressure by fetal extremities, further stimulate the cervix, causing—release more endogenous oxytocin and more contractions—(Ferguson's reflex).
• Myometrial contractions around the fetus bring the fetus, membranes, and fluid into contact with the cervix. These contractions force the fetus and the CA membrane against the dilating cervix, through which they protrude, causing the membrane to rupture. Rupture of the CA and release of allantoic fluid is commonly referred to as "breaking water" and marks the end of Stage I labor.
• If a mare is disturbed or excited during Stage I labor, the labor can sometimes terminate and parturition may be delayed for several hours or days. The urine-like allantoic fluid may play a role in lubricating the birth canal in preparation for Stage II labor. The mare commonly sniffs the allantoic fluid and displays the Flehman response.
• Rupture of the CA occurs at the cervical star (i.e., the avillous, thinner portion of the CA membrane against the internal cervical os). If it fails to rupture, the red velvet appearing CA membrane and intact cervical star emerge through the vulvar lips. In this situation, the CA, rupture because it indicates the placenta is undergoing premature separation from the uterus. If allowed to continue without assisted fetal delivery, fetal hypoxia and, possibly, fetal death may result.

Stage II

• Actual delivery of the fetus—active labor.
• As the pelvic canal soft tissues are stretched by the fetus, forceful abdominal muscle contractions are stimulated. The abdominal muscles and the diaphragm contract in synchrony, during which the glottis of the mare is closed, producing increased intra-abdominal pressure that forces the fetus through the birth canal.
• Most mares are in lateral recumbency during Stage II, but a mare standing and repositioning herself in lateral recumbency is not unusual. A few mares will foal while standing.
• As contractions continue, the transparent, bluish-white amnion can be seen at the vulvar lips. Forceful abdominal contractions and straining commonly occur in groups of 3 or 4 "efforts" followed by a 2–3 min rest period.
• During these abdominal contractions, the fetus is forced into the mare's pelvis one shoulder at a time, thus causing one forelimb to be slightly ahead of the other (by approximately 12–15 cm). This narrows the shoulder width and eases passage through the birth canal.
• The head of the fetus will lie between the carpal joints. Abdominal contractions become the most forceful when the head and then the shoulders pass through the pelvis; the chest and hips require less effort.
• When the hips of the foal pass through the vagina of the mare, straining stops, and Stage II is complete. Following delivery, the mare may lie quietly for 10–15 min, with the rear legs of the foal still in the vagina.
• The foal is usually delivered with the umbilical cord intact and the newborn covered by amnion. The amnion helps to reduce resistance to passage through the birth canal. The amnion usually is ruptured by movements of the foal; however, on occasion, one may need to quietly enter the stall, disturbing the mare as little as possible, to tear the membrane and remove any portion covering the mouth and nostrils of the foal in order to prevent asphyxia.

• Stage II labor usually is completed within 20–30 min. If the mare remains in Stage II labor for > of 30–35 min without progress, an immediate vaginal exam is essential, because the delivery may require obstetric assistance.
• The likelihood of delivering a live foal is poor if Stage II exceeds 60 min.
• The umbilical cord usually is ruptured by movement of either the foal or the mare. No significant blood flow occurs through the umbilical cord at parturition. If a neonate is weak or otherwise abnormal, blood loss from premature rupture of the cord should not be blamed.

Stage III

• Marked by expulsion of the fetal membranes/placenta.
• After delivery of the foal, the mare usually stops all obvious signs of straining; however, myometrial contractions continue. During these contractions, the vessels of the placenta collapse and the chorionic villi shrink and detach from the uterus. It is believed the myometrial contractions originate at the tip or apex of the uterine horns, and as the chorionic villi detach from the endometrial crypts of the uterus, the apex of the CA sac becomes inverted while rolling down the uterine horn.
• Inversion of the CA membrane causes the placenta to be expelled with the allantoic (i.e., fetal side) surface outermost.
• Expulsion of the placenta occurs within 0.5–3 hr after delivery.
• The mare may show signs of colic during passage of the placental membranes—restlessness, pawing, lying down, and even rolling. Mare that show excessive distress during this time may need to be walked to aid passage of the placenta. If the placenta is not passed within 3–6 hr, veterinary intervention may be necessary to avoid potentially severe side effects—metritis and toxemia.
• Retained fetal membranes occur in approximately 5–10% of foaling mares, requiring veterinary intervention.

SYSTEM AFFECTED

Reproductive

GENETICS

N/A

INCIDENCE/PREVALENCE

If normal, parturition is 100% associated with term pregnancy.

SIGNALMENT

N/A

SIGNS

Common Signs of Term Gestation/Impending Parturition:

Relaxation of the Sacrosciatic Ligaments

• Occurs late during gestation, producing an obvious sinking or depression bilaterally alongside the tail head of the mare.
• More obvious in older, multiparous mares; may be very difficult to detect in some maidens and heavily muscled mares.
• A palpable softening of the sacrosciatic ligament may be detected in some mares as parturition draws near.

Vulvar Edema and Relaxation

• During the last few weeks of gestation.
• The vulva becomes slightly edematous, and the vulvar cleft begins to lengthen.
• These changes are subtle at first, becoming most obvious when parturition is 6–8 hr away.

Mammary Gland Development

• The most reliable indicator of impending parturition, though maiden mares may be the exception, exhibiting very little/minimal change in the udder prepartum.
• Usually, mammary gland development begins 4–6 wk prepartum, with the most significant increase occurring during the last 2 wk of gestation.
• During the last 2–3 days, the mammary gland engorges with colostrum, and in about 90–95% of foaling mares, colostrum oozes from the teats to form beads of wax-like material—waxing.
• It is reasonable to expect foaling within 24–48 hr after waxing.

CAUSES

Breeding and pregnancy

RISK FACTORS

N/A

DIAGNOSIS

DIFFERENTIAL DIAGNOSIS

Hydrops Amnion/Allantois:

• No history of having been bred
• Absence of fetus and placental membranes/fluid compatible with pregnancy
• Diagnosis by transrectal palpation and ultrasound

CBC/BIOCHEMISTRY/URINALYSIS

N/A

OTHER LABORATORY TESTS

N/A

IMAGING

N/A

DIAGNOSTIC PROCEDURES

Assisted parturition/obstetric procedures are only necessary if normal time frames are exceeded or other signs of dystocia develop.

PATHOLOGIC FINDINGS

N/A

PARTURITION

TREATMENT

APPROPRIATE HEALTH CARE

N/A

NURSING CARE

N/A

ACTIVITY

- At term, most mares, because of the size of the fetus/uterus and physical discomfort, restrict their own activity.
- Activity may need to be restricted prepartum if the mare develops excessive ventral edema of the abdomen—concern regarding prepubic tendon rupture.
- Postpartum, if the neonate has physical problems (e.g., dummy foal, difficulty nursing, crooked legs), the mare and foal may require restricted activity in the stall or to turn-out in a small paddock for limited periods of time.

DIET

Pregnant mares should be on a slight plane of weight gain the last third of gestation to help with slight weight increase to support lactation, but not of an order to increase vaginal fat and the likelihood of dystocia.

CLIENT EDUCATION

- Owners must understand the importance/necessity of frequently observing prepartum mares to enable timely assistance, if needed, early in Stage II. The optimal interval to assess mares, especially during the evening hours (8 PM to 8 AM), is every 20 min.
- Have a clock in the barn, and record actual time of events (i.e., CA rupture), to ensure that critical times (Stages I, II, and III) are not exceeded and help is sought as early as possible.
- Gathered and keep, ready all necessary equipment to assist foaling mares before it is needed—towels, buckets, tail wraps, etc.

SURGICAL CONSIDERATIONS

Cesarean section may be an option in mares with dystocia if vaginal delivery is not possible.

MEDICATIONS

DRUGS OF CHOICE

N/A

CONTRAINDICATIONS

N/A

PRECAUTIONS

N/A

POSSIBLE INTERACTIONS

N/A

ALTERNATIVE DRUGS

N/A

FOLLOW-UP

PATIENT MONITORING

- Monitoring of mares within the last week of gestation can be improved by evaluation of milk calcium (to permit closer prediction of the day of parturition) and by tactile assessment of mammary content and gross development of the gland—the halves of the gland increase in size and fill over a 1–4 wk period; the teats fill within the last 1–2 days prepartum.
- Because of the forceful nature of the mare's abdominal press, equine parturition tends to be short if fetal presentation, position, and posture are normal. Thus, the optimal interval to quietly observe foaling mares at term is every 20 min.
- Many systems are available to assist owners in monitoring their mare's progress—temperature-sensitive vaginal tampons (an alarm sounds as the tampon is expelled and its sensor cools to less than body temperature); magnetic, clip, or interlocking devices (an alarm sound when the vulvar lips are parted, as with passage of the fetus into the birth canal); and in-stall cameras (to observe activity in the foaling stall from a more comfortable location).

PARTURITION

PREVENTION/AVOIDANCE
N/A

POSSIBLE COMPLICATIONS
- Dystocia, maternal and fetal compromise, and death
- Lactation failure, requiring supplemental colostrum/milk source for foal
- Maternal/fetal disease
- Postpartum metritis
- Retained fetal membranes/placenta

EXPECTED COURSE AND PROGNOSIS
- Normal course and time frames for stages I, II, and III and delivery of a live foal.
- Incidence of dystocia is <10% in mares.

MISCELLANEOUS

ASSOCIATED CONDITIONS
N/A

AGE-RELATED FACTORS
- Better if mares are not bred before 3 yr of age.
- Two-year-old fillies have a greatly increased incidence of abortion and dystocia.

ZOONOTIC POTENTIAL
N/A

PREGNANCY
Essential condition for parturition to be possible.

SYNONYMS
- Birthing
- Foaling

SEE ALSO
- Dystocia
- Eclampsia
- Fescue toxicity
- Induction of parturition
- Placentation, normal
- Placentitis
- Pseudopregnancy
- Retained fetal membranes/placenta

ABBREVIATIONS
- CA = chorioallantoic (membrane)

Suggested Reading

Card CE, Hillman RB. Parturition. In: McKinnon AO, Voss JL, eds. Equine reproduction. Philadelphia: WB Saunders, 1993;567-573.

Doarn R, Threlfall WR, Kline R. Umbilical blood flow and the effects of premature severance in the neonate horse. Therio 1987;28789-800.

Ginther OJ. Reproductive biology of the mare: basic and applied aspects. Cross Plains, WI: Equiservices, 1992.

Roberts SJ. Veterinary obstetrics and genital diseases (theriogenology). Ann Arbor, MI: Edwards Brothers, 1971;202-203.

Youngquist RS. Equine obstetrics. In: Morrow Current therapy in theriogenology, 2nd ed. DA, ed. Toronto: WB Saunders, 1986;693-699.

Author E. Ricardo Bridges

Consulting Editor Carla L. Carleton

PASTERN DERMATITIS (PD)

BASICS

DEFINITION

In mild forms, the condition is also known as scratches, cracked heels, mud fever or mud rash; the more exudative form of pastern dermatitis is called grease heel or dew poisoning. In chronic stages, mounds of granulation tissue called "grapes" occur on the caudal aspect of the lower limb. Similar to eosinophilic granuloma complex in cats, EPD should be considered a syndrome, not a diagnosis, and thus an underlying cause should be pursued whenever possible.

PATHOPHYSIOLOGY

• Infectious or non-infectious disorders that result in inflammation, ulceration, crusting or granulomatous conditions affecting the pastern region of the horse.

SYSTEMS AFFECTED

Skin

SIGNALMENT

BREED PREDILECTION

—Draft horses with feathers are more predisposed to Chorioptes
—Arabs appear to have a greater to sand irritation of the pastern
—Horses with unpigmented distal extremities are predisposed to photoaggravated disorders

MEAN AGE AND RANGE

N/A

GENETICS

N/A

PREDOMINANT SEX

N/A

SIGNS

• Dermatitis of the lower limbs (hindlimbs more often affected)
• Unpigmented skin appears predisposed
• Pruritus (Chorioptes infestation) or pain/lameness variable
• Starts at the posterior aspect of the pastern, then spreads dorsally and anteriorly
• Can be both bilaterally symmetric or involve only one limb
• Three presentations
  i) scratches—mildest/most prevalent form with scales and crusts and alopecia
    —skin may be thickened and painful +/− lameness, pruritus
  ii) grease heel—exudative dermatitis with epidermolysis
  iii) grapes—chronic form of pastern dermatitis
    —excessive granulation tissue that may become cornified
    —more often noted in draft horses

CAUSES

Primary factors
—physical and chemical irritants (most common cause)
—contact allergy; contact photosensitization, photoactivated vasculitis (clover)
—idiopathic pastern leukocytoclastic vasculitis
—dermatophytes; chorioptic mange mites (especially draft horses), chiggers
—nematodes (Pelodera strongyloides, *Strongyloides westeri larvae*)
—environmental (UV exposure, cold)

Perpetuating factors
—bacterial infections (*Staphylococcus aureus, Dermatophilus congolensis*)
—pathologic skin changes

RISK FACTORS

a) genetic (white skin and hair on lower limbs, and feathers)
b) environmental (climate, moisture, stable/pasture hygiene)
c) iatrogenic (use of irritant topical products & training devices)

DIAGNOSIS

DIFFERENTIAL DIAGNOSES

Dermatophilosis
Dermatophytosis
Staphylococcal folliculitis
Chorioptic mange
Trombiculidiasis
Contact allergic/irritant dermatitis
Photosensitivity
Photoactivated vasculitis
Canon keratosis
Cutaneous lymphoma
Cutaneous drug eruption
Idiopathic causes

CBC/BIOCHEMISTRY/URINALYSIS

—To evaluate for hepatically-induced photosensitization
—Rule-out other metabolic disorders

OTHER LABORATORY TESTS

• Bacterial culture and sensitivity to direct selection of topical/systemic antibiotics
• Fungal culture to rule out dermatophytosis

IMAGING

—May pursue radiographs to rule-out an orthopedic etiology (arthritis, boney sequestrum)

OTHER DIAGNOSTIC PROCEDURES

• History and physical examination
• Inspect environment (standing water, sand, insect burden)
• Skin scrapings to rule-out ectoparasites
• Cytology—Diff Quik or Gram's stain
  —"railroad track" (*Dermatophilus congolensis*)
  —engulfed cocci within neutrophils (*Staphylococcus* spp)

GROSS AND HISTOPATHOLOGIC FINDINGS

• Dermatopathology
  —consider if immune-mediated disorders are suspected
  —consider if immunosuppressive or expensive therapy is anticipated
  —may also be submitted for bacterial or fungal culture and sensitivity

TREATMENT

INPATIENT VERSUS OUTPATIENT

• Address underlying etiologies
• Clip hairs, especially feathers, to avoid moisture retention
• Cleanse lesions and remove crusts with antimicrobial shampoos
  —benzoyl peroxides, chlorhexidine, ethyl lactate
  —BID for 7–10 days, then taper the frequency
• Cover affected areas if dry environment not possible
  —ointments that create a moisture barrier
  —padded, water-repellent bandages (change q 24 to 48 hours)
  —Facilitator liquid bandage (Blue Ridge Pharmaceuticals)
  —hydroxyethylated amylopectin
  —cleanse wound first, pat dry
  —cover a slightly greater surface area than the lesion q 1–3 days

PASTERN DERMATITIS (PD)

ACTIVITY
- Avoid pastures/paddocks with mud, water, or sandy pastures (Arabian horses)
- Stall patient during wet weather and until morning dew has dried
- Avoid sunlight if photosensitization disorder is suspected

DIET
- Avoid clover pastures that may have a fungal organism present (e.g. rye grass rust)
- Avoid over-grazed, poor quality pasture hay containing ragwort or St. John's Wort

CLIENT EDUCATION
- The focus is to address the underlying etiology and keep the area dry and clean
- "Grease heel" is a descriptive term, not a diagnosis

SURGICAL CONSIDERATIONS
- Surgical removal of exuberant granulation tissue
  —general anesthesia
  —either electrocautery or an Esmarch bandage to control hemorrhage
  —remove to skin level (avoid excision of epithelial tissue from wound edges)
  —pressure bandage for 24 hours
  —then treat with corticosteroid/antimicrobial ointment under wrap

MEDICATIONS

DRUGS AND FLUIDS
- If exudative, use astringent solutions after cleansing such as lime sulfur (LymDyp-DVM), Domeboro solution, black tea-bag poultices
- DMSO/TBZ/Sulfa ointment
  —30 ml dimethyl sulfoxide (DMSO); antibacterial, antioxidant
  —30 g thiabendazole (TBZ) paste or powder; anti-inflammatory, antifungal
  —500 g sulfa cream or ointment; antibacterial
- Parasite-induced dermatitis
  —ivermectin @ 2-week intervals for 2–3 doses
  —topical insecticides (fipronil, flumethrin)
  —lime sulfur (LymDyp, DVM)
- Systemic antibiotics and/or steroids based on underlying etiology

CONTRAINDICATIONS
- Avoid any of the above medication if there is a history of related drug eruptions

PRECAUTIONS
- Some medications recommendations are off-label usage

POSSIBLE INTERACTIONS
N/A

ALTERNATIVE DRUGS
- Sauerkraut poultices have been described

FOLLOW-UP

PATIENT MONITORING
- Aggressive therapy initially typically results in less recurrence, once the underlying etiology has been addressed.

PREVENTION/AVOIDANCE
- See activity
- Address any asymptomatic carriers of infectious cases (Chorioptes, dermatophytes)

POSSIBLE COMPLICATIONS
- Lameness and/or proud flesh may be a sequelae if EPD not addressed aggressively

EXPECTED COURSE AND PROGNOSIS
- Prognosis and healing time of EPD depends on several factors
  —the stage of disease when treatment was begun
  —determination of the etiologic agent

MISCELLANEOUS

ASSOCIATED CONDITIONS
N/A

AGE-RELATED FACTORS
N/A

ZOONOTIC POTENTIAL
- Until a definitive diagnosis is achieved, gloves should be worn, and proper hygiene should be exercised, as several differentials are zoonotic (Chorioptes, dermatophytes)

PREGNANCY
N/A

SYNONYMS
- Scratches
- Cracked heels
- Mud fever or mud rash
- Grease heel
- Dew poisoning
- Grapes

SEE ALSO
N/A

ABBREVIATIONS
N/A

Suggested Reading

Littlewood JD. Dermatoses of the Equine Distal Limb. World Congress of Veterinary Dermatology, San Francisco, CA, Sept 1, 2000:129–133.

Stannard AA. Miscellaneous Equine Dermatoses. Veterinary Dermatology 2000; 11:217–223

Author Anthony A. Yu

PATENT DUCTUS ARTERIOSUS (PDA)

BASICS

DEFINITION

- A persistently patent vascular communication between the aorta and pulmonary artery.
- The ductus arteriosus is a vessel that allows blood to shunt from the pulmonary artery to the aorta in the fetus.
- The ductus arteriosus normally constricts after birth in response to increased local oxygen tension and prostaglandin inhibition, and closure should be complete within 4 days of birth.

PATHOPHYSIOLOGY

- When the ductus arteriosus remains patent, blood shunts from the higher-pressure aorta to the lower-pressure pulmonary artery, creating left atrial and left ventricular volume overload.
- Size of the PDA determines severity of the volume overload—with a large PDA, stretching of the mitral annulus occurs over time, and mitral regurgitation develops; as mitral regurgitation becomes more severe, left atrial pressure increases, resulting in increased pulmonary venous pressure and clinical signs of left-sided congestive heart failure.

SYSTEM AFFECTED

Cardiovascular

GENETICS

- Not yet determined in horses
- The condition is heritable in other species but rare in horses.

INCIDENCE/PREVALENCE

PDAs are rare, isolated congenital defects, but they occur more frequently in horses with complex congenital heart disease.

SIGNALMENT

- Murmurs usually are detectable at birth.
- Diagnosed most frequently in neonates, foals, and young horses but can be found at any age.

SIGNS

General Comments

May be an incidental finding, but usually is part of a more complex congenital cardiac disorder.

Historical Findings

- Exercise intolerance—medium to large PDAs
- Congestive heart failure—large PDAs

Physical Examination Findings

- A grade 3–6/6 continuous machinery murmur with PMI over the main pulmonary artery between the pulmonic and aortic valve area
- Bounding arterial pulses
- Premature beats or an irregularly irregular heart rhythm of atrial fibrillation may be present with larger PDAs.

CAUSES

Lack of constriction of the ductus arteriosus

RISK FACTORS

- Premature foal
- Hypoxia
- Neonatal pulmonary hypertension
- Neonatal respiratory distress syndrome
- Mares treated with prostaglandin inhibitors during late gestation

DIAGNOSIS

DIFFERENTIAL DIAGNOSIS

- Physiologic flow murmur (smaller PDAs)—differentiate echocardiographically.
- Ventricular septal defect with aortic regurgitation—pansystolic and holodiastolic murmur and PMI of pansystolic murmur, usually in the tricuspid valve area; differentiate echocardiographically.
- Complex congenital cardiac disease—differentiate echocardiographically.

CBC/BIOCHEMISTRY/URINALYSIS

N/A

OTHER LABORATORY TESTS

N/A

IMAGING

Electrocardiography

Atrial premature depolarizations or atrial fibrillation may be present in horses with left atrial enlargement.

Echocardiography

- Difficult to visualize
- The left atrium and ventricle are enlarged, dilated, and have a rounded appearance.
- Pulmonary artery dilatation in horses with a large shunt.
- Color-flow Doppler reveals the shunt from aorta to pulmonary artery through the PDA.
- Continuous, high-velocity, turbulent flow is detected with continuous-wave Doppler toward the main pulmonary artery.

Thoracic Radiography

- Increased pulmonary vascularity and cardiac enlargement may be detected.
- Pulmonary edema may be detected in foals or horses with congestive heart failure.

DIAGNOSTIC PROCEDURES

Cardiac Catheterization

- Right sided cardiac catheterization to directly measure pulmonary arterial and capillary wedge pressures and to sample blood for oxygen content
- Elevated pulmonary arterial and capillary wedge pressures as well as increased oxygen saturation of pulmonary arterial blood are found in affected horses.

24-Hour Holter Monitoring

Continuous monitoring is useful for establishing the diagnosis in horses with suspected atrial premature depolarizations.

PATHOLOGIC FINDINGS

- The PDA is present between the aorta and main pulmonary artery.
- Left atrial and ventricular enlargement and thinning of the left atrial and ventricular free wall in horses with a significant shunt
- Dilatation of the main pulmonary artery and right and left pulmonary arteries in those horses with a large shunt and in those with pulmonary hypertension.
- Thickened media of the pulmonary arterioles in horses with chronic pulmonary hypertension.
- Pulmonary edema in horses with congestive heart failure.

TREATMENT

APPROPRIATE HEALTH CARE

- Most newborn foals with PDAs should have the underlying pulmonary disease or pulmonary hypertension treated if present.
- Monitor affected horses on an annual basis.
- Horse with PDA and congestive heart failure could be treated for the congestive heart failure with positive inotropic drugs, vasodilators, and diuretics. Consider humane destruction, however, because only short-term, symptomatic improvement can be expected.

PATENT DUCTUS ARTERIOSUS (PDA)

NURSING CARE
N/A

ACTIVITY
• Horses with small PDAs may be able to perform successfully at lower levels of athletic competition, but they are unlikely to be able to compete at upper levels.
• Monitor affected horses echocardiographically on an annual basis to ensure they are safe to ride.
• Affected horses that develop atrial fibrillation need a complete cardiovascular examination to determine if lower levels of athletic performance are safe.
• Horses with pulmonary artery dilatation are no longer safe to ride.

DIET
N/A

CLIENT EDUCATION
• Regularly monitor the horse's rhythm; any irregularities other than second-degree AV block should prompt an electrocardiographic examination.
• Carefully monitor the horse for exercise intolerance, respiratory distress, prolonged recovery after exercise, increased resting respiratory or heart rate, or cough; if detected, obtain a cardiac re-examination.

SURGICAL CONSIDERATIONS
• Closure of the PDA is possible with a transvenous umbrella catheter or coil having a diameter large enough to close the defect.
• Surgical closure is not financially feasible or practical for obtaining an equine athlete at this time.

MEDICATIONS

DRUGS OF CHOICE
N/A

CONTRAINDICATIONS
N/A

PRECAUTIONS
N/A

POSSIBLE INTERACTIONS
N/A

ALTERNATIVE DRUGS
N/A

FOLLOW-UP

PATIENT MONITORING
Frequently monitor the horse's cardiac rate, rhythm, respiratory rate, and effort.

PREVENTION/AVOIDANCE
N/A

POSSIBLE COMPLICATIONS
Large PDA—atrial fibrillation, congestive heart failure, and pulmonary artery rupture

EXPECTED COURSE AND PROGNOSIS
• Horses with a small PDA may have a normal performance life for lower levels of athletic competition and a normal life expectancy.
• Horses with a moderate to large PDA may develop atrial fibrillation and have a guarded prognosis; these horses should have a shortened performance life at lower levels of athletic competition and a shortened life expectancy.
• Horses with pulmonary artery dilatation have a grave prognosis for life and are not safe to ride.
• Horses with associated congestive heart failure usually have a guarded to grave prognosis for life. Most horses with a PDA being treated for congestive heart failure should respond to the supportive therapy and transiently improve, but once congestive heart failure develops, euthanasia is recommended.

MISCELLANEOUS

ASSOCIATED CONDITIONS
• Complex congenital cardiac disease is the rule, rather than the exception, in affected horses.
• Mitral regurgitation can develop in horses with PDAs associated with stretching of the mitral annulus secondary to significant left atrial and ventricular volume overload.
• Pulmonary artery rupture can occur secondary to the pulmonary artery dilatation and elevated pulmonary arterial pressures.

AGE-RELATED FACTORS
Young horses are more likely to be diagnosed with this defect.

ZOONOTIC POTENTIAL
N/A

PREGNANCY
Breeding affected horses should be discouraged even though the condition is rare and the heritable nature of this defect is not known.

SYNONYMS
N/A

SEE ALSO
• Congestive heart failure—left sided
• Continuous murmurs
• Systolic murmurs

ABBREVIATIONS
• AV = atrioventricular
• PMI = point of maximal intensity

Suggested Reading

Buergelt CD, Carmichael JA, Tashjian RJ, Das KM. Spontaneous rupture of the left pulmonary artery in a horse with patent ductus arteriosus. J Am Vet Med Assoc 1970;157:313–320.

Carmichael JA, Buergelt CD, Lord PF, et al. Diagnosis of patent ductus arteriosus in a horse. J Am Vet Med Assoc 1971;158:767–775.

Glazier DB, Farrelly BT, Neylon JF. Patent ductus arteriosus in an eight-months-old foal. Irish Vet J 1974;28:12–13.

Reef VB. Cardiovascular ultrasonography. In: Reef VB, ed. Equine diagnostic ultrasound. Philadelphia: WB Saunders, 1998:215–272.

Scott EA, Kneller SK, Witherspoon DM. Closure of ductus arteriosus determined by cardiac catheterization and angiography in newborn foals. Am J Vet Res 1975;36:1021–1023.

Author Virginia B. Reef
Consulting Editor N/A

PATENT URACHUS

BASICS

OVERVIEW

A congenital or acquired failure of urachal closure, with resultant urine leakage through the umbilical stalk

SIGNALMENT

- Congenital form—seen when the urachus fails to close within 24 hours postpartum
- Acquired form—seen within the first 1–3 weeks of life in foals that underwent normal retraction and urachal closure postpartum
- No breed or sex predispositions

SIGNS

- The hallmark of this condition is urine flowing or dribbling from the umbilical remnant, which is permanently moist.
- Moist dermatitis or urine scalding may be present on the ventral abdomen or insides of the hind limbs.
- When complicated by bacterial invasion, fever, lethargy, and purulent umbilical exudate may be seen.

CAUSES AND RISK FACTORS

- Pathophysiology of the congenital form—unknown
- Acquired forms—excessive tension on the ventral abdominal musculature (e.g., prolonged recumbency, tenesmus, or abdominal distension) or umbilical inflammation (e.g., septic omphalophlebitis or generalized neonatal septicemia)

DIAGNOSIS

DIFFERENTIAL DIAGNOSIS

- Umbilical herniation may cause a similar ventral abdominal swelling, but affected animals are otherwise healthy (in uncomplicated cases), with no clinicopathologic abnormalities, a normally involuted umbilical stalk, and no urine leakage.
- The purulent nature of the umbilical drainage and systemic signs of septic inflammation differentiate umbilical abscessation; retrograde contrast cystography shows normal voiding of urine.

CBC/BIOCHEMISTRY/URINALYSIS

- Congenital form—usually no clinicopathologic abnormalities
- Complicated congenital or acquired forms involving bacterial invasion—leukocytosis with neutrophilia, toxic changes within WBCs, and hyperfibrinogenemia

OTHER LABORATORY TESTS

N/A

IMAGING

- Retrograde contrast cystoscopy—A definitive diagnosis may be reached using 100 mL of a 10-parts water to one-part iodinated radiographic contrast medium instilled into the previously catheterized bladder.
- Transabdominal ultrasonography revealing vesicourachal patency is also confirmatory; this modality also is useful in detecting abscess formation.

DIAGNOSTIC PROCEDURES

Aerobic and anaerobic bacterial cultures of aseptically collected urine samples are useful in determining appropriate antibiotic therapy, when indicated.

TREATMENT

MEDICAL

- Usually involves keeping the umbilical structures clean and disinfected using 0.5% chlorhexidine or 2% iodine solutions two or three times a day.
- Cauterizing the urachal lining using silver nitrate sticks may promote an inflammatory response and assist in closure; this technique may cause significant inflammation of the umbilical area and skin of the ventral abdomen.

SURGICAL

- Chosen in cases with no response to medical therapy after 5 days, with evidence of bacterial infection of the umbilical remnant, or in some septicemic patients.
- Complete resection of the umbilical remnant and all associated infected structures

PATENT URACHUS

MEDICATIONS

DRUGS

- Local injection of procaine penicillin two to three times daily for up to 5 days may be beneficial.
- System antibiotic therapy as dictated by results of bacterial culture and sensitivity.

CONTRAINDICATIONS/POSSIBLE INTERACTIONS

High-concentration solutions of iodine may result in inflammation and necrosis of the umbilical structures.

FOLLOW-UP

PATIENT MONITORING

- Examine patients daily for urine leakage, fever, and umbilical swelling.
- Perform repeat ultrasonography to re-evaluate the internal umbilical structures for infection.

PREVENTION/AVOIDANCE

- Other systemic problems, such as sepsis and neonatal maladjustment syndrome (hypoxic-ischemic encephalopathy), lead to prolonged recumbency, which predisposes to patent urachus.
- Attention to umbilical care, both in disinfection and in keeping structures as dry as possible.

POSSIBLE COMPLICATIONS

Septic omphalophlebitis

EXPECTED COURSE AND PROGNOSIS

- Congenital—most cases resolve quickly after medical therapy alone.
- Acquired or cases complicated by bacterial infection—patients survive more frequently and with less morbidity if treated using surgery and antibiotics than those treated using antibiotics alone.

MISCELLANEOUS

ASSOCIATED CONDITIONS

- Generalized neonatal septicemia
- Septic omphalophlebitis

SEE ALSO

- Omphalophlebitis
- Septicemia

Suggested Reading

Robertson JT, Embertson RS. Congenital and perinatal abnormalities of the urogenital tract. Vet Clin North Am Equine Pract 1988;4:359.

Author Enda Currid
Consulting Editor Mary Rose Paradis

PENILE LACERATIONS

BASICS

DEFINITION
Any wound to the penile epithelial surface.

PATHOPHYSIOLOGY
N/A

SYSTEMS AFFECTED
- Reproductive
- Urinary

SIGNALMENT
No age or breed predilection.

SIGNS
N/A

CAUSES
Trauma—Breeding accidents, improperly fitted stallion rings, kicks, jumping injuries, masturbation, and improper surgical technique.

RISK FACTORS
Aggressive stallions/colts housed or handled in unsafe conditions are more likely to injure themselves and others.

DIAGNOSIS

DIFFERENTIAL DIAGNOSIS

Differentiating Causes

- Visual inspection generally reveals the laceration.
- Paraphimosis may be present, but may be secondary to the laceration.
- Ulcerative lesions caused by neoplastic or parasitic diseases should not be considered lacerations for this discussion.

CBC/BIOCHEMISTRY/URINALYSIS
N/A

OTHER LABORATORY TESTS
N/A

IMAGING
N/A

DIAGNOSTIC PROCEDURES
N/A

TREATMENT

- Ensure urethral patency. Placement of a urinary catheter may be indicated.
- Cleanse and debride the wound as dictated by location and severity.
- Acute post-trauma lacerations can be sutured for first intention healing.
- Old or grossly contaminated lacerations may have to heal by second intention, or delayed closure can be considered.
- Support the penis and prepuce with slings, hydrotherapy, and judicious exercise to prevent or eliminate extensive dependent edema.
- Sexual stimulation is absolutely contraindicated until healing is complete.

MEDICATIONS

DRUG(S) OF CHOICE
- NSAIDs including phenylbutazone (2–4 g/450 kg/day P/O) or flunixine meglumine (1 mg/kg/day IV, IM, or P/O) for patient comfort and to decrease inflammation.
- Systemic or local antibiotics for local infections and to prevent septicemia, if indicated.

CONTRAINDICATIONS
Phenothiazine tranquilizers should never be used in the intact male.

PRECAUTIONS
N/A

POSSIBLE INTERACTIONS
N/A

ALTERNATIVE DRUGS
N/A

PENILE LACERATIONS

FOLLOW-UP

PATIENT MONITORING

- If the penis can be maintained within the prepuce without support, less frequent evaluation is necessary.
- If retraction of the penis is not possible, hospitalization may be required for frequent evaluation and care of the exposed penis.

POSSIBLE COMPLICATIONS

- Urine leakage with extensive tissue necrosis is possible if the penile urethra has been lacerated.
- Wounds that cannot be treated surgically are usually complicated by suppuration and cellulitis.
- Scar formation can result in phimosis, erectile dysfunction, impotence, or infertility.
- Hematomas generally arise from blood vessels superficial to the tunica albuginea. A hematoma that continues to enlarge is more likely attributable to a rent in the tunica albuginea, and closure of that defect is a priority.
- Paraphimosis is a common sequela to penile lacerations.
- Penile paralysis is possible as a result of the injury itself or secondary to paraphimosis.

MISCELLANEOUS

ASSOCIATED CONDITIONS

- Hemospermia
- Impotence
- Paraphimosis
- Penile paralysis
- Phimosis

AGE-RELATED FACTORS

N/A

ZOONOTIC POTENTIAL

N/A

PREGNANCY

N/A

SYNONYMS

N/A

SEE ALSO

- Erection failure
- Paraphimosis
- Penile paralysis
- Phimosis
- Semen abnormalities

ABBREVIATIONS

N/A

Suggested Reading

Schumacher J, Vaughan JT. Surgery of the penis and prepuce. In: Veterinary Clinics of North America: Equine Practice 1988;4:443-449.

Vaughan JT. Penis and prepuce. In: Equine reproduction. McKinnon AO and Voss JL, ed. Philadelphia: Lea & Febiger 1993;885-894.

Author Carole C. Miller

Consulting Editor Carla L. Carleton

PENILE PARALYSIS

BASICS

DEFINITION
Extrusion of the penis in a flaccid state.

PATHOPHYSIOLOGY
Injury to the sacral nerves that innervate the penis and/or the retractor penis muscle results in the inability to retract the penis into the prepuce.

SYSTEM AFFECTED
Reproductive

SIGNALMENT
Stallions (predominantly) or geldings of any age.

SIGNS
N/A

CAUSES
- Trauma: direct penile trauma, spinal cord injury, or disease.
- Infectious disease: EHV-1, rabies, EIA, purpura hemorrhagica, dourine (*Trypanosoma equiperdum*).
- Drug-induced: propiopromazine, acepromazine maleate, reserpine.

RISK FACTORS
- Chronic paraphimosis or priapism
- Exhaustion or starvation
- Spinal cord lesions

DIAGNOSIS

DIFFERENTIAL DIAGNOSIS

Differentiating Similar Signs
- Paraphimosis results in prolapse of the penis and prepuce, and dependent edema develops. The inability to retract the penis is generally due to the accumulated edema rather than true penile paralysis.
- Penile paralysis can be a sequela to chronic, severe paraphimosis. Long-standing penile paralysis can present as paraphimosis due to the formation of extensive dependent edema.
- Priapism, a persistent erection with engorgement of the CCP, should not be confused with penile paralysis, in which the penis is flaccid.

Differentiating Causes
- The presence of neurologic deficits other than the penile paralysis may link the penile problem with infectious causes and/or spinal cord injury as the primary problem.
- A recent history of respiratory disease (affected horse or on its farm) may implicate EHV-1 as a possible cause.

CBC/BIOCHEMISTRY/URINALYSIS
N/A

OTHER LABORATORY TESTS

EHV-1
Rising antibody titers from paired sera, collected at a 14–21 day interval; virus isolation from nasopharyngeal swabs in the acute stage of the disease.

EIA
AGID (Coggins) test

Dourine
Identification of the causative agent in urethral exudates; serologic testing by CF. Note: This disease has been eradicated from North America and Europe.

IMAGING
N/A

DIAGNOSTIC PROCEDURES
N/A

TREATMENT
- Replace the penis in the prepuce as soon as possible to prevent accumulation of dependent edema, drying of exposed surfaces, and traumatic injury. If replacement is impossible due to swelling, slings can be used to support the penis against the ventral abdominal wall.
- Lubricate the exposed mucosal surfaces with an emollient or antimicrobial ointment.
- Surgical intervention, including penile amputation or penile retraction (Bolz technique), should be considered in cases of chronic, non-responsive penile paralysis. Castration generally precedes these surgical techniques.

PENILE PARALYSIS

MEDICATIONS

DRUG(S) OF CHOICE

Anti-inflammatory medication (phenylbutazone, 2–4 g/450 kg/day, P/O) may be useful for patient comfort and to decrease inflammation.

CONTRAINDICATIONS

Phenothiazine tranquilizers should be avoided.

PRECAUTIONS

N/A

POSSIBLE INTERACTIONS

N/A

ALTERNATIVE DRUGS

N/A

FOLLOW-UP

PATIENT MONITORING

Initial management is intensive and frequent evaluation is of paramount importance. Return of the ability to maintain the penis in the prepuce is a good prognostic indicator.

POSSIBLE COMPLICATIONS

- Libido is often maintained, but if erection is impossible, it precludes live cover.
- Some affected stallions can still be trained to ejaculate into an AV or by an alternate system, e.g., application of hot compresses to the penis, semen collection into a bag.
- Possible secondary complications of paralysis:
  - Paraphimosis due to the accumulation of dependent edema.
  - Frostbite due to exposure.
  - Surface excoriations (ulcers, secondary bacterial contamination, necrosis)

MISCELLANEOUS

ASSOCIATED CONDITIONS

- Paraphimosis
- Balanoposthitis

AGE-RELATED FACTORS

N/A

ZOONOTIC POTENTIAL

N/A

PREGNANCY

N/A

SYNONYMS

N/A

SEE ALSO

- Priapism
- Paraphimosis
- Respiratory disease, infectious
- Stallion-like behavior

ABBREVIATIONS

- AGID = agar gel immunodiffusion
- AV = artificial vagina
- CF = complement fixation

Suggested Reading

Memon MA, Usenik EA, Varner DD, Meyers PJ. Penile paralysis and paraphimosis associated with reserpine administration in a stallion. Theriogenology 1988;30:411-419.

Neely DP. Physical examination and genital disease of the stallion. In: Current therapy in theriogenology. Morrow DA, ed. Philadelphia: WB Saunders Co. 1980;694-706.

Vaughan JT. Surgery of the penis and prepuce. In: Bovine and equine urogenital surgery. Walker DF and Vaughan JT, ed. Philadelphia: Lea & Febiger, 1980;125-144.

Wheat JD. Penile paralysis in stallions given propiopromazine. J Am Vet Med Assoc 1966;148:405-406.

Author Carole C. Miller

Consulting Editor Carla L. Carleton

PENILE VESICLES, EROSIONS, AND TUMORS

BASICS

DEFINITION
Any vesicular, ulcerative, or proliferative lesion associated with the penis or preputial folds.

PATHOPHYSIOLOGY
• Equine herpesvirus type 3 (EHV-3) is a relatively benign viral venereal disease of horses. The incubation period is typically 4–7 days. No proof of a non-clinically apparent carrier state exists. As with other herpes infections, virus recrudescence and formation of a new population of vesicles (infective stage) is associated with stress.
• Habronemiasis occurs when larvae of stomach nematodes are deposited on moist mucosal surfaces by stable flies. The larvae cause an influx of eosinophils to the affected tissues, resulting in granulomatous reactions and intense pruritis.
• Neoplasia—Appearance and progression vary with the type and size of neoplasia.

SYSTEMS AFFECTED
• Reproductive
• Urinary
• Lymphatic
• Dermatologic

SIGNALMENT
Any age and breed can be affected.

SIGNS
Historical Findings
Most lesions are slow-growing. Size, location, and presentation of the lesions vary. Dysuria or hematuria may be observed.

Physical Examination Findings
• Lesions may be visible on the penis, prepuce, urethral process, or in the fossa glandis. Other mucocutaneous junctions may also be affected.
• Phimosis due to stricture formation, adhesions, or tumor proliferation can be observed.
• Paraphimosis due to secondary edema formation or mechanical impedance may be present.
• Hematuria or hemospermia may be present.
• Enlargement of local lymphatics or draining sinuses may be observed.

CAUSES
• Viral infections: EHV-3
• Parasites: Habronemiasis
• Neoplasia: SCC, sarcoid, melanoma, papilloma, hemangioma
• Trauma: chronic wounds, local irritants
• Bacteria: abscessation like that associated with bastard strangles

RISK FACTORS
• Because coital exanthema is a venereal disease, natural breeding programs are more likely to have an outbreak than programs using AI. Similarly, unsanitary breeding practices can put the patients at greater risk.
• Unsanitary housing conditions or poor fly control can contribute to habronemiasis. It is more often seen in hot, humid locations in the spring or summer seasons.

DIAGNOSIS

DIFFERENTIAL DIAGNOSIS
Differentiating Causes
• EHV-3 infection: typical presentation is of multiple, circular, 1–2 mm nodules that progress into vesicles and pustules and ultimately rupture to form ulcerations 5–10 mm in diameter on the penile/preputial mucosa. Systemic involvement is rare, although lesions have been found on other mucocutaneous junctions in some cases.
• Habronemiasis: Bollinger's granules, caseous masses in the exuberant granulation tissue, are diagnostic for habronemiasis. Lesions typically are extremely pruritic. *Summer sores,* the characteristic lesion, most often occur in the area of the urethral process or on the preputial ring.
• Neoplastic lesions can be either ulcerative or proliferative: SCC is locally invasive, although it can metastasize to regional lymph nodes. Biopsy should be used to confirm possible neoplasia.
• Chronic traumatic lesions can mimic any other disease process. Diagnosis is established by history, exclusion, or response to therapy.

CBC/BIOCHEMISTRY/URINALYSIS
N/A

OTHER LABORATORY TESTS
• Virus isolation from vesicular aspirates can confirm EHV-3.
• Rising antibody titers for EHV-3 can also be detected from paired sera collected at a 14–21 day interval.

IMAGING
N/A

DIAGNOSTIC PROCEDURES
• Cytology: intranuclear inclusion bodies are indicative of EHV-3.
• Biopsy and histopathology can distinguish between the various tumor types and habronemiasis.

TREATMENT
• Coital exanthema is a self-limiting disease with a course of disease of 3–5 weeks. The lesions can be quite uncomfortable, and secondary bacterial infections can occur. Daily cleansing and the application of emollient or antimicrobial ointments may be indicated for these reasons. Sexual rest while vesicles form, rupture, and until they heal prevents transmission.
• Therapy for habronemiasis includes eradicating the infective larvae as well as controlling the local hypersensitivity reaction. Surgical resection of residual scar tissue may be necessary.
• Once diagnosed, tumors may be surgically excised, or eliminated with cryosurgery, radiation therapy, hyperthermia, reefing, or phallectomy, dependent upon their size, location, invasiveness, and type.
• Chronic wounds should be cleansed, debrided, and closed, when possible. Local irritants (i.e., povidone iodine scrub) should be thoroughly rinsed off after application, if used.
• Streptococcal infections should be treated with systemic antibiotics.

PENILE VESICLES, EROSIONS, AND TUMORS

MEDICATIONS

DRUG(S) OF CHOICE

• Habronema larvae can be eradicated using ivermectin (200 mg/kg P/O). Steroids have been used to diminish localized pruritic reactions (prednisone, 0.25–1.0 mg/kg P/O, SID initially, then decreasing to the minimum effective dose).
• NSAIDs including phenylbutazone (2–4 g/450 kg/day P/O) or flunixine meglumine (1 mg/kg/day IV, IM, or P/O) are useful for symptomatic treatment of discomfort and to reduce local inflammation.
• Systemic (Procaine penicillin G, 20,000–22,000 IU/kg IM, BID) or local (0.2% nitrofurazone ointment) antibiotics are used to treat primary or secondary bacterial infection.

CONTRAINDICATIONS

N/A

PRECAUTIONS

• Chronic steroid use can result in iatrogenic Cushing's disease and may predispose the patient to developing laminitis due to systemic vasoconstrictive action.
• Phenothiazine tranquilizers should be used with caution, or not at all, due to the possibility of their causing priapism in intact stallions.

POSSIBLE INTERACTIONS

N/A

ALTERNATIVE DRUGS

• Trichlorfon (22 mg/kg diluted in 1–2 liters 0.9% NaCl, slow IV) has been used to eliminate habronema larvae. There is risk of clinical toxicity.
• Topical application of trichlorfon in 0.2% nitrofurazone once daily to granulomatous lesions can be effective in the acute stage of habronemiasis.

FOLLOW-UP

PATIENT MONITORING

The frequency of re-evaluation depends upon the inciting cause and severity of the lesion.

POSSIBLE COMPLICATIONS

• Chronic *Habronema* spp. infection involving the urethral process can result in periurethral fibrosis; if severe, it will necessitate amputation of the urethral process.
• Paraphimosis
• Phimosis
• Metastatic lesions in local lymph or lung tissues

MISCELLANEOUS

ASSOCIATED CONDITIONS

N/A

AGE-RELATED FACTORS

• Young horses are more likely to present with papillomatous lesions.
• Gray horses are the most likely color pattern to present with melanoma.
• Lightly pigmented horses are more likely to have SCC, and geldings may be affected more often than stallions.

ZOONOTIC POTENTIAL

N/A

PREGNANCY

Coital exanthema does not cause abortion.

SYNONYMS

• EHV-3
• Equine coital exanthema
• Equine venereal balanitis
• Genital horse pox
• Habronemiasis
• Swamp cancer
• Genital bursatti
• Esponja
• Summer sores

SEE ALSO

• Equine dermatology/neoplasia
• Equine venereal diseases
• Paraphimosis
• Penile lacerations
• Phimosis

ABBREVIATIONS

• AI = artificial insemination
• EHV = equine herpesvirus
• SCC = squamous cell carcinoma

Suggested Reading

Couto MA, Hughes JP. Sexually transmitted (venereal) diseases of horses. In: Equine reproduction. McKinnon AO and Voss JL, ed. Philadelphia: Lea & Febiger, 1993;845-854.

Schumacher J, Varner DD. Surgical correction of abnormalities affecting the reproductive organs of stallions. In: Current therapy in large animal theriogenology. Youngquist RS, ed. Philadelphia: WB Saunders, 1997;24-36.

Vaughan JT. Penis and prepuce. In: Equine reproduction. McKinnon AO and Voss JL, ed. Philadelphia: Lea & Febiger, 1993;885-894.

Vaughan JT. Surgery of the penis and prepuce. In: Bovine and equine urogenital surgery. Walker DF and Vaughan JT, ed. Philadelphia: Lea & Febiger, 1980;125-144.

Author Carole C. Miller
Consulting Editor Carla L. Carleton

PENTACHLOROPHENOL (PCP) TOXICOSIS

BASICS

OVERVIEW

- PCP causes uncoupling of oxidative phosphorylation and direct irritation of the skin and respiratory tract.
- Acute and chronic intoxication syndromes have been described in animals.
- Chronic syndrome may result from PCDD and PCDF isomers in PCP.
- Restrictions on use of PCP because of environmental and toxicity concerns make exposure and toxicosis unlikely.

SIGNALMENT

N/A

SIGNS

Acute

- Hyperthermia
- Restlessness
- Tachypnea
- Increased GI motility
- Weakness
- Seizures
- Collapse

Chronic

- Anorexia
- Weight loss
- Dependent edema
- Alopecia
- Skin cracks and fissures
- Colic
- Joint stiffness
- Recurrent hoof problems
- Conjunctivitis
- Hematuria
- Secondary opportunistic infections

CAUSES AND RISK FACTORS

- Most likely source of exposure—treated wood used for fences or feedbunks
- Exposure to bedding made from treated wood

DIAGNOSIS

DIFFERENTIAL DIAGNOSIS

- Acute—infectious causes of pyrexia (CBC, bacterial culture, serology)
- Chronic—*Vicia villosa* toxicosis (skin biopsy)

CBC/BIOCHEMISTRY/URINALYSIS

- Acute—not reported for horses
- Chronic—changes consistent with hepatic dysfunction, anemia, and thrombocytopenia

OTHER LABORATORY TESTS

Acute

- Antemortem—detection of PCP in blood, serum/plasma, or urine; PCP is cleared rapidly, so measurement is useful only with acute intoxications.
- Postmortem—detection of PCP in skin, liver, or kidney

Chronic

Measurement of PCDD or PCDF isomers in plasma/serum or tissues

IMAGING

N/A

DIAGNOSTIC PROCEDURES

N/A

PATHOLOGIC FINDINGS

Acute

Not reported for horses

Chronic

- Gross findings—emaciation; alopecia; crusty, scaly dermatitis; skin cracks or fissures that exude clear, serum-like fluid; splenomegaly
- Histopathologic findings—chronic, nonsuppurative dermatitis; hepatic bile duct proliferation, inflammation, and focal necrosis; splenic hemosiderosis; multifocal renal tubular necrosis; nonregenerative bone marrow

TREATMENT

ACUTE

- Control hyperthermia.
- Remove animal from source of exposure.
- With recent oral exposure, consider GI decontamination.
- Wash exposed skin.

CHRONIC

- Remove animal from source of exposure.
- Symptomatic and supportive care

PENTACHLOROPHENOL (PCP) TOXICOSIS

MEDICATIONS

DRUGS

Acute—AC (2–5 mg/kg PO in water slurry [1 g of AC in 5 mL of water]) and either magnesium sulfate (250 mg/kg PO) or sorbitol (70%) at 3 mL/kg PO, given once with AC

CONTRAINDICATIONS/POSSIBLE INTERACTIONS

N/A

FOLLOW-UP

PATIENT MONITORING

N/A

PREVENTION/AVOIDANCE

- Avoid use of treated wood where animal contact is possible.
- Current environmental restrictions on use of PCP make clinically significant exposure and toxicosis unlikely.

POSSIBLE COMPLICATIONS

N/A

EXPECTED COURSE AND PROGNOSIS

Poor prognosis and prolonged recovery in cases of chronic intoxication caused by dioxin.

MISCELLANEOUS

ASSOCIATED CONDITIONS

N/A

AGE-RELATED FACTORS

N/A

ZOONOTIC POTENTIAL

N/A

PREGNANCY

Chronic intoxication of pregnant horses with PCDD and PCDF can result in birth of weak foals susceptible to opportunistic infections.

SEE ALSO

N/A

ABBREVIATIONS

- AC = activated charcoal
- GI = gastrointestinal
- PCDD = dibenzo-*p*-dioxin isomers
- PCDF = dibenzofuran isomers

Suggested Reading

Kerkvliet NI, Wagner SL, Schmotzer WB, Hackett M, Schrader WK, Hultgren B. Dioxin intoxication from chronic exposure of horses to pentachlorophenol contaminated wood shavings. J Am Vet Med Assoc 1992;201:296–302

Author Robert H. Poppenga
Consulting Editor Robert H. Poppenga

PERICARDITIS

BASICS

DEFINITION
An inflammation in the pericardial sac resulting in accumulation of fluid (transudate or exudate), fibrin, or both in the pericardial sac

PATHOPHYSIOLOGY
Accumulation of pericardial fluid compromises cardiac filling; beginning with compromised right atrial and ventricular filling, followed by impaired left ventricular filling and decreased cardiac output, resulting in generalized venous distention and ventral edema.

SYSTEM AFFECTED
Cardiovascular

GENETICS
N/A

INCIDENCE/PREVALENCE
N/A

SIGNALMENT
N/A

SIGNS
General Comments
Horse usually are presented for colic.

Historical Findings
- Colic
- Fever
- Exercise intolerance

Physical Examination Findings
- Depression
- Lethargy
- Tachycardia
- Other, less common findings—anorexia; weight loss; fever; generalized venous distention; ventral, pectoral, or preputial edema; weak arterial pulse; pulsus paradoxus; atrial or ventricular premature beats; muffled heart sounds; pericardial friction rubs; and dull cranioventral lung field

CAUSES
- Septic—viral or bacterial
- Bacterial infections—most frequently *Streptococcal* sp.; less frequently *Actinobacillus* sp.
- Viral infections most frequently may result in immune-mediated pericarditis
- Idiopathic—many of these also may be immune mediated
- Neoplastic—rare

RISK FACTORS
- Pleuritis or pneumonia have been reported in several horses with pericarditis.
- Pericarditis may be secondary to the primary respiratory tract infection and be septic or immune mediated.

DIAGNOSIS

DIFFERENTIAL DIAGNOSIS
- Endocarditis—many horses have a murmur, heart sounds are not muffled, and pericardial friction rubs are absent; differentiate echocardiographically.
- Congestive heart failure—murmurs of valvular insufficiency usually are detected; differentiate echocardiographically.
- Cranial mediastinal abscess/mass—heart sounds usually are not muffled; no venous distention caudally; differentiate echocardiographically and ultrasonographically.

CBC/BIOCHEMISTRY/URINALYSIS
- Neutrophilic leukocytosis and hyperfibrinogenemia frequently are detected.
- Anemia of chronic disease may be present.
- With significant cardiac compromise and low cardiac output resulting from cardiac tamponade, prerenal azotemia may be present, with mildly elevated creatinine and BUN.

OTHER LABORATORY TESTS
- Virus isolation may be performed in horses with suspected active viremia as the cause of pericarditis.
- Paired serology may be performed, looking for a fourfold increase in titer to equine viruses.
- Elevated cardiac isoenzymes (i.e., cardiac troponin I, CK-MB, HBDH, or LDH 1 and 2) may be present with concurrent myocardial disease.
- Perform cytologic evaluation of pericardial fluid along with culture and sensitivity testing.
- Perform cytological evaluation of transtracheal aspirate and pleural fluid sample along with culture and sensitivity testing of the fluid obtained with suspected concurrent pleuritis or pneumonia.

IMAGING
Electrocardiography
- Diminished amplitude of complexes occurs with significant pericardial effusion.
- Electrical alternans occurs in some horses and is thought to be secondary to swinging of the heart in the fluid-filled sac.
- Atrial or ventricular premature depolarizations occasionally occur with associated epicarditis or myocarditis.

Echocardiography
- The pericardial sac usually is distended and filled with fluid and fibrin; the fluid is usually anechoic, with hypoechoic fibrin lining the epicardial surface and pericardial sac.
- Fibrinous loculations may be present, and the pericardial sac may be thickened.
- Occasionally, horses have a noneffusive pericarditis, with only a small amount of fibrin in the pericardial sac.
- Excessive swinging of the right ventricular free wall is present in horses with pericardial effusion.

- Right atrial and ventricular diastolic collapse (first visualized in the right ventricular outflow tract) occur early with the development of pericardial effusion.
- An inspiratory increase in right ventricle diameter and decrease in left ventricle diameter also occur in horses with cardiac tamponade.
- Abrupt cessation of ventricular filling during early diastole with diastolic flattening of the left ventricular free wall indicates constrictive pericarditis—rare in horses.

Diagnostic Ultrasonography

- Evaluation of the pleural space reveals an anechoic pleural effusion in most horses with pericarditis.
- In horses with pre-existing pleuropneumonia, consolidation of the pulmonary parenchyma, a pulmonary abscess, or a composite pleural fluid may be present.

Thoracic Radiography

- A globoid cardiac silhouette is detected but cannot be differentiated from other forms of cardiac enlargement.
- Increased ventral lung field opacity and a pleural fluid line may be detected in horses with pleuropneumonia.

DIAGNOSTIC PROCEDURES

Cardiac Catheterization

- Elevated central venous pressure in all horses with cardiac tamponade
- Elevated right atrial pressure with a preserved systolic *x* descent and absence of or a diminutive diastolic *y* descent
- Right ventricular and pulmonary arterial systolic pressures usually are elevated, as are pulmonary capillary wedge pressures.

Pericardiocentesis

- Perform with ultrasound guidance to obtain a sample for cytology and culture and sensitivity testing.
- If possible, insert a large-bore chest tube (26–32-F Argyle tube), and obtain the sample obtained at that time.
- After pericardial drainage and lavage, leave the large-bore chest tube in place.
- Obtain a sample of pleural fluid, if present, for cytology and culture and sensitivity testing.
- With suspected lower respiratory tract disease (e.g., pneumonia), obtain a transtracheal aspirate for cytology and culture and sensitivity testing.

PATHOLOGIC FINDINGS

- Fibrin coating the parietal and visceral pericardial surfaces along with the pericardial effusion
- A pleural effusion usually is present.
- Concurrent fibrinous pleuritis or pneumonia in some horses

TREATMENT

APPROPRIATE HEALTH CARE

- Use of a large-bore, indwelling pericardial tube for drainage and lavage and direct instillation of antimicrobials has been so successful that the pericardial tube should be inserted immediately if there is adequate space to do so safely.
- Obtain the sample for cytology and culture and sensitivity at the time the indwelling pericardial tube is inserted.
- If there is not enough fluid for safe insertion of a large-bore pericardial tube, treat the horse with broad-spectrum antimicrobials for possible septic pericarditis, and obtain a sample as soon as the indwelling tube can be safely inserted.
- After drainage of the pericardial sac, instill 1–2 L of isotonic saline into the pericardial sac, leave in place for 30–60 minutes, drain, and then instill 1 L of isotonic saline with 10–20 million IU of sodium penicillin and/or 1 g of gentamicin. Leave this second liter of isotonic saline containing antimicrobials in place until the next drainage 12–24 hours later. Repeat the process until the initial drainage consistently recovers less fluid than is left in the pericardial sac at the time of the last instillation. At that time, the indwelling pericardial tube can be removed, and the horse should continue to improve with broad-spectrum antimicrobial coverage or systemic corticosteroids, if a septic caused has been ruled out.
- Occasionally, little or no accumulation of fluid develops, and the pericarditis resolves without drainage.

NURSING CARE

N/A

ACTIVITY

Stall rest and hand walking during treatment for pericarditis and for several weeks after discontinuation of treatment.

DIET

N/A

PERICARDITIS

CLIENT EDUCATION

Closely monitor the horse after discontinuation of treatment for tachycardia, venous distention, or exercise intolerance; if detected, seek a cardiac re-evaluation.

SURGICAL CONSIDERATIONS

• Subtotal pericardiectomy has been tried in a horse with constrictive pericarditis but was not successful in the long term.
• Direct instillation of a large-bore chest tube into the pericardial sac with repeated drainage and lavage and direct instillation of the appropriate antimicrobials is more effective than surgical resection of part of the pericardial sac.

MEDICATIONS

DRUGS OF CHOICE

• Base the selection of antimicrobials for horses with septic pericarditis on culture and sensitivity results. Initially, until these results are available, IV bactericidal drugs (e.g., penicillin, gentamicin) are recommended for broad-spectrum coverage.
• The most common causative bacterial organisms in horses are *Streptococcal* sp., which are sensitive to penicillin, and Gram-negative organisms (usually *Actinobacillus* sp.), which usually are sensitive to gentamicin. The drugs can also be directly instilled into the pericardial sac after lavage and drainage, which increases the drug concentration locally.
• Once septic pericarditis has been successfully treated or ruled out, systemic corticosteroids may be administered to horses with idiopathic pericarditis.
• If septic pericarditis is diagnosed, antimicrobial treatment for 4–6 weeks is indicated.

CONTRAINDICATIONS

Do not use corticosteroids in horses with an active bacterial or viral cause of pericarditis.

PRECAUTIONS

• Place an IV catheter before pericardiocentesis or placement of an indwelling pericardial tube so that rapid antiarrhythmic treatment can be performed, if necessary.
• Monitor the horse electrocardiographically during pericardiocentesis and placement of a large-bore, indwelling chest tube to detect any cardiac arrhythmias induced during these procedures.

POSSIBLE INTERACTIONS

N/A

ALTERNATIVE DRUGS

• Base use of alternative drugs on results of culture and sensitivity testing of the pericardial fluid.
• With suspected septic pericarditis in a horse with pleuropneumonia and no growth obtained from culture and sensitivity testing of the pericardial fluid, the results obtained from a transtracheal aspirate or pleural fluid aspirate may be used, before the organisms likely are the same.
• With pinpoint hyperechoic echoes visualized consistent with free gas, suspect an anaerobic infection, and treat with metronidazole. Anaerobic pericarditis, however, is rare in horses.

FOLLOW-UP

PATIENT MONITORING

• Monitor heart rate, which should decrease gradually and return to normal with the presence of little or no pericardial fluid.
• Monitor peripheral veins, particularly the jugular, for venous distention and its severity. The generalized venous distention and ventral edema should gradually resolve with drainage of the pericardial sac.
• Amplitude of ECG complexes should gradually increase with reduction in the pericardial fluid surrounding the heart.
• Monitor for any arrhythmias during pericardiocentesis and while the indwelling pericardial tube is in place.
• Respiratory rate and temperature should return to normal as the pericarditis and any associated pleural effusion or pleuropneumonia resolve.
• Monitor WBC count, fibrinogen, and creatinine until they return to normal.

PREVENTION/AVOIDANCE

Aggressive treatment of horses with pleuropneumonia may prevent pericarditis secondary to pleuritis.

PERICARDITIS

POSSIBLE COMPLICATIONS

Horses with fibrinous pericarditis may develop constrictive pericarditis several months later secondary to scarring of the pericardial and epicardial surfaces and subsequent restriction to ventricular filling during late diastole.

EXPECTED COURSE AND PROGNOSIS

- Most horses with pericarditis treated aggressively with placement of an indwelling chest tube in the pericardial sac, pericardial lavage and drainage, direct instillation of appropriate antimicrobials, and broad-spectrum antibiotics or corticosteroids (if indicated) have an excellent prognosis for life and return to performance.
- The indwelling pericardial tube is not removed until less fluid is recovered than was left in place for the previous 12–24 hours; in most horses, this varies from 3–5 days.
- Broad-spectrum antimicrobials are continued until cytology and culture reveal no evidence of bacterial infection, after which corticosteroid therapy is initiated.
- With septic pericarditis, the horse should remain on IV bactericidal antimicrobials for at least 7–14 days, followed by a switch to appropriate oral antimicrobials for another 2–4 weeks. In most horses, the total length of antimicrobial treatment is at least 4–6 weeks. The horse then should receive another 4 weeks rest, followed by cardiac re-evaluation before returning the horse to work.
- In most horses, any echocardiographic evidence of pericarditis is difficult to detect 1 month after discontinuation of treatment.

MISCELLANEOUS

ASSOCIATED CONDITIONS

- Pleuritis and pleuropneumonia may result in direct extension of infection into the pericardial sac.
- The pericardium also may be involved in horses with cranial mediastinal lymphosarcoma, mesothelioma, and hemangiosarcoma.

AGE-RELATED FACTORS

- Pericarditis can occur at any age.
- In old horses, a neoplastic cause, although rare, must be considered.

ZOONOTIC POTENTIAL

N/A

PREGNANCY

- Pericarditis is not likely to develop in pregnant mares. If it does, however, it may result in fetal compromise if cardiac tamponade also is present.
- Aim treatment at successful drainage of the pericardial sac and restoration of normal cardiac output and organ perfusion.

SYNONYMS

N/A

SEE ALSO

- Cranial mediastinal abscess/mass
- Congestive heart failure—right sided
- Pleuritis
- Pleuropneumonia

ABBREVIATIONS

- CK-MB = MB isoenzyme of creatine kinase
- HBDH = α-hydroxybutyrate dehydrogenase
- LDH = lactate dehydrogenase

Suggested Reading

Bernard W, Reef VB, Clark ES, et al. Pericarditis in horses: six cases (1982–1986). J Am Vet Med Assoc 1990;196:468–471.

Freestone JF, Thomas WP, Carlson GP, et al. Idiopathic effusive pericarditis with tamponade in the horse. Equine Vet J 1987;19:38–42.

Hardy J, Robertson JT, Reed SM. Constrictive pericarditis in a mare: attempted treatment by partial pericardiectomy. Equine Vet J 1992;24:151–154.

Reef VB, Gentile DG, Freeman DE. Successful treatment of pericarditis in a horse. J Am Vet Med Assoc 1984;185:94–98.

Robinson JA, Marr CM, Reef VB, Sweeney RW. Idiopathic, aseptic, effusive, fibrinous, nonconstrictive pericarditis with tamponade in a Standardbred filly. J Am Vet Med Assoc 1992;201:1593–1598.

Worth LT, Reef VB. Pericarditis in horses: a review of 18 cases (1986–1995). J Am Vet Med Assoc 1998;212:248–253.

Author Virginia B. Reef
Consulting Editor N/A

PERINEAL LACERATIONS/RECTO-VAGINAL-VESTIBULAR FISTULAS

BASICS

DEFINITION

- A laceration of the perineal body
- First-degree laceration involves the mucous membrane of the vulva and skin.
- Second-degree laceration involves the next deeper layer of the vestibule and/or the vaginal wall, extending into the perineal body and deeper layers of the vulva.
- Third-degree laceration involves full-thickness tears through the perineal body, extending through the rectal wall and anal sphincter, and full-thickness tears through the vulva.
- Recto-vaginal-vestibular fistulas are full-thickness tears through the rectal wall and, possibly, involving the perineal body, but not involving the anal sphincter or vulva.
- Recto-vestibular fistulas are much more common than recto-vaginal fistulas.

PATHOPHYSIOLOGY

- Perineal lacerations occur at parturition because of abnormal posture or position of the fetus, which predisposes the fetal extremities to be pushed more dorsal than normal, thus forcing the fetal feet into and/or through the wall of the vagina or vestibule.
- Lacerations of the rectum or vagina can occur at breeding, but perineal lacerations are rare at this time.

SYSTEM AFFECTED

Reproductive

GENETICS

Only if the mare has inherited a narrowing of the vagina

INCIDENCE/PREVALENCE

- No statistics available regarding incidence
- Not rare, but infrequent

SIGNALMENT

- All breeds
- All of breeding age

SIGNS

General Comments

- The condition is not an emergency.
- Because of the tearing, bruising, and edema occurring at and after injury, delay correction of these lacerations until the initial inflammation has subsided—generally 30 days

Historical Findings

- The mare may have a history of assisted delivery, but this is not essential.
- Because of the excessive force developed by the abdominal musculature, it is possible for the mare to deliver a live foal unassisted while creating a perineal laceration.

Physical Examination Findings

Careful physical examination of the perineum, perineal body, vagina, and rectum, including transrectal palpation and vaginal examination.

CAUSES

- Abnormal posture or position of the fetus at parturition
- Fetal extremities are pushed more dorsal than normal within the birth canal, such that they penetrate and damage maternal soft-tissue structures within the vagina, vestibule, and/or rectum.

RISK FACTORS

- Late or term gestation and parturition
- Abnormal fetal position or posture
- Because fetal posture and position can change within minutes before parturition, examinations conducted much before birthing have little value.

DIAGNOSIS

DIFFERENTIAL DIAGNOSIS

N/A

CBC/BIOCHEMISTRY/URINALYSIS

N/A

OTHER LABORATORY TESTS

N/A

IMAGING

N/A

DIAGNOSTIC PROCEDURES

N/A

PATHOLOGIC FINDINGS

- Partial to full-thickness lacerations of the vestibule and/or vagina
- Aspiration of air into the vagina and/or uterus secondary to damaged normal barrier tissues—vulvar lips; vestibular sphincter
- Fecal contamination of the vagina and vestibule, followed by inflammation of the vestibule, vagina, cervix, and possibly, the endometrium

TREATMENT

APPROPRIATE HEALTH CARE

- Confirm whether the laceration extends into the peritoneal cavity—a rare occurrence with perineal laceration or recto-vaginal fistula
- Systemic antibiotics seldom are indicated or necessary to control infection in this area; client education is imperative.
- Local medication rarely is indicated.
- Repair lacerations before attempting to rebreed.
- Boost tetanus vaccination if not recent.

NURSING CARE

N/A

ACTIVITY

No restrictions

DIET

No restrictions

CLIENT EDUCATION

- Advise regarding the importance of close/frequent observation of foaling mares.
- Many lacerations occur before a problem is detected, even in the presence of trained foaling attendants.

SURGICAL CONSIDERATIONS

General Comments

- Surgical repair once the inflammation has subsided—minimum 30 days
- Imperative after surgery that feces remain soft until healing is complete.
- Early in the spring (preoperative), place the mare on pasture, and return it to pasture immediately after surgery. Green grass has a high moisture content, which should soften stool.
- Other methods of stool softening include bran and mineral oil but are not as effective in the author's opinion.

PERINEAL LACERATIONS/RECTO-VAGINAL-VESTIBULAR FISTULAS

Two-Stage Repair

Stage 1:

- Epidural anesthesia and sedation of the mare
- The tail is wrapped and elevated over the mare and attached to a support directly above the animal.
- The rectum and vagina/vestibule are emptied of feces and thoroughly but gently cleaned. Use of irritating scrubs could stimulate postoperative straining and is contraindicated.
- Reconstruction of the perineal body—an incision is made into the remaining shelf $\cong$ 2–3 cm anterior to the cranial limit of the laceration; the incision is continued posteriorly along the sides of the existing laceration in a plane approximately equal to the original location of the perineal body; the vestibular and vaginal mucosa is reflected ventrally $\cong$ 2 cm; simple interrupted sutures are placed through the area of the perineal body so that the perineal body is reapposed and the submucosal vaginal or vestibular tissue is brought together in the same suture pattern; after placement of one or two of these sutures, a continuous suture pattern is begun in the reflected mucosal membrane to oppose the submucosal surfaces; this suture pattern continues cranial to caudal, as additional simple interrupted sutures are placed.

Stage 2:

- Completed after healing of Stage 1.
- Debride the anal sphincter and dorsal vulvar commissure, and place sutures in these tissues to reestablish the sphincters, if possible.
- Optimal success is achieved if sphincter tone is regained after repair.

One-Stage Repair

Similar to two-stage repair, except that repairs of the anal sphincter and dorsal vulvar commissure are completed with the initial surgery.

MEDICATIONS

DRUGS OF CHOICE

- Systemic antibiotics may be indicated immediately after laceration to prevent possible systemic involvement, but the laceration must be quite severe to warrant their use.
- Medications specific to accomplish the surgical repair

CONTRAINDICATIONS

N/A

PRECAUTIONS

N/A

POSSIBLE INTERACTIONS

N/A

ALTERNATIVE DRUGS

Any agent designed for sedation and analgesia can be used during surgical correction.

FOLLOW-UP

PATIENT MONITORING

An immediate examination is indicated with the possibility or concern that a laceration has occurred. If confirmed, re-examine the area in $\cong$ 2 weeks to assess degree of inflammation and formation of granulation tissue at the laceration site.

PREVENTION/AVOIDANCE

Occurrence is difficult to predict and, thus, cannot prevent by other than not breeding a mare.

POSSIBLE COMPLICATIONS

- Abscesses may develop in the laceration area, but this is uncommon, aided in part by the abundant surface area that facilitates drainage and formation of granulation tissue from the deeper layers outward.
- If the laceration is sutured immediately after the occurrence, the potential for abscessation may actually increase.

EXPECTED COURSE AND PROGNOSIS

Without surgical correction, mares with third-degree lacerations and recto-vaginal fistulas have a very low probability of conceiving and maintaining a pregnancy to term; therefore, surgical correction is strongly recommended before attempted breeding.

MISCELLANEOUS

ASSOCIATED CONDITIONS

N/A

AGE-RELATED FACTORS

N/A

ZOONOTIC POTENTIAL

N/A

PREGNANCY

Occurs only after gestation and parturition.

SYNONYMS

N/A

SEE ALSO

- Delayed uterine involution
- Dystocia
- Prolonged pregnancy
- Urine pooling/urovagina

Suggested Reading

Aanes WA. Surgical repair of third degree perineal lacerations and recto-vaginal fistulas in the mare. J Am Vet Med Assoc 1964;144:485–491.

Belknap JK, Nickels FA. A one-stage repair of third-degree perineal lacerations and rectovestibular fistula in 17 mares. Vet Surg 1992;21:378–381.

Colbern GT, Aanes WA, Stashak TS. Surgical management of perineal lacerations and recto-vestibular fistulae in the mare: a retrospective study of 47 cases. J Am Vet Med Assoc 1985;186:265–269.

Heinze CD, Allen AR. Repair of third-degree perineal lacerations in the mare. Vet Scope 1966;11:12–15.

Stickle RL, Fessler JF, Adams SB, et al. A single stage technique for repair of recto-vestibular lacerations in the mare. J Vet Surg 1979;8:25–27.

Author Walter R. Threlfall

Consulting Editor Carla L. Carleton

PERIOCULAR SARCOID

BASICS

DEFINITION
A biologically benign, locally aggressive fibroblastic tumor with variable epithelial participation

PATHOPHYSIOLOGY
- The cause is unknown, but bovine papillomavirus has been implicated.
- A C-type retrovirus was isolated in one case, but a later study suggested this was an endogenous virus unrelated to sarcoid.
- There may be a predisposition associated with the MHC, because most affected horses express an equine lymphocytic antigen (A-13).
- Flies have been implicated as vectors for transfer of sarcoid cells between animals.

SYSTEMS AFFECTED
- Eyelids and periocular skin.
- Nonophthalmic equine sarcoid can affect any cutaneous area, but approximately 32% of tumors are located on the head and neck.

GENETICS
No proven genetic basis, but genes in or near the MHC are implicated as a predisposing factor.

INCIDENCE/PREVALENCE
- The most commonly reported equine tumor, but if only ocular/periocular equine tumors are considered, SCC is the most common.
- No reported geographic distribution

SIGNALMENT

Species
Horses, donkeys, and mules

Breed Predilections
Most studies report no breed predilections, but one reported that Quarter Horses have almost twice the risk as Thoroughbreds and that Standardbreds have a much lower risk relative to all other breeds.

Mean Age and Range
- Mean age—3–6 years
- Range—1–15+ years

Predominant Sex
No proven sex predilection

SIGNS

Historical Findings
- Single or multiple, pale, firm areas of dermal thickening in the eyelids or periocular region.
- Lesions may be ulcerated, and those affecting the eyelid margins or canthi may cause secondary tearing, squinting, or ocular discharge.
- Variable growth rate

Physical Examination Findings
- Nonspecific findings—serous to mucopurulent ocular discharge, blepharospasm, and conjunctival hyperemia
- Solitary or multiple areas of linear or focal dermal thickening in the eyelids or periocular skin
- Lesions may appear as nodules, papillomas, or pedunculated masses.
- Cutaneous ulceration and infection may be present.

CAUSES
- Viral causes have been suggested.
- A predisposition associated with genes on or near the MHC has been suggested.

RISK FACTORS
- Possible genetic risk factors
- Epizootics in herds suggest an infectious risk, possibly associated with fly vectors.

DIAGNOSIS

DIFFERENTIAL DIAGNOSIS
- Other tumors—SCC, papilloma, schwannoma, adenoma, adenocarcinoma, angiosarcoma, mastocytoma, melanocytoma, plasmacytoma, fibroma, and fibrosarcoma
- Parasites—*Habronema* sp.
- Inflammatory lesions—abscesses, granulation tissue, and foreign-body reactions

CBC/BIOCHEMISTRY/URINALYSIS
Usually normal.

OTHER LABORATORY TESTS
N/A

IMAGING
Skull radiography may be required if orbital or bony involvement is suspected

DIAGNOSTIC PROCEDURES
Biopsy

PATHOLOGIC FINDINGS
- Several morphologic types of sarcoid have been described. The verrucous (i.e., "warty") sarcoid usually is <6 cm in diameter and often has cauliflower edges. Lesions may be sessile and pedunculated or papillomatous, and cutaneous ulceration and infection may be present. The fibroblastic (i.e., "proud flesh") sarcoid varies from smooth, discrete nodules to large, pedunculated masses >20 cm. The mixed sarcoid is a combination of the previous two types.
- The tumor consists of a moderate to high density of fusiform or spindle-shaped, fibroblastic cells that form whorls, interlacing bundles, and haphazard arrays with one another.
- Cells vary from slender with elongated, pointed nuclei to plump with large, irregular, pleomorphic nuclei.
- Cytoplasmic boundaries are ill-defined, and the amount of collagen varies considerably.
- Low mitotic rate
- In many sarcoids, fibroblastic cells are oriented perpendicular to the overlying epithelial basement membrane.
- The epidermis, where present, often is hyperplastic, with elongated rete pegs extending down into the tumor.

TREATMENT

APPROPRIATE HEALTH CARE
- Very small, superficial lesions may be removed while standing with sedation and local anesthesia.
- Larger, more invasive lesions or those involving the eyelid margins or canthi may require hospitalization for surgery; alternatively, lesions may be treated under sedation and local anesthesia using intralesional chemotherapy or immunotherapy.

NURSING CARE
Protect the eye from self-trauma and secondary infection with a soft or hard cup hood.

ACTIVITY
Restrict during the immediate postoperative period.

DIET
N/A

CLIENT EDUCATION
- With intralesional chemotherapy, instruct the client to wear gloves when handling the periocular region for several days after injection.
- Make the client aware of clinical signs suggesting tumor recurrence.

SURGICAL CONSIDERATIONS
- Complete surgical excision of periocular sarcoid can be difficult or impossible, and recurrence rates of 50–64% have been reported with surgical excision alone. When combined with adjunctive therapy, however, success rates range from 65–95%.
- Various adjunctive therapies include cryotherapy, hyperthermia, carbon dioxide laser photoablation, topical chemotherapy, radiotherapy, and intralesional chemotherapy and immunotherapy.
- Reconstructive eyelid surgery may be necessary after excision.
- Cryotherapy uses temperatures of −20 to −40°C in a double freeze-thaw cycle to induce cryonecrosis of sarcoid cells. Reported success rates range from 60–100%.

- Radiofrequency hyperthermia has been reported to induce tumor regression when lesions are heated to 50°C for 30 seconds using a 2-MHz radiofrequency current. Multiple treatments may be necessary to prevent recurrence.
- One study reported an 81% success rate using carbon dioxide laser photoablation. Advantages included a clean, dry surgical site and a lack of postoperative pain and swelling.
- Interstitial brachytherapy using ^{192}Ir has reported success rates ranging from 87–94%. Radium 226 and ^{60}Co have also been used, with remission rates >60%. Gold 198 has a reported a remission rate of 83% and ^{222}Rn of 92%.

MEDICATIONS

DRUGS OF CHOICE

Topical and Intralesional Immunotherapy/Chemotherapy

- Daily topical applications of podophyllum or topical 5-FU (1% TID) have been used with inconsistent results.
- Intralesional chemotherapeutics including 5-FU and cisplatin have been used with success rates of ≅80%. Intralesional cisplatin is administered in four sessions at 2-week intervals using 1 mg/cm^3 of tumor; tumors ≤20 cm^3 may be treated using 3.3 mg/mL cisplatin (10 mg Platinol in 1 mL of water and 2 mL of purified, medical-grade sesame oil). Success rates are lower for intralesional xanthate and recombinant human TNF-α.
- Immunotherapy includes autogenous vaccines and immunomodulators using mycobacterial products. Use of autogenous vaccines involves transference of sarcoid tumors, tumor homogenates, or cell-free tumor extracts, and results vary. Immunomodulation using BCG-attenuated *Mycobacterium bovis* cell wall in oil, however, has remission rates approaching 100%. Using a 25-G hypodermic needle, 1 mL of BCG/cm^2 of tumor surface area is injected into the lesion. Therapy is repeated every 2–4 weeks for up to six injections. Anaphylaxis may occur but can be minimized with pretreatment using flunixin meglumine (1.1 mg/kg IV) and corticosteroids or diphenhydramine.

Antibiotics

- Topical and systemic antibiotics may be required to prevent infection after surgical and adjunctive therapy.
- A broad-spectrum ophthalmic antibiotic such as neomycin, polymyxin B, and bacitracin (Trioptic P) may be used for prophylactic therapy if lesions involve the eyelid margins or canthi; broad-spectrum systemic antibiotics such as trimethoprim/sulfamethazone (Tribrissen) also may be used.

Analgesic/Antiinflammatory Agents

- NSAIDs may be indicated after surgical excision or adjunctive therapy.
- Banamine (1.1 mg/kg) provides analgesic and anti-inflammatory effects and may reduce the incidence of anaphylaxis associated with intralesional immunotherapy.

CONTRAINDICATIONS

N/A

PRECAUTIONS

N/A

POSSIBLE INTERACTIONS

N/A

ALTERNATIVE DRUGS

N/A

FOLLOW UP

PATIENT MONITORING

- Observe for signs of anaphylaxis immediately after injection of immunomodulating agents.
- Long-term follow up includes monitoring for tumor recurrence or failure of tumor regression.

PREVENTION/AVOIDANCE

Fly control may reduce the incidence in herds with affected animals.

POSSIBLE COMPLICATIONS

- Tumor progression may lead to eyelid deformation, possibly resulting in secondary keratitis and conjunctivitis.
- Ulceration of lesions may lead to secondary bacterial or fungal infections and possible septicemia; myiasis also may be a problem.

EXPECTED COURSE AND PROGNOSIS

- Prognosis for survival generally is good for animals with single sarcoids, because these tumors do not metastasize.
- With numerous sarcoids (seen rarely in the United States and more commonly in the United Kingdom), prognosis for survival is poor.
- Factors affecting prognosis—tumor size, tumor location, degree of local invasiveness, and the number of tumors present.
- Recurrence rates after therapy depend on the modalities used; rates approach 100% for some.

MISCELLANEOUS

ASSOCIATED CONDITIONS

N/A

ZOONOTIC POTENTIAL

No proven zoonotic potential, but multiple occurrences in some herds suggest the possibility. If so, fly vectors may be involved, possibly necessitating fly control.

PREGNANCY

N/A

SYNONYMS

N/A

SEE ALSO

- Habronemiasis
- Ocular/adnexal squamous cell carcinoma

ABBREVIATIONS

- BCG = Bacillus Calmette-Guerin
- MHC = major histocompatibility complex
- SCC = squamous cell carcinoma
- TNF = tumor necrosis factor
- 5-FU = 5-fluorouracil

Suggested Reading

Brooks DE. Equine ophthalmology. In Gelatt KN, ed. Veterinary ophthalmology. 3rd ed. Philadelphia: Lippincott Williams & Wilkins, 1999.

Author Dennis Todd Strubbe

Consulting Editor Dennis E. Brooks

PERIODONTAL DISEASE

BASICS

DEFINITION

Periodontal disease encompasses those disorders occurring in the periodontium, which consists of the tissues surrounding and supporting the tooth, namely the periodontal ligament, the alveolus, and the gingiva.

PATHOPHYSIOLOGY

Normal tooth wear and masticatory forces are required for a healthy periodontium. Abnormalities to dental wear predispose horses to periodontal disease. These abnormalities include improperly shedded deciduous premolars; step-, shear-, or wave-mouth; missing or unopposed teeth; and hooks or ramps. Abnormalities in occlusion and altered masticatory habits result in unevenly distributed forces on the teeth that in turn results in separation of adjacent teeth. Food is driven between teeth, inciting a focal gingivitis. The gingivitis can progress to the development of a gingival sulcus. Continued food impaction and bacterial activity in gingival sulci result in destruction of the periodontal ligament and the alveolar bone, and consequently decreased support for the tooth. Infection can extend to the tooth root, resulting in a periapical abscess and necrosis of the tooth.

Hoses with mandibular or maxillary fractures can develop periodontal disease as a direct result of exposure of the periodontium to food material and as an indirect result of alterations to normal mastication.

The interdental spaces most commonly affected are between the second and third premolars and molars of both arcades and between the third and fourth premolars of the maxillary arcade. The gingivae on the buccal aspect of the maxillary teeth and the lingual aspect of the mandibular teeth are most often affected.

SYSTEMS AFFECTED

- Gastro-intestinal
- Musculo-skeletal
- Respiratory (maxillary sinusitis)

GENETICS

N/A

INCIDENCE/PREVALENCE

One study found evidence of periodontal disease in approximately one-third of 500 equine skulls. The incidence and severity of periodontal disease increases with age; in one study, the majority of horses >15 yr had periodontal disease.

SIGNALMENT

Some authors consider mares to be more susceptible to periodontal disease than geldings or stallions, but objective data are not available. Periodontal disease occurs more frequently in aged animals, but periodontal disease due to trauma or retained caps may occur in younger animals. Draft animals may be predisposed.

SIGNS

Horses with periodontal disease exhibit signs due to painful mastication, including eating slowly and excessive salivation, and they may be anorectic and lose weight. Horses may also have halitosis. Quidding may indicate aberrant mastication and periodontal disease. If secondary maxillary sinusitis is present, then purulent nasal discharge and facial swelling may be seen.

CAUSES

The cause of periodontal disease is any abnormality in tooth wear or mastication resulting in abnormal forces on the occlusal surfaces of teeth.

RISK FACTORS

Fractures involving the jaws may directly or indirectly predispose horses to periodontal disease.

The period in which deciduous teeth are shed is a period of relative risk for younger horses. At this time, eruption abnormalities may cause periodontal disease.

Aging results in abnormalities of dental wear that may cause periodontal disease. Various conformational abnormalities become more common in geriatric horses; in addition, as horses age there is progressive exposure of the tapered reserve crown, and consequently a less secure fit between adjacent teeth. Feed may become impacted between teeth, causing gingival hyperplasia and periodontal disease.

A diet consisting primarily of pelleted feed may decrease the normal extent of lateral excursions of the mandible with resultant abnormalities of dental wear.

DIAGNOSIS

DIFFERENTIAL DIAGNOSIS

Differential diagnoses to consider include other causes of dental sepsis, such as tooth root abscesses and infundibular necrosis; oral neoplasia; and non-neoplastic masses such as abscesses, granulomas, phycomycosis, habronemiasis, and pharyngeal cysts. Disease of the salivary glands should also be considered, such as sialodentitis, sialolithiasis, and salivary mucoceles.

CBC/BIOCHEMISTRY/URINALYSIS

Non-specific

OTHER LABORATORY TESTS

N/A

IMAGING

Radiographs of the teeth can detect destruction of the periodontal ligament as a loss of definition of the radiolucent ligament. Changes to the alveolus include bone lysis and production as well as clubbing of tooth roots in more advanced cases. Whereas septic processes in the maxilla tend to result in radiographically evident sclerosis, the mandible is more frequently characterized by radiolucency. Other radiographic abnormalities that may be detected in the periodontal tissues includes soft-tissue densities, the production of gas from bacterial fermentation, and fluid in the maxillary sinuses if the caudal three maxillary teeth are involved. The radiographic lesions described above are seen with dental sepsis. Periodontal disease is the early stages in a continuum of dental sepsis.

Computer aided tomography has been used to increase sensitivity of radiographic imaging, and nuclear scintigraphy has also been used to localize abscessation in the mandible and maxilla.

DIAGNOSTIC PROCEDURES

A thorough oral examination is required for diagnosis of periodontal disease. Visual examination and palpation of the gingiva can identify areas of swelling (edema), hyperemia, and pain. Gingival probes may be used to measure the extent of gingival sulci. Increased mobility of a tooth may be palpated; however, significant destruction of the support structures of the tooth is required for detection of a loose tooth by peroral palpation. This is a consequence of the extensive support from adjacent teeth.

PATHOLOGIC FINDINGS

Focal gingival hyperplasia appears histologically as inflamed, well-vascularized, fibrous connective tissue covered by epitheliomatous hyperplasia. Ulcerated sections may also be present. In more advanced cases, destruction of the periodontal ligament and osteitis of the alveolus are present.

TREATMENT

APPROPRIATE HEALTH CARE

The appropriate health care depends on the stage of the disease and the treatment options chosen. Dental floating (rasping) and extraction of loose teeth may be performed on an outpatient basis. However, extraction of the cheek teeth may require general anesthesia and elective surgical management. Lavage of gingival pockets has been reported for advanced periodontal disease, but the information on efficacy of this treatment is sparse.

NURSING CARE

N/A

PERIODONTAL DISEASE

ACTIVITY
N/A

DIET
Lateral excursion of the mandible, which is important for normal dental wear, is associated with fiber length. Therefore, adequate dietary roughage is important for the prevention of this periodontal disease. However, if periodontal disease is already present and extensive, a high-energy, pelleted diet may be required to provide adequate energy intake.

CLIENT EDUCATION
Periodontal disease is very common in older horses. Routine dental prophylaxis is the best method for preventing periodontal disease, whereas treatment of affected horses is limited. Horses at risk include young horses at the time of eruption of permanent teeth and geriatric horses. These horses may benefit from biannual dental prophylaxis.

SURGICAL CONSIDERATIONS
High-quality preoperative radiographs are useful for identifying affected teeth, and intra-operative radiographs are useful for confirming correct placement of the dental punch. Following tooth repulsion, the resulting defect can be packed with dental wax or a similar preparation to prevent exposure of feed material to the alveolus. This packing should be removed in 6–8 weeks. When tooth repulsion requires entry into a sinus, a flushing system may be installed postoperatively. Postoperative radiographs are useful to confirm complete removal of the affected tooth.

MEDICATIONS

DRUG(S) OF CHOICE
Antibiotics have been tried with little data available on their success. However, antibiotics are unlikely to halt the progression of this disease, and tooth removal is the only way of resolving clinical signs.

CONTRAINDICATIONS
N/A

PRECAUTIONS
N/A

POSSIBLE INTERACTIONS
N/A

ALTERNATIVE DRUGS
N/A

FOLLOW-UP

PATIENT MONITORING
Weight gain in horses with ill-thrift should be monitored and is often impressive following treatment of periodontal disease. Otherwise, a good appetite, without evidence of quidding or undigested grain in the feces should be noted following treatment.

PREVENTION/AVOIDANCE
Regular dental prophylaxis including dental floating can prevent the formation of dental conformational abnormalities as a result of abnormal wear. Feeding diets with adequate roughage may decrease abnormal dental wear.

POSSIBLE COMPLICATIONS
With conservative therapy, progression of the disease is common. Following tooth extraction, complications may include formation of a fistula between the oral cavity and a sinus, or externally through a trephination, and formation of a sequestrum from a piece of alveolus or tooth not extracted at surgery. The dental wax may become dislodged postoperatively and require replacement. The opposing tooth requires additional floating to ensure that it does not become too long (step-mouth), causing malocclusion and further periodontal disease.

EXPECTED COURSE AND PROGNOSIS
Conservative treatment consisting of regular dental floating and a diet with sufficient high-quality roughage may successfully manage periodontal disease. However, the condition is generally considered progressive and is completely resolved following tooth extraction. When the condition is extensive, removal of several teeth may not be practicable, and management with a high-energy diet and regular dental care should be considered palliative. Periodontal disease is likely to be a life-limiting condition in wild horses.

It is possible that mild periodontal disease in younger horses, with malocclusion due to abnormalities of permanent tooth eruption or mild abnormalities of dental wear, may be reversible following resolution of the underlying cause.

MISCELLANEOUS

ASSOCIATED CONDITIONS
Ill-thrift and weight loss are commonly associated with periodontal disease.

AGE-RELATED FACTORS
As horses age, the reserve crown is exposed and the gap between adjacent teeth increases. This increases the potential for feed to become impacted between adjacent teeth.

ZOONOTIC POTENTIAL
N/A

PREGNANCY
N/A

SYNONYMS
- Periodontitis
- Alveolar periostitis
- Alveolar osteitis
- Gingivitis

SEE ALSO
- Abnormal dental wear
- Dental sepsis

ABBREVIATIONS
N/A

Suggested Reading

Crabill MR, Schumacher J. Pathophysiology of acquired dental disease of the horse. Vet Clin North Am 1998;14:291-307.

Kirkland KD, Marretta SM, Inoue OJ, Baker GJ. Survey of equine dental disease and associated oral pathology. In: Proceedings of the 40th Annual Convention of the American Association of Equine Practitioners, Vancouver, BC, 1994;119-120.

Lane JG. A review of dental disorders of the horse, their treatment and a possible fresh approach to management. Equine Vet Educ 1994;6:13-21.

Mueller POE, Lowder MQ. Dental sepsis. Vet Clin North Am 1998;14:349-363.

Author Simon G. Pearce

Consulting Editor Henry Stämpfli

PERITONITIS

BASICS

OVERVIEW

The peritoneum is the mesothelial lining of the peritoneal cavity (parietal peritoneum) and the enclosed organs (visceral peritoneum). *Peritonitis* is defined as inflammation of the peritoneal cavity. Peritonitis may be primary or secondary and diffuse or localized. Peritonitis is caused by the presence of chemicals, infectious agents, or foreign matter within the peritoneal cavity. Inflammation involves the liberation of many mediators resulting in the decrease in vascular integrity and a flux of inflammatory cells, protein, red blood cells, and electrolytes into the peritoneal cavity. These components may help control the inciting cause (such as bacteria), but may also lead to adhesion or abscess formation if the disease becomes chronic. The disease may range from mild to severe, thereby causing hypovolemic and septic/toxic shock and, ultimately, death.

SYSTEMS AFFECTED

Gastrointestinal

- Decreased borborygmi
- Alterered gastrointestinal motility (impaction, diarrhea)
- Colic
- Other signs caused by primary disease

Musculoskeletal

- Splinting/guarding of abdomen
- Reluctance to move

Behavioral

- Depressed demeanor
- Lethargy
- Inappetance

Cardiovascular

- Mild to moderate tachycardia
- Prolonged capillary refill time
- Tacky mucous membranes
- Hyperemic mucous membranes

Respiratory

- Mild tachypnea
- Shallow respiration

Hemic/Lymphatic/Immune

- Neutrophilia
- Neutropenia
- Hypoproteinemia
- Hyperproteinemia
- Immunodeficiency

Hepatobiliary

N/A (unless primary disease, such as cholelithiasis, cholangitis, or hepatitis)

Renal/Urologic

- Hypovolemia
- Primary disease

Reproductive

Primary disease

Skin/Exocrine

Sweating

SIGNALMENT

Any age, breed, or sex

SIGNS

Primary Disease

- Depressed demeanor
- Inappetance
- Fever
- Altered gastrointestinal motility
- Distended abdomen
- Splinting or guarding of abdomen
- Mild colic
- Distended viscus; serosal fibrin deposition palpated per rectum

Secondary Disease

- Signs as listed previously
- Moderate to severe colic
- Evidence of trauma

CAUSES AND RISK FACTORS

Primary

- Hematogenous spread
- Immunocompromise (failure of passive transfer, combined immunodeficiency, transient immunodeficiency)

Secondary

- Loss of gastrointestinal integrity
- Gastroduodenal ulceration, right dorsal colitis
- Proximal enteritis, typhlitis, colitis
- Gastric or intestinal rupture due to distension/devitalization
- Vascular compromise thrombosis (*S. vulgaris* migration, idiopathic) or intestinal torsion/volvulus
- Trauma—iatrogenic (abdominal paracentesis, rectal tear, surgery), foaling, foreign body
- Loss of reproductive tract (vagina, cervix, uterus) integrity
- Breeding injury (natural service, iatrogenic)
- Foaling injury
- Wounds—penetrating (foreign body or surgical)
- Surgery—castration
- Abscess rupture
- Direct extension of other infection
- Urine leakage—bladder, urethra, kidney
- Hemorrhage—rupture/tearing of spleen, liver, ovary
- Neoplasia
- Parasite migration

DIAGNOSIS

DIFFERENTIAL DIAGNOSIS

Includes any pain-causing, inflammatory, or infectious disease involving the gastrointestinal system specifically, such as abdominal pain due to spasmodic colic, gas colic, enteritis, colitis, typhlitis, or other causes of colic (gastrointestinal impaction, displacement, intussusception, torsion, volvulus). Ovulation, uterine torsion, urinary tract obstruction, cholelithiasis, and cholangitis should also be considered. Non-abdominal diseases such as pleuropneumonia may also present with similar signs.

CBC/BIOCHEMISTRY/URINALYSIS

CBC

- Neutrophilia
- Neutropenia
- Hyperproteinemia
- Hypoproteinemia

Biochemistry

- Hypoproteinemia (early loss of protein into abdominal cavity), hyperproteinemia (subacute to chronic inflammation). Albumin levels may be normal or decreased. Globulin levels may be normal, decreased, or increased.
- Urinalysis—N/A (reflect hemoconcentration)

OTHER LABORATORY TESTS

Abdominal Paracentesis

- Appearance—Normal fluid is clear, colorless, or pale yellow; turbid fluid may have elevated protein, nucleated cells, or foreign material; green or brown fluid likely contains feed or fecal material.
- Cytology (collect into EDTA tube)—Normal fluid may contain nucleated cell count up to 10×10^9 nucleated cells/L (10^4 nucleated cells/μL). With peritonitis, there may be an elevated nucleated cell count, increased proportion of neutrophils, and the presence of toxic neutrophils. There may also be an elevated protein level (>25 g/L; >2.5 g/dL). The presence of bacteria (intracellular or extracellular), feed material, and spermatazoa is also supportive of the presence of peritonitis. Puncture of the bowel while attempting to collect peritoneal fluid may result in a false-positive interpretation.
- Culture and sensitivity (collect into clot tube)—Consider Gram stain and aerobic and anaerobic culture of fluid.

IMAGING

Radiographs

Radiographs are helpful in assessing foal abdomens or searching for foreign bodies in adult horses.

Ultrasound

Ultrasound is a useful tool in evaluating foal and adult abdomens. Select areas can be evaluated. Hyperechoic fluid may have high cell count, protein level, or feed/fecal material. Can also assess presence of fibrin deposition and peripheral abscess formation.

TREATMENT

- Resolve primary problem
- Abdominal drainage or lavage (standing horse)
- Abdominal exploration and lavage (anesthetized horse)
- Fluid therapy (crystalloid fluid)
- Protein replacement (plasma, other oncotic agents)
- Laminitis prophylaxis

MEDICATIONS

DRUG(S) OF CHOICE

Antibiotic Therapy

- Broad-spectrum initially (consider parenteral penicillin, cephalosporin, and aminoglycoside); metronidazole should be used if anaerobic bacteria (especially *Bacteroides fragilis*) is suspected
- Antibiotic therapy—Adjust to sensitivity pattern of organisms isolated in culture
- Non-steroidal anti-inflammatory medications (analgesia, decrease effects of toxins)

CONTRAINDICATIONS/POSSIBLE DRUG INTERACTIONS

- Corticosteroids are contraindicated in peritonitis because a bacterial infection is usually present.
- Aminoglycoside antibiotics such as gentamicin should be used with caution because nephrotoxicity may occur in the dehydrated animal. Any fluid and metabolic deficits should be corrected and the animal monitored for urination. Periodic assessment of urine, serum creatinine, and serum BUN levels is recommended. Once-daily dosing may be advantageous.

ALTERNATIVE DRUGS

Trimethoprim–sulfonamide (enteral or parenteral); potentiated penicillins (amoxicillin/sulbactam) may be useful.

FOLLOW-UP

PATIENT MONITORING

Periodic peritoneal fluid analysis (every 2–3 days or if the patient does not show any improvement). Improvement may also be noted with normalization of blood parameters (WBC count, protein level, fibrinogen level).

POSSIBLE COMPLICATIONS

Laminitis and thrombophlebitis are the most common complications. Abscess formation and adhesion formation may also occur, resulting in a failure to thrive and colic, respectively.

MISCELLANEOUS

ASSOCIATED CONDITIONS

N/A

AGE-RELATED FACTORS

Immunodeficiency in the neonate.

ZOONOTIC POTENTIAL

N/A

PREGNANCY

Peritonitis in a pregnant animal may cause loss of the fetus. Antibiotics (gentamicin, metronidazole) and non-steroidal anti-inflammatory agents may affect the fetus.

SYNONYMS

N/A

SEE ALSO

Colic

ABBREVIATIONS

N/A

Suggested Reading

Hawkins JF et al. Peritonitis in horses: 67 cases (1985–1990). J Am Vet Med Assoc 1993;203:284-288.

Author Daniel G. Kenney

Consulting Editor Henry Stämpfli

PETECHIA, ECCHYMOSES, AND BRUISING

BASICS

DEFINITION

• Collectively—part of an increased tendency to bleed that occurs in a wide variety of clinical disorders
• Petechiae—miniscule hemorrhages into the skin, mucous membranes, or serosal surfaces
• Ecchymoses—large hemorrhages, usually >1–2 cm
• Bruise—a large, subcutaneous ecchymosis in which the hemorrhage results in the release of hemoglobin, which is converted into bilirubin and hemosiderin, resulting in a blue and green discoloration of tissue

PATHOPHYSIOLOGY

• Vessel integrity, platelets, and blood coagulation proteins are essential for normal intravascular hemostasis.
• Injury to the vessel wall occurs due to trauma, infiltrative diseases, plant and bacterial toxins, inflammatory proteins, autoimmune reactions, and viral and bacterial virulence factors.
• Platelets can be decreased in absolute numbers or have functional defects, resulting in clotting abnormalities and bleeding tendencies. Platelet abnormalities usually are first observed as petechiae, ecchymoses, or mucosal bleeding. Causes of decreased platelet numbers include excessive destruction, decreased production, and consumption; platelet function defects can be acquired (e.g., drugs and DIC) or congenital.
• Coagulation proteins interact with platelets in the formation of a blood clot, and if any of these components are impaired, hemorrhage may result. Congenital and acquired coagulation protein abnormalities have been demonstrated in the horse. Acquired disorders can result from diminished production, excessive consumption, and factor inhibition.
• Sepsis often is associated with petechia.
• Clotting factor deficiencies, DIC, and liver disease usually have ecchymoses and large bruises.

SYSTEMS AFFECTED

• Hemic/lymphatic/immune—most commonly affected and the most common underlying cause
• Cardiovascular—increased vascular permeability results in hemorrhage.
• Skin/exocrine—skin discoloration secondary to extravascular blood accumulation
• GI—hematochezia and melena; abdominal pain with significant intra-abdominal hemorrhage or primary intra-abdominal disease (e.g., neoplasia)
• Renal—hematuria
• Respiratory—increased rate and altered depth of respiration with primary underlying respiratory disease (e.g., neoplasia)

SIGNALMENT

• Unless heritable, most acquired hemostatic abnormalities have no age, sex, or breed dispositions.
• Many factor deficiencies have been identified in specific breeds—hemophilia A in Quarter Horses, Arabians, and Thoroughbreds; multiple clotting factor defects in Arabians; von Willebrand disease in Quarter Horses; and prekallikrein deficiency in Belgian and miniature horses

SIGNS

General Comments

History and clinical signs vary, depending on the underlying cause.

Historical Findings

• Sudden onset of dark discolorations to skin or mucous membranes
• Owners may report inappropriate hemorrhage.

Physical Examination Findings

• Increased bleeding tendency noted by focal, red discoloration of the skin, mucous membranes, and serosal surfaces of internal organs. With petechia, there may be focal or scattered accumulations of pinpoint hemorrhages, whereas ecchymoses are larger (1–2 cm). Frequently, larger areas of hemorrhage are associated with pressure points of skin and mucous membranes.
• Nonspecific signs—pale mucous membranes, frank hemorrhages from nose or rectum, serosanguinous discharge from nose or rectum, red discoloration of feces or urine, melena, depression, anorexia, tachypnea, tachycardia, respiratory distress, increased rectal temperature, ventral edema, edema of the peripheral limbs, splenomegaly, ascites, and pleural effusion

CAUSES

Vascular Defects

• Autoimmune—purpura hemorrhagica and vasculitis
• Viral—influenza virus and equine arteritis virus
• Bacterial—septicemia/bacteremia and *Streptococcus* sp. infections
• Parasitic—trypanosomiasis
• Toxic—snake bite
• Other—DIC

Platelet Abnormalities

• Autoimmune—immune-mediated thrombocytopenia and drug reactions
• Congenital—hemophilia A (i.e., factor VIII:C); sex-linked factor VII deficiency; recessive multiple factor deficiency of factors II, VII, VIII, IX, and XI; and Von Willebrand disease
• Viral—EIAV, influenza virus, African horse sickness virus, and Venezuelan equine encephalitis virus
• Bacterial—septicemia/bacteremia, *Streptococcus* sp. infections, salmonellosis, and *Ehrlichia equi*
• Parasitic—piroplasmosis
• Neoplastic—lymphoma, melanoma, and myeloproliferative disease
• Toxic—warfarin, sweet-clover poisoning, drug-induced thrombocytopenia, and snake bite
• Other—DIC

PETECHIA, ECCHYMOSES, AND BRUISING

Defects in Coagulation

- Congenital—hemophilia A; sex-linked factor VII deficiency; recessive multiple factor deficiency of factors II, VII, VIII, IX, and XI in Arabians; and Von Willebrand disease
- Viral—EIAV, influenza virus, and equine arteritis virus
- Bacterial—septicemia/bacteremia
- Neoplastic—lymphoma, melanoma, and myelophistic disease
- Other—DIC and liver disease

RISK FACTORS

History of any of the previously mentioned diseases

DIAGNOSIS

DIFFERENTIAL DIAGNOSIS

Trauma—ruled out by history and physical examination

CBC/BIOCHEMISTRY/URINALYSIS

Highly variable—may have anemia, thrombocytopenia, leukopenia or leukocytosis, neutropenia or neutrophilia, lymphocytosis or lymphopenia, hyperproteinemia or hypoproteinemia, hyperfibrinogenemia, and normal or abnormal liver function tests and enzymes

OTHER LABORATORY TESTS

- Platelet count, ACT, PT, APTT, fibrinogen, and FDPs to identify coagulation defects and DIC
- Prolonged bleeding time with thrombocyte disorders and deficiency; platelet aggregation tests, platelet factor 3, and platelet function tests can be performed to characterize platelet defects.
- Serology, blood smears, and cultures may be indicated to identify infectious agents.

IMAGING

- Ultrasonography of the thorax and abdomen
- Thoracic radiography

DIAGNOSTIC PROCEDURES

- Avoid invasive procedures in patients at risk of bleeding.
- Bone marrow aspirate/biopsy
- Rectal palpation

TREATMENT

- Treatment of underlying disease—antimicrobials, antiparasitics, anti-inflammatories, antineoplastics, immunomodulators, and supportive care.
- Supportive care consisting of isotonic fluids for blood volume expansion; maintenance consisting of whole blood, plasma, or platelet transfusions

MEDICATIONS

DRUGS OF CHOICE

Immune-mediated disease—dexamethasone is superior to short acting steroids.

CONTRAINDICATIONS

Aspirin and NSAIDs may impair platelet function.

PRECAUTIONS

Minimize activity to decrease risk of trauma.

POSSIBLE INTERACTIONS

N/A

ALTERNATIVE DRUGS

N/A

FOLLOW-UP

PATIENT MONITORING

Daily platelet counts to assess response to medications

POSSIBLE COMPLICATIONS

- Sudden death or acute exacerbation of morbidity
- Hypovolemic shock due to internal hemorrhage

MISCELLANEOUS

ASSOCIATED CONDITIONS

NA

AGE-RELATED FACTORS

N/A

ZOONOTIC POTENTIAL

N/A

PREGNANCY

N/A

SYNONYMS

- Bleeding
- Hemorrhagic diatheses

SEE ALSO

- DIC
- Lymphosarcoma
- Neoplasia
- *Streptococcus equi*
- Thrombocytopenia
- Vasculitis

ABBREVIATIONS

- ACT = activated clotting time
- APTT = activated partial thromboplastin time
- DIC = disseminated intravascular coagulation
- EIAV = equine infectious anemia virus
- FDP = fibrin degradation products
- GI = gastrointestinal
- PT = prothrombin time

Suggested Reading

Cotran RS, Kumar V, Robbins SL, eds. Pathologic basis of disease. 6th ed. Philadelphia: WB Saunders, 1999.

Jubb RVFK, Kennedy PC, Palmer N, eds. Pathology of domestic animals. 4th ed. San Diego: Academic Press, 1998.

Author Maureen T. Long

Consulting Editor Debra C. Sellon

PHEOCHROMOCYTOMA (PCC)

BASICS

OVERVIEW

• A tumor of the catecholamine-producing cells of the adrenal medulla
• Most reported equine PCCs have been unilateral, well-encapsulated, benign neoplasms, and almost half have been incidental findings at necropsy.
• May be functional and release catecholamines, which mainly include epinephrine, norepinephrine, or both.
• Clinical signs result from excessive catecholamine production or tumor growth; the most commonly reported in horses are sweating, tachycardia, tachypnea, abdominal pain, mydriasis, muscle tremors, and hyperglycemia.
• Organ system—endocrine and cardiovascular

SIGNALMENT

• Reported mainly in horses ≥12 years; however, one malignant PCC involving both adrenal glands has been reported in a 6-month-old foal.
• No breed or sex predilections are apparent.

SIGNS

Many clinical signs associated with functional PCC are nonspecific and may be caused by other diseases; this explains why most cases are diagnosed postmortem.

Historical Findings

• Horses may have a history of lethargy, anorexia, abdominal pain, sweating, tachycardia, diarrhea, or neurologic signs of ataxia.
• Pregnant mares may abort.
• One foal with a malignant PCC had a 4-month history of poor growth and a 5-day history of progressive ataxia.

Physical Examination Findings

• Sweating, tachycardia, tachypnea, abdominal pain, mydriasis, muscle tremors, ileus, and diarrhea are reported and attributable to excessive catecholamine production.
• A mass may be palpated rectally and medially to the left kidney.
• Signs of ataxia and paresis have been described in one case and resulted from compression of the spinal cord by the tumor's metastases.

CAUSES AND RISK FACTORS

• PCC is a benign or malignant tumor of the chromaffin cells of the adrenal medulla.
• No risk factors have yet been identified.

DIAGNOSIS

DIFFERENTIAL DIAGNOSIS

• Causes of abdominal pain and ileus (e.g., colic) should be considered.
• Clinical signs and biochemical abnormalities similar to that reported with PCC may be observed with renal disease, enteritis, colitis, hypoadrenocorticism, or other causes of cardiovascular, pulmonary, and neurologic diseases.
• Stress, hyperadrenocorticism, or diabetes mellitus, which are causes of hyperglycemia, should be considered.

CBC/BIOCHEMISTRY/URINALYSIS

• Laboratory findings are variable and nonspecific.
• Hemoconcentration and inflammatory leukogram are common.
• Hyponatremia, hyperkalemia, metabolic acidosis, hypocalcemia, hyperphosphatemia, azotemia, hyperglycemia, glucosuria, and occult hematuria are not uncommon.

OTHER LABORATORY TESTS

Assays for catecholamines and their metabolites in plasma or urine technically are difficult, and few laboratories perform these tests. Interpretation of the results may be complicated further by the intermittent nature of catecholamine release in horses with PCC and the fact that high catecholamine levels may be detected in stressed but otherwise normal horses.

IMAGING

Ultrasonography may reveal a mass medial to the kidney, along the aorta, or in the posterior vena cava.

DIAGNOSTIC PROCEDURES

Direct or indirect arterial blood pressure measurements may document hypertension.

PATHOLOGIC FINDINGS

• Usually unilateral and infrequently bilateral
• Unique or multiple nodular masses within the adrenal gland that may vary in size from a few millimeters to ≥10 cm.
• A large PCC may invade the posterior vena cava and result in extensive hemorrhage, leading to numerous blood clots in the perirenal and retroperitoneal spaces and hemoperitoneum.
• Histologically, PCCs often are necrotic and hemorrhagic, which also may result in adrenocortical hemorrhage and necrosis.

PHEOCHROMOCYTOMA (PCC)

TREATMENT

• Suspected cases should be treated on an inpatient basis.
• Medical care should be aimed at controlling pain, using fluid therapy to normalize renal function and electrolyte abnormalities, and at stabilizing cardiovascular function.
• Complete rest is recommended.
• Avoid feed intake as long as intestinal motility is impaired.
• Consider surgical resection in cases of localized nodular tumors. This procedure is difficult technically, however, and the risk of a fatal complication is high—hemorrhage, cardiac arrhythmia, or rhabdomyolysis

MEDICATIONS

DRUGS

In other species (e.g., humans, small animals), α- and β-adrenergic blocking agents may control the effects of excessive catecholamine secretion.

CONTRAINDICATIONS/POSSIBLE INTERACTIONS

N/A

FOLLOW-UP

PATIENT MONITORING

Monitor renal and cardiovascular function, electrolytes, and acid–base status.

PREVENTION/AVOIDANCE

N/A

POSSIBLE COMPLICATIONS

• Renal failure
• Hemorrhage
• Cardiac arrhythmia
• Hypotension may follow adrenalectomy.

EXPECTED COURSE AND PROGNOSIS

• No reports of functional PCC having been successfully treated in horses.
• All reported cases involved death or euthanasia within a few hours to a few days of the onset of clinical signs.

MISCELLANEOUS

ASSOCIATED CONDITIONS

N/A

AGE-RELATED FACTORS

N/A

ZOONOTIC POTENTIAL

N/A

PREGNANCY

Abortion during late gestation and death just before parturition have been reported.

SEE ALSO

N/A

Suggested Reading

Johnson PJ, Goetz TE, Foreman JH, Zachary JF. Pheochromocytoma in two horses. J Am Vet Med Assoc 1995;206:837–841.

Author Laurent Couëtil
Consulting Editor Michel Levy

PHIMOSIS

BASICS

DEFINITION
The inability to make the penis protrude from the prepuce.

PATHOPHYSIOLOGY
Constriction of either the external preputial orifice or the preputial ring can result in phimosis.

SYSTEM AFFECTED
Reproductive

SIGNALMENT
Stallions or geldings of any age.

SIGNS
Historical Findings
Urination within the preputial cavity and/or dysuria.

Physical Examination Findings
Visible or palpable thickening of the external preputial orifice or the preputial ring. May be excoriations due to urine scalding.

CAUSES
Congenital
- Stenosis of the preputial orifice
- Hermaphroditism
- Penile dysgenesis

Acquired
- Trauma: breeding injury, post-surgical edema, chronic posthitis.
- Neoplasia: sarcoid, SCC, papilloma, melanoma, hemagioma.
- Parasitism: Habronemiasis.
- Viral infections: EHV-3.

RISK FACTORS
- Poor hygiene; accumulation of excessive smegma can lead to posthitis and subsequent phimosis from the formation of scar tissue.
- Light-colored skin is associated with an increased incidence of SCC.
- Gray horses are more commonly diagnosed with melanomas.

DIAGNOSIS

DIFFERENTIAL DIAGNOSIS
Differentiating Similar Signs
Phimosis during the first 30 days of life is normal due to fusion of the internal preputial lamina to the free portion of the penis.

CBC/BIOCHEMISTRY/URINALYSIS
N/A

OTHER LABORATORY TESTS
Virus isolation using fluid from vesicular lesions may be diagnostic for EHV-3.

IMAGING
N/A

DIAGNOSTIC PROCEDURES
Cytology or biopsy (histopathology) may distinguish and/or provide a definitive diagnosis for neoplastic, granulomatous, or herpesvirus lesions.

TREATMENT
If phimosis is due to
- Post-surgical edema: hydrotherapy, massage, exercise, and diuretics are indicated. Cleansing and application of topical emollients or antibiotics may be indicated.
- Neoplastic or granulomatous lesions: surgical excision, cryosurgery, chemotherapy, or radiation, as indicated by type, location, and size.
- A stricture of the external preputial orifice: surgical removal of a triangular section of the external preputial lamina.
- A stricture at the preputial ring: incise the internal preputial fold (preputiotomy). Circumcision (reefing) may be necessary to remove the constricting tissue in its entirety.

MEDICATIONS

DRUG(S) OF CHOICE
- NSAIDs, including phenylbutazone (2–4 g/450 kg/day P/O), or flunixine meglumine (1 mg/kg/day IV, IM, or P/O) for symptomatic relief or to decrease inflammation.
- Systemic or local antibiotics if indicated to treat local infections or prevent septicemia.
- Diuretics—furosemide (1 mg/kg IV, SID, BID) may be indicated in the acute phase to reduce edema.
- Specific topical or systemic treatments for parasitic, fungal, or neoplastic conditions as indicated by test results.

PHIMOSIS

CONTRAINDICATIONS
N/A

PRECAUTIONS
Phenothiazine tranquilizers should be avoided/used with caution (see Priapism).

POSSIBLE INTERACTIONS
N/A

ALTERNATIVE DRUGS
N/A

FOLLOW-UP

PATIENT MONITORING
- Initially, daily evaluations: ensure that secondary posthitis, balanitis, balanoposthitis, urine scald, or penile/preputial excoriations are not complicating the phimosis.
- As the initial problem is effectively treated, less frequent examinations will be necessary.

POSSIBLE COMPLICATIONS
- Urination within the preputial cavity may cause inflammation of the epithelium, leading to a more extensive inflammation (posthitis, balanoposthitis) and scarring.
- Infertility or impotence can result if scarring becomes extensive.

MISCELLANEOUS

ASSOCIATED CONDITIONS
N/A

AGE-RELATED FACTORS
- Papillomas are more frequently diagnosed in young animals.
- Squamous cell carcinomas and melanomas are more frequently diagnosed in middle-age to aged horses.

ZOONOTIC POTENTIAL
N/A

PREGNANCY
N/A

SYNONYMS
N/A

SEE ALSO
- Paraphimosis
- Penile vesicles/erosions
- Venereal diseases

ABBREVIATIONS
- EHV = equine herpesvirus
- SCC = squamous cell carcinoma

Suggested Reading

Blanchard TL, Varner DD, Schumacher J. Manual of equine reproduction. St. Louis: Mosby 1998;183-184.

Schumacher J, Varner DD. Surgical correction of abnormalities affecting the reproductive organs of stallions. In: Current therapy in large animal theriogenology. Youngquist RS, ed. Philadelphia: WB Saunders Co. 1997;24-36.

Schumacher J, Vaughan JT. Surgery of the penis and prepuce. In: Veterinary Clinics of North America: Equine Practice 1988;4;473-491.

Vaughan JT. Surgery of the penis and prepuce. In: Bovine and equine urogenital surgery. Walker DF and Vaughan JT, ed. Philadelphia: Lea & Febiger 1980;125-144.

Author Carole C. Miller

Consulting Editor Carla L. Carleton

PHOSPHORUS, HYPERPHOSPHATEMIA

BASICS

DEFINITION

Serum phosphate concentration > the reference interval (e.g., >4.5 mg/dL)

PATHOPHYSIOLOGY

- Kidneys, small intestine, and skeleton are involved in phosphate homeostasis in conjunction with parathyroid hormone, calcitonin, vitamin D, and diet.
- Conditions causing decreased glomerular filtration or renal excretion, excessive intestinal absorption or dietary supplementation, or excessive bone resorption can result in hyperphosphatemia.

SYSTEMS AFFECTED

General

- Phosphorus and calcium metabolism and homeostatic mechanisms are closely linked.
- Hyperphosphatemia frequently occurs with hypocalcemia in many disorders; in these cases, effects of hyperphosphatemia on organ systems often are indirect and relate more to hypocalcemia.

Skeletal

- Skeletal effects result from concurrent hypocalcemia that occurs secondary to excessive dietary intake or imbalance of phosphorus.
- In response to hypocalcemia, calcium is mobilized from bone to maintain other metabolic functions; consequences include too little or abnormal bone formation, bone demineralization, and a skeleton more prone to injury.

Endocrine

- Hyperphosphatemia stimulates secretion of PTH.
- Effects of PTH—increased resorption of calcium from bone, kidneys, and intestine; increased renal excretion of phosphorus; the net effect is to decrease plasma phosphorus and increase plasma calcium levels.

SIGNALMENT

- Varies, depending on the underlying disease or condition.
- Neonates and young, growing animals have increased serum phosphorus levels—often 4.5–9.0 mg/dL

SIGNS

Historical Findings

History varies with the underlying cause of hyperphosphatemia, and it may reflect conditions or diseases with associated hypocalcemia or hypercalcemia.

Physical Examination Findings

- Dietary phosphorus excess or imbalance—clinical signs manifest in the skeletal system; early signs include intermittent shifting leg lameness, generalized joint tenderness, or stilted gait; as the disease progresses, abnormal bone formation and enlarged facial bones (e.g., bighead in NHP) occur.
- Hypervitaminosis D—horses may exhibit limb stiffness, with painful flexor tendons and suspensory ligaments.

CAUSES

- Neonates and young, growing animals—hyperphosphatemia commonly is seen in because of rapid bone turnover.
- Endurance exercise—transient hyperphosphatemia may be seen after long-distance endurance activity.
- Decreased glomerular filtration—common cause of hyperphosphatemia associated with prerenal, renal, or postrenal azotemia; hyperphosphatemia may be seen in some cases of acute renal failure, but equine chronic renal failure usually is accompanied by hypophosphatemia.
- Hypervitaminosis D—hyperphosphatemia and hypercalcemia result from excessive dietary supplementation with vitamin D–containing products; ingestion of plants (e.g., *Cestrum diurnum,* wild jasmine, *Solanum* sp., Hawaii) containing a vitamin D–like substance usually do not cause abnormalities in plasma phosphorus levels.
- Excessive dietary phosphorus or phosphorus imbalance—excessive phosphorus intake, dietary calcium:phosphorus imbalance, or excessive supplementation with bran, which is high in phosphorus content, inhibits absorption of calcium, thus altering calcium homeostatic mechanisms and the rate of bone turnover. This can result in calcium deficiency that may go undetected for weeks to months. In young animals, skeletal mass does not keep up with increasing body size; thus, the skeleton is more injury prone. NHP (e.g., bighead disease) occurs from excess phosphorus and low or marginal calcium intake. Secretion of PTH increases as a compensatory mechanism to correct the disturbance in mineral homeostasis induced by nutritional imbalance.

RISK FACTORS

Increased potential for soft-tissue mineralization with concurrent hyperphosphatemia and hypercalcemia

DIAGNOSIS

DIFFERENTIAL DIAGNOSIS

History is useful in determining if diet contains phosphorus excess or imbalances.

LABORATORY FINDINGS

Drugs that May Alter Lab Results

Citrate, oxalate, and EDTA anticoagulants interfere with biochemical methodology and should not be used.

Disorders that May Alter Lab Results

- Lipemia, hemolysis, and icterus may falsely elevate serum phosphorus concentrations because of interference with biochemical methodology.
- Serum is the preferred specimen for phosphate determination. Heparinized plasma can be used, but phosphate levels may be minimally lower than serum reference ranges.

Valid if Run in Human Lab?

Yes

PHOSPHORUS, HYPERPHOSPHATEMIA

CBC/BIOCHEMISTRY/URINALYSIS
- NHP—normal renal function and, depending on stage of disease, hypocalcemia, hyperphosphatemia, and elevated ALP.
- Renal failure—azotemia; isosthenuria

OTHER LABORATORY TESTS
- Dietary deficiency or imbalance—review dietary history; inspect feed, and analyze chemically for calcium and phosphorus content.
- NHP—increased urinary phosphorus and decreased urinary calcium concentrations

IMAGING
Conventional radiology has little benefit in detecting loss of skeletal mineralization until such losses exceed 30%.

DIAGNOSTIC PROCEDURES
N/A

TREATMENT
- NHP—correct dietary deficiency or imbalance by supplying the deficient nutrient; dietary calcium:phosphorus ratio must not exceed 1.5–2:1.
- Removal of vitamin D sources and time may result in recovery; however, if soft-tissue mineralization in the heart or kidney occurs, prognosis is poor.
- With suspected acute renal failure, fluid replacement and correction of electrolyte imbalances

MEDICATIONS

DRUGS OF CHOICE
Hypervitaminosis D—removal of source, fluid diuresis, corticosteroid administration, and low-calcium and -phosphorus feeds; in severe cases, treatment generally is unrewarding because of extensive soft-tissue mineralization.

CONTRAINDICATIONS
N/A

PRECAUTIONS
N/A

POSSIBLE INTERACTIONS
N/A

ALTERNATIVE DRUGS
N/A

FOLLOW-UP

PATIENT MONITORING
N/A

POSSIBLE COMPLICATIONS
N/A

MISCELLANEOUS

ASSOCIATED CONDITIONS
Hypocalcemia

AGE-RELATED FACTORS
- Hyperphosphatemia and elevated ALP levels commonly are seen in healthy, young, growing animals. Both parameters decrease with age.
- Young animals are more prone to skeletal abnormalities resulting from dietary excess or imbalances.

ZOONOTIC POTENTIAL
N/A

PREGNANCY
N/A

SYNONYMS
NHP—bighead disease, bran disease, osteodystrophia fibrosa, and Miller's disease

SEE ALSO
- Hypercalcemia
- Hypocalcemia

ABBREVIATIONS
- ALP = alkaline phosphatase
- NHP = nutritional secondary hyperparathyroidism
- PTH = parathyroid hormone

Suggested Reading

Capen CC. Nutritional secondary hyperparathyroidism. In: Robinson NE, ed. Current therapy in equine medicine. Philadelphia: WB Saunders, 1983:160–163.

Hesters NL, Yates DJ, Hunt E. Disorders of calcium metabolism: hypercalcemia. In: Smith BP, ed. Large animal internal medicine. 2nd ed. St. Louis: Mosby–Year Book, 1996:1464–1470.

Schryver HF, Hintz HF. Minerals. In: Robinson NE, ed. Current therapy in equine medicine 2. Philadelphia: WB Saunders, 1987:393–405.

Author Karen E. Russell
Consulting Editor Claire B. Andreasen

PHOSPHORUS, HYPOPHOSPHATEMIA

BASICS

DEFINITION

Serum phosphate concentration < reference interval (e.g., <2.0 mg/dL)

PATHOPHYSIOLOGY

- Phosphorus is one of the most abundant elements in the body, with >80% occurring in bone and complexed with calcium in the form of hydroxyapatite.
- Phosphorus is an important component of nucleic acids, phospholipids, and phosphoproteins.
- Maintenance of cellular integrity and metabolism depends on phosphate-containing, high-energy compounds (e.g., ATP) and many enzyme systems that require phosphorus.
- Skeletal-associated abnormalities (e.g., demineralization, deformation, poor growth) are potential consequences of hypophosphatemia.
- Depletion of ATP can affect any cell with high energy requirements; erythrocytes, skeletal muscle cells, and brain cells are especially susceptible.

SYSTEMS AFFECTED

- Skeletal—too little or abnormal bone formation, bone demineralization, and a skeleton more prone to injury
- Reproductive—anestrus, irregular estrus, or reduced conception rates
- Hematologic—severe deficiency may predispose to erythrocyte hemolysis.

SIGNALMENT

Varies with the cause.

SIGNS

General Comments

History and clinical signs reflect the underlying disease or condition rather than the serum abnormality.

Historical Findings

- Chronic renal failure—poor performance
- Dietary phosphorus deficiency—poor growth, poor reproductive history, anestrus, irregular estrus, and reduced conception rates

Physical Examination Findings

- Chronic renal failure—weight loss
- Dietary phosphorus deficiency—lameness, stiff painful gait, or pica

CAUSES

Renal Failure

Serum phosphorus in horses with chronic renal failure may be normal or low, depending on the presence and degree of hypercalcemia.

Dietary Phosphorus Deficiency

The condition is common in states of phosphate deficiency or starvation.

Primary Hyperparathyroidism

- Potential causes—parathyroid adenoma, parathyroid hyperplasia, or carcinoma
- In case reports of horses with primary hyperparathyroidism, hypercalcemia, hypophosphatemia or low-normal phosphorus concentration, and increased fractional phosphorus excretion were common findings. Vitamin D_3 concentration was not elevated.
- This condition is rare in horses but should be considered if all other causes of hypercalcemia have been excluded.

Rickets

- Young, growing animals with vitamin D deficiency may be hypophosphatemic, hypocalcemic, and have elevated ALP levels.
- Vitamin D deficiency causes defective mineralization of new bone, resulting in painful swelling of the physis and metaphysis of the long bones and costochondral junctions, bowed limbs, and stiff gait.
- Natural cases of rickets in foals probably are quite rare.

RISK FACTORS

- Severe hypophosphatemia has been associated with intravascular hemolysis and altered erythrocyte function in other species—bovine, human, and canine
- With horses in chronic renal failure that are hypercalcemic, do not feed legume hays (e.g., alfalfa, clover) or high-calcium rations, and do not treat with calcium-containing fluids.

DIAGNOSIS

DIFFERENTIAL DIAGNOSIS

- Chronic renal failure—azotemia, isosthenuria, hypercalcemia, and exposure to nephrotoxins
- History—useful in determining dietary deficiency of phosphorus or calcium.
- Primary hyperparathryoidism—hypercalcemia, hypophosphatemia, increased serum PTH concentration, increased fractional phosphorus excretion, and low to normal concentrations of vitamin D_3

LABORATORY FINDINGS

Drugs that May Alter Lab Results

- Serum is the preferred specimen for phosphate determination.
- Heparinized plasma can be used, but phosphorus levels may be minimally lower than serum reference ranges.
- Citrate, oxalate, and EDTA anticoagulants interfere with biochemical methodology and should not be used.

Disorders that May Alter Lab Results

Lipemia, hemolysis, and icterus may falsely elevate serum phosphorus concentrations.

Valid If Run in Human Lab?

Yes

CBC/BIOCHEMISTRY/URINALYSIS

- Chronic renal failure—azotemia, hypercalcemia, isosthenuria are common findings; hypophosphatemia, mild hyponatremia and hypochloridemia, and normo- or hyperkalemia also can be present.
- Moderate to marked proteinuria is common in cases of glomerulonephritis.
- Suspect urinary tract infection with the finding of moderate to many leukocytes in urine sediment.
- Primary hyperparathryoidism—renal function should be normal.
- Severe calcium or phosphorus deficiency—elevated serum ALP level

PHOSPHORUS, HYPOPHOSPHATEMIA

OTHER LABORATORY TESTS

With suspected hyperparathyroidism, fractional phosphorus excretion and immunoreactive C-terminal PTH concentration help to confirm the diagnosis.

IMAGING

Conventional radiology has little benefit in detecting loss of skeletal mineralization until such losses exceed 30%.

DIAGNOSTIC PROCEDURES

With suspected dietary phosphorus and calcium deficiencies, thorough review of dietary history, inspection of feeds, and chemical evaluation of calcium and phosphorus content in feeds are necessary.

TREATMENT

- Supplementation with appropriate mineral sources to correct deficiency or imbalance in a particular diet
- Common mineral supplements for phosphorus—defluorinated phosphate, bonemeal, dicalcium phosphate, monocalcium phosphate, or monosodium phosphate

MEDICATIONS

DRUGS OF CHOICE

N/A

CONTRAINDICATIONS

N/A

PRECAUTIONS

Dietary calcium:phosphorus ratio must not exceed 1.5–2:1.

POSSIBLE INTERACTIONS

N/A

ALTERNATIVE DRUGS

N/A

FOLLOW-UP

PATIENT MONITORING

N/A

POSSIBLE COMPLICATIONS

N/A

MISCELLANEOUS

ASSOCIATED CONDITIONS

N/A

AGE-RELATED FACTORS

Young animals may be more prone to skeletal abnormalities resulting from dietary deficiency or imbalances.

ZOONOTIC POTENTIAL

N/A

PREGNANCY

N/A

SYNONYMS

N/A

SEE ALSO

- Hypercalcemia, chronic renal failure
- Hypocalcemia

ABBREVIATIONS

- ALP = alkaline phosphatase
- PTH = parathyroid hormone

Suggested Reading

Fleming SA, Yates DJ. Disorders of phosphorus metabolism: chronic phosphorus deficiency/hypophosphatemia. In: Smith BP, ed. Large animal internal medicine. 2nd ed. St. Louis: Mosby–Year Book, 1996:1471–1474.

Frank N, Hawkins JF, Couëtil LL, Raymond JT. Primary hyperparathyroidism with osteodystrophia fibrosa of the facial bones in a pony. J Am Vet Med Assoc 1998;212:84–86.

Freestone JF, Melrose PA. Endocrine diseases. In: Kobluk CN, Ames TR, Geor RJ, eds. The horse: diseases and clinical management. Philadelphia: WB Saunders, 1995:1137–1164.

Peauroi JR, Fisher DJ, Mohr FC, Vivrette SL. Primary hyperparathyroidism caused by a functional parathyroid adenoma in a horse. J Am Vet Med Assoc 1998;212:1915–1918.

Roussel AJ, Thatcher CD. Primary hyperparathyroidism in a pony mare. Compend Contin Educ Pract Vet 1987;7:781–783.

Schryver HF, Hintz HF. Minerals. In: Robinson NE, ed. Current therapy in equine medicine 2. Philadelphia: WB Saunders, 1987;393–405.

Author Karen E. Russell

Consulting Editor Claire B. Andreasen

PHOTIC HEADSHAKING

BASICS

OVERVIEW

• Otherwise known as headtossing behavior, a condition in which, during the absence of any external stimuli other than light, a horse vigorously and violently shakes its head in horizontal, vertical, or rotary directions.
• Probably a form of optic-trigeminal nerve summation, in which retina and optic nerve stimulation produces referred sensation to the nasal cavity. The irritability in the nasal cavity causes the horse to shake its head.
• Organ systems—ophthalmic, CNS, and upper respiratory tract

SIGNALMENT

• Hunter-type horses most commonly affected
• Affected horses are 7 years old, with a mean duration of signs before referral of 8 months.
• Heritability is unknown.
• Geldings are overrepresented.

SIGNS

Excessive (and occasionally violent) rubbing, sneezing and flipping of the nose and head, either at rest or during exercise

CAUSES AND RISK FACTORS

• Sunlight may stimulate parasympathetic activity in the infraorbital nerve, resulting in irritating nasal sensations and headtossing.
• Most horses are asymptomatic during winter.

DIAGNOSIS

DIFFERENTIAL DIAGNOSIS

• Otitis media and interna and associated petrous temporal and stylohyoid bony changes
• Guttural pouch disease
• Upper respiratory tract disease
• Oral and ocular diseases

CBC/BIOCHEMISTRY/URINALYSIS

Usually normal

OTHER LABORATORY TESTS

N/A

IMAGING

Radiography of skull and cervical spine to identify changes associated with otitis media and interna

DIAGNOSTIC PROCEDURES

• Blindfold the horse or place in dark environments—improvement noted in headshakers
• Upper respiratory tract examination
• Endoscopy of the guttural pouches
• Tympanocentesis under general anesthesia may help to rule out ear disease lacking radiologic evidence.
• Thorough otic, oral, and ophthalmic examination
• Bilateral infraorbital nerve blocks

TREATMENT

• A complete workup may require overnight hospitalization; medical management can be done by the trainer/owner.
• Headshaking can occur at rest or during exercise. Most headshakers show signs shortly after the onset of activity, so working an uncontrolled photic headshaker may carry some risk.
• Medical therapy controls, but does not cure, the condition. If effective, medical treatment may be needed only during the season in which the horse exhibits headshaking behavior.
• Surgical infraorbital neurectomies are a salvage procedure.
• If a horse does not respond to medical therapy and infraorbital nerve blocks are successful, consider bilateral infraorbital neurectomy.

PHOTIC HEADSHAKING

MEDICATIONS

DRUGS

• Cyproheptadine (H_1 blocker), a serotonin antagonist that alters POMC metabolism, has the potential to alleviate clinical signs (0.3 mg/kg PO BID for 7 days initially, then continued as needed; some may require a dose up to 0.6 mg/kg PO BID).
• To mimic winter conditions physiologically, melatonin therapy (12 mg PO on a sugar cube once between 5:00 and 6:00 PM daily) also may be beneficial.

CONTRAINDICATIONS/POSSIBLE INTERACTIONS

• Avoid in hypersensitive patients.
• Additive CNS depression may be seen if combined with barbiturates or tranquilizers.
• Cyproheptadine has anticholinergic effects that may be intensified by monoamine oxidase inhibitors (e.g., furazolidone).
• Treatment of performance horses should comply with the rules of the governing organization.
• Mild lethargy, anorexia, and depression have been reported in horses treated with cyproheptadine, as have drug eruptions.

FOLLOW-UP

• A 7-day trial of cyproheptadine should determine if the patient will respond favorably to medical treatment. Therapy can be stopped periodically and reinstated if the behavior recurs and no side effects are observed.
• Horses kept in a dark environment may not show severe clinical headshaking. This type of management, however, may not be practical for the horse or its owner/trainer.
• A horse with uncontrolled headshaking may develop unwanted head trauma, and the owner/trainer may find optimal work or performance difficult for the horse.
• Long term, seasonal medical therapy can control, but not cure, this disease. Infraorbital neurectomies may eliminate headshaking signs indefinitely but should be considered only when medical therapy fails and temporary nerve blocks work.

MISCELLANEOUS

ASSOCIATED CONDITIONS

Photic sneezing in humans

PREGNANCY

No studies available on safety of cyproheptadine in pregnant mares; use with caution in such patients.

SEE ALSO

N/A

ABBREVIATION

POMC = proopiomelanocortin

Suggested Reading

Madigan JE, Kortz G, Murphy C, Rodger L. Photic headshaking in the horse: 7 cases. Equine Vet J 1995;27:306–311.

Author Daniel Biros
Consulting Editor Dennis E. Brooks

PICA

BASICS

OVERVIEW

Pica is an abnormal appetite for and consumption of non-food items, including substances such as dirt, gravel, paint, tail hairs, feces, or other inanimate objects. The pathophysiology of pica is not completely understood. It has been associated with such conditions as obesity, parasitism, malnutrition, and deficiencies in electrolytes (sodium, chloride, or phosphorus), protein, or trace mineral imbalances (copper and zinc). It may also be due to a lack of oral stimulus or boredom. Decreased roughage in the diet has been associated with wood chewing, although it is considered normal for pastured horses to eat trees and shrubs. Wood chewing has been noted to be increased in cold, wet climates. Behavior-altering diseases, such as rabies, may result in pica; stereotypies can also lead to pica.

SIGNALMENT

Miniature horses and foals appear to be more prone to pica, although no clear association with a particular signalment has been made. There is an association between stabled horses with limited pasture time, low-roughage/high-concentrate diets, and wood chewing.

SIGNS

History of eating non-food items.

CAUSES AND RISK FACTORS

Pica is frequently associated with stereotypic behavior but may be secondary to deficiencies in the diet or parasitism. Inadequate housing, exercise, stimulus, or nutrition can be associated with pica. Foals appear to be more prone to pica due to their natural coprophagic behavior and inquisitive nature. Coprophagia is considered normal behavior in young foals.

DIAGNOSIS

DIFFERENTIAL DIAGNOSIS

Deficiencies in the diet should be investigated before determining if the pica is behavioral. This disorder is usually associated with behavioral abnormalities, but may also be secondary to behavior-altering diseases, such as certain neurologic disorders (e.g., rabies), or malnutrition.

CBC/BIOCHEMISTRY/URINALYSIS

No consistent abnormalities are usually found, but should be evaluated to identify possible primary causes of pica. If no significant abnormalities are found and a complete neurologic examination reveals no abnormalities, then the problem is likely behavioral.

OTHER LABORATORY TESTS

Fecal examination for parasites and any other tests indicated by prior testing; feed evaluation, especially for trace minerals such as copper and zinc.

IMAGING

N/A

DIAGNOSTIC PROCEDURES

N/A

TREATMENT

- Treatment should be directed at any primary diseases or deficiencies identified (see section on specific diseases for treatment recommendations).
- Once other disease processes are eliminated, treatment should be directed at redirecting the behavior. This can be accomplished through:
  - limiting exposure to the items of concern
  - providing an appropriate substitute
  - increase roughage in the diet
  - alter the environmental condition causing the stereotypy (see section on behavioral abnormalities)
  - alter the desirability of the non-food item through application of repellents with an objectionable taste
  - increase level of exercise
- If behavioral in origin, once established, the behavior is difficult to discourage; therefore, prevention is recommended.

PICA

MEDICATIONS

DRUG(S) OF CHOICE
N/A

CONTRAINDICATIONS
N/A

PRECAUTIONS
N/A

POSSIBLE INTERACTIONS
N/A

ALTERNATIVE DRUGS
N/A

FOLLOW-UP

The amount of follow-up required depends on the primary disease. If no primary condition is evident, contact with the owners should be made within 2 weeks of any recommended treatment to determine if it has decreased the pica and if there is owner compliance. If the horse has made no improvements after a 2-week period, alternative recommendations should be given.

Gastrointestinal disorders such as intestinal obstruction may occur. In addition, there may be abnormal wear to the teeth, which may in turn lead to further gastrointestinal disorders.

MISCELLANEOUS

ASSOCIATED CONDITIONS
N/A

AGE-RELATED FACTORS
N/A

ZOONOTIC POTENTIAL
N/A

PREGNANCY
N/A

SYNONYMS
N/A

SEE ALSO
See specific section.

ABBREVIATIONS
N/A

Suggested Reading

Mass J. Pica. In: Smith BP, ed. Large animal internal medicine. St. Louis: Mosby, 1996;193-195.

Ralston SL. Feeding behavior. Vet Clin North Amer Equine 1986;2(3):609-621.

Houpt KA. Stable vices and trailer problems. Vet Clin North Amer Equine 1986;2(3):623-633.

Author Deborah A. Parsons

Consulting Editor Henry Stämpfli

PICA

BASICS

DEFINITION

• General—voluntary ingestion of nonfood items
• Specific—consumption of wood (i.e., wood chewing), feces (i.e., coprophagia), or the tail of another horse (i.e., tail chewing).

PATHOPHYSIOLOGY

Possible nutrient deficiency, to which the horse responds by eating "novel" foods

SYSTEMS AFFECTED

• Behavioral—pica is considered to be a behavioral problem.
• GI—consequences if too much indigestible wood or poisonous material is ingested
• Neurologic—these causes should be ruled out but rarely are the cause of pica.

SIGNALMENT

• An abnormal behavior of horses of any age
• Young, growing horses <2 years are most likely to tail chew.
• Foals are most apt to eat feces, but this is normal behavior.

SIGNS

General Comments

• Wood chewing—large scallops missing from the top rail of wooden fences (middle rail for ponies), disappearance of wooden door frames, enlargement of holes originally made by kicking, stripping of bark from trees, and ingestion of fallen tree trunks or stumps. Most apt to occur during late winter and can vary from chewing the bark off trees to eating wood shavings provided for bedding to consuming large portions of stable walls or fence rails. Lack of roughage and a variety of forages, and possibly a lack of exercise, may predispose to wood chewing. Ingestion of poisonous woody plants (e.g., yew or red-maple leaves) can be a negative or even fatal consequence.
• Coprophagia—normal foal behavior during the first 2 months, with a preference for their dam's feces. The function of this behavior is unknown. However, population of the large intestine and colon with maternal microflora has been postulated, as has the foal learning which foods are safe to eat by eating its mother's feces. The former hypothesis may be more valid and explains why some horses eat feces while recovering from GI surgery. Old horses eat feces when the diet is either deficient, lacking in long fiber, or unavailable. Coprophagia has been associated with predisposition to equine motor neuron disease.
• Tail chewing—short tails or observation of horses chewing on tails. Hair is missing from the tail bottom rather than from the dock; the latter indicates that hair loss may be the result of rubbing by the affected horses rather than of chewing by another horse.
• Ingestion of soil, rocks, and other objects without nutritional value—occurs less commonly but is much more dangerous because of the chance of obstruction. Stone eating mostly occurs during the spring. Sand colic results from inadvertent ingestion of sand with feed, especially grain. Horses can separate hay from sand with their prehensile lips but are more likely to ingest sand with the small pieces of grain; however, because such ingestion is accidental, it should be considered a management problem rather than pica.

Historical Findings

• Wood chewing may be minimal during the summer and fall but begin when snow covers the ground, reaching a peak during late winter or early spring.
• The farm or the area may have a previous history of tail chewing (e.g., California and the southwestern United States are areas in which tail chewing is prevalent).
• Coprophagia in adults usually follows an abrupt change in diet from high- to low-roughage content.

Physical Examination Findings

• Unless ingestion has led to obstruction, there may be no physical signs.
• Auscultate the abdomen to ascertain that motility is normal and that no signs of sand (i.e., sounds similar to that of sand being poured from one bucket to another) are present.
• Perform a rectal examination to identify any potential obstruction.

CAUSES

• Wood chewing—lack of long-fiber roughage, lack of grazing opportunities, and possibly, lack of exercise. Occasionally, the horse's goal is removal of a barricade between it and another horse or a food source (e.g., a horse may chew a crib feeder to gain access to the foal's feed); this is not considered to be true pica.
• Abnormal (adult) coprophagia—dietary deficiency, lack of opportunity to chew, or abnormal GI flora
• Tail chewing—unknown, but the geographic areas with the greatest prevalence indicate that lack of grazing opportunity or lack of sulfur or some other nutritional component may be a factor.
• True picas (e.g., ingestion of rocks)—unknown

RISK FACTORS

• Confinement in grass-less, snow-covered, or muddy paddocks; restricted intake, or intake of only a pelleted diet; and lack of roughage, protein, vitamins, or energy
• Dressage horses (20% wood chew) and eventing horses (15% wood chew) are at greater risk than endurance horses (9% wood chew).
• Wood chewing is seasonal, occurring mostly during late winter or cold, wet weather.
• Coprophagia sometimes occurs in horses with GI disease and may be a means of repopulating the large intestinal flora.
• Treatment with antibiotics to which GI microorganisms are sensitive may be a risk factor.

PICA

DIAGNOSIS

DIFFERENTIAL DIAGNOSIS

- Differentiate wood chewing, which causes destruction of the wood, from cribbing, which causes semicircular marks on a fence.
- Some horses bite a fence or stall wall as a sign of redirected aggression toward a horse on the far side, but little damage occurs to the wood.
- Loss of tail hair can be caused by rubbing in response to *Oxyuris equi, Culicoides* sp., or some other irritation.
- Loss of mane hair may result from rubbing in response to irritation or while trying to reach grass outside a rail fence.

CBC/BIOCHEMISTRY/URINALYSIS

Perform a chemistry screen and CBC to determine presence of an underlying disease.

OTHER LABORATORY TESTS

N/A

IMAGING

N/A

DIAGNOSTIC PROCEDURES

- Analysis of the diet will determine what deficiency might be causing coprophagia or tail chewing.
- The greatest, though rare, danger to the horse is obstruction of the GI tract due to ingestion of wood.

TREATMENT

- Most owners have dealt with wood chewing by painting horizontal surfaces with noxious substances (e.g., creosote or laundry detergent) or "hot" sauces or by putting electrified wire atop the wood. This may discourage the horse from chewing that particular surface but does not address why the horse is chewing. It also does not change a horse's motivation, so chewing may continue elsewhere.
- True treatment of pica almost always is dietary. Increasing forage helps with wood chewing. Increasing the protein level, vitamin content, or roughage level reduces coprophagia. Tail chewing has been dealt with by spreading piquant substances on the tails, but this does not change the horse's motivation or address the cause; a better approach is to provide a palatable dietary supplement.
- Correction of diarrhea or other GI problems should resolve coprophagia secondary to GI illness.
- Tree chewing can be discouraged by building a wire fence around the tree trunk.
- For truly dangerous pica (e.g., rock chewing and ingestion), remove the horse or the rocks from the environment.

MEDICATIONS

DRUGS OF CHOICE

N/A

CONTRAINDICATIONS

N/A

PRECAUTIONS

N/A

POSSIBLE INTERACTIONS

N/A

ALTERNATIVE DRUGS

N/A

FOLLOW-UP

PATIENT MONITORING

Regular follow-up after 2 weeks of treatment to evaluate the owner's compliance and the success of the treatments given

POSSIBLE COMPLICATIONS

N/A

MISCELLANEOUS

ASSOCIATED CONDITIONS

N/A

AGE RELATED FACTORS

- Coprophagia is normal in young foals.
- Tail chewing is common in weanlings and yearlings.
- Wood chewing occurs at any age, as does coprophagia if the diet is inadequate, but usually is a disease of mature horses.

ZOONOTIC POTENTIAL

N/A

PREGNANCY

N/A

SYNONYMS

- Coprophagia
- Tail chewing
- Wood chewing

SEE ALSO

Oral stereotypic behaviors

ABBREVIATIONS

GI = gastrointestinal

Suggested Reading

Houpt KA, Wooden G. Tail chewing by horses. Equine Pract 1987;9:31–32.

Jackson SA, Rich RA, Ralston SL. Feeding behavior and feed efficiency in groups of horses as a function of feeding frequency and use of alfalfa hay cubes. J Anim Sci 1984;59(Suppl 1):152–153.

Krzak WE, Gonyou HW, Lawrence LM. Wood chewing by stabled horses: diurnal pattern and effects of exercise. J Anim Sci 1991;69:1053–1058.

McGreevy PD, French NP, Nichol CJ. The prevalence of abnormal behaviours in dressage, eventing and endurance horses in relation to stabling. Vet Rec 1995;137:36–37.

Ralson SL. Common behavioral problems of horses. Comp Cont Educ Pract Vet 1982;4:S152–S159.

Author Katherine Albro Houpt

Consulting Editor Daniel Q. Estep

PIGMENTURIA (HEMATURIA, HEMOGLOBINURIA, AND MYOGLOBINURIA)

BASICS

DEFINITION

- Discoloration of urine, usually red to brown in color, from increased excretion of RBCs (hematuria), hemoglobin (hemoglobinuria), or myoglobin (myoglobinuria)
- Factitious pigmenturia may be reported when dehydrated horses pass concentrated urine that is deep amber to light brown in color or be observed as red to brown discoloration of snow or wood shavings when other porphyrins in urine are oxidized after being voided (also seen with storage of urine over time).
- Also may be observed as a side effect of medication.

PATHOPHYSIOLOGY

Hematuria

- Normal urine contains $\cong$5000 RBC/ml or $<$5 RBC/hpf on sediment examination.
- Microscopic hematuria (10,000–2,500,000 RBC/ml) can be detected as increased RBCs (10–20/hpf) on sediment examination or trace to +++ reaction on reagent strip testing of urine.
- Macroscopic or gross hematuria can be observed with $>$2,500,000–5,000,000 RBC/ml ($\cong$0.5 ml of blood per 1 L of urine).
- Throughout urination, hematuria is consistent from hemorrhage from the kidneys, ureters, or bladder. At the beginning of urination, it most often accompanies lesions of the distal urethra. At the end of urination, it usually results from lesions in the proximal urethra or bladder neck.
- Detection of RBC casts or dysmorphic RBCs (i.e., substantial variation in RBC size, shape, and hemoglobin content) on sediment examination supports glomerular bleeding. Casts are formed by RBC accumulation in renal tubules; dysmorphism results from RBC exposure to hyper- and hypotonic environments during transit through renal tubules.

Hemoglobinuria

- Hemolysis and hemoglobinuria may develop with several disorders—primary immune-mediated diseases and secondary immune-mediated hemolytic anemia with infectious disease, neoplasia, or drug administration
- Hemolysis and hemoglobinuria may develop with liver disease or exposure to toxins (e.g., acorns, red-maple leaves, onions, phenothiazines) causing oxidant injury and Heinz-body anemia.

Myoglobinuria

- Urinary excretion of myoglobin most commonly produces pigmenturia after ER, but significant rhabdomyolysis and pigmenturia also may develop with other myopathies (e.g., PSSM), postanesthetic myopathy, or infectious diseases (e.g., *Streptococcus equi*, clostridial myonecrosis).
- "Atypical myoglobinuria" has been used to describe a highly fatal syndrome of non-exertional rhabdomyolysis that has affected groups of horses and ponies on poor-quality pasture.

SYSTEMS AFFECTED

- Renal/urologic—pigmenturia, especially hematuria
- Hemic/lymphatic/immune—hemolysis; hemoglobinuria
- Hepatobiliary—hemolysis; hemoglobinuria
- Musculoskeletal—rhabdomyolysis

SIGNALMENT

Breed Predilections

- Proximal urethral defects most commonly are observed in Quarter Horses.
- Arabians appear predisposed to IRH.
- PSSM is most common in Quarter Horses but may affect draft breeds.
- ER appears more common in Quarter Horses and Thoroughbreds.
- Post-anesthetic myopathy is of greatest risk in draft breeds.

Mean Age and Range

- NI affects neonatal foals.
- Vascular malformations more commonly produce hematuria in foals
- Neoplasia usually affects old horses.

Predominant Sex

- Proximal urethral defects and habronemiasis or neoplasia of the penis and distal urethra occur in geldings and stallions.
- ER is a more significant problem in young, female racehorses.

SIGNS

Historical Findings

- Horses with pigmenturia often have obvious historical evidence of a primary problem—"tying-up", ingestion of red-maple leaves or ionophores, or dysuria from lower UTI or penile neoplasia
- In others, observation of pigmenturia may be the presenting complaint for problems—vascular anomalies, cystolithiasis, proximal urethral defects, renal or bladder neoplasia, IRH, or exercise-associated hematuria

Physical Examination Findings

- Findings in horses with hematuria are consistent with the underlying disease processes (e.g., ARF, urolithiasis, UTI, neoplasia) or may be normal (e.g., vascular malformations, proximal urethral defects, exercise-associated hematuria, IRH).
- Findings in horses with hemoglobinuria or myoglobinuria reflect the underlying disease processes—pale membranes, weakness, and anorexia with hemolytic anemia; dark-brown membranes with methemoglobinemia; icteric membranes and hepatoencephalopathy with liver disease; firm muscles and a stiff gait or reluctance to move with ER

CAUSES

Genetics

- PSSM is a genetic disease in Quarter Horses.
- Heritable forms of ER appear to affect both Quarter Horses and Thoroughbreds.

Hematuria

- ARF—microscopic hematuria is common in most cases due to either glomerular or tubular injury.
- Urolithiasis—stones anywhere in the urinary tract may have hematuria as a presenting complaint; postexercise hematuria is especially common with large cystoliths.
- UTI—infection anywhere in the urinary tract, including habronemiasis of the prepuce and distal penis, may result in hematuria.
- Neoplasia—nephroblastoma, renal adenocarcinoma, hemangiosarcoma, squamous cell carcinoma of the lower urinary tract, transitional cell carcinoma, and other bladder tumors (e.g., leiomyoma, lymphosarcoma)
- Renal vascular anomalies—arteriovenous and arterioureteral malformations may cause hematuria in young horses.
- Proximal urethral defects—consistently found at the dorsocaudal aspect of the urethra as it passes over the ischial arch; likely result from a "blowout" of the corpus spongiosum penis (i.e., cavernous vascular tissue surrounding the urethra) into the urethral lumen that develops during contraction of the bulbospongiosus and urethralis muscles, causing a dramatically increased pressure in the corpus spongiosum penis; these muscles undergo a series of contractions during ejaculation and after urination to empty the urethra of urine and can produce hemospermia or hematuria at the end of urination; once the lesion is created, it is maintained by bleeding at the end of each urination, and the surrounding mucosa heals by formation of a fistula into the vascular tissue.

PIGMENTURIA (HEMATURIA, HEMOGLOBINURIA, AND MYOGLOBINURIA)

• Exercise-associated hematuria—microscopic hematuria seems a normal physiological response to exercise due to increased blood pressure and extravasation of RBCs across glomerular capillaries; magnitude of hematuria increases with exercise intensity; an occasional horse may develop gross hematuria after exercise, when the bladder mucosa can become "bruised" due to trauma against the brim of the pelvis; horses that urinate immediately before exercise are at greatest risk, because urine in the bladder cushions against mucosal injury.
• IRH—syndrome of recurrent, potentially life-threatening hematuria of renal origin; unknown cause; diagnosis established by excluding other causes of hematuria.

Hemoglobinuria

• Primary immune disorders—NI; incompatible blood transfusions
• Secondary immune disorders—hemolysis with infectious diseases (e.g., equine infectious anemia, piroplasmosis, purpura hemorrhagica with *Streptococcus equi, Clostridium* perfringens, almost any chronic infection), neoplasia, or drug administration (e.g., penicillins).
• Exposure to toxins—acorns; red-maple leaves; onions; phenothiazines; ionophores
• Liver disease

Myoglobinuria

• Rhabdomyolysis—associated with exercise or other metabolic (e.g., PSSM) and infectious (e.g., *Streptococcus equi*) diseases
• Nutritional myopathy—selenium deficiency
• Postanesthetic myopathy—due to crush injury of muscle during anesthesia
• "Atypical myoglobinuria"—ingestion of mycotoxins is a suspected but unsubstantiated cause.

Factitious Pigmenturia

• In some, other porphyrins (of plant origin) passed in urine may discolor snow or wood shavings red to brown in color and raise owner concerns about urinary tract hemorrhage; a similar brown discoloration of urine occurs when samples are stored in a refrigerator for several days.
• Discolored urine can be observed with certain medications—orange with rifampin; dark brown to black urine with doxycycline

RISK FACTORS

• Similar to those for ARF, urolithiasis, or UTI
• Quarter Horses and Arabians appear at greater risk for proximal urethral defects and IRH, respectively.
• Multiparous mares having a previous foal with NI are at greater risk of future foals with NI; previous blood transfusions increase the risk of incompatibility in future transfusions.
• Other risk factors for hemolysis and hemoglobinuria—chronic infections, neoplasia, drug administration, ingestion of toxins, or liver disease
• A period of rest without decreased feed intake is an important risk factor for ER and myoglobinuria.
• Selenium deficiency and insufficient padding or hypotension during anesthesia are further risk factors for myoglobinuria.

DIAGNOSIS

DIFFERENTIAL DIAGNOSES

• Blood accumulation at the vulvar margins in pregnant mares may be due to hemorrhage from varicosities in the vagina rather than from the urinary tract.
• Stallions with proximal urethral defects may present for hemospermia rather than hematuria.

CBC/BIOCHEMISTRY/URINALYSIS

• Changes characteristic for ARF (azotemia and electrolyte and acid–base alterations, see *Acute Renal Failure*), urolithiasis (see *Urolithiasis*), and UTI (see *Urinary Tract Infection*) when these cause hematuria.
• Mild to moderate anemia and hypergammaglobulinemia are nonspecific findings in some cases of neoplasia; cytology of urine sediment may reveal neoplastic cells.
• Laboratory data in horses with renal vascular anomalies may be normal unless hematuria is severe and accompanied by moderate to severe anemia and prerenal azotemia.
• Mild anemia may be found in occasional horses with proximal urethral defects. Urinalysis of a sample collected via bladder catheterization may be normal, or microscopic hematuria may be found.
• Horses with exercise-associated hematuria are not anemic, but transient proteinuria accompanies hematuria.
• PCV with IRH can range from normal to $<10\%$ depending on the magnitude and duration of hematuria; hypoproteinemia and other changes consistent with hemorrhagic shock (e.g., mature neutrophilia, hyperglycemia, prerenal azotemia) may be detected.
• With primary or secondary immune-mediated hemolytic anemia, PCV is low, gross hemoglobinemia may be observed as a red discoloration of plasma after centrifugation, and serum bilirubin concentration (predominantly indirect) is increased (10–30 mg/dL). Hypergammaglobulinemia also is expected with chronic infections or neoplasia.
• Methemoglobinemia may accompany intoxication with substances causing oxidant injury to hemoglobin (most notable with ingestion of maple leaves).
• With hemoglobinuria from liver disease, elevated liver enzyme activity and serum bile acid concentration, hypoglycemia, hypertriglyceridemia, low BUN, and prolonged coagulation times may be present.
• Horses with myoglobinuria have elevated creatine kinase and aspartate aminotransferase activities from rhabdomyolysis; destruction of $\geq$200 g of muscle must occur before myoglobin can be detected in urine.

OTHER LABORATORY TESTS

• Centrifugation of urine—a simple method of differentiating hematuria from hemoglobinuria or myoglobinuria; RBCs form a red to brown pellet with clear supernatant, whereas urine remains discolored after centrifugation with hemoglobinuria or myoglobinuria.
• Urine reagent strips impregnated with orthotoluidine—react with both hemoglobin and myoglobin; RBCs adsorbed onto the pad produce a pattern of scattered red spots on the test pad, however, and this pattern may be found as long as hematuria is $<$250,000 RBCs/mL.

PIGMENTURIA (HEMATURIA, HEMOGLOBINURIA, AND MYOGLOBINURIA)

• Blondheim test—differential precipitation of hemoglobin and myoglobin with ammonium sulfate is a simple but sometimes inaccurate test of urine.
• Hemoglobin—can be differentiated from myoglobin in urine by protein electrophoresis or specific tests (e.g., radioimmunoassays, enzyme-linked immunosorbent assays) for detection of hemoglobin or myoglobin.
• Quantitative urine culture—perform in all cases of suspected hematuria to assess for concurrent UTI.
• Serum bile acid and ammonia concentrations—may useful for further evaluation of horses with liver disease.

IMAGING

• Transabdominal ultrasonography—to assess kidney size and echogenicity
• Transrectal ultrasonography—to evaluate left kidney, ureters, bladder, and proximal urethra
• Urethroscopy/cystoscopy—to confirm source of hematuria; diagnostic tool of choice for proximal urethral defects

DIAGNOSTIC PROCEDURES

• Urine collection and centrifugation—to document pigmenturia and, possibly, differentiate hematuria from hemoglobinuria or myoglobinuria
• Liver biopsy—for further evaluation of horses with liver disease
• Muscle biopsy—for further evaluation of horses with ER and other myopathies

TREATMENT

This discussion is limited to hematuria; see other sections for treatment of disorders causing hemoglobinuria and myoglobinuria.

APPROPRIATE HEALTH CARE

• ARF—see *Acute Renal Failure.*
• Urolithiasis—see *Urolithiasis.*
• UTI—see *Urinary Tract Infection.*
• Neoplasia—complete surgical excision (rarely possible) combined with topical or intralesional antineoplastic agents for bladder and urethral cancer
• Renal vascular anomalies—proper diagnosis and, when hematuria persists, appropriate surgical intervention
• Proximal urethral defects—because $\cong$50% of lesions heal spontaneously, no treatment is initially indicated; surgery is recommended for hematuria causing anemia or lasting for >1 month.
• Exercise-associated hematuria—because it is a physiological consequence of exercise that resolves within minutes after exercise stops, no treatment is indicated; bladder mucosal lesions in the rare horse with gross hematuria also usually heal without treatment, but a few days of rest may be recommended to concerned clients.
• IRH—supportive care for hemorrhagic shock, including repeated blood transfusions; nephrectomy may be attempted in select cases.

SURGICAL CONSIDERATIONS

• Unilateral nephrectomy may correct hematuria in horses with renal tumors but rarely produces long-term success; most neoplasms, especially renal adenocarcinoma, usually metastasize before a diagnosis is established.
• Nephrectomy, or renal arteriolar embolization (in foals), may be indicated for young horses with persistent hematuria from renal vascular malformation; in other foals, hematuria may be self-limiting if a thrombus forms in the malformation.
• A perineal urethrotomy approach (i.e., standing surgery with epidural or local anesthesia) into the corpus spongiosum penis, but not extending into the urethral lumen, is the treatment of choice for persistent hematuria associated with a proximal urethral defect. The procedure creates a "pressure relief valve" for the corpus spongiosum penis, allowing the urethral defect to heal while the surgical wound heals by second intention.
• Nephrectomy may be indicated in selected cases with IRH that maintain normal renal function but continue to bleed from the affected kidney; unilateral renal hemorrhage should be documented via cystoscopy on several occasions before nephrectomy is pursued. Always approach nephrectomy cautiously, because bilateral, episodic renal bleeding may occur in some cases and Arabian horses may be more predisposed to bilateral disease.

NURSING CARE

• Although a straightforward procedure, surgical treatment of proximal urethral defects should be performed on an inpatient basis, and 3–5 days of postoperative hospitalization and care are recommended—bleeding from the surgical site can be rather dramatic for the initial few days after surgery, and frequent washing of the perineum and hind limbs often is necessary.
• Horses with IRH require frequent monitoring and supportive care and, possibly, blood transfusion both before and after nephrectomy.

DIET

See *Acute Renal Failure, Urolithiasis,* and *Urinary Tract Infection.*

CLIENT EDUCATION

• Patients with urinary tract neoplasia generally have a poor long-term prognosis, but current treatments and supportive care may produce short-term survival.
• Horses with vascular malformations may have other developmental anomalies that may not be apparent until later in life. Horses with vascular malformations that resolve by spontaneous formation of a thrombus may be at risk of developing hematuria again later in life.
• Counsel patience to owners of horses with proximal urethral defects with a short duration of hematuria, because spontaneous resolution may occur. Give similar advice in cases of exercise-associated bladder mucosal damage causing gross hematuria.
• The cause of hematuria in horses with IRH is unknown, so owners of affected horses must receive considerable education before nephrectomy is considered or pursued.

PIGMENTURIA (HEMATURIA, HEMOGLOBINURIA, AND MYOGLOBINURIA)

MEDICATIONS

DRUGS OF CHOICE

• 5-Fluorouracil and triethylenethiophosphoramide are antineoplastic agents that may be used topically (at weekly or more frequent intervals) for bladder or penile neoplasms.
• Prophylactic antibiotics are recommended for horses undergoing nephrectomy (e.g., penicillin/gentamicin) or a perineal urethrotomy approach for correction of a proximal urethral defect (e.g., trimethoprim/sulfonamide combination).
• α-Aminocaproic acid (10 mg/kg IV q6h) to enhance blood clot stabilization may be used in horses with renal hematuria from neoplasia or IRH, but success has not been reported.

CONTRAINDICATIONS

Do not perform nephrectomy in patients with azotemia.

PRECAUTIONS

Always approach nephrectomy with caution, and consider it a last-resort procedure for control of refractory unilateral renal hemorrhage.

POSSIBLE INTERACTIONS

N/A

ALTERNATIVE DRUGS

N/A

FOLLOW-UP

PATIENT MONITORING

• See *Acute Renal Failure, Urolithiasis,* and *Urinary Tract Infection.*
• Assess clinical status of patients managed surgically for proximal urethral defects at least twice daily, and monitor PCV once daily, during the initial 2–4 days after surgery.
• Assess clinical status of patients managed via nephrectomy at least twice daily during the initial 2–4 days after surgery, emphasizing urine output. Serum creatinine concentration may rise by ≥50% during the initial week after surgery, but it should return to the normal range after that time.

POSSIBLE COMPLICATIONS

• Dissemination of neoplasia
• IRH from the contralateral kidney after nephrectomy

EXPECTED COURSE AND PROGNOSIS

• Prognosis for recovery after surgical correction of a proximal urethral defect generally is favorable, but the problem occasionally may recur.
• Recurrent bouts of hematuria over several years may be the expected course with IRH. Some horses may have the problem resolve; others may eventually suffer acute, fatal renal hemorrhage.
• Issue a guarded long-term prognosis for patients with renal hematuria initially treated successfully by unilateral nephrectomy due to the loss of renal functional reserve and potential for bleeding from the remaining kidney.

MISCELLANEOUS

ASSOCIATED CONDITIONS

• ARF
• Urolithiasis
• UTI
• Immune-mediated hemolytic anemia—primary and secondary
• Intoxication with agents causing hemolysis and hemoglobinuria
• Liver disease
• ER

AGE-RELATED FACTORS

• NI affects neonates during the initial 1–3 days of life.
• Vascular malformations usually result in hematuria during the first few years of life.

ZOONOTIC POTENTIAL

Leptospirosis, which may cause hematuria and ARF, has zoonotic potential; avoid direct contact with infective urine.

PREGNANCY

• Multiparous mares are at greater risk of producing alloantibodies that may lead to NI in their foals.
• Vulvar hemorrhage from varicosities can be confused with hematuria.

SYNONYMS

Azoturia (for ER)

SEE ALSO

• ARF
• UTI
• Urolithiasis

ABBREVIATIONS

• ARF = acute renal failure
• ER = exertional rhabdomyolysis
• hpf = high-power field
• IRH = idiopathic renal hematuria
• NI = neonatal isoerythrolysis
• PCV = packed cell volume
• PSSM = polysaccharide storage myopathy
• UTI = urinary tract infection

Suggested Reading

Fischer AT, Spier S, Carlson GP, et al. Neoplasia of the equine urinary bladder as a cause of hematuria. J Am Vet Med Assoc 1985;186:1294–1296.

Schott HC. Hematuria. In: Reed SM, Bayly WM, eds. Equine internal medicine. Philadelphia: WB Saunders, 1998:890–895.

Schott HC, Barbee DD, Hines MT, et al. Renal arteriovenous malformation in a Quarter Horse foal. J Vet Intern Med 1996;10:204–206.

Schott HC, Hodgson DR, Bayly WM. Haematuria, pigmenturia and proteinuria in exercising horses. Equine Vet J 1995;27:67–72.

Schumacher J, Varner DD, Schmitz DG, et al. Urethral defects in geldings with hematuria and stallions with hemospermia. Vet Surg 1995;24:250–254.

Author Harold C. Schott II
Consulting Editor Harold C. Schott II

PLACENTAL BASICS

DEFINITIONS

• Placental classification by five major systems—shape, origin of tissues, degree of invasion, vascular structure, and degree of attachment
• Shape—diffuse in mares; normal placenta covers the entire endometrial surface; for normal avillous sites, see exceptions below.
• Origin of tissues—chorioallantoic; tissues derived from fusion of fetal-derived chorion and allantoic sac
• Degree of invasion—epitheliochorial; fetal-derived tissue directly apposes maternal endometrium.
• Vascular structure—microcotyledonary/ villous; unit of exchange is villous-like maternal and placental vascular apposition.
• Degree of attachment—adeciduate; no loss of maternal tissue in placenta formation or expulsion

CHRONOLOGY

• Equine conceptus is mobile (i.e., transuterine migration) within the uterus to day 16 after conception.
• Conceptus is spheric until approximately day 35 and ellipsoid thereafter.
• Endometrial cup formation by day 36–38.
• Pregnancy maintenance by chorioallantoic placentation at approximately day 40.
• Placenta contacts the entire endometrial surface by approximately day 77.
• Placental development complete by day 150

ENDOMETRIAL CUPS

• Fetal trophoblast invasion of maternal endometrium—formation begins at approximately day 36–38; peak function of endometrial cups at approximately day 70
• Cups undergo necrosis by day 120–150.
• Cups are sloughed and become "allantochorionic pouches."
• Cups produce eCG and are responsible for formation and function of accessory CL.

EXAMINATION

• At parturition, fetus ruptures placenta at the cervical star; chorioallantois is passed inside out, with fetal surface (i.e., allantois) exteriorized.
• For complete examination, also observe chorionic surface. Lay out in the shape of an "F." To ensure none has been retained, confirm that horn tips are present, and if areas are torn, match blood vessels on the exposed allantoic surface.

VILLI

• Five normal avillous areas—location of endometrial cups, the cervical star, ostium (at tips of horns), site of umbilical attachment, and invaginated/redundant folds; appear longitudinal and symmetric
• Pathologic avillous areas—apposition of placenta in a twin pregnancy, placentitis, and endometrial fibrosis

PLACENTAL BASICS

ALLANTOCHORION

NORMAL

- Appears as "red velvet" because of the diffuse microvilli over the entire surface.
- Tip of the pregnant horn usually is thicker and edematous compared to nonpregnant horn—unknown significance.

ABNORMAL

If edematous or thickened, may indicate vascular disturbance or fescue toxicosis.

AMNION

NORMAL

- Equine amnion is completely separate from allantochorion.
- White; opaque.

ABNORMAL

- Discolored or edematous—fetal distress (e.g. fetal diarrhea).
- Thickened—amnionitis
- Extension of allantochorionitis

UMBILICAL CORD

NORMAL

- Distinct allantoic and amniotic portions (60–83 cm in length)
- Normal twists in equine cord

ABNORMAL

- Length > 100 cm increases risk of strangulation and torsion.
- Examine for fetal autolysis, vascular damage, thrombi (e.g., evidence of abnormal, excessive twisting), and urachal tearing.

ALLANTOIC FLUID

- Clear to amber—hypotonic urine and fetal excretory products
- Within the allantoic fluid—hippomane (i.e., allantoic calculus) composed of concentric layers of cellular debris
- Rubbery
- Color—dark brown, green or tan

AMNIOTIC FLUID

Opaque—respiratory and buccal secretions of the fetus.

SEE ALSO

Placentitis—bacterial; viral; fungal

ABBREVIATIONS

- CL = corpus luteum
- eCG = equine chorionic gonadotropin

Author Peter R. Morresey
Consulting Editor Carla L. Carleton

PLACENTAL INSUFFICIENCY (MARE)

BASICS

DEFINITION
- Placental exchange unit cannot meet fetal demands, resulting in fetal malnutrition.
- May result in intrauterine growth retardation, prolonged gestation, or pregnancy loss.

PATHOPHYSIOLOGY
- Physical constrictions to placental development—body pregnancy; intraluminal adhesions
- Whether caused by nonformation or separation of microcotyledonary attachments, the area available for placental villus exchange between the endometrium and fetus is decreased.
- Histiotrophe (i.e. uterine milk) exchange occurs between the microcotyledonary attachments. Its production increases during pregnancy, and sufficient histiotrophe production depends on health and number of endometrial glands.

SYSTEM AFFECTED
Reproductive

GENETICS
N/A

INCIDENCE/PREVALENCE
N/A

SIGNALMENT
- Pregnant female, usually aged or multiparous
- May have history of endometritis.
- Mares bearing twins—highlights the mare's inability to sustain two placentae and two fetuses. Classic placental lesion is at the site of apposition of the two placentae, which prevents attachment to the endometrium. Grossly visible as an avillous (pale area) at which no exchange can occur. Usual outcome is abortion of both fetuses or one dead and/or mummified; if it reaches term, the remaining twin is small for gestational age.

SIGNS

General Comments
- Preterm—abortion of small, emaciated fetus or fetuses
- Prolonged gestation or term delivery of small-for-gestational-age, dysmature fetus—underweight; silky haircoat; behavioral abnormalities; at increased risk for sepsis.

Historical Findings
- May have previously delivered in this fashion.
- Endometrial changes are irreversible. Previous endometrial biopsy commonly revealed fibrosis, glandular nesting, or decreased number of glands.

Physical Examination Findings
- Gross uterine abnormalities—intraluminal adhesions; segmental aplasia
- Histopathologic findings—see *Pathologic Findings*.

CAUSES
- Placentitis
- Degenerative endometrial changes—biopsy diagnosis

RISK FACTORS
- Age
- Chronic endometritis.
- Poor vulvar conformation.
- Uterine infection.
- Low endometrial biopsy category.

DIAGNOSIS

DIFFERENTIAL DIAGNOSIS
- Infectious causes of abortion—bacterial; viral; fungal
- Noninfectious causes of abortion—endotoxemia caused by systemic illness
- Other causes of prolonged gestation—fescue toxicosis; fetal endocrine abnormalities
- Other causes of fetal malnutrition—twinning; maternal disease

CBC/BIOCHEMISTRY/URINALYSIS
- Abnormalities reflect the systemic pathologic process, if any, in mare.
- No changes are directly attributable to placental insufficiency.

OTHER LABORATORY TESTS
N/A

IMAGING

Transabdominal Ultrasonography
- Small-for-gestational-age fetus—crown-to-rump length; fetal orbit
- IUGR—more pronounced later in gestation
- Asymmetrically affected fetal/neonatal development—long head; thin body; little body fat

Transrectal Ultrasonography
Thickness or detachment of placenta cranial to cervix—late gestation

DIAGNOSTIC PROCEDURES
N/A

PATHOLOGIC FINDINGS

Gross Findings
- Placental examination—avillous areas other than those previously described as normal (see *Placental Basics*).
- Thickened, edematous, or discolored areas
- Evidence of multiple pregnancy—mummified fetus

Histopathologic Findings
Endometrial biopsy—pronounced fibrosis; glandular nesting; lymphatic stasis of the endometrium; varying degrees of inflammation

TREATMENT
Placental insufficiency is a postpartum diagnosis.

PLACENTAL INSUFFICIENCY (MARE)

APPROPRIATE HEALTH CARE
N/A

NURSING CARE
N/A

ACTIVITY
N/A

DIET
N/A

CLIENT EDUCATION
N/A

SURGICAL CONSIDERATIONS
N/A

MEDICATIONS

DRUGS
- Progestin supplementation may be helpful to boost endometrial histiotrophe production.
- Progesterone-in-oil
- Altrenogest

CONTRAINDICATIONS
Establish viability of fetus before treatment—transabdominal fetal ultrasonography; fetal heart rate

PRECAUTIONS
N/A

POSSIBLE INTERACTIONS
N/A

ALTERNATIVE DRUGS
N/A

FOLLOW-UP

PATIENT MONITORING
- Ultrasonography
- Fetus—for viability and heart rate
- Placenta—for thickness and detachment
- Evaluation of mare when not pregnant (i.e., breeding-soundness evaluation)—endometrial biopsy to evaluate density of endometrial glands, presence of inflammation (e.g., acute, neutrophilia; chronic, plasmacytic, lymphocytic), association with pneumovagina, eosinophilia; scar tissue (e.g., periglandular fibrosis, diffuse; lymphatic, dilation, stasis).

PREVENTION/AVOIDANCE
N/A

POSSIBLE COMPLICATIONS
- Abortion
- Birth of undersized, weak neonate
- Premature placental separation at parturition

EXPECTED COURSE AND PROGNOSIS
N/A

MISCELLANEOUS

ASSOCIATED CONDITIONS
- Placentitis.
- Premature placental separation.
- Neonatal maladjustment.
- Fetal sepsis—bacterial; fungal.

AGE-RELATED FACTORS
Endometrial health declines with age and increasing parity of mares.

ZOONOTIC POTENTIAL
N/A

PREGNANCY
Abortion

SYNONYMS
N/A

SEE ALSO
N/A

ABBREVIATION
IUGR = intrauterine growth retardation

Suggested Reading

Adams R. Identification of the mare and foal at high risk for perinatal problems. In: McKinnon AO, Voss JL, eds. Equine reproduction. Philadelphia: Lea & Febiger, 1993:988–989.

Giles RC, Donahue JM, Hong CB, et al. Causes of abortion, stillbirth, and perinatal death in horses: 3,527 cases (1986–1991). J Am Vet Med Assoc 1993;203:1170–1175.

Author Peter R. Morresey
Consulting Editor Carla L. Carleton

PLACENTITIS

BASICS

DEFINITION

Inflammation of the placenta.

PATHOPHYSIOLOGY

- An infectious agent (e.g., bacterial, viral, mycotic) invades the placenta, leading to an inflammatory response.
- Placental detachment.
- Modes of entry—ascending via cervix (most common); hematogenous, as part of systemic illness; direct spread, inoculation, or recrudescence of pre-existing focus

SYSTEM AFFECTED

Reproductive

GENETICS

N/A

INCIDENCE/PREVALENCE

N/A

SIGNALMENT

Pregnant mare during late gestation.

SIGNS

- Vulval discharge—purulent; hemorrhagic
- Cervical incompetence—discharge; inflammation.
- Mammary—swelling; discharge; prepartum lactation.
- Relaxation of pelvic musculature—vulval; sacrosciatic ligament.
- Restlessness; premonitory foaling behavior.
- Placental—thickening; edema; discoloration; adenomatous hyperplasia; plaque formation, especially centered on cervical star.

CAUSES AND RISK FACTORS

Bacterial

- Throughout gestation.
- Two presentations—acute, focal or diffuse; chronic, focal or extensive.
- Acute, focal or diffuse—neutrophil infiltration; necrosis of chorionic villi; primarily early to mid gestation.
- Chronic, focal or extensive—centered around area of cervical star; eosinophilic chorionic material; necrosis of villi, adenomatous hyperplasia; mononuclear cell infiltration; primarily mid to late gestation.
- Common pathogens—*Streptococcus equi* var *zooepidemicus, Streptococcus equisimilis, Escherichia coli, Pseudomonas aeruginosa,* and *Klebsiella pneumoniae*
- Leptospira sp.—diffuse, spirochete invasion; hematogenous spread only
- Nocardioform actinomycete—horn base; Gram-positive filamentous bacillus infiltration; chronic nature

Viral

EVA—thickening of chorioallantois attributable to a longer incubation time before abortion compared with EHV-1 (either no or nonspecific placental changes)

Fungal

- Usually 300 days of gestation or later.
- *Aspergillus* sp.—chronic, focal placentitis at cervical star similar to chronic bacterial cases.
- *Candida* sp.—diffuse; necrotizing; proliferative.
- *Histoplasma* sp.—multifocal; granulomatous.

Anatomic

- Cervical incompetence—laceration; age-induced degeneration.
- Production of PGF by endotoxin release, leading to cervical relaxation.

DIAGNOSIS

DIFFERENTIAL DIAGNOSIS

- Impending parturition.
- Fescue toxicosis—placental edema; delayed parturition; decreased lactation
- Other causes of vulval discharge—vaginitis (speculum examination to assess cervical integrity/discharge); endometritis; pyometra; metritis
- Uterine trauma or hemorrhage.
- Urinary tract infection.
- Urine pooling
- Uterine or vaginal neoplasia.
- Other causes of lactation.
- Other causes of relaxation—impending parturition

CBC/BIOCHEMISTRY/URINALYSIS

- Leukocytosis with neutrophilia.
- Hyperfibrinogenemia
- Biochemistry usually normal.
- Urinalysis—normal.

OTHER LABORATORY TESTS

N/A

IMAGING

Ultrasonography:

- Transrectal; transabdominal.
- Increased uteroplacental thickness (>15 mm), especially in the cervical region.
- Areas of folding or detachment.
- Allantoic fluid debris.

DIAGNOSTIC PROCEDURES

- Microbial culture of discharge from cervix.
- Cytology—PMNs, with or without intracellular bacteria; fungal elements.

PATHOLOGIC FINDINGS

Examination of the chorioallantois.

Gross Findings

- Thickened; discolored.
- Bright red chorion becomes gray/brown, with plaques; avillous areas; exudative.

Histopathologic Findings

- Necessary to differentiate bacterial from mycotic.
- inflammatory infiltrate, fibrosis, thrombosis, edema, causative agent—bacterial or fungal elements.
- Microbiologic—bacterial/fungal/virus isolation.

TREATMENT

APPROPRIATE HEALTH CARE

- Remove inciting cause—control infectious agent (bacterial, fungal).
- Maintain fetoplacental function.
- Prevent fetal expulsion—if mare carries to 300 days, chance of fetal survival increases; stress of intrauterine environment accelerates maturity.

PLACENTITIS

NURSING CARE
Minimize material and fetal stress.

ACTIVITY
Stall rest the mare.

DIET
N/A

CLIENT EDUCATION
N/A

SURGICAL CONSIDERATIONS
N/A

MEDICATIONS

DRUGS OF CHOICE
Antibiotics
- Penicillin G; gentamicin
- Selection based on sensitivities of most likely pathogen.

Anti-inflammatories
- Decrease endotoxin production.
- Decreases luteolytic potential.
- Decrease myometrial contractility.
- Decrease incidence of laminitis.

Progestogen Supplementation
- Maintain production of histiotrophe—fetal nutrition.
- Quiets myometrium.
- To aid cervical competency.

CONTRAINDICATIONS
If Fetal death occurs:
- Discontinue progestogens and NSAIDs.
- Allow abortion to occur.
- Avoid *in utero* fetal decomposition.

PRECAUTIONS
N/A

POSSIBLE INTERACTIONS
N/A

ALTERNATIVE DRUGS
N/A

FOLLOW-UP

PATIENT MONITORING
Mare
- Vaginal speculum examination to monitor cervix—closed; relaxing
- Transrectal ultrasonography of cervix and caudal uterine body to evaluate thickness and detachment of placenta.
- Attend parturition—increased incidence of premature placental separation or decreased likelihood of thickened chorioallantois to tear readily as fetus is born; either can lead to neonatal asphyxiation.
- Preterm mammary development (especially if >30 days before parturition).
- Premature lactation.
- Placental examination—examine to ensure it remains intact no fetal membranes are retained.

Neonate
- Increased potential for sepsis.
- Prepartum lactation may have depleted colostral antibodies.

PREVENTION/AVOIDANCE
- Breeding soundness examination of the mare when not pregnant; include examination of cervical competence—best if in diestrus at examination
- Prebreeding preparation of mare and stallion—hygiene
- Keep environment and housing of pregnant mares as clean as possible.

POSSIBLE COMPLICATIONS
- Abortion
- Sick, weak neonate.

EXPECTED COURSE AND PROGNOSIS
N/A

MISCELLANEOUS

ASSOCIATED CONDITIONS
- Premature placental separation.
- Laminitis
- Fetal sepsis—bacterial; fungal.

AGE-RELATED FACTORS
Endometrial health and cervical competence decline with age and increasing parity of mares.

ZOONOTIC POTENTIAL
N/A

PREGNANCY
Abortion

SYNONYMS
N/A

SEE ALSO
Placental insufficiency.

ABBREVIATIONS
- EHV = equine herpes virus
- EVA = equine viral arteritis
- PMN = polymorphonuclear

Suggested Reading

Adams R. Identification of the mare and foal at high risk for perinatal problems. In: McKinnon AO, Voss JL, ed. Equine reproduction. Philadelphia: Lea & Febiger, 1993:988–989.

Asbury AC, Leblanc MM. Placental abnormalities. In: McKinnon AO, Voss JL, ed. Equine reproduction. Philadelphia: Lea & Febiger, 1993:514–515.

Hong CB, Donahue JM, Giles RC Jr, et al. Etiology and pathology of equine placentitis. J Vet Diagn Invest 1993;5:56–63.

Author Peter R. Morresey
Consulting Editor Carla L. Carleton

PLEURAL FLUID CYTOLOGY

BASICS

DEFINITION

- Collection of fluid from the pleural space by aspiration through a stab incision between the intercostal spaces
- Fluid usually is taken from both the right and left sides of the chest.
- Samples are collected aseptically into a sterile clot tube for bacterial culture and into EDTA for cell count, cytology, and protein determination.
- Normal equine pleural fluid is clear to yellow, with no detectable odor.
- Protein content, as measured by refractometry, usually is <2.5 g/dL in samples from normal horses. Total nucleated cell count in fluid from normal horses is reportedly 800–12,000 cells/μL, with most samples containing <8,000 cells/μL.
- Nondegenerate neutrophils (low numbers) and large mononuclear cells, including mesothelial cells and macrophages, comprise most of the cells in normal pleural fluid. A few small lymphocytes occasionally, and eosinophils rarely, are seen.
- Small numbers of RBCs commonly are present, presumably because of minor hemorrhage secondary to sampling.

PATHOPHYSIOLOGY

- Pleural fluid normally is a dialysate of the plasma, present in a small volume, and drained from the pleural cavity via lymphatic vessels.
- An increased volume of this fluid constitutes an effusion, the character of which reflects the process initiating the increased volume—inflammation, neoplasia, decreased oncotic pressure, or hemorrhage

SYSTEMS AFFECTED

- Respiratory
- Cardiovascular
- Hemic/lymphatic/immune
- Hepatobiliary

SIGNALMENT

Any breed or sex

SIGNS

- Dyspnea
- Depression
- Weight loss
- Fever
- Cough
- Nasal discharge
- Reduced lung sounds
- Exercise intolerance
- Ventral edema

CAUSES

- Pleuritis—inflammation caused by pleuropneumonia, ruptured abscess, external trauma, foreign bodies, or primary pleuritis; may be bacterial, viral, or fungal.
- Neoplasia—lymphoma, metastatic squamous cell carcinoma, metastatic adenocarcinoma, or mesothelioma
- Hemorrhage
- Decreased oncotic pressure—hypoalbuminemia
- Increased hydrostatic pressure—congestive heart failure
- Chylothorax

RISK FACTORS

N/A

DIAGNOSIS

DIFFERENTIAL DIAGNOSIS

Pleuritis

- Inflammation causes an exudate, or fluid, with an increased cell count and protein content. This most commonly is associated with pneumonia or lung abscess and often is bacterial in origin.
- A predominantly neutrophilic (≥70%) response is seen in acute inflammation.
- If bacteria are present, neutrophils may appear degenerate (with pale, swollen nuclei), and bacteria may be seen, either intracellularly or free. Some bacteria cause fewer degenerative-type changes, however, so culture is suggested when neutrophil numbers are increased, even when the morphology appears normal.
- As inflammation becomes more chronic, the proportion of large mononuclear cells increases compared to neutrophils, and these cells may appear vacuolated or actively phagocytic.
- Lymphocytes and eosinophils may be present in very small numbers in exudates.

Neoplasia

- If cells from an intrathoracic tumor are shed into the pleural fluid, a diagnosis of neoplasia may be established on the basis of cytologic examination of the fluid.
- The most common tumor causing pleural effusions is lymphoma, sometimes characterized by large lymphocytes with large nuclei, prominent nucleoli, and scant, deeply basophilic cytoplasm. Lymphoma that is not lymphoblastic is harder to diagnose cytologically, because neoplastic lymphocytes may appear morphologically normal.
- Primary mesothelioma, metastatic gastric squamous cell carcinoma, and adenocarcinoma also may exfoliate cells into the pleural fluid.
- Intrathoracic tumors not uncommonly incite inflammation, which may make establishing the diagnosis more difficult. In addition, effusions typically cause exfoliation of reactive mesothelial cells, which have some cytologic features of malignancy.

Hemorrhage

- Most hemorrhage in fluid samples is mild, iatrogenic, and occurs at the time of sampling.
- Very recent hemorrhage may be associated with platelets in the sample.
- Hemorrhage into the thorax before sampling may cause a sample to appear hemolyzed, and phagocytosis of RBCs or erythrocyte breakdown products may be seen cytologically.

PLEURAL FLUID CYTOLOGY

Decreased Oncotic Pressure

- Hypoalbuminemia may cause accumulation of a very low-protein, low-cellularity fluid in the pleural cavity because of reduced oncotic pressure in the plasma. This fluid is cytologically unremarkable, with low numbers of nondegenerate neutrophils, large mononuclear cells, and few lymphocytes.
- Mesothelial cells may appear reactive because of increased fluid volume.

Increased Hydrostatic Pressure

- Effusions that result from congestive heart failure or other causes of increased venous or lymphatic pressure usually have higher cell counts (5000–15,000 cells/μL) and protein content (2.0–5.0 g/dL) than a pure transudate.
- These modified transudates have a normal distribution of cells, including neutrophils and large mononuclear cells.

Chylothorax

This rare condition in horses has been associated with pleural fluid that was white and opaque grossly, with a predominance of small lymphocytes cytologically.

LABORATORY FINDINGS

Drugs that May Alter Lab Results

N/A

Disorders that May Alter Lab Results

N/A

Valid If Run in Human Lab?

Cell count and protein determination may be done in any lab, but interpretation of equine cytology requires special training.

CBC/BIOCHEMISTRY/URINALYSIS

- Inflammatory conditions of the pleura may be associated with leukocytosis, left shift, toxic changes in neutrophils, and hyperfibrinogenemia. These changes are not always present, however, and are not specific for pleural inflammation.
- Hypoalbuminemia on a serum biochemical panel is helpful in establishing the diagnosis of a transudate.

OTHER LABORATORY TESTS

- Culture fluid with increased numbers of neutrophils both aerobically and anaerobically.
- Bronchoalveolar lavage or transtracheal aspiration may help in establishing the diagnosis of pleuropneumonia or lung abscess.

IMAGING

Radiology and ultrasonography may help to localize pleural fluid and to characterize pathologic processes—abscesses, masses, and pneumonias

DIAGNOSTIC PROCEDURES

N/A

TREATMENT

Directed at the underlying cause of the abnormal thoracic fluid.

MEDICATIONS

DRUGS OF CHOICE

N/A

CONTRAINDICATIONS

N/A

PRECAUTIONS

N/A

POSSIBLE INTERACTIONS

N/A

ALTERNATIVE DRUGS

N/A

FOLLOW UP

PATIENT MONITORING

N/A

POSSIBLE COMPLICATIONS

N/A

MISCELLANEOUS

ASSOCIATED CONDITIONS

N/A

AGE-RELATED FACTORS

N/A

ZOONOTIC POTENTIAL

N/A

PREGNANCY

N/A

SYNONYMS

Thoracic paracentesis

SEE ALSO

N/A

Suggested Reading

Bain F. Cytology of the respiratory tract. Vet Clin North Am Equine Pract 1997;13:477–486.

Bennett DG. Evaluation of pleural fluid in the diagnosis of thoracic disease in the horse. J Am Vet Med Assoc 1986;188:814–815.

Parry BW. Pleural fluid. In: Cowell RL, Tyler RD, eds. Cytology and hematology of the horse. Goleta, CA: American Veterinary Publications, 1992:107–120.

Author Susan J. Tornquist

Consulting Editor Claire B. Andreasen

PLEUROPNEUMONIA

BASICS

OVERVIEW
Development of an inflammatory response in the lung parenchyma to bacterial pathogens, with extension to the pleural space and subsequent pleural effusion.

SIGNALMENT
- No breed or sex predilections
- All ages can be affected, but pleuritis with pneumonia is much less common in foals than the adults.

SIGNS
- Acute—fever; lethargy; anorexia; tachypnea; dyspnea; decreased bronchovesicular sounds ventrally; radiating heart sounds; pleural friction rubs; serous, serosanguinous, or mucopurulent nasal discharge; pleural pain (i.e., pleurodynia); soft cough; and ventral or limb edema.
- Subacute or chronic—fever (may be intermittent), weight loss, exercise intolerance, persistent ventral or limb edema, intermittent colic, and tachypnea and dyspnea relative to the volume of pleural effusion; cough, nasal discharge, and pleurodynia are minimal to absent.

CAUSES AND RISK FACTORS
- A single bacterial pathogen may be isolated in pleuropneumonia, but mixed infections are common.
- *Streptococcus zooepidemicus* is the primary Gram-positive pathogen.
- *Escherichia coli* and *Klebsiella pneumoniae* are the most common Gram-negative, enteric pathogens.
- *Actinobacillus* spp. and *Pasteurella* spp. are the most common Gram-negative, nonenteric pathogens.
- Anaerobic bacteria are isolated in many cases; mycoplasma has been isolated from the pleural fluid in rare cases.
- Stress, transport, exercise-induced pulmonary hemorrhage, viral disease, esophageal obstruction (i.e., choke), dysphagia, thoracic trauma, and general anesthesia.

DIAGNOSIS

DIFFERENTIAL DIAGNOSIS
- Viral pneumonia—influenza, rhinopneumonitis, or EVA
- Fungal pneumonia—coccidioidomycosis
- Neoplasia—lymphosarcoma or gastric squamous cell carcinoma
- Hemothorax
- Cardiac disease—congestive heart failure or pericarditis
- EIA
- Diaphragmatic hernia
- Thoracic auscultation, ultrasonography, and radiography indicate pleural fluid and cranioventral pulmonary consolidation and help to differentiate pleuropneumonia from uncomplicated bacterial, fungal, or viral pneumonia.
- Serologic testing can rule out coccidioidomycosis and EIC.
- Consider hemothorax or diaphragmatic hernia with historical or physical evidence of thoracic trauma.
- Jugular venous distension or pulsation combined with cardiac murmur or arrhythmia suggest cardiac disease.
- Cytology of pleural fluid is important in differentiating neoplasia.

CBC/BIOCHEMISTRY/URINALYSIS
- CBC—inflammatory leukogram (e.g., neutrophilic leukocytosis, hyperfibrinogenemia) or toxic leukogram (e.g., leukopenia with a left shift, toxic neutrophils, normal to low plasma proteins, hemoconcentration); anemia (e.g., subacute, chronic)
- Biochemistry—hypergammaglobulinemia (e.g., subacute, chronic)

OTHER LABORATORY TESTS
Arterial blood gases help to evaluate severity of hypoxemia, hypercapnia, and respiratory compromise.

OTHER DIAGNOSTIC TESTS
- The definitive diagnosis is established by cytology and microbiology of aspirates—TTA or pleural fluid sample (i.e., thoracocentesis)
- TTA often is more rewarding than thoracocentesis for positive identification of pulmonary pathogens.
- Pleural fluid glucose concentration <40 mg/dL suggests septic effusion.

IMAGING

Thoracic Ultrasonography
- Hypoechoic or anechoic fluid between the thoracic wall and the lung parenchyma
- Fluid may be loculated with significant fibrin deposition.
- Pulmonary consolidation or atelectasis can be detected.
- Pulmonary abscess can be detected if surrounded by nonaerated lung or in a subpleural location.
- Small, hyperechoic images within the pleural fluid suggest anaerobic infection.

Thoracic Radiography
- Less useful than ultrasonography for accurate detection of pleural fluid
- May be helpful after thoracocentesis and drainage of pleural fluid to reveal the extent of pneumonia.

TREATMENT

INPATIENT VERSUS OUTPATIENT
- Not all cases require hospitalization; mild cases with minimal fluid accumulation and respiratory compromise can be treated on an outpatient basis.
- Inpatient treatment is recommended in cases with significant fluid accumulation because of the need for frequent re-evaluation by ultrasonography, repeated thoracocentesis, or indwelling thoracic drainage.

SUPPORTIVE CARE
- Administer polyionic fluids with evidence of dehydration.
- Consider NSAIDs with evidence of endotoxemia or severe pyrexia.

EMERGENCY CARE
To stabilize patients in respiratory distress, nasal insufflation with oxygen and therapeutic thoracocentesis may be required.

PLEUROPNEUMONIA

MEDICATIONS

DRUGS

Antimicrobial Therapy

- Optimally, base treatment on identification of the bacterial pathogens and results of in vitro sensitivity testing; if therapy is begun without culture results, use broad-spectrum drugs because mixed infections are common.
- Choose agents that are effective against both Gram-positive and -negative as well as aerobic and anaerobic organisms.
- Penicillin is effective against the great majority of anaerobes, but *Bacteroides fragilis*, a common anaerobic isolate, often is resistant.
- A common treatment choice is penicillin or ampicillin, gentamicin or amikacin, and metronidazole.
- Table 1 lists common antimicrobial susceptibilities.

Other Drugs

- Anti-inflammatories—phenylbutazone or flunixin meglumine may be used to reduce inflammation and to provide analgesia.
- Fluids—use oral or intravenous fluids to correct dehydration and electrolyte or acid–base disturbances.
- Antithrombotics—heparin and aspirin have been used in endotoxic animals, which may be at increased risk of DIC, but their use is controversial.

CONTRAINDICATIONS/POSSIBLE INTERACTIONS

- NSAIDs inhibit prostaglandin production and, thus, can further reduce renal blood flow in dehydrated patients.
- The nephrotoxicity of aminoglycoside antibiotics may be potentiated in dehydrated patients or by concurrent administration of NSAIDs.

FOLLOW-UP

PATIENT MONITORING

- Frequent auscultation and follow-up thoracic ultrasonography are the most sensitive indicators of the patient progress.
- Repeated thoracic drainage or placement of an indwelling thoracic drain may be necessary for cases in which pleural fluid continues to accumulate.
- Diligently monitor the feet for signs of laminitis.

PREVENTION/AVOIDANCE

- Avoid or minimize risk factors.
- Vaccination against upper respiratory viruses.

POSSIBLE COMPLICATIONS

- Pulmonary or subpleural abscesses are not uncommon.
- Bronchopleural fistulas, pleural adhesions, pericarditis, and laminitis are other serious sequelae.

EXPECTED COURSE AND PROGNOSIS

- Guarded to good prognosis in cases with early diagnosis and aggressive antibacterial and supportive treatment
- Guarded to poor prognosis in cases that reach the subacute to chronic stage before an accurate diagnosis is established.

MISCELLANEOUS

ASSOCIATED CONDITIONS

N/A

AGE-RELATED FACTORS

N/A

ZOONOTIC POTENTIAL

N/A

PREGNANCY

N/A

SEE ALSO

- Aspiration pneumonia
- Expiratory dyspnea
- Heaves
- Respiratory distress syndrome
- Thoracic trauma

ABBREVIATIONS

- DIC = disseminated intravascular coagulation
- EIA = equine infectious anemia
- EVA = equine viral arteritis
- TTA = transtracheal aspirate

Suggested Reading

Byars TD, Becht JL. Pleuropneumonia. Vet Clin North Am Equine Pract 1991;7:63–77.

Chaffin MK, Carter GK. Bacterial pleuropneumonia. In: Robinson, NE, ed. Current therapy in equine medicine 4. Philadelphia: WB Saunders, 1997:449–452.

Author Joie Watson

Consulting Editor Jean-Pierre Lavoie

Table 1

Antimicrobial Susceptibilities

Organism (n)	*Penicillin (%)*	*Ampicillin (%)*	*Amikacin (%)*	*Gentamicin (%)*	*TMS (%)*	*Ceftiofur (%)*
S. zooepidemicus (14)	100	100	0	7	100	100
E. coli (74)	–	68	100	86	60	94
Klebsiella sp. (15)	–	14	100	67	67	100
Actinobacillus sp. (26)	100	89	100	100	96	100
Pasteurella sp. (6)	100	100	100	100	100	83

Reprinted with permission from Organisms isolated from non-urine sources. Microbiology Service, Veterinary Medical Teaching Hospital, University of California–Davis, 1998. Compiled by Jennifer Fitchhorn, Spencer Jang, and Dwight Hirsh.

PNEUMONIA, NEONATAL

BASICS

DEFINITION

• Inflammation of the pulmonary parenchyma in newborn foals
• The term *neonatal* is restricted to foals ≤4 weeks of age.

PATHOPHYSIOLOGY

• Causes of pneumonia in newborn foals include hematogenous spread of infection; inhalation of airborne infection; aspiration of meconium, gastric reflux, or milk; and prematurity.
• Hematogenous infection is association with septicemia. It may be acquired *in utero* from a placental infection or perinatally from another source—omphalitis or omphalophlebitis
• Inhalation of pathogens also may be a primary entry route for bacteria that results in septicemia.
• Perinatal pulmonary infections occur in foals that generally are immunocompromised as a result of failure of passive transfer.
• *Escherichia coli, Klebsiella* sp., and *Streptococcus* sp. are some of the more common bacteria involved.
• Herpes viral infection, equine arteritis virus, and adenovirus pneumonia (fatal pneumonia has been associated with combined immunodeficiency in Arabian foals) have been implicated during in utero viral infections.
• An immature ciliary apparatus and fewer alveolar macrophages in neonates compared with adults lead to decreased bacterial clearance from the lungs. Reduced complement values in neonates also may contribute to decreased humoral defense against invading bacteria.
• Aspiration of meconium occurs in utero in foals that experience fetal distress. Causes of fetal distress (e.g., in utero asphyxia, umbilical cord compression) may lead to expulsion of meconium into the amniotic fluid. The distressed foal then gasps for breath and inhales the meconium-contaminated amniotic fluid. Meconium is sterile at this time, but it creates obstruction and inflammation in the lungs at delivery.
• Postnatal aspiration of meconium most commonly occurs with upper airway dysfunction and dysphagia.
• Premature foals may not have the necessary surfactant to prevent lungs from collapsing on exhalation.
• Atelectasis and increased capillary permeability lead to pulmonary edema and RDS (see *Prematurity*).

SYSTEMS AFFECTED

Respiratory—despite the cause of the problem, the lungs are the primary organ system affected.

GENETICS

N/A

INCIDENCE/PREVALENCE

N/A

SIGNALMENT

• Foals of all breeds and sexes are susceptible.
• Arabian foals with SCID are at high risk.

SIGNS

General Comments

Clinical signs can vary depending on severity of the disease and possible associated problems—concurrent sepsis

Historical Findings

• Colostrum leakage before parturition or colostrum deprivation (e.g., poor quality or quantity) may be reported.
• Other findings—prematurity, dystocia, placental abnormalities, perinatal weakness, or milk discharge from nostrils after nursing.

Physical Examination Findings

• Early during life, localizing clinical signs of respiratory infection may be absent, even with extensive disease.
• Dyspnea—increased respiratory rate and effort
• Abnormal respiratory sounds—crackles or wheezes may be heard on auscultation; however, foals with no auscultable abnormalities may have severe pulmonary disease.
• Cyanosis—PaO_2 may be low (35–40 mm Hg) before cyanosis is observed.
• Weakness, depression, anorexia, weak or absent suckle reflex, dehydration, and fever may be present.
• Cough and nasal discharge usually are absent during the early stages.

CAUSES

• Most cases are part of a generalized septicemia caused by opportunistic pathogens infecting an immunocompromised host. The most common cause of decreased immune function is failure of passive transfer.
• Postnatal milk aspiration pneumonia usually occurs secondary to dysphagia. This may result from cleft palate, neurologic dysfunction of the pharyngeal/laryngeal muscles, and pharyngeal obstruction (see *Milk Regurgitation*).
• Premature cesarean section, induction of parturition, or premature birth secondary to placentitis may result in RDS.

RISK FACTORS

• Maternal placentitis
• Failure of passive transfer
• Unsanitary environment
• Recumbency
• Dystocia
• Dysphagia
• Septic omphalophlebitis
• Hypoxic-ischemic encephalopathy
• Premature parturition

PNEUMONIA, NEONATAL

DIAGNOSIS

DIFFERENTIAL DIAGNOSIS

Other Causes of Respiratory Distress

- Airway obstruction—guttural pouch tympany, laryngeal edema, tracheal malformation, stenotic nares, choanal atresia, and epiglottal, laryngeal, or pharyngeal cysts
- Developmental disorders—diaphragmatic hernia and pulmonary hypoplasia may present with RDS.

Nonpulmonary Causes

- Anemia—neonatal isoerythrolysis
- Congestive heart failure/primary cardiac disease
- Excitement—exercise- and excitement-induced respiratory stridor is described in foals with HYPP
- Idiopathic tachypnea
- Neuromuscular disorders—botulism, white muscle disease, and CNS lesions
- Pain
- Fever
- High environmental temperatures
- Persistent pulmonary hypertension caused by pulmonary vascular abnormalities
- Trauma—Pneumothorax; rib fracture

CBC/BIOCHEMISTRY/URINALYSIS

- CBC—neutrophilia or neutropenia, with or without left shift, can be found in bacterial infections and viral diseases; profound lymphopenia may be found in acute viral diseases and septicemia/endotoxemia.
- Lymphocyte counts—generally higher than neutrophil counts in the fetus and may reflect degree of immaturity in premature foals (e.g., neutropenia and N:L ratios <1.5 during the first 24 hours of life have been reported to indicate a poor prognosis).

OTHER LABORATORY TESTS

Arterial Blood Gas Analysis

- Samples may be taken from the great metatarsal, brachial, femoral, facial, and carotid arteries.
- Typical results as follows:

Parameter	Value (mm Hg)	Interpretation
PaO_2	>80	Normal neonatal foals reach values up to 80 mm Hg at 1 hour after birth
	60–80	Mild hypoxia; prolonged recumbency; inadequately handled sample (sealed samples may be stored on ice $\leq$6 hours without major changes in PaO_2); respiratory compromise
	<60	Hypoxemia; PaO_2 of 60 mm Hg indicates an oxygen saturation of $\cong$90%
$PaCO_2$	>60	Severe hypercapnia; may necessitate mechanical ventilation

Other Tests

- Blood cultures may help to identify the causative agent.
- Other bacterial cultures (e.g., respiratory tract sampling) and cytology—very important for confirming the diagnosis of bacterial pneumonia and development of pathogen-specific antimicrobial therapy
- Virus isolation from nasal swabs or respiratory tract sampling may be helpful. Viral serology is undependable, however, in establishing the diagnosis of neonatal viral infection, because antibodies may have been acquired from the dam's colostrum.
- Serum IgG levels, especially in cases of suspected septicemia

IMAGING

Thoracic Radiography

- Diffuse infiltrates are associated with RDS, hematogenous spread of pneumonia, pulmonary edema, and atelectasis.
- Caudoventral distribution (i.e., accessory lobe) can be seen with aspiration pneumonia.
- Primary caudodorsal distribution has been observed in several cases of suspected in utero–acquired pneumonia (significance not known).
- Distinguishing lung "immaturity" from lung pathology may be difficult in neonates, especially during the first 24 hours of life.

Thoracic Ultrasonography

Very useful in assessing pleural effusion, bronchopneumonia, or pulmonary abscessation

DIAGNOSTIC PROCEDURES

- Endoscopy—assists in assessing upper respiratory tract disorders (e.g., airway obstruction, malformation, and inflammation) and the proximal lower respiratory tract.
- Transtracheal aspiration or bronchoalveolar lavage—can be used to obtain fluid for cytology and for culture and sensitivity; use caution when performing these procedures on foals with respiratory distress.
- Pulse oximetry provides continuous measure of arterial oxygen saturation but has not been rigorously tested in foals.
- Thoracocentesis has diagnostic and therapeutic importance in cases of pleural effusion.

PNEUMONIA, NEONATAL

TREATMENT

FLUID THERAPY

- Neonatal pneumonia frequently is associated with concurrent sepsis and dehydration caused by anorexia, weakness, and depression.
- Dehydration also hinders mucociliary clearance and mobilization of secretions.
- Fluid maintenance requirements in newborns—80–100 mL/kg.
- Do not overhydrate foals.

CORRECTION OF FAILURE OF PASSIVE TRANSFER

- Transfuse equine plasma or commercial equine hyperimmune plasma (20 mL/kg).
- Check IgG levels before further transfusion.

RESPIRATORY SUPPORT/AIRWAY CLEARANCE/PHYSIOTHERAPY

- Chest coupage, a technique of loosing pulmonary secretions, is performed by slapping the chest in rapid succession with a cupped hand.
- Maintain foals in a sternal position or at least turned as frequently as possible to combat progressing atelectasis and hypoxemia.
- Nasal oxygen can be administered by placing a small feeding tube through the nostril to the back of the pharynx. Oxygen can be delivered at 5–10 L/min.
- Mechanical ventilation is important in hypercapnic foals.
- Airway suction and rapid clearance of contaminated airways is especially important with meconium aspiration.

NUTRITIONAL SUPPORT

- Enteral feeding—10% of body weight is needed for survival and 20% of body weight for growth (e.g., an average 50-kg foal needs 10 L of milk per day).
- Method—nasogastric intubation; bottle or bucket feeding
- Partial or total parenteral nutrition (*see Orphan and Sick foal Nutrition*).

MEDICATIONS

DRUGS OF CHOICE

Antibiotics

- Broad-spectrum antibiotic therapy should be used while culture results are pending—ampicillin (15–20 mg/kg IV QID) or penicillin (22,000 IU/kg IV QID) in combination with amikacin (20–25 mg/kg IV SID) is a reasonable initial empiric treatment; alternatively, a third-generation cephalosporin (e.g., ceftiofur [4 mg/kg IV BID]) may be used.
- Duration of antibiotic therapy for established pneumonia—2–5 weeks.

Inhalants

- Bronchodilators such as albuterol (one puff using an aeromask TID) and mucolytic agents (10% acetylcysteine as 30 mL nebulized during 30 minutes BID) can be considered.
- Theophylline (4–7 mg/kg PO TID or 6–10 mg/kg diluted in 100 mL given slowly IV BID, keep serum levels <15 μg/mL) and aminophylline (starting dose of 2 mg/kg, dilute in at least 100 mL of NaCl and give slowly IV, not >25 mg/min) also can be used as bronchodilators.

Gastric Protectants

Cimetidine (6–20 mg/kg PO TID or 6.6 mg/kg IV TID), ranitidine (6.6 mg/kg PO TID or 1.5 mg/kg IV TID), sucralfate (1 g PO TID), and omeprazole (1–1.5 mg/kg via nasogastric tube SID) can be used to prevent gastric ulceration secondary to stress.

NSAIDs

Ketoprofen (≤2.2 mg/kg IV) and flunixin meglumine (0.25–1.1 mg/kg IV) may become necessary to control fever and to reduce inflammation.

CONTRAINDICATIONS

Aminoglycosides in cases of renal compromise

PRECAUTIONS

- Airway clearance—continuous, strong airway suctioning can cause hypoxia and atelectasis; intermittent, short-period (2 seconds), strong suction appears to be more beneficial.
- Aminophylline/theophylline may cause CNS stimulation, cardiac dysrhythmias, and GI irritation.

- Mechanical ventilation—avoid using too much pressure or tidal volume during hand ventilation to prevent tension pneumothorax.
- NSAIDs are considered to be ulcerogenic—flunixin meglumine > ketoprofen
- Oxygen therapy may increase hypercapnia because of the onset of hypoventilation—hypoxemic stimulus for breathing is lost.

POSSIBLE INTERACTIONS

Cimetidine reduces hepatic metabolism by inhibiting the hepatic microsomal enzyme system; it also may increase serum levels and prolong half-lives of other drugs—metronidazole, lidocaine, theophylline, and diazepam

ALTERNATIVE DRUGS

- Depend on culture results and progression of clinical signs.
- Gentamicin (6.6 mg/kg IV SID) is an alternative antibiotic for Gram-negative infections.

FOLLOW-UP

PATIENT MONITORING

- Serial chest radiography is useful to monitor the progress of the respiratory condition, but radiographic changes may follow or precede the onset of clinical signs and persist after their resolution.
- Repeated arterial blood gas analysis is important when a foal is on oxygen or mechanical ventilation.

PREVENTION/AVOIDANCE

N/A

POSSIBLE COMPLICATIONS

- Nosocomial bacterial infection secondary to mechanical ventilation
- Permanent pulmonary damage that may limit future performance

EXPECTED COURSE AND PROGNOSIS

N/A

MISCELLANEOUS

ASSOCIATED CONDITIONS

- Prematurity
- Septicemia

AGE-RELATED FACTORS

N/A

ZOONOTIC POTENTIAL

N/A

PREGNANCY

N/A

SYNONYMS

N/A

SEE ALSO

- Gastric ulcers
- Neonatal sepsis
- Orphan and sick foal
- Prematurity

ABBREVIATIONS

- GI = gastrointestinal
- HYPP = hyperkalemic periodic paralysis
- N:L = neutrophil:lymphocyte
- RDS = respiratory distress syndrome
- SCID = severe combined immunodeficiency disease

Suggested Reading

Beech J. Respiratory problems in foals. Vet Clin North Am Equine Pract 1985;1:131–149.

Hondalus M, Paradis MR. Respiratory disease in foals: the initial steps toward diagnosis. Vet Med 1989;1168–1173.

Koterba AM, Paradis MR. Specific respiratory conditions. In: Koterba AM, Drummond WH, Kosch PC, eds. Equine clinical neonatology. Philadelphia: Lea & Febiger, 1990:177.

Paradis MR. Infectious disease of the equine respiratory tract: from gestation to 5 months. Vet Med 1989;1174–1177.

Author Daniela Bedenice

Consulting Editor Mary Rose Paradis

PNEUMOTHORAX

BASICS

OVERVIEW

• A rarely encountered problem that most commonly occurs following penetrating thoracic wounds or birth trauma and, occasionally, following transtracheal wash or pneumonia, which has led to a bronchopleural fistula.
• Gas usually enters the pleural cavity either from the lung via perforation of the visceral pleura or through a hole in the chest wall and perforation of the parietal pleura. Other routes include tracheal perforation and dissecting subcutaneous emphysema.
• Introduction of gas into the pleural cavity causes varying degrees of lung collapse, mechanical inability to inflate the lung, and inadequate ventilation.
• One or both hemithoraces may be involved.
• Open pneumothorax—when air freely enters and leaves the pleural cavity through a chest wound during respiration.
• Tension pneumothorax—an influx of air on inspiration without an equivalent volume of efflux on expiration, causing a build up of pressure (progressive or acute) in the pleural cavity, which occurs because a flap of tissue in a wound acts as a one-way valve.

SIGNALMENT

No age, breed, and sex predilections.

SIGNS

Historical Findings

• There may be a history of trauma.
• Recent transtracheal wash or injury.
• Neonates from primiparous mares or dystocias are predisposed.
• Foals may be lethargic and lie down in the sternal position, and they may moan and appear stiff.

Physical Examination Findings

• If the pneumothorax is not severe, no clinical signs may be evident at rest but may manifest with exercise.
• Tachypnea and superficial breathing may be evident.
• Deep, labored breathing (i.e., dyspnea) may occur in more severe and bilateral cases and can progress to severe respiratory distress in the case of a tension pneumothorax.
• Absence of lung sounds dorsally on thoracic auscultation, and increased resonance on percussion are evident.
• Reduced lung sounds ventrally and decreased resonance on percussion suggestive of hemothorax.
• Inspection and palpation of the thoracic cage may detect a penetrating wound or fractured ribs associated with birth trauma.

CAUSES AND RISK FACTORS

• Collision with an object, particularly fences, is the most common cause of penetrating thoracic wounds in horses.
• Transtracheal wash procedures
• Tracheal lacerations or trauma
• Axillary wounds
• Bronchopleural fistulae from abcedative pleuropneumonia
• Birth trauma, which occurs in 20% of Thoroughbred foals
• Newborn foals from primiparous mares or dystocia cases
• Transtracheal wash procedures

DIAGNOSIS

DIFFERENTIAL DIAGNOSIS

• Pain can cause rapid, shallow breathing.
• Diaphragmatic hernia
• Pleural effusion—hemothorax or pyothorax

CBC/BIOCHEMISTRY/URINALYSIS

Stress leukogram and leukocytosis in cases of secondary bacterial infection.

OTHER LABORATORY TESTS

Arterial blood gas analysis

IMAGING

Thoracic Radiography

• Retraction of lung margins from the thoracic wall, with varying degrees of lung collapse.
• Radiopaque foreign objects, fluid in the thorax, or fractured ribs also may be visualized.

Ultrasonography

• Air resulting from a pneumothorax appears similar to a normal, aerated lung.
• Fluid/gas interfaces permit recognition of the pneumothorax.

DIAGNOSTIC PROCEDURES

• Thoracocentesis, both as a diagnostic test and as a therapeutic measure in dyspneic animals
• Thoracoscopy can be used to evaluate pulmonary pathology and to diagnose a radiolucent foreign body.
• Tracheal endoscopy to detect tracheal laceration

TREATMENT

• Inpatient care until the horse is stabilized.
• These animals may suffer from polytrauma; an approach consisting of a first look, shock treatment, recheck, and then diagnosis is suitable in such circumstances.
• Emergency care, with continuous surveillance, is appropriate for severe cases until the problem is under control.
• Traumatic pneumothorax—temporarily close the penetrating wound using sterile gauze impregnated with antibiotic ointment; suture the wound after the patient is stabilized.

PNEUMOTHORAX

• Control of external hemorrhage and shock treatment with IV fluids is essential during the acute period.
• Administer oxygen by nasopharyngeal insufflation (15 L/min) for dyspneic and hypoxemic patients.
• IV fluid therapy for patients in cardiovascular shock. Remember, however, that the contused lung in cases of trauma is extremely sensitive to overload with IV crystalloid solutions; therefore, use sparingly.
• Decompression of the pleural cavity is necessary in cases with labored breathing at rest when the wound is sealed. Thoracocentesis is performed using a large-gauge needle or teat cannula attached to a three-way stop cock, extension set, and a 60-mL syringe. The site for aseptic air evacuation is the dorsal thoracic cavity, just in front of the ribs 12–15, to avoid the intercostal vessels along the caudal surface of the latter.
• Severe or active pneumothorax—a thoracostomy tube may be placed in the pleural cavity and attached to a Heimlich valve or, in the case of rapid reaccumulation of air, a continuous suction apparatus.
• In cases with minimal clinical signs at rest, the pneumothorax will resorb if the animal is confined.
• Stall rest is indicated until the pneumothorax resolves.
• Suture wounds whenever possible to rapidly achieve an air-tight seal.

MEDICATIONS

DRUGS

Antibiotics for wound or pneumonia

CONTRAINDICATIONS/POSSIBLE INTERACTIONS

• Avoid drugs such as xylazine or opioids, because they may reduce PaO_2.
• Check for signs of hypoventilation—increased $PaCO_2$; decreased PaO_2.

FOLLOW UP

• Monitor hourly the respiratory rate and character, mucous membranes color, and heart rate for the first 24–48 hours.
• Serial radiography and blood gas analyses reveal the effectiveness of pleural air evacuation and re-expansion of the lung.
• Thoracostomy tubes may be removed if $\leq$50 mL of air are aspirated in 12 hours.
• Full recovery is expected if the injury is not massive and the recognition and treatment of pneumothorax is prompt.

MISCELLANEOUS

ASSOCIATED CONDITIONS

N/A

AGE-RELATED FACTORS

N/A

ZOONOTIC POTENTIAL

N/A

PREGNANCY

N/A

SEE ALSO

• Diaphragmatic hernia
• Expiratory dyspnea
• Inspiratory dyspnea
• Pleuropneumonia
• Thoracic trauma

Suggested Reading

Jean DA, Laverty S, Halley J, Hannigan D, Leveille R. Thoracic trauma in newborn foals. Equine Vet J, 1999:149–152.
Laverty S. Thoracic trauma. Current therapy in equine medicine 4. Philadelphia: WB Saunders, 1997:463–465.
Laverty S, Lavoie JP, Pascoe JR, Ducharme N. Penetrating wounds of the thorax in 15 horses. Equine Vet J 1996:220–224.

Author Sheila Laverty
Consulting Editor Jean-Pierre Lavoie

PNEUMOVAGINA/PNEUMOUTERUS

BASICS

DEFINITION
Air in the vagina or uterus, generally resulting from a conformational defect of the vulva

PATHOPHYSIOLOGY
• Air accumulates subsequent to poor vulvar conformation and relaxation of the vestibular sphincter.
• The negative pressure within the lumen of the genital tract aids in movement of air into the vestibule, vagina, and uterus, which elicits a "wind-sucking" sound.
• With motion (e.g., running, rolling), air is forced back out, resulting in a characteristic expulsive sound.

SYSTEM AFFECTED
Reproductive

GENETICS
Possible genetic influence for less-than-ideal vulvar conformation, which is common

INCIDENCE/PREVALENCE
No statistics are available regarding incidence, but the condition is common and one of the major causes of equine infertility.

SIGNALMENT
• All breeds, but those breeds/individuals with less muscle in the perineal area are more severely affected.
• All of breeding age
• Older pluripara mares most commonly are affected.

SIGNS

General Comments

First described as a potential reproductive problem as early as 1937, the condition remains a major cause of infertility.

Historical Findings

• Mares may exhibit signs of chronic pneumovagina, including vaginal flatus, abnormal redness of the vaginal mucosa, and accumulation of air in the uterus, coupled with abnormal VC.
• Infertility linked with uterine infections and/or inflammation also is common.

Physical Examination Findings

• Determine if VC is normal by assessing relationship of the dorsal vulvar commissure to the pubic bone; it should lie at or below the floor of the pubis.
• Effect of poor VC on fertility would be confirmed with identification of vaginitis, pneumovagina, or pneumouterus.
• With increasing age, the anus is pulled cranially, which pulls attached soft-tissue structures forward with it—the vulva is pulled cranially over the posterior brim of the pubis.

CAUSES
Predisposing Factors:
• Changes in general conformation—sway back
• Loss of body condition—loss of vaginal fat
• Age, genetics, or trauma-related changes of VC
• Developing a weakness/stretching of the supporting soft-tissue structures in the perineal area

RISK FACTORS
• Diminishing protective barrier of a normal vulva by age, parity, genetic predisposition, and so on
• Conformation also is influenced by pregnancy, with additional stretching of the supporting tissue of this area.
• Poor nutritional condition may contribute to decreased vulvar conformation.
• The normal relaxation that occurs during estrus may slightly affect vulvar conformation.

DIAGNOSIS

DIFFERENTIAL DIAGNOSIS
N/A

CBC/BIOCHEMISTRY/URINALYSIS
N/A

OTHER LABORATORY TESTS
N/A

IMAGING
Ultrasonography—not necessary, unless confirm pneumouterus

DIAGNOSTIC PROCEDURES
N/A

PATHOLOGIC FINDINGS
• Evidence of vaginitis and endometritis are indicators of pneumovagina and/or pneumouterus. Other possible causes exist for these conditions, but with poor (i.e., decreased) VC, the diagnosis is conclusive.
• This condition may result not only in infertility but also cause abortion in pregnant mares after vaginitis and cervicitis.

TREATMENT

APPROPRIATE HEALTH CARE
Little justification to treat a mare for uterine infection or inflammation if poor VC will not be corrected.

NURSING CARE
N/A

ACTIVITY
N/A

DIET
N/A

CLIENT EDUCATION
• Advise clients to evaluate the VC of all mares.
• If conformation is less than ideal, a Caslick's surgery should be performed.

SURGICAL CONSIDERATIONS
• Surgical correction for poor VC (vulvoplasty or episioplasty) was first described by Caslick in 1937.
• First, wrap and tie the mare's tail away from the field of surgery, and thoroughly clean the perineal area with cotton and soap.
• Carbocaine or another local anesthetic is infiltrated into the mucocutaneous junction on the vulva; ≅10 mL can be used to infiltrate both sides of the vulva.

• The tissue edges are freshened before suturing, either by removing a very narrow strip of tissue from the edge or by incising at the mucocutaneous junction along the line dilated with local anesthetic—split-thickness technique; i.e. no tissue is removed.
• The split-thickness technique is tissue sparing, in that it helps to retain the normal elasticity of vulvae during labor by minimizing damage. Both described techniques can be used, however, and are acceptable.
• Use nonabsorbable suture material, with removal in ≅10 days.
• Check vaccination status for tetanus.
• Pouret technique—in cases of severe/extremely poor VC, it may be necessary to dissect the perineal body in a caudal (widest) to cranial (point), pie-shaped wedge, which permits the genital tract, ventral to the rectum, to slide caudally and away from fecal contamination as well as aspiration of air; only the skin is closed (i.e., no deep reconstruction of dissected tissue).

MEDICATIONS

DRUGS OF CHOICE
• No antibiotics are indicated.
• Selection of local anesthetic is at the discretion of the surgeon.

CONTRAINDICATIONS
N/A

PRECAUTIONS
N/A

POSSIBLE INTERACTIONS
N/A

ALTERNATIVE DRUGS
N/A

FOLLOW-UP

PATIENT MONITORING
Suture removal 10 days after surgery to prevent the possibility of stitch abscesses at the suture site

PREVENTION/AVOIDANCE
Select broodmares with excellent VC.

POSSIBLE COMPLICATIONS
Primary contraindication to vulvoplasty is the necessity to re-open the vulvar commissure ≅7–10 days before parturition to prevent tearing of the perineum at delivery; it should be replaced (i.e., incised and sutured) after breeding and confirmation of ovulation in the next season.

EXPECTED COURSE AND PROGNOSIS
Without surgical correction, mares may remain infertile or abort during pregnancy.

MISCELLANEOUS

ASSOCIATED CONDITIONS
N/A

AGE-RELATED FACTORS
High probability of this condition becoming worse with age.

ZOONOTIC POTENTIAL
N/A

PREGNANCY
Surgery may be necessary to obtain a pregnancy.

SYNONYMS
Wind sucker

SEE ALSO
• Dystocia
• Endometrial biopsy
• Endometritis
• Perineal lacerations
• Vulvar conformation

ABBREVIATIONS
VC = vulvar conformation

Suggested Reading

Aanes WA. Surgical repair of third degree perineal lacerations and recto-vaginal fistulas in the mare. J Am Vet Med Assoc 1964;144:485–491.

Caslick EA. The vulva and vulvo-vaginal orifice and its relationship to genital health of the thoroughbred mare. Cornell Vet 1937;27:178–186.

Colbern GT, Aanes WA, Stashak TS. Surgical management of perineal lacerations and recto-vestibular fistulae in the mare: a retrospective study of 47 cases. J Am Vet Med Assoc 1985;186:265–269.

Heinze CD, Allen AR. Repair of third-degree perineal lacerations in the mare. Vet Scope 1966;11:12–15.

Shipley WD, Bergin WC. Genital health in the mare. III. Pneumovagina. VM/SAC 1968;63:699–702.

Stickle RL, Fessler JF, Adams SB, et al. A single stage technique for repair of recto-vestibular lacerations in the mare. J Vet Surg 1979;8:25–27.

Author Walter R. Threlfall

Consulting Editor Carla L. Carleton

POISONING (INTOXICATION)

BASICS

DEFINITION

• A poison or toxicant is a natural or synthetic substance causing disease via its own inherent qualities.
• A toxin is a type of toxicant with a biologic origin—plants, bacteria, or animals
• Toxicosis refers to the disease caused by a poison.
• Toxicity refers to the amount of a poison that causes disease; substances with high toxicity require a lower dose to cause disease than substances with low toxicity.

PATHOPHYSIOLOGY

Mechanisms of action vary with the different toxicants and are discussed in the specific chapters dealing with those toxicants.

SYSTEMS AFFECTED

• The systems affected vary with the different toxicants.
• Some toxicants affect more than one system.

GENETICS

N/A

INCIDENCE/PREVALENCE

The occurrence of specific toxicoses can vary depending on geographic location as well as agricultural and management practices.

SIGNALMENT

Age, breed, and sex predispositions vary with the different toxicants.

SIGNS

General Comments

• Establishing the diagnosis of poisoning often is difficult, and the importance of a complete history and physical examination cannot be overstated.
• Thorough record keeping is necessary because of the possibility of legal action, especially if poisoning results from a faulty product or the negligence of others.

Historical Findings

• Establishing the history of the problem may be difficult and can require finesse by the veterinarian.
• The client may already be convinced that poisoning has occurred, even though the onset of clinical signs is only coincidental with exposure of the animal to a particular substance.
• Client may not be forthcoming with complete information if they feel guilty because poisoning resulted from their own mistakes. Conversely, clients may give biased information if they believe poisoning resulted from a faulty product, the negligence of others, or suspected malicious intent.
• The clinician should determine how many animals are at risk of poisoning and how many are actually affected.
• Collect information regarding breed, sex, reproductive status, body condition, weight, and age of the animals, because these variables can affect toxicity.
• Current or past health problems and treatments may reveal factors that can affect toxicity and influence therapeutic recommendations.
• Collect detailed information regarding the current poisoning situation—clinical signs, date of onset, time of onset, and treatments given by the owner.
• Determine how and when the animal was exposed to the toxicant.
• Record the full label name of the product, the manufacturer, and the active ingredients, including their concentrations. If the product is a pesticide, record the EPA Registration Number.
• If a potential adverse reaction to a therapeutic agent is involved, record the lot or batch number, and determine the amount of exposure to the product.

Physical Examination Findings

• Clinical signs vary with the different toxicants.
• Not all potential signs are seen in every animal.

CAUSES

Substances that cause poisoning are discussed in the specific chapters on those substances.

RISK FACTORS

• The risk of developing toxicosis depends on the toxicity of the substance, exposure dose, exposure type (e.g., acute, multiple, chronic), and exposure route (e.g., dermal, oral, inhaled, injected).
• Individual risk factors include age, breed, sex, reproductive status, body condition, weight, and previous health status.

DIAGNOSIS

DIFFERENTIAL DIAGNOSIS

• First, determine the illness actually results from poisoning rather than from a medical or surgical disease. The diagnosis may be obvious from a quick history and physical examination but usually requires more thorough investigation by the clinician.
• The foremost consideration in confirming a diagnosis of poisoning is to establish that clinical signs or lesions are compatible with a toxic exposure to the toxicant in question.
• The list of differential diagnoses varies with different toxicants. Resources to assist veterinarians in diagnosing toxicoses include diagnostic laboratories and the ASPCA National Animal Poison Control Center.

CBC/BIOCHEMISTRY/URINALYSIS

Help in defining the cause of the problem and in determining the course of treatment.

OTHER LABORATORY TESTS

• Laboratory confirmation can be made for many toxicants via sample submission to diagnostic laboratories.
• Collect whole blood, serum, and urine from live animals and liver, kidney, brain, fat, urine, and GI contents from dead animals.
• Toxicologic testing cannot be performed on formalinized samples; thus, store samples frozen.
• Collect samples of feed, water, and the suspected source material; other also samples may be necessary to confirm a diagnosis, depending on the toxicant.
• Always contact the laboratory for specific information regarding submission protocols, because incorrect samples, inadequate sample size, and improper sample storage are common causes of diagnostic testing failures.

IMAGING

N/A

DIAGNOSTIC PROCEDURES

N/A

PATHOLOGIC FINDINGS

• Gross and histopathologic findings vary depending on the specific toxicant.
• Often, lesions are nonspecific.

TREATMENT

EMERGENCY TREATMENT

- With a life-threatening situation, immediately provide life support by maintaining respiratory and cardiac function.
- Control seizures if they occur.
- Once the animal is stabilized, institute symptomatic and supportive care.

DECONTAMINATION

- The first concern is to remove the animal from the toxic source, so that further exposure does not occur.
- Before administering oral products, determine that the horse is not exhibiting gastric reflux.
- With a dermal route of exposure, bathe the animal with mild dishwashing detergent. People washing and handling the animal should take measures (e.g.., wearing gloves) to prevent contamination of themselves.
- With an ocular route of exposure, lavage the eye with copious amounts of water or normal saline.
- Many toxicants are adsorbed by AC, thereby reducing the amount of toxicant absorbed from the GI tract. AC binds many organic compounds but is relatively ineffective against inorganic compounds (e.g., heavy metals). Mix the AC (2–5 gm/kg) with warm water to form a slurry. Follow the AC with a laxative to hasten removal of the toxicant from the intestinal tract. Mineral oil (2–4 L per 500 kg) is the most commonly used equine laxative, and multiple doses of mineral oil can be given.
- Magnesium sulfate (Epsom salts) is an osmotic laxative that draws water into the intestines. The recommended dose is 250–500 mg/kg mixed in several liters of water; 70% sorbitol (3 mL/kg) or sodium sulfate (250–500 mg/kg mixed in several liters of water) are alternative cathartics.
- Ensure that the horse is adequately hydrated, because magnesium sulfate (or other cathartics) results in diarrhea at high doses.
- Some toxicants are eliminated primarily by the fecal route or undergo enterohepatic recirculation. AC followed by a laxative is the most effective means for increasing elimination of these toxicants.
- Many toxicants are eliminated by the kidneys, and in some cases, renal excretion can be enhanced by increasing urine output via fluid administration. Diuretics can be used to increase urine flow—furosemide (1 mg/kg IV); mannitol (0.25–2.0 g/kg as 20% solution by slow IV infusion)
- Manipulating the urine pH also can increase the excretion of some toxicants in the urine via ion trapping. Weak acids are ionized in alkaline urine, whereas weak bases are ionized in acidic urine. The normal range of urine pH in adult herbivores is alkaline, ranging from 7–9.

SYMPTOMATIC AND SUPPORTIVE TREATMENT

- Treat clinical signs as they occur.
- Maintain adequate hydration.
- Control acid–base imbalances.
- Maintain proper body temperature.
- Alleviate pain.
- Anticipate secondary problems that may occur from the specific toxic exposure, and provide prophylactic care.

MEDICATIONS

DRUGS OF CHOICE

- Few poisons have specific antidotes.
- Relevant medications and antidotes are discussed in those sections dealing with the specific toxicants.

CONTRAINDICATIONS

N/A

PRECAUTIONS

N/A

POSSIBLE INTERACTIONS

N/A

ALTERNATIVE DRUGS

N/A

FOLLOW-UP

PATIENT MONITORING

Potential sequelae vary with the toxicant and severity of the poisoning and are discussed in those sections dealing with specific toxicants.

PREVENTION/AVOIDANCE

Minimize the risk of intoxication by using medications and pesticides according to the label directions, storing all chemicals safely, and identifying and removing all potentially toxic plants in the animal's environment.

POSSIBLE COMPLICATIONS

N/A

EXPECTED COURSE AND PROGNOSIS

N/A

MISCELLANEOUS

ASSOCIATED CONDITIONS

Laminitis as a secondary condition

AGE-RELATED FACTORS

Vary with the specific toxicant.

ZOONOTIC POTENTIAL

N/A

PREGNANCY

- Abortion or teratogenic disease is a concern in pregnant mares depending on the toxicant and stage of pregnancy at the time of exposure.
- Some poisons can affect the fertility of mares or stallions.

SYNONYMS

Discussed in those chapters dealing with specific toxicoses.

SEE ALSO

Chapters dealing with specific toxicoses

ABBREVIATIONS

- AC = activated charcoal
- GI = gastrointestinal

Suggested Reading

Oehme FW. General principles in treatment of poisoning. In: Robinson NE, ed. Current therapy in equine medicine. 2nd ed. Philadelphia: WB Saunders, 1987.

Author Konstanze H. Plumlee

Consulting Editor Robert H. Poppenga

POLYCYTHEMIA

BASICS

DEFINITION

- Elevated PCV, RBC count, and hemoglobin concentration > reference limits.
- Can be relative or absolute.

PATHOPHYSIOLOGY

- Relative polycythemia is caused by hemoconcentration (e.g., dehydration, shock) or splenic contraction (e.g., excitement, exercise). Splenic contraction injects a mass of concentrated erythrocytes in the circulation; this polycythemia is transient and can last from 40–60 minutes to several hours, depending on the extent of excitement.
- Absolute polycythemia is an increased circulating RBC mass without any change in plasma volume. It can be further classified as primary or secondary.
- Primary absolute polycythemia is a myeloproliferative disorder associated with normal PO_2 and reduced EPO level.
- Secondary absolute polycythemia results from increased EPO production and can be physiologically appropriate, if resulting from chronic hypoxia, or inappropriate, if resulting from excessive EPO production with a normal PO_2.

SYSTEMS AFFECTED

- Cardiovascular
- Pulmonary
- Nervous
- GI
- Musculoskeletal
- Renal

SIGNALMENT

- Reference values for PCV, RBC count, and hemoglobin content vary with geographic location and breed.
- Horses have increased erythrocyte parameters at altitudes >2200 m (7200 feet).
- Thoroughbreds generally have greater RBC counts than other breeds.
- Compared with hot-blooded horses, cold-blooded horses have lower RBC counts, hemoglobin and PCV values, and blood volume.
- American miniature horse, donkeys, and ponies have lower RBC counts.

SIGNS

General Comments

- Clinical signs of relative polycythemia are associated with the primary disease process.
- Signs vary according to the degree of polycythemia.
- Poor perfusion and oxygenation, hyperviscosity, and hemostatic problems may be encountered with PCV >60%.

Historical Findings

- Transient polycythemia—excitement; vigorous exercise
- Relative polycythemia—depends on the primary disease process
- Absolute polycythemia—epistaxis, GI bleeding, laminitis, and vague signs including lethargy, weight loss, and mucosal hyperemia

Physical Examination Findings

- Relative polycythemia—dehydration caused by inadequate oral fluid intake or loss of body water in excess of absorbed water.
- Absolute polycythemia—low exercise tolerance, "muddy" mucosal hyperemia, lethargy, epistaxis, melena, and laminitis
- Primary absolute polycythemia—exceptionally rare in horses; no clear physical findings have been described.
- Appropriate secondary absolute polycythemia—signs of chronic tissue hypoxia because of altitude, congenital heart defects, or chronic pulmonary disease
- Inappropriate secondary absolute polycythemia—signs associated with neoplasia, space-occupying renal lesion, endocrine disorder, or chronic hepatic disease.

CAUSES

- Relative polycythemia (common)—dysphagia, diarrhea, overexertion and heat stress, proximal enteritis and other disease causing adynamic ileus, endotoxemia from colic or diarrhea, pleuropneumonia, or postpartum metritis
- Primary absolute polycythemia (very rare)—may occur as a single-cell disorder (i.e., primary erythrocytosis) or as a component of polycythemia vera (also includes slight leukocytosis and thrombocytosis), which are both idiopathic myeloproliferative disorders.
- Appropriate secondary absolute polycythemia—physiologically appropriate EPO production in response to chronic hypoxia caused by residence at high altitude, congenital heart defects causing right-to-left shunting (e.g., tetralogy of Fallot, ventricular septal defect), and some forms of chronic pulmonary disease
- Inappropriate secondary absolute polycythemia (exceptionally rare)—causes of inappropriate EPO secretion include renal cyst or hydronephrosis, androgenic steroid use or adrenal disorder, hepatocellular carcinoma and interstitial nephritis (one reported horse), and rarely, chronic hepatic disease.

RISK FACTORS

N/A

DIAGNOSIS

DIFFERENTIAL DIAGNOSIS

- Concurrent increase in PCV and total plasma protein suggests relative polycythemia caused by dehydration. Evidence of shock also suggests relative polycythemia.
- Secondary absolute polycythemia is caused either by diseases that produce chronic hypoxia and release of EPO or by space-occupying renal lesions, endocrine disorders, chronic hepatic disorders, or neoplasms that produce EPO or an EPO-like substance without hypoxia.
- Primary absolute polycythemia (e.g., primary erythrocytosis, polycythemia vera) is diagnosed on the basis of excluding other causes.

LABORATORY FINDINGS

Drugs that May Alter Lab Results

Fluid therapy can mask relative polycythemia—effect on PCV and total plasma protein

Disorders that May Alter Lab Results

Concurrent anemia or hypoproteinemia can influence interpretation of PCV and total plasma protein values.

Valid If Run in Human Lab?

Valid if thresholds are correctly set to analyze equine hematology when using automated analyzers.

CBC/BIOCHEMISTRY/URINALYSIS

- Standard CBC and total plasma protein determination are the basic tests to evaluate the possibility of polycythemia.
- Biochemistry is useful with suspected absolute polycythemia; creatinine, liver enzymes, and bile acid determinations are necessary.

OTHER LABORATORY TESTS

- Arterial PO_2 and EPO determinations are necessary in cases of absolute polycythemia. Unfortunately, however, demonstrating the elevated EPO may not be possible, because equine EPO must be determined by bioassay.
- Hormone assays help to assess endocrine dysfunction.

IMAGING

Thoracic radiography and echocardiography help to evaluate cardiorespiratory function.

DIAGNOSTIC PROCEDURES

Bronchoalveolar lavage can help to evaluate respiratory function.

TREATMENT

• Relative polycythemia—rehydration and specific treatment of the underlying disease are necessary.
• Absolute polycythemia—removal of erythrocytes by repeated phlebotomy to keep PCV <50% is the initial therapy to minimize complications of hypervolemia and hyperviscosity.

MEDICATIONS

DRUGS OF CHOICE

Relative Polycythemia

• Treatment is aimed at the IV fluid administration necessary to re-establish and maintain hydration as well as any therapy necessary for the primary disease process.
• Base fluid selection on proper assesment of renal function, electrolyte balance, and acid–base status.

Absolute Polycythemia

• Initial treatment is phlebotomy—remove blood (10 mL/kg) every 2–3 days until a normal PCV (<50%) is attained, then perform as needed.
• Concurrent isotonic fluid administration should prevent hypovolemia and replace the lost blood volume.
• Absolute secondary polycythemia caused by inappropriate EPO production is treated with phlebotomy and removal of the EPO source.
• Do not treat absolute secondary polycythemia caused by hypoxemia with phlebotomy, as described earlier, because it is a necessary compensatory mechanism. If needed, however, phlebotomy should be slower and less pronounced (to reach a PCV <60%), and the resulting PCV necessary to sustain life without complications must be determined by trial and error. Treatment of the cause of hypoxemia is required.
• Absolute primary polycythemia is treated with phlebotomy as needed to attain a PCV <50%; the frequency of phlebotomy eventually is reduced because of iron deficiency.
• Hydroxyurea causes reversible bone marrow suppression and has been used successfully in humans and dogs. The dose must be individualized, but 30 mg/kg per day PO for 7–10 days, followed by a maintenance dose of 15 mg/kg per day, has been suggested for dogs. No experience with hydroxyurea has been reported in horses.

CONTRAINDICATIONS

Phlebotomy may be contraindicated in patients with hypoxemia.

PRECAUTIONS

• Rapid removal of blood can cause hypotension and vascular collapse.
• No reported experience with hydroxyurea in horses

POSSIBLE INTERACTIONS

N/A

ALTERNATIVE DRUGS

N/A

FOLLOW-UP

PATIENT MONITORING

• Monitor PCV, total plasma protein, and body weight two or three times daily in severely dehydrated animals until normal hydration status is restored.
• In cases of primary absolute polycythemia, monitor PCV every 2–3 days at first and then as needed.

POSSIBLE COMPLICATIONS

Absolute polycythemia can cause hyperviscosity and then predispose to thrombosis, infarction, hemorrhage, and DIC.

MISCELLANEOUS

ASSOCIATED CONDITIONS

N/A

AGE-RELATED FACTORS

N/A

ZOONOTIC POTENTIAL

N/A

PREGNANCY

N/A

SYNONYM

Erythrocytosis

SEE ALSO

Hyperviscosity syndrome

ABBREVIATIONS

• DIC = disseminated intravascular coagulation
• EPO = erythropoietin
• GI = gastrointestinal
• PCV = packed cell volume

Suggested Reading

Jain CJ. Essentials of veterinary hematology. Philadelphia: Lea & Febiger, 1993:166–168.
Reed SM, Bayly WM, ed. Equine internal medicine. Montreal: WB Saunders, 1998:573–575.
Smith BP. Large animal medicine. 2nd ed. Toronto: Mosby, 1996:478–479.

Authors Jean-Sébastien Latouche and Anne Lanevschi
Consulting Editor Claire B. Andreasen

POLYNEURITIS EQUI

BASICS

OVERVIEW
- Multifocal polyradiculoganglioneuritis
- Cauda equina syndrome
- Granulomatous inflammatory condition involving the extradural nerve roots of the cauda equina, which may be immune mediated

SIGNALMENT
- No age or sex predilection
- Not usually seen in the very young or very old

SIGNS
- Depression, anorexia, colic, and hypersensitivity over the gluteals
- Most signs relate to neurologic involvement of the cauda equina.
- Many affected horses have decreased anal tone and, possibly, urinary and fecal retention.
- Affected cranial nerves most often include V and VII, followed by VIII, IX, X, and XII.
- Symptoms may progress more slowly than in typical herpes cases.
- Animals may be afebrile at the onset of neurologic signs, but historically, they may have been febrile or had upper respiratory disease.

CAUSES AND RISK FACTORS
- The actual cause is unknown.
- The condition is thought to be predominantly an immune-mediated event, which can be initiated by viral or bacterial infections.

DIAGNOSIS

DIFFERENTIAL DIAGNOSIS
- Consider other diseases that could be asymmetric and multifocal.
- Herpes tends to have more acute onset, to stabilize more rapidly, and to respond well to treatment. Some cases of herpes may initiate polyneuritis equi. May need CSF tap, cytology, and viral titers to differentiate.
- Rabies—IFA on tactile hairs for diagnostics
- Viral encephalitis (i.e., EEE, WEE) tend to progress more rapidly; CSF tap, cytology, and viral titers can help to differentiate.
- Equine motor neuron disease
- Equine protozoal myeloencephalitis—CSF tap, cytology, and Western blot analysis to differentiate
- Trauma—rule out by palpation.

CBC/BIOCHEMISTRY/URINALYSIS
- CBC, electrolytes, and chemistry panel may be normal, depending on the inciting cause.
- Blood work reflect any secondary disease or complications that have occurred—dehydration caused by impaction colic; urinary tract infection caused by urinary retention

OTHER LABORATORY TESTS
- Virology for herpes and encephalitis titers on CSF and serum
- CSF may be positive for antimyelin antibodies
- CSF tap—Western blot for EPM

IMAGING
N/A

DIAGNOSTIC PROCEDURES
- CSF analysis—protein may be elevated but may not as significantly as with typical herpes.
- Cytology—may have increased leukocytes, which may be lymphocytes or mononuclear cells.
- Color—tends to be within normal limits compared to horses with herpes, in which the tap may be xanthochromic.

PATHOLOGIC FINDINGS
- Necropsy is the only way to establish a definitive diagnosis.
- Cauda equina becomes thickened and covered with fibrous material.
- Axonal degeneration
- Patients may have myelin degeneration; the condition predominantly involves the cauda equina, predominantly the extradural nerve roots.
- Usually infiltrates of inflammatory cells, initially neutrophils, that later are replaced by infiltrates of plasma cells, lymphocytes, macrophages, and some giant cells in the endoneural and perineural space.

TREATMENT

• Supportive
• If cranial nerve signs are present and animals are having difficulty eating, mash may need to be fed—bran mash if fecal retention is a problem; otherwise, use complete feed or other feed for mash
• May need to place a urinary catheter.
• May need to evacuate feces manually.

MEDICATIONS

DRUGS

• Antibiotics for secondary urinary tract infections
• Steroids (0.1 mg/# BID–SID, depending upon severity of signs). The dose can be tapered depending on progression. Steroids prolong life but, historically, have not improved mortality.

CONTRAINDICATIONS/POSSIBLE INTERACTIONS

N/A

FOLLOW-UP

• Monitor for choke, impaction colics, and fecal and urinary incontinence.
• The disease usually progresses, and the long-term prognosis is poor.
• Most affected animals are euthanized.

MISCELLANEOUS

ASSOCIATED CONDITIONS

N/A

AGE-RELATED FACTORS

N/A

ZOONOTIC POTENTIAL

N/A

PREGNANCY

N/A

SEE ALSO

N/A

ABBREVIATIONS

• CSF = cerebrospinal fluid
• EEE = eastern equine encephalitides
• EPM =
• IFA = immunofluorescent antibody
• WEE = western equine encephalitides

Suggested Reading

Equine current veterinary therapy. 3rd ed.

Author S.G. Witonsky
Consulting Editor Joseph J. Bertone

POLYURIA (PU) AND POLYDIPSIA (PD)

BASICS

DEFINITION
- PU—urine output >50 mL/kg per day
- PD—fluid intake >100 mL/kg per day

PATHOPHYSIOLOGY
- Production of concentrated or dilute urine results from permeability of the collecting ducts to water (controlled by ADH activity) and the concentration gradient from the renal cortex to the inner medulla.
- Rather modest increases in plasma tonicity (≅3 mOsm/kg) stimulate production and release of ADH by the posterior pituitary and increase water permeability and reabsorption in the collecting ducts.
- Decreases in plasma tonicity inhibit ADH release. As a result, collecting ducts become impermeable to water, and dilute urine is produced. Thus, PU may be a normal physiologic response to eliminate excess body water.
- Transient PU may be a desired or undesired effect of drug administration or loss of the medullary concentration gradient—medullary washout
- Persistent PU generally results from a number of disease processes—CRF, Cushing's disease, DI, DM, and endotoxemia
- Two important stimuli for thirst—an increase in plasma tonicity, and hypovolemia.
- PD may be a physiologic response to PU (to prevent dehydration), a consequence of drug administration (e.g., corticosteroids), or a primary problem of excessive water intake. In horses, the latter problem usually is behavioral in origin (primary PD) but also may accompany excessive salt intake.
- Urine production and water consumption vary with age, diet, workload, environmental temperature, and GI water absorption. Urine production increases 50%–100% when diet is changed from a grass to a legume hay; similarly, horses in heavy exercise, stabled in hot climates, or with chronic diarrhea may have a water intake in excess of 100 L/day yet produce normal urine volumes.

SYSTEM AFFECTED
- Renal/urologic—excessive urine production
- Endocrine/metabolic—Cushing's disease; DM
- Nervous—hypothalamic injury resulting in central DI

SIGNALMENT
Breed Predilections
Cushing's disease appears more common in Morgans and ponies.

Mean Age and Range
- Foals consuming a predominantly milk diet (first 3 months of life) normally are polyuric. Daily fluid intake may approach 250 mL/kg per day (fivefold greater than adults), and a urine specific gravity <1.008 should be expected.
- Cushing's disease occurs in old (typically > 20 years) horses and ponies.

Predominant Sex
Familial nephrogenic DI in Thoroughbred colts

SIGNS
Historical Findings
- Horses with mild to moderate PU/PD often go undetected by owners, or complaints may include stopping to urinate while being ridden or excessive thirst after exercise.
- With more substantial PU/PD (e.g., with primary PD), the magnitude of PU typically is dramatic, with owners reporting that horses drink two- to threefold more water than stablemates and that stalls can be flooded with urine.

Physical Examination Findings
- Consistent with the underlying disease processes (e.g., CRF, Cushing's disease) or normal (e.g., primary PD, excessive salt ingestion).
- Patients with CRF, DI, or DM may become dehydrated rapidly if deprived of water, so careful assessment of hydration status is important in evaluation for PU/PD.

CAUSES
Primary PD
- Primary or "psychogenic" PD probably is the most common cause of PU/PD in adults for which clients will have a primary complaint of excessive urination.
- Cause unknown
- In some, it appears to be a stable vice reflecting boredom; in others, it may develop after a change in environmental conditions, stabling, diet, or medication administration.
- Anecdotally reported to be more common in southern states during periods of high temperature and humidity.

Excessive Salt Consumption
- Occasionally in apparent primary PD, PU/PD may be attributed to excessive salt consump-
tion and is manifested by an increased fractional sodium clearance.
- Such "psychogenic salt eaters" appear to be less common than "psychogenic water drinkers"; salt intake may have to exceed 5%–10% of dry matter intake before PU/PD becomes apparent.

Drug Administration
Administration of PO or IV fluids, diuretics, α_2-agonists, and corticosteroids

CRF
- These horses cannot concentrate urine beyond the isosthenuric range (specific gravity, 1.008–1.014).
- The degree of PU is modest compared to primary PD or DI, so it is a client complaint only in ≅50% of afflicted horses.

Cushing's Disease
- May lead to PU/PD by several mechanisms
- An osmotic diuresis when plasma glucose concentration exceeds the renal threshold, leading to glucosuria
- Antagonism of the action of ADH on collecting ducts by cortisol
- A primary dipsogenic effect of excessive cortisol
- Compression of the posterior pituitary by growth of the adenoma leading to central DI.

DI

- May occur because of inadequate secretion of ADH (i.e., neurogenic or central DI) or decreased sensitivity of the epithelial cells of the collecting ducts to circulating ADH (i.e., nephrogenic DI).
- An acquired form of central DI has been described in horses and is idiopathic in nature or secondary to encephalitis.
- Nephrogenic DI has been described in sibling Thoroughbred colts, suggesting an inherited form may occur.

DM

- A state of chronic hyperglycemia usually accompanied by glucosuria
- The resultant osmotic diuresis occasionally causes PU/PD.

Sepsis/Endotoxemia

- PU/PD occasionally is observed in horses with sepsis or endotoxemia.
- The mechanism is unclear, but PU/PD may result from endotoxin-induced prostaglandin production. Prostaglandin E_2 is a potent renal vasodilating agent that also can antagonize the effects of ADH on collecting ducts, producing medullary washout.

DIAGNOSIS

DIFFERENTIAL DIAGNOSIS

N/A

CBC/BIOCHEMISTRY/URINALYSIS

- Changes characteristic for CRF when that is the cause of PU/PD—mild anemia, azotemia, isosthenuria, and electrolyte and acid–base alterations in more advanced cases; see *Chronic Renal Failure.*
- With Cushing's disease, mild anemia and a mature neutrophilia are characteristic CBC findings. Hyperglycemia and mild increases in hepatic enzyme activity may be found in more advanced cases. Glucosuria may be present and, if so, supports osmotic diuresis as the causative mechanism.
- With primary PD, CBC and serum chemistry results are normal, but urine specific gravity typically is <1.005. Fractional sodium clearance is increased (>1%) when excessive salt intake is the cause.
- With DI, CBC and serum chemistry usually are normal but may reflect dehydration, and urine specific gravity is <1.005
- With DM, hyperglycemia and glucosuria
- When sepsis/endotoxemia is the cause of PU/PD, CBC and serum chemistry abnormalities reflect the underlying disease process.

OTHER LABORATORY TESTS

- Measurement of plasma cortisol and adrenocorticotropin concentrations in horses with Cushing's disease
- Measurement of fractional sodium clearance (fractional excretion of sodium) in horses with primary PD
- Measurement of plasma ADH concentration would be useful in cases of DI to differentiate neurogenic (low ADH) from nephrogenic (high ADH when dehydrated) forms, but this assay is not commercially available.

IMAGING

Transabdominal ultrasonography—to assess kidney size and echogenicity (should be normal, except with CRF)

DIAGNOSTIC PROCEDURES

- Urine collection—to document low specific gravity and determine fractional sodium clearance
- Dexamethasone suppression test in horses with suspected Cushing's disease
- Overnight water deprivation probably is the most useful test to determine ability to concentrate urine. Horses with primary PD should concentrate urine to a specific gravity of 1.025–1.030); horses with CRF and DI fail to concentrate urine to a specific gravity of >1.012–1.014. Approach water deprivation cautiously in horses with suspected DI, and do not perform when azotemia is detected (with CRF). Measure body weight before water deprivation; extending the test beyond the time needed to lose 5% of body weight (may be <12 hours in horses with DI) has no benefit.
- In horses with suspected DI based on failing to concentrate urine during water deprivation, exogenous ADH (synthetic ADH; 60 IU, IM, or SC q6h) can be used to differentiate neurogenic (will concentrate urine) from nephrogenic (will not concentrate urine) DI.

TREATMENT

APPROPRIATE HEALTH CARE

- CRF—see *Chronic Renal Failure.*
- Cushing's disease—medical treatment (pergolide) with other necessary supportive care (nutrition, foot care and analgesia for laminitis, antibiotics for secondary infections)
- Primary PD—gradual restriction of water intake (initially to 100 mL/kg per day, which is approximately twice maintenance needs in a temperate climate, followed by a decrease to 75 mL/kg per day after several days) with careful monitoring of body weight and hydration status along with "trial and error" management changes; removal of supplemental salt when excessive consumption is the cause of PD
- DI—mild water restriction (to 100 mL/kg per day with careful monitoring of body weight and hydration status) and use of medications may help in limiting PU/PD; discontinue water restriction if dehydration or >5% loss of body weight occurs.
- DM—exogenous insulin replacement therapy
- Sepsis/endotoxemia—appropriate antibiotic treatment and supportive care (including judicious fluid therapy) for the underlying disease process

NURSING CARE

Long-term survival of horses with Cushing's disease likely improves with close monitoring, prompt recognition, and appropriate treatment of complications—flare-ups of laminitis and secondary infections

DIET

- See *Chronic Renal Failure* for dietary recommendations in horses with CRF.
- Horses with Cushing's disease usually are aged and may have dental problems, requiring feeding of complete pelleted rations.
- Increasing the amount of forage in the diet may help to decrease excessive water intake by horses with primary PD.
- Limit availability of supplemental salt to horses with excessive salt consumption as the cause of primary PD.

POLYURIA (PU) AND POLYDIPSIA (PD)

CLIENT EDUCATION

• Inform clients that provision of adequate fresh water at all times is imperative to prevent dehydration with all pathologic causes of PU/PD.
• Horses with primary PD may need "trial and error" management changes (e.g., increasing turn- out time, increasing exercise, provision of a stablemate or other diversions in the stall) along with gradual water restriction
• When excessive salt consumption is the cause of PD, removing salt availability usually is corrective.
• The magnitude of PU/PD with inherited forms of DI may be reduced with mild salt and water restriction and medical therapy. With acquired forms of DI, especially nephrogenic DI from reversible renal disease or drug treatment, PU/PD may last for weeks to months but often may resolve over time.
• Some horses with DM are managed successfully with insulin replacement therapy, but most have a guarded to poor prognosis for long-term survival. Inform owners of the indications for euthanasia—loss of appetite and body condition; progressive weakness

MEDICATIONS

DRUGS OF CHOICE

Cushing's Disease

The dopamine agonist pergolide (2–6 μg/kg PO q24h) is the drug of choice.

DI

• With neurogenic DI, hormone replacement therapy with desmopressin (a potent ADH analogue administered as eye drops) has been successful in small-animal patients but has not been described in horses and may be cost prohibitive.
• With nephrogenic DI, replacement hormone therapy is ineffective; the only practical treatment is to restrict sodium and water intake and to administer thiazide diuretics.

DM

• Insulin replacement therapy in horses with low serum insulin concentrations—type I DM
• Exogenous insulin therapy may have some benefit to horses with elevated serum insulin concentrations—insulin-resistant or type II DM

CONTRAINDICATIONS

Gradual water restriction is contraindicated in horses with CRF, Cushing's disease, DM, or sepsis/endotoxemia.

PRECAUTIONS

Perform water restriction with caution in horses with primary PD and DI to avoid significant dehydration.

POSSIBLE INTERACTIONS

N/A

ALTERNATIVE DRUGS

N/A

FOLLOW-UP

PATIENT MONITORING

• Closely monitor all patients with PU/PD at all times to minimize the risk of dehydration; horses with DI are at greatest risk of developing significant dehydration, even during short periods (hours) of water deprivation.
• See *Chronic Renal Failure* for specific follow-up recommendations in horses with CRF.
• See *Cushing's disease* for specific follow-up recommendations in horses with this condition.

POLYURIA (PU) AND POLYDIPSIA (PD)

POSSIBLE COMPLICATIONS
Moderate to severe dehydration may develop when horses with CRF, DI, or DM are unintentionally deprived of water for short periods.

MISCELLANEOUS

ASSOCIATED CONDITIONS
- CRF
- Cushing's disease
- DM

AGE-RELATED FACTORS
- During the first 3 months of life, foals consuming a predominantly milk diet normally are polyuric.
- Cushing's disease occurs in old (typically > 20 years) horses and ponies.

ZOONOTIC POTENTIAL
N/A

PREGNANCY
N/A

SYNONYMS
N/A

SEE ALSO
- CRF
- Cushing's syndrome

ABBREVIATIONS
- ADH = antidiuretic hormone
- CRF = chronic renal failure
- DI = diabetes insipidus
- DM = diabetes mellitus
- GI = gastrointestinal
- PU = polyana
- PD = polydipsia

Suggested Reading

Browning AP. Polydipsia and polyuria in two horses caused by psychogenic polydipsia. Equine Vet Educ/AE 2000;2:231–236.

Genetzky RM, Loparco FV, Ledet AE. Clinical pathological alterations in horses during a water deprivation test. Am J Vet Res 1987;48:1007–1011.

Schott HC. Polyuria and polydipsia. In: Reed SM, Bayly WM, eds. Equine internal medicine. Philadelphia: WB Saunders, 1998:895–901.

Schott HC, Bayly WM, Reed SM, Brobst DF. Nephrogenic diabetes insipidus in sibling colts. J Vet Intern Med 1993;7:68–72.

Author Harold C. Schott II
Consulting Editor Harold C. Schott II

POST ANAGEN DEFLUXION (PAD) AND TELOGEN EFFLUVIUM (TE)

BASICS

OVERVIEW

PAD is characterized by the loss of anagen hairs within a few days of stressful situations, such as a systemic illness associated with a high fever. It is a recognized condition in small animals and may also occur in humans.

Similar conditions such as TE, also known as telogen defluxion or defluvium, can occur when synchronous loss of telogen hairs occurs several months after similar types of stress. After-pregnancy it has been referred to as post-partum telogen effluvium.

ORGAN SYSTEM

Dermatologic

SIGNALMENT

No age, breed, sex predilections

SIGNS

- Multifocal/patchy to generalized alopecia
- Can involve the mane and tail
- Non-inflammatory, non-pruritic

CAUSES AND RISK FACTORS

Pathogenesis (PAD)

- Stresses such as antimitotic drugs, endocrine disorders,infectious or metabolic disease interfere with the anagen phase resulting in hair loss and breaking of the anagen phase hairs at the epidermal surface within days to weeks of the insult
- The hairs are lost in anagen defluxion due to dysplastic changes such as narrowing or damaging of the hair shafts
- The hair shafts are structurally weak at narrow sites and break off to leave ragged points.

Pathogenesis (TE)

- A stress (high fever, pregnancy, shock, surgery, anesthesia, sever illness) result in abrupt cessation of anagen hair growth
- Sudden synchrony of hair follicles entering into catagen and telogen results in a simultaneous shedding or hair loss, usually 2–3 months after the stressful event

DIAGNOSIS

DIFFERENTIAL DIAGNOSES

- Alopecia Areata
- Dermatophytosis
- Linear alopecia
- Mercury poisoning
- Hypothyroidism
- Normal shed

CBC/BIOCHEMISTRY/URINALYSIS

N/A

OTHER LABORATORY TESTS

N/A

IMAGING

N/A

POST ANAGEN DEFLUXION (PAD) AND TELOGEN EFFLUVIUM (TE)

DIAGNOSTIC PROCEDURES

- Trichogram
  - —PAD hairs are characterized by irregularities and dysplastic changes; shaft diameter may be narrowed/deformed resulting in breaking at stress points
  - —TE hairs are characterized by uniform shaft diameter and a clubbed, non-pigmented root with no root sheath
- Dermatopathology
  - —PAD will reveal apoptosis and fragmented nuclei in the hair matrix of anagen hair follicles, along with eosinophilic dysplastic hair shafts within the pilar canal
  - —TE will reveal a predominance of telogen hairs or synchronized anagen with no other abnormalities, depending on the timing of the biopsy.

TREATMENT

MEDICATIONS

DRUGS

- Identify underlying etiology and address accordingly
- No specific pharmaceutical therapy to promote hair regrowth

CONTRAINDICATIONS/POSSIBLE INTERACTIONS

N/A

FOLLOW-UP

EXPECTED COURSE AND PROGNOSIS

- Both PAD & TE spontaneously resolve when the underlying stress is removed
- No drug treatment is needed other than elimination of potential inciting drugs

MISCELLANEOUS

SEE ALSO

N/A

ABBREVIATIONS

See Above

Suggested Reading

Stannard AA. Alopecia in the Horse. Vet Derm 2000 vol 11(3):191–193.

Author Anthony A. Yu

POSTPARTUM METRITIS

BASICS

DEFINITION

• Acute metritis resulting from RFM (i.e., retained placenta) or contamination of the uterus after parturition or dystocia
• Marked by concurrent septicemia/endotoxemia and, possibly, laminitis.

PATHOPHYSIOLOGY

• Because of difficult foaling, RFM, or heavy bacterial contamination of the uterus during foaling, coupled with septicemia/endotoxemia, the uterus is flaccid and thin walled compared with the normal involuting uterus—thick walls and longitudinal rugae present as it rapidly involutes postpartum.
• Accumulated fluid and debris provide favorable conditions for bacterial growth, inflammation, and toxin release.
• Toxins are easily absorbed into the maternal circulation (i.e., endotoxemia) because of the highly vascularized and thin-walled postpartum uterus.

SYSTEMS AFFECTED

• Reproductive
• Hemic/lymphatic/immune
• Musculoskeletal

GENETICS

N/A

INCIDENCE/PREVALENCE

N/A

SIGNALMENT

• Postpartum mare
• Signs of abdominal pain or depression after dystocia, RFM, or extensive intrapartum uterine contamination
• Also can occur after normal delivery when the mare does not exercise, which aides clearance of postpartum debris and fluid accumulation—mare with a foal with limb deformity needing exercise restriction.

SIGNS

• Metritis may become evident by 12–24 hours postpartum, characterized by depression, abdominal pain, and anorexia.
• Depression is associated with shock or endotoxemia.
• Fever, elevated pulse and respiratory rate, and congested or toxic mucous membranes
• Uterus is enlarged, flaccid, and baggy from accumulation of fetid, dark-red to chocolate-colored fluid.
• Attachment of RFM usually at/in the previously nonpregnant horn. The RFM may comprise a large portion of the total and be seen hanging through the vulvae or be limited to only a small piece.
• Signs of laminitis (e.g., bounding digital pulses, lameness) may appear 12 hours to 5 days postpartum.

CAUSES AND RISK FACTORS

• Mares with a history of placentitis, RFM, dystocia, prolonged or assisted delivery, fetotomy, or cesarean section are at greater risk of postpartum metritis.
• Postpartum complications depend on the amount and type of bacteria in the reproductive tract. A dirty foaling environment or excessive manipulation at parturition often are associated.
• In addition to aerobic Gram-positive and -negative bacteria such as *Streptococcus zooepidemicus and other B-hemolytic Streptococci, Staphylococcus* sp., *Escherichia coli, Pseudomonas aeruginosa,* and *Klebsiella pneumoniae,* the anaerobe *Bacteroides fragilis* frequently is involved.
• Autolytic RFM, in concert with bacterial contamination, results in endometritis and metritis.
• Left untreated, can lead to septicemia, endotoxemia, and laminitis.

DIAGNOSIS

DIFFERENTIAL DIAGNOSIS

Other Causes of Postpartum Abdominal Pain/Depression

• Normal uterine involution and placental expulsion
• Uterine artery rupture, with or without internal hemorrhage—a clot forms between the myometrium and serosa; the uterus/broad ligament usually is enlarged and painful at palpation, and the hematocrit may be normal or decreased; if the clot is not contained within the broad ligament, abdominocentesis may reveal increased RBCs, PMNs, and some bacteria.
• Uterine torsion.
• Uterine rupture—may be difficult to identify at transrectal palpation; abdominocentesis reveals PMN, bacteria, and elevated protein.
• Rupture of cecum or right ventral colon—strong abdominal contractions during parturition can rupture or bruise the large bowel if it is distended by gas or ingesta or becomes trapped between the uterus and the pelvis; abdominocentesis reveals ingesta in the peritoneal cavity.

Other Causes of Postpartum Vaginal Discharge

Normal postpartum ($\leq$6 days postpartum) lochia—odorless, dark red-brown vaginal discharge associated with a palpable, normally involuting uterus, with thickening and corrugation (i.e., transrectal palpation description) of uterine wall

CBC/BIOCHEMISTRY/URINALYSIS

• Marked leukopenia ($\leq$2000 cells/μL) with toxic PMN and left shift—response to treatment is evaluated by the return of WBC to normal values (5000–12,000 cells/μL).
• Fibrinogen may increase to $\geq$500 mg/dL during the acute phase but usually returns to normal values ($\leq$400 mg/dL) 2–3 days after WBC count returns to the normal range.

OTHER LABORATORY TESTS

• Bacterial identification—obtain a sample of uterine contents using a guarded swab; plate the sample on blood and McConkey agar; blood agar will support growth of Gram-positive, select Gram-negative, and some yeasts, whereas McConkey will only support growth of Gram-negative organisms; incubate plates at 37°C; examine at 24 and 48 hours.
• For anaerobes, streak swabs onto two Wilkins-Chalgren anaerobe agar plates and incubate in an atmosphere of 10% hydrogen, 10% CO_2, and 80% N_2 at 37°C; examine at 24 and 48 hours.
• Culture before instituting antibiotic therapy, if possible, but do not wait for culture results before beginning treatment. Initiate treatment immediately with broad-spectrum antibiotics, metronidazole, IV fluids, and antiendotoxic doses of anti-inflammatory drugs if metritis is suspected based on clinical signs, CBC, history of dystocia, RFM ($\geq$8–12 hours) or contamination/trauma has occurred. Adjust therapy when the culture and sensitivity results come back, switching to other, more appropriate antibiotics if indicated.

IMAGING

Ultrasonography:
• Large amounts of fluid may accumulate in the uterus after 24–48 hours postpartum.
• Degree of echogenicity generally relates to the amount of debris or inflammatory cells in the fluid.
• Uterine wall appears thick and edematous.

DIAGNOSTIC PROCEDURES

N/A

PATHOLOGIC FINDINGS

Postpartum acute inflammatory response extending from the endometrium to the deeper regions (i.e., stratum compactum, stratum spongiosum, to and including the myometrium [full- thickness, uterine wall disease]) contrast with endometritis and routine uterine infections/reaction in the mare, endometritis, and luminal infection.

TREATMENT

APPROPRIATE HEALTH CARE

• Endotoxemia is prevented/treated by IV fluids for circulatory support and anti-endotoxic doses of flunixin meglumine. Polymyxin-B is used to neutralize circulating endotoxins.
• Administer systemic, broad-spectrum antibiotics and metronidazole to control uterine bacterial overgrowth and to prevent endotoxemia.
• Only after the mare is medically stable should physical evacuation of bacteria and inflammatory debris from the uterine lumen begin—perform uterine lavage with large volumes of warm saline solution; 3–6 L are infused at each treatment period through a sterile nasogastric tube; uterine contents then are siphoned off, and the lavage is repeated until the recovered fluid is clear; repeat 2–3 times daily based on transrectal palpation and ultrasound findings.
• Finding a thickened, corrugated uterine wall at palpation indicates a positive response to treatment and stimulation of uterine involution.
• Unresponsive mares have flaccid, thin uterine walls and accumulate large amounts of fluid between treatments. Treatment is discontinued when intrauterine fluid is clear or slightly cloudy.
• Begin with a smaller volume (1 L) if a uterine tear is suspected.
• Administer oxytocin routinely to aid uterine evacuation or if fluid remains after lavage.
• Laminitis—treat with anti-inflammatory drugs, 3M pads to reduce pressure on the lamina, and nitroglycerin ointment to promote digital circulation.

POSTPARTUM METRITIS

NURSING CARE
N/A

ACTIVITY
Exercise—turn out time twice a day.

DIET
N/A

CLIENT EDUCATION
N/A

SURGICAL CONSIDERATIONS
N/A

MEDICATIONS

DRUGS OF CHOICE

Fluids
- Use polyionic solutions—Normosol.
- Estimate dehydration based on clinical signs (e.g., skin turgor), hematocrit (normal, 32%–53%), and total protein (normal, 5.7–7.9 g/dL).
- Calcium gluconate (125 mL of 23% solution) and oxytocin (40 IU) may be added to every other 5-L bag of Normosol.
- Mild colic or discomfort will result from uterine contractions stimulated by treatment.
- Discontinue or slow the rate of administration if signs of severe colic occur.

Systemic Antibiotics
- Potassium penicillin for Gram-positive organisms—loading dose of 44,000 IU IV, followed by 22,000 IU IV QID
- Combine with gentamicin for Gram-negative organisms—2.2 mg/kg IV QID or 6.6 mg/kg IV SID
- For oral administration, use 15 mg/kg of trimethoprim sulfa (broad-spectrum) BID.
- Metronidazole, for anaerobes, should be always combined with IV or PO therapy—loading dose of 15 mg/kg PO, followed by 7.5 mg/kg PO QID.

Uterotonic Drugs
- Oxytocin—different protocols have been used.
- 10 IU IV or 20 IU IM after uterine lavage
- 40 IU added to IV fluids
- 10 IU IV QID

NSAIDs
- Flunixin meglumine (Banamine)—antiendotoxic dose, 0.25 mg/kg IV or IM TID; anti-inflammatory dose, 1mg/kg IV or IM BID
- Phenylbutazone—2.2–4.4 mg/kg IV or PO BID; at the onset of laminitis, recommended loading dose is 8.8 mg/kg IV.
- Polymyxin B—administer 6000 U/kg IV in 1 L of sterile saline over 30–60 min; recommended BID for 1–2 days.
- Nitroglycerin ointment—apply 15–20 mg to each digital vessel SID.

CONTRAINDICATIONS
N/A

PRECAUTIONS
- NSAIDs may cause bone marrow dyscrasia and GI ulceration.
- Aminoglycosides can be nephro- and ototoxic; assure good hydration during treatment.
- Nitroglycerin—wear gloves when applying.
- Polymyxin B—potentially nephrotoxic at therapeutic doses

POSSIBLE INTERACTIONS
N/A

ALTERNATIVE DRUGS
N/A

FOLLOW-UP

PATIENT MONITORING
- Monitor CBC every 48–72 hours for signs of endotoxemia or response to treatment.
- Monitor for signs of laminitis by early and repeated evaluation of digital pulses, signs of weight shift, and radiographs of the distal phalanx—rotation or sinking
- Monitor for postpartum constipation or postsurgical/dystocia ileus. Mineral oil (0.5–1.0 gallon) or Bran mash may be used to prevent or treat ileus; fluid therapy also is helpful.

PREVENTION/AVOIDANCE
N/A

POSSIBLE COMPLICATIONS
- Delayed uterine involution.
- Septicemia/endotoxemia
- Laminitis
- Death

EXPECTED COURSE AND PROGNOSIS
- Prognosis depends on severity, duration, and secondary complications caused by metritis.
- Rapid response to therapy indicates a favorable prognosis.
- Laminitis after endotoxemia carries a guarded to grave prognosis.

MISCELLANEOUS

ASSOCIATED CONDITIONS
N/A

AGE RELATED FACTORS
N/A

ZOONOTIC POTENTIAL
N/A

PREGNANCY
N/A

SYNONYMS
- Metritis/laminitis/septicemia complex
- Toxic metritis

SEE ALSO
- Delayed uterine clearance
- Dystocia
- Endometritis
- Laminitis
- RFM
- Uterine torsion

ABBREVIATIONS
- GI = gastrointestinal
- PMN = polymorphonuclear/WBC
- RFM = retained fetal membranes

Suggested Reading

Asbury AC. Care of the mare after foaling. In: Mackinnon AO, Voss JL, ed. Equine reproduction. Philadelphia: Lea & Febiger, 1993:976–980.

Threlfall WR, Carleton CL. Treatment of uterine infections in the mare. In: Morrow DA, ed. Current therapy in theriogenology. Philadelphia: WB Saunders, 1986:730–737.

Author Maria E. Cadario

Consulting Editor Carla L. Carleton

POTASSIUM, HYPERKALEMIA

BASICS

DEFINITION

Serum potassium concentration > the laboratory reference range—generally >4.8 mEq/L.

PATHOPHYSIOLOGY

- Potassium is the main intracellular cation.
- Cell uptake is favored by insulin and epinephrine.
- Horses ingest a large quantity of K^+ daily; however, efficient renal K^+ secretion by distal tubules prevents cardiotoxic hyperkalemia.
- Aldosterone promotes K^+ tubular secretion, which also is influenced by tubular fluid flow rate, tubular sodium delivery rate, acid–base state, ADH, and unreabsorbable anions.
- Some K^+ is lost in sweat and feces.
- Renal failure and uroperitoneum are two important causes of hyperkalemia. A shift of K^+ from the ICF to ECF compartment is associated with hyperkalemia during metabolic acidosis.
- HPP is seen in Quarterhorses and Quarterhorse cross-breeds.
- Most of the body K^+ is located in skeletal muscles. During exercise, K^+ is released from muscles, and transient hyperkalemia can be seen.
- Extensive tissue necrosis can lead to hyperkalemia.
- RBCs also contain high levels of K^+, and false hyperkalemia can develop in vitro because of hemolysis or prolonged storage (i.e., leakage of K^+) of more than 120 minutes. Markedly elevated leukocytes or platelet counts will have the same effect.
- Also seen in potassium chloride poisoning.

SYSTEMS AFFECTED

Cardiovascular

- ECG abnormalities when $K^+ > 6$ mEq/L; severe changes at 8 mEq/L < K^+ <10 mEq/L.
- The most consistent change is a broadening and flattening of the P wave.
- Ventricular asystole or fibrillation can occur.
- Heart block develops when extracellular K^+ reaches threefold or more the normal values.
- The heart stops in diastole.

Musculoskeletal

- Muscular weakness
- Hyperkalemia decreases membrane potential and causes hyperexcitability.

SIGNALMENT

HPP in Quarterhorses and related breeds—Paints and Palominos

SIGNS

Historical Findings

- Muscular fasciculations—shivering
- Spasms and myoclonus
- Weakness—swaying and staggering
- Involuntary recumbency
- Collapse
- Death

Physical Examination Findings

In addition to those described above, cardiac dysrhythmias and ECG abnormalities

CAUSES

- Pseudohyperkalemia—in vitro artifact caused by hemolysis or leakage of K^+ into serum from RBC, WBC, and platelets if the sample is not analyzed or the serum separated quickly.
- Hypovolemia with renal shutdown, renal disease, and uroperitoneum
- Shift of intracellular K^+ caused by metabolic acidosis or vigorous exercise
- HPP in Quarterhorses and cross-breeds
- Tissue necrosis; severe intravascular hemolysis
- Diabetes mellitus; Addison's disease
- High potassium intake from oral or parenteral potassium supplements

RISKS FACTORS

- HPP—homozygotes are more severely affected than heterozygotes; male horses seem more affected than females. Crisis may be precipitated by PO or IV administration of K^+, irregular feeding schedules, drastic changes in ration composition, weather changes, trailer rides, and general anesthesia.

DIAGNOSIS

DIFFERENTIAL DIAGNOSIS

- Rule out other causes of muscular spasms—colic, tetanus, seizures, and exertional rhabdomyolysis
- Investigate causes of electrolyte abnormalities—chronic renal failure
- Investigate other causes of sudden death—cardiovascular (e.g., aortic ring rupture, CNS embolism, massive internal hemorrhage), metabolic (e.g., hypocalcemia, eclampsia), infectious and parasitic (e.g., anthrax, babesiosis), and toxic
- Evaluate renal function.

LABORATORY FINDINGS

Drugs that May Alter Lab Results

K_3-EDTA contamination increases K^+ concentrations.

Disorders that May Alter Lab Results

Thrombocytosis >1,000,000 platelets/μL or leukocytosis >200,000 cells/μL increases K^+ concentration; hemolysis leads to the same result.

Valid If Run in Human Lab?

Yes

CBC/BIOCHEMISTRY/URINALYSIS

- Consider renal disease or uroperitoneum in animals with azotemia
- Consider Addison's disease in animals with low sodium levels.
- Consider muscular injury in animals with elevated CK and AST levels; rule out hemolysis and pseudohyperkalemia.

OTHER LABORATORY TESTS

HPP

- DNA blood testing to detect mutation in the Na^+ channel gene and to assess if the horse is homozygous or heterozygous for this mutation.
- Potassium chloride provocation test carries risk in horses with HPP, cardiac disease, renal disease, or impaired adrenocortical function.

Postmortem Analysis of Vitreous K^+ Concentration

May be useful to determine if death was associated with hyperkalemia.

IMAGING

N/A

DIAGNOSTIC PROCEDURES

Electromyography—indicates membrane irritability.

TREATMENT

- Depends on the underlying cause
- Promote renal K^+ elimination, and initiate supportive treatment while pursuing a diagnosis.
- In severe cases, as indicated by ECG and clinical signs, initiate aggressive therapy.
- Remove hay with high K^+ content (e.g., alfalfa) from the diet.

POTASSIUM, HYPERKALEMIA

MEDICATIONS

DRUGS OF CHOICE

- Moderate hyperkalemia—fluid therapy with potassium-free isotonic fluid. Administer IV saline (0.9%) in 5–10-L volumes every 30–60 hours; water requirements for maintenance in horses are ≅10–15 L.
- Severe hyperkalemia—calcium gluconate (23%; 0.2–0.4 mL/kg diluted in 1–2 L of 5% dextrose IV) gives good results; sodium bicarbonate (1–2 mEq/kg IV) or 5% dextrose (6 mL/kg IV) also can be used.
- Acetazolamide (2–4 mg/kg PO q6–12h), a carbonic anhydrase inhibitor diuretic, can be used daily to control HPP episodes.

CONTRAINDICATIONS

- Potassium-containing fluids or oral supplements
- Fluids causing hyponatremia, acidosis, or hypocalcemia
- Drugs interfering with potassium elimination

PRECAUTIONS

Acetazolamide can induce a hyperchloremic acidosis, but at a higher dose (30 mg/kg PO BID) than that used in HPP.

POSSIBLE INTERACTIONS

N/A

ALTERNATIVE DRUGS

- Hydrochlorothiazide, though it is less efficient than acetazolamide.
- Furosemide, by inducing diuresis, natriuresis, and chloruresis. Normal prostaglandin metabolism within the kidneys is needed for its effect, however, and furosemide is inhibited by administration of NSAIDs.

FOLLOW-UP

PATIENT MONITORING

- Recheck potassium and other electrolytes; frequency is dictated by the underlying cause and the severity of the clinical signs.
- Monitor ECG in severe cases until return to normal.

POSSIBLE COMPLICATIONS

Severe hyperkalemia can lead to death.

MISCELLANEOUS

ASSOCIATED CONDITIONS

N/A

AGE-RELATED FACTORS

N/A

ZOONOTIC POTENTIAL

N/A

PREGNANCY

N/A

SYNONYMS

N/A

SEE ALSO

See *Causes*.

ABBREVIATIONS

- ADH = antidiuretic hormone
- AST = aspartate aminotransferase
- CK = creatine kinase
- ECF = extracellular fluid
- HPP = hyperkalemic periodic paralysis
- ICF = intracellular fluid

Suggested Reading

Carlson GP. Clinical chemistry tests. In: Smith BP, ed. Large animal internal medicine. 2nd ed. St. Louis: Mosby, 1996.

Carlson GP. Fluid, electrolyte, and acid–base balance. In: Kaneko JJ, Harvey JW, Bruss ML, eds. Clinical biochemistry of domestic animals. 5th ed. New York: Academic Press, 1997.

Foreman JH. The exhausted horse syndrome. Vet Clin North Am Equine Pract 1998;14:205–219.

Hyyppä S, Pösö AR. Fluid, electrolyte, and acid–base responses to exercise in racehorses. Vet Clin North Am Equine Pract 1998;14:121–136.

Schmall LM. Fluid and electrolyte therapy. In: Robinson NE, ed. Current therapy in equine medicine 4. Philadelphia: WB Saunders, 1997.

Authors Valerie O. Guilpin and E. Duane Lassen

Consulting Editor Claire B. Andreasen

POTASSIUM, HYPOKALEMIA

BASICS

DEFINITION

- Serum K^+ concentration <2.8 mEq/L
- May reflect an internal redistribution of K^+ or whole-body K^+ deficiency.

PATHOPHYSIOLOGY

- Potassium is the main intracellular cation.
- Cellular uptake is favored by insulin and epinephrine.
- Shift of K^+ from the ECF to ICF compartment during IV administration of glucose-containing solutions can lead to hypokalemia; a similar process is seen with alkalosis and IV administration of sodium bicarbonate.
- As horses ingest large amounts of K^+ in their ration, renal K^+ elimination (i.e., secretion by distal tubules) is increased.
- Aldosterone promotes K^+ tubular secretion, which also is influenced by tubular fluid flow rate, tubular sodium delivery rate, acid–base state, ADH, and presence of unreabsorbable anions.
- Some K^+ is lost in sweat and feces.
- Because several days may pass before onset of renal K^+ conservation mechanisms, whole-body deficiency can develop when horses are fed a low-K^+ diet or are unable or unwilling to eat. During this period, K^+ is lost in urine despite development of whole-body K^+ depletion.
- Whole-body K^+ deficiency also can result from urinary K^+ loss in tubular renal diseases.
- Through the GI tract, K^+ can be lost via diarrhea or fluid sequestration.
- Sweat contains as much as 10-fold more K^+ than blood, so excessive sweating can lead to K^+ depletion as well.

SYSTEMS AFFECTED

- Cardiovascular—cardiac arrhythmias and ECG abnormalities
- Musculoskeletal—with hypokalemia, an increased membrane potential leading to decreased muscle irritability; muscular weakness, muscle hypoxia, and predisposition to exertional myopathies
- GI—intestinal ileus
- Renal—renal dysfunction

SIGNALMENT

N/A

SIGNS

- History of decrease food intake or dietary change.
- Acute hypokalemia usually does not lead to clinical signs unless the serum K^+ concentration is <1.8 mEq/L.
- Muscular weakness
- Paralysis
- Exertional myopathies
- Colic

CAUSES

- GI losses with diarrhea or gut sequestration
- Renal losses from decreased potassium intake or renal disease
- Shift of K^+ into cells because of IV administration of bicarbonate or glucose-containing solution
- Excessive sweating after prolonged exercise
- Diabetes mellitus

RISK FACTORS

Sudden switch from a high-K^+ to a low-K^+ diet

DIAGNOSIS

DIFFERENTIAL DIAGNOSIS

- History to rule out decreased intake, excessive sweating, and administration of IV fluid leading to a shift of K^+ from the ECF to ICF compartment
- Investigate renal disease.
- Rule out intestinal obstruction and diarrhea.
- Investigate other causes of muscular weakness or paralysis.
- Investigate other causes of cardiac arrhythmias.

LABORATORY FINDINGS

Drugs That May Alter Lab Results

A K_3-EDTA contamination increases the K^+ concentration.

Disorders That May Alter Lab Results

- Thrombocytosis >1,000,000 platelets/μL or leukocytosis >200,000 cells/μL increase the K^+ concentration.
- Hemolysis leads to the same result.

Valid If Run in Human Lab?

Yes

CBC/BIOCHEMISTRY/URINALYSIS

- Electrolyte abnormalities in horses with diarrhea or intestinal obstruction
- Increased HCO_3^- as an indicator of metabolic alkalosis
- Increased BUN and creatinine associated with electrolyte abnormalities in horses with renal disease.
- Urine specific gravity and pH are useful in establishing the diagnosis of renal tubular disease.
- Increased CK in horses with muscle injury
- Myoglobinuria in horses with rhabdomyolysis
- Persistent hyperglycemia and glucosuria in horses with diabetes mellitus

OTHER LABORATORY TESTS

Urinary fractional excretion of K^+ increases with renal dysfunction.

IMAGING

N/A

DIAGNOSTIC PROCEDURES

N/A

TREATMENT

- Varies with the underlying cause.
- Promote intake of high-K^+ hay.
- Oral supplementation is sufficient in mild cases, but initiate both oral and parenteral treatment to correct electrolyte abnormalities in severe cases. Also correct acid–base disorders.
- Assessing K^+ deficiency is difficult, and currently, no accurate way exists to determine whole-body K^+ content.

POTASSIUM, HYPOKALEMIA

MEDICATIONS

DRUGS OF CHOICE
- The oral route is a safe method with which to administer a large dose of K^+. Oral administration of 40 g of potassium chloride diluted in 4–6 L of water can be performed twice a day.
- IV administration of potassium chloride (20–40 mEq/L, not to exceed 100–150 mEq/hour)
- Generally, K^+ supplementation is not needed once the horse is able to eat.

CONTRAINDICATIONS
- If possible, avoid sodium bicarbonate– and glucose-containing fluids.
- Diuretics—furosemide; acetazolamide

PRECAUTIONS
Osmotic diarrhea can be induced when potassium chloride and sodium bicarbonate are administrated orally.

POSSIBLE INTERACTIONS
N/A

ALTERNATIVE DRUGS
Potassium iodide (2–20 g PO SID)

FOLLOW-UP

PATIENT MONITORING
Recheck potassium and other electrolytes; frequency of monitoring varies with the underlying cause and severity of the condition.

POSSIBLE COMPLICATIONS
Cardiac arrhythmias

MISCELLANEOUS

ASSOCIATED CONDITIONS
N/A

AGE-RELATED FACTORS
N/A

ZOONOTIC POTENTIAL
N/A

PREGNANCY
N/A

SYNONYMS
N/A

SEE ALSO
See *Causes.*

ABBREVIATIONS
- ADH = antidiuretic hormone
- CK = creatine kinase
- ECF = extracellular fluid
- GI = gastrointestinal
- ICF = intracellular fluid

Suggested Reading

Carlson GP. Clinical chemistry tests. In: Smith BP, ed. Large animal internal medicine. 2nd ed. St. Louis: Mosby, 1996.

Carlson GP. Fluid, electrolyte, and acid-base balance. In: Kaneko JJ, Harvey JW, Bruss ML, eds. Clinical biochemistry of domestic animals. 5th ed. New York: Academic Press, 1997.

Foreman JH. The exhausted horse syndrome. Vet Clin North Am Equine Pract 1998;14:205–219.

Hyyppä S, Pösö AR. Fluid, electrolyte, and acid-base responses to exercise in racehorses. Vet Clin North Am Equine Pract 1998;14:121–136.

Schmall LM. Fluid and electrolyte therapy. In: Robinson NE, ed. Current therapy in equine medicine 4. Philadelphia: WB Saunders, 1997.

Authors Valerie O. Guilpin and E. Duane Lassen

Consulting Editor Claire B. Andreasen

POTOMAC HORSE FEVER (PHF)

BASICS

DEFINITION

Potomac horse fever (PHF) is an acute enterotyphlocolitis of horses caused by infection with the monocytotropic rickettsia *Ehrlichia risticii.*

PATHOPHYSIOLOGY

The pathophysiology of PHF is poorly understood. *Ehrlichia risticii* is an obligate intracellular parasite with a predilection for blood monocytes and tissue macrophages. Within days of infection, *E. risticii* can be found in blood monocytes, although readily phagocytosed by monocytes. *Ehrlichia risticii* survives within phagosomes in macrophages by inhibiting phagosome–lysosome fusion. The ehrlichemia persists throughout the clinical period.

The pathogen has a predilection for the cecum and large colon, but is occasionally found in the jejunum and small colon. Colonic and small intestinal epithelial cells, colonic mast cells, and macrophages are the targets of infection. Even mild cases of PHF without diarrhea have evidence of colitis. The major clinical signs observed resemble those of salmonellosis and/or endotoxemia. It is possible that many pathophysiologic changes observed in horses with PHF are secondary to effects by altered colonic flora (diarrhea, endotoxemia, etc.).

SYSTEMS AFFECTED

- Gastrointestinal—predominantly cecum and large colon
- Cardiovascular—dehydratration and shock may develop in severe cases.
- Reproductive—occasional cause of abortion

GENETCS

N/A

INCIDENCE/PREVALENCE

In Ohio, 13–20% of horses on racetracks had serologic evidence of exposure to *E. risticci,* although only 10–20% of the seropositive horses had clinical signs of the disease.

Geographic Disribution

PHF has been reported from most areas of the mainland of the United States and some areas of Canada.

SIGNALMENT

All breeds and all ages may be affected; however, horses younger than 1 yr rarely develop PHF. Clinical cases of PHF generally occur sporadically, with rarely more than 5% of horses on any one affected farm. Only when an area is experiencing significant epizootic infection does the attack rate on individual farms become high (20–50%).

SIGNS

There is a considerable variation in severity of the clinical manifestations of PHF. The manifestation of colitis is common in all cases; however, not all cases of colitis show colic or diarrhea.

- Depression (90%)
- Anorexia (80%)
- Fever (70%) (variable, biphasic): initially a transient fever of 39.4°–41.1°C (103°–106°F) followed in 3–7 days by a second, more persistent febrile episode.
- Injected or congested mucous membranes (70%)
- Mild to severe gastrointestinal signs, ranging from mild colic and soft manure to profuse diarrhea
- Ileus (70%): decreased frequency and amplitude of intestinal sounds (reduced or absent borborygmal sounds) with intermittent, loud, high-pitched sounds ("tinkling") heard on abdominal auscultation. Signs of ileus are one of the most consistent clinical findings.
- Diarrhea (<60%): mild, cow-like consistency to profuse, watery, pipe-stream diarrhea present in 45–60% of cases. Course of diarrhea ranges 1–10 days.
- Colic (30%)
- Dehydration
- Laminitis develops in about 20–25% of PHF cases
- Mortality rate from PHF: 5–30%
- Some horses show only mild signs of anorexia, depression, and fever
- Clinical course is usually 5–10 days without treatment
- Abortion may occur, although an infrequent occurrence

CAUSES AND RISK FACTORS

Causes

Infection with *E. risticii.* The organism is an obligate intracellular parasite. Different strains of *E. risticii* have been identified, not all of which appear to be pathogenic.

The means by which horses become infected is unknown. There is no evidence for the spread of PHF by arthropod vectors such as ticks; however, there are recent reports from California that snails may be involved as vectors of PHF-causing organisms.

Risk Factors

Endemic areas, in which PHF occurs in successive years, have been identified. *Ehrlichia risticii* infection has been strongly associated with rivers or other aquatic habitats. Increased risk is associated with horses grazing pastures bordering rivers and irrigation ditches; horses coming from an area with a high PHF prevalence or a farm with history of PHF; or travel to an area with a high incidence of PHF.

Season

There is a definite seasonal pattern, with most clinical cases of PHF occuring during the summer months. The majority of clinical PHF cases occur in July, August, and September in the Northern Hemisphere.

POTOMAC HORSE FEVER (PHF)

DIAGNOSIS

DIFFERENTIAL DIAGNOSIS

Differential diagnoses for PHF include other causes of colitis [e.g., acute salmonellosis, clostridial colitis, cyathostomes (small strongyles), antibiotic-induced colitis, non-steroidal anti-inflammatory drug (NSAID) toxicity, cantharidin toxicity]; peritonitis; and dietary changes.

CBC/BIOCHEMISTRY/URINALYSIS

- Hematology is highly variable during the early phases of clinical signs.
- The most consistent abnormalities are an elevated packed cell volume (PCV) and total plasma protein (TPP) concentrations that develop when diarrhea occurs.
- Leukopenia with a neutropenia and lymphopenia may be initially present in some cases, and within a few days a marked leukocytosis may occur.
- Hyponatremia
- Hypochloremia
- Hypokalemia
- Metabolic acidosis
- Pre-renal azotemia may be present and is directly proportional to the degree of dehydration.

OTHER LABORATORY TESTS

N/A

IMAGING

N/A

OTHER DIAGNOSTIC PROCEDURES

Serology is the most commonly used method of diagnosing PHF. The indirect fluorescent-antibody (IFA) test is presently the most widely used diagnostic test for PHF; however, the interpretation of results can be difficult. PHF is diagnosed by demonstrating a four-fold or greater increase or decrease in IFA titers between acute and convalescent serum samples. The acute sample should be collected as soon as first clinical signs are observed; the convalescent sample should be collected 5–7 days later. This is necessary because PHF-infected horses have a rapid rise in antibody titer that usually begins before the onset of clinical signs. Clinical signs of PHF may be delayed as long as 14 days after infection. As a consequence, paired titers may demonstrate a rise, a decline, or no change. Due to the need for paired serum samples, serology is used for retrospective diagnosis of PHF in individual cases and for establishing the presence of PHF in an area or on a particular farm.

Failure to seroconvert does not rule-out PHF. The expected antibody titer of naturally affected horses is >1:80. Persistence of high antibody titers (1:2560) for more than a year has been noted in clinical and subclinical cases after natural infection.

Other available tests include an enzyme-linked immunosorbent assay (ELISA), and a nested polymerase chain reaction (PCR) technique has been developed that detects the partial 16S rRNA gene of *E. risticii* and appears to be as sensitive as blood culture for detecting infection with *E. risticii*. Isolation of *E. risticii* by blood culture is the most definitive method of diagnosis of PHF. Requires collecting 100–400 mL heparinized blood and harvesting buffy coat for culture.

PATHOLOGIC FINDINGS

There is gross distension of the cecum and large colon with fluid contents. Histologically the lesions are mild, with no inflammatory response or necrosis in the wall of the affected bowel. This is in marked contrast to the other causes of acute enterotyphylocolitis seen in the horse (e.g., enteric salmonellosis and clostridiosis). There may be mucus depletion of the goblet cells of the colon, with shortening and basophilia of the mucosal epithelial cells.

TREATMENT

APPROPRIATE HEALTH CARE

Mild cases can be managed on the farm, but severely affected animals may require in-patient intensive care. As other causes of some of the clinical signs are potentially highly infectious (e.g., salmonellosis), animals should be managed in isolation. The clinical signs of most cases of PHF are not sufficient to make a definitive diagnosis, and serologic confirmation of the diagnosis is available only after 7–10 days have passed since the onset of clinical signs. However, early, appropriate treatment gives the best chance for a successful outcome, and therefore therapy must be started based on limited data. In endemic areas during the seasons of peak incidence it is common practice to assume that many horses exhibiting clinical signs consistent with PHF do indeed have PHF, and to treat accordingly. Failure to respond to therapy is often a diagnostic clue that the horse does not have PHF.

ACTIVITY

Stall rest during the course of therapy is recommended.

POTOMAC HORSE FEVER (PHF)

DIET
A grass hay diet is recommended until fecal consistency is normal.

CLIENT EDUCATION
N/A

SURGICAL CONSIDERATIONS
N/A

MEDICATIONS

DRUGS
- Oxytetracycline 6.6 mg/kg IV q24hr for 3–5 days is treatment of choice. A rapid recovery and dramatic decrease in fatality rate is observed when oxytetracycline therapy is commenced within 24 hr after the development of fever. A response to therapy (decreased temperature and improved attitude, appetite, and intestinal sounds) can be observed within 12 hr.
- Oral erythromycin estolate (25 mg/kg q12hr) and rifampin (10 mg/kg q12hr) combination is also effective when given early in the clinical course; however, the clinical response is not as rapid as intravenous oxytetracycline.
- Non-steroidal anti-inflammatory drugs, such as flunixin meglumine, may be useful to treat endotoxemia.

FLUIDS
Intravenous fluid and electrolyte replacement therapy is important to maintain fluid and electrolyte balance.

CONTRAINDICATIONS
N/A

PRECAUTIONS
Diarrhea may occur in horses receiving erythromycin/rifampin.

POSSIBLE INTERACTIONS
N/A

ALTERNATIVE DRUGS
N/A

FOLLOW-UP

PATIENT MONITORING
Relapses rarely occur following the cessation of intravenous oxytetracyline therapy. If relapse occurs, administer a second course of intravenous oxytetracycline.

PREVENTION/AVOIDANCE
- Contact with recovered or currently ill animals is not associated with the development of PHF.
- Natural infection with PHF induces a protective immunity for as long as 20 months.
- Horses do not remain chronic carriers of *E. risticii.*
- Horses in endemic areas may be vaccinated with an inactivated, partially purified cell vaccine between early spring and early summer.
- Require two-dose primary series 3–4 weeks apart; peak protection is reached 3–4 weeks after second dose.
- Revaccination at 6- to 12-month intervals is dependent on whether in highly endemic area.
- Vaccination should occur 1 month before the first cases of PHF are expected.
- Vaccine failure (89%) has been reported in endemic areas and has been attributed to poor antibody response to PHF vaccination and heterogeneity of strains of *E. risticii* isolates.
- There have been anecdotal reports of reduced severity of clinical signs in vaccinated horses.

POSSIBLE COMPLICATIONS

- Acute or chronic laminitis in 20–25% of PHF cases
- Thrombophlebitis
- Disseminated intravascular coagulation

EXPECTED COURSE AND PROGNOSIS

Horses with mild signs and that are treated aggressively and early in the course of the disease show a dramatic response to therapy and can be clinically normal in 3–5 days. Horses with more severe and long-standing problems require a longer period of therapy, and if secondary problems such as laminitis and hypoproteinemia are present, then the clinical course may be much longer and the outcome less favorable.

MISCELLANEOUS

SYNONYMS

- Equine monocytic ehrlichosis
- Equine ehrlichial colitis
- Acute equine diarrheal syndrome

ABBREVIATIONS

- PHF = Potomac horse fever
- IFA = indirect fluorescent-antibody
- ELISA = enzyme-limited immunosorbent assay
- PCV = packed cell volume
- TPP = total plasma protein
- PCR = polymerase chain reaction

Suggested Reading

Dutta SK, Vemulapalli R, Biswas B. Association of deficiency in antibody response to vaccine and heterogeneity of *Ehrlichia risticii* strains with Potomac horse fever vaccine failures in horses. J Clin Microbiol 1998;36:506-512.

Mott J, Rikihisa Y, Zhang Y, Reed SM, Yu CY. Comparison of PCR and culture to the indirect fluorescent-antibody test for diagnosis of Potomac horse fever. J Clin Microbiol 1997;35:2215-2219.

Palmer JE. Potomac horse fever. Vet Clin N Am Equine Pract 1993;9:399-410.

Reubel GH, Barlough JE, Madigan JE. Production and characterization of *Ehrlichia risticii,* the agent of Potomac horse fever, from snails (Pleuroceridae: *Juga* spp.) in aquarium culture and genetic comparison to equine strains. J Clin Microbiol 1998;36:1501-1511.

Author John D. Baird

Consulting Editor Henry Stämpfli

PREGNANCY DIAGNOSIS

BASICS

DEFINITION

- Pregnancy—the condition after fertilization of an embryo or fetus developing and maturing in utero
- Pregnancy diagnosis—determination of a pregnant state based on clinical signs, laboratory results, and physical examination findings, including transrectal palpation and ultrasonography.

PATHOPHYSIOLOGY

N/A

SYSTEM AFFECTED

- Reproductive
- Other systems may be affected during abnormal pregnancy.

GENETICS

N/A

INCIDENCE/PREVALENCE

N/A

SIGNALMENT

- Nonspecific
- Puberty occurs between 12–24 months in equine females.
- Pregnancy may occur in mares anytime after puberty until advanced age.

SIGNS

Historical Findings

Failure of a mare that has been bred to return to estrus 16–19 days after ovulation

Physical Examination Findings

- Early in pregnancy, little physical change may be noted.
- As pregnancy advances, most mares develop recognizable abdominal distention and weight gain.
- In the final 2–4 weeks before parturition, most mares have increased development of the mammary gland, with secretion of fluid from the nipples ranging from thin and straw-colored to sticky and creamy.

CAUSES

Mating

RISK FACTORS

N/A

DIAGNOSIS

DIFFERENTIAL DIAGNOSIS

Other Causes of Failure to Cycle

- Seasonal anestrus—transrectal palpation and ultrasonography reveal little ovarian activity; uterine and cervical tone is flaccid.
- Behavioral anestrus—serial transrectal palpation/ultrasonography distinguishes mares in estrus from those in diestrus or pregnancy.
- Prolonged luteal lifespan—evidence of corpus luteum at ultrasonographic examination of the ovary or progesterone assay; responds to $PGF_{2\alpha}$ treatment.
- Granulosa–theca cell tumor—abnormally enlarged, multicystic ovary and small contralateral ovary; confirmed by elevated serum inhibin concentrations.
- Chromosomal abnormalities (e.g., gonadal dysgenesis, testicular feminization)—karyotype determination

Other Ultrasonographic Findings Resembling Early Pregnancy

Uterine Cysts:

- Ultrasonography before pregnancy can aid in determining presence, number, size, and shape of uterine cysts.
- Permanent record of cystic structures can be beneficial in distinguishing uterine cysts from early embryonic vesicles.

CBC/BIOCHEMISTRY/URINALYSIS

N/A

OTHER LABORATORY TESTS

Progesterone Assay

- Assay for serum or milk progesterone concentrations using ELISA and RIA.
- High concentrations of progesterone 18–21 days after ovulation imply functional luteal tissue.
- This is a presumptive, not a diagnostic, test for pregnancy.
- May be a useful adjunct to other methods of early pregnancy diagnosis—transrectal palpation without ultrasonography
- Confirmation of pregnancy using an assay such as estrone sulfate is advisable if early pregnancy was diagnosed solely by progesterone assay.

eCG Assay

- The hormone eCG is secreted by endometrial cups in the pregnant mare uterus.
- Endometrial cups form between ≅36–37 days of gestation, when chorionic girdle cells from the trophoblast actively invade the endometrial epithelium.
- Cups attain maximum size and hormone output between 55–70 days of gestation.
- Cups generally regress between 80–120 days of gestation, and eCG secretion ceases at that time.
- eCG is measured using ELISA.
- False-positive reactions can occur if a mare has persistent endometrial cups and a nonviable fetus or fetal loss.
- False-negative results are possible in samples evaluated before endometrial cup formation (<36 days of gestation) or after endometrial cup regression (>120 days of gestation).

Estrogen Assay

• Estrogens are secreted by the fetoplacental unit.
• Total estrogens or estrone sulfate (i.e. conjugated estrogen) can be measured from plasma or urine to diagnose pregnancy after 60 days of gestation using RIA.
• Estrone sulfate concentrations in milk are diagnostic for pregnancy after 90 days of gestation.
• Fetal death (and subsequent compromise to the fetoplacental unit) results in an immediate decline of estrogen concentrations.

IMAGING

Transrectal Ultrasonography

• Pregnancy diagnosis can be determined as early as 9 days after ovulation with a 5-MHz transducer and a high-quality ultrasound scanner.
• Optimal time to scan for early pregnancy is 13–15 days after ovulation.
• The embryonic vesicle is an anechoic, spheric yolk sac averaging 12–20 mm in height.
• Detection of an embryonic vesicle is more reliable during this period, and twin embryonic vesicles can be consistently located at this time.
• Early diagnosis of twin pregnancies increases the probability of successfully reducing twins to a singleton pregnancy using the manual reduction technique.
• Ultrasonographic appearance of the vesicle becomes more triangular by 18 days of gestation, when the embryonic vesicle becomes less turgid.
• The embryo proper often can be visualized by 20–21 days of gestation, and a heartbeat can be seen as early as 24 days.
• The allantoic sac is visible ventral to the embryo by 24 days of gestation.
• As the allantois develops and the yolk sac regresses, the embryo appears to be lifted from the ventral aspect of the vesicle and to migrate dorsally.
• The embryo is visualized midvesicle by 28–30 days of gestation and is in the dorsal aspect of the vesicle by 35 days.
• The umbilical cord forms and attaches at the dorsal aspect of the vesicle around 40 days of gestation.
• As the cord elongates, the fetus migrates toward the ventral aspect of the allantoic sac.
• Descent to the ventral wall normally is complete by 48 days of gestation.
• The fetus generally can be visualized using transrectal ultrasonography until approximately 70–75 days of gestation, depending on the age and parity of the mare. During this time period, the weight of the developing pregnancy pulls the uterus over the brim of the pelvis.

Fetal Sexing

• Determination of fetal gender is best accomplished between 60–70 days of gestation.
• The technique is very useful in both horses and cattle, but high-resolution ultrasound equipment and experience are necessary for accurate identification of fetal sex.
• Fetal sex is determined by locating the position of the genital tubercle during its developmental migration. The genital tubercle is the precursor to the clitoris in females and the penis in males, is located on the ventral midline, and is imaged as a hyperechoic, bilobed structure ≅2 mm in diameter. The tubercle migrates from between the rear legs caudally toward the tail in female and cranially toward the umbilicus in male fetuses.
• The location and orientation of the fetus must be determined. Fetal position can be determined by locating the mandible, which points ventrally and caudally. The heart is imaged on the ventral midline of the thorax. Examining the fetus cranially to caudally, the abdominal attachment of the umbilicus is located. Immediately caudal to the umbilical attachment is the male genital tubercle. The female tubercle is best visualized at the caudalmost aspect of the fetus under the tailhead. The optimal image of the female tubercle appears within a triangle formed by the tailhead and the distal tibias or hocks.
• At 95 days of gestation, the fetus may move more dorsally within the pregnant uterus and can be imaged for fetal sex.
• From 95–130 days of gestation, fetal sex can be determined by locating external genital structures, such as the mammary gland, teats, and clitoris in the female and the penis, prepuce, and scrotum in the male.

DIAGNOSTIC PROCEDURES

Behavioral Assessment

• A mare teased to a stallion should begin to show signs of behavioral estrus 16–18 days after ovulation if not pregnant.
• Response of a mare to a stallion is a non-specific indicator of pregnancy. This method should be used only as an adjunct to more reliable means—transrectal palpation and ultrasonography
• False positive—failure to show estrus even as the mare returns to heat; pregnancy loss occurs after formation of endometrial cups; prolonged luteal activity but no pregnancy
• False negative—mare continues to exhibit signs of behavioral estrus when pregnant.

Vaginal Speculum Examination

• Under the influence of progesterone, the cervix is tightly closed, pale, and dry.
• This test is not diagnostic for pregnancy, because functional luteal tissue (i.e., diestrus) in a cycling mare has the same effect on the cervix.
• Often, this examination is an adjunct to transrectal evaluation of the reproductive tract.

Transrectal Palpation of the Reproductive Tract

15–18 Days After Ovulation:

• The tubular tract becomes toned, and the "v" shape of the uterine bifurcation often is distinctly palpable.
• Palpation of a vesicular bulge in the uterine horn has been reported as early as 15 days; however, palpation of a true bulge at this stage is difficult in all but maiden mares with small uterine horns.
• The cervix generally is tightly closed, narrow, and elongated.
• Both ovaries often are actively producing follicles during early pregnancy.

PREGNANCY DIAGNOSIS

• False diagnosis of pregnancy, based on transrectal palpation findings, may occur at this stage because of EED or persistent/prolonged luteal activity.

25–30 Days of Gestation:
• Uterine tone is very distinct (i.e., elevated), and the cervix is narrow and elongated.
• Follicular activity is present.
• A bulge the size of a small hen's egg can be appreciated at the caudoventral aspect of a uterine horn, adjacent to the uterine bifurcation.
• The uterine wall is slightly thinner over the fluid-filled, resilient vesicle.

35–40 Days of Gestation:
• The uterus still demonstrates increased tone, the cervix is closed and elongated, and the ovaries are active.
• A tennis ball–sized bulge can be noted at the base of the uterine horn.
• Uterine tone begins to drop at/around the enlarging bulge.
• Greatly increased uterine tone remains present in the nonpregnant horn.

45–50 Days of Gestation:
• The palpable bulge increases to the size of a softball.

60–65 Days of Gestation:
• The vesicle begins to expand into the uterine body, and the palpable bulge resembles the shape of a child-sized football.
• The wall of the uterine horn is distinctly thinner, and the pregnancy begins to lose some of its resiliency.
• Good uterine tone often is maintained in the nongravid horn and the tip of the gravid horn.
• The increasing size of the pregnancy begins to pull the uterus ventrally.

75–120 Days of Gestation:
• The pregnancy occupies more of the uterus, and the uterine tone diminishes.
• The pregnancy expands dorsally and resembles the size of a basketball.
• The pregnant uterus can be confused with a full urinary bladder. To distinguish the two, the fluid-filled uterus can be traced back to the closed cervix at its caudal aspect. Additionally, as the uterus continues to drop deeper into the abdomen, the ovaries are drawn ventrally and toward the midline.
• Occasionally, the fetus may be ballotted during the latter aspect of this time period; however, this can prove difficult or impossible.

150–210 Days of Gestation:
• Uterine descent into the ventral abdomen is complete, and the ovaries often are found at the midline.
• The fetus may be consistently ballotted within the fluid-filled uterus.

≅250 Days of Gestation To Term:
• Tremendous fetal growth occurs.
• Ratio of the fluid volume of the pregnancy to the fetus decreases, because fetal growth is rapid and the fetus occupies a greater percentage of the uterus late in gestation.

TREATMENT

APPROPRIATE HEALTH CARE
N/A

NURSING CARE
N/A

ACTIVITY
N/A

DIET
N/A

CLIENT EDUCATION
N/A

SURGICAL CONSIDERATIONS
N/A

MEDICATIONS

DRUGS OF CHOICE
N/A

CONTRAINDICATIONS
N/A

PRECAUTIONS
N/A

POSSIBLE INTERACTIONS
N/A

ALTERNATIVE DRUGS
N/A

FOLLOW-UP

PATIENT MONITORING
• Pregnant mares are routinely examined during the last trimester of gestation to verify fetal viability.
• The most common method of pregnancy diagnosis at this stage is transrectal palpation with ballottement of the fetus.
• Transabdominal ultrasonography can be used to measure fetal parameters—heart rate, aortic diameter, activity, and fluid quality

PREVENTION/AVOIDANCE
N/A

POSSIBLE COMPLICATIONS
- Embryonic or fetal loss
- Twins
- Placentitis
- Abortion
- Ruptured prepubic tendon
- Abdominal wall herniation
- Hydrallantois
- Hydramnion
- Uterine torsion
- Uterine rupture
- Prolonged gestation
- Dystocia

EXPECTED COURSE AND PROGNOSIS
N/A

MISCELLANEOUS

ASSOCIATED CONDITIONS
N/A

AGE-RELATED FACTORS
N/A

ZOONOTIC POTENTIAL
N/A

PREGNANCY
N/A

SYNONYMS
N/A

SEE ALSO
- Abortion
- Conception failure
- Dystocia and parturient complications
- EED
- Fetal sexing
- Placenta
- Twinning

ABBREVIATIONS
- eCG = equine chorionic gonadotropin
- EED = early embryonic death
- ELISA = enzyme-linked immunoadsorbent assay
- RIA = radioimmunoassay

Suggested Reading

Ginther OJ. Reproductive biology of the mare. 2nd ed. Cross Plains: Equiservices, 1992.

Ginther OJ. Ultrasonic imaging and reproductive events in the mare. Cross Plains: Equiservices, 1986.

McKinnon AO. Diagnosis of pregnancy. In: McKinnon AO, Voss JL, eds. Equine reproduction. Philadelphia: Lea & Febiger, 1993.

Author Margo L. Macpherson
Consulting Editor Carla L. Carleton

PREMATURE PLACENTAL SEPARATION

BASICS

OVERVIEW

• Premature disassociation (i.e., detachment) of the chorioallantoic membrane from the endometrium before delivery of the term fetus
• The chorioallantois is responsible for supplying the fetus with oxygen and nutrients and for removing its waste products; with premature detachment (e.g., late stage I, early stage II), the fetus dies from hypoxia if immediate assistance is unavailable to aid in delivery
• Proposed origins—alterations in the chorioallantoic membrane in the area of the internal os of the cervix; abnormal attachment of the chorioallantoic membrane to the endometrium, which predisposes to premature separation; secondary to cervical relaxation (hormonal, ascending infection, cervical incompetency) and development of low-grade placentitis, which compromises the normal relationship of chorioallantois and the endometrium.
• Incidence increases significantly with induction of parturition.
• Incidence of <1% in medium to large breeds of horses, but higher in Miniature Horses.

SIGNALMENT

• All breeds, with increased occurrence in Miniature Horses.
• All females of breeding age.

SIGNS

• This is an emergency.
• Because of the abrupt reduction in oxygen delivery to the fetus, immediate delivery assistance is essential as soon as the chorio-allantoic membrane protrudes through the vulvar lips.
• Although it may happen for the first time at any parity, a history of premature placental separation often is found.
• Closely observe any mare with a history of premature placental separation.
• Physical examination findings are normal.
• Chorioallantoic membrane, when presented at the vulva, may appear to be characteristically velvety and roughened.

CAUSES AND RISK FACTORS

• Miniature Horses
• Induction of parturition
• Older mares

DIAGNOSIS

DIFFERENTIAL DIAGNOSIS

• Evagination of the vaginal wall.
• Eversion of the urinary bladder.
• Prolapse of the vaginal wall.
• Lacerations of the vaginal wall and prolapse of the intestines.

CBC/BIOCHEMISTRY/URINALYSIS

N/A

OTHER LABORATORY TESTS

N/A

IMAGING

Ultrasonography:
• Prepartum ultrasonography may reveal an area of detachment cranial to the cervix, which also may indicate a mare at risk for placentitis.
• Intrapartum appearance of the chorioallantoic membrane protruding through the vulvar lips (i.e., "red velvet") is diagnostic in itself.

DIAGNOSTIC PROCEDURES

Best diagnostic method—visual examination of the tissue when exposed

PREMATURE PLACENTAL SEPARATION

TREATMENT

Client Education:

• Knowledge regarding the normal appearance of placenta at parturition
• With normal parturition, the first membrane observed at the vulvae should be smooth and white, opaque, or perhaps, pale pink.
• Any reddish or roughened protruding membrane indicates a problem requiring immediate action.
• This is a true emergency. Because of fetal hypoxia, insufficient time is available to seek outside assistance and still deliver a live foal.
• Normal placenta serves as an excellent teaching tool to educate clients regarding what is normal and abnormal.
• If observed and client can't/won't tear CA and assist in delivery, instruct client to walk mare until you arrive; may aid in decreasing further/full abdominal contractions and thus < further/full separation (still only partial usefulness for a few minutes until DVM arrives).

MEDICATIONS

DRUGS

N/A

CONTRAINDICATIONS/POSSIBLE INTERACTIONS

Oxytocin is contraindicated.

FOLLOW-UP

PATIENT MONITORING

• Mares do well after delivery.
• The potential problem is with the fetus and its inability to exchange oxygen and (with the neonate) permanent damage from oxygen deprivation that occurred during delivery.

PREVENTION/AVOIDANCE

• No known method to prevent this condition.
• Observe parturition for any mare with a history of a previous delivery involving premature placental separation.

POSSIBLE COMPLICATIONS

• Mare—none.
• Fetus—death caused by lack of oxygenation; dummy foal postpartum.

EXPECTED COURSE AND PROGNOSIS

Delayed delivery results in fetal death.

MISCELLANEOUS

ASSOCIATED CONDITIONS

N/A

AGE-RELATED FACTORS

N/A

ZOONOTIC POTENTIAL

N/A

PREGNANCY

Only occurs at the end of gestation.

SYNONYMS

• Red bag
• Red bagging

SEE ALSO

• Dystocia
• Prolonged pregnancy

Suggested Reading

Asbury AC, LeBlanc MM. The placenta. In: McKinnon AO, Voss JL, eds. Equine reproduction. Philadelphia: Lea & Febiger, 1993:513.

Roberts SJ. In: Veterinary obstetrics and genital diseases (theriogenology). Woodstock, VT: published by the author, 1986:251–252.

Whitwell KE, Jeffcott LB. Morphological studies on the fetal membranes of the normal singleton foal at term. Res Vet Sci 1975;19:44–55.

Author Walter R. Threlfall
Consulting Editor Carla L. Carleton

PREMATURITY

BASICS

DEFINITION

• Difficult to define in foals because of the highly variable gestational length (320–365 days) in some mares
• Generally, foals with a gestational age <320 days, but foals taken by cesarean section or induced before labor begins or before colostrum is present in the udder are likely to present with all the problems of prematurity even with 340 days of gestation. This is the concept of "readiness for birth," which is different for each foal.

PATHOPHYSIOLOGY

• Can affect foals in several ways.
• Respiratory development is crucial to survival of the foal. Depending on the degree of lung maturity, the foal may experience mild problems or may die. This often is determined by how much maternal/fetal stress the foal undergoes in utero. A foal born at 310 days from a mare carrying twins may experience little lung problems, whereas one taken at 330 days by cesarean section because the mare has an inoperable acute colic may die of respiratory failure.
• This difference in outcome results from the presence and maturity of surfactant in the foal's lungs. Surfactant is a microaggregate of lipoproteins consisting of phospholipids, proteins, and neutral lipids and reduces the surface tension of the alveolar lining of the lungs and, thereby, prevents collapse of the airspaces. Production of surfactant and, therefore, maturation of fetal lungs occurs during late gestation. Animals born before their lungs have reached maturity are at high risk for respiratory problems (e.g., RDS) during the first few days of life. Chronic maternal/fetal stress hastens maturation of surfactant; hence, a foal from a mare carrying twins or from a mare with chronic placentitis may have more mature surfactant.
• The skeletal structure of premature foals is not fully developed. Normal cartilage templates of the cuboidal bones begin to ossify late during gestation. At birth, these bones are 42–62% calcified. Premature foals with gestational ages <315 days may have only 20–40% ossification.

SYSTEMS AFFECTED

• Respiratory—surfactant, a lung phospholipid that decreases surface tension, begins to mature during late gestation. Premature foals may be born without surfactant, which leads to respiratory failure and death, or they may have immature surfactant, which presents as hypoxemia.
• Musculoskeletal—premature foals often lack calcified carpal and tarsal bones, which may lead to angular limb deformities and bone malformation.
• Behavioral—premature foals may be slower to stand and nurse than normal-term foals and may have poor co-ordination and weak suckle response.
• Endocrine/metabolic—premature induced foals have low serum cortisol levels at birth compared with term foals; prematurely induced foals also exhibited hypoglycemia and slow insulin response to IV glucose.
• GI—the intestinal tract may not be ready for an oral diet.
• Hemic/lymphatic—premature foals may have persistent, low WBC count, with a N:L ratio <2:1.

SIGNALMENT

• Newborn foals with a gestational age <320 days or that have been delivered (cesarean section or induction) before colostrum has developed or labor begins
• No breed or sex predilections

SIGNS

Historical Findings

• Mares may exhibit signs of early parturition, with precocious udder development.
• Mares with placentitis may have fever and vulvar discharge.
• Cases with *Erhlichia equi* or herpes viral infection may have no historical signs.

Physical Examination Findings

• General weakness; takes longer to stand and nurse.
• Small size
• Thin, fine, silky haircoat; pliant ears
• Increased respiratory rate and effort
• Overextended or lax tendons
• Angular limb deformities
• Dome-shaped head

CAUSES

Early parturition in mares—twin pregnancies, placentitis, herpes viral infection, *E. equi* infection, and body pregnancy

RISK FACTORS

N/A

DIAGNOSIS

DIFFERENTIAL DIAGNOSIS

Small Size

• Small size of the foal must be distinguished as being from prematurity or small for gestational age.
• Close evaluation of breeding dates determines gestational age.
• Examination of the placenta may aid in determining whether small size is secondary to placental insufficiency.

Respiratory Abnormalities

• Foals that present with increased respiratory rate and effort must be evaluated further for bacterial pneumonia, which could result from hematogenous spread by sepsis or aspiration pneumonia secondary to an upper airway abnormality.
• Foals born with herpes viral infection exhibit severe signs of respiratory distress.

Angular and Flexural Limb Deformities

• Occur in term foals but generally do not result from incomplete ossification of the carpal or tarsal bones.
• Radiography helps to distinguish the degree of ossification.

CBC/BIOCHEMISTRY/URINALYSIS

• Leukopenia, with a N:L ratio <2:1, may be seen.
• Hypoglycemia is common.

OTHER LABORATORY TESTS

• Arterial blood gases help to determine the degree of respiratory compromise.
• Premature foals lacking surfactant have respiratory acidosis with hypercapnia and hypoxemia; foals with immature surfactant may exhibit only hypoxemia.
• Fibrinogen levels >400 mg/dL suggest in utero infection.

IMAGING

Thoracic Radiography

- In foals lacking surfactant, pulmonary lesions progress from a diffuse, interstitial pattern to a diffuse, alveolar pattern.
- Foals with immature surfactant initially may have a diffuse, interstitial pattern that shows improvement over time.

Carpal and Tarsal Radiography

- Incomplete ossification of the carpal and tarsal bones in premature foals can be graded on a scale of 1–4.
- Grade 1—some cuboidal bones show no ossification.
- Grade 2—all cuboidal bones show some ossification.
- Grade 3—cuboidal bones are small and rounded.
- Grade 4—cuboidal bones have a mature configuration.

DIAGNOSTIC PROCEDURES

N/A

TREATMENT

- Generally, premature foals are high-risk foals and may require intensive care at an inpatient facility.
- Orally administer high-quality colostrum within 2 hours of birth. Because these foals are slower to stand, feed colostrum by bottle in those that can suckle or by nasogastric intubation in that that cannot. If colostrum is not available, transfuse with plasma (1–3 L, depending on the product's immunoglobulin concentration and the foal's size).
- Administer supplemental oxygen in hypoxic foals through a nasopharnygeal tube or an intratracheal catheter.
- Mechanical ventilation in foals with $PaCO_2$ >55.
- Supplemental surfactant has been helpful in premature human infants, but no controlled studies have been done on premature foals.
- Because of incomplete ossification of the carpal and tarsal bones, premature foals may need to have their limbs placed in splints or tube casts to allow the legs to develop normally. These supports should extend from the distal metacarpus/metatarsus to the elbow or stifle, respectively, and the fetlock and pastern should be able to move freely.
- Because foals may have difficulty rising while wearing splints/casts, pay special attention to nutrition; these foals may need assistance in standing and nursing.
- Stall rest

MEDICATIONS

DRUGS OF CHOICE

- Prophylactic antibiotics in foals with a high risk of sepsis (e.g., cases of premature birth secondary to placentitis or foals placed on ventilators).
- Ampicillin (10–20 mg/kg IV QID) or penicillin (22,000 IU/kg IV QID) in combination with amikacin (20–25 mg/kg IV SID) provide broad-spectrum coverage.

CONTRAINDICATIONS

N/A

PRECAUTIONS

- Prolonged use of high levels of oxygen (80–100%) produce oxygen toxicity in human infants; this could be a problem in foals on ventilators.
- High ventilator pressures may result in barotrauma to the lungs.
- Aminoglycosides can cause renal toxicity, and amikacin has a prolonged serum half-life in premature, hypoxic foals. Careful monitoring is essential.

POSSIBLE INTERACTIONS

N/A

FOLLOW-UP

PATIENT MONITORING

- Monitor lung status with arterial blood gases and thoracic radiography.
- Repeat radiography of the cuboidal bones every 5–7 days to monitor progress of bone ossification.
- Monitor renal parameters if an aminoglycoside is used in treatment.

POSSIBLE COMPLICATIONS

- Foals lacking surfactant have a grave prognosis for life; most die of respiratory failure.
- Foals with less severe respiratory problems have a guarded prognosis.
- Increased plasticity of the incompletely ossified cuboidal bones may lead to microtrauma and deformation of the cartilage template, which in turn may lead to permanent angular limb deformities.

MISCELLANEOUS

ASSOCIATED CONDITIONS

- Foals born prematurely because of bacterial placentitis are at high risk of septicemia. This also becomes a problem in premature foals that do stand and ingest high-quality colostrum.
- Angular limb deformities also are associated with incomplete ossification of cuboidal bones.

AGE-RELATED FACTORS

N/A

ZOONOTIC POTENTIAL

N/A

PREGNANCY

N/A

SYNONYMS

N/A

SEE ALSO

- Angular limb deformities
- Flexural deformities
- Neonatal pneumonia
- Neonatal sepsis

ABBREVIATIONS

- GI = gastrointestinal
- N:L = neutrophil:lymphocyte
- RDA = respiratory distress syndrome

Suggested Reading

Green SL, Conlon PD. Clinical pharmacokinetics of amikacin in hypoxic premature foals. Equine Vet J 1993;276–280.

Kosch PC, Koterba AM, Coons TJ, Webb AI. Developments in management of the newborn foal in respiratory distress. 1: evaluation. Equine Vet J 1984;16:312–318.

Paradis MR. Lecithin/sphingomyelin ratios and phosphatidylglycerol in term and premature equine amniotic fluid. Proc Am Coll Vet Intern Med 1987.

Webb AI, Coons TJ, Koterba AM, Kosch PC. Developments in management of the newborn foal in respiratory distress. 2: treatment. Equine Vet J 1984;16:319–323.

Author Mary Rose Paradis

Consulting Editor Mary Rose Paradis

PREPUBIC TENDON RUPTURE

BASICS

DEFINITION

Separation of the prepubic tendon from its attachment to the pubis

PATHOPHYSIOLOGY

- The weight of the mare's abdomen, in addition to that of the enlarging fetus, the increasing quantity of fetal fluids and membranes, and the accumulation of ventral abdominal edema, places pressure on the prepubic tendon's attachment to the pelvis that surpasses the tendon's load limit.
- Separation occurs (e.g., partial tear, half, or full rupture), and the ventral abdominal wall falls ventrally as the tendon's attachment tears away from the pubis.

SYSTEM AFFECTED

Reproductive

GENETICS

N/A

INCIDENCE/PREVALENCE

Extremely low

SIGNALMENT

- All breeds; all of breeding age.
- Older mares at increased risk.
- Predominant sex—female; rupture occurs in the late/near-term pregnant mare because of excessive weight of the fetus, uterine fluid and membranes, and ventral edema.
- The male's prepubic tendon may rupture after severe trauma.

SIGNS

General Comments

- Mares usually have advanced pregnancy with twins, hydrops, or other reason for a uterus enlarged beyond normal limits.
- Prepubic tendon rupture may occur after severe trauma—being struck by a car.

Historical Findings

- Mares usually present with an abdomen that has slowly enlarged to where excessive size is quite noticeable.
- Discomfort is associated with size of the abdomen, difficulty breathing with short shallow respirations, or reluctance to lie recumbent.

Physical Examination Findings

- Dependent edema of the ventral abdomen; may involve the legs.
- Characteristic appearance of the ventral abdomen after rupture (one of the best indicators)—a distinct profile when viewing the abdomen from the side; the ventral line appears flat, with no rise in the flank region by the udder; the udder loses its normal orientation, with the anterior aspect slanting steeply down and lying at a lower point than the posterior aspect; normal definition between udder and abdominal wall is absent.
- Transrectal palpation of the rupture may not be possible while the mare is pregnant.
- Identifying intestines immediately below the skin outside the abdominal musculature indicates rupture of the tendon or abdominal wall.

CAUSES

Excessive pressure and weight on the abdominal wall, usually from excessive uterine size, exceeding the physiologic limit that the attachment can withstand.

RISK FACTORS

- Mares pregnant with twins or triplets
- Those with excessive fluid accumulation, extra-abdominally from edema or intra-abdominally with conditions such as hydrops, are predisposed.

DIAGNOSIS

- Physical examination usually reveals dependant edema of the ventral abdomen, which may involve the legs.
- Side profile of the dam is flat from the front limbs to, and including, the udder.
- Definition between the udder and abdominal wall is lacking.
- Intestines may be palpated immediately underlying the skin in the absence of the abdominal wall.

DIFFERENTIAL DIAGNOSIS

- Abdominal wall rupture.
- Tearing of the muscles near the prepubic tendon—may be impossible to distinguish from actual tendon rupture.

CBC/BIOCHEMISTRY/URINALYSIS

N/A

OTHER LABORATORY TESTS

N/A

IMAGING

Abdominal ultrasonography—may help to confirm abdominal viscera immediately underlying the skin near the udder.

DIAGNOSTIC PROCEDURES

See physical examination.

PATHOLOGIC FINDINGS

Tearing or rupture of the prepubic tendon

TREATMENT

APPROPRIATE HEALTH CARE

- With complete rupture, the mare cannot expel the fetus at term.
- Once assisted delivery is complete, a better assessment can be made to determine if any surgical options are realistic.

NURSING CARE

- Keep the mare off surfaces that could lead to falling and/or further damage—slippery; angled; uneven
- Prevent the mare from rolling, if possible.
- Maintain close observation for intestinal obstruction or parturition—dystocia
- Consider use of trusses or supportive devices carefully. Additional problems may result from transferring all the weight of the abdomen and its contents onto the mare's back and from pressure on the ventral abdomen and its contents that have lost their normal orientation.

ACTIVITY

Restrict exercise to hand walking to prevent additional tearing of the ruptured tendon.

DIET

Changes in diet may be indicated to reduce additional bulk within the abdominal cavity.

CLIENT EDUCATION

- Because the condition occurs primarily during late gestation, educate the client regarding of the mare's impaired ability to participate in active labor without an intact abdominal wall musculature.
- Advise owners to seek veterinary advice if a mare appears to exceed a reasonable abdominal size during pregnancy.

SURGICAL CONSIDERATIONS

- Dependent on the degree of tissue damage as determined postpartum and on the value of the mare.
- Reproductive life of the mare will be limited to ET, if repair is possible.
- Surgery is contraindicated if the mare is to carry any subsequent pregnancies.

MEDICATIONS

DRUGS OF CHOICE

- Diuretics (e.g., furosemide) may aid with reducing edema in the dependent areas.
- Phenylbutazone, but only if the possibility of ulcer induction in the foal has been considered.

CONTRAINDICATIONS

Avoid any medications that may have detrimental fetal effects.

PRECAUTIONS

- Care of the mare aims for medical stabi-lization.
- Preparation and observation of the mare for an induced parturition.

POSSIBLE INTERACTIONS

N/A

ALTERNATIVE DRUGS

N/A

FOLLOW-UP

PATIENT MONITORING

- Close observation of affected mares is essential.
- Ensure that assistance will be available at parturition.

PREVENTION/AVOIDANCE

Termination of pregnancy in seriously at-risk mares before prepubic tendon rupture, especially if with excessive abdominal size and/or ventral dependent edema during late pregnancy

POSSIBLE COMPLICATIONS

Mares may die prepartum or postpartum from GI complications or rupture of the uterine or middle uterine arteries.

EXPECTED COURSE AND PROGNOSIS

- Mares have a high probability of survival, if managed properly.
- Many do well after delivery without surgical repair, if they are not rebred.
- Do not recommend rebreeding of any mare that has had a partial prepubic tendon rupture; the rupture will worsen with additional pregnancies.

MISCELLANEOUS

ASSOCIATED CONDITIONS

- Conceptus—twins; triplets; hydrops pregnancy.
- Mare origin—thick accumulation of dependent edema of the ventral abdomen; history of partial tearing of the prepubic tendon or excessive ventral edema during late gestation.
- Any other condition that increases size and weight of the pregnant uterus.

AGE-RELATED FACTORS

- Increasing age
- Old mares that have had multiple pregnancies.

ZOONOTIC POTENTIAL

N/A

PREGNANCY

- Usually associated with the late-pregnant mare.
- May occur in any horse that has suffered a severe, traumatic abdominal injury.

SYNONYMS

N/A

SEE ALSO

- Dystocia
- Prolonged pregnancy

ABBREVIATIONS

- ET =
- GI = gastrointestinal

Suggested Reading

Löfstedt R: Miscellaneous diseases of pregnancy and parturition. In: McKinnon AO, Voss JL, eds. Equine reproduction. Philadelphia: Lea & Febiger, 1993:596–603.

Roberts SJ: Veterinary obstetrics and genital diseases (theriogenology). Woodstock, VT: published by the author, 1986:229–230, 347–352.

Tulleners E, Fretz P. Prosthetic repair of large abdominal wall defects in horses and food animals. J Am Vet Med Assoc 1983;192: 258–262.

Author Walter R. Threlfall

Consulting Editor Carla L. Carleton

PRIAPISM

BASICS

DEFINITION
Persistent erection, with engorgement of the corpus cavernosum penis (CCP), in the absence of sexual arousal.

PATHOPHYSIOLOGY
• The smooth muscles of the arteries that supply and the veins that drain the CCP are under the control of the pudendal nerves. Parasympathetic stimulation of the pudendal nerves causes arterial dilation and venous constriction to/from the CCP to promote erection. Parasympathetic control also allows relaxation of the retractor penis muscles (causing penile prolapse) and the smooth muscle cells located in the walls of the CCP (allowing them to fill with blood).
• Detumescence is less well understood, but it is thought to be under sympathetic control. Adrenergic stimulation decreases arterial blood flow to the CCP and causes constriction of the smooth muscle cells lining the CCP. Agents or conditions that interfere with sympathetic stimulation are thought to directly or indirectly block detumescence.
• When detumescence fails, CO_2 tension in the CCP increases, causing increased blood viscosity and RBC sludging, and further occluding venous outflow from the CCP.
• Prolonged erection may then lead to secondary problems, including paraphimosis or penile paralysis, damaging the retractor penis muscles and/or the pudendal nerves proper.

SYSTEMS AFFECTED
Reproductive

SIGNALMENT
• Predominantly seen in stallions, although geldings can also be affected.
• It has been proposed that serum testosterone levels may contribute to the development of priapism.
• An alternative explanation may be that the lack of testosterone in geldings causes atrophy of the smooth muscles of the CCP, decreasing the size of the cavernous spaces available for filling with blood during the process of erection.

SIGNS
N/A

CAUSES
• Phenothiazine-derivative tranquilizer administration*, including propiopromazine hydrochloride, chlorpromazine hydrochloride, and acepromazine maleate.
• Spinal cord injury or disease.
• Other causes that have been reported, but are rare, include neoplasia, infectious diseases (i.e., purpura hemorrhagica), post-surgical complications (castration), and severe debilitation or starvation.

RISK FACTORS
Most cases of priapism occur subsequent to administration of phenothiazine tranquilizer to stallions. Avoid using this class of drugs in intact male equids.

DIAGNOSIS

DIFFERENTIAL DIAGNOSIS

Differentiating Similar Signs
• Paraphimosis is the prolapse of the penis and prepuce, with extensive edema of those tissues. Paraphimosis may occur secondary to priapism, but paraphimosis may occur without a history of priapism. It is significant if the history includes the administration of phenothiazine tranquilizer or the presence of erection prior to edema formation.
• Penile paralysis is differentiated by the fact that in that case the prolapsed penis is flaccid, not erect or partially erect as is seen in priapism.

Differentiating Causes
• History of phenothiazine tranquilizer administration to an intact stallion.
• If there is evidence of debilitation, starvation, or systemic illness, these merit further investigation and can contribute to the development of priapism.
• A complete neurologic exam is indicated to rule out spinal cord injury or disease as the inciting cause of priapism.

CBC/BIOCHEMISTRY/URINALYSIS
N/A

OTHER LABORATORY TESTS
N/A

IMAGING
N/A

DIAGNOSTIC PROCEDURES
N/A

TREATMENT
• As with paraphimosis (see text), penile support in the form of slings, massage, application of emollient dressings to the penis and prepuce, and hydrotherapy are advocated.
• With the horse under anesthesia, manual compression of the erect penis and physically replacing it in the prepuce have been successful in some cases.
• Flushing the CCP with heparinized saline (10 units sodium heparin/mL 0.9% saline) using 12g needles has been used in intractable cases of priapism.
• A surgical procedure successfully used in men has been to create a vascular shunt between the CCP and the corpus spongiosum penis.
• Chronic cases that ultimately undergo detumescence may need surgery in the form of circumcision (reefing) or retraction (Bolz technique) to retain the penis within the prepuce; in some cases, penile amputation has been necessarry.

MEDICATIONS

DRUG(S) OF CHOICE
• Superficial or deep lacerations secondary to exposure may require topical or systemic antibiotics.
• Anti-inflammatory medication (phenylbutazone at 2–4 g/450 kg/day P/O) is indicated if secondary paraphimosis or intractable inflammation exists.

PRIAPISM

CONTRAINDICATIONS
Phenothiazine tranquilizers are absolutely contraindicated.

PRECAUTIONS
N/A

POSSIBLE INTERACTIONS
N/A

ALTERNATIVE DRUGS
A cholinergic blocker (benztropine mesylate, 8 mg IV) has been used successfully in reduction of priapism in one gelding. It was administered within 24 hr of the onset of priapism.

FOLLOW-UP

PATIENT MONITORING
- Due to initial intensive patient management, hospitalization may be indicated to allow frequent re-evaluation.
- Pain and discomfort are managed with physical therapy (massage, hydrotherapy, support) or pharmacologically.
- Successful reduction of the erection and return of the penis to the prepuce are considered good prognostic indicators.

POSSIBLE COMPLICATIONS
- Chronic priapism may cause inflammation of the pudendal nerve where it passes over the ischium. The pudendal nerve innervates the retractor penis muscle. Damage to the pudendal nerve can cause malfunction of the retractor penis muscles, resulting in permanent penile paralysis.
- Secondary paraphimosis may develop as dependent edema accumulates.
- Impotence (inability to achieve an erection) can occur as a result of desensitization of the glans penis from nerve damage or fibrosis of the CCP.

MISCELLANEOUS

ASSOCIATED CONDITIONS
- Paraphimosis
- Penile paralysis

AGE-RELATED FACTORS
N/A

ZOONOTIC POTENTIAL
N/A

PREGNANCY
N/A

SYNONYMS
N/A

SEE ALSO
- Paraphimosis
- Penile paralysis

ABBREVIATION
- CCP = corpus cavernosum penis

Suggested Reading

Blanchard TL, Schumacher J, Edwards JF, Varner DD, Lewis RD, Everett K, and Joyce JR. Priapism in a stallion with generalized malignant melanoma. J Vet Med Assoc 1991;198:1043-1044.

Blanchard TL, Varner DD, Schumacher J. Surgery of the stallion reproductive tract. In: Manual of equine reproduction. St. Louis: Mosby 1998;182-185.

Pearson H, Weaver BMQ. Priapism after sedation, neuroleptanalgesia and anaesthesia in the horse. Equine Vet J 1978;10:85-90.

Schumaker J, Hardin DK. Surgical treatment of priapism in a stallion. Vet Surg 1987;16:193-196.

Schumacher J, Vaughan JT. Surgery of the penis and prepuce. In: Vet Clin North Am, Equine Pract 1988;4:473-491.

Author Carole C. Miller

Consulting Editor Carla L. Carleton

PRIMARY HYPERPARATHYROIDISM (HP)

BASICS

OVERVIEW

- Caused by excessive parathyroid hormone (PTH) secretion by hyperplastic or neoplastic parathyroid cells, which results in increased calcium resorption from bones leading to hypercalcemia and clinical signs of fibrous osteodystrophy.
- Hypophosphatemia and hyperphosphaturia result from low renal tubular reabsorption of phosphate secondary to increased PTH secretion.
- Excessive PTH may originate from parathyroid hyperplasia, adenoma, or adenocarcinoma.
- Organ systems—endocrine and musculoskeletal

SIGNALMENT

- Any sex or breed
- Reported only in old equids.

SIGNS

- Intermittent weakness
- Weight loss
- Anorexia
- Enlargement of facial bones
- Shifting-leg lameness
- Difficult mastication

CAUSES AND RISK FACTORS

Excessive, uncontrolled secretion of PTH by chief cells of one or more parathyroid glands

DIAGNOSIS

DIFFERENTIAL DIAGNOSIS

- Fibrous osteodystrophy commonly has been reported as resulting from nutritional secondary HP in horses fed low concentrations of calcium and excess phosphorus; however, hypocalcemia (or normocalcemia) and hyperphosphatemia characterize nutritional HP.
- Other causes of hypercalcemia—chronic renal failure, hypervitaminosis D, and neoplastic disease.
- Normal serum BUN, creatinine concentration, and urine specific gravity rule out chronic renal failure.
- Ingestion of oxalate-containing plants and vitamin D toxicosis can be eliminated based on history; in addition, vitamin D toxicosis is characterized by hyperphosphatemia.
- Certain neoplastic tissues produce a PTH-related protein with identical biologic properties to PTH that results in pseudo-HP, but ruling out neoplastic disease in live horses may be difficult. Measurements of intact PTH, using an immunoradiometric assay that does not cross-react with PTH-related protein, may help in differentiation.

CBC/BIOCHEMISTRY/URINALYSIS

- Hypercalcemia, hypophosphatemia, and hyperphosphaturia are characteristic.
- Hyperchloremic metabolic acidosis has been associated.

OTHER LABORATORY TESTS

- Fractional excretion of phosphorus (reference range, 0.04–0.16%) and serum PTH are abnormally elevated.
- PTH may be measured by immunoradiometric assay for immunoreactive PTH (detects C-terminal portion) or for intact PTH (detects both C- and N-terminal portions); however, the latter assay does not measure PTH-related protein, which often is elevated in cases of pseudo-HP

IMAGING

- Skull radiography may reveal osseous proliferation of the facial bones and loss of the lamina dura surrounding the premolars and molars.
- Detection of parathyroid neoplasia may be attempted with nuclear scintigraphy using ^{99m}Tc sestamibi.

DIAGNOSTIC PROCEDURES

Horses have two pairs of parathyroid glands, one cranial pair adjacent to the cranial pole of the thyroid gland, and one caudal pair variably located along the neck anywhere from the thoracic inlet to the cranial third of the trachea; therefore, if a mass is identified in that part of the neck, biopsy may be attempted.

PATHOLOGIC FINDINGS

- Parathyroid gland hyperplasia, adenoma, or adenocarcinoma
- Equine parathyroid glands may be difficult to distinguish from surrounding tissues.
- With parathyroid neoplasia, atrophy of the nonaffected parathyroid tissue is expected.
- Single or multiple glands may be affected.

PRIMARY HYPERPARATHYROIDISM (HP)

TREATMENT

• Removal of the affected parathyroid gland, and medical treatment for hypercalcemia
• Eliminate exogenous sources of vitamin D and calcium.
• Successful surgical removal of a parathyroid adenoma has been reported in a pony.
• Disease progression may be slow; one pony has been reported to still be clinically normal 2 years after diagnosis.

MEDICATIONS

DRUGS

IV fluid therapy, diuretics, and corticosteroids may promote calcium excretion.

CONTRAINDICATIONS/POSSIBLE INTERACTIONS

N/A

FOLLOW-UP

• Monitor electrolytes, acid–base status, and bone ossification.
• Possible complications—difficulty chewing because of loosening teeth; lameness secondary to osteopenia

MISCELLANEOUS

ASSOCIATED CONDITIONS

N/A

AGE-RELATED FACTORS

N/A

ZOONOTIC POTENTIAL

N/A

PREGNANCY

N/A

SEE ALSO

N/A

ABBREVIATIONS

• HP = hyperparathyroidism
• PTH = parathyroid hormone

Suggested Reading

Frank N, Hawkins JF, Couëtil LL, Raymond JT. Primary hyperparathyroidism with osteodystrophia fibrosa of the facial bones in a pony. J Am Vet Med Assoc 1998; 212:84–86.

Author Laurent Couëtil
Consulting Editor Michel Levy

PROGRESSIVE ETHMOIDAL HEMATOMA (PEH)

BASICS

OVERVIEW
• An uncommonly encountered, slowly expanding, nonneoplastic mass originating in the submucosa of the ethmoid labyrinth
• The mass slowly expands into the nasal passage, paranasal sinuses, or nasopharynx, causing destruction of adjacent tissue.
• Occasionally bilateral

SIGNALMENT
• Any age, but rare in horses <3 years (median age, ≅10 years)
• Predilection for Arabians and Thoroughbreds
• No difference in prevalence between males and females or between geldings and stallions

SIGNS
• Most common—intermittent, serosanguineous discharge, not associated with exercise, from the affected nasal passage
• Other signs—halitosis, abnormal respiratory noise, dyspnea, coughing, head shaking, and facial deformity
• The mass may be visible at the nostril.
• Small lesions may cause no clinical signs.

CAUSES AND RISK FACTORS
Cause unknown

DIAGNOSIS

DIFFERENTIAL DIAGNOSIS
• Other conditions that may cause epistaxis—mycosis of the guttural pouch; nasal trauma; neoplasia of the larynx, pharynx, paranasal sinuses, or lungs; exercise-induced pulmonary hemorrhage; and septic pneumonia
• Lesions of the nasal passages that resemble PEH endoscopically—polyps, fungal masses, and neoplasms

CBC/BIOCHEMISTRY/URINALYSIS
Usually normal, but may reveal anemia.

OTHER LABORATORY TESTS
N/A

IMAGING
• If confined to the nasal passage, the mass appears radiographically as an abnormal opacity of soft-tissue density with smooth margins ventral to the eye and rostral to the ethmoid labyrinth.
• Masses may protrude into the adjacent paranasal sinuses, and if so, fluid lines in the compartments of the paranasal sinuses may be noted.
• Positive-contrast sinusography or CT may allow more complete evaluation of lesion extent in the paranasal sinuses.

DIAGNOSTIC PROCEDURES
• Endoscopy of the nasal passages reveals a yellow-red-green mass that appears to originate from the nasal portion of the ethmoid labyrinth.
• White colonies of *Aspergillus* spp. may be present on the lesion.
• The origin of the mass may be obscured from view because of the size of the mass.
• The mass may protrude caudally around the nasal septum into the contralateral nasal passage, obscuring the contralateral ethmoid labyrinth and giving the impression of two masses; less commonly, the mass may originate from the portion of the ethmoid labyrinth within the paranasal sinus, in which case it is not seen at endoscopy of the nasal passage unless it protrudes into the nasal passage through the nasomaxillary aperture.
• A mass within the paranasal sinuses may distort the nasal passage.
• Always examine both nasal passages, because masses can occur bilaterally.
• The diagnosis often is established on the basis of the location and endoscopic appearance of the lesion, but biopsy of the lesion is confirmatory.

PATHOLOGIC FINDINGS
• The lesion is covered by respiratory epithelium, which overlies submucosal fibrous tissue as well as old and recent hemorrhage.
• The hemorrhage contains hemosiderin-filled macrophages and multinucleated giant cells.

TREATMENT
• Affected horses can be treated by surgical ablation of the mass, paranasal cryotherapy, transendoscopic laser therapy, and transendoscopic injection an aqueous solution of 4% formaldehyde into the lesion.
• Surgical ablation is performed, with the horse anesthetized, through an osteoplastic frontonasal flap. The nasal portion of the ethmoid labyrinth is exposed, if necessary, by perforating the floor of the dorsoconchal sinus, and the lesion and diseased portion of the ethmoid labyrinth are excised. Perforation of the dorsoconchal sinus and excision of the mass usually are associated with severe hemorrhage; other complications include encephalitis, dehiscence of the wound, and suture periostitis.
• Application of a cryogen (e.g., liquid nitrogen) to ablate the mass causes minimal hemorrhage and can be performed with the horse both conscious and standing. This method, however, is only used for small lesions.
• The mass can be ablated transendoscopically using a laser with the horse both conscious and standing. Laser therapy usually requires multiple treatments, however, and the cost of the equipment may limit its availability.

PROGRESSIVE ETHMOIDAL HEMATOMA (PEH)

MEDICATIONS

DRUGS

- Transendoscopic ablation using a 4% aqueous solution of formaldehyde can be performed with the horse both conscious and standing. A lesion in the paranasal sinuses can also be injected, via the endoscope, through a trephine hole into the caudal maxillary or conchofrontal sinus.
- Injection of only the nasal portion of a lesion extending from the nasal portion of the ethmoid labyrinth into the adjacent paranasal sinuses may cause the entire lesion to resolve. Lesions are injected until they distend and begin to leak formaldehyde solution.
- Horses are retreated at 3–4-week intervals until the lesion is either eliminated or so small and deep within the ethmoid labyrinth that injection no longer is possible.
- Treatment of small lesions that do not protrude beyond the external lamina of the ethmoid bone may not be possible or necessary.
- Laminitis may be a rare complication of injection with formaldehyde solution. Systemic administration of am NSAID before intralesional injection may be warranted to help avoid this complication.

CONTRAINDICATIONS/POSSIBLE INTERACTIONS

N/A

FOLLOW-UP

- Regardless of the treatment method, prognosis for long-term cure is guarded to poor.
- The incidence of recurrence has been reported to range from 14–45% but may be even higher.
- The incidence of recurrence seems to be much higher in bilaterally affected horses.
- Even when the condition appears to have resolved, re-examine horses periodically with endoscopy to determine if the lesion has reappeared. Always examine both nasal passages.

MISCELLANEOUS

ASSOCIATED CONDITIONS

N/A

AGE-RELATED FACTORS

N/A

ZOONOTIC POTENTIAL

N/A

PREGNANCY

N/A

SEE ALSO

- Exercise-induced pulmonary hemorrhage
- Guttural pouch mycosis
- Hemorrhagic nasal discharge

Suggested Reading

Bell BTL, Baker GJ, Foreman JH. Progressive ethmoid hematoma: background, clinical signs, and diagnosis. Compend Contin Educ Pract Vet 1993;15:1101–1110.

Bell BTL, Baker GJ, Foreman JH. Progressive ethmoid hematoma: characteristics, cause, and treatment. Compend Contin Educ Pract Vet 1993;15:1391–1398.

Author Jim Schumacher

Consulting Editor Jean-Pierre Lavoie

PROGRESSIVE RETINAL ATROPHY

BASICS

OVERVIEW

• Includes a number of genetic diseases with degeneration of the photoreceptor or RPE cells.
• Because of their important functional relationship with photoreceptor cells, RPE cell degeneration eventually leads to loss of vision resulting from secondary death of photoreceptor cells.
• Organ system—ophthalmic

SIGNALMENT

Observed in Thoroughbreds.

SIGNS

• Progressive visual impairment combined with multifocal depigmented areas and hyperpigmented centers primarily in the nontapetal retina
• Nyctalopia (i.e., night blindness) may occur early and optic nerve atrophy late in the disease process.

CAUSES AND RISK FACTORS

• Unknown
• As in dogs, it may be a retinal biochemical abnormality based on genetic mutations.

DIAGNOSIS

DIFFERENTIAL DIAGNOSIS

• Chorioretinitis
• Congenital defects of the retina or optic nerve

CBC/BIOCHEMISTRY/URINALYSIS

N/A

OTHER LABORATORY TESTS

N/A

IMAGING

N/A

DIAGNOSTIC PROCEDURES

Electroretinography to assess functionality of the retina

PATHOLOGIC FINDINGS

Depend on the retinal cell type that is primarily affected

PROGRESSIVE RETINAL ATROPHY

TREATMENT

No treatment

MEDICATIONS

DRUGS

N/A

CONTRAINDICATIONS/POSSIBLE INTERACTIONS

N/A

FOLLOW-UP

EXPECTED COURSE AND PROGNOSIS

As the cause is unknown, the prognosis for vision is poor.

MISCELLANEOUS

ASSOCIATED CONDITIONS

N/A.

AGE-RELATED FACTORS

N/A

ZOONOTIC POTENTIAL

N/A

PREGNANCY

N/A

SEE ALSO

- Chorioretinitis
- Optic neuropathy
- Recurrent uveitis
- Retinal detachment
- Stationary night blindness

ABBREVIATION

- RPE = retinal pigment epithelium

Suggested Reading

Brooks DE. Equine ophthalmology. In: Gelatt KN, ed. Veterinary ophthalmology. 3rd ed. Philadelphia: Lippincott Williams & Wilkins, 1999.

Author Andras M. Komaromy

Consulting Editor Dennis E. Brooks

PROLIFERATIVE OPTIC NEUROPATHY

BASICS

OVERVIEW

- A slowly enlarging, white mass protruding from the optic disc into the vitreous
- The lesion generally is fixed (i.e., does not move when the eye moves).
- Organ system—ophthalmic

SIGNALMENT

Primarily horses >15 years

SIGNS

- No or minimal effect on vision
- Normal PLR
- Generally unilateral
- No signs of pain

CAUSE AND RISK FACTORS

Unknown

DIAGNOSIS

DIFFERENTIAL DIAGNOSIS

- Tumors—astrocytoma, medulloepithelioma, and neuroepithelioma
- Granuloma
- Abscess

CBC/BIOCHEMISTRY/URINALYSIS

N/A

OTHER LABORATORY TESTS

N/A

IMAGING

N/A

DIAGNOSTIC PROCEDURES

N/A

PATHOLOGIC FINDINGS

- Histologically resembles a schwannoma in many cases, but also may be similar to an astrocytoma or xanthoma.
- Schwannomas are well-circumscribed masses attached to peripheral nerves, cranial nerves, or spinal nerve roots and contain areas of densely packed spindle cells intermixed with looser, myxoid regions.

TREATMENT

N/A

PROLIFERATIVE OPTIC NEUROPATHY

MEDICATIONS

DRUGS
No therapy for this condition

CONTRAINDICATIONS/POSSIBLE INTERACTIONS
N/A

FOLLOW-UP

PATIENT MONITORING
Observe for vision changes.

POSSIBLE COMPLICATIONS
N/A

EXPECTED COURSE AND PROGNOSIS
- No effect on vision
- Size—slowly progressing

MISCELLANEOUS

ASSOCIATED CONDITIONS
N/A

AGE-RELATED FACTORS
Primarily horses >15 years

ZOONOTIC POTENTIAL
N/A

PREGNANCY

SEE ALSO
- Exudative optic neuritis
- Ischemic optic neuropathy
- Traumatic optic neuropathy

ABBREVIATIONS
PLR = pupillary light reflex

Suggested Reading

Brooks DE. Equine ophthalmology, In: Gelatt KN, ed. Veterinary ophthalmology. 3rd ed. Philadelphia: Lippincott Williams & Wilkins, 1999.

Author Maria Källberg
Consulting Editor Dennis E. Brooks

PROLONGED DIESTRUS

BASICS

DEFINITION

Persistence of a CL post-ovulation such that the normal return to estrus is delayed.

PATHOPHYSIOLOGY

- After ovulation, the CL forms and begins progesterone production. In the mare, a CL is unresponsive to prostaglandin administration within 4–5 days after ovulation.
- Endogenous prostaglandin, produced by the endometrium, is released approximately 14–16 days post-ovulation to initiate luteolysis in the non-pregnant mare.
- The life-span of the CL is prolonged when prostaglandin release is inhibited or when the CL fails to respond to prostaglandin that is released.

SYSTEM AFFECTED

Reproductive

SIGNALMENT

Mares of any age and breed.

SIGNS

Historical Findings

Failure to return to estrus at the expected time interval in the cycling mare.

Physical Examination

- The general physical examination is usually normal.
- Transrectal palpation may reveal some ovarian activity (complete inactivity could indicate anestrus and is addressed elsewhere), a normal or enlarged uterus, and a closed cervix.
- With transrectal ultrasound, a CL (one or more) may be present. A mature CL appears as a uniform hyperechoic area within the ovary. It appears round or tear-drop shaped. The periphery of a recent ovulation may appear as expected, but the center of the CH/CL may be hypoechoic or mottled. It is possible to identify one or more CL if a mare is prone to multiple ovulations. While scanning the ovaries, look for uterine luminal fluid or pregnancy.
- Vaginoscopy can confirm transrectal palpation findings regarding the degree of cervical relaxation, as well as the presence of uterine or cervical discharge.

CAUSES

Idiopathic/Spontaneous Persistence of the CL

Associated with normal diestrous ovulations (after day 10 of the cycle), resulting in an immature CL being present at the time of normal luteolysis (typically day 14). Persistent CL have also been related to fescue ingestion.

Pregnancy

CL function continues in the presence of a conceptus.

EED

Maternal recognition of pregnancy occurs by day 14 postovulation. Embryonic death after this time results in a delayed return to estrus, i.e., a longer than expected interestrus interval. If embryonic death occurs after the formation of endometrial cups (35–40 days post-ovulation), the mare will not return to estrus until the cups regress and production of eCG (until day 120–150 post-ovulation) by the cups ceases.

Uterine Infections/Endometrial Degeneration

Because endogenous $PGF_{2}\alpha$ is of endometrial origin, endometritis, infection, or other decline of uterine health can result in ineffective prostaglandin formation or release.

Iatrogenic

Administration of progesterone or NSAIDs can result in prolonged diestrus.

Lactation

A CL may persist following the first, or *foal heat,* ovulation. This may be more likely in mares that are in less than optimal body condition (caloric deficit).

RISK FACTORS

N/A

DIAGNOSIS

DIFFERENTIAL DIAGNOSIS

Differentiating Similar Signs

Diagnosis is based on finding a normal, non-pregnant, diestrus reproductive tract coupled with a history of failing to show estrus behavior more than 2 weeks post-ovulation and a serum progesterone concentration of >4 ng/mL. This assumes some ovarian activity has previously been observed and is therefore not being mistaken for anestrus. Regular teasing, serial transrectal palpation, and ultrasonography are the cornerstones to proper interpretation of the reproductive cycle of an individual mare.

Differentiating Causes

- Pregnancy and/or EED can occur without any history of a scheduled breeding, if access to any stallion/colt is remotely possible in the mare's environment. Therefore, it is essential to palpate a mare before doing any invasive vaginal procedures (uterine culture or biopsy) or administering prostaglandin to short-cycle a mare in a prolonged diestrus.
- Pyometra and endometritis are typically diagnosed on the basis of transrectal palpation, ultrasonography, uterine culture, and biopsy. See uterine disease, endometritis, pyometra.
- History of a normal foal heat followed by reproductive quiescence can be due to either prolonged diestrus or lactational anestrus. Ovarian activity and serum progesterone concentrations allow differentiation of the two.

CBC/BIOCHEMISTRY/URINALYSIS

N/A

OTHER LABORATORY TESTS

- Serum progesterone concentrations. Basal levels of <1 ng/mL indicate no mature luteal tissue is present. Mature CL function is associated with levels of >4 ng/mL.
- Measurement of serum eCG levels may be useful in cases of suspected EED after endometrial cups had formed, especially if there is no evidence of pregnancy at the time of the examination.

IMAGING

N/A

DIAGNOSTIC PROCEDURES

Uterine cytology, culture, and endometrial biopsy are useful to diagnose and treat pyometra and endometritis properly.

PROLONGED DIESTRUS

TREATMENT

• Prolonged diestrus, if the presence of a CL is confirmed, is treated with prostaglandin. Luteolysis is the goal of treatment, whether the release of endogenous prostaglandin is accomplished with uterine manipulation or exogenous prostaglandin is administered to the mare (see Drug(s) of Choice).
• Endogenous prostaglandin release can be stimulated by intrauterine infusion of sterile saline at ambient temperature or warmed to <120°F/48°C, maintain aseptic techniques, use a volume of 500–1000 mL.
• Endometrial biopsy or uterine culture may infrequently stimulate endogenous prostaglandin release.

MEDICATIONS

DRUG(S) OF CHOICE

• $PGF_2\alpha$ (1 mg/100#, IM, Lutalyse™, Upjohn, Kalamazoo, MI) or its analogs are used to stimulate luteolysis. Mares with a functional CL typically exhibit estrus 2–4 days post-injection and ovulate 6–12 days after treatment.
• Two doses of $PGF_2\alpha$, given 14–15 days apart, are useful if transrectal palpation cannot easily or safely be accomplished. This regimen ensures that immature/non-responsive luteal tissue present at the time of the first injection has ample time to mature and be able to respond to the second $PGF_2\alpha$ injection.

CONTRAINDICATIONS

Mares with subacute or acute respiratory or GI tract disease should not be subjected to natural prostaglandin administration. Analogs of prostaglandin have fewer or less severe side-effects, and may be safer to use in a mare that is prone to colic or has a history of heaves.

PRECAUTIONS

• Exogenous prostaglandins should never be administered intravenously.
• Prostaglandin administration causes pregnant mares to abort, and should not be administered until pregnancy has been definitively ruled out.
• Symptoms of colic can occur following the administration of prostaglandin.
• The most common side effect observed is sweating, which begins within 15–20 min of administration. A mare should be monitored after injection and treated symptomatically if her level of discomfort persists beyond 1–2 hr.
• Pregnant women should handle prostaglandins with extreme caution.

POSSIBLE INTERACTIONS

NSAIDs can interfere with endogenous prostaglandin release and function.

ALTERNATIVE DRUGS

Equimate (fluprostenol sodium, Miles), 250 μg or 0.55 μg/kg, IM, is a prostaglandin analog. This product is used in similar fashion as the natural prostaglandin. Although approved for use in the horse, it is currently unavailable/out of production.

FOLLOW-UP

PATIENT MONITORING

• Serial (three times weekly) teasing, transrectal palpation, and ultrasonography is recommended to evaluate the mare's reproductive tract for evidence of estrus.
• Serum progesterone concentrations, measured twice weekly for 2 weeks post-$PGF_2\alpha$ administration, can be used to determine the effectiveness of treatment and/or persistence of functional luteal tissue.

POSSIBLE COMPLICATIONS

Prolonged non-pregnant periods and/or infertility.

MISCELLANEOUS

ASSOCIATED CONDITIONS

N/A

AGE-RELATED FACTORS

N/A

ZOONOTIC POTENTIAL

N/A

PREGNANCY

• Administration of prostaglandin causes abortion in pregnant mares. It should not be administered until pregnancy has been definitively ruled out.
• Prostaglandin can also terminate a human pregnancy, and caution must always be taken with its use.

SYNONYMS

eCG = PMSG or pregnant mare serum gonadotropin

SEE ALSO

• Anestrus
• Early embryonic death
• Endometritis
• Estrus, Abnormal intervals
• False pregnancy
• Pyometra
• Uterine disease

ABBREVIATIONS

• CH = corpus hemorrhagicum
• CL = corpus luteum
• eCG = equine chorionic gonadotropin
• EED = early embryonic death
• $PGF_2\alpha$ = natural prostaglandin

Suggested Reading

Daels PF, Hughes JP. The abnormal estrous cycle. In: Equine reproduction. McKinnon AO and Voss JL, ed. Philadelphia: Lea & Febiger, 1993;144-160.

Hinrichs K. Irregularities of the estrous cycle and ovulation in mares. In: Current therapy in large animal theriogenology. Youngquist RS, ed. Philadelphia: WB Saunders Co. 1997;166-171.

Löfstedt RM. Some aspects of manipulative and diagnostic endocrinology of the broodmare. Proc Soc Therio 1986;67-93.

Sharp DC. Early pregnancy in mares: Uncoupling the luteolytic cascade. Proc Soc Therio 1996;236-242.

Van Camp SD. Prolonged diestrus. In: Current therapy in equine medicine. Robinson NE, ed. Philadelphia: WB Saunders Co. 1983;401-402.

Author Carole C. Miller
Consulting Editor Carla L. Carleton

PROLONGED PREGNANCY

BASICS

OVERVIEW

• Gestation exceeding the normal range for the mare; gestation that appears to be lengthened by abnormal characteristics of the fetus.
• Normal range of gestation is 320–355 days, but it is not rare for gestational length to fall outside this range.
• Multifactorial—individual variation, placental function or dysfunction, and hormonal changes; could also involve damage to the endometrium, thus reducing the nutrient supply to the fetus; still able to sustain life, but resulting in fetal growth retardation.
• No statistics are available regarding incidence, but it is not a major reproductive problem.

SIGNALMENT

• Females
• All breeds
• All of breeding age

SIGNS

General Comments

• Differs from other domestic species, in which prolonged pregnancy is linked with iodine deficiency, increased progesterone, and inheritance.
• May be caused by abnormal fetal pituitary and adrenal development or by lack of hypothalamic maturity at term.

Historical Findings

Usually appears to be a fetal problem, so historical information may have limited value.

Physical Examination Findings

• Mare—no abnormalities of the mare unless excessive uterine fluid has accumulated.
• Fetus—postpartum examination usually reveals a dead or very weak fetus; smaller than normal; may appear undernourished.

CAUSES AND RISK FACTORS

• Hormonal—pituitary or adrenal; most common.
• Not a mare problem; mares can be bred again with little concern for recurrence.

DIAGNOSIS

• Accurate history combined with transrectal palpation.
• Outward gross appearance of the mare.
• Appearance of the fetus—prepartum, postpartum, and/or necropsy.

DIFFERENTIAL DIAGNOSIS

Hydrops:

• Prolonged pregnancy with a hydrops is invariably shorter than the lengthened gestation associated with a fetus having a higher center defect.
• Known breeding and ovulation dates facilitate differentiation.

CBC/BIOCHEMISTRY/URINALYSIS

N/A

OTHER LABORATORY TESTS

Peritoneal tap:

• To determine the location of excessive fluid accumulation.
• To differentiate prolonged pregnancy from hydrops.

IMAGING

To determine if:

• Excessive fluid is present.
• The endometrium is thickened.
• Fetal extremities are smaller than normal.

DIAGNOSTIC PROCEDURES

Perform an endometrial biopsy to determine the endometrial status.

PATHOLOGIC FINDINGS

• The uterus may or may not be larger than normal.
• The fetus should be necropsied to determine if the adrenals, pituitary, and hypothalamus are normal.

PROLONGED PREGNANCY

TREATMENT

• Parturition induction is an option. However, it is essential that the breeding date is accurate, and that records can confirm its validity.
• Remind owners that fetal survival after a prolonged gestation is in question. The actual circumstances of survival may not be known until after delivery.
• Routine care for the mare during the postpartum period.
• Emphasize to owners that prolonged pregnancies can occur, and that most affected mares have normal foals.
• Remind owners that gestational length may fall outside the normal range and still be normal for that individual.

MEDICATIONS

DRUGS

None required or indicated

CONTRAINDICATIONS/POSSIBLE INTERACTIONS

N/A

FOLLOW-UP

PATIENT MONITORING

• Monitor mares once they are suspected to be "overdue."
• Take no action unless pregnancy goes beyond the expected due date without external evidence of advancing gestation and approaching parturition.
• A pluriparous mare should be close to a previous "term gestation" length in which she delivered a normal foal before considering inducing parturition.

PREVENTION/AVOIDANCE

Unknown, because the major causes involve abnormal fetal pituitary, adrenals, or hypothalamus.

POSSIBLE COMPLICATIONS

Prolonged pregnancy could result in dystocia. Because the fetus usually is smaller than normal and has no ankylosis of joints, however, this usually is not a problem.

EXPECTED COURSE AND PROGNOSIS

Postpartum:
• Normal postpartum examination of the mare
• The fetus is expected to be smaller than normal and has a low probability of survival.

MISCELLANEOUS

ASSOCIATED CONDITIONS

N/A

AGE-RELATED FACTORS

N/A

ZOONOTIC POTENTIAL

N/A

PREGNANCY

Occurs only during gestation.

SEE ALSO

• Parturition induction
• Postpartum care

Suggested Reading

Vandeplassche M. Obstetrician's view of the physiology of equine parturition and dystocia. Equine Vet J 1980;12(2):45–49.

Author Walter R. Threlfall
Consulting Editor Carla L. Carleton

PROTEIN, HYPERFIBRINOGENEMIA

BASICS

DEFINITION

- High fibrinogen concentration (>400 mg/dL)
- Associated with a wide variety of inflammatory diseases, and may be the only indicator of inflammation if the accompanying leukogram is normal.
- Plasma fibrinogen concentration generally is believed to return to normal as inflammation subsides and often is used to indicate resolving inflammation.

PATHOPHYSIOLOGY

- Fibrinogen is an acute-phase glycoprotein derived solely from the liver that increases during inflammation.
- Cytokines manufactured early during an inflammatory process because of cell and tissue injury reduce hepatic synthesis of certain plasma proteins, including albumin, prealbumin and transferrin (i.e., negative acute-phase proteins), and increase synthesis of other proteins, including fibrinogen, complement, haptoglobin, and C-reactive protein.
- During inflammation, plasma proteins, including fibrinogen, exude into an inflammatory focus. Subsequent precipitation of fibrinogen and fibrin monomers provides a scaffolding for in-growth of fibroblasts and capillary buds, which eventually mature into vascularized and well-organized connective tissue serving to wall off the inflammatory process.

SYSTEM AFFECTED

N/A

SIGNALMENT

- Fibrinogen concentrations increase in normal foals during the first 5 months of age. The cause has been attributed to maturing hepatic function and is not associated with subclinical disease (see *Age-Related Factors*).
- Pregnant mares experience a dramatic increase in fibrinogen during pregnancy and after parturition (see *Pregnancy*).

SIGNS

- Hyperfibrinogenemia itself is not responsible for clinical signs.
- A multitude of inflammatory diseases, from mild viral infections to severe colic, can result in hyperfibrinogenemia.
- Establishing the diagnosis of the primary inflammatory condition is of utmost importance.

CAUSES

- Cardiovascular—pericarditis; endocarditis
- Metabolic—dehydration (relative increase)
- GI—colic, acute or chronic GI disease, colitis, enteritis, peritonitis, parasites, salmonellosis, endotoxemia, chronic internal abscessation, neoplasia, chronic wasting diseases, and surgical tissue trauma
- Hemic/lymphatic/immune—leukemia, purpura hemorrhagia, lymphangitis, equine infectious anemia, equine viral arteritis, and neoplasia
- Hepatobiliary—acute hepatic failure (i.e., Theiler's disease), cholangitis, hepatitis, and neoplasia
- Musculoskeletal—*Corynebacterium pseudotuberculosis* (i.e., pigeon fever), tissue trauma, exertional rhabdomyolysis, myositis (e.g., infectious, postanesthetic), and neoplasia
- Ophthalmic—uveitis, trauma or injury to eye, and neoplasia
- Renal/urologic—chronic renal failure, acute renal failure, neoplasia, pyelonephritis, and cantharidin poisoning
- Reproductive—pregnancy (see below); pyometra
- Respiratory—bacterial pneumonia, *Streptococcus equi* (e.g., strangles, chronic internal abscessation), pneumonia, pleuropneumonia, and guttural pouch disease (i.e., empyema)
- Skin/exocrine—neoplasia; abscessation

RISK FACTORS

- Hyperfibrinogenemia can be associated with any acute or chronic illness that has an inflammatory component.
- Fibrinogen levels also can be elevated in foals (see *Age-Related Factors*) and pregnant mares (see *Pregnancy*).

DIAGNOSIS

DIFFERENTIAL DIAGNOSIS

- The challenge lies in identifying the primary cause of hyperfibrinogenemia in a patient with no overt clinical signs of disease.
- A thorough physical examination is essential.
- Ancillary diagnostic aids (e.g., CBC and chemistry panel, abdominal or pleural fluid evaluation, radiography, endoscopy) often are employed to determine the origin of inflammation.

LABORATORY FINDINGS

Drugs that May Alter Lab Results

N/A

Disorders that May Alter Lab Results

- Fibrinogen concentrations may be falsely lowered if the blood has clotted before determination. Laboratories that determine concentration using methods dependent on normal clotting (i.e., Clauss method, as found in many human labs); hemolyzed, icteric, or lipemic specimens; heparin contamination; and over- or underfilling of citrated collection tubes are sources of analytic error.
- Hyperproteinemia caused by dehydration or hypoproteinemia caused by marked protein loss can falsely increase or decrease, respectively, plasma fibrinogen concentrations. Perform the plasma protein:fibrinogen ratio for proper interpretation of the fibrinogen values when these metabolic disturbances are present; this ratio is calculated as (total plasma protein [g/dL])−fibrinogen [g/dL])/fibrinogen (g/dL). Ratios >15 are normal; ratios from 10–15 demonstrate a relative increase in plasma fibrinogen and suggest inflammation. Clinical impression and other diagnostic aids must be employed in these cases to determine if the ratio is significant. Ratios <10 are abnormal and indicate active inflammation.

Valid If Run in Human Lab?

- Yes, but various techniques may require different sample types.
- Laboratories using the heat precipitation method can utilize blood collected in a standard EDTA tube for fibrinogen quantification.
- Commonly, a thrombin-initiated clotting rate assay is used in human labs to determine fibrinogen concentration. In this test, fibrinogen quantification is based on the rate of clot formation in dilute, citrated plasma after addition to thrombin. For this assay, blood must be submitted in sodium citrate.
- Human labs also may use an immunologic assay for fibrinogen that quantitates an immunoprecipitate formed by specific antifibrinogen antisera. The high degree of immunologic cross-reactivity for fibrinogen between species suggests this may be a valid assay for horses; however, other methods should be used until this assay has been validated for use with equine plasma.

CBC/BIOCHEMISTRY/URINALYSIS

Without overt clinical signs of inflammation (e.g., external abscessation, pneumonia), CBC, chemistry panel, and urinalysis are essential profiles to screen specific organ systems for abnormalities.

OTHER LABORATORY TESTS

N/A

IMAGING

Radiography or ultrasonography may identify an inflammatory focus e.g., pleuropneumonia or focal abscessation

DIAGNOSTIC PROCEDURES

- Ancillary diagnostic tests (e.g., tracheal wash, bronchoalveolar lavage, peritoneal or pleural fluid analysis) may identify an inflammatory focus.
- Bacteriology and serology may identify specific pathogens.
- Consult specific laboratories for appropriate sample submission protocols.

TREATMENT

- Identifying the underlying, primary disease process is the only course of treatment.
- Hyperfibrinogenemia is highly correlated with septic inflammatory processes; thus, prophylactic antibiotics may be useful in some circumstances while awaiting results or while a more extensive diagnostic workup is being pursued

MEDICATIONS

DRUGS OF CHOICE

N/A

CONTRAINDICATIONS

N/A

PRECAUTIONS

N/A

POSSIBLE INTERACTIONS

N/A

ALTERNATIVE DRUGS

N/A

FOLLOW-UP

PATIENT MONITORING

- Fibrinogen concentrations often are monitored to identify resolution of an inflammatory process. This is especially advantageous when leukocyte numbers have never changed or have returned to normal concentrations.
- Fibrinogen concentrations peak within 72–96 hours after the onset of inflammation, and resolution of hyperfibrinogenemia may be lengthy if the inflammatory focus persists.
- In one study, fibrinogen concentrations did not return to normal even 15 days after surgical tissue trauma.

POSSIBLE COMPLICATIONS

Severity of disease resulting in death or euthanasia is correlated with higher plasma fibrinogen concentrations.

MISCELLANEOUS

ASSOCIATED CONDITIONS

N/A

AGE-RELATED FACTORS

Fibrinogen increases in normal foals during the first 5 months of age and can exceed normal adult concentrations. Ranges of 260 ± 60 mg/dL in 1-day-old foals to 460 ± 70 mg/dL in 1–3-month-old foals have been reported. This trend is a consistent finding, suggesting that subclinical disease is not present. Maturing hepatic enzyme systems that may possibly overreact to newly encountered environmental stimuli, causing induced acute-phase reactants, has been suggested as the cause.

ZOONOTIC POTENTIAL

N/A

PREGNANCY

- In one study, fibrinogen concentrations dramatically increase (>40%) in prepartum mares.
- These concentrations can further increase by >10% between 12–36 hours postpartum, but can return to prepartum concentrations by 14 days after foaling.

SYNONYMS

N/A

SEE ALSO

N/A

ABBREVIATIONS

GI = gastrointestinal

Suggested Reading

Allen BV, Kold SE. Fibrinogen response to surgical tissue trauma in the horse. Equine Vet J 1988;20:441–443.

Andrews DA, Reagan WJ, DeNicola DB. Plasma fibrinogen in recognizing equine inflammatory disease. Compend Contin Educ 1994;16:1349–1356.

Duncan JR, Prasse KW, Mahaffey EA. Veterinary laboratory medicine: clinical pathology. 3rd ed. Ames, IA: Iowa State University Press, 1994:115.

Gentry PA, Feldman BF, O'Neill SL, Madigan JE, Zinkl JG. Evaluation of the haemostatic profile in the pre- and postparturient mare, with particular focus on the perinatal period. Equine Vet J 1992;24:33–36.

Taylor FGR, Hillyer JH. Diagnostic techniques in equine medicine. London: WB Saunders, 1997.

Author Dina A. Andrews

Consulting Editor Claire B. Andreasen

PROTEIN, HYPERPROTEINEMIA

BASICS

DEFINITION

• Higher-than-normal concentration of all plasma proteins (i.e., panhyperproteinemia), absolute increase in globulins (i.e., hyperglobulinemia), or increase in fibrinogen (i.e., hyperfibrinogenemia)
• Globulin proteins include α_1, α_2, β_1, β_2, and γ globulins. The γ globulins include the immunoglobulins.
• Paraproteins are immunoglobulins produced by neoplastic immune cells, such as plasma cells in cases of multiple myeloma.

PATHOPHYSIOLOGY

Panhyperproteinemia

• Most commonly results from loss of the fluid component of blood because of decreased fluid intake or excessive fluid loss, such as dehydration, which causes hyperproteinemia with an associated increase in PCV.
• A hemoconcentrated patient that is concurrently anemic has hyperproteinemia with a normal or decreased PCV.
• Dehydration initially causes a shift of tissue fluid into the intravascular space as the body attempts to maintain adequate blood volume. As dehydration persists, however, intravascular fluid is lost, resulting in hemoconcentration with a relative increase in total protein.
• If renal function is adequate, urine output decreases to compensate for the fluid loss, and urine concentration increases.
• Water is absorbed from the GI tract, assuming that GI function is normal.
• Dehydration secondary to decreased fluid intake can occur with restricted access to water, dysphagia, or lack of thirst caused by depression or toxemia. More commonly, dehydration occurs after excessive fluid loss, particularly with diarrhea, or loss from the vascular space via excessive sweating, fluid sequestration subsequent to intestinal obstruction, polyuria with renal failure, and exudation from extensive skin wounds—burns.
• With hyperproteinemia in a patient having normal hydration, hyperglobulinemia should be anticipated, because hyperalbuminemia only occurs after dehydration.

Hyperglobulinemia

• Relative (i.e., secondary to hemoconcentration) or absolute
• The absolute form occurs in animals with immunostimulation resulting in hepatic synthesis of acute-phase proteins and plasma cell synthesis of immunoglobulins.
• Serum protein electrophoresis is required to quantitate the individual protein fractions.
• Most commonly caused by an increased γ globulin concentration—polyclonal gammopathy. This arises from the activity of plasma cells producing several immunoglobulins, usually in response to chronic antigenic stimulation.
• IgM migrates in the β-globulin region, and polyclonal increases in β globulins usually are associated with increased γ globulins.
• Abscessation, chronic infection, amyloidosis, and neoplasia typically result in increased γ globulins.
• A marked increase in γ-globulin concentration often is noted with hepatic abscessation, chronic hepatitis, and highly suppurative disease processes reflecting the severity of the disease and intensity of the antigenic response. A concomitant decrease in albumin commonly occurs.

Neoplastic Diseases

• Animals with neoplastic diseases that synthesize a single type of immunoglobulin in large quantities develop a monoclonal gammopathy, in which serum protein electrophoresis reveals a monoclonal peak as sharp as, or sharper than, the albumin peak. This represents a single clone of plasma cells producing an increased amount of immunoglobulin.
• Monoclonal gammopathies can be caused by multiple myeloma, lymphocytic leukemia, and lymphosarcoma; however, lymphosarcoma and other tumors can result in either monoclonal or polyclonal gammopathies.

Fibrinogen

• A large-molecular-weight protein synthesized by the liver that serves primarily as substrate for thrombin to form fibrin during hemostasis.
• As an acute-phase reactant protein, fibrinogen increases in concentration during active inflammation and provides a useful marker for assessment of the inflammatory response.
• Plasma fibrinogen almost always increases during severe inflammatory disease and may increase with mild to moderate inflammation not associated with leukocytosis or neutrophilia.
• Chronic inflammation is associated with increased fibrinogen concentrations as long as the inflammation is active; however, the degree of hyperfibrinogenemia does not always correlate with the severity of disease.

SYSTEMS AFFECTED

N/A

SIGNALMENT

Hyperglobulinemia associated with a monoclonal gammopathy secondary to neoplasia is more likely in older animals.

SIGNS

General Comments

• No pathognomonic signs for hyperproteinemia
• Physical findings associated with dehydration, chronic infection, or neoplasia warrant hematologic and serum chemistry evaluation, which may demonstrate hyperproteinemia.

Historical Findings

• Fever, decreased appetite, cough, nasal discharge, respiratory distress, exercise intolerance, poor performance, diarrhea, GI dysfunction, and weight loss may be noted by owners.
• A history of any of the above warrants further diagnostic evaluation.

PROTEIN, HYPERPROTEINEMIA

Physical Examination Findings

Clinical signs of dehydration include decreased capillary perfusion, as demonstrated by increased capillary refill time in the oral mucous membranes, decreased pulse pressure, tachycardia, decreased skin elasticity, and decreased urine output.

CAUSES

Panhyperproteinemia

- Dehydration
- Acute toxic colitis
- Salmonellosis
- Potomac horse fever
- Intestinal clostridiosis
- Intestinal strangulating obstruction
- Proximal enteritis
- Gram-negative sepsis/endotoxemia
- Botulism
- Esophageal obstruction—"choke"
- Chronic renal failure
- Chronic hepatic disease
- Guttural pouch mycosis with dysphagia
- EPM
- Salt toxicity
- Toxic plant ingestion
- Lead toxicity
- Yellow star thistle poisoning—dysphagia
- Dysphagia—idiopathic

Hyperglobulinemia

- Abdominal (mesenteric) abscess
- Chronic peritonitis
- Pulmonary abscess
- Chronic pleuritis
- Purpura hemorrhagica
- Strangles
- EIA
- Chronic hepatic disease
- Strongylosis
- Lymphosarcoma
- Immune-mediated disease
- Chronic inflammation

Hyperfibrinogenemia

- Abscessation
- Peritonitis
- Pleuritis
- Pneumonia
- Osteomyelitis
- Septic arthritis
- Cholelithiasis
- Neoplasia with associated inflammation
- Vasculitis—equine purpura hemorrhagica
- Cellulitis
- GI inflammation
- Salmonellosis

RISK FACTORS

Hyperproteinemia is associated with dehydration, inflammation, or neoplasia

DIAGNOSIS

DIFFERENTIAL DIAGNOSIS

- Evidence of dehydration (e.g., decreased capillary refill time, dry mucous membranes, decreased skin turgor, sunken eyes) supports relative hyperproteinemia.
- Signs of inflammation or infection suggest hyperglobulinemia and hyperfibrinogenemia as the causes of the hyperproteinemia.
- Weight loss in old patients warrants consideration of neoplasia.

LABORATORY FINDINGS

Drugs that May Alter Lab Results

N/A

Disorders that May Alter Lab Results

- Dehydration and hemoconcentration increase globulins and albumin.
- Hyperlipemia and hyperlipidemia increases globulins.

Valid If Run in Human Lab?

- Globulin values are accurate; albumin determination is not.
- Human labs often do not routinely include fibrinogen determination.

PROTEIN, HYPERPROTEINEMIA

CBC/BIOCHEMISTRY/URINALYSIS

- Increased PCV, albumin concentration, and urine specific gravity support dehydration.
- Normal or decreased PCV may indicate concomitant anemia with dehydration or infectious/inflammatory disease.

OTHER LABORATORY TESTS

- Serum protein electrophoresis to quantitate individual protein fractions encountered in hyperglobulinemic patients and to differentiate polyclonal from monoclonal gammopathies.
- Immunoelectrophoresis to identify specific immunoglobulins in patients demonstrating monoclonal gammopathy
- Appropriate tests for infectious or inflammatory diseases that can cause hyperproteinemia may be necessary to establish a definitive diagnosis.
- Fibrinogen level can be valuable in detecting newborn foals that have been infected or exposed to inflammatory placental disease in utero. In these cases, fibrinogen levels at birth may be $\geq$1000 mg/dL (normal $\leq$300 mg/dL), whereas during the early stages of postnatal acquired infections, levels may be only mildly increased (400–500 mg/dL). With chronicity, the inflammatory process causes dramatic increases in fibrinogen. In contrast to other species, horses with DIC commonly have normal to increased fibrinogen concentrations.

IMAGING

Ultrasonography and radiography of the thorax, abdomen, or soft tissue may help to identify the cause or to direct further diagnostic evaluations necessary to establish a definitive diagnosis.

DIAGNOSTIC PROCEDURES

- Abdominocentesis, thoracocentesis, transtracheal aspiration or bronchoalveolar lavage, endoscopy, laparoscopy, bone marrow aspiration, CSF evaluation, biopsy, and histopathology
- Selection of these diagnostic procedures depends on physical examination and laboratory findings.

TREATMENT

- Severity of dehydration and electrolyte imbalances dictate whether patients are candidates for PO versus IV fluid administration and the aggressiveness of the therapy administered.
- Address sources of fluid loss (e.g., diarrhea, intestinal obstruction, pleuropneumonia) with appropriate medical or surgical treatment.

MEDICATIONS

DRUGS OF CHOICE

N/A

CONTRAINDICATIONS

N/A

PRECAUTIONS

N/A

POSSIBLE INTERACTIONS

N/A

ALTERNATIVE DRUGS

N/A

FOLLOW-UP

PATIENT MONITORING

- Clinical evaluation of hydration status using mucous membrane color and capillary refill time three to four times daily in critical cases
- Laboratory evaluation using PCV and total protein determination twice daily
- Adjust frequency of monitoring based on severity of the case and clinical response to therapy.

POSSIBLE COMPLICATIONS

Complications directly relate to the cause of the hyperproteinemia.

PROTEIN, HYPERPROTEINEMIA

MISCELLANEOUS

ASSOCIATED CONDITIONS

Hyperglobulinemia commonly is associated with hyperalbuminemia.

AGE-RELATED FACTORS

- Passive transfer of immunoglobulins during colostrum absorption increases the total protein concentration of newborns; with time, the passively absorbed immunoglobulins decrease through natural catabolic degradation.
- Adult protein concentrations remain relatively stable.

ZOONOTIC POTENTIAL

N/A

PREGNANCY

- Fetal development stresses the maternal protein reserve, resulting in an increased globulin concentration with a concomitantly decreased albumin concentration.
- Serum immunoglobulin concentrations increase in the dam until ≅1 month before term, when the proteins rapidly leave the plasma to form colostrum in the mammary gland. Immunoglobulins are not produced locally in the mammary gland.
- Most immunoglobulin in equine colostrum is IgG.
- At birth, foals have specialized enterocytes in the GI tract that allow absorption of large molecules (e.g., immunoglobulins) by pinocytosis. This absorptive ability only lasts from birth to 18–24 hours of age and is greatest during the first 6–12 hours. The specialized enterocytes then are shed from the GI lining and replaced by more mature cells.

SYNONYMS

- Gammopathy
- Hypergammaglobulinemia

SEE ALSO

Refer to individual conditions and diseases causing hemoconcentration (i.e., dehydration), hyperglobulinemia, and hyperfibrinogenemia.

ABBREVIATIONS

- CSF = cerebrospinal fluid
- DIC = disseminated intravascular coagulation
- EIA = equine infectious anemia
- EPM = equine protozoal myelitis
- GI = gastrointestinal
- PCV = packed cell volume

Suggested Reading

Kobluk CN, Ames TR, Geor RJ, eds. The horse: diseases and clinical management. Philadelphia: WB Saunders Company, 1995.

Meyer DJ, Coles EH, Rich LJ. Veterinary laboratory medicine. Philadelphia: WB Saunders, 1992.

Smith BP. Large animal internal medicine. St. Louis: CV Mosby, 1990.

Author Kent A. Humber

Consulting Editor Claire B. Andreasen

PROTEIN, HYPOPROTEINEMIA

BASICS

DEFINITION

• A lower-than-normal concentration of all plasma proteins (i.e., panhypoproteinemia), an absolute decrease in globulins (i.e., hypoglobulinemia), or a decrease in fibrinogen (i.e., hypofibrinogenemia)
• Globulin proteins include alpha$_1$, alpha$_2$, beta$_1$, beta$_2$, and gamma globulins.
• Gamma globulins include the immunoglobulins.
• Hypoalbuminemia is discussed as a separate topic (see *Albumin*).

PATHOPHYSIOLOGY

Panhypoproteinemia

• Most commonly results from vigorous fluid therapy or excess water intake, resulting in dilution of plasma proteins.
• The condition frequently occurs in animals with acute protein-losing colitis/enteritis treated with IV fluids.
• Horses that lose large amounts of sodium in diarrhea and then drink fresh water may become hyponatremic because of a relative water excess.

Acute Blood Loss

• Results in loss of plasma proteins from the vascular compartment in addition to dilution of the remaining protein by rapid movement of interstitial fluid into the intravascular space to help maintain a sufficient circulatory volume.
• This dilutional effect is exacerbated by the excess water intake that commonly occurs after acute blood loss.
• Rule out acute hemorrhage secondary to trauma, epistaxis, or internal vascular erosion, or rupture out in hypoproteinemic, anemic patients.

GI Blood Loss

• Can result from GI ulceration, blood-sucking parasites, viral or bacterial infection, azotemia, neoplastic invasion, or exposure to caustic chemicals.
• Use of NSAIDs can result in hemorrhage or exudation of plasma with resultant hypoproteinemia.
• Strangulating GI obstructions and infarctions may cause mucosal necrosis with leakage of plasma proteins into the gut lumen.
• Protein-losing enteropathy initially results in hypoalbuminemia, but panhypoproteinemia eventually will occur.

Urinary Trace Blood Loss

• Can occur from congenital vascular disorders, renal trauma, renal calculi, pyelonephritis, neoplasia, or cystic calculi.
• Coagulation dysfunction (e.g., DIC or immune-mediated thrombocytopenia) also may cause blood loss.

Congestive Heart Failure

• Results in dilution of extracellular fluid by retained sodium and water, with concomitant loss of plasma protein into the interstitial spaces, ascitic fluid, and GI tract.
• Reduced food intake, inadequate protein absorption, and inadequate hepatic synthesis contribute to hypoproteinemia.
• Acute severe peritonitis or pleuritis with massive protein exudation can result in hypoproteinemia.

Infectious Disease

• Can occur from failure of the host defense systems and from overwhelming external challenge.
• The role of host defense mechanisms should be explored in patients with repeated infections or chronic symptoms.
• Successful protection from disease results from numerous cell types and soluble serum factors.

T and B Cells

• Required for cell-mediated immune responses that protect against fungal, protozoal, intracellular bacterial, and many viral infections.
• Regulate the immune response through the action of helper T cells and suppressor T cells, which augment and depress immune responses, respectively.
• B lymphocytes are the precursors of plasma cells and produce immunoglobulins. Classes of immunoglobulins produced by horses are IgG, IgM, IgA, and IgG(T), which provide defense against extracellular bacterial and some viral infections.
• Deficiency of functional T cells, B cells, and/or nonspecific components predispose to infection and, possibly, death.
• Clinical features associated with immunodeficiencies include infections during the first 6 weeks of life, repeated infections that respond poorly to standard therapy, increased susceptibility to low-grade pathogens, infection with organisms rarely observed in immunocompetent individuals, systemic illness after vaccination, and persistent deficiencies in leukocyte levels—lymphopenia or neutropenia
• Laboratory or special in vivo testing is required to confirm and to define an immunodeficiency disorder, because clinical signs are nonspecific.

PROTEIN, HYPOPROTEINEMIA

Normal Foals

• Immunocompetent at birth but immunologically naïve, because they have not had any exposure to antigens or mounted any type of protective immune response.
• Essentially devoid of immunoglobulins, except for a small amount of IgM normally produced in utero.
• Immunoglobulins are detected within 1–2 weeks after birth and reach significant levels by 2 months of age.
• Temporary protection against infection is provided by passively transferred antibody in colostrum. No transplacental transfer of immunoglobulins occurs in horses. Presuckle serum, therefore, normally does not contain IgG, IgG(T), or IgA.

Fibrinogen

• A large-molecular-weight protein synthesized by the liver
• Serves primarily as substrate for thrombin to form fibrin during hemostasis.
• Hypofibrinogenemia may result from increased consumption or decreased production.
• Severe, diffuse liver damage (e.g., cases of pyrrolizidine alkaloid toxicity) causes decreased fibrinogen, whereas mild to moderate inflammatory disease usually causes increased fibrinogen.
• Hypofibrinogenemia is not common in horses with DIC, because inflammatory disease often is the initiating cause of a compensatory increase in fibrinogen production, which masks increased fibrinogen consumption.
• Rapid removal of fibrinogen from the circulation rarely occurs because of primary hyperfibrinolysis.
• Falsely decreased fibrinogen levels should be suspected if fibrinogen concentrations are quantitated from samples containing clotted blood.

SYSTEM AFFECTED

Hypoglobulinemia may reflect immunodeficiency and warrants further diagnostic evaluation.

SIGNALMENT

• Neonates with hypoproteinemia, particularly hypoglobulinemia, should be investigated for FPT.
• Without obvious hemorrhage, adult horses with a history of chronic infections or "poor doers" should be evaluated for immunodeficiency.

SIGNS

General Comments

• No pathognomonic signs for hypoproteinemia
• Physical findings associated with colitis/enteritis, peritonitis, pleuritis, hemorrhage, and weight loss warrant hematologic and serum chemistry evaluation, which may demonstrate hypoproteinemia.

Historical Findings

Fever, decreased appetite, cough, nasal discharge, respiratory distress, exercise intolerance, poor performance, diarrhea, GI dysfunction, dysuria, weight loss, or a history of prolonged NSAID administration warrants further diagnostic evaluation.

Physical Examination Findings

• Findings reflect the underlying cause and contributing factors.
• Abnormal findings are not specific.

CAUSES

Panhypoproteinemia

• Excessive fluid therapy or water intake
• Acute blood loss
• GI ulceration
• Strangulating GI obstruction/infarction
• Protein-losing enteropathy
• Acute severe peritonitis
• NSAID toxicity
• Acute severe pleuritis
• Glomerulonephritis
• Parasitism
• Intestinal lymphosarcoma
• Urinary blood loss—congenital vascular disorders, renal trauma, renal calculi, pyelonephritis, neoplasia, or cystic calculi
• DIC
• Immune-mediated thrombocytopenia
• Congestive heart failure

Hypoglobulinemia

• FPT
• Combined immunodeficiency
• Selective IgM deficiency
• Transient hypogammaglobulinemia
• Agammaglobulinemia
• Adult acquired immunodeficiency

Hypofibrinogenemia

• Impaired hepatic synthesis—rare
• DIC—fibrinogen levels usually normal or increased
• Primary hyperfibrinolysis—rare
• Uncompensated loss during massive hemorrhage

Hypoalbuminemia

See *Albumin.*

RISK FACTORS

Often associated with aggressive IV fluid therapy, FPT, or immunodeficiency.

PROTEIN, HYPOPROTEINEMIA

DIAGNOSIS

DIFFERENTIAL DIAGNOSIS

• In hypoproteinemic newborn foals, rule out FPT.
• In adults with chronic infection, consider immunodeficiency.
• Consider infectious diseases causing accumulation of protein-containing fluids in body cavities (e.g., pleuritis, peritonitis) or protein loss (e.g., protein-losing enteropathy).

LABORATORY FINDINGS

Drugs That May Alter Lab Results

N/A

Disorders That May Alter Lab Results

N/A

Valid If Run in Human Lab?

• Globulin values will be accurate; albumin determination will not.
• Human labs often do not routinely include fibrinogen determination.

CBC/BIOCHEMISTRY/URINALYSIS

A compensatory increase in albumin often is noted with decreased globulin concentrations.

OTHER LABORATORY TESTS

• Characterization of the equine immune system is limited to quantitation of immunoglobulins, detection of specific antibody response to immunization, skin testing, quantitation of peripheral lymphocyte numbers, and histopathologic examination of lymphoid organs.
• The only practical tests of B-cell function are quantitation of immunoglobulins and measurement of specific antibody responses.
• Methods are available to quantitate or semiquantitate immunoglobulin levels.
• Semiquantitative methods are useful to demonstrate conditions such as FPT but do not provide information on specific immunoglobulin classes.
• Test kits based on precipitation of immunoglobulins with specific concentrations of salts are available commercially.
• Serum electrophoresis is used to quantitate gamma globulins, which are primarily immunoglobulins.
• Other methods based on antigen–antibody reactions that use latex bead agglutination or enzyme immunoassay are available commercially.
• Radial immunodiffusion quantitates specific classes of immunoglobulins.
• Specialized immunologic evaluation using techniques such as fluorescent-antibody labeling and in vitro blastogenesis are available at many veterinary schools and research facilities.
• Occult blood tests can be used to demonstrate blood in feces when not grossly apparent.
• Appropriate tests for infectious or inflammatory diseases may be necessary to establish a definitive diagnosis.

IMAGING

Ultrasonography and radiography of the thorax, abdomen, or soft tissue may be helpful in identifying a cause or directing further diagnostics necessary to establish at a definitive diagnosis.

DIAGNOSTIC PROCEDURES

• Abdominocentesis
• Thoracocentesis
• Transtracheal aspiration or bronchoalveolar lavage
• Endoscopy
• Laparoscopy
• Bone marrow aspiration
• CSF evaluation
• Biopsy
• Histopathology
• Select based on physical examination and laboratory findings

TREATMENT

• Address sources of blood or protein loss (e.g., hemorrhage, diarrhea, intestinal obstruction, pleuropneumonia) with appropriate medical or surgical treatment.
• FPT requires administration of colostrum or plasma, depending on patient age.
• Therapy for immunodeficient patients is supportive, because no specific treatment is available.

MEDICATIONS

DRUGS OF CHOICE

• Oral colostrum is suggested before closure of the specialized enterocytes in the GI tract in cases of FPT.
• If equine colostrum is unavailable, bovine colostrum, equine plasma, or lyophilized equine IgG can be administered PO.
• IV administration of equine plasma is required after closure of the enterocytes.

CONTRAINDICATIONS

N/A

PRECAUTIONS

• Anaphylactic reactions can occur during IV plasma administration.
• Give a test dose of plasma slowly IV, and monitor patients closely during treatment.

POSSIBLE INTERACTIONS

N/A

ALTERNATIVE DRUGS

N/A

PROTEIN, HYPOPROTEINEMIA

FOLLOW-UP

PATIENT MONITORING
• Perform clinical evaluation three to four times daily in critical cases.
• Laboratory evaluation using PCV and total protein determination is recommended twice daily.
• Adjust frequency of monitoring based on severity of the case and clinical response to therapy.

POSSIBLE COMPLICATIONS
• Complications relate directly to the cause.
• Dependent and pulmonary edema is possible in cases of hypoalbuminemia (see **Hypoalbuminemia**).

MISCELLANEOUS

ASSOCIATED CONDITIONS
Often associated with hypoalbuminemia

AGE-RELATED FACTORS
• Neonates have lower protein levels than adults.
• Specific evaluation of immunoglobulin status may be necessary to determine if a pathologic process is present.

ZOONOTIC POTENTIAL
N/A

PREGNANCY
N/A

SYNONYMS
• Gammopathy
• Hypogammaglobulinemia

SEE ALSO
• Refer to individual conditions and diseases causing hypoglobulinemia and hypofibrinogenemia.
• Hypoalbuminemia

ABBREVIATIONS
• CSF = cerebrospinal fluid
• DIC = disseminated intravascular coagulopathy
• GI = gastrointestinal
• PCV = packed cell volume

Suggested Reading

Kobluk CN, Ames TR, Geor RJ, eds. The horse: diseases and clinical management. Philadelphia: WB Saunders, 1995.
Meyer DJ, Coles EH, Rich LJ. Veterinary laboratory medicine. Philadelphia: WB Saunders, 1992.
Smith BP. Large animal internal medicine. St. Louis: C V Mosby, 1990.

Author Kent A. Humber
Consulting Editor Claire B. Andreasen

PROTEIN-LOSING ENTEROPATHY (PLE)

BASICS

OVERVIEW

Normally, the intestinal capillary endothelium allows a small amount of protein to enter the mucosal interstitium; however, the movement of protein and fluid into the intestinal lumen is restricted by the tight intercellular bridges between the mucosal epithelial cells. Plasma proteins such as albumin are present in low concentrations in normal gastrointestinal secretions, and protein usually undergoes complete degradation within the intestinal lumen. In the protein-losing enteropathies (PLEs), the normal intestinal protein losses are substantially increased. The pathophysiologic mechanisms of gastrointestinal protein loss include mucosal ulceration and plasma exudation, lymphatic obstruction with leakage and rupture of dilated lacteals, passive diffusion through intracellular spaces, active secretion by mucosal cells, intracellular loss, increased permeability of capillaries and venules, and disordered cell metabolism.

The excessive loss of proteins into the gastrointestinal tract causes hypoproteinemia, especially hypoalbuminemia. If severe, hypoalbuminemia may result in the development of subcutaneous edema of the ventral thorax, abdomen, and distal extremities. The early intestinal protein loss in PLE involves relatively larger quantities of albumin than globulins. In the later stages of the disease, all protein fractions may be lost. Feces are frequently normal in consistency, especially if large colon function is not impaired.

PLE is usually a progressive condition; however, accelerated protein leakage can occur in acute gastrointestinal diseases such as salmonellosis.

SIGNALMENT

- Granulomatous enteritis (GE) and eosinophilic gastroenteritis are most common in young adult horses (range 1–5 yr). Standardbreds are more frequently affected with GE.
- Intestinal lymphosarcoma and intestinal parasitism may occur in horses of all ages.
- Gastric squamous cell carcinoma affects mainly older horses.
- Ponies and young animals are reportedly more susceptible to NSAID toxicity.
- *Lawsonia intracellularis* in weanling foals
- Severe gastric ulceration in young (1–3 yr) racehorses

SIGNS

The clinical signs of PLE depend on the nature of the gastrointestinal disease and the severity of the hypoproteinemia. Affected animals show some of the following signs:

- Chronic, progressive weight loss
- Dependent edema (involving ventral thorax, ventral body wall, distal extremities)
- Depression
- Anorexia
- Reduced performance
- Lethargy
- Intermittent colic (variable)
- Diarrhea is not present in PLE cases with lesions primarily in the small intestine because the colon can effectively absorb electrolytes and water
- Focal alopecia and a thin or rough haircoat may be present
- Enlarged peripheral lymph nodes in some cases
- Acute colic and signs of endotoxemia may occur in horses with intestinal parasitism or NSAID toxicity
- On perrectal examination, may be able to palpate enlarged mesenteric lymph nodes and thickened bowel wall in some PLE cases
- Occasionally, pharyngeal and laryngeal edema may develop in severely hypoproteinemic animals and may produce an upper airway obstruction.
- Pain after eating may be observed in some horses with gastric squamous cell carcinoma.

CAUSES AND RISK FACTORS

Diseases that have been most commonly associated with PLE include granulomatous enteritis, gastrointestinal neoplasia (lymphosarcoma, squamous cell carcinoma), chronic eosinophilic gastroenteritis, parasitic thrombosis of the cranial mesenteric artery (Strongylus vulgaris), cyanthostomiasis (occurs when third- and fourth-stage larvae of small strongyles are embedded in the mucosa of the cecum or colon), non-steroidal anti-inflammatory drug (NSAID) toxicity, acute salmonellosis, other causes of acute enterocolitis, and congestive heart failure.

DIAGNOSIS

DIFFERENTIAL DIAGNOSIS

The diagnosis of PLE is usually made after protein loss through other routes (e.g. urine, into body cavities such as thorax and abdomen) and inability to synthesize protein (liver disease) are ruled out.

CBC/BIOCHEMISTRY/URINALYSIS

- Hypoalbuminemia
- Decreased, normal, or increased plasma globulin concentrations
- Serum protein electrophoresis is the preferred test for quantifying protein fractions
- Panhypoproteinemia
- Hypocalcemia may occur in conjunction with hypoalbuminemia because a large portion of serum calcium is protein bound
- Anemia

OTHER LABORATORY TESTS

- Fecal examination for parasitic ova and larvae
- Fecal occult blood test may be positive in horses with gastrointestinal blood loss from gastric squamous cell carcinoma, intestinal parasitism, or iatrogenic following rectal examination
- Oral D-xylose absorption test (0.5 g/kg as a 10% solution) is preferable to the oral glucose tolerance test (1 g/kg as a 20% solution) as an indicator of small intestine absorptive function
- Abdominocentesis—cytology to check for evidence of neoplasia. Intestinal lymphosarcoma occasionally exfoliates into the peritoneal fluid. A normal abdominal fluid does not rule out neoplasia.

PROTEIN-LOSING ENTEROPATHY (PLE)

IMAGING

N/A

OTHER DIAGNOSTIC PROCEDURES

- Immunoelectrophoresis
- Fiberoptic gastroduodenoscopy to visualize stomach and duodenum
- Rectal mucosal biopsy maybe useful in the diagnosis of granulomatous enteritis, eosinophilic enteritis, or lymphosarcoma
- Exploratory laparotomy and intestinal biopsy often necessary for definitive diagnosis
- Increased fecal radioactivity following of [^{51}Cr] albumin documents gastrointestinal protein loss. However, this can be a difficult test to conduct due to the restrictions associated with the use of radiolabeled compounds and the difficulties in the disposal of radioactive feces and urine.

TREATMENT

Because the condition is usually well advanced when the first clinical signs are recognized, the prognosis for recovery is poor and treatment is frequently unrewarding.

MEDICATIONS

Treatment depends on the primary disease causing PLE or treating the hypoproteinemia.

DRUG(S) OF CHOICE

- Plasma transfusion is usually indicated when total plasma protein concentration is or falls below 40 g/L (4 g/dL). The effect may be minimal due to the continued protein losses.
- If horse is receiving NSAIDs, therapy should be discontinued.
- When internal parasites are suspected as the cause of PLE, administer larvicidal anthelmintics (moxidectin 0.4 mg/kg PO; ivermectin 0.2 mg/kg PO; or fenbendazole 10 mg/kg SID PO for 5 days).
- Total parenteral nutrition may be indicated in valuable horses.

DIET

Dietary management—feed pelleted feed and restrict roughage. Provide palatable, easily assimilated, high-energy and -protein sources supplying electrolyte mixtures to include calcium, magnesium, and to a lesser extent, zinc, copper, and iron, and supplementing fat- and water-soluble vitamins.

CONTRAINDICATIONS/POSSIBLE INTERACTIONS

N/A

FOLLOW-UP

- Monitor total serum protein and albumin concentrations
- Monitor body weight

MISCELLANEOUS

ABBREVIATION

- GE = granulomatous enteritis
- PLE = protein-losing enteropathy

Suggested Reading

Morris DD, Vaala WE, Sartin E. Protein-losing enteropathy in a yearling filly with subclinical disseminated intravascular coagulation and autoimmune hemolytic disease. Compend Contin Educ Pract Vet 1982;4:S542-S546.

Roberts MC. Protein-losing enteropathy in the horse. Compend Contin Educ Pract Vet 1983;5:S550-S556.

Author John D. Baird

Consulting Editor Henry Stämpfli

PROTOZOAL MYELOENCEPHALITIS (PM)

BASICS

DEFINITION
An often debilitating, multifocal, neurologic disease caused by protozoal infection of the CNS

PATHOPHYSIOLOGY
- The primary causative agent is *Sarcocystis neurona.*
- Infection results from ingestion of the infective stage of the parasite (i.e., sporocysts) in food or water contaminated by the feces of infected opossums, the definitive host.
- Sporocysts excyst in the horse's small intestine, releasing sporozoites that penetrate the intestinal lining and enter the bloodstream. Parasites appear to gain access to the CNS by direct penetration of the blood–brain barrier. Passive entry within WBCs also may occur.
- Individual parasites (i.e., merozoites) multiply within neurons and leukocytes, resulting in cell death.
- Clinical signs result from direct neuronal loss and inflammation and swelling, which disrupt normal CNS architecture, compromise blood flow, and reduce oxygen delivery.
- Severity of clinical signs depends on the number and location of parasitic foci and the horse's ability to limit protozoal multiplication.

SYSTEMS AFFECTED
- Nervous—multifocal CNS infection results in variable sensory, motor, and cognitive dysfunction.
- Neuromuscular—discrete, neurogenic muscle atrophy and weakness are common; various cranial nerve deficits
- Musculoskeletal—occasional secondary injuries and soreness from ataxia and asymmetric muscle weakness/atrophy
- Skin—discrete areas of sensory loss and sweating
- GI—cranial nerve signs associated with prehension, mastication, and swallowing; loss of anal tone
- Respiratory—laryngeal hemiplegia and pneumonia secondary to dysphagia
- Ophthalmic—loss of ocular reflexes and blindness
- Renal/urologic—urinary incontinence

GENETICS
Unknown

INCIDENCE/PREVALENCE
- A New World disease; not reported in horses native to the Eastern Hemisphere
- Seroprevalence studies indicate that ≅45% of horses from the west coast and eastern half of the United States have been exposed to *S. neurona.* Nonetheless, the incidence of clinical disease appears to be <1%.

SIGNALMENT

Species
Horses

Breed Predilection
All breeds are susceptible to infection, but Thoroughbreds and Standardbreds most frequently are affected.

Mean Age and Sex
- Horses may be affected at any age, but 60% of cases confirmed at postmortem have involved horses younger than 4 years.
- Recent retrospective and case-controlled prospective studies indicate that the average age among clinically affected horses approaches 8 years.

Predominant Sex
N/A

SIGNS

General Comments
Clinical signs may be peracute to chronic, mild to severe, and are highly variable, depending on the location of infected foci within the CNS.

Historical Findings
- Apparent lameness from asymmetric ataxia and muscle weakness is the most common clinical complaint.
- Muscle atrophy, sore back, and various cranial nerve signs (e.g., headtilt, facial paralysis) also may be reported.

Physical Examination Findings
- A complete neurologic examination frequently reveals asymmetric ataxia from proprioceptive and motor deficits.
- Additional signs—localized muscle atrophy, various cranial nerve signs (e.g., headtilt, facial paralysis, diminished ocular reflexes, poor prehension, mastication or dysphagia, laryngeal hemiplegia), urinary incontinence, localized sweating, seizure
- Affected horses usually are bright and alert.

CAUSES
- *S. neurona*
- *Neospora caninum*

RISK FACTORS
- Stress
- Corticosteroid use

DIAGNOSIS

DIFFERENTIAL DIAGNOSIS
- EPM may mimic any equine neurologic disease and often must be differentiated from lameness.
- CSM affects young male horses, has similar breed predilection, and usually produces symmetric ataxia.
- Trauma frequently causes neurologic dysfunction, but external evidence of injury and anatomic localization to a single area of the CNS are common.
- EDM, which is common in the northeastern United States, causes progressive, symmetric ataxia (frequently posterior) and weakness in horses younger than 2 years.
- Equine herpes myeloencephalopathy typically affects more than one horse in a group and often follows respiratory disease. It produces symmetric, posterior ataxia and weakness, bladder dysfunction, and loss of tail and anal tone.
- Additional diseases that infrequently may require differentiation—Lyme disease, botulism, leukoencephalomalacia, otitis media/interna, temporohyoid osteoarthropathy, epilepsy, narcolepsy, verminous encephalomyelitis, EMND, cauda equina syndrome, polyneuritis equi, viral encephalitides, rabies, bacterial or fungal CNS infections, hepatic encephalopathy, epidural abscess, neoplasia, and ingestion of toxic plants or chemicals

CBC/BIOCHEMISTRY/URINALYSIS
Standard laboratory tests typically are within normal limits.

OTHER LABORATORY TESTS

- Biochemical and cellular analysis of CSF typically is within normal limits.
- Serum may be tested for *S. neurona*–specific antibodies by immunoblot analysis (i.e., EPM test). Serum antibodies indicate exposure to *S. neurona,* but not necessarily clinical disease.
- The positive predictive value of the EPM test for serum samples from a population of 295 horses that died from neurologic disease was only 72% because of a high *S. neurona* exposure rate among horses in the group with other neurologic diseases. The negative predictive value was 88%.
- The positive predictive value of the EPM test for CSF samples from the same population of horses was 89%. The negative predictive value for CSF samples was 92%. Sensitivity and specificity for the test were both 89%. Note that the positive predictive value was derived from a population of horses with a 40% incidence of EPM.
- The reliability of the positive predictive value of any test depends on the incidence of the disease in the population tested. The expected positive predictive value for any test with 89% sensitivity and specificity in a population with a 1% incidence of disease is approximately 8%. Therefore, appropriate interpretation of positive CSF test results from normal horses is not possible (incidence of EPM <1%). The negative predictive value, however, remains very high.
- The primary reason for false-positive CSF test results among horses with neurologic disease is contamination with serum antibodies. Total albumin in CSF, albumin quotient ([CSF albumin]/[serum albumin]), and IgG index ([CSF IgG]/[serum IgG] × [serum albumin]/[CSF albumin]) should be performed to help assess CSF quality and to aid subsequent interpretation of EPM test results.
- A PCR test for detection of *S. neurona* DNA in CSF is available but lacks sensitivity because of the infrequent presence of parasite DNA in the CSF of affected horses.

IMAGING

- EPM does not produce radiographic changes, but several neurologic diseases may be differentiated with radiography of the head and neck.
- Myelography often is important for an accurate diagnosis of CSM.
- CT and MRI are useful in the diagnosis of EPM, but their availability for equine diagnostic use is severely limited.
- Nuclear scintigraphy, ultrasonography, and thermography are useful to differentiate lameness.

DIAGNOSTIC PROCEDURES

- Neurologic disease may be confirmed at EMG and EEG, but specific changes associated with EPM are unknown.
- Biopsy of the spinal accessory nerve may help to confirm EMND.
- Local and regional nerve blocks help to differentiate lameness.

PATHOLOGIC FINDINGS

- Gross lesions occur infrequently. When present, small areas of hemorrhage to pale discoloration may be observed most commonly in the gray and white matter of the brainstem and spinal cord.
- Histopathologic changes include focal to diffuse areas of nonsuppurative inflammation and necrosis, with perivascular infiltration of mononuclear cells, axonal degeneration, and neovascularization.

TREATMENT

APPROPRIATE HEALTH CARE

Severely affected horses may be recumbent and require constant care or hospitalization.

NURSING CARE

Severely ataxic horses should be confined in a heavily bedded box stall.

ACTIVITY

- The amount of appropriate activity varies for each horse, but prolonged inactivity does not enhance recovery.
- Light exercise is appropriate as improvement warrants.
- Work may be increased gradually as the horse improves and therapy is completed.
- Avoid overworking horses undergoing treatment.
- Premature return to heavy work may prolong the time to recovery and promote relapse.

DIET

- Standard medication may result in bone marrow suppression and anemia.
- Folinic acid helps to prevent these side effects in other species, but the cost of supplemental administration for horses is prohibitive.
- High-quality pasture and alfalfa hay are excellent sources of folinic acid and highly recommended during treatment.
- Folic acid is poorly absorbed by the horse. Therefore, folic acid supplementation for prevention or treatment of anemia while administering standard EPM medication is not recommended.
- If life-threatening anemia develops, discontinue standard medication for 2–3 weeks to allow recovery or switch to an alternative medication.

CLIENT EDUCATION

N/A

SURGICAL CONSIDERATIONS

N/A

PROTOZOAL MYELOENCEPHALITIS (PM)

MEDICATIONS

DRUGS OF CHOICE

- The most common medications currently recommended are contained in a commercially prepared, liquid PO formulation of sulfadiazine and pyrimethamine that delivers 20 mg/kg of sulfadiazine and 1.0 mg/kg of pyrimethamine at the recommended dose once daily.
- A second daily dose of sulfadiazine at 20 mg/kg PO 12 hours later has been recommended by some, but whether this has an appreciable effect on response to treatment is unclear.
- Many veterinarians now recommend 1.5–2.0-fold the standard dose of pyrimethamine for the initial treatment or after 30 days without satisfactory progress.
- Sulfa–pyrimethamine combinations should be given on an empty stomach to prevent interference with absorption from the gut. Withhold feed for at least 2 hours before and 1 hour after administration.
- Oral potentiated sulfas (e.g., sulfadiazine, sulfamethoxazole-trimethoprim) at 15–30 mg/kg (combined dose) BID and pyrimethamine at 1.0 mg/kg SID also are effective.
- The need for trimethoprim has been questioned, but many veterinarians believe that horses respond faster and have fewer relapses when trimethoprim is included.
- Medication should be continued for a least 1 month after the horse stops showing further improvement. The average length of treatment based on this rule-of-thumb is approximately 4 months. This regimen appears to work reasonably well, but relapse may occur. According to current estimates, neurologic signs may return within a few weeks or months of therapy in 10%–25% of horses treated.
- Administration of NSAIDs the first 1–2 weeks of treatment and anytime the condition appears to worsen should help to minimize further damage due to parasite death and the host response. Flunixin meglumine (1.1 mg/kg BID) or phenylbutazone most frequently are used. Dimethyl sulfoxide (1.0 g/kg in 10% saline IV SID for 3 days) often is helpful. Severely affected horses often receive moderate doses of dexamethasone parenterally (0.05 mg/kg BID) for 1–3 days; longer-term use may cause immunosuppression. Oral vitamin E supplementation (10–20 IU/kg daily) is recommended to promote CNS healing.

CONTRAINDICATIONS

Known sensitivity to sulfa drugs

PRECAUTIONS

- Increasing the dosage of pyrimethamine may increase the potential for anemia, low WBC counts, and short-term depression.
- Some have suggested that abortion and decreased stallion fertility may occur using standard therapy, but controlled studies have not been done. Avoid higher doses in pregnant mares until more is known regarding the effects of therapy.
- Corticosteroid use should not exceed 1–3 days to avoid exacerbating the disease.

POSSIBLE INTERACTIONS

Use of potentiated sulfas and pyrimethamine may increase the potential for side effects.

ALTERNATIVE DRUGS

Recently, diclazuril and toltrazuril (5–10 mg/kg PO SID for 28 days) have been used to treat horses with EPM. Preliminary trials indicate that the effectiveness of this therapy is comparable to standard therapy and may result in fewer relapses.

FOLLOW-UP

PATIENT MONITORING

- Neurologic examination of affected horses is recommended at monthly intervals during treatment.
- Many veterinarians have attempted to reduce the relapse rate by continuing medication until CSF samples test negative for parasite-specific antibodies. These antibodies should clear the CSF within a few weeks of parasite elimination, but some horses remain CSF positive for an extended period after full recovery or stabilization. The most likely explanation is continued presence of parasites in the CNS. The relapse rate among horses with negative CSF at the time that treatment is stopped has been extremely low; however, not all horses taken off treatment with positive CSF tests will relapse.
- When using standard medication, monthly CBCs are recommended to monitor anemia. It also may be useful to monitor serum folate concentration at monthly intervals.

PROTOZOAL MYELOENCEPHALITIS (PM)

PREVENTION/AVOIDANCE

• A healthy, fit horse is the best protection against many equine diseases. The stress associated with other diseases may provide an ideal opportunity for *S. neurona.* Development of clinical signs appears to relate to the number of sporocysts ingested, but a horse's ability to resist infection should determine the number of sporocysts required. Therefore, all routine preventive health care recommendations apply (e.g., routine vaccinations, regular deworming, proper nutrition, adequate exercise, routine foot care, preventive dental care). Whenever possible, owners should avoid management decisions that introduce significant changes into the horse's physical and social environment.

• The condition and layout of physical facilities can help to avoid injuries and reduce exposure to *S. neurona.* Horse-friendly design and construction as well as routine maintenance help to prevent physical stress from injury and bacterial infection.

• Limit the access of opossums and other wildlife to the horse's environment as much as possible. Individual opossums cover a fairly small territory during their lives (≅1 square mile), are prolific, and have an average life span of 3 years. Because a single female can produce as many as 30 offspring per year, local populations may become dense. Keep the area clean, because opossums eat virtually anything. Keep pet food, garbage, and anything edible (e.g., dead birds and rodents) inaccessible. Store livestock feeds, including hay and grain, away from opossums.

• Long trailer rides are extremely stressful and commonly mentioned in clinical histories of affected horses. Make plans in advance to avoid travel stress. Kepp vaccinations up to date to help avoid stress associated with various contagious diseases, and minimize corticosteroid use to avoid immune suppression. Feed and water supplies at various destinations may be contaminated. Consider the potential for exposure under these circumstances, and plan ahead to avoid them.

POSSIBLE COMPLICATIONS

• Secondary injuries may occur from ataxia.
• The stress associated with pregnancy precludes breeding until after recovery.
• Keep performance animals out of training during therapy to avoid relapse.

EXPECTED COURSE AND PROGNOSIS

• Referral centers using standard therapy have reported up to a 75% response rate and a full-recovery rate of <25%. Mildly affected horses treated early in the course of infection have a much greater opportunity for complete recovery. Prompt aggressive therapy is essential. Improvement often is observed during the first week of therapy and frequently progresses steadily for several weeks. The rate of improvement typically slows, however, as the horse gradually improve over many weeks, until a plateau is reached. Chronic signs of CNS damage (e.g., muscle atrophy) rarely improve.

• If relapse occurs, double the dose of pyrimethamine used to re-treat. The population of parasites causing the problem are descendants of the parasites remaining from the first round of therapy, so it is unreasonable to assume the same dosage will remain as effective. Immunostimulants may be helpful, but the amount of CNS inflammation may be increased, causing further immunopathology. Few choices remain when horses relapse repeatedly—indefinite treatment, an even higher dose of standard medication, use of alternative drugs, and drug combinations

MISCELLANEOUS

ASSOCIATED CONDITIONS

Secondary injuries

AGE-RELATED CONDITIONS

The average age of clinically affected horses is ≅8 years.

ZOONOTIC POTENTIAL

N/A

PREGNANCY

Avoid high doses of standard medication in pregnant mares until more is known regarding the validity of suggested side effects.

SYNONYMS

Protozoal equine myeloencephalitis

SEE ALSO

N/A

ABBREVIATIONS

• CSF = cerebrospinal fluid
• CSM = cervical stenotic myelopathy
• EDM = equine degenerative myeloencephalopathy
• EEG = electroencephalography
• EMG = electromyography
• EMND = equine motor neuron disease
• GI = gastrointestinal
• MRI = magnetic resonance imaging
• PCR = polymerase chain reaction

Suggested Reading

Granstrom D. Equine protozoal myeloencephalitis: parasite biology, experimental disease, and laboratory diagnosis. In: International Equine Neurology Conference Proceedings, Cornell University, Ithaca, New York, July 11–13, 1997:4–6.

Granstrom D. Understanding EPM. Lexington, KY: Bloodhorse Publications, 1997.

Granstrom D, Saville W. Equine protozoal myeloencephalitis. In: Reed S, Bayley W, eds. Equine internal medicine Philadelphia: WB Saunders, 1998:486–491.

Author David E. Granstrom
Consulting Editor Joseph J. Bertone

PSEUDOPREGNANCY

BASICS

DEFINITION

• Condition existing after the loss of a pregnancy between 15–140 days of gestation
• Affected mares fail to show estrus (type I, early loss) and genital tract tone (although not uterine horn diameter) is consistent with that of pregnancy.
• Type II occurs after formation of endometrial cups and persists until these cups regress.

PATHOPHYSIOLOGY

Characterized by two types, I and II, occurring during different stages of gestation.

Type I

• Occurs when the conceptus is lost between days 15–36 of gestation.
• Recognition of pregnancy normally occurs by 12–14 days after ovulation. The embryo blocks uterine release of prostaglandin and signals the CL to maintain its function—production of progesterone

Type II

• Occurs when pregnancy is lost between 37–140 days of gestation.
• Production of eCG by the cups is an independent process that does not require a viable fetus to continue.
• Characterized by the continued eCG production until the endometrial cups regress.
• Production of eCG begins at ≅36–37 days of gestation in a normal pregnancy and continues until ≅120–140 days.
• Source of eCG in mares is the endometrial cups of the placenta.
• The major function of eCG is to stimulate development of accessory CLs, which provide additional progesterone for pregnancy maintenance from day 40 to ≅120–140 days of gestation.
• Clinical features—obvious lack of a conceptus within the uterus, as detected at ultrasonography or transrectal palpation; uterine and cervical tone mimic that of pregnancy; mare may show two distinct reproductive behavior patterns: recurrent periods of estrus with follicular development and nonovulatory luteinization of these follicles, and continued progesterone production or prolonged periods of anestrus with small, inactive ovaries

SYSTEM AFFECTED

Reproductive

GENETICS

Occurs in all breeds.

INCIDENCE/PREVALENCE

• ≅10%–15% occurrence in the general broodmare population
• Occurrence may be much higher (25%) in old mares (18–20+ years).

SIGNALMENT

• See *Incidence/Prevalence.*
• Type I—10%–15% of general broodmare population <15–18 years
• Type II—≅25% of mares >18–20+ years

SIGNS

No overt clinical signs other than lack of conceptus in uterus, as would be detected at transrectal palpation and ultrasonography.

CAUSES

• Type I—stress (e.g., colic); embryo defects; negative energy deficit.
• Type II—stress; uterine disease (e.g., delayed uterine clearance, lymphatic stasis, chronic endometritis, fibrosis); body pregnancy

RISK FACTORS

Type II—aged mares.

DIAGNOSIS

DIFFERENTIAL DIAGNOSIS

N/A

CBC/BIOCHEMISTRY/URINALYSIS

N/A

OTHER LABORATORY TESTS

N/A

IMAGING

Ultrasonography:
• Identification of retained CL, prolonged function, in the face of pregnancy loss
• Type I—inappropriate embryonic vesicle size (i.e., reduced conceptus volume) for known gestational length, increased echogenicity of the embryonic vesicle, and loss of normal embryonic architecture.

DIAGNOSTIC PROCEDURES

Transrectal Palpation:
• Detects disappearance of the palpable bulge of pregnancy because of fluid resorption.
• Other characteristics of early pregnancy remain—tightly closed, narrow and elongated cervix, and excellent uterine tone.

PATHOLOGIC FINDINGS

Chronic endometrial fibrosis and endometrial cysts, particularly in type II aged mares.

PSEUDOPREGNANCY

TREATMENT

APPROPRIATE HEALTH CARE

- Types I and II breeding management techniques to reduce the chance of EED
- Proper breeding hygiene—washing of mare and stallion
- AI, using appropriate semen extender
- Pre- and postbreeding intrauterine infusions/flushes
- Postovulatory uterine treatment—antibiotic and/or oxytocin

NURSING CARE

N/A

ACTIVITY

N/A

DIET

N/A

CLIENT EDUCATION

See *Appropriate Health Care.*

SURGICAL CONSIDERATIONS

N/A

MEDICATIONS

DRUGS OF CHOICE

- $PGF_2\alpha$ to lyse the existing CL and initiate ovarian activity
- Exogenous progestogens (Regu-mate® for 15 days) to induce renewed cyclic activity

CONTRAINDICATIONS

N/A

PRECAUTIONS

N/A

POSSIBLE INTERACTIONS

N/A

ALTERNATIVE DRUGS

N/A

FOLLOW-UP

PATIENT MONITORING

- Monitor pregnancy via transrectal palpation and ultrasonography.
- Possible benefit from using exogenous progesterone (such benefits remain a source of controversy).

PREVENTION/AVOIDANCE

N/A

POSSIBLE COMPLICATIONS

N/A

EXPECTED COURSE AND PROGNOSIS

- Prognosis for mare is good.
- Pregnancy has been terminated.
- Likelihood for recurrence is good in some aged mares suffering from chronic, irreversible uterine disease—fibrosis; endometrial cysts

MISCELLANEOUS

ASSOCIATED CONDITIONS

- EED
- Pregnancy

AGE-RELATED FACTORS

N/A

ZOONOTIC POTENTIAL

N/A

PREGNANCY

By definition, this is a pregnancy-related condition.

SYNONYMS

- False pregnancy
- Pseudocyesis
- Spurious pregnancy

SEE ALSO

- EED
- Endometritis
- Pregnancy diagnosis

ABBREVIATIONS

- AI = artificial insemination
- CL = corpus luteum
- eCG = equine chorionic gonadotropin
- EED = early embryonic death

Suggested Reading

England GCW. Problems during pregnancy. In: Sutton JB, Swift ST, eds. Allen's fertility and obstetrics in the horse. London: Blackwell Science Ltd., 1996:127–129.

Ginther OJ. Reproductive biology of the mare: basic and applied aspects. Cross Plains, WI: Equiservices, 1992:228–229.

McKinnon AO, et al. Reproductive examination of the mare. In: McKinnon AO, Voss JL, eds. Equine reproduction. Philadelphia: Lea & Febiger 1993:297.

Author E. Ricardo Bridges

Consulting Editor Carla L. Carleton

PSYCHOGENIC SEXUAL BEHAVIOR DYSFUNCTION

BASICS

DEFINITION

- Includes slow or variably inadequate precopulatory behavior, sexual arousal, erection, or copulatory behavior.
- Particular preferences and aversions for mares, handlers, breeding locations, procedures, or equipment have also been demonstrated; can also be general or specific to certain conditions.
- In stallions, can be chronic or intermittent and can include certain aberrant precopulatory or copulatory behaviors—excessive biting or licking, savaging the mare or handler, or premature dismount

PATHOPHYSIOLOGY

In stallions, can be the result of single or multiple factors—genetic predisposition, inadequate social maturation, simple inexperience, suboptimal breeding stimuli, or aversive experience associated with sexual behavior, breeding, or general handling

SYSTEMS AFFECTED

- Behavior—other behavior problems, including aggression stereotypies, can follow unresolved or ill-handled sexual behavior dysfunction; it is not uncommon for managers to physically abuse stallions for failure to perform sexually.
- Reproduction—subfertility or infertility

SIGNALMENT

Novice and experienced breeders of any age, breed, or performance type

SIGNS

Historical Findings

- Current and past general health, attitude, and temperament? Early socialization experience?
- Training and performance history?
- What is the stallion fed, including supplements?
- Any current medications?
- Current work and performance schedule?
- How is the stallion housed?
- Breeding experience?
- Age of first use?
- Libido and temperament?
- General behavior in stall and at pasture?
- Step-by-step details of behavior in sexual situation?
- Past and current breeding schedules and results?
- Natural cover or collection of semen?
- Stimulus and mount mares used?
- How is the stallion handled for breeding?
- Experience of personnel?
- Behavior of any other stallions at same facility?

Physical Examination Findings

Usually normal, but take care to identify any evidence of possible past sources of discomfort (e.g., stallion ring, other scars).

CAUSES

- Inexperience
- Pain associated with breeding—legs, feet, chest, shoulder, stifle, back, penis, testicles, cord torsion, or inguinal testicle
- Punishment associated with sexual behavior
- Antimasturbatory devices or practices
- Injudicious punishment or rough or inconsistent handling during breeding, particularly intolerance of normal sexual behavior or overhandling of the head
- Breeding accidents—slipping during breeding, hitting the head on a low ceiling when mounting, or being kicked by a mare
- Overuse as a breeding stallion or overwork in performance
- Abuse
- Suboptimal stimulus mare
- Innate mare preferences
- Suboptimal breeding environment—poor footing, low ceilings, or noise and distractions
- Suboptimal artificial vagina or dummy mount conditions or techniques
- Too rigid or too flexible breeding organization

RISK FACTORS

- Age <2 years
- Novice breeders >5 years
- Sire with low or temperamental libido
- Heavy training or work
- Exposure to anabolic steroids and other performance-enhancing medications and feed supplements
- Discipline for showing normal sexual behavior
- Heavy breeding schedule
- Poor general health
- Physical abuse
- Handrearing, particularly if isolated from other horses during development
- Housing conditions—deliberate or inadvertent sensory, exercise, and social deprivation
- Injudicious, rough, or inconsistent handling during breeding
- Any musculoskeletal or genital pain, discomfort, or instability
- Fear of people or a particular person
- Obesity
- Severely underweight
- Extreme hot or cold environmental temperatures
- Change in environment, housing conditions, or management, which can suppress sexual response
- Self-serve dummy mounts

DIAGNOSIS

DIFFERENTIAL DIAGNOSIS

Medical differentials must be ruled out before a primary psychogenic diagnosis can be established.

CBC/BIOCHEMISTRY/URINALYSIS

Should be normal

OTHER LABORATORY TESTS

- Endocrinology—stallion panel (i.e., testosterone, estradiol, LH, FSH, T3, T4, insulin, and cortisol) should be normal. For old stallions or those with suspected testicular degeneration, hCG and GnRH challenge tests may be useful. Use challenge and sampling protocols of an equine endocrine laboratory with a large stallion database and knowledge regarding interpretation of their protocol results.
- Semen—can be evaluated for signs of infection or hemospermia that might suggest urogenital lesions causing discomfort.

IMAGING

Radiography, scintigraphy, ultrasonography, and endoscopy to identify or rule out any sources of present or past musculoskeletal or urogenital pain

DIAGNOSTIC PROCEDURES

- Cardiovascular examination to rule out aortic iliac disease that may affect breeding ability
- Musculoskeletal and neurologic examinations on the ground and during breeding
- Video surveillance in the stall to observe erection and penile movement during normal, spontaneous erections
- Video surveillance of the stallion in the stall next to a mare or turned out at liberty with or near a mare to determine stallion-like behavior under less-controlled conditions
- Video or direct observation of breeding procedures and stallion handling

TREATMENT

MANAGEMENT AND ENVIRONMENT

- To the extent possible, correct obvious housing, handling, and breeding environment deficiencies, providing optimal stimulus mares and physical facilities for breeding—excellent footing, ample head room, and plenty of space
- Establish a feeding and exercise program to maximize fitness for breeding and to minimize fatigue and pain.
- Establish a breeding schedule to maximize libido and breeding performance; for stallions with low or variable libido, a breeding schedule of two or three times weekly usually maximizes arousal and performance.

PSYCHOGENIC SEXUAL BEHAVIOR DYSFUNCTION

• To the extent possible, identify and abide any specific preferences or aversions of the animal.

BEHAVIOR MODIFICATION

• Provide as much uncontrolled access to mares as possible; this likely will increase endogenous male hormones and build confidence in responding to mares.
• For slow-starting, novice breeders, continue daily exposure to breeding, with patient and gentle handling and a variety of stimulus mares; pasture breeding opportunities can build confidence and naturally train a stallion to breed.
• When people are present, they can encourage and positively reinforce sexual arousal and response.
• Educate handlers to use positive reinforcement–based stallion handling procedures to encourage spontaneous erection and masturbation.

MEDICATIONS

DRUGS OF CHOICE

• Analgesics, acupuncture, and related therapies for management of any potential sources of physical discomfort or instability during breeding
• Anxiolytics as a training aid to overcome past, negative breeding experiences—diazepam (0.05 mg/kg [to maximum of 20 mg] slow IV 5–7 minutes before breeding; extralabel use)
• Unless androgen levels are greater than the normal range, administer GnRH (50 μg SC 2 hours and again 1 hour before breeding; extralabel use) to boost endogenous androgens, which often increases sexual interest and arousal and appear to make genital tissues more sensitive to stimulation.
• If quick results are needed, short-term treatment with aqueous testosterone (50–80 mg SC every other day for at least 1 week; extralabel use) can effectively increase circulating testosterone and boost libido; the greatest improvement in libido typically occurs after 4–7 days of treatment.
• Imipramine hydrochloride (500–800 mg for each 1000 lb PO 2–3 hours before breeding; extralabel use) to lower the ejaculatory threshold and reduce the amount of work needed to breed.
• Drug-induced ejaculation regimens (extralabel use) are available as substitutes for in copula breeding or collection of semen.

PRECAUTIONS

• Benzodiazepine anxiolytics release innate aggressive as well as sexual behavior. Caution handlers to expect and to prepare for possibly increased aggressive behavior before or during the increased sexual behavior. Similarly, increasing male hormone levels with GnRH or androgens also likely increases aggressive behavior. If the aggression is not skillfully directed or abided, mare or handler interaction with the stallion can be counter-productive. Increasing the dose of testosterone often is tempting, but possible adverse side effects on pituitary gonadal function are a concern.
• At certain levels, imipramine hydrochloride can inhibit rather than enhance ejaculation, disturb bladder neck function, and cause premature flaring of the glans penis. Should these occur, a lower dose usually is more effective at enhancing ejaculation without these side effects.

POSSIBLE INTERACTIONS

N/A

ALTERNATIVE DRUGS

N/A

FOLLOW-UP

PATIENT MONITORING

• Once to twice weekly follow-up for at least 1 month, with monthly follow-up thereafter during the current breeding season to monitor and fine-tune improvements and medications
• Re-examination near the end of the current breeding season and near the beginning of the next breeding season, or with change in environment or health status

POSSIBLE COMPLICATIONS

• Best results occur if everyone involved with the care and handling of the horse communicate positively among each other and with the clinician toward a positive outcome for the stallion.
• Counter-productive blaming or failure of all to co-operate or comply with the treatment plan

MISCELLANEOUS

ASSOCIATED CONDITIONS

• Some stallions become "sour" if continually failing at breeding and may develop self-mutilation or tendencies to savage the mare or handlers.
• Many stallions with low libido actually began high-energy, unruly stallions that, in association with discipline, became uninterested or slow to respond.
• Subclinical lameness, neurologic disease, or aortic iliac disease that may specifically disturb pelvic circulation or cause hindlimb pain or weakness during copulation

AGE RELATED FACTORS

• Inadequate sexual interest and response in young novice stallions more likely is primarily psychogenic than a libido problem in old experienced stallion that has been breeding successfully for years.
• Most healthy, sound stallions maintain stable libido through their mature years and into old age. However, with advancing age and accumulated minor physical deterioration, once tolerable musculoskeletal discomfort or disabilities may become more problematic for breeding stallions.
• Cardiac pathology, particularly with advancing age, often is associated with reduced libido, apparent anxiety on exertion during breeding, and delayed or urgent dismount.

ZOONOTIC POTENTIAL

N/A

PREGNANCY

N/A

SYNONYMS

• Libido problem
• Erection dysfunction
• Breeding dysfunction
• Sexual behavior dysfunction
• Poor breeding performance

SEE ALSO

• Aggression
• Fears and phobias
• Self-mutilation

ABBREVIATIONS

• FSH = follicle-stimulating hormone
• GnRH = gonadotropin-releasing hormone
• hCG = human chorionic gonadotropin
• LH = luteinizing hormone
• T3 = triiodothyronine
• T4 = thyroxine

Suggested Reading

Martin BB, McDonnell SM, Love CC. Effects of musculoskeletal and neurologic disease on breeding performance in stallions. Compend Cont Educ Pract Vet 1998;20:1159–1169.
McDonnell SM. Ejaculation: physiology and dysfunction. Equine Pract 1992;8:57–70.
McDonnell SM. Normal and abnormal behavior. Equine Pract 1992;8:71–89.
McDonnell SM. Sexual behavior dysfunction of stallions. In: Robinson NO, ed. Current therapy in equine medicine 3. 1992;3:633–637.
McDonnell SM. Treatment of libido, erection, and ejaculatory dysfunction in stallions. Compend Cont Educ Pract Vet 1999;21:XXX–XXX.

Author Sue M. McDonnell
Consulting Editor Daniel Q. Estep

PTERIDIUM AQUILINUM (BRACKEN FERN) TOXICOSIS

BASICS

OVERVIEW

- *Pteridium aquilinum* (bracken fern) is a dark green, herbaceous, perennial plant that grows from a single, stout, long, blackish, horizontal rhizome.
- The fern has bipinnate leaves that are scattered, erect, coarse, and have curved-under edges and, when reproductive, sporangia lining the undersurface margins.
- The leaves may appear elongated or broadly triangular in shape.
- The rhizomes and leaves grow to ≅1 m in length, and the plant reaches 1–2 m in height.
- The fern is common to upland or unimproved pastures, open woodlands, and woodland meadows, being most abundant on dry, sandy, or gravelly soils.
- Numerous varieties of the plant are distributed worldwide, and all are equally toxic.
- In the U.S., serious losses have been reported in the northeastern, southeastern, Great Lakes, midwestern, and far western states.
- A heat-sensitive thiaminase and heat-stable antithiamine component (suspected to be caffeic acid) are toxic to horses; toxicity is retained after drying.
- The neuromuscular syndrome (i.e., staggers) exhibited by intoxicated horses is typical of thiamine (i.e., vitamin B_1) deficiency.
- Thiamine acts as a cofactor in cellular decarboxylation reactions. A deficiency impairs the oxidation of α-ketoglutarate to succinyl-CoA in the Kreb's cycle and the conversion of pyruvate to acetyl-CoA. The increased concentration of cellular metabolites and impairment of energy pathways results in neuromuscular dysfunction—CNS, cardiac muscle, and skeletal muscle
- Typically, clinical signs of intoxication do not become evident until ≅30 days after continuous ingestion of forage (e.g., pasture, hay) containing significant amounts of the fern.
- Milk from mares ingesting the fern is not believed to be a significant source of thiaminase or of antithiamine toxins for nursing foals; however, other plant toxins are eliminated in the milk of other lactating animals.
- Bracken fern intoxication is also known as pteridism.

SIGNALMENT

Horses ingesting significant dietary amounts of the fern are at risk.

SIGNS

- Neuromuscular signs can occur as soon as 2–3 days or as long as 2–3 months after ingestion.
- Horses exhibit inco-ordination, staggering gait, arched back, widespread hindlimbs, and variable but visible muscle tremors.
- Without treatment, recumbency rapidly ensues.
- Additional signs include cardiac arrhythmia (initially bradycardia, with tachyarrhythmia occurring late in the disease), severe muscle tremors, tonic-clonic seizures, and opisthotonos.
- Untreated horses usually die 2–10 days after the onset of signs.

CAUSES AND RISK FACTORS

- Intoxication usually occurs during the autumn months, when other desirable forages are less available, or during the late winter months, when good-quality hay is unavailable.
- Horses with ongoing hepatic disease may have a slightly higher risk.
- Low dietary copper, together with high dietary sulfur, has been reported to induce thiamine deficiency, thus increasing susceptibility to intoxication.

DIAGNOSIS

DIFFERENTIAL DIAGNOSIS

- Horsetail (*Equisetum* spp.) intoxication—*Equisetum* plants also contain a thiaminase; therefore, signs of horsetail intoxication are identical to those of bracken fern intoxication. With suspected intoxication, search for access to horsetail plants.
- Ryegrass (*Lolium perenne*) intoxication—ryegrass staggers are caused by ingestion of endophytic fungal toxins (e.g., lolitrem B, paxilline) associated with ryegrass infected with *Acremonium lolii.* With suspected intoxication, search for access to endophyte-infected ryegrass forage and associated toxins.
- Moldy corn intoxication—*Fusarium* molds produce fumonisin, a mycotoxin that is responsible for ELEM. With suspected moldy corn intoxication, dietary concentrations of fumonisin are >5 ppm, and brain lesions are characteristic.
- Lead intoxication—whole-blood lead values >0.3 ppm
- EPM—antibody to *S. neurona* in the CSF.
- EHV-1—xanthochromic CSF with a protein concentration >80 mg/dL or characteristic paired serum samples (fourfold or greater increase, or single sample >1:400) for EHV-1 antibody.

CBC/BIOCHEMISTRY/URINALYSIS

Moderate thrombocytopenia and mild depression of other hematopoietic elements may be present.

PTERIDIUM AQUILINUM (BRACKEN FERN) TOXICOSIS

OTHER LABORATORY TESTS

- Low thiamine levels in the blood (<3 ng/mL; normal reference range, 5–23 ng/mL) and urine
- High serum levels of pyruvate (>10 mg/dL; normal reference range, 2–3 mg/dL) and lactate (>20.0 mg/dL, normal reference range, 2.5–15.5 mg/dL)

IMAGING

N/A

DIAGNOSTIC PROCEDURES

N/A

PATHOLOGIC FINDINGS

- Cardiomegaly with pulmonary and hepatic congestion (signs consistent with heart failure) may be present at necropsy.
- No specific histopathologic lesions

TREATMENT

- GI decontamination
- Symptomatic and supportive care

MEDICATIONS

DRUGS

- Decontamination with AC (2–5 g/kg PO in a water slurry) and a cathartic (e.g., magnesium sulfate [250–500 mg/kg PO as a 20% solution]) followed by vitamin B_1 supplementation is recommended.
- Thiamine HCl for injection (100 or 200 mg/mL) is available under various generic labels.
- For adult horses, the recommended initial dose is 2500 mg (5 mg/kg) given by slow IV injection followed by daily doses of 125–250 mg (0.25–0.5 mg/kg) given by slow IV or by IM injection for a minimum of 7 days.
- To control seizure activity in adults, diazepam can be administered at a dose of 25–50 mg (0.05–0.1 mg/kg) given by slow IV injection; repeat at 30-minute intervals as needed.

CONTRAINDICATIONS/POSSIBLE INTERACTIONS

Atropine is not beneficial in treatment of cardiac arrhythmia associated with bracken fern toxicosis, stops intestinal peristalsis, and prolongs elimination of toxic material.

FOLLOW-UP

PATIENT MONITORING

- Horses often respond dramatically to treatment with thiamine.
- Alleviation of clinical signs within 12–24 hours after treatment often aids in establishing a diagnosis.

PREVENTION/AVOIDANCE

- Monitor for the fern in pasture or hay.
- Consider dietary vitamin supplementation.

POSSIBLE COMPLICATIONS

N/A

EXPECTED COURSE AND PROGNOSIS

Prognosis is good if thiamine is administered early.

MISCELLANEOUS

ASSOCIATED CONDITIONS

N/A

AGE-RELATED FACTORS

N/A

ZOONOTIC POTENTIAL

N/A

PREGNANCY

N/A

SEE ALSO

N/A

ABBREVIATIONS

- AC = activated charcoal
- CoA = coenzyme A
- CSF = cerebrospinal fluid
- ELEM = equine leukoencephalomalacia
- EHV = equine herpes virus
- EPM = equine protozoal myelitis
- GI = gastrointestinal

Suggested Reading

Cheeke PR. Natural toxicants in feeds, forages, and poisonous plants. 2nd ed. Danville, IL: Interstate Publishers, 1998:423–430.

Author William R. Hare
Consulting Editor Robert H. Poppenga

PTYALISM

BASICS

OVERVIEW

Excessive salivation (ptyalism) arises either through excessive production of saliva or saliva that cannot be swallowed. Saliva is produced continuously from the salivary glands and is secreted into the oral cavity. Any condition that causes dysphagia may produce ptyalism through inhibiting swallowing of saliva [see causes of dysphagia, (e.g., oral pain), neurologic conditions, obstruction of the esophagus]. Increased production of saliva may occur following the ingestion of forage or hay contaminated with *Rhizoctonia leguminicola.* This produces a mycotoxin, slaframine, that has parasympathomimetic properties. It is an alkaloid that requires hepatic activation. The active compound is thought to either cause the release of histamine or have direct histaminergic effects. Heavy-metal toxicity, parasympathomimetic poisoning, neurologic disease, and stomatitis (e.g., vesicular stomatitis) may also increase saliva production. Gastroesophageal reflux secondary to gastroduodenal ulceration is also associated with ptyalism, particularly in foals.

Primary diseases of the salivary glands are uncommon and can include sialoadenitis, salivary calculi, salivary mucocele, trauma, neoplasia (adenocarcinomas, acinar cell tumors, melanomas), or infection (e.g., *Streptococcus equi,* rabies). Some of these may also be associated with increased production of saliva. Horses have relatively high levels of salivary chloride and low levels of bicarbonate. Therefore, loss of saliva causes a transient metabolic alkalosis due to loss of the chloride.

SIGNALMENT

Dependent on the primary problem.

Foals

- Esophageal disorders due to dysmaturity, septicemia, botulism, and congenital disorders
- Increased risk of gastroduodenal ulceration

Young Horses

Esophageal disorders due to improper chewing during tooth eruption.

Aged Horses

- Esophageal disorders due to neoplasia or improper chewing of feed due to poor teeth
- Feeding practices and pica can increase likelihood of foreign body obstruction or choke with feed material.
- Feeding mold-infected legumes such as red clover increase likelihood of slaframine toxicity.

SIGNS

Increased saliva from the mouth. Other signs are associated with the primary disease and include:

- Enlargement of the esophageal area with cervical esophageal obstruction
- Signs of dysphagia include coughing during swallowing, frequent swallowing motions, extension of the neck, and regurgitation of feed material out the nostrils. Should be able to differentiate choke due to the mixture of feed material with the saliva.
- Salivation following slaframine ingestion usually occurs within 30–60 min and may persist for 24 hr. May also be accompanied by diarrhea, anorexia, polyuria, or abortion. Clinical signs resolve within 28 hr of removing the infected feed.
- Gastroduodenal ulceration frequently accompanied by bruxism and decreased appetite, especially for grain.

CAUSES AND RISK FACTORS

- Secondary to stomatitis—Vesicular stomatitis, irritants, caustic chemicals, yellow bristle grass, foxtails, NSAID toxicity, erosions secondary to point on teeth
- Decreased ability to swallow the saliva produced may be secondary to esophageal disorders such as obstruction or disorders in motility or structure secondary to obstructions.
- Secondary to botulism or sepsis
- Secondary to pharyngeal trauma as a result of improper administration of bolus medication
- Secondary to other causes of dysphagia; neurogenic, obstructive
- Toxin ingestion
- NSAID administration leading to gastroduodenal ulceration

DIAGNOSIS

DIFFERENTIAL DIAGNOSIS

Determine the primary conditions resulting in ptyalism:

- Neurogenic dysphagia
- Pharyngeal obstruction
- Esophageal disorders
- Gastric/gastroduodenal ulceration
- Toxin ingestion

CBC/BIOCHEMISTRY/URINALYSIS

- Results of the CBC are often normal, but may reflect the primary disease (neonatal septicemia, *S. equi* infection)
- Stress leukogram
- Biochemical analysis may be normal or may reflect changes consistent with the primary disease. After prolonged ptyalism, horse may develop metabolic alkalosis due to loss of chloride in the saliva.

OTHER LABORATORY TESTS

N/A

IMAGING

Radiographs of the skull if trauma is suspected, or to localize foreign bodies, temporomandibular joint (TMJ) disease, or retropharyngeal masses.

DIAGNOSTIC PROCEDURES

Oral Examination

It should be remembered that rabies is a possible cause, and therefore care should be taken to wear gloves when examining the mouth and limit exposure of non-vaccinated individuals/animals.

Nasogastric Intubation

- Endoscopsy—pharynx, guttural pouches, esophagus, stomach, duodenum
- Postmortem immunofluorescent antibody testing on brain tissue for rabies, if suspected
- Examination of hay source or pasture

TREATMENT

- Treat the primary condition (see section on specific conditions)
- Symptomatic treatment rarely attempted
- Treat any fluid and acid–base disorders that may have resulted from chronic loss of saliva
- Remove any feed material that may contain *R. legumincola*

MEDICATIONS

DRUGS AND FLUIDS

The appropriate crystalloid fluid should be given intravenously to treat any existing dehydration or acid–base disorders that may have developed.

CONTRAINDICATIONS/POSSIBLE INTERACTIONS

N/A

ALTERNATIVE DRUGS

N/A

FOLLOW-UP

- Monitor for signs of aspiration pneumonia or rupture of the esophagus
- Possible complications include aspiration pneumonia, dermatitis, and dehydration and electrolyte disorders

MISCELLANEOUS

N/A

SEE ALSO

- Stomatitis
- Esophageal disorders
- Gastroduodenal ulceration
- Dental eruptions and disorders
- Dysphagia
- Rabies
- Mycotoxicosis
- Fracture of the mandible or maxilla

ABBREVIATIONS

- EPM = equine protozoal myelitis
- TMJ = temporomandibular joint

Suggested Reading

Easley KJ. Salivary glands and ducts. In: Smith BP, ed. Large animal internal medicine. St. Louis: Mosby, 1996;697.

Schmitz DG. Toxicological problems. In: Reed SM, Bayly WM, eds. Equine internal medicine. Philadelphia: WB Saunders Co., 1998:988-989.

Sockett DC, Baker JC, Stowe CM: Slaframine (*Rhizoctonia leguminicola*) intoxication in horses. J Am Vet Med Assoc 1982;181:606

Author Deborah A. Parsons

Consulting Editor Henry Stämpfli

PULMONARY ASPERGILLOSIS

BASICS

OVERVIEW

• An uncommon fungal pneumonia, frequently life-threatening and caused by a member of the genus *Aspergillus.*
• *Aspergillus* sp. are ubiquitous in nature; thus, horses have constant exposure to this opportunistic agent.
• Infections usually are seen in immunocompromised horses or in those with overwhelming exposure to the organism.
• The conidial diameter of *Aspergillus* sp. is ideal for inhalation and deposition in the respiratory tract, but the GI tract also is a frequent portal causing embolic mycotic lung disease.
• The pathogenic mechanism in most horses is postulated to be immunocompromise from profound neutropenia associated with colitis, followed by invasion of *Aspergillus* sp. from disrupted intestinal mucosa.

SIGNALMENT

No age, breed, or sex predilections

SIGNS

• Abnormal breath sounds
• Tachypnea
• Abnormal (often foamy) nasal discharge
• Abnormal pleural sounds
• Hemoptysis
• Dyspnea
• Nasal plaques
• Many horses show no definitive signs of respiratory tract disease.

CAUSES AND RISK FACTORS

• The most common species for infections is *A. fumigatus.*
• Other pathogenic species—*A. flavus, A. niger, A. nidulans, A. clavatus, A. deflectus, A. ochraceus,* and *A. terreus.*
• Risk factors—acute enterocolitis, immunosuppression (e.g., prolonged neutropenia, depressed neutrophil function) from debilitating disease, prolonged use of corticosteroids or antibiotics, and massive exposure to the spores.

DIAGNOSIS

DIFFERENTIAL DIAGNOSIS

• Heaves—fungal organisms are seen in tracheal aspirate, but horse is not sick.
• Interstitial pneumonia—no fungal elements in tracheal aspirate or BAL

CBC/BIOCHEMISTRY/URINALYSIS

No consistent changes reported

OTHER LABORATORY TESTS

Currently, anti-*Aspergillus* antibody tests to detect disease are not helpful, because serum titers are present in both diseased and normal horses.

IMAGING

• Radiography may reveal virtually any infiltrative or miliary pattern.
• The most common initial radiographic finding is a patchy bronchopneumonia—multiple focal sites are common, and lesions tend to be peripheral in distribution.
• Lesions, though multiple and diffuse, usually are small in size and not detectable by ultrasonography.

DIAGNOSTIC PROCEDURES

• Antemortem diagnosis is difficult.
• Most *Aspergillus* sp. grow on routine fungal media within 48 hours.
• Fungal hyphae often are present in tracheal aspirates from healthy horses. Fungal elements in the tracheal aspirate or BAL should be present in large numbers and be involved in the inflammatory process within the lung.
• Percutaneous lung biopsy might confirm the diagnosis.
• Biopsy of a nasal erosion or ulcer that reveals organisms histologically is highly predictive of concomitant or future invasive pulmonary aspergillosis.
• Awareness of the possibility for infection in the appropriate clinical and epidemiologic setting is perhaps the most important step.
• Recovery of *Aspergillus* sp. isolated from a transtracheal wash of healthy horse is not uncommon.
• Given the appropriate setting, multiple isolations should be considered suggestive of the invasive disease.

PATHOLOGIC FINDINGS

Gross Findings

Multiple, frequently black nodules scattered throughout the lungs

Histologic Findings

• Multiple septate, branching hyphae with congestion, necrosis, inflammatory cells, hemorrhage, and/or edema in the lung parenchyma
• Fungal hyphae radiating from the center of vessels, effacing pulmonary parenchyma, and tending to invade all surrounding blood vessels
• Necrotic and hemorrhagic parenchyma in which fungi penetrate blood vessels and fungal balls grow in airways
• Fungal organisms commonly are seen in tissues other than the lung in many horses—intestine, CNS, and nasal mucosa

TREATMENT

• Treatment is difficult.
• Inpatient or outpatient medical management with stall rest.

PULMONARY ASPERGILLOSIS

MEDICATIONS

DRUGS

Specific and fungal agents currently being used—fluconazole (4 mg/kg PO SID), itraconazole (3 mg/kg PO BID), or amphotericin B (day 1: 0.3 mg/kg; day 2: 0.4 mg/kg; day 3: 0.5 mg/kg; day 4: no drug; and day 5: 0.5 mg/kg; this dose is given every 2 days for 1 month)

CONTRAINDICATIONS/POSSIBLE COMPLICATIONS

- Corticosteroids
- Any immunosuppressive medications

FOLLOW-UP

PATIENT MONITORING

Monitor clinical signs daily.

PREVENTION/AVOIDANCE

- Prevention of invasive fungal pneumonia is difficult.
- Avoidance of large, inhaled inocula is impossible in horses because of their environmental conditions. Horses that are recumbent for long periods inhale even greater numbers of spores, even in well-ventilated stables. Improving ventilation and minimizing exposure to inspired spores is most beneficial. Air filters sometimes are placed in stables, but they frequently are inadequate for the size of the area and/or inadequately maintained. Negative ionizers may enhance killing of airborne bacteria but do little to lower the levels of fungal spores from moldy hay.
- The most important method of disease prevention is decreasing environmental exposure, prompt and effective treatment of predisposing illnesses, and possibly, judicious avoidance of overusing corticosteroids and broad-spectrum antibiotics.
- Horses with enteritis, colitis, typhlitis, or other GI diseases resulting in mucosal compromise and showing clinical respiratory disease, particularly if nonresponsive to antimicrobial therapy, should be considered prime candidates for pulmonary aspergillosis.
- Medications predisposing to enteritis or colitis should be viewed as also predisposing to disseminated mycoses associated with fungal translocation across the bowel lesions. Antibiotics are the most commonly implicated medication associated with the onset of diarrhea, but NSAIDs, particularly at higher doses, can be responsible for loss of bowel integrity.

POSSIBLE COMPLICATIONS

Disseminated aspergillosis

EXPECTED COURSE AND PROGNOSIS

- Even with an antemortem diagnosis, the prognosis remains grave despite intensive treatment.
- Invasive aspergillosis has a high mortality rate.

MISCELLANEOUS

ASSOCIATED CONDITIONS

Enteritis, colitis, typhlitis, or other GI diseases resulting in mucosal compromise frequently are associated.

AGE-RELATED FACTORS

N/A

ZOONOTIC POTENTIAL

This disease does not spread from horses to humans.

PREGNANCY

N/A

SEE ALSO

- Aspiration pneumonia
- Expiratory dyspnea
- Heaves
- Inspiratory dyspnea
- Pleuropneumonia
- Pulmonary abscesses

ABBREVIATIONS

- BAL = bronchoalveolar lavage
- GI = gastrointestinal

Suggested Reading

Sweeney CR, Habecker PL. Pulmonary aspergillosis in horses: 29 cases (1974–1997). J Am Vet Med Assoc, 1999;214(6):808–811.

Author Corinne R. Sweeney
Consulting Editor Jean-Pierre Lavoie

PURPURA HEMORRHAGICA

BASICS

DEFINITION

- An acute vasculitis that can be a sequel to infection or vaccine administration
- Specific diseases usually are associated with suppuration or necrosis.
- Most resembles Henoch-Schönlein syndrome in humans, an acute, anaphylactoid purpura in which antibody–antigen complexes fix complement in the vessel walls or lumens (i.e., Arthus reaction)

PATHOPHYSIOLOGY

- Complement fixation results in chemotaxis and localization of neutrophils. Complex deposition and localization of neutrophils result in damage to vessel walls, and hemorrhagic diathesis ensues.
- As in humans, clinicopathologic components suggest an immune-mediated phenomenon. Immune complex deposition, hypersensitivity, and autoimmunity have been implicated, but the pathophysiology has not been completely elucidated.
- Infection with and vaccination against *Streptococcus equi* most commonly are associated with this syndrome; circulating immune complexes containing IgA and IgM and antigen of *Streptococcus* sp. have been demonstrated.

SYSTEMS AFFECTED

- Hemic/lymphatic/immune—usually an immune-mediated condition associated with a type III hypersensitivity reaction to an infectious agent
- Cardiovascular—leakage of blood or blood components from small vessels, resulting in hemorrhage or edema

GENETICS

N/A

INCIDENCE/PREVALENCE

Reported incidence varies from 0.5 to 5% of horses with signs of *S. equi* var. *equi* infection.

SIGNALMENT

- No breed, sex, or age predilections
- Mares are over-represented in studies involving generalized vasculitis.

SIGNS

General Comments

Signs commence within 2–4 weeks of infection or vaccination.

Historical Findings

- History of exposure to or infection with respiratory pathogens frequently reported
- Exposure to *S. equi* is common.
- Vaccinal exposure to antigens may precede disease.

Physical Examination Findings

- Frequently, head edema is the initial sign, with swelling beginning around the nostrils; the edema then progresses over the whole face, limbs, and ventral midline, with well-demarcated areas of hot, sensitive swellings.
- Petechia and ecchymotic hemorrhages appear on light-skinned areas and mucous membranes.
- Pharyngeal and laryngeal mucosa may become hyperemic and develop purpura; dysphagia and upper airway obstruction can occur from the swelling and pain.
- Large areas of skin often ooze serum and eventually may slough. Mucosa also can slough and ulcerate, and necrotic laryngitis can result.
- If edema and hemorrhage are associated with the GI tract, abdominal pain and ileus can occur.

CAUSES

- No inciting cause found in some cases, but has been associated with *S. equi* var. *equi* and *S. equi* var. *zooepidemicus.*
- Influenza virus infection, equine herpevirus-1 infection, severe myositis, and prolonged drug administration have been implicated.

RISK FACTORS

Exposure to antigens from the previously mentioned pathogens

DIAGNOSIS

DIFFERENTIAL DIAGNOSIS

- Immune-mediated thrombocytopenia—may be difficult to differentiate; most cases of PH have normal to only slightly decreased platelet counts.
- Hypersensitivity vasculitis—biopsy
- Viral arteritis—virus isolation from buffy coat or seroconversion after infection
- EIA—anemia and thrombocytopenia with only mild edema; ruled out by serology (Coggins test)
- Ehrlichiosis (caused by *Ehrlichia equi*)—may be difficult to differentiate; horses with ehrlichiosis are febrile, with limb edema, anorexia, depression, and reluctance to move; usually leukopenia and thrombocytopenia with monocytosis; a blood smear may reveal evidence of ehrlichial inclusions within neutrophils and eosinophils; *E. equi* serology or PCR performed on the buffy coat are diagnostic procedures.
- Warfarin toxicity—because vitamin K–dependent clotting factors are important, increases in PT and, ultimately, APTT are seen; first signs usually are epistaxis and bleeding into joints.
- Moldy sweet clover—similar to warfarin; bleeding is a major sign.

CBC/BIOCHEMISTRY/URINALYSIS

- Anemia—decreased RBC count and hemoglobin
- Leukocytosis—with or without left shift
- Normal platelet count
- Hyperfibrinogenemia
- Hypergammaglobulinemia

OTHER LABORATORY TESTS

Increased C3 levels; serology to various infectious agents

IMAGING

- Thoracic radiography for evidence of lower respiratory tract infection
- Endoscopy of upper airways for *S. equi* var. *equi* lymphadenopathy
- Abdominal ultrasonography

DIAGNOSTIC PROCEDURES

- Biopsy of skin and mucous membranes
- Rectal examination for abdominal masses and lymphadenopathy
- Immunofluorescent antibody testing on frozen and fixed tissues for equine globulin deposition along vessels
- Blood culture
- Culture of any abscesses
- Thoracocentesis
- Abdominocentesis

PATHOLOGIC FINDINGS

- Numerous, discrete, hemorrhagic areas of necrosis throughout the cutis, submucosa, musculature, pharynx, or respiratory and GI tracts on gross postmortem examination. These areas frequently are raised, and the overlying mucosa can be ulcerated, with gray borders. Serosal surfaces frequently are affected similarly.
- Microscopic examination—massive necrosis of affected tissues and leukoclastic vasculitis.
- Neutrophils frequently surround vessels, and tissue lesions contain neutrophils, with frequent pyknotic nuclei.
- Stains for bacteria and fungal elements—negative

PURPURA HEMORRHAGICA

TREATMENT

APPROPRIATE HEALTH CARE
Frequently requires long term medical therapy and supportive care

NURSING CARE
- Supportive care— hydrotherapy and wrapping of limbs, tracheostomy for upper airway–associated dyspnea and respiratory distress, and provision of soft feeds to minimize pharyngeal swelling and damage.
- Local treatment with topical wound ointments over sloughed areas
- Isotonic fluid administration to maintain hydration

ACTIVITY
Limited; hand walking may be useful to increase peripheral circulation, especially in cases with significant edema of the limbs.

DIET
Soft feeds may be necessary in cases with pharyngeal swelling and damage.

CLIENT EDUCATION
Depends on the inciting disease process (e.g., discuss *S. equi* if strangles precipitated PH).

SURGICAL CONSIDERATIONS
N/A

MEDICATIONS

DRUGS OF CHOICE
- Corticosteroids—dexamethasone (0.05–2.0 mg/kg IV or IM q12h to q24h) or prednisolone (0.5–1.0 mg/kg IM q12h) are continued but very gradually decreased during a period of 14–21 days.
- Anti-inflammatories for pain and swelling
- Antibiotics for any underlying condition

CONTRAINDICATIONS
N/A

PRECAUTIONS
High-dose corticosteroid therapy occasionally is associated with laminitis or secondary infections.

POSSIBLE INTERACTIONS
N/A

ALTERNATIVE DRUGS
N/A

FOLLOW-UP

PATIENT MONITORING
- Truncated therapy can result in recurrence of clinical signs that are more severe than the initial episode.
- Sequela—sloughing of skin over affected areas of severe edema; glomerulonephritis progressing to chronic renal failure
- Evaluate BUN, Cr, and urine protein at weekly intervals.

PREVENTION/AVOIDANCE
- Minimize exposure to *S. equi.*
- Avoid vaccination of horses recently exposed to *S. equi.*

POSSIBLE COMPLICATIONS
Sloughing of large areas of skin, especially on the distal extremities

EXPECTED COURSE AND PROGNOSIS
- Prognosis depends on the severity and extent of the condition; extensive skin sloughing, evidence of internal organ involvement, or development of laminitis are poor prognostic indicators.
- Most uncomplicated cases recover if treated early and aggressively with immunosuppressive drugs.

MISCELLANEOUS

ASSOCIATED CONDITIONS
Streptococcus equi (i.e., strangles) or other respiratory infections frequently precede development of PH.

AGE-RELATED FACTORS
N/A

ZOONOTIC POTENTIAL
N/A

PREGNANCY
N/A

SYNONYMS
- Immune-mediated vasculitis
- Leukocytoclastic vasculitis

SEE ALSO
- EIA
- Equine viral arteritis
- *Streptococcus equi* (strangles)
- Vasculitis

ABBREVIATIONS
- APTT = activated partial thromboplastin time
- Cr = creatinine
- EIA = equine infectious anemia
- GI = gastrointestinal
- PCR = polymerase chain reaction
- PH = purpura hemorrhagica
- PT = prothrombin time
- C3 = third component of complement

Author Maureen T. Long
Consulting Editor Debra C. Sellon

PURULENT NASAL DISCHARGE BASICS

BASICS

DEFINITION
Fluid discharge of varying turbidity, color, amount, frequency, and odor from one or both nostrils

PATHOPHYSIOLOGY
- Composed of combinations of leukocytes and varying amounts of fluid and/or mucous from any location in the respiratory tract
- Production originates from an inflammatory process incited by traumatic, immune, allergic, infectious, or noxious stimuli; thus, the discharge can be septic or nonseptic.
- Color varies—white, yellow, green, reddish, or brown depending on the presence of bacteria, ingesta, blood, or necrotic tissue
- Malodorous discharge is associated with anaerobic infections, foreign bodies, necrotic bone, and tooth root abscesses.

SYSTEMS AFFECTED
- Respiratory—lower tract, consisting of alveoli, bronchioles, bronchi, and trachea; upper tract, consisting of nasopharynx, guttural pouches, larynx, turbinates, nasal passages, paranasal sinuses, and false nostrils
- GI—oropharynx and esophagus

SIGNALMENT
- Young horses or any immunocompromised animal more prone to infections
- Neonates with milk in the discharge may have cleft palate and aspiration pneumonia.
- Old horses—heaves tooth infections, and neoplasia

SIGNS

Historical Findings
- Nasal discharge accompanied by coughing, fever, reluctance to eat, dyspnea, respiratory noise, or odor
- Discharge that is continuous or intermittent, spontaneous, and/or associated with exercise or eating
- Discharge may be copious or scant, unilateral or bilateral.
- Previous signs of respiratory disease or exposure to other animals with disease
- Previous treatments and management changes and responses
- Seasonal correlation with worsening or alleviation may indicate allergic disease.
- Exercise intolerance
- Facial swelling or bony remodeling is indicative of a chronic sinus problem.

Physical Examination Findings
- Ongoing discharge or dried material at nares
- Normal or decreased airflow with upper airway obstruction
- Fever—consistent with infectious agent
- Lymphadenopathy with swelling and inflammation of retropharyngeal and/or submandibular lymph nodes with *Streptococcus equi* or *S. zooepidemicus* infection
- Guttural pouch distention with empyema or chondroids
- Dull areas on percussion and auscultation of paranasal sinuses indicate exudate or cystic structure.
- Evidence of dental disease is associated with sinusitis.
- Odor with tooth root infection, bony necrosis (i.e., neoplasia), foreign body, or gram-negative lung abscessation
- Abnormal lung sounds consistent with pneumonia, pleuropneumonia, or heaves; may be exacerbated or elicited with use of a rebreathing bag.
- Percussion of lung field—dull areas are indicative of pleural fluid, abscess, or consolidated lung.
- Auscultation of fluid in trachea with exudate in pneumonia or heaves.
- Dysphagia with esophageal obstruction, guttural pouch disease (resulting neuropathy), or episodes of hyperkalemic periodic paralysis
- Milk in discharge with cleft plate in neonates, severe depression, botulism, or nutritional myopathy
- Depression—severe illness with severe pneumonia or pleuropneumonia

CAUSES
- Viral/bacterial infections
- Bacterial infections—*S. equi* lymphadenitis, guttural pouch empyema, sinusitis, lung abscessation, and pleuropneumonia
- Foreign bodies or trauma with subsequent inflammation/infection
- Heaves associated with airway inflammation, with or without secondary bacterial infection
- Esophageal obstruction or pharyngeal dysfunction

RISK FACTORS
- Viral infections—influenza and equine herpesvirus
- Exposure to animals infected with upper respiratory virus or strangles
- Lack of vaccination against respiratory pathogens
- Immunodeficiency—FPT, SCIDS, and steroid therapy
- Environmental—indoors, dust, molds, air pollutants, and smoke inhalation
- Transport—subsequent pleuropneumonia
- Dental disease

DIAGNOSIS

DIFFERENTIAL DIAGNOSES
- Unilateral discharge suggests a problem affecting the upper airways; bilateral discharge may originate from either the upper or the lower airway.
- Presence of food may indicate esophageal obstruction or pharyngeal dysfunction.
- Infectious—bacterial, viral, and fungal
- Immune-mediated—allergic
- Trauma—foreign body
- Abscessation
- Inflammation
- Neoplasia

PURULENT NASAL DISCHARGE BASICS

CBC/BIOCHEMISTRY/URINALYSIS

- May or may not have an inflammatory leukogram with neutrophilia and hyperfibrinogenemia if localized or extensive.
- Leukogram may be degenerative, with left shift and toxic cells depending on severity (especially with lower airway disease or pneumonia).

OTHER LABORATORY TESTS

- Serum immunoglobulin levels for FPT or immunodeficiency
- Serum/plasma *S. equi* titers and upper respiratory virus titers
- Arterial blood gases—PaO_2 for lower airway disease or pneumonia

IMAGING

- Endoscopy—nasal passages, pharynx, and trachea
- Radiography—sinuses, teeth, guttural pouches, pharynx, and lungs
- Ultrasonography—thorax

DIAGNOSTIC PROCEDURES

- Culture and sensitivity of exudate or nasal swab for bacterial infections often obtain very mixed growth due to contamination; useful for early detection of strangles.
- Bronchoalveolar lavage—cytology in diffuse lower airway disorders
- Transtracheal wash—culture and cytology
- Lymph node (if affected) aspiration—culture and cytology
- Sinus aspiration/trephination—culture and, occasionally, cytology
- Thoracocentesis—culture and cytology

TREATMENTS

- Removal of foreign body
- Antimicrobial regimen based on culture and sensitivity results
- Surgical drainage trephination of the sinuses.
- Surgical tooth expulsion
- Flushing of affected sinuses or guttural pouches
- Heaves—environmental management

MEDICATIONS

DRUGS OF CHOICE

- COPD— steroids with or without bronchodilators, inhalants, and expectorants
- Bacterial pneumonia/abscessation—appropriate antimicrobials depending on age and disease process, preferably based on culture and sensitivity results; NSAIDs; with or without bronchodilation; supportive oxygen/fluid therapy.

CONTRAINDICATIONS

N/A

PRECAUTIONS

N/A

POSSIBLE INTERACTIONS

N/A

ALTERNATIVE DRUGS

N/A

FOLLOW-UP

PATIENT MONITORING

N/A

POSSIBLE COMPLICATIONS

Aspiration pneumonia if dysphagia

MISCELLANEOUS

ASSOCIATED CONDITIONS

N/A

AGE-RELATED FACTORS

N/A

ZOONOTIC POTENTIALS

N/A

PREGNANCY

N/A

SYNONYMS

N/A

SEE ALSO

- Aspiration pneumonia
- Heaves (COPD)
- Pleuropneumonia
- Sinusitis

ABBREVIATIONS

- COPD = chronic obstructive pulmonary disease
- FPT = failure of passive transfer of immunity
- GI = gastrointestinal
- SCIDS = severe combined immunodeficiency syndrome

Suggested Reading

Colahan PT. Nasal discharge. In: Colahan PT, Merritt AM, Moore JN, Mayhew IG, eds. Equine medicine and surgery. 5th ed. St. Louis: Mosby, 1999:30–31.

Traub-Dargatz J. Field examination of the equine patient with nasal discharge. Vet Clin North Am 1997;13:561–588.

Wilson WD, Lofstedt J. Alterations in respiratory function. In: Smith BP, ed. Large animal intern medicine. 2nd ed. St. Louis: Mosby, 1996:46–99.

Author Wendy Duckett

Consulting Editor Jean-Pierre Lavoie

PYOMETRA

BASICS

DEFINITION
Accumulation of a purulent exudate within the uterus.

PATHOPHYSIOLOGY
- Frequently a sequela to metritis, cervicitis, or cervical adhesions/trauma.
- Associated with severe endometrial inflammatory changes, loss of epithelium, and permanent gland atrophy.
- Signs of systemic disease are rare.

SYSTEM AFFECTED
Reproductive

GENETICS
N/A

INCEDENCE/PREVALENCE
No geographic distribution.

SIGNALMENT
Aged pluriparous mares are predisposed to recurrent uterine infections because of anatomic defects and failing mechanical uterine defense mechanisms—poor VC, pendulous uterus, aging, and cervical/uterine trauma or adhesions.

SIGNS

General Comments
- The mare may cycle regularly or remain in a prolonged diestrus.
- Prolonged diestrus is associated with inability of the uterus to secrete or of the CL to respond to endogenous prostaglandin because of extensive endometrial destruction.

Historical Findings
- Purulent vaginal discharge may be continuous, intermittent (i.e., open pyometra), or absent (i.e., closed pyometra) depending on cervical patency and stage of the estrous cycle.
- Contact dermatitis and alopecia of the inner thighs and hocks may be evident.
- Can be an incidental finding on routine examination.

Physical Examination Findings
- External conformation may be normal.
- Chronic or intermittent purulent vaginal discharge.
- Transrectal palpation reveals an enlarged, fluid-filled uterus that may be further described with ultrasonography. A large fluid volume (0.5–60 L) may have accumulated within the uterine lumen.
- Digital cervical examination often reveals adhesions or other abnormalities.
- Culture and cytology results show bacteria and fungi similar to those associated with infectious endometritis. Bacterial isolation ranges from a mixed population of organisms to no bacterial growth.

CAUSES AND RISK FACTORS

Infectious
- Bacteria do not cause pyometra in mare but are opportunists.
- Most common isolates—*Streptococcus zooepidemicus, Escherichia coli, Actinomyces* sp., *Pasteurella* sp., and *Pseudomonas* sp.

Noninfectious
- Mechanical impairment preventing normal uterine drainage.
- Physical obstruction of the cervical canal that inhibits uterine evacuation—trauma, cervical fibrosis/induration that prevents either complete closure or dilation, and obstruction of the cervical lumen by adhesions.
- Extrauterine impairment caused by abdominal adhesions to the uterus may prevent the uterus from involuting or evacuating completely.
- Chronic uterine distention also impairs ability of the uterus to contract and evacuate its contents.
- Age and parity—multiparous; > 14 years of age.
- Conformational abnormalities—history of postpartum metritis/cervicitis; history of cervical laceration, trauma, or incomplete cervical dilation.

DIAGNOSIS

DIFFERENTIAL DIAGNOSIS

Pregnancy
- The uterine walls in pyometra lack the characteristic tone and responsiveness associated with pregnancy; in comparison, the uterine walls may become thickened and with the purulent exudate cause the uterus to feel "doughy."
- Ultrasonographic findings provide additional differentiating characteristics of pyometra with appearance/characteristics of/in the uterine fluid.

Pneumouterus
- Associated with abnormal VC and poor uterine tone, resulting in wind-sucking—pneumovagina.
- Poor tone of the vestibulovaginal sphincter allows air to pass through the cervix and into the uterus. This most commonly occurs during estrus because of vulvar/cervical relaxation and also after administration of sedatives—acepromazine.

Mucometra
Mucoid exudate accumulation associated with cystic endometrial hyperplasia in old mares is a very rare condition.

Placentitis
- May be characterized by a purulent vaginal discharge in a pregnant mare.
- Ascending placentitis occurs late in gestation and is localized at the cervical star.
- Premature mammary development also may be present.

Distended Bladder
Distinguish the uterus from the bladder by the ability to locate ovaries and/or trace along either the uterine horns or the cervix during transrectal palpation.

Other Causes of Vaginal Discharge
See *Endometritis*.

CBC/BIOCHEMISTRY/URINALYSIS
Mild normocytic, normochromic anemia and/or neutropenia in some mares.

OTHER LABORATORY TESTS
For Infectious Causes:

Bacteria
- Endometrial cells and intraluminal contents may be obtained by scraping the endometrial surface with the swab tip or cap (if using a Kalayjian® culture swab). The sample is then stained with Diff-Quik®. The presence of neutrophils indicates active inflammation.
- Evaluation of the endometrial contents for bacteria is obtained using a guarded swab. The sample should be cultured in blood agar and MacConkey's at 37°C and examined at 24 and 48 hours. Blood agar will support growth of Gram-positive, select Gram-negative, and some yeasts, whereas MacConkey will support only the growth of Gram-negative organisms. Therefore, both should be used.

Yeasts
- Samples obtained for bacterial culture can also be used to isolate *Candida* and *Aspergillus* sp., because these organisms grow in blood agar.
- Branching hyphae can be identified in stained smears or wet mounts.
- For fungal-specific culture, the sample is inoculated in Sabouraud agar and incubated for 4 days at 37°C.

IMAGING
Ultrasonography:
- Intrauterine fluid can be categorized by its presence, quantity, and quality.
- Depending on the amount of accumulated debris and inflammatory cells, the exudate may be moderately to highly hyperechoic.

PYOMETRA

DIAGNOSTIC PROCEDURES

Endometrial Biopsy

• An important prognostic tool.
• Collect the initial sample before treatment.
• Evacuate uterine content before performing the biopsy to lessen what is a slight likelihood of rupturing/penetrating the uterine wall during the procedure.

Endoscopy

• May reveal intrauterine adhesions that are precluding effective uterine drainage.
• Purulent exudate may be attached to the walls and/or found free in the lumen.

PATHOLOGIC FINDINGS

• Wide range of findings, depending on the severity and duration of the condition.
• Especially pronounced in old mares—severe endometrial inflammatory changes; glandular atrophy.
• Atrophy may be permanent and confers an extremely poor prognosis for the mare's reproductive life.

TREATMENT

APPROPRIATE HEALTH CARE

• Mechanical evacuation of purulent contents by repeated uterine lavage (daily or alternate days) followed by administration of an ecbolic drug (oxytocin or prostaglandin) using a nasogastric tube and warm saline for the lavage. The uterus is then infused with antibiotics based on culture and sensitivity results.
• **NOTE:** antibiotics should be infused 45–60 min after oxytocin administration to avoid their premature evacuation.
• Administer a luteolytic dose of $PGF_{2\alpha}$ if a persistent corpus luteum is suspected.

NURSING CARE

N/A

ACTIVITY

N/A

DIET

N/A

CLIENT EDUCATION

N/A

SURGICAL CONSIDERATIONS

• If the option is to forego further breeding, treatment may be left undone, or hysterectomy, although not often used, is an option.
• Do not consider hysterectomy as a simple, elective procedure; if performed, the uterus must be emptied as completely as possible before surgery.

MEDICATIONS

DRUGS OF CHOICE

• See *Endometritis.*
• $PGF_{2\alpha}$—dinoprost tromethamine (Lutalyse®; 5–10 mg total IM)

CONTRAINDICATIONS

See *Endometritis.*

PRECAUTIONS

Infuse fluid for uterine lavage carefully into the distended and friable uterus, beginning with relatively low volumes to avoid rupture.

POSSIBLE INTERACTIONS

N/A

ALTERNATIVE DRUGS

N/A

FOLLOW-UP

PATIENT MONITORING

• Transrectal palpation and ultrasonography to evaluate response to treatment—uterine size and tone; amount of intrauterine fluid.
• Biopsy and/or endoscopy after treatment for endometrial visualization, evaluation of response to treatment, and prognosis.

PREVENTION/AVOIDANCE

N/A

POSSIBLE COMPLICATIONS

N/A

EXPECTED COURSE AND PROGNOSIS

• Recurrence is common.
• Prognosis for fertility is poor.
• The prognosis for fertility is grave in cases with severe uterine or cervical adhesions.

MISCELLANEOUS

ASSOCIATED CONDITIONS

Cervical adhesions may obliterate the cervical lumen and keep it from opening and closing properly.

AGE-RELATED FACTORS

Repeated stretching associated with pregnancy results in a uterus suspended low in the abdomen, predisposing to fluid accumulation and increased risk for pyometra.

ZOONOTIC POTENTIAL

N/A

PREGNANCY

N/A

SYNONYMS

N/A

SEE ALSO

• Cervical lesions
• Endometritis/DUC
• Postpartum metritis
• Vulvar conformation

ABBREVIATIONS

• CL = corpus luteum
• DUC = delayed uterine clearance
• VC = vulvar conformation

Suggested Reading

Murray WJ. Uterine defense mechanisms and pyometra in mares. Compend Contin Educ Pract Vet 1991;13:659–663.
Hughes JP, Stabenfeldt GH, Kindahl H, et al. Pyometra in the mare. J Reprod Fertil Suppl 1979;27:321–329.

Author Maria E. Cadario
Consulting Editor Carla L. Carleton

PYRROLIZIDINE ALKALOID (PA) INTOXICATION

BASICS

DEFINITION

• A disease associated with chronic ingestion of plants containing PAs, which are a distinct group of structurally similar molecules found in ≅6000 different species worldwide.
• Hundreds of different alkaloids, defined as saturated or unsaturated, exist, along with their corresponding *N*-oxide forms.
• Some PAs are hepatotoxic; some are not.
• Alkaloid composition and concentration as well as toxicity vary tremendously among plants. The alkaloid concentration varies with respect to stage of plant maturity and part of the plant.
• Three plant families (i.e., Compositae, Leguminosae, and Boraginaceae) account for most PA-containing plants. The most common plant genera responsible for clinical disease in the U.S. are *Senecio, Amsinckia, Cynoglossum,* and *Crotalaria.*
• Economic losses caused by these plants once were estimated at ≅$20 million per year in the Pacific Northwest alone. Because of widespread recognition of the problem and effective livestock management and biologic control measures (particularly with *S. jacobaea*), however, intoxications resulting from these plants are much less common.
• Intoxications usually occur when horses graze paddocks or pastures heavily contaminated with these plants or consume contaminated hay during a period of several weeks to months.
• Acute intoxications are rare, primarily because of the large amount of plant material a horse would need to ingest at any one feeding.

PATHOPHYSIOLOGY

• PAs are rapidly absorbed from the GI tract and undergo extensive hepatic metabolism by mixed-function oxidases.
• Some are detoxified to harmless metabolites, primarily by ester hydrolysis and conversion to *N*-oxides, which then are eliminated via the urine or bile. Others are activated by conversion to toxic metabolites, primarily by dehydrogenation, yielding highly toxic pyrrole derivatives.
• Pyrroles alkylate double-stranded DNA, thus inhibiting cell mitosis. Nuclear and cytoplasmic cell masses expand because of the impaired ability to divide, thus forming megalocytes. As megalocytes die, they are replaced by fibrous connective tissue.
• Pyrroles also bind to cellular constituents in lung and kidney tissues, either because of systemic distribution of reactive pyrroles from the liver or in situ metabolism of the parent PA.

SYSTEMS AFFECTED

• Hepatobiliary—interference with cell replication leads to hepatocytomegaly and necrosis with bile duct proliferation and fibrosis; endothelial proliferation in centrilobular and hepatic veins occurs.
• Renal/Urologic—pyrrole-bound molecules can lead to megalocytosis of the proximal convoluted tubules, atrophy of glomeruli, and tubular necrosis; however, this has not been described in horses.
• Respiratory—pyrrole-bound molecules can lead to alveolar hemorrhage and edema, progressive proliferation of alveolar walls, pulmonary arteritis, and hypertension; however, this is rare in horses.
• Cardiovascular—right ventricular hypertrophy and cor pulmonale have been documented experimentally, most likely secondary to PA-induced lung damage.

GENETICS

N/A

INCIDENCE/PREVALENCE

• Most intoxications occur during late spring, summer, and early fall, when there is access to the growing plant; however, intoxications can occur at any time because of the persistent toxicity of these alkaloids in baled hay.
• Most recently reported cases have occurred in the northwestern U.S.—Washington, Oregon, Idaho, Montana, and Colorado

SIGNALMENT

N/A

SIGNS

General Comments

• Most affected horses suffer chronic weight loss and debilitation associated with hepatic insufficiency, which can be subtle in nature; this is referred to as the chronic-delayed form.
• In the chronic-delayed form, clinical signs can appear quite suddenly, despite exposure and liver lesions having been chronic and progressive.
• The extent of hepatic damage depends greatly on the daily amount of alkaloid consumption, degree of pyrrole conversion, age of the animal, and metabolic and mitotic status of the target cells.
• Food intake and nutritional status also can modify the effects of PAs.
• Most affected patients, particularly those suffering from the chronic-delayed form, exhibit neurological signs attributable to hepatoencephalopathy.

PYRROLIZIDINE ALKALOID (PA) INTOXICATION

Physical Examination Findings

- Loss of appetite and weight
- Weakness and sluggishness
- Photodermatitis
- Icterus
- Behavioral abnormalities—mania, derangement, yawning, aimless walking, head pressing, drowsiness, blindness, and ataxia
- Inspiratory dyspnea—related to paralysis of the pharynx and larynx
- Gastric impaction
- Ascites
- Diarrhea with tenesmus

CAUSES

- Plants incriminated in the U.S.—*Senecio jacobaea* (tansy ragwort), *S. vulgaris* (common groundsel), *S. douglasii* var *longiilobus* (threadleaf groundsel), *S. riddelli* (Riddell's groundsel), and *Cynoglossum officinale* (hound's-tongue)
- Depending on the plant, stage of maturity, environmental conditions, and age of the horse, most animals must ingest 1–5% of body weight in plant material daily before effects are observed. Sometimes as much as 50% is required before clinical signs become apparent.
- With tansy ragwort, some authors suggest a chronic lethal dose for horses of 0.05–0.2 kg/kg. Thus, for a 500-kg horse, ingestion of one dried hound's-tongue plant per day for 2 weeks can cause clinical disease.
- *Amsinckia* and *Crotalaria* spp. rarely cause problems, because the highest percentage of alkaloid is present in the seed.
- Most intoxications result from ingestion of contaminated grain or cakes; however, horses have been poisoned after chronic ingestion of *Amsinckia* spp.–contaminated hay.

RISK FACTORS

Intoxication occurs from grazing heavy stands of the plants or eating contaminated hay for extended periods of time (2–4 weeks to several months).

DIAGNOSIS

DIFFERENTIAL DIAGNOSIS

- Alsike clover (*Trifolium hybridum*) or red clover (*T. pratense*) intoxication
- Acute hepatitis—Theiler's disease
- Cholangiohepatitis
- Liver abscess
- Cholelithiasis
- Viral encephalitis
- Nigropallidal encephalomalacia
- Leukoencephalomalacia
- Equine protozoal encephalomyelitis
- Miscellaneous hepatotoxic chemicals—more acute in nature; causing more necrosis (e.g. carbon tetrachloride, chlorinated hydrocarbons, pentachlorophenols, coal-tar pitch, phenol, iron, phosphorus)
- Aflatoxin intoxication—rare

CBC/BIOCHEMISTRY/URINALYSIS

- Elevations in GGT and ALP
- Hyperbilirubinemia
- Hypoalbuminemia
- Hypoproteinemia
- Inflammatory leukogram
- Hyperammonemia

OTHER LABORATORY TESTS

- Prolonged BSP clearance time
- Elevated bile acids
- Abnormal liver biopsy

IMAGING

Ultrasonography may detect extensive liver fibrosis.

DIAGNOSTIC PROCEDURES

- Detection of pyrrole metabolites in blood or hepatic tissue
- Identification of PA-containing plants on premise or in hay or stomach contents
- Identification and quantification of the active PA in feed or stomach contents
- Liver biopsy to detect characteristic lesions

PATHOLOGIC FINDINGS

- Poor body condition; loss of body fat
- Jaundice
- Ascites and generalized edema
- Small, pale, firm liver with a mottled, cut surface
- Megalocytosis, with mild necrosis
- Fibrosis—centrilobular and periportal
- Veno-occlusive lesions
- Biliary hyperplasia
- Pulmonary edema
- Interstitial pneumonia
- Brain status spongiosus
- Other, less recognized lesions—myocardial necrosis, cecal and colonic edema and hemorrhage, and adrenal cortical hypertrophy

PYRROLIZIDINE ALKALOID (PA) INTOXICATION

TREATMENT

APPROPRIATE HEALTH CARE

• No specific treatment
• Primary goal—to provide supportive therapy until enough liver tissue can regenerate and function adequately for the intended use of the horse
• Most PA-poisoned patients respond poorly to treatment, because by the time the disease is diagnosed, adequate liver regeneration no longer is possible.

NURSING CARE

• IV fluids to correct dehydration often are necessary.
• Photodermatitis can be treated with an appropriate combination of cleansing, hydrotherapy, and debridement, along with restricting exposure to sunlight.

ACTIVITY

Plenty of rest, with reduction of stress, is important.

DIET

• Replace contaminated feed with a high-nutrient diet (i.e., highly digestible, high in calories, low in protein) divided into 4–6 daily feedings.
• One suggested diet includes 1–2 parts beet pulp and 0.25, 0.50, or 1 part cracked corn mixed with molasses and fed at a rate of 2.5 kg per 100 lb. Sorghum or milo can be substituted for beet pulp.
• Oat or grass hay is a good source of roughage.
• Avoid alfalfa and other legumes because of their high protein content.
• Oral pastes and IV preparations containing high concentrations of branched-chain amino acids and antioxidants have been used, but with questionable success.
• Consider weekly vitamin B_1, folic acid, and vitamin K_1 supplementation.

CLIENT EDUCATION

• Recognize PA-containing plants of concern in the geographic area, and prevent access by the horse.
• Provide adequate forage and prevent overgrazing to limit ingestion of toxic plants.

SURGICAL CONSIDERATIONS

N/A

MEDICATIONS

DRUGS OF CHOICE

• Horses with neurological signs may require diazepam (foals: 0.05–0.4 mg/kg IV; adults: 25–50 mg IV; may be necessary to repeat) or xylazine (1.1 mg/kg IV or 2.2 mg/kg IM).
• With septic photodermatitis, consider oral, broad-spectrum antibiotics—cephalosporins
• With low blood glucose, a continual 5% dextrose drip may be administered IV at a rate of 2 mL/kg per hour. Dilute the dextrose 0.5-strength normal saline or LRS if the infusion will last longer than 24–48 hours.
• Oral neomycin (50–100 mg/kg QID for 1 day), lactulose (0.3 mL/kg QID), or mineral oil have been used to decrease blood ammonia concentrations, but with varying results.

CONTRAINDICATIONS

N/A

PRECAUTIONS

• Diarrhea is a common sequela after neomycin or lactulose therapy.
• Neomycin can predispose to salmonellosis.
• Exercise care when administering any medication that undergoes extensive hepatic metabolism.

POSSIBLE INTERACTIONS

N/A

ALTERNATIVE DRUGS

N/A

FOLLOW-UP

PATIENT MONITORING

• Monitor appetite, weight, serum liver enzymes, and bile acids every 2–4 weeks.
• Magnitude of the elevation of serum hepatic enzymes does not always correlate with degree of hepatic impairment.

PREVENTION/AVOIDANCE

• Recognize PA-containing plants, both in the field and in hay.
• Use good management practices and appropriate herbicide control to avoid overexposure of horses to these plants.
• Sheep are relatively resistant and can be used to graze heavily contaminated land.

POSSIBLE COMPLICATIONS

Pneumonia and chronic wasting are the most common sequelae.

EXPECTED COURSE AND PROGNOSIS

- Most affected horses are given a poor prognosis and often euthanized because of severe debilitation or nonresponsive neurologic signs.
- Some animals can recover after several months of care but generally cannot regain their former fitness or activity level.

MISCELLANEOUS

ASSOCIATED CONDITIONS

N/A

AGE-RELATED FACTORS

Although not documented, foals or young ponies may be at slightly greater risk because of their small body mass, less discriminating eating habits, higher metabolic activity, and higher susceptibility of tissues in which cells are rapidly dividing.

ZOONOTIC POTENTIAL

N/A

PREGNANCY

- PAs have been detected in milk collected from PA-exposed cattle and goats, but the levels have been considered clinically insignificant.
- PAs cross the placenta in other species, causing various fetotoxic effects.

SYNONYMS

- Walking disease
- Yawning disease

SEE ALSO

N/A

ABBREVIATIONS

- ALP = alkaline phosphatase
- BSP = bromosulfophthalein
- GGT = γ-glutamyltransferase
- GI = gastrointestinal
- LRS = lactated Ringer solution

Suggested Reading

Barton MH, Morris DD. Diseases of the liver. In: Reed SM, Bayly WM, eds. Equine internal medicine. Philadelphia: WB Saunders, 1998:707–738.

Craig AM, Pearson EG, Meyer C, Schmitz JA. Clinicopathologic studies of tansy ragwort toxicosis in ponies: sequential serum and histopathological changes. Equine Vet Sci 1991;11:261.

Divers TJ. Therapy of liver failure. In: Smith BP, ed. Large animal internal medicine. St. Louis: CV Mosby, 1996:948–950.

Knight AP, Kimberling CV, Stermitz FR, Roby MR. Cynoglossum officinale (hound's-tongue)—a cause of pyrrolizidine alkaloid intoxication in horses. J Am Vet Med Assoc 1984;185:647.

Mendel VE, Witt MR, Gitchell BS, et al. Pyrrolizidine alkaloid-induced liver disease in horses: an early diagnosis. Am J Vet Res 1988;49:572.

Pearson EG. Liver failure attributable to pyrrolizidine alkaloid toxicosis and associated with inspiratory dyspnea in ponies: three cases (1982–1988). J Am Vet Med Assoc 1991;198:1651.

Author Patricia A. Talcott

Consulting Editor Robert H. Poppenga

QUERCUS SPP. (OAK) TOXICOSIS

BASICS

OVERVIEW

- This plant genera contains a variety of species, including trees and shrubs.
- Species more commonly associated with poisoning—Gambel's oak (*Quercus gambelii*), Havard or shinnery oak (*Q. havardii*), and white shin oak (*Q. durandii* var. *brevilobata*).
- Other species implicated in poisoning—wavyleaf oak (*Q. undulata*), Emory oak (*Q. emoryi*), shrub live oak (*Q. turbinella*), and silverleaf oak (*Q. hypoeucoides*).
- All *Quercus* spp. should be considered toxic.
- Ingestion of large quantities of leaves, leaf buds, or acorns results in severe GI/nephrotoxic syndrome.
- Poisoning most commonly is associated with ingestion of new leaf buds, hence the common name "oak-bud poisoning."
- Gallotannins are the toxic principles; ingested tannins react with dietary and tissue proteins, rendering them nonfunctional.
- Toxicosis generally occurs when oak comprises >50% of the diet.
- Poisonings most commonly occur during early spring, with ingestion of new leaf buds, or during late fall, with ingestion of acorns.

SIGNALMENT

- Poisoning is rare in horses but can occur at any age.
- Male and female horses are equally susceptible.

SIGNS

- Abdominal pain
- Depression
- Anorexia
- Constipation (early), followed by hemorrhagic diarrhea
- Peripheral edema
- Diphtheritic membranes in feces
- Weakness
- Polydipsia/polyuria
- Tachycardia
- Prostration
- Death

CAUSES AND RISK FACTORS

- Intoxication often is associated with lack of available forage or dietary supplementation.
- Drought or conditions inhibiting other forages from growth predispose to ingestion of oak.
- Most common during the early spring, when leaf buds are developing, and during the late fall, when acorns are dropping.

DIAGNOSIS

CBC/BIOCHEMISTRY/URINALYSIS

- Increased BUN and creatinine
- Hyposthenuria
- Proteinuria
- Hematuria
- Hyperphosphatemia
- Hypocalcemia
- Increased AST

OTHER LABORATORY TESTS

N/A

IMAGING

N/A

DIAGNOSTIC PROCEDURES

N/A

PATHOLOGIC FINDINGS

Gross Pathology

- Subcutaneous edema
- Mucoid or hemorrhagic enteritis
- Pseudomembranous enteritis
- Edema of mesenteric lymph nodes
- Hydropericardium
- Perirenal edema
- Swollen and pale kidneys
- Ascites
- Petechial hemorrhage of the kidneys
- Hepatic congestion

Histopathologic Findings

- Kidneys—numerous pink to brown casts in the proximal tubules; proximal tubular necrosis; medullary congestion
- GI—pseudomembranous, necrotizing enteritis, with hemorrhage and ulceration
- Other—vascular congestion in the liver and lungs; generalized tissue congestion

QUERCUS SPP. (OAK) TOXICOSIS

TREATMENT

- Prevent further exposure by removing horses from access to oaks.
- Minimize further GI and renal damage with general decontamination and supportive care; decontamination may decrease the duration and severity of signs.
- AC may bind tannins in the GI tract, rendering them unabsorbable, but this is not proven.
- Decreased GI transit time with cathartics—mineral oil; magnesium sulfate (i.e., Epsom salt).
- Use gastric demulcents or sucralfate for severe GI damage.
- Use IV normal saline to keep the horse hydrated and to maintain flow of urine.

MEDICATIONS

DRUGS

- AC (2–5 g/kg PO once in a water slurry)
- Magnesium sulfate (250–500 mg/kg PO once as a 20% solution)
- Sucralfate (2 mg/kg PO TID)

CONTRAINDICATIONS/POSSIBLE INTERACTIONS

- Do not give AC with mineral oil, because the oil prevents binding of compounds to AC.
- Do not give AC with evidence of severe GI mucosal damage, because AC can imbed in mucosal erosions.

FOLLOW-UP

PATIENT MONITORING

Monitor renal function daily; maintenance of renal function is a good indicator of treatment efficacy.

PREVENTION/AVOIDANCE

- Avoid pasturing horses in areas containing oaks, unless other adequate forage is available.
- Supplementation with calcium hydroxide (15% pellet) to inactivate tannins has been beneficial in other species, but its effectiveness in horses is unknown.

POSSIBLE COMPLICATIONS

With severe GI ulceration and necrosis, scarring and strictures are possible.

EXPECTED COURSE AND PROGNOSIS

Recovery may require 2–3 weeks of intense care.

MISCELLANEOUS

ASSOCIATED CONDITIONS

N/A

AGE-RELATED FACTORS

N/A

ZOONOTIC POTENTIAL

N/A

PREGNANCY

N/A

SEE ALSO

N/A

ABBREVIATIONS

- AC = activated charcoal
- AST = aspartate aminotransferase
- GI = gastrointestinal

Suggested Reading

Harper KT, Ruyle GB, Rittenhouse LR. Toxicity problems associated with the grazing of oak in the intermountain and southwestern U.S.A. In: James LF, Ralphs MH, Nielsen DB, eds. The ecology and economic impact of poisonous plants on livestock production. Boulder, CO: Westview Press, 1988:197–206.

Author Jeffery O. Hall
Consulting Editor Robert H. Poppenga

QUINIDINE TOXICOSIS

BASICS

OVERVIEW

Dose-related and idiosyncratic adverse reactions can occur that affect the cardiovascular, dermatologic, respiratory, GI, and musculoskeletal systems, including sudden death.

SIGNALMENT

No age, breed, or sex predispositions

SIGNS

- Urticaria, diarrhea, colic, upper respiratory mucosal edema and associated respiratory difficulty, laminitis, tachycardia with weak pulse caused by hypotension, and sudden death
- ECG changes—various degrees of AV block, SA block, or ventricular fibrillation; prolonged PR, QRS, or QT intervals

CAUSES AND RISK FACTORS

- Patients receiving quinidine
- Some signs are idiosyncratic and unpredictable.
- IV administration is associated with greater risk than PO administration.
- Pre-existing ventricular tachycardia
- Concurrent or previous digoxin administration may reduce the effective dose and increase toxic potential.

DIAGNOSIS

DIFFERENTIAL DIAGNOSIS

- Cardiovascular signs may be similar to some signs associated with the primary disease being treated.
- Sequential monitoring of ECG, sequential therapeutic drug monitoring and coincidental occurrence of laminitis, diarrhea, or colic assist in differentiation.

CBC/BIOCHEMISTRY/URINALYSIS

No pathognomonic changes

OTHER LABORATORY TESTS

ECG abnormalities

IMAGING

N/A

DIAGNOSTIC PROCEDURES

TDM—therapeutic concentrations range from 0.5–3.0 μg/mL of plasma.

TREATMENT

- Assess benefits/risks of treatment relative to those of the condition being treated.
- Discontinue administration of quinidine when QRS interval is increased >25%.
- Consider GI decontamination if the drug is orally administered.
- Supportive care—cardiovascular support with IV polyionic fluids; analgesics as needed

QUINIDINE TOXICOSIS

MEDICATIONS

DRUGS

- AC (2–5 g/kg in a water slurry) via nasogastric intubation.
- AC PO may be useful after IV administration of quinidine, because it may adsorb drug distributed to the GI tract and serve as a drug "sink."
- Sodium bicarbonate (0.5–1 mEq/kg IV)

CONTRAINDICATIONS/POSSIBLE INTERACTIONS

- See *Causes and Risk Factors.*
- Avoid exacerbation of hypotension by analgesics.

FOLLOW-UP

PATIENT MONITORING

Monitor ECG.

PREVENTION/AVOIDANCE

N/A

POSSIBLE COMPLICATIONS

Laminitis

EXPECTED COURSE AND PROGNOSIS

Prognosis is good with appropriate therapeutic intervention.

MISCELLANEOUS

ASSOCIATED CONDITIONS

N/A

AGE-RELATED FACTORS

N/A

ZOONOTIC POTENTIAL

N/A

PREGNANCY

N/A

SEE ALSO

N/A

ABBREVIATIONS

- AC = activated charcoal
- AV = atrioventricular
- GI = gastrointestinal
- SA = sinoatrial
- TDM = therapeutic drug monitoring

Suggested Reading

Brumbaugh GW. Toxicity of pharmacological agents. In: Robinson NE, ed. Current therapy in equine medicine. 3rd ed. Philadelphia: WB Saunders, 1992:353–358.

Author Gordon W. Brumbaugh
Consulting Editor Robert H. Poppenga

RABIES

BASICS

DEFINITION

Rabies is a virally induced neurologic disease of mammals presenting with a wide variety of clinical signs. Although uncommon in the horse, it should be considered in all cases of acute neurologic disease because of its zoonotic potential. In 1996, 574 cases of rabies virus infection were reported in domestic animals within the United States. Of these, 46 involved horses, mules, or donkeys.

PATHOPHYSIOLOGY

The rabies virus is a single-stranded RNA virus of the genus *Lyssavirus,* family Rhabdoviridae. It is a large, cylindrical, bullet-shaped neurotropic virus that is heat-labile and susceptible to most disinfectants. The reservoir hosts in the United States are skunks, racoons, and red fox. Horses are thought to be most commonly infected by the bite of an infected carnivore or insectivorous bat carrying the virus. Domestic dogs, cats, and others horses may transmit the virus via bite wounds, and may also be transmitted by droplet inhalation, orally, and transplacentally. Initially, the virus replicates within infected myocytes at the site of introduction. It may remain quiescent and undetected for months before moving centrally, then traverses neuromuscular and neurotendinous spindles to infect peripheral nerves and replicate within the dorsal and ventral root ganglia. When it reaches the CNS, the virus spreads rapidly by multiplication within neurons of the brain, spinal cord, and sympathetic trunk and glial cells. The virus can also spread passively via cerebrospinal fluid. Tissues outside the CNS are infected as the virus travels peripherally along nerve axons.

The incubation period is reported to be from 9 days to 1 year in horses. This period is affected by site of innoculation, dose of innoculum, virus strain, and host species. Shorter incubation periods may be associated with the virus entering peripheral nerves directly rather than replicating in local myocytes. Studies using specific rabies antibody immunohistochemistry techniques have clearly demonstrated that histologic lesion severity and the presence of rabies virus antigen do not necessarily correlate, suggesting that mechanisms other than direct, virally induced cytolysis may be involved in the pathogenesis of the disease.

SYSTEM(S) AFFECTED

Nervous System

All components of the central and peripheral nervous system may be affected.

Extraneural Tissues

Although extraneural tissues—specifically, corneal epithelium, salivary glands, and epidermis—of other species such as skunk and fox reportedly contain rabies virus antigen, this finding was not present in a study of five naturally infected horses.

GENETICS

N/A

SIGNALMENT

Horses of any age or use may be affected, although the virus is more common in adult horses with potential exposure to wildlife.

SIGNS

General Comments

Infected animals may be asymptomatic for up to 1 year, making it difficult to identify the source of exposure. There are no pathognomonic signs for rabies in horses, and clinical signs at presentation can range from lameness to sudden death.

Historical Findings

A bite wound is usually not found, but owners may uncommonly report that animals have been in close proximity to known rabid animals or that they found a bite wound on the animal days to months previously. Owners may also report a slow progression of signs from a mild lameness to recumbency. Alternatively, they may report an acute onset of bizarre behavior. It is important to remember that any horse presenting with neurologic signs of less than 10 days' duration is a rabies suspect until proved otherwise. In one study, rabies was confirmed in horses that had been vaccinated against rabies within 2 years of the onset of clinical signs.

Physical Examination

- Exercise intolerance, lameness, hyperesthesia, paresis or paralysis, recumbency, anorexia, colic, behavior change, and sudden death have all been reported as presenting complaints for confirmed cases of rabies.
- A bite wound is rarely found.
- Horses may be afebrile.
- The neurologic signs are dependent on the portion of the CNS affected, and are classified according to neuroanatomic location.
- Aggressive behavior, hyperesthesia, muscle tremors, convulsions, photophobia, and hydrophobia are associated with the so-called furious form of rabies that has a cerebral localization.
- Depression, anorexia, circling, ataxia, dementia, dysphagia, and facial paralysis may be associated with the "dumb" form of rabies, in which lesions predominate in the brainstem.
- Finally, shifting lameness with hyperesthesia, self-mutilation, ataxia, and progessive ascending paralysis has been associated with the "paralytic" or "spinal" form of the disease. As the virus is widespread throughout the CNS, a single case may present with any or all of the above signs, and new signs may develop at any time throughout the clinical course.
- Death usually occurs within 2–3 days of onset of central signs.

DIAGNOSIS

DIFFERENTIAL DIAGNOSIS

All diseases resulting in rapidly progressive or diffuse central and peripheral nervous system signs should be considered. These diseases include, but are not limited to:

- equine protozoal encephalomyelitis
- equine herpes virus-1
- nigropallidal encephalomyelitis
- Eastern, Western and Venezuelan encephalomyelitis
- Japanese B encephalitis
- Borna disease
- St. Louis virus
- West Nile virus
- Powassan virus
- Main Drain virus
- bacterial meningitis
- trauma
- lead poisoning
- botulism
- space-occupying lesions
- otitis media-interna
- cauda equina neuritis (peripheral polyneuritis)

CBC/BIOCHEMISTRY/URINALYSIS

CBC and serum biochemistry findings are non-specific and non-diagnostic. Urinalysis is usually within normal limits.

OTHER LABORATORY TESTS

In animals that survive for longer than 10–14 days, acute and convalescent serum titers for specific etiologic agents may provide diagnostic clues, particularly for viral associated diseases.

DIAGNOSTIC PROCEDURES

CSF analysis may be abnormal, but results are non-specific and not diagnostic. Increased protein and white blood cell counts may be noted. CSF is frequently within normal limits. Positive Western blot analysis for EPM should be interpreted with caution. It has been suggested that facial skin biopsies and corneal biopsies be tested for rabies virus antigen using fluorescent antibody imaging to achieve an antemortem diagnosis of rabies. Given the failure of one study to demonstrate rabies virus antigen in either of these locations using immunoperoxidase histochemistry techniques, neither test can be considered reliable or potentially beneficial.

PATHOLOGIC FINDINGS

There may be no gross lesions on examination of the spinal cord and brain. Focal hemorrhage was reported as a gross finding in one study, but was not observed in another later study. Histologically, cases are characterized by a nonsuppurative polioencephalomyelitis with ganglionitis. A mild to severe, almost exclusively lymphocytic perivascular infiltrate with rare plasma cells is present. Intravascular lymphocytosis and monocytosis with lymphocytic diapedesis can be observed. Multifocal to diffuse gliosis with microglia and prominent astrocytic nuclei predominate in the gray matter.

Glial nodules may be present, associated with hyperemic vessels. Vacuolation of white matter and neurons may be present. In the brainstem, axonal fragmentation and swelling associated with lymphocytic infiltrate and gliosis is present. In horses, only approximately 30% of cases have the characteristic Negri body formation. The spinal cord can contain moderate to severe, bilateral, assymetric perivascular infiltrate within the gray matter, usually more severe in the dorsal gray column. Perivascular cuffing may extend into the white matter, with associated mild perivascular hemorrhage and multifocal Wallerian degeneration. Spinal cord lesions are frequently segmental. The brain is positive for rabies virus antigen when tested using fluorescent antibody techniques or immunoperoxidase histochemistry.

IMAGING

N/A

TREATMENT

APPROPRIATE HEALTH CARE

There is no specific treatment for rabies in horses. Symptomatic and supportive treatment may prolong the clinical course and allow for completion of ante-mortem diagnostic testing. The horse may be cared for in-hospital or at home, if facilities permit. Consideration should be given to the ability of the owner to transport the horse safely and to the potential for exposure.

NURSING CARE

Horses that have been exposed to rabies by the bite of a rabid animal should have all wounds cleaned, debrided, and lavaged aggressively with iodine or quarternary ammonium compounds. The area surrounding the wound should be instilled with rabies antiserum. Affected horses should be kept in quiet, well-bedded, and padded surroundings. Head protection and leg wraps may be used in down horses or in horses likely to harm themselves. Because of the zoonotic potential, contact with rabies suspects by humans and other animals should be minimized.

ACTIVITY

Horses suspected of having rabies should be maintained as quietly as possible and activity limited by stall confinement.

DIET

Horses with anorexia or dysphagia may require tube feeding at frequent intervals with a commercially prepared diet or with an alfalfa meal slurry.

CLIENT EDUCATION

- The client should be informed that rabies victims do not survive, and that continuing to treat the animal and pursue diagnostics is in the hope that the horse has another, treatable, disease.
- Personnel regularly handling the horse should be educated regarding rabies and vaccinated against rabies.
- All handlers, regardless of vaccination status, should wear gloves, eye protection, and masks when handling the patient or any biological samples from the patient.
- Animals suspected of being exposed to the rabies virus must be quarantined for 6 months and observed for neurologic abnormalities. Unvaccinated exposed horses should not receive rabies prophylaxis until after the period of quarantine. It is important to check with local authorities, as requirements for quarantine and other precautions may vary with locality.

SURGICAL CONSIDERATIONS

N/A

MEDICATIONS

DRUG(S) OF CHOICE

- All treatments are supportive and palliative, and are only justified if there is doubt regarding the diagnosis.
- Broad-spectrum antimicrobial therapy of the clinician's choice may be administered as a protective measure against secondary bacterial infection of wounds or due to aspiration.
- Dysphagic, anorexic, depressed, or maniacal patients may require intravenous fluid support to maintain hydration.
- Sedation may be required in horses that are hyperesthetic or excitable. Drugs that lower the seizure threshold should be avoided.
- Anti-inflammatory agents such as flunixin meglumine, phenylbutazone, or DMSO may be administered. If CNS edema is suspected, intravenous mannitol boluses may be given.

CONTRAINDICATIONS/PRECAUTIONS/ POSSIBLE INTERACTIONS/ ALTERNATIVE DRUGS

Avoid the use of drugs that may lower the seizure threshold.

FOLLOW-UP

PATIENT MONITORING

N/A

PREVENTION/AVOIDANCE

Exposed clients should contact their personal physician and local health authorities.

It is recommended that horses in high-risk areas be vaccinated annually. Two inactivated diploid vaccines (Imrab-1, Pittman-Moore, Inc., Terre Haute, IN; and Rabgard, Norden Laboratories, Inc., Lincoln, NB) are available and approved for use in horses. The dose is 2 mL administered intramuscularly in the semimembranosus or semitendinosus muscle groups.

The client is to be cautioned that there have been documented cases of rabies in vaccinated horses.

MISCELLANEOUS

ABBREVIATION

- EPM = equine protozoal encephalomyelitis

Suggested Reading

Del Piero F, Wilkins PA, deLahunta A, Trimarchi C, Dubovi EJ. Rabies in horses in New York State: Clinical, pathological, immunohistochemical and virological findings. Suppl. Equine Vet J In press. 1998.

Green SL, Smith LL, Vernau W, Beacock SM. Rabies in horses: 21 cases (1970–1990). J Vet Med Assoc 1992:200(8):1133-1137.

Hamir AN, Moser G, Rupprecht CE. A five year (1983–1988) retrospective study of equine neurological diseases with special reference to rabies. J Comp Path 1992;106:411-421.

Keane DP, Little PB. Equine viral encephalomyelitis in Canada: a review of known and potential causes. Can Vet J 1987;28:497-504.

Krebs JW, Smith JS, Rupprecht CE, Childs JE. Rabies surveillance in the United States during 1996. J Am Vet Med Assoc 1997;211(12):1225-1239.

Author Pamela A. Wilkins

Consulting Editor Corinne R. Sweeney

RABIES ENCEPHALITIS

BASICS

DEFINITION
A lethal encephalitis caused by a bullet-shaped, neurotropic, single-stranded RNA virus in the family Rhabdoviridae, genus *Lyssavirus*

PATHOPHYSIOLOGY
- Usually transmitted by salivary contamination of a bite wound, but infection by inhaled, oral, or transplacental routes has been demonstrated in the laboratory.
- The virus may amplify in muscle tissue before invading the peripheral nervous system. It is not known how the virus enters the peripheral nerves.
- The virus moves to the CNS by axoplasmic flow. Spread and multiplication into the CNS is rapid.
- The virus ultimately affects almost all nerves in the body as well as the eye and salivary glands. Salivary secretion of virus precedes the onset of clinical signs by as much as 30 days.
- The incubation period in horses varies from 2 weeks to several months.
- Clinical signs and survival time depend on proximity of the bite wound to the brain, dose, and pathogenicity of the viral strain.

SYSTEM AFFECTED
CNS

SIGNALMENT
Any breed, sex, and age

SIGNS

Historical Findings
Horses may be in areas where rabies is more common, but location does not rule out the diagnosis.

Physical Examination Findings
- Presenting signs and clinical course are extremely variable but can be related to severe diffuse or multifocal CNS disease initially localized to the brain or spinal cord.
- Presenting signs (singly or in combination)—anorexia, ataxia, colic, depression (i.e., dumb rabies), blindness, hyperesthesia, lameness, dementia, mania (i.e., furious rabies), muscle-twitching, paresis, paralysis, urinary incontinence, and sudden death
- Regardless of the presenting signs, progression is rapid and results in death 3–10 days after onset.

CAUSE
- The disease is caused by serotype 1 rabies virus, which is a bullet-shaped, neurotropic, single-stranded RNA virus of the genus *Lyssavirus* and family Rhabdoviridae.
- This family includes ≅25 viruses, but only serotype 1 is pathogenic.
- Rabies has two cycles, which include canine (i.e., urban) and wildlife (i.e., sylvatic) rabies.
- Most wildlife vectors are small omnivores, such as skunks and raccoons in the United States.
- Extension occurs into domestic animals, which are essentially dead-end hosts.
- Horse to human transmission appears to be very rare.

RISK FACTORS
Horses in enzootic areas

DIAGNOSIS

DIFFERENTIAL DIAGNOSIS
- Consider any disease associated with progressive gray-matter disruption.
- Togaviral encephalitides, heavy-metal toxicity, neuritis of the cauda equina, acute protozoal myeloencephalitis, sorghum-sudan grass poisoning, hepatoencephalopathy, CNS trauma, moldy corn poisoning, and probably many other disorders

CBC/BIOCHEMISTRY/URINALYSIS
No specific abnormalities

OTHER LABORATORY TESTS
CSF often is normal but may have moderate elevations in protein and mononuclear cell numbers.

IMAGING
N/A

DIAGNOSTIC PROCEDURES
- Fluorescent antibody staining of the muzzle tactile hair follicles (containing nervous tissue) of suspect horses may be a useful antemortem test, but false-negative results will occur.
- Antemortem diagnosis is difficult.
- Consider the disease in any horse with rapidly progressive CNS signs, especially (but not solely) in areas where rabies is enzootic.
- Half of the brain should be kept cool and transported to a diagnostic laboratory with rabies diagnostic capabilities (e.g., fluorescent antibody test with fluorescein-conjugated rabies antiserum) that can identify rabies antigen in the tissue. The other half should be fixed in 10% formalin for histopathologic examination if the rabies diagnostic tests are negative.

PATHOLOGIC FINDINGS

• Diffuse, mild to severe, nonsuppurative polioencephalomyelitis predominates.
• Large, eosinophilic cytoplasmic inclusions (i.e., Negri bodies) occur in ganglion cells and neurons, but not in all cases.
• Results of fluorescent antibody tests are confirmed by mouse inoculation of brain homogenates intrathecally.

TREATMENT

None

MEDICATIONS

DRUGS OF CHOICE

N/A

CONTRAINDICATIONS

N/A

PRECAUTIONS

N/A

POSSIBLE INTERACTIONS

N/A

ALTERNATIVE DRUGS

N/A

FOLLOW UP

POSSIBLE COMPLICATIONS

N/A

PREVENTION/AVOIDANCE

• Avoid exposure to affected nervous and other tissues.
• Horses in enzootic areas may be immunized with annual vaccination beginning at 6 months of age with commercial, inactivated vaccine.
• Horses previously immunized and bitten by suspect rabid animals can be given a three-booster immunization series over 7 days and should be quarantined for a minimum of 90 days.

MISCELLANEOUS

ASSOCIATED CONDITIONS

N/A

AGE-RELATED FACTORS

N/A

ZOONOTIC POTENTIAL

N/A

PREGNANCY

N/A

SYNONYMS

N/A

SEE ALSO

N/A

ABBREVIATIONS

CSF = cerebrospinal fluid

Suggested Reading

Green SL. Equine rabies. Vet Clin North Am Equine Pract 1993;9:337–347.

Hamir AN, et al. A five year (1985–1989) retrospective study of equine neurological diseases with special reference to rabies. J Comp Pathol 1992;106:411–421.

King AA, Turner GS. Rabies: a review. J Comp Pathol 1993;108:1–39.

Author Joseph J. Bertone

Consulting Editor Joseph J. Bertone

RECTAL PROLAPSE

BASICS

DEFINITION

Rectal prolapse is the evagination of the rectal mucous membrane and its associated structures through the external anal sphincter and can be categorized into four types, depending on the tissues displaced:

- Type 1 = rectal mucosa + submucosa
- Type 2 = full-thickness rectal wall (mucosa, submucosa, muscularis, and serosa) + rectal ampulla (=retroperitoneal rectal dilatation within the pelvic girdle)
- Type 3 = full-thickness rectal wall + invagination of the terminal small colon
- Type 4 = full-thickness rectal wall + intussusception of the peritoneal rectum and varying lengths of the small colon

PATHOPHYSIOLOGY

Rectal prolapse results from an increase in pressure gradient between the abdominal cavity and the anus, such as that which develops with tenesmus. With sufficient increase in pressure gradient, the rectal mucosa and submucosa glide backward over the muscularis layer to produce the typical rectal protrusion. Unreduced prolapses become edematous and cyanotic due to compromise of venous outflow secondary to tension on affected vessels. The anal sphincter also compromises blood flow by constricting around the exteriorized tissues. With types 3 and 4 prolapses, the entire rectum disengages from the perirectal tissues, resulting in complete displacement of the rectum as well as the distal small colon. Because the mesocolon of the distal small colon is relatively short, caudal displacement and tearing of the mesocolon during prolapse often results in avulsion of the colonic blood supply. If the blood supply to the small colon is disrupted, ischemic necrosis ensues.

SYSTEMS AFFECTED

Gastrointestinal

Rectal impaction, peritonitis, or small colon necrosis can occur subsequent to rectal prolapse and may contribute to ileus.

Behavioral

Horses may exhibit signs of tenesmus or of mild to moderate abdominal pain associated with prolapse or rectal impaction.

Cardiovascular

Circulatory shock may be evident in horses with thrombosis or rupture of the small colonic vasculature.

GENETICS

N/A

INCIDENCE/PREVALENCE

N/A

SIGNALMENT

Breed Predilections

N/A

Mean Age and Range

Seen most often in adults.

Predominant Sex

Affects mares more often than stallions or geldings.

SIGNS

Historical Findings

Prolonged or dramatic tenesmus.

Physical Examination Findings

Palpation and inspection are simple means of differentiating between the four types of rectal prolapses. Types 1, 2, and 3 are continuous with the mucocutaneous junction of the anus. Characteristic findings include:

- Type 1—a circular, doughnut-shaped, edematous swelling at the anus that is usually most prominent ventrally
- Type 2—a larger, cauliflower-shaped swelling that is often thicker ventrally than dorsally
- Type 3—appears similar to type 2, but is firmer due to the presence of invaginated peritoneal rectum or small colon
- Type 4—a palpable trench exists between the prolapse and the anus, and can be appreciated by sliding a finger underneath the prolapse and past the normal mucocutaneous junction

CAUSES

Rectal prolapse is most often associated with tenesmus* secondary to a variety of conditions:

- Parturition
- Dystocia
- Uterine prolapse
- Diarrhea
- Constipation
- Colitis
- Proctitis
- Rectal masses: neoplasms (leiomyoma, lipoma), foreign bodies, abscesses, polyps, hematomas
- Grade 2 rectal tears
- Intestinal parasitism
- Urethral obstruction: urolithiasis

In many cases, however, a cause cannot be identified.

RISK FACTORS

Any condition that induces tenesmus. Prolapse may occur more readily in horses in poor body condition due to loss of tone in the anal sphincter, or to the presence of loose attachments between the rectal mucosa/submucosa and the muscularis, or between the rectum and perirectal tissues. Type 1 rectal prolapses are often seen in horses with severe diarrhea, and type 4 rectal prolapses are most often associated with dystocias in broodmares.

DIAGNOSIS

DIFFERENTIAL DIAGNOSIS

Prolapsed tissues may be mistaken for a neoplastic mass. Visual inspection and palpation can differentiate between the two conditions. Evaginated rectal tissues are obvious with a prolapse, whereas a neoplasm arises from a localized aspect of the rectal or perirectal tissues.

CBC/BIOCHEMISTRY/URINALYSIS

Systemic abnormalities corresponding to the inciting cause may be identified. Early in the course of types 3 and 4 prolapses, leukocytosis and neutrophilia with a left shift may be observed, as well as increases in PCV, fibrinogen, TP, sodium, and potassium levels. With intensified demand and depletion of WBC reserves, leukopenia and neutropenia ensue. Chronicity may lead to decreases in potassium, sodium, and chloride levels and increases in BUN, creatinine, and bilirubin.

OTHER LABORATORY TESTS

Abdominocentesis is useful for evaluation of compromise to the small colon and its blood supply. Peritoneal fluid in horses with types 3 or 4 prolapses may have an increase in WBC count or TP level. The presence of degenerate neutrophils, bacteria, or plant material on cytologic examination of the peritoneal fluid is indicative of septic inflammation of the peritoneal cavity and is associated with a poor prognosis. Culture and sensitivity of peritoneal fluid may help direct systemic antibiotic therapy.

IMAGING

N/A

DIAGNOSTIC PROCEDURES

Evaluation of the location, degree of trauma, and vascular compromise to the small colon in type 4 prolapses can be performed via a flank laparotomy, a ventral midline celiotomy, or laparoscopy. In the standing horse, laparoscopy provides superior visualization and selection of the most appropriate surgical procedure in a minimally invasive manner.

TREATMENT

APPROPRIATE HEALTH CARE

Relief of tenesmus is of paramount importance to the successful treatment of rectal prolapses. The specific cause of the prolapse should therefore be identified and addressed. Epidural anesthesia is an effective means of alleviating tenesmus. Alternatively, heavy sedation, use of lidocaine gel, a lidocaine enema, or infiltration of the inflamed tissues with local anesthetic may provide some relief.

Types 1 and 2 rectal prolapses without extensive edema, trauma, or contamination usually respond to conservative therapy aimed at reduction of tissue edema, manual reduction of the prolapse, and placement of a purse-string suture in the anus. The suture should consist of a large (size 1–3), nonabsorbable (nylon, polypropylene, umbilical tape, caprolactam) material and be placed using four wide bites located 1–2 cm from the anus. Following placement, the external anal sphincter should be dilatable to a diameter of 4–6 cm to permit defecation. Epidural anesthesia/analgesia should be maintained to prevent straining against the suture. The suture should be removed within 24–48 hr to minimize complications.

Types 1 and 2 prolapses that are chronic in nature or that have failed to respond to conservative therapy can be treated successfully by submucosal resection or by rectal amputation. Both procedures can be performed in the standing, sedated horse using epidural anesthesia. Submucosal resection is preferred over rectal amputation because the rectal vasculature and muscular layers are preserved, an aseptic peritoneal environment is maintained, there is decreased risk of postoperative peri-rectal abscess formation or of rectal stricture, and postoperative tenesmus is decreased.

Submucosal resection involves placement of two 6- to 8-inch long 18 gauge spinal needles at right angles through the external anal sphincter to anchor the prolapsed tissues in position. Two circumferential incisions are made at the junction between healthy and unhealthy mucosal layers, one at the outermost aspect of the prolapse and one at the anal sphincter. These two incisions are joined by a longitudinal incision, and the mucosa is dissected from the submucosa. The incised edges are apposed with size 0 to size 1 monofilament absorbable suture in a simple interrupted pattern or in a simple continuous pattern interrupted at three equidistant points around the circumference. Once suturing is complete, the spinal needles are removed and the prolapse can be reduced without difficulty.

Rectal amputation is usually reserved for cases with advanced necrosis of the rectal mucosa and submucosa. Rectal amputation involves placement of spinal needles through the anal sphincter in a similar fashion, thus dividing the prolapsed tissues into quadrants. The entire prolapse is resected and the layers are anatomically reconstructed with size 0 to size 1 monofilament absorbable suture material in a simple continuous pattern. When the spinal needles are removed, the sutured rectal tissues readily retract through the anus. Types 3 and 4 rectal prolapses require referral to a surgical facility.

RECTAL PROLAPSE

NURSING CARE

Placement of a caudal epidural catheter can allow continued administration of agents to alleviate straining and provide analgesia/anesthesia. It can also prevent difficulties encountered with repeated attempts at epidural injection.

Emollients and lubricants may be used to soften and soothe prolapsed tissues.

Hyperosmotic compounds such as magnesium sulfate, mannitol, 50% dextrose, and anhydrous glycerin may be applied to prolapsed tissues to decrease mucosal edema.

Fecal softeners such as mineral oil or dioctyl sodium sulfosuccinate (DSS) can be administered via nasogastric tube to facilitate passage of feces. Fecal softening within the rectum can be achieved using mineral oil enemas.

Balanced polyionic intravenous fluid therapy may be required by horses with types 3 or 4 prolapses for treatment of hypovolemia or endotoxemic shock. The fluid rate should be based on the horse's hydration status and clinical condition.

ACTIVITY

Horses should be restricted to a stall for appropriate monitoring and postoperative care. The animal should also be kept standing if possible to avoid increases in abdominal pressure associated with recumbency.

DIET

Feed should be withheld for 12–24 hr following treatment. A low-bulk laxative diet consisting of green pasture, a complete pelleted ration, or alfalfa pellets soaked in water is then recommended for the next 10 days.

CLIENT EDUCATION

Horses with type 4 rectal prolapse have a serious condition carrying a guarded to poor prognosis for survival. Depending on the length of intussuscepted tissues, chronicity of the prolapse, the horse's medical status and value, and the owner's intentions for the horse, euthanasia may be warranted. If the owner wishes to pursue treatment, factors that require discussion include cost, the need for extensive postoperative care, and multiple possible complications following resection/anastamosis or colostomy. Horses undergoing colostomy require a second procedure for revision; the second procedure necessitates general anesthesia, incurs additional costs, and provides additional opportunities for complications to arise.

SURGICAL CONSIDERATIONS

Notable hemorrhage may occur during submucosal resection or rectal amputation, but can be controlled with electrocautery or ligation.

MEDICATIONS

DRUGS OF CHOICE

Sedation may be achieved with xylazine (0.2–1.1 mg/kg IV) or detomidine (0.005–0.02 mg/kg IV). Both duration and quality of sedation may be enhanced by the co-administration of butorphanol tartrate (0.1 mg/kg IV).

Epidural administration of a variety of agents may provide anesthesia for initial evaluation and treatment, as well as analgesia for prevention of postoperative tenesmus (for details and dosages, see the chapter entitled Rectal Tear).

CONTRAINDICATIONS

N/A

PRECAUTIONS

N/A

POSSIBLE INTERACTIONS

N/A

ALTERNATIVE DRUGS

N/A

FOLLOW-UP

PATIENT MONITORING

Following treatment, the patient should be observed regularly for evidence of tenesmus, rectal impaction, or relapse. Purse-string sutures should be removed within 24–48 hr to minimize complications.

PREVENTION/AVOIDANCE

Prompt recognition and treatment of factors predisposing to tenesmus reduces the likelihood of rectal prolapse.

RECTAL PROLAPSE

POSSIBLE COMPLICATIONS
- Rectal impaction
- Reprolapse
- Dehiscence of suture lines
- Perirectal abscess formation
- Rectal stricture
- Ischemic necrosis of the small colon
- Complications associated with colostomy, celiotomy, or resection/anastomosis procedures

EXPECTED COURSE AND PROGNOSIS
The prognosis for types 1 and 2 rectal prolapses is favorable, whereas the prognosis for types 3 and 4 prolapses is guarded to poor.

MISCELLANEOUS

ASSOCIATED CONDITIONS
- Endotoxemia
- Laminitis
- Uterine prolapse

AGE-RELATED FACTORS
N/A

ZOONOTIC POTENTIAL
N/A

PREGNANCY
N/A

SYNONYMS
N/A

SEE ALSO
See individual factors listed under Causes.

ABBREVIATIONS
- BUN = blood urea nitrogen
- CBC = complete blood count
- DSS = dioctyl sodium sulfosuccinate
- PCV = packed cell volume
- TP = total protein
- WBC = white blood cell

Suggested Reading

Ragle CA, Southwood LL, Galuppo LD, et al. Laparoscopic diagnosis of ischemic necrosis of the descending colon after rectal prolapse and rupture of the mesocolon in two postpartum mares. J Am Vet Med Assoc 1997;210:1646-1648.

DeBowes RM. Standing rectal and tail surgery. Vet Clin North Am Eq Pract 1991; 7(3):649-667.

Meagher DA. Rectal surgery. In: White NA, Moore JN, eds. Current practice of equine surgery. Philadelphia: JB Lippincott Co., 1990.

Rick MC. Management of rectal injuries. Vet Clin North Am Eq Pract 1989; 5(2):407-428.

Turner TA, Fessler JF. Rectal prolapse in the horse. J Am Vet Med Assoc 1980; 177(10):1028-1032.

Author Annette M. Sysel

Consulting Editor Henry Stämpfli

RECTAL TEAR

BASICS

DEFINITION

A partial- to full-thickness disruption of the wall of the retroperitoneal or peritoneal rectum.

PATHOPHYSIOLOGY

Most tears result from rupture of the rectal wall as it contracts around the examiner's forearm rather than from direct penetration of the wall with fingertips. They occur 25- to 30-cm from the anus in the dorsal aspect of the rectum positioned between 10 and 2 o'clock. They are classified according to the tissue layers involved:

- Grade 1—Tearing of the rectal mucosa + submucosa, palpable as a defect in the rectal wall.
- Grade 2—Disruption of the muscular layer of the rectum, with prolapse of the mucosa and submucosa through the defect to create a diverticulum, which may act as a pocket for fecal impaction. Grade 2 tears do not produce luminal bleeding or an appreciable change in the texture of the rectal lining. They are palpable as a mucosa-lined dimple in the rectal wall.
- Grade 3(a)—Involvement of the rectal mucosa, submucosa, and muscularis layers resulting in a palpable void in the rectal wall that exposes the serosa.
- Grade 3(b)—Disruption of all layers of the rectal wall without involvement of the mesorectum. This tear is palpable as a defect in the rectal wall that exposes the fat-filled mesorectum. Grade 3 tears can cause formation of a retroperitoneal space within the pelvic cavity that can become impacted, then rupture and convert to a grade 4 tear. The presence of intact serosa or mesorectum prevents contamination of the abdominal cavity with fecal material; however, movement of bacteria through these tissues may induce local peritonitis.
- Grade 4—Tearing of all layers of the rectum as well as the mesorectum. As a result, direct communication exists between the rectum and the abdominal cavity, and peritoneal surfaces become contaminated with fecal material. This type of tear results in development of endotoxemia and circulatory shock.

SYSTEM AFFECTED

Gastrointestinal

Local and diffuse peritonitis may develop within 2 hr of a rectal tear. Ileus secondary to diffusion of bacteria and toxins may follow. Abdominal discomfort and straining may accompany rectal impactions, especially in horses with grade 2 rectal tears.

Behavioral

Signs of abdominal pain secondary to peritonitis and ileus may be present initially, but progress to signs of depression and endotoxic shock.

Cardiovascular

Vascular collapse secondary to endotoxemic shock may be evident within 2 hr following a rectal tear.

GENETICS

N/A

INCIDENCE/PREVALENCE

N/A

SIGNALMENT

Breed Predilections

- Arabians
- Miniature horses and other small breeds
- Ponies

Mean Age/Range

Rectal tears may be seen in horses of any age. Young horses that have a small rectal diameter or those that are unaccustomed to rectal examination may be predisposed.

Predominant Sex

May occur more often in males than females.

SIGNS

General Comments

Tearing of the rectum during a rectal examination may not be sensed by the palpator, but should be suspected if a significant amount of blood is evident on the rectal sleeve or in the feces following rectal examination.

Historical Findings

Horses with grades 1 or 2 rectal tears rarely demonstrate signs relative to the tear. Grade 2 tears are often not identified until signs of rectal impaction develop; frequently, these tears are identified during an unassociated rectal examination. More severe rectal tears are often associated with signs of sweating, pawing, a splinted abdomen, or tachycardia within 2 hr following breeding or rectal palpation.

Physical Examination Findings

Rectal findings are summarized under Pathophysiology.

CAUSES

- Rectal palpation of the gastrointestinal or urogenital system*
- Misdirected intromission of a stallion's penis during breeding*
- Enema administration
- Meconium extraction with forceps
- Dystocia
- External trauma
- Fractures of the pelvis or vertebrae
- Sodomy
- Displaced granulosa cell tumors
- Ruptured small colon hematomas
- Spontaneous

RISK FACTORS

Any condition that necessitates repeated rectal examination.

RECTAL TEAR

DIAGNOSIS

DIFFERENTIAL DIAGNOSIS

Mild mucosal irritation may result in a few flecks of blood or blood-tinged fluid on the palpation sleeve following rectal examination. Colitis or conditions that compromise the vascular supply of the small colon, with or without compromise to its lumen, may produce bloody or malodorous brown fluid on rectal examination.

CBC/BIOCHEMISTRY/URINALYSIS

Leukocytosis and neutrophilia with a left shift, as well as increases in PCV, fibrinogen, TP, sodium, and potassium occur early in the course of grades 3 and 4 rectal tears, and leukopenia; neutropenia; decreases in potassium, sodium, and chloride levels; and increases in BUN, creatinine, and bilirubin may occur later.

OTHER LABORATORY TESTS

An increase in peritoneal fluid, WBC count, or TP level is consistent with a diagnosis of peritonitis. The presence of degenerate neutrophils, bacteria, or plant material on cytologic examination is indicative of septic peritonitis and is associated with a poor prognosis.

IMAGING

Abdominal ultrasound may be useful in assessment of quantity and quality of peritoneal fluid.

DIAGNOSTIC PROCEDURES

Bare-armed evaluation of the rectum is useful in ruling out the presence of a rectal tear. The veterinarian's arm should be lubricated copiously with a water-soluble gel and the feces gently removed from the rectum. Rectal tears can be identified through circumferential palpation of the rectum cranially from the anus in 3- to 4-inch (6- to 10-cm) increments. The rectal tear should be assessed for depth of penetration, size, position, and distance from the anus.

A vaginal speculum may be used for visualization of the tear, but infolding of the mucosa around the end of the speculum often hampers adequate assessment.

The severity of damage to the rectal wall can be assessed endoscopically.

Laparoscopy may be performed in horses with severe grades 3 or 4 tears to determine presence and degree of fecal contamination of the abdominal cavity. Laparoscopy may also permit direct visualization and assessment of tears of the peritoneal rectum.

PATHOLOGIC FINDINGS

See Pathophysiology.

TREATMENT

APPROPRIATE HEALTH CARE

If a rectal tear is suspected, straining and rectal peristalsis should be reduced by sedation, epidural anesthesia, and/or parasympatholytic drugs. A lidocaine enema (12–25 mL of 2% lidocaine in 50 mL water) or lidocaine jelly may be used. Fecal softeners and a laxative diet are valuable in the management of all rectal tear cases. Grade 1 rectal tears usually respond well to a 3-5 day course of anti-inflammatory and broad-spectrum antibiotic therapy. Periodic cleaning and delicate debridement with gauze squares may be needed to hasten healing and prevent abscess formation, a permanent diverticulum, or a rectal stricture. In addition to the above, grade 2 rectal tears may be treated with a combination of flushing and drainage of the diverticulum. Grades 3(a) and (b) and grade 4 rectal tears should be considered emergencies that require referral to a surgical facility. Prior to transport, the rectal tear should be packed with 3-inch (7.5-cm) stockinette filled with moistened roll cotton. This should be sprayed with povidone–iodine and lubricated with surgical gel and inserted to a point 10 cm proximal to the tear. The tear should not be packed. The packing may be secured by closing the anus with towel clamps or a purse-string suture. Epidural anesthesia should be maintained to prevent straining during transport. Parenteral anti-inflammatory and broad-spectrum antibiotic therapy should be initiated, and intravenous fluids should be administered to horses in shock. Feed should be withheld, and fecal softeners should be administered via nasogastric tube.

ACTIVITY

Horses that have undergone surgical treatment should be confined to a stall for appropriate postoperative monitoring and management.

DIET

All horses with rectal tears should be fed a low-bulk laxative diet, such as green grass, a complete pelleted ration, or alfalfa pellets soaked in water.

CLIENT EDUCATION

The owner should be informed of the presence of a rectal tear or a suspected tear immediately. If treatment is pursued, the owner should be advised of the cost, extensive postoperative care, and multiple complications that can be associated with surgical treatment.

RECTAL TEAR

MEDICATIONS

DRUG(S) OF CHOICE

• Parasympatholytic agents such as propantheline bromide (0.014 mg/kg IV or IM) or atropine (0.44–0.1 mg/kg IM or SC) decrease rectal peristalsis and prevent straining during transport.
• Sedation may be achieved with xylazine (0.2–1.1 mg/kg IV) or detomidine (0.005–0.02 mg/kg IV). Both duration and quality of sedation may be enhanced by the co-administration of butorphanol tartrate (0.1 mg/kg IV).
• Epidural administration of a variety of agents (e.g., lidocaine, xylazine, detomodine) may provide anesthesia for initial evaluation and treatment as well as analgesia for prevention of postoperative tenesmus. A caudal epidural catheter allows repeated administration of agents to alleviate straining and provide analgesia/anesthesia to the perineal region
• Broad-spectrum antibiotic therapy is recommended for 3–10 days with grades 1 and 2 rectal tears. Extensive broad-spectrum antibiotic therapy is required for grades 3 and 4 tears.
• Tetanus prophylaxis should be considered.
• Flunixin meglumine therapy is recommended in horses with endotoxemia.

CONTRAINDICATIONS

• Acepromazine is contraindicated for sedation of hypovolemic horses.
• Indiscriminate use of atropine can result in gastrointestinal complications, such as prolonged ileus with tympanic distention of the bowel, mild to moderate abdominal pain, and tachycardia.

PRECAUTIONS

Administration of epidural lidocaine may be associated with ataxia.

POSSIBLE INTERACTIONS

If sedatives have been administered by the intramuscular or intravenous route, the epidural dosage of xylazine or detomidine should be adjusted to avoid excessive cumulative sedation.

ALTERNATIVE DRUGS

N/A

FOLLOW-UP

PATIENT MONITORING

• Horses with grade 1 rectal tears should be monitored closely for 4–8 days, with serial CBC's, fibrinogen levels, and peritoneal fluid analyses.
• Rectal palpation should be avoided for 30 days. Most grades 1 and 2 tears heal within 7–14 days.
• Horses with grades 3 and 4 rectal tears should be monitored for complications associated with the surgical procedure(s) performed. These horses should be assessed with serial CBC's, fibrinogen levels, and peritoneal fluid analyses.

PREVENTION/AVOIDANCE

Rectal examination of horses should be reserved for veterinarians. Rectal examinations should be done only when necessary, and the history of the problem as well as the size and temperament of the patient should be considered. Appropriate restraint and careful technique should be used.
Appropriate supervision during breeding may reduce the likelihood of inadvertent tearing by the stallion.

POSSIBLE COMPLICATIONS

• Progression of the tear
• Fecal contamination of the tear or of the abdomen
• Peritonitis
• Extensive cellulitis
• Abscess formation
• Rectoperitoneal fistula formation
• Rectal impaction or stricture
• Ileus
• Abdominal adhesions
• Complications associated with primary closure: excessive tissue trauma; incomplete closure; inadvertent suturing of mucosal folds leading to stricture
• Complications associated with temporary liner placement: tearing of the liner; retraction of the liner into the rectum to uncover the tear; premature sloughing
• Complications associated with colostomy: dehiscence; adhesions; abscessation; herniation/prolapse; rupture of mesenteric vessels; infarction; spontaneous closure

EXPECTED COURSE AND PROGNOSIS

Chances for survival improve with adequate and immediate first aid. Grades 1 and 2 rectal tears have a good prognosis; grade 3(a) tears have a fair to guarded prognosis; grade 3(b) tears have a guarded to poor prognosis because of the likelihood of greater tissue damage and undermining; grade 4 tears have a poor to grave prognosis because gross fecal contamination of the abdomen predisposes to massive adhesion formation and fatal peritonitis.

RECTAL TEAR

MISCELLANEOUS

ASSOCIATED CONDITIONS
- Peritonitis
- Endotoxemia
- Laminitis
- Abdominal adhesions

AGE-RELATED FACTORS
N/A

ZOONOTIC POTENTIAL
N/A

PREGNANCY
Broodmares left with permanent colostomies are prone to intestinal herniation in advanced pregnancy, and at parturition due to unusual abdominal pressures placed against the colonic stoma.

SYNONYMS
N/A

SEE ALSO
See also Associated Conditions.

ABBREVIATIONS
- BUN = blood urea nitrogen
- PCV = packed cell volume
- TP = total protein

Suggested Reading

Baird AN. Rectal tears. In: Robinson NE, ed. Current therapy in equine medicine, 3rd ed. Philadelphia: WB Saunders Co., 1992.

Freeman DE, Martin BB. Rectum and anus. In: Auer JA. Equine surgery. Philadelphia: WB Saunders Co., 1992.

Meagher DA. Rectal surgery. In: White NA, Moore JN, eds. Current practice of equine surgery. Philadelphia: JB Lippincott Co., 1990.

Rick MC. Management of rectal injuries. Vet Clin North Am Eq Pract 1989; 5(2):407-428.

Watkins JP, Taylor TS, Schumacher J, et al. Rectal tears in the horse: an analysis of 35 cases. Eq Vet J 1989;21(3):186-188.

Author Annette M. Sysel

Consulting Editor Henry Stämpfli

RECURRENT UVEITIS

BASICS

DEFINITION

Equine recurrent uveitis (ERU) is a common cause of blindness in horses. It is a group of immune-mediated diseases of multiple origins. Recurrence of anterior uveitis due to immunologic mechanisms is the hallmark of ERU.

PATHOPHYSIOLOGY

The causes of ERU are not completely understood. ERU can occur as a late sequelae to systemic infection with ocular signs developing 12 to 15 months post-inoculation. Hypersensitivity to infectious agents such as *Leptospira interrogans* are suspected with corresponding antibodies found in serum, tears, and aqueous humor. The presence of living *Leptospira* organisms is not necessary for disease production. Not all horses positive for *Leptospira* have uveitis.

SYSTEM AFFECTED

Ophthalmic

GENETICS

Unknown, but some genetic predisposition is possible.

INCIDENCE/PREVALENCE

Unknown

SIGNALMENT

Breed Predilection

Leptospira interrogans seropositive Appaloosas were 8.3 times as likely to develop uveitis as other breeds, and 3.8 times more likely than other breeds to lose vision following development of uveitis.

Mean Age and Range

All ages can be affected.

Predominant Sex

None

SIGNS

- The clinical signs of acute *Leptospira* infections are generally rather benign and self-limiting, although inappetence, fever, icterus, or abortions may be seen.
- Horses with ERU display increased lacrimation, blepharospasm, and photophobia. Subtle amounts of corneal edema, conjunctival hyperemia, and ciliary injection are present initially, and can become prominent as the condition progresses. Aqueous flare, hyphema, intraocular fibrin, and hypopyon may be observed. Miosis is usually a prominent sign and can result in a misshapen pupil and posterior synechiae. Delayed or failure to achieve pharmacologic mydriasis is common when uveitis is active. Intraocular pressure (IOP) is generally low, but ERU may be associated with intermittent and acute elevations in IOP. Fibrin and iris pigment may be deposited on the anterior lens capsule. Cataract formation may occur if the inflammation does not subside quickly.
- Severe anterior segment inflammation often prevents an adequate fundic exam of the acutely affected eye. As the pupil dilates and the ocular media clears with successful treatment, one should evaluate the fundus for evidence of active or inactive chorioretinitis. Choroiditis may be associated with leakage of plasma or blood from choroidal and retinal blood vessels to result in focal or diffuse, nontapetal, exudative retinal detachments. Retinal vascular congestion can occur. The vitreous may develop haziness due to leakage of proteins and cells from retinal vessels. The optic nerve head can appear congested.
- In chronic cases, corneal vascularization, permanent corneal edema, synechiation, cataract formation, and iris depigmentation or hyperpigmentation can result. Secondary glaucoma and phthisis bulbi can occur. Vitreous liquefaction, and retinal degeneration indicated by focal to generalized peripapillary regions of depigmentation in the nontapetum can result. Irreversible blindness is a common sequelae to ERU and is due to retinal detachment, cataract formation, or severe chorioretinitis.

CAUSES

Although the pathogenesis is clearly immune-mediated, the causes are often unknown. Hypersensitivity to infectious agents such as *Leptospira interrogans* serovar *pomona* are commonly implicated as the possible cause. Other serovars discussed include *grippotyphosa, icterohaemorrhagiae, canicola, hardjo,* and *sejroe.* Toxoplasmosis, brucellosis, salmonellosis, *Streptococcus, Escherichia coli, Rhodococcus equi,* borreliosis, intestinal strongyles, onchocerciasis, parasites such as *Halicephalobus deletrix,* and viral infections (e.g., equine influenza virus, herpesvirus 1 and 4, arteritis virus, infectious anemia virus) have also been implicated as causes of ERU with no consistency in isolation of these organisms from affected horses. Dead or dying microfilaria of *Onchocerca cervicalis* may release antigens to incite ERU following migration of living microfilaria via vascular migration to the eye. Blunt or penetrating ocular trauma, mechanical trauma, and systemic lymphosarcoma are also incriminated as causes of ERU.

RISK FACTORS

Leptospira infections in horses occur with exposure to urine or urine-contaminated feed or water. Horses with insufficient vaccination or parasite prevention are more prone for viral and parasitic infections. See Prevention/Avoidance for more risk factors.

DIAGNOSIS

DIFFERENTIAL DIAGNOSIS

It is imperative to immediately differentiate a painful eye in a horse as a result of ulcerative keratitis or stromal abscessation from the pain associated with ERU by employing a fluorescein dye test. Although corticosteroids are the treatment of choice for ERU, they can lead to the rapid demise of an eye with a corneal ulcer. Infectious endophthalmitis, hypermature cataracts, and intraocular melanomas can have clinical signs of ERU.

CBC/BIOCHEMISTRY/URINALYSIS

Serum biochemical profiles and CBC may detect major organ abnormalities and/or active systemic infection.

OTHER LABORATORY TESTS

Conjunctival biopsies for examination for *Onchocerca* microfilaria may be performed, although detection of live microfilaria does not necessarily indicate a causal relationship. Serologic testing for leptospirosis, brucellosis, and toxoplasmosis should be considered. Aqueous humor antibody titer determinations can reveal intraocular antibody production, although aqueous paracentesis can be difficult to perform in horses without general anesthesia. Results of serology can be difficult to interpret as many horses have positive titers with no evidence of ocular or systemic diseases. Leptospiral titers for *pomona, bratislava,* and *autumnalis* should be requested in the United States. Positive titers for serovars of 1:400 or greater are of importance. A higher titer in the aqueous humor than the serum is indicative of antibody production, and supports a leptospiral etiology for the uveitis.

IMAGING

N/A

DIAGNOSTIC PROCEDURES

N/A

PATHOLOGIC FINDINGS

Histologic lesions depend on the stage of the disease. In acute stages, lymphocytic infiltration with some neutrophils can be found in the uveal tract, resulting in edema and plasmoid vitreous. In addition, fibrin and leukocytes are present in the anterior chamber, which manifests clinically as aqueous flare. The vessels of the iris, ciliary body, choroid, and retina can be cuffed by lymphocytes and plasma cells. The chronic stages manifest by corneal scarring, cataract formation, and peripapillary chorioretinitis with retinal degeneration and loss of photoreceptors.

TREATMENT

APPROPRIATE HEALTH CARE

The major goals of treatment of ERU are to preserve vision, decrease pain, and prevent or minimize the recurrence of attacks of uveitis. Specific prevention and therapy is often difficult as the etiology is not identified in each case. Treatment should be aggressive and prompt in order to maintain the transparency of the ocular structures. Therapy can last for weeks or months, and should not be stopped abruptly or the uveitis may recur. Medications should be slowly reduced in frequency once clinical signs abate.

NURSING CARE

N/A

ACTIVITY

Activity should be reduced pending resolution of clinical signs.

DIET

Diet should be appropriate for the degree of activity.

CLIENT EDUCATION

Treatment of the disease can be both time consuming and expensive, but it is worth attempting to save vision as long as possible. The owner should be educated immediately about the potential recurrence, the blinding nature of this disease, and the possibility of enucleation to remove a painful eye if vision is lost.

SURGICAL CONSIDERATIONS

- In addition to medical treatment, pars plana vitrectomy in horses with ERU has been used successfully to remove vitreal debris in order to improve vision and delay the progression of the clinical signs.
- Radiation therapy to the sclera may be beneficial in severe, refractory cases, but has a risk of other ocular side effects.

RECURRENT UVEITIS

MEDICATIONS

DRUG(S) OF CHOICE

• Anti-inflammatory medications—specifically, corticosteroids and nonsteroidal drugs—are used to control the generally intense intraocular inflammation that can lead to blindness. Medication can be administered topically as solutions or ointments, subconjunctivally, orally, intramuscularly, and/or intravenously.
• Prednisolone acetate (1%) or dexamethasone (0.1%) should be applied a minimum of 4–6 times per day initially. When the frequent application of topical steroids is not practical, subconjunctival corticosteroids may be used. Methylprednisolone acetate (40 mg q1–3 weeks) and triamcinolone acetonide (40 mg q1–3 weeks) are commonly utilized subconjunctivally in the horse. Systemic corticosteroids may be beneficial in severe, refractory cases of ERU, but pose some risk of inducing laminitis and should be used with caution.
• The NSAIDs, such as topical flurbiprofen, indomethacin, diclofenamic acid, and suprofen (BID to TID), can provide additive anti-inflammatory effects to the corticosteroids and are effective at reducing the intraocular inflammation when a corneal ulcer is present. Cyclosporine A, an immunosuppressive drug, can be effective topically BID for ERU.
• Flunixin meglumine (0.25–1.0 mg/kg BID, PO), phenylbutazone (1 g BID, IV or PO), or aspirin (25 mg/kg BID, PO) are frequently used systemically to control intraocular inflammation. Some horses become refractory to the beneficial effects of these medications, and it may be necessary to switch to one of the other NSAIDs to ameliorate the clinical signs of ERU.
• Mydriatic and cycloplegic medications minimize synechiae formation by inducing mydriasis, and alleviate some of the pain of ERU by relieving spasm of ciliary body muscles (cycloplegia). These drugs also narrow the capillary inter-endothelial cell junctions to reduce capillary plasma leakage. Although topically administered atropine can last several days in the normal equine eye, its effect may be only a few hours in duration in the inflamed ERU eye. A combination of topically administered phenylephrine (2.5%) and atropine (1%) can also be used to attempt to obtain maximum dilation in the inflamed ERU eye. Injectable atropine can be administered subconjunctivally for a repository effect (5–10 mg/injection) in horses difficult to manage, although this may increase the risk of reduction in gut motility. The ease with which mydriasis can be achieved with intermittent use of atropine is an important indication as to the stimulus intensity of the ERU. Failure to achieve mydriasis with atropine indicates the stimulus for the ERU is quite prominent, and/or indicates the presence of synechiation.
• The use of systemically of topically administered antibiotics is often recommended for ERU. Antibiotics should be broad spectrum and appropriate for the geographic location of the patient. Topical antibiotics are indicated in cases of uveitis due to penetrating ocular trauma or ulcerative keratitis. Antibiotic treatment for horses with positive titers for *Leptospira* remains speculative, but streptomycin (11 mg/kg IM BID) may be a good choice for horses at acute and chronic stages of the disease. Penicillin G sodium (10,000 U/kg IV or IM, QID) and tetracycline (6.6–11 mg/kg IV BID) at high dosages may be beneficial during acute leptospiral infections.

CONTRAINDICATIONS

N/A

PRECAUTIONS

• A complete ophthalmic examination should be performed to determine if the uveitis is associated with a corneal ulcer. The presence of a corneal ulcer precludes the use of topical corticosteroids, but not topical nonsteroidal drugs.
• Gut motility should be strictly monitored by abdominal auscultation and observation of signs of abdominal pain when using topically administered atropine in adult horses and foals, as gut motility can be markedly reduced by atropine in some horses. Should gut motility decrease during treatment with topically administered atropine, one can either discontinue the drug or change to the shorter-acting tropicamide.

ALTERNATIVE DRUGS

Homeopathic remedies (e.g., poultices of chamomile and oral methylsulfonylmethane) for ERU have been discussed. Acupuncture at ST1 (stomach 1, intersection of the nasal and middle one-third of the lower eyelid), and BL1 (bladder 2, at the supraorbital foramen) every 3 days has been used to treat active ERU.

RECURRENT UVEITIS

FOLLOW-UP

PATIENT MONITORING

Repeated examination of the anterior and (if possible) the posterior eye segment should be performed to monitor effect of treatment.

PREVENTION/AVOIDANCE

Reduction of exposure to potential antigens by appropriate parasite control programs, eliminating environmental contact with cattle and wildlife, exclusion of horses from ponds and swampy areas, limiting rodent access to horse feed, decreasing incidence of bacterial and viral respiratory and systemic infections, and maintaining a quality feed supply can be beneficial in reducing ERU. Multivalent bovine leptospiral vaccines have been used in horses to treat intractable cases of ERU and to suppress herd outbreaks of leptospiral ERU, but their routine use as a preventative for ERU is controversial.

POSSIBLE COMPLICATIONS

ERU can potentially blind the horse.

EXPECTED COURSE AND PROGNOSIS

Recurrence of anterior uveitis due to immunologic mechanisms is the hallmark of ERU. Overall, the prognosis for ERU is usually poor for a cure to preserve vision, but the disease can be controlled.

MISCELLANEOUS

ASSOCIATED CONDITIONS

Systemic infection by the ERU-causing organism.

AGE-RELATED FACTORS

N/A

ZOONOTIC POTENTIAL

Infectious agents such as *Leptospira* or *Brucella* can be a health risk for people, especially if basic hygienic principals are disregarded.

PREGNANCY

Leptospira infection may lead to abortion. The potential side effects of the medications (especially glucocorticoids and NSAIDs) must be considered.

SYNONYMS

Periodic ophthalmia, moon blindness, iridocyclitis.

SEE ALSO

- Equine Corneal Ulcerations
- Equine Stationary Night Blindness
- Equine Chorioretinitis
- Equine Retinal Detachment
- Systemic Infectious Diseases

ABBREVIATIONS

- ERU = equine recurrent uveitis
- IOP = intraocular pressure
- ST1 = stomach 1
- BL2 = bladder 2

Suggested Reading

Brooks DE. Equine ophthalmology. In: Gelatt KN, ed. Veterinary ophthalmology. 3nd ed. Philadelphia: Lippincott, Williams & Wilkins 1999; chapter 30.

Schwink KL. Equine uveitis. Vet Clin North Am Eq Pract 1992;8:557-574.

Author Andras M. Komaromy

Consulting Editor Dennis E. Brooks

REGURGITATION/DYSPHAGIA

BASICS

DEFINITION

Regurgitation is a rare condition in horses that is associated with a poor prognosis. It is defined as the backward flow of pharyngeal, esophageal, or gastric contents through the mouth or nares.

PATHOPHYSIOLOGY

Eating or drinking can be divided into prehension and deglutition. Prehension is the process of taking food into the oral cavity, whereas deglutition is the process of passing food from the oral cavity to the level of the stomach. Regurgitation reflects an abnormality in the deglutition process. Failure of the functional neurologic or motor control at the level of the oral cavity, oropharynx, nasopharynx, esophagus, or stomach, may result in regurgitation. In addition, any physical obstruction at any of these levels may also result in regurgitation.

SYSTEMS AFFECTED

The gastrointestinal system is primarily affected. Involvement of the cardiovascular system is possible in cases where the regurgitation is secondary to a persistent right aortic arch. The respiratory system may be affected, with the development of aspiration pneumonia. The nervous system may also be affected in cases where the regurgitation is secondary to neurologic disorders, such as tetanus or rabies.

SIGNALMENT

Signalment is variable, depending on the primary condition.

SIGNS

Historical Findings

The owner should be questioned about possible exposure of the horse to poisonous plants, snakes, or other toxins. Information about the time of regurgitation in relation to feeding may further localize the anomaly. Usually, regurgitation immediately following feeding is due to an obstruction of the oral cavity or pharynx. A prolongation in the time between feeding and regurgitation indicates an obstruction of the esophagus or stomach.

Physical Exam Findings

Adult horses have bilateral nasal discharge consisting of feed and saliva. Depending on the severity and duration of clinical signs, dehydration may be evident. Nursing foals have a nasal discharge consisting of milk. All foals should be examined for the presence of a cleft palate or signs of septicemia. Horses may show signs of respiratory disease, including tachypnea, coughing, and increased lung sounds. Other clinical signs are specific to the cause of regurgitation.

CAUSES

The location of the defect may be oral, pharyngeal, esophageal, or gastric. The physical defects may be caused by a physical obstruction (i.e., an intraluminal mass or a cleft palate), whereas the functional defects may involve a disruption in the nervous or muscular control of swallowing (i.e., tetanus). These causes may be congenital or acquired.

RISK FACTORS

Specific risk factors exist depending on the primary underlying condition. Please refer to specific chapters for details.

DIAGNOSIS

DIFFERENTIAL DIAGNOSIS

Differential diagnoses include:

- Esophageal obstruction
  - Choke
  - Atresia,* agenesis*
  - Stenosis*
  - Persistent right aortic arch*
- Neurologic disorders
  - Tetanus
  - Rabies
  - Equine protozoal myeloencephalitis
  - Head trauma
  - Bacterial meningitis*
  - Hydrocephalus*
- Gastric rupture
- Gastric ulceration
- Cleft palate*
- Guttural pouch tympany* or mycosis
- Weakness in neonatal foals with a poor suckle reflex (transient)*
- Foreign body or mass of the oral cavity, pharynx, esophagus, or stomach
- Diaphragmatic hernia
- Megaesophagus
- Subepiglottic or pharyngeal cysts
- Dorsal displacement of the soft palate
- Rostral displacement of the palatopharyngeal arch
- Severe inflammatory condition of the oral cavity, pharynx, esophagus, or stomach
- Various plant toxins (including oleander)
- Various other toxins (including snake bite venom, lead, arsenic)

CBC/BIOCHEMISTRY/URINALYSIS

The CBC and biochemistry profile may be normal or show evidence of dehydration (elevated PCV, TP, BUN, and creatinine). The profile may also reveal hypochloremia and metabolic alkalosis secondary to loss of saliva.

*More commonly observed in young horses or foals.

OTHER LABORATORY TESTS

These are variable, depending on the primary condition. Please refer to specific chapters for details.

IMAGING

Cranial Gastrointestinal Radiography

Radiography of the oral cavity, pharynx, esophagus, and/or stomach may be performed to further localize and define the cause of regurgitation. Disorders such as a mass, foreign body, guttural pouch tympany, esophageal impaction, or diaphragmatic hernia may be diagnosed using plain radiography.

Fluoroscopy is a valuable diagnostic modality in which barium is administered orally followed by fluoroscopic examination.

Abnormalities in transit and clearance times may be estimated. In foals, normal emptying of contrast from the stomach occurs in <2 hr and reaches the large intestine within 3 hr.

Irregularities, including luminal obstructions or esophageal dilatation, can be identified.

Extraluminal masses may be discovered due to displacement of the esophagus from its normal anatomic position. An "hour-glass" appearance of the dilated esophagus has been described. In this case, the esophagus is constricted, either by fibrous tissue at the level of the thoracic inlet or by vasculature.

DIAGNOSTIC PROCEDURES

Passage of a Stomach Tube

A stomach tube assesses the patency of the pharynx and esophagus and indicates the presence of fluid or gas under pressure in the stomach.

Endoscopy

Endoscopic evaluation of the pharynx, esophagus, trachea, and guttural pouches may be performed. Cleft palate, gastric and esophageal ulcerations, intraluminal masses or foreign bodies, and guttural pouch disorders may be identified. The integrity of the gastrointestinal tract should be determined, as any ulceration or rupture will worsen prognosis.

REGURGITATION/DYSPHAGIA

TREATMENT

Patients with regurgitation should be treated as an intensive-care medical inpatient in most cases. Balanced polyionic fluids with or without chloride supplementation should be considered. Total (in foals) or partial parenteral nutrition may be considered. The patient should be stall rested until it is stabilized. In most cases the horse should be held off feed to prevent further regurgitation and possible aspiration. The owner should be aware of the severe complication of aspiration pneumonia. Surgical options exist for certain primary conditions that cause regurgitation; please refer to specific chapters for details.

MEDICATIONS

DRUG(S) OF CHOICE

Drugs prescribed are variable depending on the primary condition.

CONTRAINDICATIONS

N/A

PRECAUTIONS

N/A

POSSIBLE INTERACTIONS

N/A

ALTERNATIVE DRUGS

N/A

FOLLOW-UP

PATIENT MONITORING

Monitoring is variable depending on the primary condition.

POSSIBLE COMPLICATIONS

Common complications include aspiration pneumonia, dehydration, electrolyte abnormalities, and malnutrition.

MISCELLANEOUS

ASSOCIATED CONDITIONS

- Aspiration pneumonia
- Dehydration
- Colonic impaction
- Malnutrition
- Septicemia (in young animals)

AGE-RELATED FACTORS

The most likely differential diagnosis for an adult horse with regurgitation is an esophageal obstruction or neurologic disorder, whereas congenital defects such as cleft palate or persistent right aortic arch are seen only in foals.

ZOONOTIC POTENTIAL

Some differential diagnoses, especially neurologic disorders such as rabies, must be ruled out. The necessary precautions should be undertaken during handling and management of these cases.

PREGNANCY

The most significant consideration in a pregnant animal with regurgitation is the often poor prognosis for survival of the mare. Under special circumstances, caesarian section may be considered in order to attempt salvage of a near-term fetus.

SYNONYMS

- Pharyngeal dysphagia
- Esophageal dysphagia

SEE ALSO

- Esophageal obstruction (choke)
- Cleft palate
- Dysphagia
- Gastric ulceration
- Specific neurologic disorders (tetanus, EPM)
- Specific toxins (lead, oleander)

ABBREVIATIONS

N/A

Suggested Reading

Barton MH. Nasal regurgitation of milk in foals. Comp Cont Ed 1993;15:81-91,93.

Greet TRC. Observations on the potential role of oesophageal radiography in the horse. Equine Vet J 1982;14:73-79.

Milne E. Differential diagnosis of dysphagia. In Robinson NE (ed): Current therapy in equine medicine. Philadelphia: WB Saunders. 1997:141-143.

Smith BP. Regurgitation/vomiting. In Smith BP (ed): Large animal internal medicine. St. Louis: Mosby. 1996:132-134.

Author Mollie C. M. Ferris

Consulting Editor Henry Stämpfli

RETAINED DECIDUOUS TEETH

BASICS

OVERVIEW

The deciduous teeth of the second, third, and fourth premolars are shed at approximately 2.5, 3, and 4 yr of age, respectively. The first, second, and third incisors erupt according to a similar schedule. The permanent teeth erupt under the roots of the deciduous teeth, depriving them of a blood supply and forcing them to be shed into the mouth. Deciduous premolars (called *caps*) may remain attached to the permanent teeth, which then can cause soft-tissue lacerations. Alternatively, retained deciduous premolars or incisors may cause mal-eruption of the permanent teeth. Eruption of permanent teeth may be delayed and they may become impacted or the erupting teeth may be displaced caudally for incisors or lingually for premolars. The fourth premolar is the last deciduous tooth to be shed, and also the most commonly retained tooth.

Progressive lysis of the alveolar bone surrounding an impacted tooth results in an eruption cyst with symmetric bony swelling and a characteristic radiographic appearance. If the impaction is of sufficient severity, the bony swelling can be inflamed and painful. The tooth pulp at this stage is susceptible to hematogenous bacterial colonization termed *anachoretic pulpitis*. This can progress to a periapical abscess and a draining fistulous tract to the mandible or maxilla.

SIGNALMENT

Eruptions of teeth occur at defined times (see previous section), which determines the age of affected horses. Breed and sex predilections have not been reported, although horses with smaller heads and relative overcrowding of the teeth may be predisposed.

SIGNS

Pain associated with laceration of gums from caps can be associated with head shy behavior and resistance to the bit. In addition, mal-eruption and tooth impaction can cause oral discomfort with headshaking while eating, quidding, hemorrhage from the oral cavity, and rubbing of incisors against fixed objects. Retained caps may also cause abnormal mastication, uneven dental wear, and weight loss.

CAUSES AND RISK FACTORS

Retained deciduous teeth are relatively common and may be caused by abnormalities to mastication either as a result of inadequate roughage in the diet or other causes of abnormal dental wear. Overcrowding of the dental arcades can also cause retention of deciduous teeth. Hooks or ramps in young animals may cause a displacement of the opposing dental arcade with a resultant overcrowding of the premolars. Also an excessively large first premolar (wolf tooth) or supernumary teeth (polyodontia) may cause overcrowding.

DIAGNOSIS

DIFFERENTIAL DIAGNOSIS

There are few differential diagnoses, as the characteristic age and the presence of dental caps or mal-erupted teeth are pathognomonic. However, periapical abscess formation may need to be differentiated from sepsis caused by trauma, infundibular necrosis, or (less commonly) neoplasia. Any painful condition of the mouth resulting from trauma (e.g., tongue laceration), infection (e.g., vesicular stomatitis), or neurologic dysfunction can cause some of the signs seen with retained deciduous teeth.

CBC/BIOCHEMISTRY/URINALYSIS

N/A

OTHER LABORATORY TESTS

N/A

IMAGING

Radiographic projections of the cheek teeth may assist in the diagnosis of retained premolars. The characteristic findings of an eruption cyst include a cystic extension of the periodontal ligament (lamina dura) with a regular outline and the absence of sclerosis and periosteal reaction. Eruption cysts are also associated with an erupting tooth.

DIAGNOSTIC PROCEDURES

A thorough oral examination should reveal the presence of caps, which are also palpable when the border between the permanent and deciduous tooth extends above the gingiva. An oral examination should also reveal malerupted teeth in the premolar or incisor arcades. Radiographs are also useful as outlined above.

TREATMENT

Deciduous teeth should not be removed until the corresponding permanent tooth has erupted through the gingiva. Caps are removed using a dental elevator or similar instrument. Retained incisors are usually easily elevated and removed. Molar or cap removal forceps may assist in removal of retained premolars. Some authors consider removal of caps that are not causing clinical signs to be unnecessary, whereas other authors believe that once the permanent teeth have erupted, caps should be removed prophylactically. A further opinion is that once a deciduous tooth is shed, the remaining three corresponding sites should be checked and the caps removed. This should only be done provided that the permanent tooth has erupted through the gingiva.

It is possible to leave behind a fragment of the root from retained deciduous teeth after removal, and the site should be inspected carefully to ensure that these fragments are removed, as these sharp shards of tooth root can cause soft-tissue lacerations to the tongue or the gums.

MEDICATIONS

DRUGS

Antimicrobial therapy may be useful in cases of impacted teeth to prevent formation of anachoretic pulpitis. Antimicrobials used early in the course of a periapical infection in young horses have been reported to be successful. However, resolution of the infection commonly requires extraction of the affected tooth.

CONTRAINDICATIONS/POSSIBLE INTERACTIONS

N/A

FOLLOW-UP

PREVENTION/AVOIDANCE

Adequate dental care for younger horses may decrease abnormal dental wear and resultant overcrowding of the dental arcades. Regular dental care should also identify retained deciduous teeth prior to their causing significant problems.

EXPECTED COURSE AND PROGNOSIS

Removal of retained deciduous teeth usually results in the normal alignment and development of the permanent teeth. When abnormal conformation of the arcades remain, this should be corrected.

MISCELLANEOUS

ASSOCIATED CONDITIONS

Associated conditions include abnormal dental wear and periapical abscesses.

AGE-RELATED FACTORS

The age at which the permanent teeth erupt (between 2.5 and 4 yr) are the times at which deciduous teeth become retained. The actual age of eruption is variable, and the deciduous teeth of the lower arcade are usually shed before the upper arcade. One report suggests that 2 yr 8 months, 2 yr 10 months, and 3 yr 8 months may be a more accurate eruption schedule for premolars two, three, and four than outlined previously.

Suggested Reading

Crabill MR, Schumacher J. Pathophysiology of acquired dental diseases of the horse. Vet Clin North Am Equine Pract. 1998:14;291-307.

Author Simon G. Pearce

Consulting Editor Henry Stämpfli

RETAINED FETAL MEMBRANES (RFM)

BASICS

DEFINITION

Fetal membranes are defined as retained if they have not been passed within 3 hours postpartum.

PATHOPHYSIOLOGY

Suggested Causes:

• Pathologic sites of adherence between the endometrium and chorion with the first occurrence that may recur during future pregnancies.
• Infections between the endometrium and chorion.
• Any debilitating condition—excessive fatigue, poor conditioning, unhygienic environment, or advanced age.

SYSTEM AFFECTED

Reproductive

GENETICS

N/A

INCIDENCE/PREVALENCE

• The most common postpartum condition in mares, with an incidence of 2%–10%.
• Incidence is reported to increase after dystocia or cesarean section, in draft mares, with hydrops pregnancy, and after prolonged pregnancy.

SIGNALMENT

• All breeds.
• All females of breeding age.

SIGNS

General Comments

• The portion of RFM visible at the vulvar lips is not a reliable indicator of the proportion that may yet be attached (i.e., retained) within the uterus.
• As mares move about immediately post-partum, portions of the membranes may be torn or break free. A careful look through stall bedding may yield the balance and lessen concern regarding a portion otherwise thought to be retained.

Historical Findings

• Previous history of partial or complete failure to pass the fetal membranes.
• Higher occurrence after dystocia, prolonged pregnancy, or abortion.
• Incidence increases in mares of > 15 years.
• No effect of previous reproductive status, maiden, barren, or foaling the previous year.
• No effect attributed to breeding by AI versus natural (i.e., live) cover the previous year.
• No affect from sex of foal or birth of a weak or dead fetus.

Physical Examination Findings

• Transrectal examination to determine size and tone of the uterus and to gauge amount of fluid in the uterine lumen.
• Vaginal examination may be necessary, but is not always essential, depending on condition of the placenta and the uterus.

CAUSES

See *Pathophysiology.*

RISK FACTORS

See *Historical Findings.*

DIAGNOSIS

DIFFERENTIAL DIAGNOSIS

• Uterine infection.
• Delay or failure of postpartum involution.

CBC/BIOCHEMISTRY/URINALYSIS

N/A

OTHER LABORATORY TESTS

N/A

IMAGING

N/A

DIAGNOSTIC PROCEDURES

N/A

PATHOLOGIC FINDINGS

See *Pathophysiology.*

TREATMENT

APPROPRIATE HEALTH CARE

• Treat primarily with oxytocin—best results.
• Initiate oxytocin treatment <3 hours postpartum if membranes have not passed; repeat every 90–120 minutes for the first 12–18 hours postpartum.
• After 12–18 hours, if membranes still have not passed, may treat intrauterine with irritants or antibiotics or systemically with antibiotics.
• Use of systemic antibiotics is not necessary unless systemic disease develops subsequent to the RFM.
• Flushing the uterus can have great value if a portion of the placenta is retained.
• Insufflation—If the membranes are by-in-large intact, place fluid within the innermost aspect of the fetal membranes, sufficient to expand the uterus and stimulate uterine activity; gather the exposed portion of placenta, and tie around it outside of the vulvae to maintain fluid within the uterus and placenta for a brief time; this maintains the expansion, stretching to facilitate release of the microvilli; cost of this larger-volume treatment may be more expensive but yields a modest increase in benefit.

NURSING CARE

• Administer oxytocin postpartum to all mares with a history of RFM. Such mares are at higher risk for recurrence.
• Examine all membranes after passage to determine that all portions are present.

ACTIVITY

Affected mares should have normal exercise.

DIET

No changes are indicated.

RETAINED FETAL MEMBRANES (RFM)

CLIENT EDUCATION

- RFM is relatively common and should be treated if not passed within 3 hours post-partum, regardless of the time at which foaling occurred.
- Advisable for owners to maintain a supply of oxytocin, with administration beginning only after 3 hours have passed.

SURGICAL CONSIDERATIONS

N/A

MEDICATIONS

DRUGS OF CHOICE

Oxytocin (≤20 IU per injection, with injections repeated at 60–120-minute intervals).

CONTRAINDICATIONS

Higher doses of oxytocin may lead to uterine prolapse.

PRECAUTIONS

- Oxytocin may induce uterine cramping.
- The mare may go down, with potential to cause harm to the foal.

POSSIBLE INTERACTIONS

N/A

ALTERNATIVE DRUGS

None as effective as oxytocin.

FOLLOW-UP

PATIENT MONITORING

- Examine the mare to determine if placenta has been expelled.
- Evaluate uterine size and tone to determine if they are normal relative to the number of days postpartum.

PREVENTION/AVOIDANCE

- Exercise and dietary supplementation with selenium may have value.
- Avoid pasturing mares on fescue near term.

POSSIBLE COMPLICATIONS

- Septic metritis.
- Laminitis

EXPECTED COURSE AND PROGNOSIS

- Of mares treated with oxytocin, >90% pass the RFM without any other problem, and the prognosis is excellent.
- RFM passed without secondary involvement have no affect on foal heat breeding conceptions.
- Affected mares treated with intrauterine antibiotics have higher rates of conception and pregnancy termination.

MISCELLANEOUS

ASSOCIATED CONDITIONS

See *Historical Findings*.

AGE-RELATED FACTORS

Old mares have a higher incidence on some farms.

ZOONOTIC POTENTIAL

N/A

PREGNANCY

- Follows parturition.
- May increase with induction of parturition.

SYNONYMS

Retained afterbirth

SEE ALSO

N/A

ABBREVIATION

AI = artificial insemination

Suggested Reading

Alexander RW. Excessive retainment of the placenta in the mare. Vet Rec 1971;89:175–176.

Burns SJ, Judge NG, Martin JE, Adams LG. Management of retained placenta in mares. Proc Am Assoc Equine Pract 1977;381–390.

Provencher R, Threlfall WR, Murdick PW, Wearly WK. Retained fetal membranes in the mare. A retrospective study. Can Vet J 1988;29:903–910.

Threlfall WR. Retained placenta. In: McKinnon AO, Voss JL, eds. Equine reproduction. Philadelphia: Lea & Febiger, 1993:614–621.

Threlfall WR, Carleton CL. Treatment of uterine infections in the mare. In: Morrow DA, ed. Current therapy in theriogenology. 2nd. Philadelphia: WB Saunders, 1986:730–737.

White TE. Retained placenta. Mod Vet Pract 1980;61:87–88.

Author Walter R. Threlfall

Consulting Editor Carla L. Carleton

RHABDOMYOLYSIS

BASICS

DEFINITION

• A complex syndrome with numerous causes, some of which are understood and many of which are not.
• Characterized by varying degrees of muscular dysfunction, ranging from mild stiffness to rigid immobility and, occasionally, recumbency.
• Individual episodes often are acute, but in many animals, the condition is recurrent.

PATHOPHYSIOLOGY

• A single pathophysiologic theory is unlikely to explain all occurrences, because the triggering factors and clinical course can vary significantly from case to case.
• Often, only one horse is affected in a group, even though its management and work schedule may not differ from its peers.
• This implies affected individuals have an underlying metabolic or structural abnormality predisposing to the condition; indeed, some specific conditions have been identified in some groups and breeds of horse (see *Causes*).

SYSTEMS AFFECTED

• Musculoskeletal—primarily affects type II muscle fibers.
• Renal/urologic—pigmenturia (from myoglobin) may be seen during the acute phase of severe cases, and this may give rise to renal damage, particularly with significant circulatory problems (e.g., hypotension, dehydration).

GENETICS

• In Thoroughbreds, probably inherited as an autosomal dominant trait, with variable expression.
• In Quarter Horses and those with Quarter Horse lineage, rhabdomyolysis due to polysaccharide storage myopathy has a familial basis, with an autosomal recessive inheritance.

INCIDENCE/PREVALENCE

• Worldwide incidence, with no apparent limited geographic distribution
• In a 1995 study of 984 Thoroughbreds in training, 59 (6%) had a least one episode of rhabdomyolysis.

SIGNALMENT

Breed Predilections

• No reported breed predilection
• Heavily built horses are suggested to have a higher incidence, with a potential bias toward Thoroughbreds.

Mean Age and Range

Predominantly seen in horses of working age (2 to ≅15 years), but may occur at any age.

Predominant Sex

Said to be more common in females, particularly young fillies in training.

SIGNS

Historical Findings

• Clinical signs range from mild to very severe and usually develop soon after (or sometimes during) exercise, often after a period of 1–2 days of rest.
• A bilaterally stiff gait, particularly affecting the hind limbs, may be seen; in severe cases, the horse may be reluctant or unable to move.
• Because the condition is painful, horses may sweat excessively relative to the workload and be tachypneic.
• Myoglobinuria may be seen.
• Often a history of recurrent episodes.

Physical Examination Findings

• Affected muscles may be firm, swollen, and painful on palpation.
• Pulse rate may be elevated, often >80 bpm in severe cases.

CAUSES

In most cases, the underlying cause is not identified. These cases should, perhaps, be classified as idiopathic, but this might imply a common cause for all of these cases, which is unlikely.

Polysaccharide Storage Abnormality

• Increased, elevated muscle glycogen content and polysaccharide storage inclusions in type II muscle fibers
• Polysaccharide is stored in a nonbioavailable form.
• Reported as a familial condition in Quarter Horses, but has been diagnosed in many other breeds, including Percherons and Belgians.

Abnormal Sarcolemmal Function

In vitro muscle twitch and contracture testing of horses with rhabdomyolysis has shown some to have abnormal sarcolemmal function.

Electrolyte Abnormalities

• The exact role of electrolyte abnormalities as a cause is poorly understood and implied from indirect assessments of electrolyte status or from the response to dietary supplementation.
• Low urinary fractional excretion of sodium or potassium or high fractional excretion of phosphorous have been associated with this syndrome.
• Appropriate dietary supplementation has reduced the recurrence of rhabdomyolysis in this group of horses.

Hypothyroidism

No data support hypothyroidism as a cause.

EHV-1

One report in which a high incidence of muscle stiffness and apparent myopathy was associated with an outbreak of EHV-1 infection in a U.K. training yard

Vitamin E/Selenium

Though once thought to have a significant role in the cause of this problem, no data show any correlation the vitamin E/selenium status of affected animals.

RISK FACTORS

- Changes in work regimen—commonly reported to occur in horses that are in regular work, then rested for 1–2 days, and then returned to work.
- Excessive dietary carbohydrate
- High dietary potassium
- Weather—inclement weather (both hot and cold) has been implicated.
- Overwork of unfit horses

DIAGNOSIS

DIFFERENTIAL DIAGNOSIS

Laminitis

- Affected horses also may have a stiff gait or be reluctant or unable to move.
- Usually, horses are more severely affected on the forelimbs, but in some cases, all four feet are equally affected.
- Usually, prominent pulsation of the digital arteries is noted, with increased heat in the affected feet.
- Usually pain on percussion of the wall and soles of the feet; radiographic changes also may be noted.
- Serum enzyme concentrations characteristic of rhabdomyolysis usually are absent in laminitis, but occasional cases of severe rhabdomyolysis may develop laminitis as well.

Aortoiliac Thrombosis

- Usually recurrent and occurs each time the horse is exercised, whereas rhabdomyolysis often is intermittent but recurrent.
- Usually unilateral
- Rectal and external physical examination may confirm the obstructed artery and reduced venous filling on the affected limb.
- The marked elevations in serum enzymes seen in rhabdomyolysis usually are absent in this condition.

Spinal Cord Diseases

- A variety of spinal cord conditions, including cervical stenosis, trauma, and protozoal myelitis, could produce some signs similar to those of rhabdomyolysis.
- These signs would be present all the time, however, and not be associated with recent exercise or resolve with rest.
- Again, serum enzymology assists in differentiation.

Pigmenturia

- May be caused by a variety of conditions, most of which give rise to hemoglobinuria or hematuria.
- Specific clinical and laboratory tests separate the potential causes.

CBC/BIOCHEMISTRY/URINALYSIS

CBC

Usually normal, but evidence of stress may be noted on the leukogram.

Serum CK

- Rises rapidly after myolysis, peaking 3–15 hours after onset of the problem.
- Values in the tens of thousands of U/L often are reported.
- Depending on severity and duration of the problem, levels return to baseline within 1–7 days.
- Height of the elevation relates somewhat to the clinical signs, but considerable variation may be noted.

Serum AST and LDH

- Levels of AST and LDH (particularly of LDH 4 and LDH 5), will be elevated, peaking at 24 hours.
- LDH returns to baseline in ≅5–10 days and AST in 2–4 weeks.

Urinalysis

- Pigmenturia may be noted.
- Distinguishing myoglobinuria from hemoglobinuria requires special testing but usually is not needed if clinical signs and serum enzyme elevations are consistent with myolysis.

RHABDOMYOLYSIS

OTHER LABORATORY TESTS
NA

IMAGING
N/A

DIAGNOSTIC PROCEDURES
Muscle Biopsy:
- May be valuable for establishing a retrospective diagnosis and be particularly valuable in horses with suspected polysaccharide storage myopathies.
- Contact the laboratory before taking samples to determine if any particular sites are preferred or any special preservation or sample handling is required.

PATHOLOGIC FINDINGS
Gross Findings
- Changes can be extensive and involve the dorsal and central lumbar muscles, gluteals, and quadriceps.
- Affected muscles may be pale and swollen, with some scattered hemorrhage.

Histopathologic Findings
- Variable, which may reflect the possible multiple forms of this condition.
- In many cases, the most obvious changes are seen in type II fibers.
- Acute cases may have hypercontracted fibers and lysis.
- Macrophages invade the affected areas, and myoblasts appear as repair is initiated.
- Both regenerating fibers and some mature ones may have central nuclei.
- Horses with polysaccharide storage myopathy have many intensely para-aminosalycylate–positive fibers and some atrophied fibers.

TREATMENT

APPROPRIATE HEALTH CARE
- Management protocols depend on severity of the problem.
- Mild cases often can be managed at the farm or stable with minimal intervention.
- Severe cases may be medical emergencies requiring aggressive interventions and the support of a referral hospital.
- In severe cases, there may be the dilemma of getting the horse to the facility. Obviously, the animal should not be walked any significant distance, because this will exacerbate the problem. Even transportation for long distances in a horse trailer can induce more damage, however, because the horse must use significant muscle function to handle the swaying motion of the trailer. Thus, some severe cases may need to be managed at the location where the problem occurred. This is particularly true for recumbent horses.

NURSING CARE
- Severe cases and those involving dehydration require fluid therapy—balanced electrolyte fluid (e.g., IV lactated Ringer solution)
- In some cases, fluids can be given by indwelling nasogastric tube. This is less expensive and can be done by the owner once the tube is placed.
- Fluid therapy is particularly important if large amounts of myoglobin have been released, and a volume diuresis should be sustained until the pigmenturia has stopped.
- Recumbent horses should be on deep bedding and turned every few hours.

ACTIVITY
- Restrict activity to stall rest at first.
- Return to activity depends on clinical improvement of the horse and return of serum CK to near-baseline levels. This period will be from 1–10 or more days.
- Return to exercise should be gradual, with turn out initially for a short period in a paddock.

DIET
- Initial diet should be low energy—grass hay and water
- During the next few days, depending on progress of the case, the energy level should be gradually increased to ≅80% of maintenance.
- Maintain adequate fluid intake.

CLIENT EDUCATION
- If this is the first bout of myopathy for the horse, warn the client about the recurrent nature of the problem and that life-long preventative measures will be necessary.

SURGICAL CONSIDERATIONS
N/A

MEDICATIONS

DRUGS OF CHOICE
- NSAIDs for analgesia as required—phenylbutazone (2–4.4 mg/kg BID); flunixin meglumine (1.1 mg/kg BID)
- Some horses in severe pain may need butorphanol (0.02–0.1 mg/kg q3–4 h) as needed.
- In some cases, acepromazine (0.04–0.1 mg/kg BID), both for its tranquilizing effects and promotion of increased muscle blood flow.
- Dantrolene sodium (1.5 mg/kg IV on the first day, then 2 mg/kg PO for the next 2 days) has been reported to decrease recovery time, but the IV form is not readily available.
- DMSO (0.9 g/kg as a 20% solution IV) has been used, purportedly as a free radical scrounger, but all reports of its benefit are anecdotal.

CONTRAINDICATIONS
N/A

PRECAUTIONS
Use NSAIDs with caution in dehydrated animals.

POSSIBLE INTERACTIONS
N/A

ALTERNATIVE DRUGS
N/A

RHABDOMYOLYSIS

FOLLOW-UP

PATIENT MONITORING

• Monitor hydration status in severely affected cases.
• Assess serum CK every 2–3 days to determine if myolysis has stopped and, hence, as a gauge for when to start limited exercise.

PREVENTION/AVOIDANCE

• Once the horse has recovered from an initial bout, instigate a regimen of regular exercise. Avoid breaks, even of only 1–2 days.
• Diet should be balanced to work load, and any reduction in work should be accompanied by a reduction in feed intake.
• Dantrolene (2 mg/kg via stomach tube for 3–5 days, then every third day for a month) has been suggested, as have other regimens (e.g., 500 mg PO for 3 days, then 300 mg every third day). Because this drug is hepatotoxic, long-term therapy is not recommended, and liver function should be monitored regularly.
• In some horse with abnormal sarcolemmal function, phenytoin (8–12 mg/kg BID for 3 days, then 10 mg/kg TID for 1 week) may have benefit. Training can then be started with a dosage of 5–6 mg/kg TID. (Remember many drugs are not permitted in most equestrian sports.)
• In horses with polysaccharide storage myopathy, decreasing the dietary energy derived from carbohydrate and increasing that from fat is recommended. As much as 20% of the diet can be from fat, using corn oil or rice bran. This regime also may benefit horses with rhabdomyolysis of unknown cause.

POSSIBLE COMPLICATIONS

Rarely, acute renal failure may result from myoglobin-induced nephropathy in severe cases.

EXPECTED COURSE AND PROGNOSIS

• The course often depends on severity of the condition; generally, the most severely affected horses take longer to recover.
• Again, prognosis depends on severity of the problem.
• Many horses, particularly those with an established underlying metabolic defect, have the potential for recurrent bouts.
• In many cases, the long-term prognosis depends on the success of preventative and management protocols.

MISCELLANEOUS

ASSOCIATED CONDITIONS

N/A

AGE-RELATED FACTORS

N/A

ZOONOTIC POTENTIAL

N/A

PREGNANCY

N/A

SYNONYMS

• Tying up
• Monday morning disease
• Paralytic myoglobinuria
• Azoturia

SEE ALSO

N/A

ABBREVIATIONS

• AST = aspartate aminotransferase
• CK = creatine kinase
• DMSO = dimethyl sulfoxide
• EHV-1 = equine herpes virus 1
• LHD = lactate dehydrogenase

Suggested Reading

Beech J. Chronic exertional rhabdomyolysis. Vet Clin North Am Equine Pract 1997;13:145–168.
MacLeay JM, Valberg SJ, Sorum SA, Kassube T, Santcshi EM, Mickelson JR, Geyer CJ. Habitability of recurrent exertional rhabdomyolysis in Thoroughbred racehorses. Am J Vet Res 1999;60:259–256.
Valberg SJ, Cardinet GH, Carlson GP, DiMauro S. Polysaccharide storage myopathy associated with recurrent exertional rhabdomyolysis in horses. Neurosmusc Disord 1992;2:351–359.
Valberg SJ, Mickelson JR, Gallant EM, MacLeay JM, Lentz L, de la Court F. Exertional rhabdomyolysis in Quarter Horses and Thoroughbreds: one syndrome, multiple etiologies. Equine Vet J Suppl 1999;30:533–538.

Author Christopher M. Brown
Consulting Editor Christopher M. Brown

RHODOCOCCUS EQUI

BASICS

DEFINITION

Rhodococcus equi is an important cause of pneumonia in foals less than 6 months of age. Infection with *R. equi* may also result in diarrhea, joint sepsis, intra-abdominal abscessation, and multifocal abscesses throughout the body.

PATHOPHYSIOLOGY

Rhodococcus equi is a gram-positive pleomorphic intracellular facultative organism that normally inhabits soil. Inhalation of dust containing the organism is thought to be the primary route of exposure for both the horse and humans. *Rhodococcus equi* then resides within the alveolar macrophages, replicates, and can produce a severe, potentially life-threatening pyogranulomatous bronchopneumonia as necrosis and destruction of lung parenchyma occurs. Intestinal forms of the disease include ulcerative colitis and abdominal lymphadenitis. Associated gastrointestinal infections likely arise from infected foals swallowing sputum containing the organism. Peyer's patches become infected and ulcerated and, with time, significant mesenteric lymphadenitis can occur. *Rhodococcus equi* may disseminate to other body sites and produce septic arthritis, serositis, vertebral body abscesses, and cutaneous ulcerative lymphangitis. Other extra-thoracic manifestations of the disease include immune-mediated polysynovitis, uveitis–keratouveitis, immune-mediated hemolytic anemia, immune-mediated thrombocytopenia, hyperthermia associated with erythromycin–rifampin, hyperlipemia, and telogen effluvium.

SYSTEMS AFFECTED

- Respiratory
- Gastrointestinal
- Musculoskeletal
- Hemic/lymphatic/immune
- Ophthalmic
- Renal
- Skin
- Hepatobiliary
- Nervous

GENETICS

N/A

SIGNALMENT

Foals 1–6 months of age. Most foals show clinical signs before 4 months of age. *Rhodococcus equi* infection has been reported in immuno-compromised adults or adults with concurrent illness.

SIGNS

Fever, cough, lethargy, depression, anorexia, poor weight gain, exercise intolerance, diarrhea, respiratory distress, joint distention, and sudden death. Foals may have abnormal thoracic auscultation and percussion findings, although severely affected foals may not have ausculatable abnormalities.

DIAGNOSIS

DIFFERENTIAL DIAGNOSIS

Primary differentials are other causes of pneumonia in foals, including: *Streptococcus equi* var *equi, S. equi* var *zooepidemicus,* parasite migration, and viral respiratory infections. There has been a suggestion that equine herpesvirus type 2 (EHV-2) infection may predispose foals to *R. equi.* Definitive diagnosis is based on culture of *R. equi.*

CBC/BIOCHEMISTRY/URINALYSIS

CBC is characterized by leukocytosis with a mature neutrophilia. Fibrinogen is increased. Serum protein may be increased. Foals with severe disease may have anemia and thrombocytopenia. Foals with diarrhea may have electrolyte abnormalities, including hyponatremia and hypochloremia. Creatinine and BUN may be increased in foals with dehydration secondary to diarrhea or respiratory distress. Urinalysis is usually normal, excepting cases with renal and/or urinary tract involvement.

OTHER LABORATORY TESTS

Agar gel immunodiffusion serology (AGID) for detection of precipitating antibody for equi-factors and exoenzymes produced by *R. equi.* Enzyme-linked immunosorbent assay (ELISA) serology for detection of antibody to cell surface *R. equi* antigen.

DIAGNOSTIC PROCEDURES

Transtracheal Aspirate (TTA)

Cytology reveals gram-positive to gram-variable pleomorphic ("chinese character") intracellular rods. Culture positive for *R. equi.*

Bronchoalveolar Lavage

Results similar to TTA. May recognize concurrent infection with *Pneumocystis carinii,* requires specialized stain (silver stain). Caution: Either TTA or bronchoalveolar lavage may be detrimental to a foal with significant respiratory disease.

PATHOLOGIC FINDINGS

Findings are related to the organ system involved. Characteristic finding at necropsy is bilateral bronchopneumonia with severe coalescing abscess formation. Ventral lung field involvement is generally more severe. Abscesses may range in size from a few millimeters to more than 10 cm. Generalized miliary abscess formation is also common. Pulmonary parenchyma surrounding pulmonary abscesses is usually congested or consolidated. Bronchial and mediastinal lymphadenopathy with abscessation is common. Pleural empyema can occur. Pleural inflammation is unusual unless empyema secondary to abscess rupture has occurred.

Gastrointestinal lesions are variable and may involve the entire GI tract. Lesions include: mucosal villous atrophy, mucosal necrosis, diphtheritic membrane formation, ulcerative enterocolits, and mesenteric lymphadenopathy with abscess formation. Pulmonary histology abnormalities are predominately pyogranulomatous. Abscesses have a necrotic central core with surrounding degenerate neutrophils. Adjacent areas are infiltrated with macrophages, lymphocytes, and occasional giant cells. There is congestion, edema, and alveolar infiltration by macrophages and neutrophils, acute suppurative bronchitis, and peribronchitis. Organisms may be identified using H & E and/or gram stains. Some organisms demonstrate acid-fast characteristics. There are reports of concurrent infection with *Pneumocystis carinii.* Identification of concurrent infection is facilitated by the use of silver stains. Gastrointestinal histology abnormalities are characterized by infiltration of phagocytic cells into the lamina propria. Necrosis of the villi and submucosa and mucosal ulceration are prominent. Peyer's patches are frequently involved.

IMAGING

Ultrasonography

Consolidation of lung parenchyma; pulmonary and intra-abdominal abscessation. Lesions deep within pulmonary parenchyma and not in contact with pleura will not be recognized.

Radiography

Abnormalities range from increased interstitial density to dense patchy areas of alveolar pattern to areas of consolidation and abscessation in the thorax. Radiographs may be useful in monitoring response to therapy and determining the severity of pulmonary involvement.

TREATMENT

APPROPRIATE HEALTH CARE

Affected foals may be treated at the farm. Severely affected foals may benefit from treatment at a referral facility with climate-controlled environments. Foals being sent to such facilities should be transported during cool times of the day and stress should be minimized. Foals with *R. equi* infection should not be transferred from an endemic farm to a farm with no previous history of *R. equi* infection.

NURSING CARE

The most important aspect of nursing care is minimizing stress. Provision of climate-controlled environments, air conditioning, and good ventilation may improve the short-term prognosis with severely affected foals.

ACTIVITY

Exercise should be restricted. Stall confinement is not necessary as long as turn-out is in a small area only. Affected foals should be completely restricted from exercise during the hot periods of the day.

DIET

There are no specific dietary considerations. Severely affected foals experiencing weight loss and anorexia may benefit from parenteral nutrition.

CLIENT EDUCATION

Rhodococcus equi probably infects all horse farms to some degree. The difference in disease appearance is related to differences in environments, management techniques, and virulence of the isolate. On enzootic farms, *R. equi* infections result in huge economic losses associated with costs of prevention, treatment, and the death of some foals.

Most foals treated for *R. equi* infection recover. Severely affected foals are less likely to survive. Severely immunocompromised humans have been diagnosed with *R. equi* infection. It then becomes important to inform people with diseases resulting in immunodeficiency that *R. equi* is endemic on certain farms, and that they may be at risk of developing this disease if they either reside or work at these farms.

SURGICAL CONSIDERATIONS

Surgical drainage of easily accessible abscesses may be reasonable. However, surgical removal of abdominal abscesses is unlikely to be rewarding.

MEDICATIONS

DRUG(S) OF CHOICE

Erythromycin (10–37.5 mg/kg BID to QID PO) and rifampin (5–10 mg/kg SID to BID PO) is standard therapy. Treatment continues until CBC, fibrinogen, and clinical presentation are normal. If possible, pneumonia should be resolved radiographically.

CONTRAINDICATIONS/PRECAUTIONS/ POSSIBLE INTERACTIONS/ ALTERNATIVE DRUGS

Some foals receiving the above-mentioned drug combination may develop severe diarrhea. Decreasing the erythromycin dose may resolve the problem.

Mares housed with foals receiving the combination have developed severe fatal colitis, thought to be associated with *Clostridum difficile* infection secondary to ingestion of small amounts of erythromycin from the foal.

Idiosyncratic hyperthermia and tachypnea has been reported in foals receiving erythromycin. Use of the estolate form of the drug may decrease this adverse response. Aminophylline should not be used in combination with erythromycin due to potential toxicity.

Foals diagnosed very early in the clinical course of infection may respond to trimethoprim–sulpha combinations.

Rifampin-resistant strains of *R. equi* have been identified. Rifampin should never be used alone due to the rapidity of development of resistance.

FOLLOW-UP

PATIENT MONITORING

Response to therapy can be monitored by resolution of clinical signs, normalization of CBC and fibrinogen, and radiographic improvement. Treatment should be continued until all recognized abnormalities have resolved.

PREVENTION/AVOIDANCE

Several strategies for prevention of *R. equi* infection exist. Decreasing the size of infective challenge by good housing and management practices and isolation of affected foals is important.

Early recognition of infection is important. This can be facilitated by serologic (AGID and/or ELISA) monitoring, daily temperature monitoring of foals, frequent routine physical examinations, and frequent thoracic ultrasound examinations.

Passive immunization by the intravenous administration of *R. equi* hyperimmune plasma has been shown to be an effective preventative technique. Timing of this treatment is important and depends on expected exposure; it is typically administered during the first month of life.

To date, no active immunization protocol has been effective.

EXPECTED COURSE AND PROGNOSIS

In well-established pulmonary cases, therapy may extend over 3–5 weeks.

MISCELLANEOUS

ABBREVIATIONS

- AGID = agar gel immunodiffusion
- EHV-2 = equine herpesvirus 2
- TTA = transtracheal aspirate

Suggested Reading

Ainsworth DM, Yeagar AE, Eiker SW, Erb HE, Davidow E. Athletic performance of horses previously infected with *R. equi* pneumonia as foals. Proc 43rd Annu Conv Am Assoc Eq Pract 1997:81-82.

Chaffin MK, Martens RJ. Extrapulmonary disorders associated with *Rhodococcus equi* pneumonia in foals: retrospective study of 61 cases (1998–1996). Proc 43rd Annu Conv Am Assoc Eq Pract 1997:79-80.

Giguere S, Prescott JF. Strategies for control of *Rhodococcus equi* infections on enzootic farms. Proc 43rd Annu Conv Am Assoc Eq Pract 1997:65-70.

Hondalus MK. *Rhodococcus equi:* pathogenesis and virulence. Proc 43rd Annu Conv Am Assoc Eq Pract 1997:71-78.

Wilkins PA, Lesser FR, Gaskin JM. *Rhodococcus equi* infection in foals: comparison of AGID and ELISA serology on a commercial Thoroughbred breeding farm. Proc 38th Annu Conv Am Assoc Eq Pract 1992:289.

Author Pamela A. Wilkins

Consulting Editor Corinne R. Sweeney

RIGHT AND LEFT DORSAL DISPLACEMENT OF THE COLON

BASICS

DEFINITION

Right Dorsal Displacement

• An anatomic relocation of the colon because of rotation around the root of the colonic mesenteric attachment.
• Rotation can be either clockwise or counterclockwise.
• The pelvic flexure often is located at the diaphragm, and the colon is located between the cecum and the body wall.

Left Dorsal Displacement

An anatomic relocation of the colon such that it is located (i.e., entrapped) between the body wall and the nephrosplenic (i.e., renosplenic) ligament

PATHOPHYSIOLOGY

• Highly speculative, as with other intestinal displacements.
• Parietal attachments of the right ventral and dorsal colon, and attachment of the ventral to the dorsal colon (i.e., mesocolon) are such that the left ventral and dorsal colon (and pelvic flexure) are easily displaced and the right ventral and dorsal colon follow to a limited degree.

Right Dorsal Displacement

• Can occur in two directions—clockwise and counterclockwise
• Clockwise (as viewed from above) displacement occurs more frequently than counterclockwise displacement and consists of the pelvic flexure being displaced between the cecum and the body wall in a cranial-to-caudal direction. The pelvic flexure then often continues in a clockwise direction and is located near the diaphragm.
• Counterclockwise displacement consists of the pelvic flexure being displaced lateral to the cecum in a caudal-to-cranial direction.

Left Dorsal Displacement

• A result of the pelvic flexure passing through the nephrosplenic space in a cranial-to-caudal direction or of the left dorsal and ventral colon passing lateral to the spleen in a ventral-to-dorsal direction.
• The colon ascends dorsally between the spleen and the body wall. The dorsal colon is proposed to fall into the nephrosplenic space first, followed by the ventral colon.
• The entrapped colon often is rotated 180° in the nephrosplenic space, lending credence to the theory of ventral-to-dorsal mechanism for left dorsal displacement.
• The left colon can be palpated between the spleen and the body wall in resolving left dorsal displacements, suggesting this route is important in the pathogenesis of the condition.

Vascular Compromise

Vascular compromise is usually minor. It is associated with torsion of the colon at the root of the mesentery for right dorsal displacements and with torsion at the site of entrapment over the nephrosplenic ligament in left dorsal displacements.

SYSTEMS AFFECTED

GI

• The colon is displaced, and other sections of the abdominal GI tract can be displaced as a result—especially the cecum, but also the small colon and small intestine.
• Mechanical traction on the mesentery can result in considerable pain.
• Vascular obstruction results in compromise of the colon, resulting in colonic necrosis.

Cardiovascular

With long duration or vascular compromise, dehydration and fluid shifts may lead to circulatory compromise.

GENETICS

N/A

INCIDENCE/PREVALENCE

• In one study of exploratory celiotomies, 14% of cases were diagnosed as nonstrangulating colonic displacements.
• In another study, 23% of all colic cases presented to a referral practice were large colon displacements.

SIGNALMENT

No particular signalment. Mares, particularly following parturition may be predisposed to displacement of the ascending colon.

SIGNS

• Referable to the amount of colonic distension and any vascular compromise.
• Mild to moderate abdominal discomfort after 12–24 hours.
• Colic usually responds to analgesia initially but returns when the analgesic efficacy decreases.
• Acute escalation of signs is associated with increased colon distension or bowel compromise.
• Gastric reflux is inconsistent and usually caused by mechanical obstruction of the proximal small intestine.
• Heart rate often is less than might be expected from the degree of pain displayed (Left dorsal displacement).

CAUSES

• Possible causes include alteration to the intestinal motility and changes in the weight of the colon because of excess gas formation or mild impactions.
• Changes in intra-abdominal volume and GI activity after parturition may predispose postpartum mares to colonic displacement.
• Left dorsal displacement—in addition to the above, gastric distension resulting in displacement of the spleen from the body wall, splenic contraction, and displacement of the spleen because of adhesions between the spleen and previous ventral midline celiotomy incisions

RISK FACTORS

• Adhesions of the spleen to midline because of previous celiotomies, previous colonic displacements, and other forms of colic that may cause a horse to roll.
• Sudden dietary changes

RIGHT AND LEFT DORSAL DISPLACEMENT OF THE COLON

DIAGNOSIS

DIFFERENTIAL DIAGNOSIS

- Colonic/cecal tympany
- Colonic impaction
- Colonic volvulus
- Enterolithiasis
- A diagnosis of left dorsal displacement may be established on the basis of rectal examination by identifying the colon running across the dorsal aspect of the nephrosplenic ligament in conjunction with characteristic ultrasound images.
- Right dorsal displacement is more problematic, because excessive distension of the colon may preclude a thorough rectal examination of the caudal abdomen; however, the need for surgery is based on the degree of colon distension, tight bands, edematous bowel wall, and the lack of response to analgesia.

CBC/BIOCHEMISTRY/URINALYSIS

- CBC and biochemistry may be normal, with mild alkalosis to mild acidosis in cases of nonstrangulating displacements.
- Decreased hematocrit may result from sequestration of RBCs in the spleen.
- If strangulation of the colon occurs, significant dehydration, with a relatively decreased protein and metabolic acidosis, is common.

OTHER LABORATORY TESTS

- Peritoneal fluid usually is normal, unless the bowel is compromised.
- Abdominoparacentesis may result in perforation of the spleen in patients with left dorsal displacement, because the spleen is forced medially and ventrally.

IMAGING

- Ultrasound of right dorsal displacement may reveal large intestine distended with gas and fluid. Ultrasonography of a left dorsal displacement is characterized by failure to visualize the left kidney because of gas in the large colon and a flat, horizontal border of the dorsal spleen, which is displaced ventrally.
- A false-positive diagnosis can result from a gas-distended viscus near the left kidney, obstructing visualization of the kidney.
- A false-negative diagnosis can result from lack of gas in the entrapped colon.
- One study reported a correct diagnosis in 89% of cases of nephrosplenic entrapment, with no false-positive results.

DIAGNOSTIC PROCEDURES

- Abnormal findings on rectal examination for right dorsal displacement—transverse tight bands in the caudal abdomen, gas distension of the large intestine, and inability to palpate the cranially displaced cecum. If the cecum is palpable, it may be distended, and the colon may be palpable between the cecum and the right body wall. Sections of impacted colon may be palpable as well.
- Abnormal findings on rectal examination for left dorsal displacement—distended large bowel on the left, with tight bands coursing craniodorsally toward the nephrosplenic space; medial or caudal displacement of the spleen; and gas distension of the cecum. The colon above the nephrosplenic ligament may be clearly palpable in some horses. Correct rectal diagnosis of left dorsal displacement varies, with one report claiming a definitive diagnosis in 32% of cases and another that nephrosplenic entrapment was correctly diagnosed in 61% of cases (false-positive results not included).

PATHOLOGIC FINDINGS

Left dorsal displacement—sometimes a focal area of bowel necrosis associated with the site of entrapment.

TREATMENT

APPROPRIATE HEALTH CARE

- Right dorsal displacement—surgical correction is often required; correction of non-strangulating colonic displacements may occur with conservative therapy, but these cases monitored carefully and delay may worsen the prognosis.
- Left dorsal displacement—surgical correction, rolling the horse under general anesthesia, administration of phenylephrine (with or without forced exercise) and conservative management as for RDD.
- Choice of treatment depends on several factors—certainty of the diagnosis, degree of colonic distension, and financial limitations of the client.
- If the diagnosis is not certain or colonic distension is marked, rolling and forced exercise may be contraindicated.
- Reported success rates for conservative regimes vary widely and may relate to the accuracy of the original diagnosis.

NURSING CARE

- Vital
- Exploratory celiotomy—large deficits in fluid volume need to be addressed before surgery, as do acid–base and electrolyte imbalances.
- Abdominal distension restricting respiratory tidal volume—supplemental oxygen therapy may be required. In addition, deflation of a markedly distended large intestine via percutaneous trocarization may be beneficial but may cause leakage of intestinal contents; therefore, administer prophylactic antibiotics if performed.
- Passage of a nasogastric tube and decompression of the stomach are vital when a mechanical obstruction of the small intestine results in gastric distension.

Right and Left Dorsal Displacement of the Colon

ACTIVITY

• Forced exercise may assist resolution of left dorsal displacement of the colon.
• Uncontrolled rolling may convert a nonstrangulating to a strangulating displacement.

DIET

Discontinue oral intake until the condition resolves.

CLIENT EDUCATION

• Counsel owners on the decision of whether to treat left dorsal displacement conservatively, either by close monitoring alone, rolling, or with forced exercise or phenylephrine.
• Stress that treatment without surgery has obvious benefits, but that risks are associated with conservative treatment—rupture or further strangulation of a markedly distended viscus

SURGICAL CONSIDERATIONS

When the colon is not strangulated, the condition usually is straightforward to correct.

MEDICATIONS

DRUGS OF CHOICE

• Administer standard analgesia for colic—see *Acute Abdominal Pain.* Drug usage and dosage vary depending on the nature of the colic and the therapy to be instituted.
• Left dorsal displacement—phenylephrine. The rationale is that phenylephrine causes splenic contraction and may facilitate conservative therapy aimed at dislodging the colon from the nephrosplenic space. Commonly used dosages include 3–5 μg/kg per minute infused over 15 minutes or a bolus of 45 μg/kg injected slowly.

CONTRAINDICATIONS

Acepromazine sometimes is used for mild colic but is contraindicated in hypotensive patients and has negligible analgesic properties. Hypotension can be exacerbated in stressed animals.

PRECAUTIONS

N/A

ALTERNATIVE DRUGS

N/A

FOLLOW-UP

PATIENT MONITORING

• Routine postoperative monitoring after surgery or conservative therapy.
• Recurrence of displacement is well recorded for some horses, but data regarding the frequency of recurrence are difficult to find.

PREVENTION/AVOIDANCE

• The cause of displacement is poorly understood; therefore, avoidance is difficult.
• Management that may alter colonic activity, production of excess gas, and formation of impactions should be minimized; therefore, institute nutritional changes gradually.
• Prevent horses from rolling when showing signs of mild colic.

POSSIBLE COMPLICATIONS

Displacement can progress such that the colon becomes strangulated; at this stage, horses can rapidly succumb to cardiovascular shock from endotoxemia and hypovolemia or to colonic rupture from devitalization of the colon.

RIGHT AND LEFT DORSAL DISPLACEMENT OF THE COLON

EXPECTED COURSE AND PROGNOSIS

- The prognosis is good, provided there has been no volvulus or significant vascular insult to the colon.
- In one study, long-term survival of horses with nonstrangulating displacements was >70%.

MISCELLANEOUS

ASSOCIATED CONDITIONS

- Cholestasis
- Colonic volvulus
- GI impaction

AGE-RELATED FACTORS

N/A

ZOONOTIC POTENTIAL

N/A

PREGNANCY

- The colon is held in place largely by its association with surrounding organs, and the gravid uterus, as well as the empty abdomen in postfoaling mares, may predispose to displacement.
- Volvulus rather than dorsal displacement is more commonly associated with the postpartum mares.

SYNONYMS

Left dorsal displacement is also called nephrosplenic ligament entrapment.

SEE ALSO

- Large colon impaction
- Large colon volvulus

ABBREVIATION

GI = gastrointestinal

Suggested Reading

Hackett RP. Nonstrangulating colonic displacement in horses. J Am Vet Med Assoc 1983;182:235–240.

Johnston JK, Freeman DE. Diseases and surgery of the large colon. Vet Clin North Am Equine Pract 1997;13:317–340.

Santschi EM, Slone DE Jr, Frank WM. Use of ultrasound in horses for diagnosis of left dorsal displacement of the large colon and monitoring its nonsurgical correction. Vet Surg 1993;22:281–284.

Author Simon G. Pearce

Consulting Editor Henry R. Stämpfli

RIGHT DORSAL COLITIS IN HORSES

BASICS

DEFINITION

Localized ulcerative inflammation of the right dorsal colon (RDC), some cases of which have been associated with administration of high dosages of phenylbutazone and hypovolemia or deprivation of water.

PATHOPHYSIOLOGY

As a nonsteroidal anti-inflammatory drug (NSAID), phenylbutazone inhibits cycloxygenase activity. This drug is a competitive antagonist for both the constitutive cycloxygenase 1 (cox 1), which is responsible for the production of prostaglandins involved in physiologic functions, and for the inducible cycloxygenase 2 (cox 2), which is involved in inflammatory pathways. Intestinal mucosal cell production of prostaglandin E_2 and prostaglandin F_2alpha is decreased by the inhibition of the constitutive cox 1 activity. Subsequent loss of the prostaglandin-mediated protective effect on the intestinal mucosa results. The integrity of the intestinal mucosa may be compromised to the point that local bacterial invasion of the mucosa and luminal endotoxin absorption become possible. Plasma proteins may leak into the intestinal lumen, resulting in hypoproteinemia.

Phenylbutazone toxicity is potentiated in hypovolemic or water-deprived horses, because the prostaglandin-mediated local vascular changes, which guard against ischemic injury and intestinal mucosal cell atrophy from blood flow decrease, are inhibited.

SYSTEM AFFECTED

Gastrointestinal Tract

The RDC is the main portion of the gastro-intestinal tract to be affected by this condition.

SIGNALMENT

Breed

N/A

Sex

N/A

Age

N/A

SIGNS

Historical Findings

Most cases have a history of chronic administration or an overdose of oral or parenteral phenylbutazone, which is usually administered for a problem not related to the gastrointestinal tract, most frequently for a painful musculoskeletal conditions. Many cases also have a history of systemic dehydration, due to either a systemic illness or an inabililty to maintain proper hydration.

Physical Examination Findings

Horses with acute disease may have clinical signs that include depression, lethargy, partial or complete anorexia, fever, colic, and shortly thereafter, diarrhea, which can be profuse and watery, and severe dehydration and congestion of the mucous membranes is seen. Horses with more chronic disease may have clinical signs that include intermittent colic; soft, unformed feces; weight loss; and ventral edema.

CAUSES

The exact cause is uknown and it is not understood why the histopathologic lesions are localized to the RDC.

RISK FACTORS

A degree of hypovolemia and exposure to NSAIDs such as phenylbutazone are frequent prerequisites for the development of this condition.

DIAGNOSIS

DIFFERENTIAL DIAGNOSES

For the acute form of right dorsal colitis, severe medical conditions of the gastrointestinal tract, such as salmonellosis, intestinal clostridiosis, and Potomac horse fever (PHF) should be included in the differential diagnoses. However, in right dorsal colitis, seronegative status to *Ehrlichia risticii* (PHF) is observed, direct smear and Gram stain of feces do not reveal *Clostridium*-like organisms and no specific organisms such as *Salmonella* are cultured from the diarrheic feces.

For the chronic form of the disease, all disorders resulting in chronic abdominal pain, chronic diarrhea, or weight loss in the horse should be included in the differential diagnosis. Making a definitive diagnosis depends on the history of the case, a complete physical examination, and appropriate auxillary testing.

CBC/BIOCHEMISTRY/URINALYSIS

Complete Blood Count

Hematologic abnormalities include mild to moderate toxic neutrophil changes with either a regenerative or degenerative left shift. Neutropenia is occasionally seen. Hemoconcre-ntation characterized by an increased PCV is frequently observed in acute cases. In chronic cases a mild anemia may be present.

Biochemistry Profile

Biochemistry abnormalities may include absolute hypoproteinemia, hypochloremia, azotemia, and metabolic acidosis. Hypoprotei-nemia is observed in spite of hemoconcen-tration. Hypoalbuminemia is usual, but when total protein concentration is below 4.5 g/dL (45 g/L) panhypoproteinemia is observed.

Urinalysis

May reveal mild proteinuria.

OTHER LABORATORY TESTS

Abdominocentesis

Elevation of protein and nucleated cell count may be observed in abdominal fluid.

Fecal Occult Blood Test

May be positive

IMAGING

Gastroscopy

Because similar clinicopathologic findings can be observed in horses with gastric and small intestinal ulceration caused by NSAIDs, gastroscopy should be performed to differentiate the two conditions.

Ultrasonography

Thickening of the wall of the RDC may detected in some cases by abdominal ultrasonography via the right paralumbar fossa.

OTHER DIAGNOSTIC PROCEDURES

Exploratory Celiotomy

A tentative diagnosis of this condition can be made when gross findings of marked edema, thickening, or reduction in diameter of the intestinal tract are restricted to the RDC.

Intestinal Biopsy

The definitive diagnosis of the condition is made by histopathologic examination of a biopsy of the RDC collected during celiotomy.

PATHOLOGIC FINDINGS

A variable area of the right wall of the RDC-wall is thickend and the mucosal surface ulcerated. Histologically, the lesions are characterized by multifocal to coalescing ulceration in the wall of the RDC. Islands of mucosal regeneration may be observed. Lesions can be subacute or chronic. Subacute lesions are characterized by a fibrinonecrotic ulcerative colitis. In chronic cases, fibrous connective tissue is present in the lamina propria underlying the ulcerated mucosa. In chronic severe cases, colonic stenosis with ingesta impaction and subsequent necrosis and rupture of the colon can be observed.

RIGHT DORSAL COLITIS IN HORSES

TREATMENT

Acute Right Dorsal Colitis

Horses with acute disease are treated with supportive treatment, including intravenous fluids (lactated Ringer's solution), systemic broad-spectrum antibiotics, and analgesics. Flunixin meglumine should be used with caution. When hypoproteinemia is severe (plasma protein concentration <4 g/dL (40 g/L)), plasma transfusion should be instituted.

Chronic Right Dorsal Colitis

Horses with chronic disease can be managed with feeding and environmental adjustments and avoidance of treatment with NSAIDs. Dietary management consists of frequent feeding of a complete pelleted concentrate that contains 30% dietary fiber and 14% protein. Pelleted feed is advocated because it decreases the mechanical and physiologic load of the large colon. Roughage is eliminated or restricted to small amounts of fresh grass for at least 3 months. The concentrate is fed according to manufacturer's recommendations. The diet change is gradually completed over a period of 8 days. The first day, 25% of the recommended amount of pelleted feed is offered, then the amount is increased by 25% every other day. Once on the new diet, the recommended amount of pelleted feed is divided into 4–6 equal parts and the horse is fed every 4–6 hr. Actions to decrease stress include discontinuing or decreasing workloads such as strenous exercise.

Surgery

Sugical treatment is advocated when RDC cannot be controlled with medical treatment. It consists of either by-passing or resecting the diseased RDC. Side-to-side colocolostomy between the proximal intact part of the RDC and the small colon can be performed to by-pass the diseased part of the RDC. End-to-end colocolostomy after resection of the diseased RDC can also be performed. The prognosis for horses that undergo surgery is guarded.

MEDICATION

DRUG(S) OF CHOICE

Supportive treatment for horses with acute disease include:

- Lactated Ringer's solution (6–12 mL/kg/hr, IV) as a fluid volume replacement.
- Broad-spectrum systemic antibiotics (sodium penicillin G, 20,000 IU/kg, IV, q6hr, and gentamicin sulfate, 6.6 mg/kg, IV, q24hr; or ceftiofur, 2.2 mg/kg, IV, q12hr , or trimethoprim–sulphamethoxazole, 5 mg–25 mg/kg, IV, q12hr)
- Analgesics such as xylazine (0.2–0.5 mg/kg, IV) alone or in combination with butorphanol (0.02 mg/kg, IV) can be administered.
- Flunixin meglumine (0.25 mg/kg, IV, q6hr) to suppress prostaglandin-mediated effects of endotoxemia.

PRECAUTION

NSAIDs such as flunixin meglumine should be used with caution because they may also be involved in the pathogenesis of the disease. Aminoglycoside and flunixin meglumine should be used with caution when clinical signs of severe dehydration (prerenal azotemia) are present.

FOLLOW-UP

PATIENT MONITORING

Hematocrit and plasmatic protein concentration should be monitored when intravenous fluid therapy is administered. If plasma protein concentrations decrease to <4 g/dL (40 g/L) during fluid therapy, plasma transfusion should be instituted.

POSSIBLE COMPLICATION

Horses with acute disease can develop a persistent diarrhea with progressive edema, laminitis, or renal disease. The chronic disease can be complicated with continuous weight loss, hypoproteinemia, colic, and loose feces.

EXPECTED COURSE AND PROGNOSIS

Both acute and chronic forms have a guarded prognosis. If acute cases are recognized early and appropriate actions are taken, then the prospects of a sucessful outcome are increased. Chronic, well-established cases respond poorly to medical management, and surgical intervention is only feasable in a limited number of cases. Even in these cases the prognosis is guarded.

MISCELLANEOUS

ABBREVIATIONS

- RDC = right dorsal colon
- PCV = packed cell volume

Suggested Reading

Karcher LF, Dill SG, Anderson WI, King JM. Right dorsal colitis. J Vet Int Med 1990; 4:247-253.

Author Ludovic Bouré

Consulting Editor Henry Stämpfli

ROBINIA PSEUDOACACIA (BLACK LOCUST) TOXICOSIS

BASICS

OVERVIEW
- *Robinia pseudoacacia* (black locust) toxicosis results from an unknown toxin found in all portions of the plant except the flowers.
- A glycoprotein called robin is the putative toxin.
- The tree is widely distributed east of the Mississippi River.
- Signs relate to GI and cardiovascular effects of the toxin.
- Among domestic livestock species, horses may be the most susceptible.

SIGNALMENT
No known breed, age, or genetic susceptibilities

SIGNS
- Depression
- Colic
- Diarrhea or constipation
- Decreased intestinal peristalsis
- Weakness
- Cardiac dysrhythmias
- Hyperexcitability
- Dyspnea
- Laminitis

CAUSES AND RISK FACTORS
- Leaves are palatable and will be eaten if other forage is of poor quality or unavailable.
- Clinical signs have been reported in horses ingesting as little as 70 g of bark.

DIAGNOSIS

DIFFERENTIAL DIAGNOSIS
- Ionophore intoxication—differentiated by detection of an ionophore in feed.
- *Eupatorium rugosum* (white snakeroot) intoxication—evidence of plant consumption.
- Other causes of colic—appropriate physical examination and imaging (e.g., ultrasonography; radiography)

CBC/BIOCHEMISTRY/URINALYSIS
- Hypocalcemia was noted in two ill horses after leaf ingestion.
- Recumbent horses have increased serum CK concentrations.

OTHER LABORATORY TESTS
N/A

IMAGING
N/A

DIAGNOSTIC PROCEDURES
ECG may demonstrate cardiac dysrhythmias, but the types of dysrhythmias are not well documented.

PATHOLOGIC FINDINGS

Gross Findings
- Plant material (e.g., bark, leaves, pods) in stomach contents
- Watery and hemorrhagic intestinal contents

Histopathologic Findings
Enteritis characterized by diffuse villus-tip necrosis and hemorrhage

TREATMENT
- Decontamination with AC and saline cathartic or mineral oil
- Treat dysrhythmias.
- Analgesics for abdominal discomfort
- Balanced electrolyte fluids

MEDICATIONS

DRUGS
- AC (2–5 g/kg PO in water slurry [1 g of AC in 5 mL of water])
- One dose of cathartic PO with AC if no diarrhea or ileus—70% sorbitol (3 mL/kg) or sodium or magnesium sulfate (250 mg/kg), with the latter two in a water slurry
- NSAIDs—flunixin meglumine (1.1 mg/kg IV or IM as necessary)

CONTRAINDICATIONS/POSSIBLE INTERACTIONS
- Use NSAIDs with caution in dehydrated patients.
- Do not give mineral oil concurrently with AC because of impaired binding ability of AC.

ROBINIA PSEUDOACACIA (BLACK LOCUST) TOXICOSIS

FOLLOW-UP

PATIENT MONITORING

N/A

PREVENTION/AVOIDANCE

Prevent access to black locust; if not practical, provide good-quality diet in adequate amounts.

POSSIBLE COMPLICATIONS

N/A

EXPECTED COURSE AND PROGNOSIS

- Guarded prognosis in symptomatic animals
- No long-term sequelae are expected in recovered animals.

MISCELLANEOUS

ASSOCIATED CONDITIONS

N/A

AGE-RELATED FACTORS

N/A

ZOONOTIC POTENTIAL

N/A

PREGNANCY

N/A

ABBREVIATIONS

- AC = activated charcoal
- CK = creatine kinase
- GI = gastrointestinal

Suggested Reading

Burrows GE, Tyrl RJ, Rollins D, Thedford TR, McMurphy W, Edwards WC. Poisonous plants of Oklahoma and the southern plains. OSU Cooperative Extension Publication E-868, 24.

Author Robert H. Poppenga
Consulting Editor Robert H. Poppenga

SALMONELLOSIS

BASICS

DEFINITION

Salmonellosis refers to clinical syndromes that result from infection with species of the bacterial genus *Salmonella.*

PATHOPHYSIOLOGY

Exposure to *Salmonella* bacteria is usually through the alimentary tract. *Salmonella* bacteria can invade the pharyngeal, intestinal, and colonic mucosa. Bacteria attach to the mucosa, invade epithelial cells, and spread through the mucosa to lymphoid tissue and into the bloodstream. Virulence factors that promote infection and disease in an exposed host include the ability of the bacteria to invade tissues of the host; production of toxins that damage cells of the host; production of toxins that stimulate fluid secretion in the gastrointestinal tract; lipopolysaccharide, which can cause severe cardiovascular impairment; and factors that stimulate the host's inflammatory response, which can cause further tissue damage and signs of toxemia.

SYSTEMS AFFECTED

The gastrointestinal tract is the principal system affected. *Salmonella* bacteria can enter the blood and disseminate to other organs, including bone, lung, liver, and kidneys.

GENETICS

N/A

INCIDENCE/PREVALENCE

The incidence of salmonellosis is low in non-hospital settings. Epizootics of salmonellosis occasionally occur on farms, stables, sales facilities, and veterinary hospitals. The prevalence of fecal shedding of *Salmonella* bacteria by clinically normal horses has been reported to be as low as 1.5% and as high as 20% using fecal culture and polymerase chain reaction (PCR) methods. The prevalence of fecal shedding of *Salmonella* bacteria by horses with a gastrointestinal disorder is higher than in clinically normal horses.

SIGNALMENT

N/A

SIGNS

Typical cases of salmonellosis are characterized by fever, lethargy, diarrhea, and often abdominal discomfort. Cardiovascular function can be severely compromised because of dehydration that accompanies diarrhea and the systemic effects of endotoxin and pro-inflammatory cytokines. Animals with salmonellosis have tachycardia, injected mucous membranes, and delayed capillary refill time. Affected animals may also have cold extremities due to impaired circulation. Hypoproteinemia typically accompanies the severe intestinal inflammation with salmonellosis, and peripheral edema may be evident.
Neonatal foals may present with non-specific signs of septicemia, and subsequently any organ system may be involved. Young foals may present with lameness from primary musculoskeletal involvement, such as septic arthritis or osteomyelitis, or pneumonia caused by *Salmonella* bacteria. Atypical cases of salmonellosis in adult horses present with fever and often abdominal discomfort, but without diarrhea. Some cases may present with small colon impaction.

CAUSES

The most frequently isolated serotypes from horses include *Salmonella typhimurium, S agona, S anatum,* and *S krefeld.*

RISK FACTORS

The protective processes in the gut that prevent salmonellae from attaching can be perturbed in many ways, including antimicrobial administration, gastrointestinal disease ("colic"), transportation, high-density confinement or housing, and high-intensity training.

DIAGNOSIS

DIFFERENTIAL DIAGNOSIS

- Diarrhea may be referable to many other disorders, particularly Potomac Horse Fever, intestinal clostridiosis, and idiopathic colitis.
- Signs of endotoxemia can occur with many gastrointestinal disorders.
- Signs of colic may be referable to many other disorders.
- Peripheral edema may result from congestive heart failure, vasculitis, other protein losing enteropathy, and glomerulonephritis.

CBC/BIOCHEMISTRY/URINALYSIS

CBC

- Hemoconcentration
- Decreased (<5.0 g/dL; <50g/L) to normal (with dehydration) total solids
- Leukopenia
- Leukocytosis can occur in horses with colitis of several days' duration and with infectious thrombophlebitis.
- White blood cells can have highly reactive appearance secondary to stimulation by pro-inflammatory cytokines.
- +/− hyperfibrinogenemia

Serum Chemistries

- Azotemia (creatinine >2.0 mg/dL; >176.8 μmol/L)
- Hypoalbuminemia (albumin <2.5 g/dL; <25 g/L)
- Hyponatremia, hypochloremia, hypokalemia, hypocalcemia (ionized)
- Metabolic acidosis

Urine Analysis

Hyposthenuria (sp. gr. <1.020) may result from renal insult from toxemia.

OTHER LABORATORY TESTS

- Arterial blood gas analysis
- Fecal culture for *Salmonella* bacteria
- Fecal PCR for *Salmonella* bacteria
- Fecal clostridial toxin test

IMAGING

Trans-abdominal or transrectal ultrasonography may be used to determine whether there is intestinal or colon thickening (infiltrative disease, edema) or excessive peritoneal fluid accumulation.

DIAGNOSTIC PROCEDURES

Exploratory laparotomy with biopsy for bacterial culture is infrequently done to confirm a suspected case of salmonellosis in which repeated fecal cultures are negative.

PATHOLOGIC FINDINGS

In horses that die or are euthanized because of salmonellosis, lesions predominate in the cecum and large colon. The serosal surfaces often appear congested and purple. The mucosa may be thickened, sometimes markedly. The small colon may have a similar appearance. Colon infarction and perforation occur infrequently. Gross lesions in the kidneys, such as infarctions, may be found in severe cases. Also, immunocompromise may occur in severe cases, resulting in disseminated bacterial or fungal infection in multiple organs, particularly the lungs.

TREATMENT

APPROPRIATE HEALTH CARE

N/A

NURSING CARE

Restoration and maintenance of fluid volume is the most important treatment goal in salmonellosis patients with severe diarrhea. Horses with profuse diarrhea can present with 7–10% dehydration, which in a 500-kg horse represents a 35–50 L fluid deficit. Maintenance requirements can be 5 mL/kg/hr or more. Polyionic fluids should be used for replacement and maintenance, but if there are specific electrolyte deficits (sodium, chloride, potassium, calcium), supplemental solutions can be given. Hypertonic saline solution (8% NaCl) can be given for pronounced hyponatremia (<125 mEq/L). Potassium chloride (up to 40 mEq/L) can be added to polyionic fluids. Calcium gluconate can be administered separately, although recent research results might indicate that calcium supplementation could be disadvantageous in animals with endotoxemia.

Catheter selection, placement, and care are critical, as complications such as thrombophlebitis frequently occur in these patients.

ACTIVITY

Horses that recover from salmonellosis should have their activity restricted proportionate to the severity of illness. In horses with severe salmonellosis and resultant weight loss, this may require several weeks.

DIET

Dietary management depends on the severity of the intestinal disease. Generally, concentrate feed is withheld in acute cases of salmonellosis because of possible adverse effects on the already perturbed intestinal microflora. Hay and pellets are likely to be poorly digested in horses with colitis because of changes in the microflora, but acetic acid produced by fermentation of cellulose may be beneficial in cecal and colonic mucosal healing. Horses that are anorectic should be fed by stomach tube or intravenously because the severely ill colitis patient can quickly become nutritionally debilitated.

The caloric requirements of a typical adult horse confined to a stall are approximately 15 Mcal per day (30 kcal/kg/day), and this can increase substantially with severe salmonellosis.

CLIENT EDUCATION

Clients should be informed about the potential for fecal shedding of *Salmonella* bacteria into the environment. This varies, with potentially substantial fecal shedding from horses with diarrhea to much less shedding from horses with formed manure that are convalescing. Isolation procedures, specific for the facility, should be considered, particularly with a diarrheic horse. The zoonotic potential of salmonellosis should also be discussed with clients.

SURGICAL CONSIDERATION

N/A

SALMONELLOSIS

MEDICATIONS

DRUG(S) OF CHOICE

Opinions differ as to whether antimicrobials should be given to adult horses with salmonellosis. Foals with salmonellosis, particularly with concurrent septicemia, are routinely treated with antimicrobial drugs.

Reasons for the use of antimicrobials include:

- May kill existing *Salmonella* bacteria
- May prevent spread of *Salmonella* bacteria in gastrointestinal tract to other organs
- May prevent spread of enteric bacteria through damaged intestinal mucosa to other organs

Reasons against the use of antimicrobials include:

- Probably will not kill existing *Salmonella* bacteria
- Killing gram-negative bacteria may release additional lipopolysaccharide into the system
- May prolong fecal shedding of *Salmonella* bacteria

Antimicrobials used in the treatment of salmonellosis include combinations of penicillin and gentamicin; ceftiofur and gentamicin; and fluoroquinolones such as enrofloxacin and orbifloxicin.

Flunixin meglumine and ketoprofen have been shown to ameliorate the effects of endotoxemia and are often used in salmonellosis patients. Flunixin can be given at a dose of 0.25–0.5 mg/kg q6hr, and ketoprofen at 0.5 mg/kg q6hr.

Products that contain antibody to lipopolysaccharide (LPS) or that neutralize circulating LPS, such as polymyxin B, have also been used with varying results.

Dimethylsulfoxide (DMSO) is used by some clinicians because it scavenges oxygen radicals and has anti-inflammatory effects in some models of gastrointestinal disease.

Plasma therapy may be required if there is severe hypoproteinemia and edema. The amount of plasma given depends on the severity of hypoproteinemia and the response to treatment, but an adult horse with a serum protein <3.5 g/dL; <35 g/L may require 5–20 L. Some clinicians add heparin, 40–80 U/kg, to plasma to activate antithrombin III.

Gastric ulcer prophylaxis with an acid-suppressive drug is recommended because gastric ulcers typically occur in horses with salmonellosis because of disturbed gastrointestinal function and anorexia.

CONTRAINDICATIONS

N/A

PRECAUTIONS

If glomerular filtration is impaired, administering drugs that depend on renal clearance, particularly aminoglycosides, should be done judiciously.

POSSIBLE INTERACTIONS

N/A

ALTERNATIVE DRUGS

N/A

FOLLOW-UP

PATIENT MONITORING

- Heart rate—should progressively decrease toward normal (32–40 BPM)
- Rectal temperature
- Peripheral leukocyte count
- Leukocyte morphology—should progressively change from highly reactive appearance ("toxic") to normal
- Attitude, appetite
- Fecal *Salmonella* culture/PCR
- Weight gain
- Serum protein concentration
- Serum creatinine

PREVENTION/AVOIDANCE

Thorough cleaning of areas where fecal contamination is likely and preventing mechanical distribution of contaminated material are the most important measures that should be taken. Extensive use of disinfectants may not be necessary if cleaning measures are adequate. Cleaning must include removal of organic debris, which can be accomplished with several products designed for that task. Areas that require particular attention are stalls, including water buckets or automatic waterers, drains, and cracks in the floors and wall; stall implements; and for veterinary hospitals surgical areas, including drains, and nasogastric tubes and pumps.

If a diarrheic horse is in the environment, it should be isolated to the degree possible. Bedding material should be removed frequently to minimize accumulation of potential enteropathogens. Personnel entering the stall should be restricted to the professional staff, and they should wear disposable plastic boots. Footbaths with disinfectant are probably not effective, because they quickly accumulate organic material, which negates the disinfecting potential of the footbath. Once a horse vacates a stall, the stall should be thoroughly cleaned, allowed to dry, disinfected (we prefer a 1:30 dilution of chlorine bleach), and determined to be negative for *Salmonella* by culturing selected sites in the stall (floor, drain, waterer). Personnel should use common sense when dealing with diarrheic cases. If bedding is being blown about by wind or mechanical blowers are used to clean aisles, then potential enteric pathogens may readily be spread to other horses.

POSSIBLE COMPLICATIONS

- Laminitis
- Colon infarction
- Disseminated bacterial infection
- Chronic diarrhea
- Chronic, recurrent colic
- Chronic poor body condition

EXPECTED COURSE AND PROGNOSIS

Horses that have profuse diarrhea and toxemia require intensive care; the prognosis for survival is approximately 50%. Horses that survive typically show substantial improvement within 7 days, and horses that do not substantially improve in 7–10 days have a very poor prognosis for survival.

MISCELLANEOUS

ASSOCIATED CONDITIONS

- Laminitis
- Venous thrombophlebitis
- Catheterized veins
- Spontaneous

AGE-RELATED FACTORS

N/A

ZOONOTIC POTENTIAL

Salmonellosis has a high zoonotic potential that should be communicated to all personnel involved in the care of an affected patient. Personnel on antimicrobial treatment, immunosuppressive treatment, or who have immunocompromising illnesses should not come into contact with salmonellosis patients.

PREGNANCY

Abortion caused by *Salmonella* bacteria is rare. Pregnancy may be affected by the severity of illness of a mare with salmonellosis.

SYNONYMS

N/A

SEE ALSO

- Potomac Horse Fever
- Intestinal Clostridiosis

ABBREVIATIONS

N/A

Suggested Reading

Cohen ND, Martin LJ, Simpson, RB, Wallis, DE, et al. Comparison of polymerase chain reaction and microbiologic culture for detection of salmonellae in equine feces and environmental samples. Am J Vet Res 1996;57:780-786.

Hartmann FA, Control of an outbreak of salmonellosis caused by drug-resistant *Salmonella anatum* in horses at a veterinary hospital and measures to prevent future infections. J Am Vet Med Assoc. 1996;209:629-631.

Mainar-Jaime RC, House JK, Smith BP, Hird DW, House AM, Kamiya DY. Influence of fecal shedding of *Salmonella* organisms on mortality in hospitalized horses. J Am Vet Med Assoc 1998;213:1162-1166.

Murray, MJ. Epidemiologic considerations with *Salmonella* infection in horses. J Am Vet Med Assoc 1996;209:558-560.

Walker RL, Madigan JE, Hird DW, et al. An outbreak of equine neonatal salmonellosis. J Vet Diagn Invest 1991;3:223-227.

Author Michael J. Murray
Consulting Editor Henry Stämpfli

SAND IMPACTION AND ENTEROPATHY

BASICS

DEFINITION

Gravitational sedimentation of ingested sand in the large intestine causing colonic impaction and mucosal irritation.

PATHOPHYSIOLOGY

Horses ingest sand while grazing on loose sandy soil or while eating from the ground in sandy stalls or paddocks. Some horses, particularly foals, develop pica and intentionally eat sand or fine grit contained in decomposed granite used for stall or paddock floors in many areas. Under the influence of gravity ingested sand sediments and accumulates in the large colon until impaction and partial or complete obstruction may occur. Fine sand tends to accumulate in the ventral colon, whereas coarse sand or grit may also accumulate in the dorsal colon. Abdominal pain is caused by colonic distension from the impaction or from ingesta and gas accumulating proximally, and by reflex intestinal spasms stimulated by distension. Chronic irritation of the bowel wall and reduction in the absorptive surface area by accumulated sand may interfere with normal water absorption in the colon and give rise to diarrhea.

SYSTEM(S) AFFECTED

The gastrointestinal system is the only system affected.

GENETICS

N/A

INCIDENCE/PREVALENCE

Sand impaction has a worldwide distribution, but is much more common in geographic locations with loose sandy soil or in areas where horses are frequently kept in sandy paddocks or stalls and fed on the ground. Underfed horses and horses on closely grazed overstocked pastures appear to be at greatest risk.

SIGNALMENT

There is no breed predilection, and horses of any age can be affected.

SIGNS

Historical Findings

Feeding hay and/or grain on the ground or grazing on pastures with sandy soil are typical features of the history. Recurrent or chronic colic of mild to moderate severity, intermittent or chronic diarrhea, weight loss, and ill-thrift in spite of a good appetite are frequent historical findings.

Physical Examination Findings

Typical signs in horses with sand impaction reflect mild to moderate colic. Scant or absent feces are typical, although watery to "cow pie" diarrhea, often containing sand, may accompany or precede the onset of colic and may be the major presenting sign. Other signs include anorexia, lethargy, depression, abdominal distension, prolonged capillary refill time, and tachypnea. Auscultation of the colon over the most dependent portion of the abdomen for 1–5 min reveals typical "sand sounds" that result from sand/sand and mucosal/sand friction induced by mixing contractions. These occur at a rate of 2–5 per min and last for 2–5 sec. Sounds also arise from propulsive–retropulsive contractions that occur at intervals of 2–3 min and last for 15–30 sec and sound like the sound generated by slowly rotating sand in a partially filled paper bag. Except in horses with hypomotility or ileus, sand sounds are sensitive and reliable indicators of sand accumulation.

In thin horses that lack muscle tone and have massive accumulations of sand in the colon, external palpation and ballotment of the ventral and ventrolateral abdomen may reveal a firm, heavy viscus. Rectal examination usually reveals distinct distension of the large colon and/or cecum. However, definitive diagnosis of sand impaction is achieved in only about 15% of cases because affected portions of the bowel are often beyond reach. Fecal sand may be detected as "gritty" feeling during rectal examination.

CAUSES

See Pathophysiology

RISK FACTORS

See Pathophysiology

DIAGNOSIS

DIFFERENTIAL DIAGNOSIS

All other causes of colic (see relevant section), but particularly those that cause chronic or recurrent colic, including enterolithiasis, thromboembolic colic, internal abdominal abscess, gastric ulcer, peritonitis, abdominal neoplasia, cholelithiasis, and nephrolithiasis. Of the many causes of chronic diarrhea and ill-thrift, the most important differentials for sand enteropathy include parasitism, inflammatory bowel disease with malabsorption, intestinal neoplasia, and abnormal fermentation associated with non-inflammatory bowel disease or antibiotic use.

CBC/BIOCHEMISTRY/URINALYSIS

Changes are non-specific for sand impaction or enteropathy.

OTHER LABORATORY TESTS

Feces may contain frank or occult blood.

IMAGING

Abdominal radiography may demonstrate sand in craniovantral abdominal visera, particularly in foals, ponies, and small horses.

DIAGNOSTIC PROCEDURES

The sand sedimentation test is performed by breaking up three or four fecal balls collected during rectal examination in a rectal sleeve and mixing them with water to form a slurry. The open end of the sleeve is then tied off and suspended to allow the sand to settle inside the tips of the fingers. A sediment of more than 1/4 inch (0.6 cm) of sand remaining in the fingertips indicates that the horse is passing excessive quantities of sand in feces. In a more quantitative test, the finding of more than a teaspoon (5 g) of sand in the bottom of a bucket after suspending six fecal balls with water and allowing organic matter to float out is considered abnormal.

PATHOLOGIC FINDINGS

N/A

SAND IMPACTION AND ENTEROPATHY

TREATMENT

Horses with well-formed impactions or profuse diarrhea benefit from intragastric administration of water and electrolytes or intravenous administration of balanced electrolyte solutions. The choice of analgesics and the frequency of administration are dictated by the degree of pain.

Withholding of food for 24 hr or more and intragastric administration of mineral oil and water promotes lubrication and dissolution of the feed impaction that frequently complicates sand impaction. Re-suspension and removal of sand is best accomplished by intragastric administration of lubricating, motility-stimulating bulk laxatives containing *Psyllium hydrophila* mucilloid (0.25–0.5 kg/500 kg). Because psyllium gels quickly when mixed with water and may occlude the nasogastric tube, it is best administered mixed with 2 L of mineral oil, followed by 4 L of water. Continued daily administration of 0.25–0.5 kg of psyllium orally mixed with grain or sweet feed or administered by nasogastric tube for 10–14 consecutive days is recommended. Thereafter, further treatment is based on an assessment of whether all of the accumulated sand has been removed from the large colon, as determined by abdominal auscultation and repeated fecal sand sedimentation tests. Medical treatment is most likely to be successful in horses with good intestinal motility, modest accumulations of sand, low levels of abdominal pain, and pain that is easily controlled.

APPROPRIATE HEALTH CARE

Initial evaluation and treatment of horses with sand colic is handled appropriately on an outpatient basis. Transportation to a referral center is usually necessary for radiographic confirmation of the diagnosis and surgical management of horses that do not respond to medical therapy.

NURSING CARE

Prevention of rolling and self-induced trauma, provision of analgesia, and maintenance of hydration are important elements of nursing care. Placement of an indwelling nasogastric tube and fluid therapy is recommended before referral and during transportation for horses requiring surgical treatment.

ACTIVITY

Horses being treated for sand colic should be stall rested and hand-walked as necessary until the sand impaction has resolved.

DIET

Feed should be withheld during medical treatment for sand colic until the impaction has broken down, significant quantities of feces have been passed, and signs of abdominal pain have abated.

CLIENT EDUCATION

Feeding practices must be modified to prevent further accidental or intentional ingestion of sand.

SURGICAL CONSIDERATION

Affected horses with persistently reduced or absent intestinal motility, those with large accumulations of sand and horses that fail to respond to medical treatment within 48–72 hr, have uncontrollable pain, abdominal distension, gaseous distension of the bowel palpable on rectal examination, repeated gastric reflux, bowel displacement, a rising white cell count in peritoneal fluid, or sudden worsening of clinical signs are candidates for surgical intervention.

MEDICATION

DRUG(S) OF CHOICE

See section titled Treatment.

CONTRAINDICATIONS

Acepromazine is contraindicated in affected horses showing evidence of shock.

PRECAUTIONS

Repeated use of potent analgesics such as flunixin meglumine or ketoprofen to control colic pain should be avoided unless appropriate diagnostic and therapeutic intervention is also pursued.

POSSIBLE INTERACTIONS

N/A

ALTERNATIVE DRUGS

N/A

SAND IMPACTION AND ENTEROPATHY

FOLLOW-UP

PATIENT MONITORING

Repeat physical examinations including abdominal auscultation and sand sedimentation–testing of feces should be repeated at weekly intervals for 2–4 weeks to monitor the effectiveness of treatment in removing accumulated sand. Thereafter, abdominal auscultation and sand sedimentation tests should be performed at intervals of 3–6 months during routine health examinations.

PREVENTION/AVOIDANCE

Prevention involves identification and evacuation of accumulated sand from the large colon and modification of feeding and management practices to minimize further ingestion of significant quantities of sand. Auscultation of the ventral abdomen during routine physical examinations frequently identifies horses with significant accumulations of sand before overt clinical signs become apparent. The likely source of sand and causes of pica should be identified, and horses should not be fed on the ground and pastures should not be grazed too short. Feeders should be placed above a solid, sand-free surface or provided with a solid bottomt to prevent accidental ingestion of sand. Feeders made from two tractor tires bolted on top of each other and to a plywood base have proved to be very effective for feeding horses in dry paddocks when feeders cannot be placed on a solid base of concrete or similar material. Sufficient feeder space should be provided for all horses in order to discourage them from pulling hay out of the feeder and eating it from the ground. Horses should receive appropriate quantities of feed on a regular schedule and fresh water should be freely available. Pastures should be rotated to prevent overgrazing. Overgrazed bare pastures should be rested, fertilized, irrigated, and, when necessary, re-seeded to promote lush growth before reintroducing horses. Avoiding sand as the flooring material for stalls and paddocks occupied by horses that habitually eat sand or dirt may also be necessary because, these horses are difficult to manage.

If management practices cannot be modified to prevent ingestion of sand, intermittent "purge" treatments with psyllium-containing products marketed for equine use is recommended. Daily oral administration of 0.25 kg of psyllium for 7 consecutive days each month has proved to be effective.

POSSIBLE COMPLICATIONS

Complications include chronic diarrhea, bowel perforation, peritonitis, and bowel displacement, with or without strangulation.

EXPECTED COURSE AND PROGNOSIS

Medical therapy is usually successful in resolving sand impaction and relieving signs of colic within 1–4 days if bowel displacement is not a complicating factor. However, complete removal of accumulated sand often takes several weeks. Prognosis is good for those horses in which sand impaction is diagnosed at an early in stage because these cases generally respond rapidly to medical treatment. More chronic, high-volume sand impactions respond more slowly and are more likely to require surgical intervention, in which case prognosis is guarded, although survival after surgery is reported to be 75–90%. The long-term prognosis depends on preventing re-accumulation of sand and on the degree of mucosal injury and scarring resulting from the original episode of sand impaction. Some horses, presumably those with extensive mucosal injury, may show diarrhea and ill-thrift for extended periods after evacuation of the offending sand.

SAND IMPACTION AND ENTEROPATHY

MISCELLANEOUS

ASSOCIATED CONDITIONS

Chronic diarrhea, ill-thrift, colonic displacement, colonic rupture, septic peritonitis, endotoxemia, and the other post-operative complications listed above have been recognized in association with sand impaction.

AGE-RELATED FACTORS

Sand impaction can occur in horses of any age, including foals as young as a few weeks old.

ZOONOTIC POTENTIAL

N/A

PREGNANCY

Pregnant mares requiring surgical treatment for sand colic are likely at increased risk for abortion. Prophylactic use of nonsteroidal anti-inflammatory drugs (flunixin meglumine) and progestagens such as altrenogest are indicated in pregnant mares.

SYNONYMS

- Sand impaction
- Sand colic
- Sand enteritis
- Sand enteropathy

SEE ALSO

Colic

ABBREVIATIONS

N/A

Suggested Reading

Ragle CA, Meagher DM, Schrader JL, Honnas CM. Abdominal auscultation in the detection of experimentally induced gastrointestinal sand accumulation. J Vet Int Med. 1989;3:12-14.

Ferraro GL. Diagnosis and treatment of sand colic in the horse. Vet Med/Small Anim Clin. 1973;68:736.

Jones SL, Snyder JR, Spier SJ. Obstructive conditions of the Large Intestine. In Equine internal medicine (Reed S, Bayly W, eds.). Philadelphia: W B Saunders Co. 1998;682-694.

Bertone JJ, Traub-Dargatz JL, Wrigley RW, Bennett DG, Williams RJ. Diarrhea associated with sand in the gastrointestinal tract of horses. J Am Vet Med Assoc. 1988;193:1409-1412.

Ragle CA, Meagher DM, Lacroix CA, Honnas CM. Surgical treatment of sand colic: results in 40 horses. Vet Surg. 1989;8:48-51.

Author W. David Wilson

Consulting Editor Henry Stämpfli

SCRAMBLING IN TRAILERS

BASICS

DEFINITION

• A horse that leans its shoulder, hip, or barrel against the side wall of a trailer or against an interior partition and that moves its feet rapidly in a treading motion as if attempting to regain a normal standing posture and balance; the treading motion can be any locomotor pattern and usually involves the feet slipping across the contact surface.
• Severe scrambling may involve the horse leaning against one wall of a trailer and moving its feet against the opposite wall rather than on the floor, which may result in the fall of the horse.
• Can occur while the trailer is stationary or in motion.
• Signs of anxiety, active escape, or aggressive behaviors are seen in some cases.

PATHOPHYSIOLOGY

Most cases are not caused by disease; however, impaired vision or balance may contribute.

SYSTEMS AFFECTED

• Behavioral—signs range from mild anxiety with locomotor involvement to severe fear responses with corresponding involvement of organ systems.
• Cardiovascular—signs may be consistent with sympathetic stimulation (e.g., tachycardia and vasodilation).
• Endocrine/metabolic—sympathetic stimulation, increases in ACTH and cortisol concentrations, perspiration, and defecation
• Respiratory—increased respiration rate

SIGNALMENT

Any age, sex, or breed

SIGNS

• Historical findings—the horse may be unfamiliar with the confinement of the trailer or van or have had an unpleasant experience or injury involving a trailer.
• Physical examination findings—unremarkable, unless the horse has been injured by falling or hitting the sides of the trailer.

CAUSES

• Innately, horses are claustrophobic, desire to remain standing during stress-producing situations, and initiate flight responses to maintain their balance; scrambling involves a vicious cycle in which the horse perceives it is slipping, or actually slips, and then rapidly moves its feet to regain its balance, thus causing more slipping and more frantic attempts to regain an upright posture.
• Unpleasant experiences and injuries involving trailering can create anxiety about confinement in a trailer or van.
• Trailers that are too small, have slippery flooring, a poor design, or an inexperienced driver can contribute to the problem.

RISK FACTORS

• Trailers that are too small or have slippery flooring
• Poor trailer-driving skills (e.g., sudden starts and stops or sharp turns)

DIAGNOSIS

DIFFERENTIAL DIAGNOSIS

• Scrambling usually is behavioral in nature.
• Evaluate for normal vision, balance, and kinesis (ruling out confounding conditions, e.g., spinal ataxia, equine protozoal myelitis, myositis, lameness, etc.); if no abnormalities are found, the problem probably is behavioral.

CBC/BIOCHEMISTRY/URINALYSIS

N/A

OTHER LABORATORY TESTS

N/A

IMAGING

N/A

DIAGNOSTIC PROCEDURES

N/A

TREATMENT

GENERAL COMMENTS

• Adjust the trailering situation so the horse experiences less anxiety and can better maintain its balance.
• Tranquilizers may alleviate anxiety but generally are contraindicated due to their influence on the locomotor system.

MILD PROBLEMS

• Modify the trailer to make it easier for the horse to maintain its balance; generally, a horse that can spread its legs apart and brace against the movement of the trailer does not scramble.
• Rubber mats to make the floors nonslip
• Reduce the vertical width of the interior partitions so the trailer is open from the horse's stifle to the floor, allowing room for a wide stance, or either remove the interior partition or swing it to one side and secure it.
• Use a trailer with larger interior dimensions.
• Use a trailer in which individual stalls are situated diagonally to the direction of travel
• Tie the horse's head so it has enough range of motion to help maintain its balance but cannot turn its neck around completely.
• Train the driver of the tow vehicle to execute slow, smooth turns as well as controlled accelerations and decelerations.

SCRAMBLING IN TRAILERS

SEVERE PROBLEMS

- Problems in which the horse becomes self-destructive may require major modifications.
- The best treatment is to use an open stock trailer and turn the horse loose in the trailer; generally, the more freedom the horse has, the less anxiety and the less scrambling.
- Most horses loose in an open trailer quickly assume a position with their body diagonal to the long axis of the trailer and facing the rear; horses that travel facing the rear generally show less anxiety and maintain their balance more easily than horses facing forward.
- A trailer with a center of gravity close to the coupling with the tow vehicle reduces the amount of sway, which in turn reduces the occurrences of the horse losing its balance laterally.
- A tow vehicle and braking system designed to support and control the weight of the trailer also reduces lateral sway.

MEDICATIONS

DRUGS OF CHOICE

N/A

CONTRAINDICATIONS

N/A

PRECAUTIONS

N/A

ALTERNATIVE DRUGS

N/A

FOLLOW-UP

PATIENT MONITORING

Consult with the owner after a reasonable time to see if trailer modifications were attempted and successful at alleviating the problem.

POSSIBLE COMPLICATIONS

N/A

MISCELLANEOUS

ASSOCIATED CONDITIONS

Aversion to loading

AGE-RELATED FACTORS

N/A

ZOONOTIC POTENTIAL

N/A

PREGNANCY

N/A

SYNONYMS

N/A

SEE ALSO

Trailer loading/unloading problems

Suggested Reading

Clark DK, Friend TH, Dellmeier G. The effect of orientation during trailer transport on heart rate, cortisol and balance in horses. Appl Anim Behav Sci 1993;38:179–189.

Creiger SE. Reducing equine hauling stress: a review. Equine Vet Sci 1982;2:187–198.

Author Cynthia A. McCall

Consulting Editor Daniel Q. Estep

SEIZURES, COMA IN FOALS

BASICS

DEFINITION

• Seizures are a clinical sign of cerebral dysfunction and are classified as focal/multifocal clonic, tonic, and subtle.
• Clonic and focal tonic convulsions are epileptiform seizures with a distinct EEG signature. Rigid, jerking motions that cannot be suppressed by restraint characterize clonic convulsions.
• Focal tonic seizures describe sustained, asymmetric posturing of the trunk or limbs, accompanied by deviation of the eyes, nystagmus, apnea, and occasionally, clonus.
• Subtle seizures are called motor automatisms and are characterized by a variety of paroxysmal events, including eye blinking, strabismus, nystagmus, peddling movements, an array of oral-buccal-lingual movements, and other vasomotor changes (e.g., apnea; elevated blood pressure; changes in pulse, respiration, and pupil size). Subtle seizures are nonepileptiform seizures without any consistent EEG signature.
• Coma is characterized by loss of consciousness.

PATHOPHYSIOLOGY

• Seizures may result from any event that lowers the seizure threshold, which is the sum of events controlling neuronal excitability. Changes in the neuronal membrane, the concentration of neurotransmitters, alterations in the perineuronal environment, local tissue injury, or systemic illness can affect the seizure threshold.
• The most common cause of seizures in foals is asphyxia, which results in HIE associated with brain edema, necrosis, and less commonly, hemorrhage. Asphyxia-induced disruption of endothelial cell tight junctions leads to vasogenic brain edema.
• Elevated extracellular concentrations of excitatory amino acids, aspartate and glutamine, are neurotoxic and lead to an influx of calcium into brain cells, resulting in delayed cell death.
• Difficult deliveries, meconium-stained fetal fluids and fetus, and heavy, edematous placentas are peripartum events associated with birth hypoxia.
• Bacterial meningitis also can cause seizures and should be suspected in foals with systemic signs of sepsis.

SYSTEM AFFECTED

• Nervous—the primary system involved
• Behavioral—altered to varying degrees, from mild depression and decreased suckle to complete lose of consciousness
• Respiratory—tf the respiratory center in the brain is affected, paroxysmal breathing and apnea may occur.
• GI/renal—can be affected if affected foals become hypotensive either during or after seizures.

SIGNALMENT

• No sex or breed predilections for seizures caused by asphyxia or sepsis
• Seizures or coma resulting from asphyxia usually appear in foals within 72 hours of delivery.
• Seizures resulting from meningitis are associated with generalized septicemia, which is most common in foals <2 weeks of age.

SIGNS

Historical Findings

• Peripartum events associated with asphyxia—severe prepartum maternal illness, including endotoxemia, hypoproteinemia, hypotension, and colic; dystocia, placentitis; heavy; edematous placenta weighing >10% of foal's birth weight; premature placental separation; hydrops; oligohydramnios; twinning; meconium-stained fetal fluids and fetus; cesarean section; and early umbilical cord rupture
• Events associated with neonatal sepsis—vaginal discharge in the dam, placentitis, weakness, and failure of passive transfer

Physical Examination Findings

• Clonic seizures are moderately slow, rhythmic jerking motions of the facial, limb, or axial musculature that cannot be suppressed by restraint or repositioning.
• Tonic posturing involves symmetric hyperextension or flexion of extremities and may be accompanied by eye movements and apnea. Stimulation can provoke tonic posturing.
• Subtle seizures include paroxysms of roving eye movement, strabismus, repetitive blinking, oral-buccal-lingual movements (e.g., tongue protrusion, grimacing, drooling, sucking), rhythmic limb movements (e.g., pedaling, marching), and abnormal breathing (e.g., apnea, hyperpnea). Tactile stimulation can elicit subtle seizures.
• Foals with meningitis often exhibit rigid opisthotonus.
• The problem may be progressive, with the foal first appearing depressed. It may wander from its dam and lose its suckle reflex, which further progresses to recumbency and seizures, with coma being the end point. As the foal recovers, it usually regresses back through these signs in a stepwise manner.

CAUSES

• HIE—caused by peripartum asphyxia and generally is secondary to severe maternal illness, including endotoxemia, colic, severe anemia or hypoproteinemia; placental insufficiency associated with placentitis, placental edema, premature placental separation, twinning, hydrops, or oligohydramnios; dystocia; induction of labor; cesarean section; postterm pregnancy caused by placental insufficiency; early cord rupture with excessive hemorrhage; or severe neonatal cardiopulmonary disease, including pneumonia, persistent fetal circulation associated with intracardiac shunts (e.g., PDA, patent foramen ovale), or cardiac defects (e.g., VSD).

SEIZURES, COMA IN FOALS

• Metabolic disorders—hypocalcemia, hypomagnesemia, hypoglycemia, hyponatremia, hypernatremia, hyperosmolality, azotemia, and hepatoencephalopathy may result in cerebral disorders.
• Cranial trauma—can result in intracranial hemorrhage or swelling.
• Developmental conditions—CNS malformations, including internal hydocephalus, agenesis of the corpus callosum, and cerebellar abiotrophy (most common in Arabians)
• Infectious—septic meningoencephalitis, usually associated with Gram-negative sepsis; septicemia; endotoxemia; and viral meningitis associated with EHV-1 infection all may present with seizures or coma.
• Toxins and drug-induced—drug withdrawal after prolonged barbiturate administration; methlyxanthine administration

RISK FACTORS

• Placental insufficiency and difficult labor are closely associated with development of asphyxia-induced seizures.
• Failure of passive transfer of colostral antibodies, delay in first colostrum ingestion, umbilical infection, and early infectious neonatal pneumonia or enteritis are associated with development of Gram-negative septicemia, which increases the risk of septic meningitis.

DIAGNOSIS

DIFFERENTIAL DIAGNOSIS

• Paddling and whinnying observed during REM sleep can be confused with seizures; however, once the foal is aroused, this behavior quickly ceases.
• Muscle rigidity associated with WMD might be confused with seizures; however, WMD is accompanied by markedly elevated CK concentrations.
• Extensor rigidity caused by tetanus is very rare in foals but could be confused with convulsions. Poor maternal vaccination history, failure of passive transfer, a source of *Clostridia tetani* toxin (e.g., an open wound), and induced prolapse of the nictitans should increase the index of suspicion for tetanus.

CBC/BIOCHEMISTRY/URINALYSIS

• Leukopenia, neutropenia with a N:L <1, toxic changes in the neutrophils, IgG <400–800 mg/dL, hyperfibrinogenemia, are hematologic changes associated with sepsis.
• Azotemia in newborn foals (creatine >3–4 mg/dL) often is associated with placental insufficiency and peripartum asphyxia.
• Serum electrolyte concentrations help to rule out metabolic causes.
• Blood glucose <40 mg/dL can be associated with abnormal mentation and seizures.
• Markedly elevated concentrations of liver enzymes (e.g., AST, GGT, SDH) and elevated ammonia and bilirubin levels with concurrently low glucose and BUN concentrations are serum chemistries associated with hepatic failure and hepatoencephalopathy.
• Bacteriuria at urinalysis suggests bacteremia and septicemia in newborns.

OTHER LABORATORY TESTS

• Perform blood culture to look for evidence of sepsis.
• With suspected EHV-1 infection submit serum for viral titers. Positive titers in presuckle foal blood is highly suggestive of in utero infection.
• Plasma IgG levels <400–800 mg/dL indicate failure of passive transfer.

IMAGING

• Ultrasonography—lack of open fontanelles in foals precludes use of cranial/coronal ultrasonography to evaluate the brain.
• CT and MR imaging can be used, if available, to evaluate hypoxic brain damage and congenital defects and to look for hemorrhage.

DIAGNOSTIC PROCEDURES

• EEGs and brainstem auditory-evoked responses have been used primarily as research tools to document brain damage in foals.
• Perform a CSF tap in foals with suspected septic meningitis—foal CSF values: WBC <5 cells/μL, TP <150 mg/dL, RBC <500 cells/μL.

TREATMENT

• Seizing foals are difficult to treat on the farm and should be hospitalized to permit effective control of seizures and to prevent self-trauma. Wrap the foal's legs and use protective headgear if convulsions are severe and recurrent, but human restraint is the most effective method of reducing self-trauma. Place the foal on soft, absorbent bedding (e.g., a fleece-lined mattress, inside a sleeping bag) to reduce the risk of pressure sores. Medicate the eyes with artificial tears to reduce the risk of traumatic corneal ulceration.
• If the foal cannot nurse from the mare or bottle but has a functional GI tract, initiate nasogastric tube feeding. Ideally, foals should receive 10–25% of body weight in milk per day, divided into feedings given every 1–2 hours. In sick neonates, begin enteral feeding slowly, at 10% of body weight. If gut function is questionable, use parenteral nutrition.
• Evaluate plasma IgG and colostrum or plasma administered to increase the foal's serum immunoglobulin levels to >800 mg/dL.

MEDICATIONS

DRUGS OF CHOICE

Seizures

• Diazepam (0.11–0.44 mg/kg IV) is used initially because of its rapid onset. the dose can be repeated in 30 minutes. Do not store in plastic syringes, and protect from light.
• If seizures recur, use phenobarbital (2–10 mg/kg IV given slowly q12h), and monitor serum levels. High doses and rapid administration are associated with respiratory depression. Pentobarbital (2–10 mg/kg IV) is an alternative.

SEIZURES, COMA IN FOALS

CNS Edema

• Mannitol (0.25–1.0 g/kg IV as a 20% solution over 15–20 minutes and repeated twice daily)

• DMSO (0.5–1.0 g/kg IV given as a 20% solution slowly over 1–2 hours); use cautiously in hypotensive patients.

• Naloxone (0.01–0.02 mg/kg IV), an opiate antagonist, has been used to diminish CNS depression.

• Thiamine (0.5–5.0 mg/kg) can be added to IV fluids to help preserve aerobic brain metabolism.

• With seizure-associated respiratory depression, methylxanthines can be given to treat periodic apnea and to improve diaphragmatic contractility—caffeine (loading dose: 10 mg/kg PO SID; maintenance dose: 2.5–3.0 mg/kg PO SID)

Broad-Spectrum, Bactericidal Antibiotics

• Give agents such as amikacin (20–25 mg/kg IV SID) and potassium penicillin (22,000 U/kg IV QID) to recumbent, compromised foals to prevent sepsis.

• With suspected bacterial meningitis, consider a third-generation cephalosporin because of their improved CSF penetration—cefotaxime (20–40 mg/kg IV TID–QID).

Antiulcer Medication

Use of ranitidine, cimetidine, omeprazole, or sucralfate is recommended.

CONTRAINDICATIONS

• Avoid acepromazine, because it lowers the seizure threshold.

• Avoid xylazine, especially in cases with head trauma, because it causes transient hypertension that can exacerbate CNS hemorrhage.

PRECAUTIONS

Mannitol may exacerbate severe intracranial hemorrhage; observe for deterioration in CNS status after administration.

POSSIBLE INTERACTIONS

N/A

ALTERNATIVE DRUGS

• Low doses of magnesium sulfate (25–50 mg/kg diluted to 1% and given slowly IV) have been used to control seizures.

• With septic meningitis, ceftiofur (5–10 mg/kg TID–QID) or chloramphenicol succinate (25–50 mg/kg q4h) can be tried.

SEIZURES, COMA IN FOALS

FOLLOW-UP

PATIENT MONITORING

Serial neurologic evaluations to assess response to treatment.

POSSIBLE COMPLICATIONS

Permanent CNS Deficits

• Cases with suspected bacterial or viral meningitis have a grave prognosis for intact neurologic survival.
• Severe CNS malformations also carry a grave prognosis for survival.
• Foals with the poorest prognosis fail to show improvement in CNS function within the first 5 days of life, remain comatose, and experience severe, recurrent seizures that are refractory to barbiturate therapy.
• Foals with HIE have a 70–75% recovery rate if sepsis does not intervene.

Self-Trauma

Frequently includes pressure sores and corneal ulceration.

MISCELLANEOUS

ASSOCIATED CONDITIONS

• Hypoxic lung injury
• Hypoxic-ischemic necrotizing enterocolitis
• Ischemic renal failure injury

AGE-RELATED FACTORS

Premature foals tend to show more tonic posturing.

ZOONOTIC POTENTIAL

N/A

PREGNANCY

N/A

SYNONYMS

• Barker foal
• Dummy foal
• HIE
• Neonatal maladjustment syndrome
• NMS
• Wanderer foal

SEE ALSO

Neonatal septicemia

ABBREVIATIONS

• AST = aspartate aminotransferase
• CK = creatine kinase
• CSF = cerebrospinal fluid
• DMSO = dimethyl sulfoxide
• EHV = equine herpes virus
• GGT = γ-glutamyltransferase
• GI = gastrointestinal
• HIE = hypoxic ischemic encephalopathy
• MR = magnetic resonance
• N:L = neutrophil:lymphocyte
• NMS = neonatal maladjustment syndrome
• PDA = patent ductus arteriosus
• REM = rapid eye movement
• SDH = sorbitol dehydrogenase
• TP = total protein
• VSD = ventricular septal defect
• WMD = white muscle disease

Suggested Reading

Green SL, Mayhew IG. Neurologic disorders. In: Koterba AM, et al., eds. Equine clinical neonatology. Philadelphia: Lea & Febiger, 1990:496–530.

Vaala WE. Peripartum asphyxia. Vet Clin North Am Equine Pract 1994;10:187–218.

Author Wendy E. Vaala
Consulting Editor Mary Rose Paradis

SELECTIVE IgM DEFICIENCY

BASICS

OVERVIEW

Decreased or absent serum IgM with no abnormalities of other immunoglobulins or immune functions

SIGNALMENT

- Predominantly seen in Arabians; also described in other breeds (Thoroughbred, Standardbred, Quarter Horse, Paso Fino).
- Typically seen in horses <2 years of age; can occur in a secondary form in old horses.
- No apparent sex predilections

SIGNS

- Presentation occurs in three forms.
- Severe pneumonia, arthritis, or enteritis leading to death in foals <10 months of age
- Recurrent respiratory and alimentary infections in horses <2 years of age, associated with poor growth rates and stunting.
- Associated with lymphoreticular neoplasia in horses 2–5 years of age; ill thrift, weight loss, or chronic recurrent infections may occur.

CAUSES AND RISK FACTORS

- Genetic basis—suspected but unproven
- Secondary (i.e., adult) form is commonly associated with lymphosarcoma and may involve other immune system abnormalities.

DIAGNOSIS

DIFFERENTIAL DIAGNOSIS

- Agammaglobulinemia—primary differential consideration; seen exclusively in males; diagnosis supported by absent or significantly decreased serum IgA, IgG, and IgM.
- With selective IgM deficiency, only IgM is decreased; other globulins are normal to increased.
- SCID—typically seen in young foals, with an associated lymphopenia not seen in selective IgM deficiency.
- Failure of passive transfer—observed in neonates; age of onset for IgM deficiency is older.

CBC/BIOCHEMISTRY/URINALYSIS

- Hemogram—normal or reflects infection/inflammation (leukocytosis, neutrophilia, hyperfibrinogenemia)
- Biochemistry profile—nonspecific changes, depending on the presence of chronic inflammation and the organ systems involved
- Urinalysis—unremarkable

OTHER LABORATORY TESTS

- Serum IgM is <2 SD below age-matched normal (4–8 months, <15 mg/dL; >8 months, <25 mg/dL).
- Normal serum IgG and IgA
- Specific tests of cellular immune function are normal.

IMAGING

N/A

DIAGNOSTIC PROCEDURES

As needed for lymphosarcoma in the secondary form of the disease.

PATHOLOGIC FINDINGS

Lymphoid tissue—grossly and histologically normal

SELECTIVE IGM DEFICIENCY

TREATMENT

- No specific treatment is available.
- Plasma transfusion provides only short-term benefit.

MEDICATIONS

DRUGS

Treat infections with appropriate antibiotics.

CONTRAINDICATIONS/POSSIBLE INTERACTIONS

N/A

FOLLOW-UP

- Prognosis is poor to grave, although rare cases have spontaneously recovered.
- Confirm diagnosis by repeat IgM assay.

MISCELLANEOUS

ASSOCIATED CONDITIONS

N/A

AGE-RELATED FACTORS

N/A

ZOONOTIC POTENTIAL

N/A

PREGNANCY

N/A

SEE ALSO

- Lymphosarcoma
- SCID

ABBREVIATIONS

- SCID = severe combined immune deficiency
- SD = standard deviation

Suggested Reading

Perryman L, McGuire T. Evaluation for immune system failure in horses and ponies. J Am Vet Med Assoc 1980;176:1374.

Author Martin Furr

Consulting Editor Debra C. Sellon

SELENIUM TOXICOSIS

BASICS

OVERVIEW

- Acute selenosis almost invariably results from oversupplementation, either via treated feedstuffs or parenteral medications.
- Plant species that accumulate sufficient selenium to be acutely toxic are so unpalatable that horses will starve rather than eat them.
- Clinical signs involve the respiratory, cardiovascular, hematologic, and GI systems.
- Chronic selenosis is associated with naturally contaminated forages or hay.
- The most obvious clinical signs involve the epithelium.
- Research during the last two decades indicates that the condition described as "blind staggers" does not exist but is, in fact, a potpourri of other maladies mistakenly ascribed to selenium toxicosis.

SIGNALMENT

- No known breed, age, or sex predilections
- Horses are somewhat more sensitive to chronic selenosis than ruminants and, thus, may be poisoned on pastures not affecting cattle.

SIGNS

Acute Selenosis

- Can present as sudden death with few, if any, clinical signs.
- When clinical signs occur, they progress rapidly.
- Affected horses exhibit lassitude, muscular weakness, anorexia, and progressively worsening dyspnea beginning 1–24 hours after exposure.
- Colic and diarrhea may occur.
- Heart rate and respiration are elevated, pulse is weak, and animals frequently are cyanotic.
- Fever, polyuria, and hemolytic anemia have been reported in some cases.
- Lethally poisoned animals usually become comatose and die with 12–48 hours.

Chronic Selenosis

- Sometimes called alkali disease.
- Usually requires chronic (30–90 days) exposure to seleniferous forages or pastures.
- In rare cases, the condition may result from shorter exposures but still requires $\cong$30 days to manifest clinical signs
- The most obvious clinical manifestations are bilaterally symmetric alopecia and dystrophic hoof growth.
- Alopecia typically involves the mane and tail but, in severe cases, may involve other parts of the body.
- Hoof lesions begin as lameness, erythema, and swelling of the coronary bands. These subside only to be followed in a few days to weeks by a circumferential crack parallel and just distal to the coronet. Hoof separation and lameness increase until the damaged claw is displaced from underneath by new growth and subsequently sloughs. In many cases, however, the damaged claw is not shed but remains attached, resulting in an extended, upwardly curled toe that places abnormal stresses on the appendicular skeleton. Affected animals become so lame that they cannot eat or drink and, thus, starve.

CAUSES AND RISK FACTORS

- Selenium- or vitamin E–deficient animals are more susceptible to acute selenosis.
- Chronic selenosis usually is associated with naturally seleniferous vegetation; as such, specific geographic localities.
- Plants may be classified as indicator species, which occur only on seleniferous soils and may contain as much as 50,000 ppm of selenium; as accumulator species, which grow anywhere and accumulate selenium to a lesser extent; or as nonaccumulators, which never accumulate more than 20–30 ppm.
- Nonaccumulaters include most of the commonly used forage species and actually constitute the most important source of selenium, because the indicator and accumulator species are extremely unpalatable.

DIAGNOSIS

DIFFERENTIAL DIAGNOSIS

- Acute—heavy metal (e.g., arsenic) intoxication, endotoxemia, and blister beetle intoxication
- Chronic—leucana (*Leucaena leucocephala*) intoxication, ergotism, laminitis, and thallium intoxication

CBC/BIOCHEMISTRY/URINALYSIS

- Hematology and serum enzymes in horses with acute selenosis suggest stress and damage to the heart, liver, and GI tract, but there are no pathognomonic findings.
- Uncomplicated chronic selenosis does not usually produce any deviation from normal in routine clinical laboratory tests.

OTHER LABORATORY TESTS

- Tissue selenium concentrations are less reliably predictive of damage than with other toxic elements.
- Blood and liver concentrations <1.0 ppm usually rule out selenosis; the only exception might be a chronic case in which the first samples are not taken until several weeks after the onset of signs.
- Higher concentrations may indicate excessive exposure but, by themselves, do not prove selenosis.

IMAGING

N/A

SELENIUM TOXICOSIS

DIAGNOSTIC PROCEDURES

N/A

PATHOLOGIC FINDINGS

Acute Selenosis

- The most obvious gross lesions occur in the thorax and GI tract.
- The heart may be pale or mottled and flaccid.
- Petechial or ecchymotic hemorrhages are found within the myocardium and throughout the thoracic viscera.
- The lungs are wet, heavy, and congested, with prominent septal edema and froth in the airways.
- Congestive heart failure manifests as hydrothorax and ascites.
- The intestinal tract may be hyperemic or hemorrhagic, especially after oral exposure, and usually is edematous.
- Hepatic centrilobular necrosis or renal proximal tubular necrosis often occur but seldom are recognizable grossly.

Chronic Selenosis

- The most distinctive gross lesions involve the integument, specifically the hoof and hair follicles.
- Alopecia of the mane and tail, and separation of the wall of the hoof
- Histologically, hoof damage begins as ballooning degeneration and necrosis of keratinocytes near the tips of the primary laminae. Neutrophils and dyskeratotic debris accumulate around the tips of the epidermal papillae and in the lumen of keratin tubules.
- Alopecia results from atrophy of the primary hair follicles. Most atrophic follicles are collapsed and lack a hair shaft. The inner root sheath is atrophic or absent, and the outer sheath contains dyskeratotic keratinocytes. Accessory follicular structures (e.g., sebaceous glands, erector pili muscles) are unaffected.

TREATMENT

- No proven therapies for acute selenosis
- Uncomplicated chronic selenosis has been successfully treated with palliative measures—heart-bar shoes, therapeutic trimming, and nursing care

MEDICATIONS

DRUGS

- No specific drugs for treating acute selenosis
- Analgesics and NSAIDs are essential in keeping a horse with chronic selenosis both mobile and eating.

CONTRAINDICATIONS/POSSIBLE INTERACTIONS

N/A

FOLLOW-UP

PATIENT MONITORING

N/A

PREVENTION/AVOIDANCE

- Prevention consists of avoiding excess selenium exposure.
- Total dietary concentrations as low as 5 ppm of dry matter are potentially (but not always) toxic.
- Avoid selenium-containing mineral supplement if possible in seleniferous areas.
- Low dietary protein levels potentiate selenium toxicity, but there is some question whether extremely high protein levels are protective.

POSSIBLE COMPLICATIONS

N/A

EXPECTED COURSE AND PROGNOSIS

- Poor prognosis with acute selenosis
- Prolonged recovery with chronic selenosis

MISCELLANEOUS

ASSOCIATED CONDITIONS

N/A

AGE-RELATED FACTORS

N/A

ZOONOTIC POTENTIAL

N/A

PREGNANCY

Most research seems to indicate that selenium is not teratogenic in mammals; the author has seen several normal foals born to mares recovering from chronic selenosis.

SEE ALSO

N/A

ABBREVIATION

GI = gastrointestinal

Suggested Reading

O'Toole D, Raisbeck MF, Case JC, Whitson TD. Selenium-induced "blind staggers" and related myths. A commentary on the extent of historical livestock losses attributed to selenosis on western rangelands. Vet Pathol 1996;33:104–116.

Author Merl F. Raisbeck
Consulting Editor Robert H. Poppenga

SELF-MUTILATION

BASICS

DEFINITION

Biting directed at the horse's own flanks, chest, or limbs

PATHOPHYSIOLOGY

- The cause of self-mutilation of psychic origin is believed to be frustration, particularly of sexual and aggressive behaviors.
- Endogenous opiates are believed to be released, resulting in sufficient analgesia that the horse does not feel pain when biting itself; this hypothesis is based on the finding that opiate blockers temporarily inhibit the behavior.
- Stallions with olfactory, auditory, or visual access to mares but that cannot reach them and also have olfactory, auditory, and visual access to rival stallions but can not reach them may redirect their aggression toward themselves.
- The cause of the behavior in geldings may be similar and seems to be aggravated by housing with the dam. Horses avoid consanguineous mating, so the presence of a mare in heat that is attractive (because she is in heat) but to be avoided (because she is socially dominant and a close relative) may lead to a redirected behavior, aggression. Sometimes the aggression is directed toward the mare, but a gelding more often directs the aggression toward itself.
- Complete isolation of the stallion or the gelding may help.

SYSTEMS AFFECTED

- Behavioral—behavior is definitely abnormal, because in the most serious cases, the horse is causing tissue damage.
- GI—these problems must be ruled out as a cause.
- Skin—these problems must be ruled out as a cause; skin lesions are created when the horse bites itself.
- Reproductive—usually a behavior problem in stallions, which castration ameliorates; uterine pain or granulosa cell tumors may cause mares to bite their flanks.
- Neurologic—these problems must be ruled out as a cause.

SIGNALMENT

- Stallions are affected most often, geldings occasionally, and mares rarely.
- Reported in Arabians and Quarter horses, American Saddlebreds, Thoroughbreds, Standardbreds, and Morgans.
- Usually >1 year of age

SIGNS

General Comments

- The horse bites at its flanks, chest, limbs, or rarely, tail; this usually is accompanied by vocalization or kicking.
- In some cases, the behavior is preceded by circling, grasping objects, and head and mouth movements.

Historical Findings

- First manifests in response to very specific stimuli (e.g., sight of the dam) and then may generalize to any horse or large moving object, etc.
- Severity of the biting may increase with time.

Physical Examination Findings

Can vary from ruffled, saliva-coated hair to mild hair loss to laceration of the skin and underlying tissue of the flank, chest, or limbs.

CAUSES

- Frustration, usually sexual, or re-directed aggression is the main cause.
- Separation from companions—frustration of the desire to be with the herd.
- Attention-getting—owners respond by examining the horse and giving it positive attention.

RISK FACTORS

- Breed and genetic predisposition
- Underworked stallions kept alone in a stall or a paddock, especially when housed with other stallions and with intermittent exposure to mares.
- Because of the genetic predisposition, environmental factors do not affect all stallions, only those that are genetically susceptible.
- A stallion or gelding housed with its dam
- With foals, temporary or permanent separation from the mother
- Weaning

DIAGNOSIS

DIFFERENTIAL DIAGNOSIS

- Differentiate self-mutilation of psychic origin from a dermatologic (e.g., allergic irritant induced dermatitis), external or internal parasitic, or painful condition of the skin or underlying tissues and from peripheral neuritis or a central neural lesion.
- Most self-mutilation is directed at the flanks, so an abdominal cause must be ruled out.
- Testicular torsion has been associated with one case.
- CNS problems—rabies or Lyme disease; hyperesthesia rather than self-mutilation is more common with the latter.

CBC/BIOCHEMISTRY/URINALYSIS

- Perform a chemistry screen and CBC to determine presence of an underlying disease and whether medication can be administered safely.
- Perform urinalysis to rule out kidney or bladder stones as a source of pain.

OTHER LABORATORY TESTS

Blood test geldings for testosterone levels indicative of incomplete castration. Basal testosterone levels usually indicate whether the gelding is cryptorchid, but a stimulation test can be performed in equivocal cases. After an initial blood sample, administer hCG (2500 IU IV), and perform another blood test 90 minutes later. Testosterone levels >200 pg/mL indicate presence of testicular tissue.

IMAGING

Only necessary to rule out CNS, GI, or reproductive tract problems

DIAGNOSTIC PROCEDURES

Test for Lyme disease.

SELF-MUTILATION

TREATMENT

- Castration of stallions usually reduces or eliminates the behavior
- Cradles for flank and bibs for chest biters prevent damage to the skin, but neither changes the horse's motivation or reduces the squealing and kicking that accompany the behavior. The kicking is a distinct threat to handlers.
- Creating a naturalistic environment for the stallion by housing him in a pasture with a mare or mares.
- Increasing exercise, increasing available forage, and decreasing grain can greatly reduce the frequency of the behavior.
- Remove geldings from contact with mares, and provide more exercise and less grain.
- Do not allow the horse to lose too much weight; oil can be substituted for carbohydrate calories if necessary.

MEDICATIONS

DRUGS OF CHOICE

Opiate blockers such as nalmefene (0.08–1.2 mg/kg IM) have been used to inhibit the behavior, but these drugs are too expensive and too short acting to be practical.

CONTRAINDICATIONS

Mares during late pregnancy

PRECAUTIONS

GI side effects, including diarrhea, inappetence, and behavior indicative of colic, are seen after naloxone administration.

POSSIBLE INTERACTIONS

N/A

ALTERNATIVE DRUGS

- Oral tryptophan
- Acupuncture

FOLLOW-UP

PATIENT MONITORING

Regular follow-up after 2 weeks to evaluate the owner's compliance and the success of the treatments given.

POSSIBLE COMPLICATIONS

N/A

MISCELLANEOUS

ASSOCIATED CONDITIONS

N/A

AGE-RELATED FACTORS

- Usually a disease of sexually mature stallions, but it can occur in foals separated from their dams.
- Young horses usually do not actually mutilate themselves.

ZOONOTIC POTENTIAL

N/A

PREGNANCY

A mare in labor may bite at her flanks, presumably because of pain.

SYNONYMS

Flank biting

SEE ALSO

Psychogenic sexual behavior dysfunction

ABBREVIATIONS

- GI = gastrointestinal
- hCG = human chorionic gonadotropin

Suggested Reading

Dodman NH, Normile JA, Shuster L, Rand W. Equine self-mutilation syndrome (57 cases). J Am Vet Med Assoc 1994;204:1219–1223.

Dodman NH, Shuster L, Court MH, Patel J. 1988. Use of a narcotic antagonist (nalmefene) to suppress self-mutilative behavior in a stallion. J Am Vet Med Assoc 1988;192:1585–1587.

Houpt KA. Self-directed aggression: a stallion behavior problem. Equine Pract 1983;5(2):6–8.

Kamerling SG, Hamra JG, Bagwell CA. Naloxone induced abdominal distress in the horse. Equine Vet J 1990;22:241–243.

Murray MJ, Crowell-Davis SL. Psychogenic colic in a horse. J Am Vet Med Assoc 1985;186:381–383.

Author Katherine Albro Houpt

Consulting Editor Daniel Q. Estep

SEMEN EVALUATION: NORMAL STALLION

BASICS

DEFINITION

• Stallion semen is evaluated to determine semen quality before the breeding season, as part of a prepurchase examination, and to investigate presumptive subfertility.
• Semen evaluation is not a predictor of future fertility but, rather, a means to determine semen quality on the day of examination.

PATHOPHYSIOLOGY

N/A

SYSTEM AFFECTED

Reproductive

GENETICS

N/A

INCIDENCE/PREVALENCE

N/A

SIGNALMENT

• Stallions, all breeds.
• Prevalence of Thoroughbred, Standardbred, Quarter Horse, and Warmblood breeds.

SIGNS

• Normal fertility.
• Normal physical examination findings.

CAUSES

N/A

RISK FACTORS

N/A

DIAGNOSIS

DIFFERENTIAL DIAGNOSIS

N/A

CBC/BIOCHEMISTRY/URINALYSIS

Not a usual component of a BSE, but may be indicated if multisystemic disease is present.

OTHER LABORATORY TESTS

Sperm Motility

• Best evaluated using phase-contrast microscopy.
• Assess at least 10 fields at ×200–400.
• Stallion semen is easily cold-shocked. Ensure that anything (e.g., slides, coverslips, pipettes) that comes into contact with sperm is prewarmed to 37°C.
• Estimate of sperm motility is the ratio TM:PM.
• With experience, can estimate sperm velocity or vigor and subjectively categorize the sample using a scale of 0–4 (i.e., 0, nonmotile; 4, rapidly motile).
• Motility and velocity can be evaluated objectively using a CASA system. Several commercial units are available, all of which are quite expensive.
• Sperm motility is acceptable if PM exceeds 60% in all fields.

Sperm Morphology

• Evaluate using one of several commercial stains—eosin-nigrosin background staining (adequate method); evaluation of unstained sperm fixed using 10% buffered formol saline and phase-contrast microscopy (optimal method); both methods are recommended by the Society for Theriogenology.
• Defects are characterized as major or minor (formerly primary and secondary, respectively).
• Major defects—those likely to relate to fertility problems and thought to occur during spermatogenesis.
• Defects of the sperm head and midpiece most likely relate to fertility problems.
• Most relevant parameter—percentage of normal sperm; should exceed 60% in ejaculated semen from most normal, fertile stallions.
• At minimum, 100–200 cells should be evaluated.

Sperm Concentration

• Estimated using raw semen and a 1:100 dilution, WBC Unopette system and a hemocytometer.
• Fill both grid chambers under the cover slip, then allow a few minutes for sperm settling.
• Count sperm heads on both grids, take an average of the two, and count all central squares—25 small boxes within each grid.
• Number of sperm heads is multiplied by 1×10^6, which is the number of sperm per milliliter of raw semen.
• Multiply this number by the total gel-free semen volume (ml). This is the total number of sperm in the horse's ejaculate.
• Sperm concentration also can be determined using a commercial sperm densitometer.

Semen Volume

• Measure after the semen gel fraction has been removed—in-line separation, with the filter positioned between the AV and the collection bag or bottle.
• Use nylon- or cotton-mesh filters.
• Prewarmed (37°C), sterile, disposable or glass graduated cylinders or specimen cups can be used.

Semen pH

• Measure with a pH meter or pH paper.
• Powdered or liquid color indicators are inappropriate, because semen contamination and lethal sperm damage can result.
• Alterations of semen pH can indicate contamination of ejaculated semen by urine, purulent material, or blood.

Calculation of Semen Breeding Dose

• The recommended minimum number of PM to be inseminated near the time of ovulation when using fresh extended semen is 500 million PM.
• Some veterinarians factor in the MN, which provides a more conservative estimation of inseminated sperm and ensures more sperm per insemination.

SEMEN EVALUATION: NORMAL STALLION

- Whenever possible, more sperm than the minimum should be inseminated, but the concentration should not exceed 50 million sperm/mL.
- Semen should be diluted (i.e. extended) to 25–50 million sperm/mL to optimize sperm motility and buffering capacity.
- If a concentration of 25 million sperm/mL is used, then 20 mL of extended semen would provide 500 million sperm (25 million/mL × 20 ml = 500 million).
- If morphology is considered, then with 75% MN, 75% of 25 million sperm/mL (18.75 million/mL) are present, and 500 million/18.75 = 26 mL (i.e. 26 mL are needed to provide 500 million normal, motile cells).
- If the sample contained only 50% PM, then 20 mL contain only 250 million PM, and the volume should be doubled to contain 500 million PM (i.e. a 40-mL insemination volume).
- To calculate an insemination dose of stallion sperm for a desired final concentration of 50×10^6 sperm/mL, considering PM:
  1. Concentration of raw sperm/(50×10^6) = dilution factor (dilute raw semen by this factor)
  2. 500 million/%PM = number of sperm required to provide 500 million PM
  3. Number of sperm required to provide 500 million PM/Concentration of raw sperm = volume of raw sperm to use for insemination
  4. Multiply the calculated volume (obtained in step 3) by the dilution factor (from step 1) to find the total milliliters of insemination volume in which to add the raw semen.
- If the original ejaculate contains 75% PM and 50% MN and a concentration of 150 million sperm/mL, then to calculate an insemination dose of stallion sperm to have 500 million PM and MN spermatozoa per mare:
  1. 500 million/(%PM × %MN) = number of sperm required for 500 million PM spermatozoa
  2. 500/(.75PM × .5MN) = 1333, which is the number of total sperm needed to provide 500 PM/MN sperm for breeding a mare

IMAGING
See *Subfertile Stallion.*

DIAGNOSTIC PROCEDURES
See *Subfertile Stallion.*

PATHOLOGIC FINDINGS
See *Subfertile Stallion.*

TREATMENT

APPROPRIATE HEALTH CARE
N/A

NURSING CARE
N/A

ACTIVITY
N/A

DIET
N/A

CLIENT EDUCATION
N/A

SURGICAL CONSIDERATIONS
N/A

MEDICATIONS

DRUGS OF CHOICE
N/A

CONTRAINDICATIONS
N/A

PRECAUTIONS
N/A

POSSIBLE INTERACTIONS
N/A

ALTERNATIVE DRUGS
N/A

FOLLOW-UP

PATIENT MONITORING
N/A

PREVENTION/AVOIDANCE
N/A

POSSIBLE COMPLICATIONS
N/A

EXPECTED COURSE AND PROGNOSIS
N/A

MISCELLANEOUS

ASSOCIATED CONDITIONS
See *Subfertile Stallion.*

AGE-RELATED FACTORS
See *Subfertile Stallion.*

ZOONOTIC POTENTIAL
N/A

PREGNANCY
N/A

SYNONYMS
N/A

SEE ALSO
Semen Evaluation: Subfertile Stallion

ABBREVIATIONS
- AV = artificial vagina
- BSE = breeding soundness examination
- CASA = computer-assisted sperm analysis
- MN = morphologically normal sperm (%)
- PM = progressively motile sperm (%)
- TM = total motility (%)

Suggested Reading

Kenney RM, Hurtgen J, Pierson R, Witherspoon D, Simons J. Clinical fertility evaluation of the stallion. In: Society for theriogenology manual, volume IX, part II. 1983.

Varner DD, Schumacher J, Blanchard TL, Johnson L. Diseases and management of breeding stallions. Goleta, CA: American Veterinary Publications, Inc., 1991.

Author Stuart A. Meyers
Consulting Editor Carla L. Carleton

SEMEN EVALUATION: SUBFERTILE STALLION

BASICS

DEFINITION

- Presentation of a stallion for infertility to determine if a perceived problem is associated with semen quality or ability to deliver an adequate number of normal spermatozoa in an ejaculate.
- Careful attention must be given to both semen evaluation and physical examination.
- Additional diagnostics may be indicated to determine the cause.

PATHOPHYSIOLOGY

N/A

SYSTEMS AFFECTED

- Reproductive
- Musculoskeletal
- Nervous
- Endocrine/metabolic
- Behavioral

GENETICS

N/A

INCIDENCE/PREVALENCE

Prevalence of Thoroughbred, Standardbred, Quarter Horse, and Warmblood breeds

SIGNALMENT

- Stallions
- All breeds

SIGNS

- Mares returning to estrus at regular intervals (e.g., conception failure, EED) after breeding
- Pain or reluctance to breed or mount
- Premature dismount—before or during ejaculation
- Hemospermia; pyospermia
- Endometritis in exposed mares

CAUSES

- Testicular degenerative atrophy—testicular degeneration
- Testicular trauma, inflammation, and ensuing thermal damage to the scrotum
- Anabolic steroid drugs—boldenone, decadurabolin, and testosterone
- Aging/senescence
- Musculoskeletal instability or pain
- Hereditary factors
- Infectious venereal disease
- Poor breeding/AI hygiene

RISK FACTORS

- Kick injuries
- Infectious disease
- Management—no isolation facilities as new horses arrive into farm population, poor housing, and pasture breeding versus hand-breeding or use of a phantom mare to protect stallion from injury
- Poor hygiene in the breeding shed
- History of any drugs administered, especially during training

DIAGNOSIS

DIFFERENTIAL DIAGNOSIS

- Mare subfertility can appear similar clinically but tends to be more sporadic. Subsequent breeding of a subfertile mare to a different stallion would not yield a different benefit.
- Infectious infertility/EED also may appear similar; an affected mare's cycle length can vary, with some exhibiting short (<17 days) or long (>24 days) interestrus intervals.

CBC/BIOCHEMISTRY/URINALYSIS

Indicated with suspected multisystemic disease.

OTHER LABORATORY TESTS

Paired Serology

- Mares
- To rule out infectious embryonic loss

BSE

- Mares
- To rule out a mare basis for low pregnancy rates

Sperm Motility

- To determine if sperm quality is a cause of subfertility
- Sperm movement patterns may be associated with decreased fertilization potential if displaying excessive spermatozoal circling (>10%) or decreased total (<70%) and progressive motility (<60%).
- Decreased sperm longevity (<10% progressive motility at ambient temperature at <6 hours) could be consistent with lowered fertility.

Sperm Morphology

- To determine if a low percentage of normal sperm (<60%) can be implicated in lowered fertilization rate.
- Stallions with low percentages (0%–30%) of normal sperm often, but not always, are subfertile because of low numbers of normal sperm arriving at the oviductal site of fertilization.
- Decreases of sperm motility or the percentage normal morphology usually are associated with decreased fertility or reproductive efficiency.
- Stallions ejaculating large numbers of sperm are thought to compensate for a lowered percentage of normal sperm by having an adequate number of normal, motile sperm in their ejaculates.
- Single sperm defects in excess of 20% may be associated with subfertility and indicate abnormal spermatogenesis or sperm maturation.
- Common sperm abnormalities consistent with stallion subfertility—midpiece defects such as swollen and frayed midpieces, bent midpieces, and reflected midpieces (i.e. hairpins)
- Sperm defects associated with subfertility—abnormally shaped heads, detached heads, proximal cytoplasmic droplets, and coiled or sharply bent tails
- Effect of individual sperm abnormalities is less well understood for stallions than for bulls.
- Abnormal acrosomes are consistent with subfertility, but evaluation of these cell organelles requires special stains or fluorescence microscopy.

Sperm Concentration and Semen Volume

Not associated with stallion subfertility.

Semen pH

Can be lowered by hemospermia or urospermia and elevated by pyospermia.

Testicular Biopsy

May have value in rare circumstances to rule out depressed or absent spermatogenesis as a cause of azoospermia or oligospermia.

Sperm Chromatin Structure Assay

- Has been useful in cases of decreased fertility to diagnose abnormal sperm chromatin packing in sperm nuclei.
- Has been associated with subfertility in human, bovine, and equine sperm.
- Specialized test performed by a few reference labs; requires flow cytometry.

Karyotype/DNA Index

Specialized test performed by a few reference labs providing cytogenetics testing.

SEMEN EVALUATION: SUBFERTILE STALLION

IMAGING

Scintigraphy

- To rule out musculoskeletal or spinal problems in difficult cases.
- Technetium 99 most often is used as the radiolabel.

Ultrasonography

Testicular ultrasonography to assess testicular parenchyma, spermatic cord integrity, accessory sex gland structures (e.g., prostate, ampullae, seminal vesicles, pelvic urethra, ductus deferens), and aortic and iliac branches (for thrombotic foci).

Radiography

To assess for the source of cervical instability and fore- or hindlimb lameness.

DIAGNOSTIC PROCEDURES

Urethral Endoscopy

May be diagnostic for the cause of hemospermia, pyospermia, and urethral strictures in cases of hemo- or pyospermia or seminal vesiculitis.

DSO

- Approximated from daily semen collections for 7–10 days.
- Total sperm numbers of the last three ejaculates are averaged to estimate DSO.
- Evaluate semen at optimal production efficiency; thus, stallions should have semen collected daily until DSO is approached.
- May require hospitalization for frequent semen collection.
- Alternate method—calculate DSO using ultrasonographic testicular measurements as testicular volume $= 4/3\pi \times abc$, where a is testicular height/2, b is testicular width/2, and c is testicular length/2 (for each testicle). This equation shortens to height × width × length × 0.5333 = volume of each testicle. Thus, predicted DSO $= (0.024 \times$ volume of both testicles$) - 0.76 = 10^9$ sperm/day.

TREATMENT

- Fertilization rates on farms can be increased with improved ovulation detection and breeding or AI close to or before ovulation.
- Mares should be reproductively sound.
- Breeding should be performed using minimal contamination technique and excellent hygiene.

MEDICATIONS

DRUGS OF CHOICE

- Appropriate antibiotics, with selection based on microbial isolation and sensitivity results
- Phenylbutazone for musculoskeletal pain
- Diazepam (5 mg IV before semen collection) for anxiety- or aggression-associated ejaculation difficulty

CONTRAINDICATIONS

N/A

PRECAUTIONS

N/A

POSSIBLE INTERACTIONS

- Though very few drugs have been proven to affect spermatogenesis, erection, and ejaculation, exercise caution when treating stallions.
- Anabolic steroids have reversible as well as irreversible detrimental effects on sperm production, testicular size, and libido.
- Do not use phenothiazine tranquilizers (particularly acepromazine) in stallions, because they can cause severe penile trauma as a result of penile paralysis, paraphimosis, and priapism.

ALTERNATIVE DRUGS

N/A

FOLLOW-UP

PATIENT MONITORING

- Spermatogenesis requires ≅60 days, followed by 10–14 days of epididymal transit time.
- Monitor patients for improvements in semen quality at 30–60-day intervals, especially if a specific injury or insult has occurred.

PREVENTION/AVOIDANCE

- Adequate nutrition
- Routine preventive health care—regular dental care, vaccinations, and deworming
- Annual semen evaluation and testicular palpation/ultrasonography to establish baseline parameters and monitor for any developing abnormalities in semen, genitalia, or behavior.

POSSIBLE COMPLICATIONS

N/A

EXPECTED COURSE AND PROGNOSIS

N/A

MISCELLANEOUS

ASSOCIATED CONDITIONS

- Spondylopathies
- Arthritis
- May cause incomplete ejaculation.
- Neoplasia—see testicular tumors

AGE-RELATED FACTORS

- Testicular degenerative atrophy
- Spondylopathies
- Arthritis

ZOONOTIC POTENTIAL

N/A

PREGNANCY

N/A

SYNONYMS

Infertility and sterility are more severe forms than subfertility.

SEE ALSO

- Abnormal scrotal enlargement
- Epididymitis
- Estrus, abnormal intervals
- Hemospermia
- Orchitis
- Spermatocele
- Testicular neoplasia
- Testicular torsion
- Varicocele
- Venereal diseases

ABBREVIATIONS

- AI = artificial insemination
- BSE = breeding soundness examination
- DSO = daily sperm output
- EED = early embryonic death

Suggested Reading

Kenney RM, Hurtgen J, Pierson R, Witherspoon D, Simons J. Clinical fertility evaluation of the stallion. Society for Theriogenology Manual Vol. IX, Part II, 1983.

Varner DD, Schumacher J, Blanchard TL, Johnson L. Diseases and management of breeding stallions. Goleta, CA: American Veterinary Publications, Inc., CA, 1991.

Author Stuart A. Meyers
Consulting Editor Carla L. Carleton

SEPTIC ARTHRITIS, NEONATAL

BASICS

DEFINITION

A bacterial infection of one or more joints that involve synovial structures, adjacent bone, or both.

PATHOPHYSIOLOGY

- Nearly always associated with septicemia.
- Hematogenous spread of bacteria inoculates the joints.
- Infection is modulated by virulence of the organism (associated with binding ability to collagen and ability to secrete destructive enzymes) and by host production of plasmin in the joint fluid.
- Inflammatory mediators (e.g., interleukins, eicosanoids, TNF, free radicals) are produced locally in response to bacteria or may enter the capsule from the blood because of a generalized breakdown of the blood–synovial barrier slightly later in the disease.
- Neutrophils are attracted to the joint and release lysozyme, elastase, collagenase, and other enzymes, which are activated and amplified by plasmin and further incite synoviocytes to release collagenase and the chondrocytes to release a variety of matrix metalloproteinases that have a catabolic effect on cartilage. Additionally, activated chondrocytes decrease their production of proteoglycans, which in turn decreases the compressive stiffness of the cartilage and further potentiates damage to cartilage already weakened by collagenase.
- Catabolic enzymes in the joint digest the long, spring-like HA molecules, which decreases cushioning and the boundary lubrication normally provided by this molecule under cartilage compression. This loss of full-length HA is thought to produce the lack of viscosity in synovial fluid seen during this disease.
- The increased TP sometimes measured in infected joints results from breakdown of the blood–synovium barrier rather than from a change in HA content.
- Increased intra-articular pressure and joint distension cause pain, reduce blood flow to the synovium, and may cause ischemia. Subchondral bone, which also receives its blood via this route, may be similarly affected.
- Slowing of blood flow may potentiate deposition of bacteria to these areas. Additionally, fibrin deposition within the joint decreases the flow of synovial fluid, thereby decreasing the nutrition delivered to cartilage and providing a medium for further adherence and protection of bacteria.

SYSTEM AFFECTED

Musculoskeletal—both soft tissue and bones may be infected in septic arthritis, resulting in synovitis, osteomyelitis, or both.

GENETICS

N/A

INCIDENCE/PREVALENCE

This condition occurred in 0.5% of foals during a prospective study in Texas, accounting for 2.1% of illness in foals <18 months of age.

SIGNALMENT

- Appears to occur in two separate groups of foals—neonates (<30 days), and old foals (1–6 months)
- Average age of affected foals is ≅40 days.
- Colts and fillies are equally represented.

SIGNS

Historical Findings

- Foal unable to suckle
- Mare that leaked colostrum before parturition or that produces low-quality colostrum
- Prolonged stage II labor
- Prematurity
- History (or concurrent episode) of bacterial infection (e.g., pneumonia, omphalitis)
- Lameness

Physical Examination Findings

- Severe lameness, swelling and heat of joint, and pain on palpation or movement of the joint
- Most foals have more than one focus of infection (e.g., multiple joints, joint plus something else), but fever or other signs of systemic involvement are not always apparent.
- Stifle, hock, carpus, and fetlock are the joints most often affected.
- Because of the pain, foals are recumbent for long periods of time, which often results in development of decubital skin ulceration skin over bony prominences.

CAUSES

- Septicemia
- Commonly reported bacteria infecting the joint—*Escherichia coli, Klebsiella sp., Staphylococcus* sp., *Streptococcus* sp., *Actinobacillus* sp., and *Salmonella* sp.

RISK FACTORS

- Omphalitis
- Omphalophlebitis
- Failure of passive transfer
- Unhygienic birthing conditions
- High sepsis score
- Pneumonia
- Hypogammaglobulinemia

DIAGNOSIS

DIFFERENTIAL DIAGNOSIS

The main differential diagnosis is trauma, with or without periarticular edema mimicking a swollen joint; differentiate on the basis of degree of lameness, sepsis score, ultrasonography, and arthrocentesis.

SEPTIC ARTHRITIS, NEONATAL

CBC/BIOCHEMISTRY/URINALYSIS

- Peripheral WBC levels are variable.
- With acute or overwhelming sepsis, neutropenia is the predominant finding.
- Later in the disease, foals become neutrophilic, and increased fibrinogen usually is present.

OTHER LABORATORY TESTS

- Blood culture and sensitivity—delay in results should not delay treatment; provide important information for later use if the primary antibiotic choice is not effective.
- IgG level—usually <800 mg/dL

IMAGING

Radiography

- Increased soft-tissue swelling surrounding the joint.
- Primarily used for detection of osteomyelitis, which worsens the prognosis.
- Osteomyelitis presents as lytic areas in the epiphysis, physis, or diaphysis of the bones of the limbs.
- Contrast radiology better delineates periarticular soft-tissue involvement (i.e., tenosynovitis) in cases with suspected trauma.

Ultrasonography

- Distinguishes articular from periarticular effusion.
- Can detect cartilage erosions.
- Evaluation of the umbilical structures is important, because omphalophlebitis is a risk factor in these foals.

DIAGNOSTIC PROCEDURES

- Arthrocentesis and joint fluid analysis—essential; WBC >500 cells/μL is abnormal, but usually >10,000 cells/μL are found; >90% neutrophils in active septic arthritis (normally, PMNs are <10%); TP in joint fluid usually is elevated; mucin clot is poor.
- Culture and sensitivity—performed by inoculating $\leq$5 mL of synovial fluid into a blood culture bottle and plating at 1 and 7 days.
- Synovial biopsy—perform if the foal goes to surgery; culturing the synovial membrane has a greater success rate than joint fluid culture because of the adherence of bacteria to the synovium.
- Arthroscopy—used to assess cartilage damage; has the advantage of doubling as a treatment modality through fibrin removal, debridement, and joint lavage.

PATHOLOGIC FINDINGS

- Distended joints; suppurative joint fluid, with poor mucin clot and high fibrin content; and possible articular cartilage erosion
- Histopathology shows joint capsule thickening, with possible infiltration of immune system cells in longer-standing infections.
- Osteomyelitis may be grossly visible as easily separable physes, discoloration of the bone, and suppurative bone cavities.

TREATMENT

APPROPRIATE HEALTH CARE

Hospitalize affected foals.

NURSING CARE

Plasma Transfusion

Indicated in cases with failure of passive transfer.

IV Fluid Therapy

Important in foals with sepsis

Padding/Bandaging

- Application to the bony prominences may lessen the chance of decubital ulcer development.
- If ulcers are present, they should be cleaned and bandaged daily.
- Foals with septic arthritis spend much of their time recumbent.

Joint Lavage

- Essential
- Can be accomplished with a 14-G needle in a through-and-through lavage under sedation.
- Use 1–2 L of isotonic fluid.
- Repeat lavage every other day until the synovial fluid is normal and the foal is more comfortable.

SEPTIC ARTHRITIS, NEONATAL

Intra-articular Injection of Antibiotics

• Administration after the lavage increases the concentration of antibiotic at the site of infection.
• May add HA to decrease inflammation inside the joint capsule after the last lavage.

Regional Perfusion with Antibiotics

• Achieves high concentration of antibiotic in the joint without trauma to the joint capsule.
• Apply a tourniquet above the affected joint, and place a catheter in the venous system of that joint. Antibiotics are delivered through the catheter under pressure.
• The disadvantage of this technique alone is that it does not provide the flushing action of joint lavage.

ACTIVITY

Limited to stall rest initially, with physical therapy after initial stabilization.

DIET

Foals may have difficulty standing to nurse; if so, assist with standing to nurse on an hourly basis.

CLIENT EDUCATION

• Make owners aware regarding the importance of colostral management.
• Take routine hygiene measures at the time of parturition.
• Dip navels in 2% iodine or 0.5% chlorhexidine.

SURGICAL CONSIDERATIONS

• If the large amounts of fibrin are in the infected joint, arthroscopy or arthrotomy is necessary to achieve a thorough joint lavage. Visualization of the joint surfaces is another advantage to these techniques.
• Occasionally, open drainage of the joint must be established, which is done by creating a small incision into the joint that is left open and allowed to drain into a sterile bandage.
• With evidence of omphalophlebitis, remove infected structures.

MEDICATIONS

DRUGS OF CHOICE

Antibiotics

• Many cases result from mixed infections, which must be treated immediately, before culture results are obtained. Therefore, a broad-spectrum combination of antibiotics must be given.
• Gram-negative organisms (commonly Enterobacteriaceae)—amikacin (20–25 mg/kg IV SID)
• Gram-positive organisms (*Streptococcus* sp.)—ampicillin (10—20 mg/kg IV or IM QID) or potassium penicillin (20,000–40,000 IU/kg IV QID)
• Intra-articular administration of aminoglycosides achieves a much higher concentration but also increases the risk of introducing more bacteria and of increasing capsular reaction and fibrosis.
• High (100× MIC) local concentrations of antibiotic significantly aid in elimination of the organism.

NSAIDs

Ketoprofen (2.2 mg/kg IM or IV) is preferred in foals, because it is less ulcerogenic than phenylbutazone.

CONTRAINDICATIONS

N/A

PRECAUTIONS

Use aminoglycoside therapy with caution if renal malfunction is suspected (possibly secondary to septicemia) or dehydration exists.

POSSIBLE INTERACTIONS

N/A

ALTERNATIVE DRUGS

• Flunixin meglumine or phenylbutazone for pain, but be cautious of gastric ulceration and overuse of the affected joint by the foal, which promotes cartilage damage.
• Gentamicin may be given instead of amikacin, but resistance studies indicate it is becoming less effective.

FOLLOW-UP

PATIENT MONITORING

- Repeat radiography every 7–10 days during the course of the problem to monitor the extent of bony involvement.
- Joint fluid aspiration and analysis as necessary to monitor response to treatment.
- Alter antibiotic therapy as indicated by culture and sensitivity results.
- Monitor for depression, elevated temperature, or other signs of sepsis and for decubital ulcers.
- Lack of appetite may indicate gastric ulceration.
- Monitor disease progression by assessing patient comfort and repeated WBC counts on synovial fluid.

PREVENTION/AVOIDANCE

A clean birthing area, good quality colostrum (which may be frozen), and prompt attention to any decrease in suckling during the first 18 hours of life

POSSIBLE COMPLICATIONS

- Proteolytic enzymes, which are the byproducts of inflammation, can cause irreversible damage to cartilage.
- If tendon sheaths are involved, permanent fibrosis can lead to lasting lameness.

EXPECTED COURSE AND PROGNOSIS

- Outcome and future soundness depend most on the speed and aggressiveness of treatment. The longer the inflammatory process progresses inside the joint, the greater the chance for permanent cartilage damage.
- In one study, 45% of foals with septic arthritis were discharged from the hospital, but 18 of 66 underwent immediate euthanasia without treatment. Days of hospitalization ranged from 0.5–34 (average = 10.4, $n = 48$), and 52% of foals had radiographic evidence of osteomyelitis—13 of the physis, 13 of the epiphysis, and 8 of both.
- Prognosis is better in old than in young foals.

MISCELLANEOUS

ASSOCIATED CONDITIONS

- Diarrhea
- OCD
- Omphalitis
- Osteomyelitis
- Physitis
- Pneumonia
- Tenosynovitis

AGE-RELATED FACTORS

- Synovitis without concurrent osteomyelitis most often occurs in systemically ill foals only a few days of age.
- Foals with associated osteomyelitis (either physitis or epiphysitis) tend to be somewhat older (mean age for physitis = 38 days).

ZOONOTIC POTENTIAL

N/A

PREGNANCY

N/A

SYNONYMS

- Joint ill
- Navel ill
- Polyarthritis
- Septic epiphysitis
- Septic physitis
- Septic polyarthritis

SEE ALSO

- Septic omphalophlebitis
- Septicemia

ABBREVIATIONS

- HA = hyaluronic acid
- MIC =
- PMN = polymorphonucleotides
- TNF = tumor necrosis factor
- TP = total protein

Suggested Reading

Bertone A. Infectious arthritis. In: Schneider CW, Bramlage RL, Moore R, Mecklenberg C, Kohn C, Gabel A, eds. Joint disease in the horse. 1996.

Cohen N. Causes of and farm management factors associated with disease and death in foals. J Am Vet Med Assoc 1994;204:1644–1651.

Firth E. Current concepts of infectious polyarthritis in foals. Equine Vet J 1983;15:5–9.

Martens RJ, Auer K, Carter. Equine pediatrics: septic arthritis and osteomyelitis. J Am Vet Med Assoc 1986;188:582–585.

Author Jessie McCoy

Consulting Editor Mary Rose Paradis

SEPTIC MENINGOENCEPHALOMYELITIS

BASICS

DEFINITION

Bacterial-associated inflammation of the CNS

PATHOPHYSIOLOGY

- Bacterial meningoencephalomyelitis most commonly is associated with hematogenous extension of a suppurative process or results from traumatic penetration of the CNS.
- It is most commonly associated with neonatal foal sepsis.
- The associated diffuse neurologic deficits are a manifestation of the extensive involvement of the superficial parenchyma and nerve roots.
- CNS edema or secondary obstructive hydrocephalus may profoundly affect the clinical presentation.

SYSTEMS AFFECTED

CNS

SIGNALMENT

Most often young foals, but rarely, adult horses may be affected.

SIGNS

Historical Findings

- See *Foal Sepsis.*
- Possible history of CNS trauma

Physical Examination Findings

- Fever, lethargy, behavioral changes (e.g., aimless walking, depression, abnormal vocalization, lack of affinity for the mare) characterize the prodromal period of septic meningitis.
- Later, hyperesthesia, muscular rigidity, and tremors may occur.
- CNS pain often manifests by reluctance to move the head or neck and trismus—spasms of the muscles of mastication.
- Signs progress rapidly to loss of the suckling reflex, cranial nerve abnormalities, ataxia, paresis, blindness, and hypalgesia.
- Recumbency, coma, seizures, and death quickly follow.

CAUSES

- Bacterial meningoencephalomyelitis most commonly is associated with hematogenous extension of a suppurative process or results from traumatic penetration of the CNS.
- The bacteria involved most commonly are those associated with neonatal sepsis.
- Organisms that commonly affect foals include hemolytic streptococci, *Actinobacillus equuli, Escherichia coli, Klebsiella pneumoniae,* coagulase-positive staphylococci, and *Salmonella* sp.
- Meningitis in adult horses has been associated with *Streptococcus equi* and *Actinomyces* sp.

RISK FACTORS

- Those associated with septic conditions of foals
- Maternal uterine infection, premature placental separation, poor hygiene during parturition, failure of passive transfer of maternal immunoglobulins, adverse environmental conditions in early life, all have been associated with this condition.

DIAGNOSIS

DIFFERENTIAL DIAGNOSIS

- Viral encephalitis
- Intoxication

CBC/BIOCHEMISTRY/URINALYSIS

No pathognomonic abnormalities occur.

OTHER LABORATORY TESTS

None indicated

IMAGING

Radiography to identify sites of trauma

DIAGNOSTIC PROCEDURES

- Early diagnosis and aggressive treatment are essential for affected animals to survive.
- Clinical signs alone obligate the initiation of aggressive therapy.
- The diagnosis is confirmed by bacteria or inflammatory cell effusions in CSF and is supported by elevated protein and decreased glucose concentrations.
- Make efforts to identify the causative organism. This information may not be necessary for a positive outcome, however, and will not reduce the chances of mortality.
- Evaluate CSF by Gram stain and culture, and culture blood as well.
- Antimicrobial therapy should be guided by CSF Gram-stain results and, subsequently, by bacterial culture and antimicrobial sensitivity tests. Whether these data are available, appropriate doses of broad-spectrum antimicrobials are essential.

TREATMENT

- Supportive treatment is essential in any impaired foal.
- Caloric, fluid, electrolyte, respiratory, and thermic support may be required for a successful outcome.

SEPTIC MENINGOENCEPHALOMYELITIS

MEDICATIONS

DRUGS OF CHOICE

Antimicrobials

- The hallmark of treatment
- Bactericidal drugs probably are advised over bacteristatic antimicrobials.
- These drugs must reach sufficient levels in the CSF. Normally, aminoglycosides and penicillins poorly cross the blood–CSF barrier. However, meningeal inflammation improves drug distribution.
- The low toxicity of penicillins allows use of increased doses to achieve high CSF levels. In general, cephalosporins have these same characteristics, with an enhanced spectrum of activity.
- Enrofloxacin may be recommended, but the adverse effects on cartilage metabolism must be weighed against use of fluoroquinolone antibiotics in foals.
- Antimicrobial administration cannot wait for sensitivity testing. Penicillin (22,000 IU/kg IV q6h), ceftiofur (2.2 mg/kg IV q8h), or cephazolin (15 mg/kg IV q8h) plus amikacin (21 mg/kg IV q24h) or gentamicin (6.6 mg/kg IV q24h) provide a good initial spectrum.
- Continue antimicrobial therapy for at least 7 days after resolution of clinical signs.

Seizures

- Manage with diazepam (5–20 mg IV, repeated as necessary in 50-kg foals), but intractable seizures may require phenobarbital (10–20 mg/kg diluted in saline and administered slowly over 15 minutes IV q12h). Time to peak effect is 15–30 minutes.
- Phenytoin also may be useful (initial dose of 5–10 mg/kg, followed by 1–5 mg/kg every 2–4 hours).
- Pentobarbital and xylazine can be used when other drugs are not available, but cardiovascular and respiratory depression likely will occur with these formulations.

Other Drugs

Consider DMSO (1 gm/kg IV administered as a 10% solution in 5% dextrose or normal saline), corticosteroids (e.g., dexamethasone [0.05–0.1 mg/kg or equivalent]), or both when progression is rapid.

CONTRAINDICATIONS

N/A

PRECAUTIONS

N/A

POSSIBLE INTERACTIONS

N/A

ALTERNATIVE DRUGS

Consider drugs intended to resolve secondary problems—antiulcer medications, ocular preparations, and so on

FOLLOW-UP

PATIENT MONITORING

- Foals need continuous monitoring and support.
- See *Septicemia.*

POSSIBLE COMPLICATIONS

Prognosis in foals with septic meningitis is poor; even with appropriate intensive treatment, >50% will die.

MISCELLANEOUS

ASSOCIATED CONDITIONS

Neonatal sepsis

AGE-RELATED FACTORS

Young foals are affected most often.

ZOONOTIC POTENTIAL

N/A

PREGNANCY

N/A

SYNONYMS

N/A

SEE ALSO

Neonatal sepsis

ABBREVIATIONS

- CSF = cerebrospinal fluid
- DMSO = dimethyl sulfoxide

Author Joseph J. Bertone
Consulting Editor Joseph J. Bertone

SEPTICEMIA, NEONATAL

BASICS

DEFINITION

Systemic disease associated with the presence and persistence of pathogenic microorganisms or their toxins in the blood

PATHOPHYSIOLOGY

- The condition implies a massive, whole-body insult, which can emanate from single or multiple sources of infection.
- Gram-negative bacteria most commonly are involved, with *Escherichia coli* and *Klebsiella* sp. predominating.
- Approximately 50% of infections also involve Gram positive bacteria, with streptococcal species being most common; 30% involve anaerobic bacteria.
- Clinical signs, especially those of septic shock, largely result from endotoxin generated by Gram-negative infection. Endotoxin stimulates macrophages to liberate a vast array of cytokines (e.g., TNF, IL-1, IL-6) as well as activating phospholipase A_2. Together, these mediators cause signs of inflammation—fever, vasodilation, accelerated procoagulant activity, myocardial depression, hypertension, hypoglycemia, V/Q mismatches, and eventually, DIC.
- Hypoperfusion results in metabolic acidosis, with associated tachypnea and tachycardia.
- Shock, dehydration, acidemia, hypoxia, hypovolemia, hypercapnia, and hypoglycemia all combine to cause depression.

SYSTEMS AFFECTED

- Behavioral—depression caused by systemic disease is the most common sign.
- Respiratory—pneumonia and V/Q mismatch cause hypoventilation, with hypoxemia and hypercapnia.
- Cardiovascular—shock, hypovolemia, and myocardial depression may result from sepsis.
- GI—diarrhea, intestinal stasis, denuding of villi, and loss of ability to absorb nutrients can occur.
- Musculoskeletal—bacteria can infect joints and bones, resulting in septic arthritis and osteomyelitis.
- CNS—depression, meningitis, and seizures all may be manifestations of sepsis.
- Umbilical remnants—omphalophlebitis or omphalitis may be the source of the bacteria involved.
- Renal—pyelonephritis (especially from *Actinobacillus equi* infections) and endotoxin-mediated renal cortical and tubular necrosis can be sequelae of sepsis.
- Ophthalmic—uveitis results from direct systemic infection; entropion/corneal ulceration results from catabolism of fat around the eye globe and trauma.
- Hepatobiliary—hyperbilirubinemia can occur secondary to endotoxemic hepatic insult.
- Endocrine—adrenal necrosis can be a sequela of endotoxic shock; rarely, surviving foals may become addisonian.

GENETICS

N/A

INCIDENCE/PREVALENCE

Accounts for 30% of foal mortality.

SIGNALMENT

- Can occur in many species.
- No sex or breed predilections
- Most foals are septic at birth from in utero infections or become septic postnatally, within the first week of life.

SIGNS

General Comments

Clinical signs largely depend on the organ systems primarily involved and whether the animal is evaluated during the acute or chronic stage.

Historical Findings

- Owners often report the foal was slow at birth and did not stand and suckle within the first 3 hours.
- Owners may report the mare leaked milk before foaling or had a systemic illness or placentitis.
- Depression may be first clinical sign noted by owners.

Physical Examination Findings

- Most common—mild to severe depression, dehydration, hypothermia, tachycardia, tachypnea, scleral injection, hyperemic mucous membranes with poor capillary refill time, poor suckle reflex, and petechiation of mucous membranes or insides of pinnae
- Variable—diarrhea, respiratory distress, colic, seizures, uveitis, entropion, corneal ulceration, joint distention, lameness, and umbilical enlargement

CAUSES

FPT

- Mares may have leaked colostrum before foaling or have produced inferior colostrum.
- Foals may have failed to ingest enough colostrum.

Massive Exposure to Pathogens

- Entry routes of bacteria in foals—in utero exposure, inhalation, ingestion, and spread from the umbilical stump
- Ingestion has been implicated because the intestinal tract is "open" to absorb immunoglobulins from birth until 24 hours of age; translocation of bacteria is possible at the same time.

RISK FACTORS

From Mares

- Elderly mares may produce inferior colostrum.
- Systemically ill mares or mares with placentitis
- Premature placental separation
- Premature lactation

At Birth

- Prematurity/dysmaturity
- Dystocia
- Birth asphyxia

Environmental

- Overcrowding
- Poor ventilation
- Cold environment
- High pathogen load in the environment

Intrinsic

Immature immune system

SEPTICEMIA, NEONATAL

DIAGNOSIS

DIFFERENTIAL DIAGNOSES

- Prematurity—look for attributes of prematurity (e.g., domed head, silky haircoat, incomplete ossification of carpal and tarsal bones)
- HIE (neonatal maladjustment syndrome)—low sepsis score; premature foals and those with HIE may be depressed to obtunded, lack a suckle reflex, and be unwilling to stand; distinguishing these conditions as being uncomplicated by septicemia is difficult; sepsis score evaluation is valuable.
- White muscle disease—massively elevated CK, AST and LDH levels
- GI—intussusception, volvulus, lactose intolerance, dietary indiscretion, viral diarrhea, and bladder rupture
- Neurologic—HIE, neonatal isoerythrolysis, hydrocephalus, and hepatic encephalopathy may present, with depression and weakness; low sepsis score and CBC/biochemistry profiles help to distinguish from sepsis.
- Respiratory—choanal atresia, aspiration pneumonia, persistent fetal circulation, atelectasis, and pneumothorax can be eliminated with thoracic radiography and upper airway endoscopy.
- Musculoskeletal—trauma often is cited as the cause of lameness in foals; radiography and arthrocentesis of the affected joint are important.

CBC/BIOCHEMISTRY/URINALYSIS

- WBC may be normal, increased or decreased.
- Leukopenia with neutropenia and left shift are most common.
- Toxic changes and Döhle bodies often are seen in neutrophils.
- Look for an inverted N:L ratio if total numbers normal.
- High fibrinogen at birth indicates congenital infection.
- Hypoglycemia and azotemia are common.
- Electrolytes depend on the organ systems involved—may see increased bilirubin, mildly increased muscle enzymes (i.e., CPK, AST, LDH), and mildly increased liver enzymes (i.e., GGT, SDH, AST).
- Urinalysis—less useful; may see bacteriuria or pyuria.

OTHER LABORATORY TESTS

- Blood gases—hypoxemia; hypercapnia; mixed metabolic/respiratory acidosis
- Immunology—test IgG levels in all sick neonates; <200 mg/dL indicates complete FPT; 200 to <400 mg/dL indicates partial FPT; ≤800 mg/dL is ideal.
- Blood cultures—help to direct therapy if the animal does not respond to initial treatment; positive in 60–80% of cases.
- Sepsis score—helps to synthesize laboratory results into coherent whole; sensitivity of 93%; specificity of 89%; still treat if clinically suspicious, because 7% are false negatives.

IMAGING

Thoracic Radiography

- Always indicated, because auscultation and clinical signs are unreliable.
- Findings compatible with pneumonia, atelectasis, and pulmonary edema.

Abdominal Radiography

Findings consistent with enteritis or intestinal stasis—gas-distended bowel may be found.

Distal Limb Radiography

Important in the evaluation of osteomyelitis.

Ultrasonography

- Umbilical—always indicated, because internal infections are not palpable.
- Joints—excessive, turbid fluid consistent with septic arthritis
- Chest—lung consolidation; pleural effusion; abscessation
- Abdomen—dilated small intestine; ascites; hepatic abscessation

DIAGNOSTIC PROCEDURES

- CSF tap if neurologic signs are seen; however, use caution (or avoid) if signs of increased intracranial pressure are noted.
- Arthrocentesis if joint distension is noted.

PATHOLOGIC FINDINGS

Findings are nonspecific and referable to the clinical signs the animal was showing.

TREATMENT

APPROPRIATE HEALTH CARE

- Emergency, inpatient, intensive care management is preferred for septic neonates.
- A center that provides on-site laboratory testing, environmental control, and 24-hour nursing care is the best choice.

NURSING CARE

Intravenous Fluids

- Foals may require 80–100 mL/kg per day of maintenance fluids after shock doses of fluids have been given.
- Use polyionic isotonic crystalloid fluids.
- Because many foals also are hypoglycemic, 100 mL of 50% dextrose can be added to 900 mL of one of the above-mentioned fluids to make a 5% dextrose solution.

Acid–Base Correction

- A mixed metabolic/respiratory acidosis may be present.
- Administration of an isotonic bicarbonate solution helps the metabolic acidosis but may increase the respiratory acidosis; in these cases, initiate mechanical ventilation to decrease the $PaCO_2$ before administering bicarbonate.

SEPTICEMIA, NEONATAL

Immunologic Support
• IgG <800 mg/dL requires 0.5–2.0 L of hyperimmune plasma.
• Colostrum supplementation in addition to plasma is desirable in foal <12 hours of age.
• Consider treatment with hyperimmune antiendotoxin serum.

Supportive Care
• Maintain adequate body temperature with heat lamps and circulating hot-water blankets.
• Maintenance of sternal recumbency decreases pulmonary atelectasis.
• Prevent decubitus ulcers by keeping foals well padded and dry.

Intra-articular Therapy
If septic arthritis is present (see Septic Arthritis)

Respiratory Care
• Most foals benefit from nasal insufflation of oxygen if they are recumbent and hypoxic.
• Mechanical ventilation is important in hypercapnic foals.

Ophthalmic Care
• Entropion requires mattress suture of the lower eyelid.
• Ocular lubricant helps to prevent self-induced ocular trauma.

ACTIVITY
• Often self-limited
• Stall rest necessary

DIET
• Placement of a nasogastric tube for enteral feeding often is necessary in foals that cannot or will not nurse.
• Foals require at least 20% of their body (in kg) of mare's milk or milk replacer per day, with feedings every 1–2 hours.
• Consider TPN or PPN in debilitated foals.

CLIENT EDUCATION
• Treatment is expensive and emotionally exhausting for owners.
• Owner should understand that new problems may develop every day.

SURGICAL CONSIDERATIONS
• With omphalophlebitis or ruptured bladder, surgery is necessary once the patient is stabilized.
• Arthrotomy or arthroscopy may be needed for septic arthritis.

MEDICATIONS

DRUGS OF CHOICE

Antimicrobials
• Antibiotic coverage cannot wait for sensitivity testing.
• Use of a broad-spectrum agent with good Gram-negative coverage is necessary.
• Usually, a penicillin (22,000 IU/kg IV QID) plus amikacin (20–25 mg/kg IV SID) provide good initial coverage.
• Metronidazole (10–15 mg/kg PO or IV TID) may be necessary if clostridial infection is suspected.

Gastric Ulcer Therapy
Consider in every sick neonate (see *Gastric Ulcers*).

Ophthalmic Medications
With corneal ulceration, treat with atropine, a topical NSAID, and a broad-spectrum topical antimicrobial.

NSAIDs
Consider use of antiprostaglandin drugs—flunixin meglumine (0.25 mg/kg IV QID) or ketoprofen (2.2 mg/kg IM BID).

PRECAUTIONS
• Use aminoglycosides and NSAIDs with caution in dehydrated animals.
• Monitor urine output and clinical hydration status, creatinine levels, and therapeutic drug levels, if possible.
• Use topical atropine with caution—may cause ileus.
• Consider every-other-day use.

POSSIBLE INTERACTIONS
Cimetidine may potentiate toxicities of drugs that rely on the hepatic microsomal P450 system for breakdown—lidocaine; metronidazole

ALTERNATIVE DRUGS
• Gentamicin is considerably less expensive than amikacin, but disadvantages include increased bacterial resistance and questionably increased nephrotoxicity.
• Ketoprofen may be less ulcerogenic than flunixin meglumine.

FOLLOW-UP

PATIENT MONITORING
• Initially, foals require 24-hour care and monitoring, because their condition can change quickly.

- Check vital signs every 2–4 hours.
- Frequent analysis of blood glucose levels in foals not eating on their own.
- Monitor PCV and TP to prevent dehydration or overhydration.
- Record urine and fecal output.
- Monitoring may be required for specific body systems—repeat chest radiography and blood gas analyses with pneumonia; repeat distal limb radiography with suspected osteomyelitis or septic arthritis

PREVENTION/AVOIDANCE

- During future foalings, monitor prenatal health of the mare.
- If mares leak colostrum before foaling, have good-quality colostrum from another mare available to give to the foal.
- Make sure foals nurse within 3 hours of birth.
- Test colostrum quality.
- Test the foal's IgG at 12–24 hours of age.
- Keep the environment clean.

POSSIBLE COMPLICATIONS

Foal may have decreased athletic performance because of permanent damage to lungs or joints.

EXPECTED COURSE AND PROGNOSIS

- Guarded prognosis
- Recovery depends on severity of the problem and manifestations of the infection.
- Septic meningitis has a grave prognosis.
- Septic pneumonia has ≅40% survival rate; septic arthritis has a 50–60% survival rate.
- Expect a minimum of 1–4 weeks of intensive care.
- Expect frequent short-term complications.
- With aggressive treatment and if the foal has only one major focus of infection, the foal may reach its expected athletic level.

MISCELLANEOUS

ASSOCIATED DISEASES

- Colic
- Corneal ulceration
- Decubital ulceration
- Gastroduodenal ulceration
- Patent urachus
- Ruptured bladder

AGE-RELATED FACTORS

Septicemia is seen during the first week of life.

ZOONOTIC POTENTIAL

N/A

PREGNANCY

N/A

SYNONYMS

- Bacteremia
- Navel ill
- Sepsis

SEE ALSO

- FPT
- Neonatal pneumonia
- Orphan and sick foals
- Seizures and coma
- Septic arthritis
- Shock

ABBREVIATIONS

- AST = aspartate aminotransferase
- CK = creatine kinase
- CPK = creatine phosphokinase
- CSF = cerebrospinal fluid
- DIC = disseminated intravascular coagulation
- FPT = failure of passive transfer
- GGT = γ-glutamyltransferase
- GI = gastrointestinal
- HIE = hypoxic-ischemic encephalopathy
- IL = interleukin
- LDH = lactate dehydrogenase
- N:L = neutrophil/lymphocyte
- PCV = packed cell volume
- PPN = partial parenteral nutrition
- SDH = sorbitol dehydrogenase
- TNF = tumor necrosis factor
- TP = total protein
- TPN = total parenteral nutrition
- V/Q = ventilation/perfusion

Suggested Reading

Brewer BD, Koterba AM. Development of a scoring system for the early diagnosis of equine neonatal sepsis. Equine Vet J 1988;20:18–22.

Koterba AM, Drummond WH, Kosch PC. Equine clinical neonatology. Philadelphia: Lea & Febiger, 1990.

Lavoie JP. Hemodynamic, clinical pathologic, haemotologic and behavioral changes during endotoxin infusion in equine neonates. Equine Vet J 1990;22:23.

Paradis MR. Neonatal septicemia. In: Robinson NE, ed. Current therapy in equine medicine. 4th ed. Philadelphia: WB Saunders, 1997:595–603.

Paradis MR. Update on neonatal septicemia. Vet Clin North Am Equine Pract 1994;10:109–135.

Author Melissa R. Mazan

Consulting Editor Mary Rose Paradis

SEVERE COMBINED IMMUNE DEFICIENCY (SCID)

BASICS

OVERVIEW

• An inherited disease of Arabian foals causing an immune deficiency characterized by the lack of functional T and B lymphocytes, resulting in the lack of humoral and cell-mediated immune responses
• The genetic defect is a mutation in the DNA-dependent protein kinase gene; deficiency of DNA-dependent protein kinase prevents lymphocytes from properly maturing.

SIGNALMENT

• Arabian and Arabian cross-bred foals
• Clinical signs develop by 2 months of age.
• Most foals die by 5 months of age.

SIGNS

• Affected foals appear physically normal at birth.
• Most owners seek veterinary attention for secondary infectious disease resulting from the immunocompromised state of the affected foal; many different body systems can be affected.
• Infectious agents isolated from SCID foals (e.g., adenoviral and *Pneumocystis carinii* pneumonia) do not typically cause disease in immunocompetent foals.
• Pneumonia is the most commonly reported disease in affected foals.
• Recurrent pyrexia and clinical signs of enteritis, arthritis, and peritonitis are other common presentations.

CAUSES AND RISK FACTORS

• Autosomal recessive inherited disease
• An estimated 16–25% of Arabian horses are carriers of the recessive gene, and 1–3% of Arabian foals are affected.

DIAGNOSIS

DIFFERENTIAL DIAGNOSIS

• A major challenge is determining if the infectious disease in the foal is the primary problem or secondary to an immunodeficient state.
• Failure of passive transfer occurs at birth and is characterized by lack of maternal antibodies, which is verified by a low serum IgG concentration in foals >24 h of age. Most foals with failure of passive transfer have normal lymphocyte counts; most foals with SCID have normal serum IgG concentrations after birth until >3 weeks of age.
• Foals with selective IgM deficiency tend to develop infections at an older age; lymphocyte counts and PHA test usually are normal.
• Agammaglobulinemia has not been reported in Arabian foals to date. Foals with primary agammaglobulinemia tend to acquire secondary infections at an older age and survive for many months or even years. Lymphocyte counts and PHA test usually are normal.
• Foals with transient hypogammaglobulinemia tend to acquire secondary infections at an older age; lymphocyte counts and PHA test are normal.

CBC/BIOCHEMISTRY/URINALYSIS

• Lymphopenia (<1000 lymphocytes/μL) is persistent and must be documented by obtaining several absolute lymphocyte counts over 1–2 weeks, because immature or severely ill foals can be transiently lymphopenic.
• Total WBC and neutrophil counts can be low, normal, or high depending on secondary infections.
• Biochemistry and urinalysis usually are unremarkable.

OTHER LABORATORY TESTS

• DNA test that identifies the mutant SCID gene *definitively* diagnoses both affected and carrier foals.
• Serum IgM is absent in affected Arabian foals sampled before colostrum consumption or >4 weeks of age.

IMAGING

N/A

DIAGNOSTIC PROCEDURES

• Before availability of the DNA test, a confirmed diagnosis was based on persistent lymphopenia, absence of serum IgM, and hypoplastic lymphoid tissue at histopathology.
• PHA intradermal test is negative in affected foals, indicating an absence of cell-mediated immune responses.
• Immunohistochemistry using monoclonal antibodies for various equine lymphocytic cell-surface antigens reveals that most lymphocytes in the thymus and lymph nodes of affected foals have a unique phenotype characterized as $EqCD3^{-}EqCD4^{-}EqCD8^{+}$.

PATHOLOGIC FINDINGS

• Small or grossly undetectable thymus and small lymph nodes are gross lesions suggesting SCID.
• Histologically, the thymus consists of small, hypocellular lobules with no corticomedullary differentiation and contains epithelial cells and Hassall's corpuscles, with a few, widely dispersed lymphocytes. Within the lymph nodes, follicles and germinal centers are absent, and the cortex has small accumulations of lymphocytes.

SEVERE COMBINED IMMUNE DEFICIENCY (SCID)

TREATMENT

• Therapy is supportive and directed at acquired secondary infections.
• Successful bone marrow transplant has been reported in one foal but is not a practical therapy at this time.

MEDICATIONS

DRUGS

Antimicrobials for treatment of acquired secondary infections

CONTRAINDICATIONS/POSSIBLE INTERACTIONS

N/A

FOLLOW-UP

• Prognosis is grave, even with intensive conventional therapy; most foals die from acquired infections by 5 months of age.
• Prevention can be accomplished by DNA testing both stallions and mares before breeding. Ideally, only SCID gene–negative animals should be bred. Breeding a SCID gene carrier with a SCID gene–negative horse produces a foal that is free of SCID disease but that has a 50% chance of being a carrier.

MISCELLANEOUS

ASSOCIATED CONDITIONS

N/A

AGE-RELATED FACTORS

N/A

ZOONOTIC POTENTIAL

N/A

PREGNANCY

N/A

SEE ALSO

• Agammaglobulinemia
• Selective IgM deficiency

ABBREVIATIONS

• EqCD = equine cluster determinant
• PHA = phytohemagglutinin

Suggested Reading

Shin EK, Perryman LE, Meek. Evaluation of a test for identification of Arabian horses heterozygous for the severe combined immunodeficiency trait. J Am Vet Med Assoc 1997;211:1268–1270.

Author J. Trenton McClure
Consulting Editor Debra C. Sellon

SEVERE COMBINED IMMUNODEFICIENCY (SCID)

BASICS

OVERVIEW

- A genetic disease of Arabian horses in which both functional B and T lymphocytes are deficient
- Characterized by lymphopenia, absence of immunoglobulin production and cell-mediated immunity, and thymic and lymph node hypoplasia
- Autosomal recessive mode of inheritance
- Affected foals secondarily succumb to infectious diseases, with the pulmonary system the most frequently affected.

SIGNALMENT

- A disease of the Arabian breed, with no sex predilection
- Foals are affected at birth but, because of colostral protection, usually demonstrate no signs of infection until colostrally derived antibodies are consumed (i.e., 2–5 months of age).
- Because of the autosomal inheritance mode, an affected foal's parents are both nonaffected heterozygotes; breeding of heterozygous animals carries a 25% chance of producing an affected foal.
- ≅8.29% of tested Arabian foals in 1997 were *SCID* gene carriers.

SIGNS

- History—foals may appear normal from birth until 2–5 months; as the colostral antibodies decrease, the foal shows signs of an infection that is nonresponsive to antibiotic treatment.
- Fever
- Respiratory system—nasal discharge, cough, and increased respiratory sounds on auscultation usually are present.
- GI—diarrhea
- Neurologic—meningitis, ataxia, and depression

CAUSES AND RISK FACTORS

- Affected foals have a DNA-dependent protein kinase deficiency caused by the absence of 5 bp in the gene encoding for this.
- Breeding two animals that are heterozygous for this defect

DIAGNOSIS

DIFFERENTIAL DIAGNOSIS

- Affected foals can have any of the normal infections. Respiratory infection is a common problem of 2–5-month-old foals; in nonimmunocompromised foal, pathogens include *Streptococcus zooepidemicus, S. equi,* and *Rhodococcus equi.*
- Foals without SCID have a normal to increased neutrophil count, with normal lymphocyte numbers. Enlarged intermandibular lymph nodes may be present, and they generally are responsive to appropriate antibiotic treatment.
- GI signs may appear in normal and SCID foals. Causes of diarrhea in both groups include rotavirus infection, salmonellosis, and clostridial diarrhea; however, SCID foals are nonresponsive to treatment.
- Infection secondary to FPT must be distinguished from SCID. Foals with FPT generally have a normal lymphocyte count and some IgM.

CBC/BIOCHEMISTRY/URINALYSIS

Severe lymphopenia (i.e., 1000 lymphocytes).

OTHER LABORATORY TESTS

- Presuckle serum or serum from a 2–3-week-old affected animal has no IgM.
- Genetic testing (VetGen LLC, Ann Arbor, MI) to determine carrier, clear, or SCID-affected status is now available.

IMAGING

Thoracic radiology—depending on severity of the secondary infection, bronchopneumonia and consolidation may be present.

DIAGNOSITIC PROCEDURES

N/A

PATHOLOGIC FINDINGS

- Postmortem examination—evidence for a variety of bacterial and/or viral infections, thymic hypoplasia, and markedly reduced lymph nodes and splenic lymphocytes

SEVERE COMBINED IMMUNODEFICIENCY (SCID)

TREATMENT

Once identified, affected foals should be euthanized because of the grave prognosis.

MEDICATIONS

DRUGS

N/A

CONTRAINDICATIONS/POSSIBLE INTERACTIONS

N/A

FOLLOW-UP

PREVENTION/AVOIDANCE

- Test Arabian broodmares and stallions for the genetic defect.
- Avoid breeding two heterozygous animals.
- Breeding a carrier with a noncarrier does not produce an affected foal but could perpetuate the genetic defect in the population.

EXPECTED COURSE AND PROGNOSIS

All affected foals develop a fatal infection; the timing of death generally relates to the amount of colostral protection the foal received at birth.

MISCELLANEOUS

ASSOCIATED CONDITIONS

Pneumonia, diarrhea, and meningitis

AGE-RELATED FACTORS

Signs of infection vary in both timing and type, but foals are affected at birth.

ZOONOTIC POTENTIAL

N/A

PREGNANCY

N/A

SEE ALSO

- Diarrhea
- FPT
- Pneumonia

ABBREVIATIONS

FPT = Failure of passive transfer

Suggested Reading

Perryman LE, Torbeck RL. Combined immunodeficiency of Arabian horses: confirmation of autosomal recessive mode of inheritance. J Am Vet Med Assoc 1980;1250–1251.

Poppie MJ, McGuire TC. Combined immunodeficiency in foal of Arabian breeding: evaluation of mode of inheritance and estimation of prevalence of affected foals and carrier mares and stallions. J Am Vet Med Assoc 1977;31–33.

Shin EK, Perryman LE, Meek K. Evaluation of a test for identification of Arabian horses heterozygous for the severe combined immunodeficiency trait. J Am Vet Med Assoc 1997;1268–1270.

Author Mary Rose Paradis

Consulting Editor Mary Rose Paradis

SHIVERS (SHIVERING)

BASICS

OVERVIEW

• A nervous or neuromuscular disease characterized by involuntary movements of the limbs and tail.
• Hind limbs primarily are affected, but forelimbs and tail may be involved.

SIGNALMENT

Most often observed in Belgians and Clydesdales, but other breeds may be affected.

SIGNS

• Mild cases may be difficult to detect because of clinical signs occurring at irregular intervals, but in most cases, clinical signs are characteristic.
• Signs usually are noticed when an attempt is made to back or turn the affected horse or when the affected horse is forced to step over an object. The affected limb is held off the ground in a flexed and abducted manner, and muscles of the upper limb and tail may quiver. After a short time the quivering ceases, and the affected limb and tail return to a normal position. The horse then appears to be normal, but clinical signs reappear if additional attempts are made to turn or back the affected horse.

CAUSE AND RISK FACTORS

The exact cause is unknown, but some cases have developed following influenza, strangles, or other systemic diseases.

DIAGNOSIS

DIFFERENTIAL DIAGNOSIS

• Shivering should be distinguished from stringhalt, upward fixation of the patella, and equine protozoal myelitis.
• Horses with upward fixation of the patella often drag the front of the hoof while moving forward, with the affected limb locked. In shivering, no locking and releasing of the patella is observed.
• Equine protozoal myelitis may be ruled out by an absence of *Sarcocystis neurona* antibodies in the CSF.

CBC/BIOCHEMISTRY/URINALYSIS

N/A

OTHER LABORATORY TESTS

N/A

IMAGING

N/A

DIAGNOSTIC PROCEDURES

N/A

TREATMENT

No effective treatment at present

SHIVERS (SHIVERING)

MEDICATIONS

DRUGS
N/A

CONTRAINDICATIONS/POSSIBLE INTERACTIONS
N/A

FOLLOW-UP

- Because the disease is slowly progressive, the prognosis for affected horses is poor.
- Improvement occurs with rest, but the condition returns when work is resumed.
- Mildly affected individuals may be worked in some cases.

MISCELLANEOUS

ASSOCIATED CONDITIONS
N/A

AGE-RELATED FACTORS
N/A

ZOONOTIC POTENTIAL
N/A

PREGNANCY
N/A

SEE ALSO
N/A

Suggested Reading

Adair HS. Common lameness problems of the draft horse. In: Robinson NE, ed. Current therapy in equine medicine. 3rd ed. Philadelphia: WB Saunders, 1992:85.
Frank ER. Veterinary surgery. 7th ed. Minneapolis: Burgess Publishing, 1964:333.
Stashak TS. Adam's lameness of horses. 4th ed. Philadelphia: Lea & Febiger, 1987:725.

Author Steven T. Grubbs
Consulting Editor Joseph J. Bertone

SHOCK AND RESUSCITATION IN FOALS

BASICS

DEFINITION

Three types of shock are recognized in neonatal foals—cardiogenic (i.e., heart failure), hypovolemic/anemic (i.e., dehydration, blood loss, hemolysis), and distributive shock (i.e., septic shock, SIRS)

PATHOPHYSIOLOGY

Cardiogenic Shock

Rare in neonatal foals and usually can be excluded, except in cases with significant congenital heart disease or significant hypoxic-ischemic asphyxial insults to the myocardium, resulting in significant arrhythmias.

Hypovolemic/Anemic Shock

Generally seen in neonates secondary to blood loss, severe neonatal isoerythrolysis, or acute fluid loss—high-volume diarrhea; high-volume gastric reflux

Distributive Shock

- Occurs when loss of vascular control is coupled with unusual tissue demands, resulting in a maldistribution of perfusion.
- The most common form of shock in neonatal foals and often initiated by release of inflammatory mediators in response to sepsis, resulting in septic shock.
- Septic shock is the clinical manifestation of SIRS, the cause of which may be severe hypoxic-ischemic asphyxial disease, trauma with extensive tissue damage, extensive burns, or sepsis—bacterial, viral, or fungal.
- A commonly held misconception is that endotoxin is the exclusive link between sepsis and shock. In actuality, SIRS may be initiated by four different components of Gram-negative bacteria (i.e., endotoxin, formyl peptides, exotoxins, proteases), five different components of Gram-positive bacteria (i.e., exotoxins, enterotoxins, hemolysins, peptidoglycans, lipoteichoic acid), viral pathogens, protozoal pathogens, and fungal pathogens.

SYSTEMS AFFECTED

Cardiovascular

- Cardiogenic shock involves a decrease in cardiac output.
- Hypovolemic/anemic and distributive shock generally involve an increase in cardiac output and redirection of perfusion to vital organs during early states (i.e., compensated shock), then a decrease in cardiac output and, finally, refractory hypotension leading to death during late stage (i.e., uncompensated shock).

Respiratory

- During cardiogenic shock, pulmonary edema develops.
- During late distributive shock or SIRS, acute respiratory distress syndrome develops, with widespread pulmonary damage and failure.

Endocrine/Metabolic

- Both adrenocortical and adrenomedullary hormones are important during the early response (i.e., compensation); adrenal exhaustion is common during the late phases.
- Excessive catabolic demands outrun the ability to meet those demands, resulting in hypoglycemia early in the disease.

Renal/Urologic

- Prerenal azotemia leading to renal parenchymal disease is common.
- Infarcts, microvasculature occlusion, and septic emboli also cause renal damage.

GI

Disruption of the mucosal barrier secondary to hypoperfusion and occlusion of the microvasculature commonly lead to translocation of bacterial or fungal pathogens and absorption of excessive amounts of bacterial toxins.

Nervous

- Hypoperfusion, hypoxia, hypoglycemia, loss of vascular control, and damage to the vascular epithelium lead to compromise of the blood–brain barrier and diffusion of toxins.
- Neurologic disruption and microvasculature occlusion lead to hypoxic-ischemic encephalopathy.

Hemic/Lymphatic/Immune

- Stimulation results in release of a cascade of mediators.
- Profound leukopenia is a consistent finding.
- Inhibition of the host's immune response occurs.

Hepatobiliary

Hypoperfusion, metabolic demands, and loss of vascular integrity lead to disruption of liver function.

SIGNALMENT

Neonates are most susceptible during the first 72 hours of life; however, the condition can occur anytime during the neonatal period.

SIGNS

Historical Findings

- Loss of suckle
- Lethargy
- Weakness
- Central depression, progressing to recumbency and unresponsiveness

Physical Examination Findings

- Fever/hypothermia
- Tachycardia
- Tachypnea
- Cold legs
- Bounding pulses, followed by weak to imperceptible pulses
- Decreased or increased CRT
- Decreased urine output
- Injected sclera/oral membranes
- Petechia—oral, scleral, and aural
- Hyperemic coronary bands

SHOCK AND RESUSCITATION IN FOALS

CAUSES

- Bacterial sepsis—*Escherchia coli, Enterobacter* sp., *Enterococcus* sp., *Staphylococcus* sp., *Actinobacillus* sp., *Klebsiella* sp., *Acinetobacter* sp., *Streptococcus* sp., *Pasteurella* sp., *Salmonella* sp., *Clostridia* sp., *Bacillus* sp., and others
- Viral sepsis—equine herpes virus; equine viral arteritis
- Fungal sepsis—*Candida* and *Aspergillus* sp.
- Hemorrhage—uncontrolled umbilical bleeding, either external or internal; fractured ribs resulting in hemothorax; necrotizing enterocolitis resulting in luminal bleeding; fulminant von Willebrand's disease; and others
- Hemolysis—severe isoerythrolysis
- Dehydration—secretory diarrheas, excessive gastric reflux without IV replacement therapy, and intestinal crisis

RISK FACTORS

- Hypoxic-ischemic disease
- Prematurity
- Placentitis
- Traumatic birth
- Traumatic umbilical cord rupture
- Failure of passive transfer
- History of neonatal isoerythrolysis
- Hypothermia
- Poor nutrition
- Poor husbandry

DIAGNOSIS

DIFFERENTIAL DIAGNOSIS

- Severe hypoglycemia
- Severe hypoxic-ischemic disease
- Acidosis not associated with hypoperfusion—renal tubular acidosis

CBC/BIOCHEMISTRY/URINALYSIS

- Leukopenia with neutropenia, lymphopenia, and thrombocytopenia often are found on the CBC of foals with distributive shock.
- Depending on the organ system affected, laboratory evidence of liver disease, coagulopathy, hypoglycemia, hyperglycemia, electrolyte imbalances, and azotemia may be found.

OTHER LABORATORY TESTS

- Analyze arterial blood gas samples frequently to follow pulmonary function and acid–base balance.
- Blood culture results may be helpful in retrospect.

IMAGING

Pulmonary infiltrates may be evident at radiography or ultrasonography.

DIAGNOSTIC PROCEDURES

Direct or indirect blood pressure monitoring helps in recognizing hypotension.

TREATMENT

KEY INTERVENTIONS

- Treat the underlying infection.
- Provide hemodynamic support.
- Maximize oxygen delivery.
- Block proinflammatory mediators.

OXYGEN THERAPY/VENTILATION

- All cases, regardless of the PaO_2 may benefit from supplemental intranasal oxygen, which decreases the work of breathing and helps to avoid hypoxemia as mismatching develops secondary to positioning and early pulmonary problems.
- The work of breathing accounts for 24% of oxygen consumption in cases of SIRS, so beginning positive-pressure ventilation early in the course of disease generally is beneficial to spare this oxygen consumption (so that other tissues benefit).

FLUID RESUSCITATION

- Provide 20 mL/kg over 20 minutes, then reassess.
- Repeat as often as necessary to obtain adequate perfusion, as indicated by clinical findings.
- Patients may require 80–120 mL/kg.
- Fluid of choice—normal saline

MAINTENANCE FLUID ADMINISTRATION

- Amount infused over 24 hours = excessive fluid loss + maintenance (based on the formula 100 mL/kg per 24 hours for the first 10 kg + 50 mL/kg per 24 hours for the second 10 kg + 25 mL/kg per 24 hours for weight >20 kg)
- Calculating maintenance fluids using this formula is useful in neonates and results in delivery of an amount of fluid at the low end of requirements, helping to avoid fluid overload.
- Calculation of fluid intake should include PO and IV fluids.

IV GLUCOSE THERAPY

- Even normoglycemic or hyperglycemic, the foal will be catabolic and in need of additional calories.
- Begin with dextrose (4 mg/kg per minute, increasing to 8 mg/kg per minute within 3 hours if blood glucose <180 mg/dL; if blood glucose <80 mg/dL, continue to increase infusion rate; 20–25 mg/kg per minute may be needed).
- The lower the blood glucose, the more rapidly the infusion should be increased.
- To prevent fluid overload, dextrose may need to be concentrated, but it should not exceed 15%.

SHOCK AND RESUSCITATION IN FOALS

PLASMA THERAPY

- Use whole plasma.
- Hyperimmune plasma with a high titer of antiendotoxin antibody may be most beneficial.
- When available, plasma may be used as a replacement fluid during resuscitation or maintenance phases, except when capillary leak syndrome is well advanced, in which case it is contraindicated.

WHOLE-BLOOD THERAPY

- The most important goal in treating shock is to increase oxygen delivery to tissues.
- When shock is caused by anemia secondary to massive blood loss or massive hemolysis, perform blood transfusion immediately, without waiting for cross-match results.
- When shock is not as severe and the foal can be stabilized before transfusion, perform a full cross-match, with attention to both hemolysins and agglutinins in the major and minor group reactions.
- Give serious consideration to transfusion in foals with PCV <24%.
- Amount of whole blood needed =

$$\frac{Body\ wt(kg) \times Blood\ volume(ml/kg) \times (PCV\ desired - PCV\ observed)}{PCV\ donor}$$

where blood volume of a 2-day-old foal = 150 mL/kg and of a 2-week old-foal = 100 mL/kg. The amount required usually ranges from 2–4 L.

COLLOID THERAPY

- The most effective colloid is whole blood.
- A readily available second choice is plasma.

SODIUM BICARBONATE REPLACEMENT THERAPY

- Replacement therapy is useful in reversing metabolic acidosis if the $PaCO_2$ is normal or low.
- Contraindicated in cases of hypoventilation.
- Take care to avoid hypernatremia and sudden osmotic changes by using isotonic infusions—1.3%

ELECTROLYTE REPLACEMENT THERAPY

- Pay special attention to potassium, ionized calcium, ionized magnesium, and chloride relative to sodium.
- Neonatal foals generally have lower ionized calcium than adults, except at birth, when their values generally are higher.

ORAL FEEDING

In most cases, oral nutrition is contraindicated because of hypoperfusion of the intestinal tract, metabolic instability, and local damage that has occurred during shock.

MEDICATIONS

DRUGS OF CHOICE

In all cases, assumed there is bacterial sepsis, either as the initiating event or a secondary complication.

Antimicrobials

- Treat all cases aggressively with IV antimicrobials.
- Penicillin (40,000 IU/kg IV by slow infusion QID)
- Amikacin (20–25 mg/kg IV SID); monitor with peak and trough levels.
- Ceftiofur (0 mg/kg IV by slow infusion QID)
- Cefotaxime (50–100 mg/kg IV by slow infusion QID)
- Ticarcillin/clavulanic acid (50–100 mg/kg IV by slow infusion QID)
- Imipenem (10–20 mg/kg IV by slow infusion QID)

Pressors/Inotropes

- The goal of pressor/inotrope therapy is to increase effective perfusion.
- Generally, blood pressures in neonates are much lower than those in old animals, making it important to use signs of effective perfusion (e.g., urine production, warm legs, good peripheral pulses, good mental status, good borborygmi) as an indication of perfusion.

- These drugs must be delivered by a very accurate IV pump to control their effect.
- As a practical matter, when preparing inotropes or pressors for IV infusion, use the "rule of six" (6 wt [kg] = mg of drug to be added to 100 mL, so that each 1 mL/hour delivers 1 μg/kg per minute of drug; use 0.1 this amount for epinephrine and norepinephrine, so that each 1 mL/hour delivers 0.1 μg/kg per minute of drug).
- Dopamine (5–20 μg/kg per minute; usual starting dose, 10 μg/kg per minute)
- Dobutamine (5–40 μg/kg per minute; usual starting dose, 10 μg/kg per minute)
- Norepinephrine (0.05–2 μg/kg per minute; usual starting dose, 0.5 μg/kg per minute)
- Epinephrine (0.1–3 μg/kg per minute; usual starting dose, 0.5 μg/kg per minute)
- Methylene blue (0.5–2 mg/kg as a bolus or infusion)—blocks NO production, which may help to reverse hypotension; NO has many actions, however, so nonspecific suppression may be harmful; decrease inotropes/pressors as infusion continues.
- Naloxone—blocks endorphin-mediated hypotension, especially in hemorrhagic shock; increases myocardial sensitivity and responsiveness to adrenergics in septic shock; may differentially affect vascular resistance.

CONTRAINDICATIONS

Because of the potential for hypotension, drugs that cause hypotension (e.g., acepromazine) are contraindicated in foals with shock.

PRECAUTIONS

Use aminoglycoside antibiotics and NSAIDs with caution because of possible nephrotoxicity, especially in hypotensive situations.

POSSIBLE INTERACTIONS

N/A

ALTERNATIVE DRUGS

N/A

FOLLOW-UP

PATIENT MONITORING

- These patients require intensive monitoring and intensive therapy until resolution of shock.
- Monitoring should include frequent assessment of PCV, TP, and glucose.
- Measurement of percentage-oxygen saturation with use of pulse oximetry is useful.
- Continuing assessment of hydration and urine production is necessary to determine fluid needs.

POSSIBLE COMPLICATIONS

Multiple organ dysfunction syndrome—may be signs of damage or failure in any organ system.

MISCELLANEOUS

ASSOCIATED CONDITIONS

N/A

AGE-RELATED FACTORS

Increased susceptibility during the neonatal period.

ZOONOTIC POTENTIAL

Depends on the pathogen involved.

PREGNACY

N/A

SYNONYMS

- Endotoxemia
- Septic shock
- SIRS

SEE ALSO

- Neonatal isoerythrolysis
- Septicemia

ABBREVIATIONS

- CRT = capillary refill time
- GI = gastrointestinal
- NO = nitric oxide
- PCV = packed cell volume
- SIRS = systemic inflammatory response syndrome
- TP = total protein

Suggested Reading

Drummond WH. Neonatal shock: pathophysiology and management. In: Koterba AM, Drummond WH, Kosch PC, eds. Equine clinical neonatology. Philadelphia: Lea & Febiger, 1990:106–123.

Author Jonathan E. Palmer
Consulting Editor Mary Rose Paradis

SLAFRAMINE TOXICOSIS

BASICS

OVERVIEW

- Slaframine, commonly called slobber factor, is a mycotoxin produced by *Rhizoctonia leguminicola.*
- As the species name indicates, this fungus is a pathogen of legumes, usually red clover (*Trifolium pratense*); other, less likely substrates include alfalfa (*Medicago sativa*) and Ladino or white clover (*T. repens*).
- Slaframine has a high affinity for the muscarinic-receptor subtype that regulates the secretory glands.
- It has been suggested that the slobbers syndrome involves other physiologically active compounds (e.g., swainsonine) also produced by *R. leguminicola.*

SIGNALMENT

- All horses are susceptible.
- No breed, age, or sex predispositions

SIGNS

- Onset of hypersalivation within hours of ingestion is the hallmark.
- Polydipsia results from fluid loss.
- Less common signs—anorexia, excessive lacrimation, polyuria, and diarrhea.

CAUSES AND RISK FACTORS

- Black patch is the fungal disease responsible for slaframine production.
- This plant pathogen is most likely to grow on clovers during wet, humid weather; a moist, humid environment with a temperature of 25–29°C and a substrate pH of 5.9–7.5 is needed to support growth.
- The fungus appears as dark spots or concentric rings on diseased leaves and stems.
- Contaminated seed spreads the fungus. Consumption of infected pastures or second-cutting forage usually is associated with intoxication.

DIAGNOSIS

DIFFERENTIAL DIAGNOSIS

- Excessive salivation can be induced by dental disease, stomatitis, or foreign objects lodged in the pharynx.
- Ptyalism may result from inflammation of the oral mucosa or salivary glands by penetrating wounds or plant awns—foxtail
- Hypersalivation in organophosphate and carbamate poisoning is associated with more life-threatening signs of dyspnea, colic, and diarrhea.

CBC/BIOCHEMISTRY/URINALYSIS

N/A

OTHER LABORATORY TESTS

- The diagnosis is established on the basis of rapid onset of profuse salivation associated with consumption of legume forage infected with *R. leguminicola.*
- Chemical analysis of suspect forage confirms the presence of slaframine.
- Plant pathologists can confirm black patch disease on suspect forages.

IMAGING

N/A

DIAGNOSTIC PROCEDURES

N/A

SLAFRAMINE TOXICOSIS

TREATMENT

Although specific antidotes are not available or, in most cases, even necessary, introduction of uncontaminated forage resolves the condition in 1–3 days.

MEDICATIONS

DRUGS

Response to atropine is questionable—empiric evidence suggests atropine given before exposure prevents hypersalivation; administration after the onset of hypersalivation is not particularly effective; use with caution in horses.

CONTRAINDICATIONS/POSSIBLE INTERACTIONS

N/A

FOLLOW-UP

PATIENT MONITORING

N/A

PREVENTION/AVOIDANCE

- Storage of contaminated hay for several months produces a significant reduction in toxicity; in one report, red-clover hay containing 50–100 ppm of slaframine contained $\cong$7 ppm after 10 months of storage.
- Reseeding with newer clover varieties resistant to *Rhizoctonia* sp. infection can solve persistent problems.

POSSIBLE COMPLICATIONS

N/A

EXPECTED COURSE AND PROGNOSIS

Resolution of the problem occurs when horses are provided uncontaminated forage, which in uncomplicated recovery is 1–3 days.

MISCELLANEOUS

ASSOCIATED CONDITIONS

N/A

AGE-RELATED FACTORS

N/A

ZOONOTIC POTENTIAL

N/A

PREGNANCY

N/A

SEE ALSO

N/A

Suggested Reading

Croom WJ, Hagler WM, Froetschel MA, Johnson AD. The involvement of slaframine and swainsonine in slobbers syndrome: a review. J Anim Sci 1995;73:1499–1508.

Author Stan W. Casteel

Consulting Editor Robert H. Poppenga

SLEEP DEPRIVATION AND PERIODIC COLLAPSE

BASICS

DEFINITION

A disorder associated with inappropriate periods of somnolence secondary to a lack of willingness by the animal to rest, which may result from discomfort associated with lying down and/or herd behavior.

PATHOPHYSIOLOGY

- Neurologically, these horses are normal, in contrast to horses with narcolepsy and cataplexy.
- Periodic collapse and sleep deprivation most often are associated with other diseases that prevent horses from lying down or rising, which precludes these horses from accumulating deep rest.
- Abdominal and thoracic adhesions, enterolithiasis, abscesses, and most commonly, musculoskeletal abnormalities have been associated with the collapse syndrome.
- In some cases, I have seen lone horses (i.e., housed in an isolated environment) that experienced periods of collapse. Soon after companion (i.e., sentinel) animals were reintroduced into the environment, however, the affected horses were seen frequently resting, and the episodes of collapse disappeared. Presumably, this response is associated with herd behavior where sentinel animals are not present.
- Periods of added anxiety in the environment (e.g., thunder- and windstorms, fireworks, excessive and intermittent motor noise) also can be associated with sleep deprivation and collapse.

SYSTEM AFFECTED

N/A

SIGNALMENT

No specific signalment, but in my experience, old horses with more chronic pain syndromes seem to dominate.

SIGNS

Historical Findings

- Collapse under restful circumstances is common.
- Horses seem to perform normally but may have episodes of collapse or near-collapse when standing, with or without a rider.
- Collapse in cross-ties or while being groomed also occurs.
- In some cases, owners recall that the time the episodes began coincided with an injury or reduced frequency of the horse being seen lying down.

Physical Examination Findings

- In horses with sufficient duration of signs, trauma to the fetlocks from collapse or near-collapse frequently is evident.
- Other abnormalities may be associated with the site of pain—musculoskeletal abnormalities
- Horses may present as unthrifty as well.

CAUSES

See *Pathophysiology.*

RISK FACTORS

See *Pathophysiology.*

DIAGNOSIS

- Historical characteristics can identify the syndrome, but the specific cause may be more difficult to determine.
- A detailed husbandry evaluation is essential to rule out behavior or management issues.
- Further examination should extend to a musculoskeletal and abdominal visceral evaluation.
- In some cases, administration of an anti-inflammatory drug (i.e., flunixin meglumine or phenylbutazone) may be followed in the next 48 hours by decreased episodes of collapse and the horse being found lying down and sleeping deeply.

DIFFERENTIAL DIAGNOSIS

- Narcolepsy
- Seizure syndrome
- Cardiac arrhythmia

CBC/BIOCHEMISTRY/URINALYSIS

No specific abnormalities

OTHER LABORATORY TESTS

N/A

IMAGING

May be useful to identify suspect areas of pain.

DIAGNOSTIC PROCEDURES

As indicated by physical examination findings

PATHOLOGIC FINDINGS

Depend on the associated cause.

SLEEP DEPRIVATION AND PERIODIC COLLAPSE

TREATMENT

- Depends on the primary problem.
- Pain control, addition of herdmates, and resolution of the primary problem may be required.

MEDICATIONS

DRUGS OF CHOICE

Depend on the primary disease.

CONTRAINDICATIONS

N/A

PRECAUTIONS

N/A

POSSIBLE INTERACTIONS

N/A

ALTERNATIVE DRUGS

N/A

FOLLOW-UP

PATIENT MONITORING

N/A

POSSIBLE COMPLICATIONS

N/A

EXPECTED COURSE AND PROGNOSIS

Excellent once the primary cause is identified and resolved to the degree that the horse can rest.

MISCELLANEOUS

ASSOCIATED CONDITIONS

N/A

AGE-RELATED FACTORS

N/A

ZOONOTIC POTENTIAL

N/A

PREGNANCY

N/A

SYNONYMS

N/A

SEE ALSO

Sleep attack syndrome

Suggested Reading

Guilleminault C, Anagnos A. Narcolepsy. In: Kryger M, Roth T, Dement W, eds. Principle and practices of sleep medicine. 3rd ed. Philadelphia: WB Saunders, 2000:676–686.

Author Joseph J. Bertone
Consulting Editor Joseph J. Bertone

SMALL INTESTINAL OBSTRUCTION

BASICS

DEFINITION

Impaired aboral transit of digesta between the stomach and cecum

PATHOPHYSIOLOGY

- May be physical or functional in origin.
- Physical impairment may result from intraluminal/extraluminal and strangulating/nonstrangulating factors.
- Following physical obstruction, peristaltic waves produce strong, spasmodic contractions in the region of obstruction, resulting in local stretching of the bowel wall and activation of pain receptors.
- Following blockage of the intestinal ingesta, saliva and secretions from the stomach, liver, pancreas, and bowel accumulate orally to the obstruction. These fluids, along with the gas produced by intestinal bacteria, produce increased intraluminal hydrostatic pressure and further bowel distention.
- Once intraluminal hydrostatic pressure rises above 15 cm H_2O, absorption of water by the intestinal mucosa ceases, and net water flow ensues from the mucosa into the intestinal lumen, contributing to hypovolemia. The increased pressure and expanding volume of fluid forces intestinal fluids into the stomach, creating gastric distention and compounding abdominal pain and hypovolemia, after which ileus ensues.

SYSTEMS AFFECTED

- GI
- Behavioral—activation of pain receptors is associated with clinical signs of abdominal pain; with progressive distention, depression may ensue.
- Cardiovascular—collapse occurs secondary to hypovolemia, endotoxemia, and altered electrolyte status; with gastric distention, pressure on the vena cava decreases cardiac return.
- Respiratory—decreased pulmonary function may be secondary to pressure on the diaphragm from gastric distention or diaphragmatic herniation.
- Endocrine/metabolic—affected patients frequently demonstrate metabolic alkalosis secondary to loss of hydrochloric acid in gastric reflux; as the condition progresses and hypovolemia ensues, metabolic acidosis develops.
- Hemic/lymphatic/immune—once tissue pressures exceed venous portal pressures, the small veins, venules, and lymphatics that drain the affected intestine collapse, and net fluid movement into the bowel is potentiated.
- Renal/urologic—hypovolemia is associated with decreased glomerular filtration rate, renin release, angiotensin II production, and aldosterone secretion.

SIGNALMENT

- Any age, sex, or breed
- Ascarid impactions frequently are seen in foals/weanlings/yearlings.
- Small intestinal intussusception and volvulus occur most often in horses <3 years.
- Abdominal tumors usually are identified in horses >5 years.
- Strangulating lipoma and epiploic foramen entrapment most often occur in horses >7 years.
- Scrotal hernias are observed in stallions.
- Proximal enteritis may occur more commonly in stallions.
- Gastrosplenic ligament incarceration of the small intestine has been described most often in male horses.
- Mesoduodenal rents and diaphragmatic hernias can be seen in mares during late gestation.
- Warmbloods, Standardbreds, Tennessee Walking Horses, and American Saddlebreds appear to be predisposed to inguinal herniation.

SIGNS

Historical Findings

- Horses with partial obstruction may display subacute, intermittent signs of abdominal pain or vague signs of lethargy, weakness, or weight loss. Transient episodes of abdominal pain may recur over a period of weeks to months and may progress in severity with time.
- Complete small intestinal obstruction is associated with signs of severe, persistent abdominal pain and ileus. Horses may display a dog-sitting posture with distention of the stomach.
- Recent abdominal surgery may indicate abdominal adhesions.
- Recent anthelmintic treatment contributes to ascarid impaction.
- Prolonged or high-dose NSAID therapy may indicate duodenal ulceration.
- Previous infection with *Streptococcus equi* can result in abscessation within the small intestinal mesentery.

Physical Examination Findings

- Clinical signs depend on the lesion present and the location, duration, and severity of that lesion.
- Most common signs—abdominal discomfort, tachycardia, discolored mucous membranes, prolonged capillary refill time, clinical dehydration, decreased to absent small intestinal borborygmi, reflux from the small intestine (yellow-brown, fetid odor, pH 6–8), and distended loops of small intestine on rectal examination.

CAUSES

Physical, Nonstrangulating, Intraluminal

- Impaction—feed, trichobezoar, ascarids, or tapeworms
- Foreign body
- Healed duodenal ulcer, with scarring and stricture
- Granulomatous enteritis

SMALL INTESTINAL OBSTRUCTION

Physical, Nonstrangulating, Extraluminal

- Tension on duodenocolic ligament secondary to distention or displacement of the large colon
- Adhesions—ischemic bowel, peritonitis, prolonged distention, excessive or traumatic surgical manipulation, anastomotic leakage, tissue dehydration, and inappropriate suture or technique
- Ileal muscular hypertrophy
- Ileal neurogenic stenosis
- Ileocecal valve edema or infarction secondary to migrating strongyle larvae
- Diverticula—traction, pulsion, or Meckel's
- Mesenteric abscess
- Neoplasia—pedunculated lipoma, lymphosarcoma, leiomyosarcoma, or carcinoid
- Intramural hematoma

Physical, Strangulating

- Volvulus
- Herniation—inguinal/scrotal, umbilical, diaphragmatic, epiploic foramen, gastrosplenic, renosplenic, or tears in mesentery/omentum/ligaments/fibrous bands/adhesions
- Intussusceptions
- Vaginal evisceration

Functional (Ileus)

- Intestinal distention
- Intestinal ischemia
- Intestinal inflammation—enterocolitis, surgical manipulation, or resection/anastomosis
- Endotoxemia
- Peritonitis
- Pain—GI, musculoskeletal, etc.
- Drugs—α-adrenergic agonists, opioids, etc.
- General anesthesia
- Hypovolemia/hypotension
- Electrolyte imbalances—hypocalcemia secondary to massive sweat loss
- Parasitism

RISK FACTORS

Diet

- Sudden changes in feed or feeding practices
- Moldy hay or grain
- Poor-quality or low-grade roughage
- Decreased roughage intake over 24 hours
- Coastal Bermuda hay—ileal impaction
- Pelleted feed—impaction
- Decreased water intake or availability—impaction

Management

Poor deworming program—ascarid/tapeworm impaction, large strongyle migration, and infarction

Body Condition

Obesity—pedunculated lipoma

Geographic Location

Southeastern U.S.—ileal impaction and proximal enteritis

Genetic

Inflammatory bowel disease—granulomatous enteritis and eosinophilic gastroenteritis

DIAGNOSIS

DIFFERENTIAL DIAGNOSIS

Differentiating Similar Signs

GI reflux usually is pathognomonic for small intestinal lesions but may be present secondary to large colon lesions that compress the small intestine or place tension on the duodenocolic ligament.

Differentiating Causes

The ability to differentiate between causes depends on the severity of clinical findings, which may be influenced by location of the lesion, length of intestine involved, and stage of disease.

Abdominal Pain

- In affected horses, some degree of gastric distention usually is present, which contributes to signs of abdominal pain.
- Decompression of gastric contents allows assessment of pain originating from the small intestine.
- Abdominal pain may be absent in foals with umbilical or inguinal hernias.
- Biphasic abdominal pain has been associated with ileal impaction.
- Severe, acute abdominal pain usually is associated with strangulating lesions—volvulus
- Ileocecal intussusception is accompanied by severe, acute abdominal pain, which subsides in 8–12 hours to mild, intermittent pain that can persist for weeks to months, until complete obstruction occurs.

Clinical Findings

- Intestinal involvement in an umbilical hernia usually is evident on palpation—pain on palpation of the hernia may indicate a strangulating hernia.
- Scrotal hernias may be accompanied by mild to severe scrotal swelling, palpable loops of intestine within the scrotum, and decreased scrotal temperature because of vascular obstruction.

Rectal Palpation

- Only the caudal 30–40% of the abdomen is palpable on rectal evaluation, but distension usually pushes affected intestinal segments into reach.
- Any distended loops should be evaluated for position, degree of distension, wall thickness, gas versus fluid content, and pain on palpation.
- A thick, tubular structure palpable in the center of the abdomen may indicate ileal impaction, jejunal intussusception, or ileal intussusception.
- Resentment to palpation of the ileocecal region often accompanies ileocecal intussusception.

SMALL INTESTINAL OBSTRUCTION

- Asymmetric inguinal rings, intestine or mesentery extending into an inguinal ring, or inability to identify one inguinal ring represent palpation findings in horses with inguinal herniation.
- If ileum is involved in inguinal herniation, the edematous antimesenteric ileocecal band may be palpable entering the ring on the affected side.

CBC/BIOCHEMISTRY/URINALYSIS

- The WBC count usually is not affected by acute intestinal strangulation or obstruction.
- Leukocytosis/neutrophilia with a left shift may be observed with peritonitis, proximal enteritis, or mesenteric abscessation.
- Leukopenia/neutropenia may develop secondary to intestinal necrosis or endotoxemia.
- Most cases are accompanied by an increased PCV and TP because of fluid sequestration within the bowel.
- Hypoproteinemia may develop as the disease progresses.
- Hypoalbuminemia may be observed with proximal enteritis or mesenteric abscessation.
- Hypergammaglobulinemia may be found with mesenteric abscessation or lymphosarcoma—β- and γ-fractions
- Decreased potassium and chloride levels occur with loss into the bowel, and decreased sodium and calcium levels occur secondary to extracellular fluid shifts.
- Loss of hydrochloric acid with gastric reflux results in metabolic alkalosis.
- Acute strangulating obstructions associated with release of endotoxin, increased production of lactic acid, and hypoperfusion result in metabolic acidosis.
- If small intestinal obstruction occurs in the region of the hepatopancreatic ampulla, increases in total bilirubin, ALP, and GGT may be observed

OTHER LABORATORY TESTS

N/A

IMAGING

- Abdominal ultrasonography can be used to assess small intestinal wall thickness and movement.
- With strangulating obstructive lesions, the intestinal wall becomes thickened, and motility is absent.
- Intestinal intussusception may display a characteristic concentric ring or "bull's eye" appearance.
- Abdominal radiography may be useful in distinguishing small from large intestinal problems in foals.

DIAGNOSTIC PROCEDURES

Abdominocentesis

- As peritonitis and intestinal ischemia progress, the fluid becomes increasingly sanguineous and cloudy as the cellularity and protein levels increase.
- WBC:TP ratios <3 and RBC:TP ratios <15 represent nonstrangulating obstructions or proximal enteritis; ratios >3 or 15, respectively, indicate strangulating lesions.
- Peritoneal fluid may be evaluated cytologically for neoplastic cells.

Endoscopy

- May be used to identify duodenal ulcers.
- A 2.5–3.0-m endoscope is needed to visualize this region in adults.

Laparoscopy and Celiotomy

May be performed to diagnose and correct the cause of obstruction or for intestinal biopsy.

TREATMENT

- Most affected horses require referral to a hospital facility for further evaluation and treatment.
- Horses with strangulating lesions are candidates for surgery.
- Before transport, nasogastric decompression is vital. Horses may be transported with nasogastric tubes left in place.
- Surgical intervention is necessary if a surgical lesion can be identified at rectal examination or abdominocentesis, if abdominal pain becomes uncontrollable, or if there is a lack of response to medical therapy.
- IV fluid therapy is important to maintain hydration and tissue perfusion and to correct electrolyte and acid–base abnormalities. Balanced polyionic IV solutions (e.g., lactated Ringer solution) are ideal; rate and quantity depend on the horse's status.
- The decision whether to administer IV fluids before transport depends on horse's condition. Often, rehydration increases the volume of gastric reflux, so gastric decompression may need to be performed more frequently.
- Hyperimmune serum may benefit horses with endotoxemia.
- Medical alteration of intestinal motility in cases of functional obstruction may not be possible if severe ischemia or chronic distention have occurred.

SMALL INTESTINAL OBSTRUCTION

MEDICATIONS

DRUGS OF CHOICE

• Sedation and analgesia may be achieved with xylazine (0.2–1.1 mg/kg IV) or detomidine (0.005–0.02 mg/kg IV); both duration and quality of sedation or analgesia may be enhanced by coadministration of butorphanol tartrate (0.1 mg/kg IV).
• NSAIDs such as flunixin meglumine (1.1 mg/kg IM or IV BID) or phenylbutazone (2.2–4.4 mg/kg PO or IV BID) may be used for analgesic and anti-inflammatory effects as well as to mediate the effects of endotoxin.
• Endotoxemia also may be mediated with polymixin B (6000 U/kg diluted in 0.5–1.0 L of saline IV BID) or pentoxifylline (8.5 mg/kg PO BID).
• Specific therapies for ileus, sepsis, gastric ulcers, and laminitis are discussed elsewhere.

CONTRAINDICATIONS

Acepromazine for sedation in hypovolemic horses

PRECAUTIONS

• Continued monitoring after administration of analgesics is important to ensure the drug is not masking signs of pain while the disease process progresses.
• Certain drugs (e.g., xylazine, detomidine) decrease GI motility.
• Gentamicin, amikacin, and polymixin B are nephrotoxic drugs.

POSSIBLE INTERACTIONS

N/A

ALTERNATIVE DRUGS

N/A

FOLLOW-UP

PATIENT MONITORING

Depends on cause of obstruction and method of treatment.

POSSIBLE COMPLICATIONS

• Gastric rupture
• Intestinal necrosis
• Abdominal adhesions
• Thrombophlebitis
• Laminitis

MISCELLANEOUS

ASSOCIATED CONDITIONS

• Endotoxemia
• Ileus
• Impaction of the large or small colon secondary to dehydration
• Laminitis

AGE-RELATED FACTORS

N/A

ZOONOTIC POTENTIAL

N/A

PREGNANCY

Outcome of pregnancy is determined more by cardiovascular and metabolic status of the mare and fetus than by the specific cause of the condition.

SYNONYMS

N/A

SEE ALSO

• Endotoxemia
• Ileus
• Proximal enteritis

ABBREVIATIONS

• ALP = alkaline phosphatase
• GGT = γ-glutamyltransferase
• GI = gastrointestinal
• PCV = packed cell volume
• TP = total protein

Suggested Reading

Doran R, Allen D, Orsini JA. Small intestine. In: Auer JA, ed. Equine surgery. Philadelphia: WB Saunders, 1992.
White NA. Examination and diagnosis of the acute abdomen. In: White NA, ed. The equine acute abdomen. Philadelphia: Lea & Febiger, 1990.

Author Annette M. Sysel
Consulting Editor Henry R. Stämpfli

SMOKE INHALATION

BASICS

OVERVIEW

• May produce several upper and lower respiratory tract injuries.
• Two principal mechanisms lead to respiratory and systemic dysfunction—direct thermal injury and intoxication by noxious agents in smoke.
• Three stages of pulmonary dysfunction after inhalation injury—acute pulmonary failure, pulmonary edema, and bronchopneumonia
• Acute pulmonary failure—caused by both carbon monoxide toxicity and heat injury; usually observed during the initial 36-hour period.
• Pulmonary edema—results from chemical injury and is most severe during the first 24 hours after severe smoke inhalation.
• Bronchopneumonia—occurs at the end of the first week after injury; impaired mucociliary clearance and alveolar macrophage function, together with the effects of smoke inhalation, predispose patients to bacterial infection. Pneumonia generally is caused by gram-negative bacteria.

SIGNALMENT

N/A

SIGNS

• Clinical signs depend on the amount and type of smoke inhaled, duration of exposure, and inhalation of specific poisonous gases.
• Burns around the face, oral and nasal inflammation, soot-stained nasal discharge, and the smell of smoke suggest inhalation exposure; observe asymptomatic patients closely for 1 week after exposure to smoke.
• Affected horses may show signs of severe hypoxemia and be depressed, irritable, or even moribund and comatose.
• Fever may be observed a short time after exposure but does not necessarily relate to infection.
• Signs of shock may be present.
• Heat and chemical injuries may cause tachypnea, inspiratory dyspnea, cough, or nasal discharge.
• Cyanosis and dehydration may be observed.
• Upper airway edema may be progressive and lead to airway obstruction.
• Thoracic auscultation may reveal decreased lung sounds, crackles, or wheezes.
• Signs of multiple organ failure may be present in severe cases—acute renal failure, cardiac failure, etc.
• Clinical findings may be similar to bronchopneumonia, but persistent fever is unusual.
• Worsening of clinical signs after initial improvement suggests secondary bacterial bronchopneumonia.

CAUSES AND RISK FACTORS

N/A

DIAGNOSIS

DIFFERENTIAL DIAGNOSIS

• The diagnosis is established based on history and physical examination findings; however, in humans, these criteria have led to underestimation of the incidence of pulmonary injury.
• Several diagnostic aids are available to confirm and to document equine smoke inhalation—hematology, bronchoscopy, thoracic radiography, blood gas analysis, transtracheal fluid cytology and culture, and measurement of blood carboxyhemoglobin levels.

CBC/BIOCHEMISTRY/URINALYSIS

• Leukocytosis and hyperfibrinogenemia indicate an inflammatory process.
• Anemia and hypergammaglobulinemia may reflect chronic inflammation.
• Severe cases may reveal increased creatinine and BUN, suggesting prerenal or renal failure.

OTHER LABORATORY TESTS

• Sequential arterial blood gas analyses are good indicators of respiratory function and prognosis. Carboxyhemoglobin levels in venous blood samples may be measured in most human hospitals; carbon monoxide toxicity and smoke exposure are suspected with carboxyhemoglobin levels >10%.
• Cytology of transtracheal fluid may reveal carbon particles in phagocytic cells.
• Perform bacterial culture and sensitivity testing of transtracheal fluid to document bronchopneumonia.

IMAGING

• The most common radiographic abnormalities include diffuse bronchial and peribronchial lesions or diffuse, patchy interstitial infiltration, which are suggestive of edema.
• Radiographic lesions may not correlate with the severity of pulmonary dysfunction.
• Radiographic findings indicative of pneumothorax, pneumomediastinum, and emphysema may be found in severe cases.

DIAGNOSTIC PROCEDURES

Endoscopy may reveal airway edema and inflammation, mucosal necrosis, and soot in the lower respiratory tract.

SMOKE INHALATION

TREATMENT

• Aimed at providing a patent airway, reversing bronchospasms and hypoxemia, decreasing pulmonary inflammation and edema, providing ventilatory support, and controlling other toxic effects (if multiple organ failure).
• Supplemental humidified oxygen may be needed if impaired pulmonary ventilation and hypoxemia is severe.
• Perform a tracheotomy if signs suggest upper airway obstruction; patients maintained with tracheal tubes require careful and frequent nursing care to prevent obstruction of the tube by secretions.

MEDICATIONS

DRUGS

• Early use of bronchodilators to control bronchospasm and airway obstruction—β2-adrenergic agonists (e.g., clenbuterol [0.8–3.2 μg/kg PO BID], terbutaline sulfate [0.02–0.06 mg/kg PO BID], and albuterol [1–2 μg/kg]) may be administered safely to most horses; aminophylline (5–10 mg/kg PO or IV BID) may be associated with toxic side effects (e.g., tachycardia, hyperesthesia, excitement).
• Furosemide (1–2 mg/kg IM or IV) may be given for treatment of upper airway or pulmonary tract edema.
• IV fluid administration is indicated in most horses, because dehydration and renal failure often are present. Administered with caution, however, to prevent exacerbation of pulmonary edema and overhydration. Fluid selection is based on the serum electrolyte disturbances and acid-base status of the affected horse.
• Dimethyl sulfoxide (1.0 g/kg in a 20% solution IV [slowly] SID or BID) may be potentially effective.
• Antibiotic prophylaxis in affected horses is controversial, because it may lead to development of bacterial resistance. In severe cases, however, early antibiotic treatment with broad-spectrum activity may be justified.
• NSAIDs (e.g., phenylbutazone [4.4 mg/kg PO or IV SID) may be beneficial in decreasing mediator release and controlling fever.

CONTRAINDICATIONS/POSSIBLE INTERACTIONS

• Concurrent treatment with aminophylline may potentiate the diuretic effect of furosemide.
• Corticosteroid therapy is controversial and associated with increased septic complications in people (e.g., bacterial bronchopneumonia); avoid such therapy if possible.

FOLLOW-UP

• Favorable prognosis if the horse survives the initial injury.
• The time required for complete recovery after the initial insult varies with the severity of the injury; several months may be needed before the animal can return to work.
• Owner should modify the environment to reduce dust, molds, and other irritants to avoid development of airway hypersensitivity.

MISCELLANEOUS

ASSOCIATED CONDITIONS

N/A

AGE-RELATED FACTORS

N/A

ZOONOTIC POTENTIAL

N/A

PREGNANCY

N/A

SEE ALSO

• Inspiratory dyspnea
• Pleuropneumonia
• Pneumothorax

Suggested Reading

Beech J. Smoke inhalation: miscellaneous lung and pleural injuries. In: Beech J, ed. Equine respiratory disorders. Philadelphia: Lea & Febiger, 1991:216–217.

Geor RJ, Ames TR. Smoke inhalation injury in horses. Compend Cont Educ Pract Vet 1991;13:1162–1169.

Kemper T, Spiers S, Barratt-Boyes SM, Hoffman R. Treatment of smoke inhalation in five horses. J Am Vet Med Assoc 1993,202:91–94.

Author Daniel Jean
Consulting Editor Jean-Pierre Lavoie

SNAKE ENVENOMATION

BASICS

DEFINITION

- Disease associated with bites from two families of venomous snakes in the U.S.—Elapidae, which includes the eastern coral snake (*Micrurus fulvius fulvius*) and Texas coral snake (*M. fulvius tenere*); and Crotalidae (pit viper), which includes the genera *Agkistrodon* (copperheads and cottonmouth water moccasins), *Crotalus* (rattlesnakes), and *Sistrurus* (pygmy and massasauga rattlesnakes).
- Coral snakes have a relatively small head, black snout, and round pupils. Their color pattern consists of fully encircling bands of red, yellow, and black. Coral snakes are not only shy and nocturnal but have fixed front fangs of the upper jaw, which makes them less of a threat to large livestock.
- Pit viper characteristics include bilateral pits between the nostril and eye, elliptical pupils, two well-developed and retractable maxillary fangs, and an undivided row of ventral scales caudal to the cloaca. The hollow, hinged front fangs rotate forward for striking and delivering the venom.
- Copperheads are stout and orange/brown; their head typically is a solid copper tone.
- Cotton-mouths are brown to black, thick-bodied, aggressive snakes with a white oral mucosa they display when agitated.

PATHOPHYSIOLOGY

- Pit viper venom is a complex mixture of enzymes and nonenzymatic polypeptides.
- These proteins include myotoxins, proteases, hyaluronidase, bradykinin-releasing enzyme, and phospholipase A_2, and they primarily are responsible for significant local tissue destruction—myonecrosis, edema, hemorrhage, and inflammation at the bite site.
- These enzymes, in addition to other nonenzymatic proteins, cause an increase in capillary permeability, with subsequent loss of plasma volume and peripheral pooling of blood. The sequelae of these events are decreased cardiac output, hypoproteinemia, hypotension, and a metabolic acidosis that, if not corrected, can lead to complete respiratory and circulatory collapse.
- Other toxins are associated with hemolysis, thrombocytopenia, and alterations in the coagulation cascade.
- Hemorrhagins are responsible for hemorrhage observed either at the bite wound or systemically.

SYSTEMS AFFECTED

- Cardiovascular—interference with vascular endothelial intercellular cement substance, RBC lysis, vasodilation, enhanced degradation of fibrinogen to fibrin, enhanced activation of factor X to Xa, enhanced production of degradation products, enhanced platelet aggregation, and hypoxia
- Skin/exocrine/musculoskeletal—dilatation of the sarcoplasmic reticulum; inhibition of the calcium ion pump; hydrolysis of peptide linkages of amino groups of aliphatic, hydrophobic amino acids; disruption of connective tissue viscosity by depolymerizing hyaluronic acid; hydrolysis of the ester bond at C-2 of lecithin, which results in release of histamine, serotonin, bradykinin, and prostaglandins
- Respiratory—direct damage to alveolar membranes; hemorrhage of the pulmonary capillary bed
- Neuromuscular—neurotransmitter decrease, resulting in neuromuscular junction dysfunction and respiratory center paralysis
- Renal/urologic—nephrotoxic effects of myoglobinuria, hemoglobinuria, defibrination syndrome, DIC-like syndrome, direct toxic effect, and hypovolemic shock
- Nine rattlesnake species have subpopulations with venom containing Mojave toxin, a potent neurotoxin that interrupts neurotransmission at the neuromuscular junction. This can lead to loss of control of skeletal musculature, including the diaphragm, resulting in flaccid paralysis and respiratory failure.
- Coral snake venom also contains a potent neurotoxin that causes an irreversible decrease of acetylcholine release at the neuromuscular junction. Possible sequelae include bulbar paralysis and respiratory collapse from paralysis of the diaphragm. Other systemic effects from coral snake venom include RBC lysis and rhabdomyolysis.

GENETICS

N/A

INCIDENCE/PREVALENCE

- Most snakebites occur from April to October and result from accidental encounters.
- Several hundred horses are bitten each year by pit vipers, mostly rattlesnakes in the western US.
- Coral snakes are small and shy, and bites from these snakes are infrequent.
- Pit vipers are found in all states, except for Maine, Hawaii, and Alaska.
- Eastern coral snakes range from North Carolina to the north, southern Florida to the south, and the Mississippi River to the west.
- Texas coral snakes are found in Arkansas, Louisiana, and Texas.
- Arizona coral snakes are small, nocturnal, and burrowing; they are not considered medically significant in veterinary medicine.

SIGNALMENT

N/A

SIGNS

General Comments

- Most horses are bitten on or near the muzzle, which results in severe local tissue destruction that often leads to head swelling and airway obstruction during the acute phase.
- A smaller percentage of horses receive bites on the limbs below the carpus or tarsus; bites to the trunk are rare.
- Less than half of bitten horses develop multiple or severe manifestations of envenomation.
- In addition to airway obstruction, hemolytic anemia or coagulopathies can be acute, life-threatening problems.
- Determining the species of pit viper involved is not necessarily important, but determining whether the snake delivered sufficient venom is.
- Most venomous bites elicit local signs of edema within 60 minutes.
- Onset of systemic signs may be delayed for up to 6 hours; monitor the patient for at least this time period.
- Lack of local signs does not preclude life-threatening problems from occurring, particularly with bites from a pit viper, whose venom contains neurotoxins.

- Coral snake venom is primarily neurotoxic, and envenomations that elicit neurologic signs in the victim carry a poor prognosis.
- Horses bitten by coral snakes may show a lag phase of up to 18 hours between the bite and onset of clinical signs; however, once neurologic signs appear, they are difficult to reverse.

Physical Examination Findings

Pit Vipers:

- Painful soft-tissue swelling with hemorrhage at the bite marks; possible ecchymosis and petechiation
- Dyspnea and tachypnea caused by upper airway obstruction, pulmonary edema, or hemorrhage
- Cardiac abnormalities—tachycardia; dysrhythmias
- Fever
- Epistaxis
- Other signs—lethargy, diarrhea, salivation caused by dysphagia, flaccid paralysis, incontinence, tremors, clotting abnormalities, laminitis, colic, coma, and shock.

Coral Snakes:

- Puncture wounds—usually small and without hemorrhage
- Salivation caused by dysphagia
- Bulbar paralysis—flaccid paralysis
- Respiratory arrest

CAUSES AND RISK FACTORS

- Primary factors determining severity of a venomous snakebite—species of snake, circumstances of the bite, age of the snake, and venom composition
- The snake controls the degree of envenomation—defensive bites tend to be less severe than offensive and agonal bites.
- Decapitated heads can reflexively bite for up to 1 hour after decapitation.
- Larger snakes generally inject more venom than smaller snakes.
- Venom from young snakes tends to contain a high peptide fraction, so although tissue slough may not be as severe, systemic effects may be worse.
- Peptide fractions have been reported by some to have higher concentrations in venoms during the spring, thus causing more serious problems.
- Bite site location can affect the speed of systemic uptake of the venom.
- Size of the victim and their activity level after envenomation influence the extent of venom systemic circulation and severity of the toxicosis.
- Time from bite to medical intervention can significantly alter the prognosis.

DIAGNOSIS

DIFFERENTIAL DIAGNOSIS

- Angioedema secondary to insect sting/bite
- Trauma
- Foreign body/abscess
- Botulism
- *Centaurea solstitialis* (yellow star thistle) or *C. repens* (Russian knapweed) poisoning
- Purpura hemorrhagica

CBC/BIOCHEMISTRY/URINALYSIS

Elevated CPK, AST, and SDH and immediate hemoconcentration, followed by a hemolytic or coagulopathy-induced anemia, leukocytosis with an inflammatory leukogram, hyper- or hypofibrinogenemia, hypoproteinemia, thrombocytopenia, hyperglobulinemia, azotemia, and nonspecific abnormal renal changes

OTHER LABORATORY TESTS

- Prolonged clotting times—ACT, PT, and PTT
- High FDP
- Metabolic acidosis

IMAGING

Echocardiography to assess cardiac dysfunction

DIAGNOSTIC PROCEDURES

Electrocardiography to assess cardiac dysfunction

PATHOLOGIC FINDINGS

- Extensive soft-tissue edema, hemorrhage, and myonecrosis at and around the bite
- Generalized congestion, with petechiation of major organs
- Hepatocellular necrosis
- Possible myocardial inflammation and fibrosis with pleural and pericardial effusions
- Laminitis, pneumonia, and chronic changes associated with wound complications—osteomyelitis
- Secondary clostridial infections

TREATMENT

APPROPRIATE HEALTH CARE

- Immediate attention is critical.
- First-aid measures—calm the patient, and immediately transport to a veterinary facility for appropriate monitoring
- Inpatient medical management may last for several days; short-term goals include preventing or controlling shock, neutralizing the venom, minimizing tissue necrosis, and preventing secondary bacterial infections.
- Establishing a patent airway is essential; horses with bites on the head and accompanying head and neck swelling may require tracheotomy.
- Some form of rigid tubing can be sutured into the nostrils to keep the nasal passages patent.

SNAKE ENVENOMATION

NURSING CARE
• IV crystalloid fluids to combat shock and hypotension and to increase tissue perfusion and maintain hydration; alternatively, whole blood or blood products to correct anemias, thrombocytopenias, and clotting abnormalities
• Local wound management—continuous cleansing, hydrotherapy, and debridement
• Administer tetanus toxoid or antitoxin as appropriate.

ACTIVITY
Calm the patient to decrease distribution of the venom.

DIET
N/A

CLIENT EDUCATION
• Size and condition of the wound site may not correlate with severity of the systemic signs.
• Avoid first-aid techniques such as tourniquets, cryotherapy, lancing, suction, and electroshock.
• Systemic signs may be delayed by several hours, so immediate treatment is essential.

SURGICAL CONSIDERATIONS
Fasciotomies are not indicated, except for extremely rare circumstances with documented, elevated compartmental pressures.

MEDICATIONS

DRUGS OF CHOICE
• Pay attention to use of specific antivenin against pit viper or coral snake envenomations—*M. fulvius* (equine origin, for coral snakes, Wyeth); Antivenin (Crotalida) polyvalent, equine origin (Wyeth).
• Consider antivenin for bites in foals; small, young horses; and ponies because of their smaller body mass.
• Adult horses have some innate protection from envenomations because of their large body mass, but fatalities do occur.
• Antivenin is most effective shortly after envenomation has occurred. This is especially true in combating local tissue necrosis and neurologic sequela.
• Initial dose of antivenin should be 5 vials IV. The total number of vials used depends on the clinical signs, progression of the syndrome, degree of hypotension, and the bite site.
• Do not administer Antivenin IM or into the bite site itself.
• All animals should receive a broad-spectrum antibiotic (e.g., cephalosporin) for at least 7–10 days.
• NSAIDs (e.g., flunixin meglumine) can be used 24 hours after the bite for control of pain and swelling.
• Approach use of pain-control medications conservatively, and take care using compounds that interfere with platelet function.

CONTRAINDICATIONS
• Heparin
• Dimethyl sulfoxide

PRECAUTIONS
• Use of corticosteroids (e.g., dexamethasone) is debatable. Avoid long-term, high dose of corticosteroids, which depress immune response to the venom and alter clinically relevant laboratory parameters that are useful in monitoring progression of the syndrome. Corticosteroids also may interfere with effectiveness of the antivenom and have little effect on local tissue response to snake venom.
• Antihistamines are of no benefit.

POSSIBLE INTERACTIONS
N/A

ALTERNATIVE DRUGS
N/A

FOLLOW-UP

PATIENT MONITORING

- Patient monitoring is critical to a successful outcome.
- Assess CBC, serum chemistry panel, clotting panel, and fibrinogen every 12–24 hours at minimum and more often if the patient is deteriorating.
- Close observation of vital signs along with the respiratory and cardiovascular systems is recommended.

PREVENTION/AVOIDANCE

N/A

POSSIBLE COMPLICATIONS

Common chronic problems after rattlesnake bites include cardiac dysfunction, liver disease, pneumonia, colitis, laminitis, pharyngeal paralysis, and various wound complications.

EXPECTED COURSE AND PROGNOSIS

- Clinical signs can last as long as 2 weeks, with close inpatient monitoring.
- Poor prognosis after coral snake bites results from the neuromuscular effects of the venom, leading to respiratory collapse as the most common cause of death.
- Estimated mortality rate after rattlesnake bites is ≅10–30%.

MISCELLANEOUS

ASSOCIATED CONDITIONS

N/A

AGE-RELATED FACTORS

Young foals or ponies are at greatest risk because of their small body mass.

ZOONOTIC POTENTIAL

N/A

PREGNANCY

N/A

SYNONYMS

N/A

SEE ALSO

N/A

ABBREVIATIONS

- ACT = activated clotting time
- AST = aspartate aminotransferase
- CPK = creatine phosphokinase
- DIC = disseminated intravascular coagulation
- FDP = fibrin degradation products
- SDH = sorbitol dehydrogenase
- PT = prothrombin time
- PTT = partial thromboplastin time

Suggested Reading

Dickinson CE, et al. Rattlesnake venom poisoning in horses: 32 cases (1973–1993). J Am Vet Med Assoc 1996;208:1866–1871.

Hudelson S, Hudelson P. Pathophysiology of snake envenomation and evaluation of treatments—part I. Compend Contin Educ Pract Vet 1995;17:889–898.

Hudelson S, Hudelson P. Pathophysiology of snake envenomation and evaluation of treatments—part II. Compend Contin Educ Pract Vet 1995;17:1035–1041.

Hudelson S, Hudelson P. Pathophysiology of snake envenomation and evaluation of treatments—part III. Compend Contin Educ Pract Vet 1995;17:1385–1396.

Authors Patricia A. Talcott and Michael Peterson

Consulting Editor Robert H. Poppenga

SODIUM, HYPERNATREMIA

BASICS

DEFINITION

A serum sodium concentration > the upper limit of normal horses—generally >144 mEq/L.

PATHOPHYSIOLOGY

- Sodium is the major extracellular cation in the body and, therefore, is critical for maintenance of the extracellular space.
- Serum Na^+ concentrations reflect the ratio of total-body sodium to total-body water. Thus, knowledge of the hydration state is important for accurate interpretation of serum sodium concentrations.
- Hypernatremia usually reflects an absolute or relative water deficiency.

SYSTEM AFFECTED

Nervous—hypernatremia may lead to hyperosmolality and intracellular water loss from neurons, in turn leading to CNS shrinkage.

SIGNALMENT

No breed, sex, or age predilections

SIGNS

- Lethargy
- Weakness
- Seizures
- Coma
- Death
- Severity of signs depends on the duration and degree of hypernatremia.
- Other findings depend on the underlying cause.

CAUSES

- High total-body sodium—excessive intake of sodium chloride (rare); IV administration of hypertonic saline or sodium bicarbonate solutions
- Normal total-body sodium with excessive free-water loss—decreased water intake because of unavailable water source or physical abnormality causing decreased ingestion; central and nephrogenic DI (i.e., lack of ADH effect in the kidneys); prolonged hyperventilation associated with exercise during hot weather or pulmonary disease, acidosis, or severe anemia; evaporative loss from extensive burns; exhausted horse syndrome
- Low total sodium and hypotonic fluid loss—loss of sodium-containing fluid without compensatory water replacement
- Urinary loss—osmotic diuretic administration (i.e., mannitol)
- Gastrointestinal loss—early stages of diarrhea, before the point of compensatory water intake occurs

RISK FACTORS

Intense exercise in hot weather with inadequate access to water

DIAGNOSIS

DIFFERENTIAL DIAGNOSIS

- DI
- Hypertonic dehydration associated with decreased water intake or excessive free-water loss
- Prolonged panting
- Salt ingestion (rare)

LABORATORY FINDINGS

Drugs That May Alter Lab Results

Sodium salts of EDTA, fluoride, and heparin can result in pseudohypernatremia.

Disorders That May Alter Lab Results

Sample dehydration can result in pseudohypernatremia.

Valid If Run in Human Lab?

Yes

CBC/BIOCHEMISTRY/URINALYSIS

- High serum sodium concentration
- DI—hyposthenuria
- Exhausted horse syndrome—stress neutrophilia and lymphopenia; occasionally leukopenia Decreased potassium, chloride, calcium, and magnesium

OTHER LABORATORY TESTS

- Vasopressin concentration in conjunction with water deprivation—nephrogenic DI, vasopressin ≥3 normal; neurogenic DI, vasopressin normal
- ADH response test—vasopressin administered IV, and urine osmolality measured at 2-hour intervals; if urine osmolality increases to ≥1.025, neurogenic DI is present.

IMAGING

N/A

DIAGNOSTIC PROCEDURES

N/A

SODIUM, HYPERNATREMIA

TREATMENT

• Treatment of the underlying cause and adequate water availability in most transient causes (**NOTE:** long-standing hypernatremia should be corrected gradually
• DI—low-sodium diets and adequate water availability
• Exhausted horse syndrome—immediate cooling (e.g., shade, fans, cold water poured over the body), large volumes of lactated Ringer's solution, NSAIDs for pain

MEDICATIONS

DRUGS OF CHOICE

• Correct severe, long-standing hypernatremia gradually
• Central DI—ADH

CONTRAINDICATIONS

N/A

PRECAUTIONS

The combination of hypernatremia and dehydration is a therapeutic dilemma, because rapid reduction of serum sodium concentrations can lead to cerebral and pulmonary edema.

POSSIBLE INTERACTIONS

N/A

ALTERNATIVE DRUGS

N/A

FOLLOW-UP

PATIENT MONITORING

• Electrolytes, urine output, and body weight
• DI—monitor water intake.

POSSIBLE COMPLICATIONS

• Seizures/convulsions
• Probable permanent neurologic damage in severe, long-standing cases

MISCELLANEOUS

ASSOCIATED CONDITIONS

N/A

AGE-RELATED FACTORS

N/A

ZOONOTIC POTENTIAL

N/A

PREGNANCY

N/A

SYNONYMS

N/A

SEE ALSO

• DI
• Exhausted horse syndrome
• Hyposthenuria

ABBREVIATION

• DI = diabetes insipidus

Suggested Reading

Carlson GP. Clinical chemistry tests. In: Smith BP, ed. Large animal internal medicine. St. Louis: Mosby, 1996.
Johnson PJ. Electrolyte and acid-base disturbances in the horse. Vet Clin North Am Equine Pract 1995;11:491–514.
Schmall LM. Fluid and electrolyte therapy. In: Robinson NE, ed. Current therapy in equine medicine 4. Philadelphia: WB Saunders, 1997.

Authors Wendy S. Sprague and E. Duane Lassen
Consulting Editor Claire B. Andreasen

SODIUM, HYPONATREMIA

BASICS

DEFINITION

A serum sodium concentration < the lower limit of normal horses—generally <132 mEq/L

PATHOPHYSIOLOGY

- Sodium is the major extracellular cation in the body and, therefore, is critical for maintenance of the extracellular space.
- Serum sodium concentration reflects the ratio of the total-body sodium to total-body water; therefore, knowledge of the hydration state is important for accurate interpretation of serum sodium concentrations.
- Hyponatremia usually results from relative water excess and usually is not clinically significant until serum sodium concentrations are <122 mEq/L.

SYSTEMS AFFECTED

- Nervous—cerebral edema (also seen with rapid correction of severe hyponatremia)
- Renal—medullary washout
- Hematopoietic—intravascular hemolysis

SIGNALMENT

No breed, sex, or age predilections

SIGNS

- Lethargy
- Central blindness
- Seizures
- Tremors
- Abnormal gait
- Other findings depend on the underlying cause.

CAUSES

- Loss of sodium-containing fluid—diarrhea, pronounced sweating, hemorrhage, sequestration of fluid in the GI tract (e.g., obstruction, ileus), protein-losing gastroenteropathies, chronic/subacute colitis, GI fluid drainage by nasogastric intubation, and acute renal disease (usually in foals)
- Adrenal insufficiency—iatrogenic (from acute withdrawal of glucocorticoids in race horses) or adrenal exhaustion (a poorly characterized syndrome)
- Sequestration of fluid—peritonitis, ascites, ruptured bladder (usually in foals), and gut torsion or volvulus
- Water retention with normal circulating fluid volume (rare)—heart failure, chronic hepatic fibrosis, severe hypoalbuminemia, psychogenic polydipsia, renal disease, and inappropriate ADH secretion
- Iatrogenic—oral administration of hypotonic fluids, inappropriate fluid therapy (i.e., excessive administration of 5% dextrose solution)
- Furosemide causes natriuresis, which infrequently may result in hyponatremia.

RISK FACTORS

N/A

DIAGNOSIS

DIFFERENTIAL DIAGNOSIS

- Azotemia and hyperkalemia in foals—consider renal disease and ruptured bladder
- Lethargy and weight loss in young race horses—consider iatrogenic hypoadrenocorticism and adrenal exhaustion
- Other clinical signs can help to differentiate causes—diarrhea, abdominal pain, and ascites

LABORATORY FINDINGS

Drugs That May Alter Lab Results

Mannitol can cause pseudohyponatremia.

Disorders That May Alter Lab Results

- Hyperlipidemia and hyperproteinemia can cause pseudohyponatremia unless an ion-specific electrode is used for measurement.
- Marked hyperglycemia causes dilution of circulating sodium concentration by osmotic water movement.

Valid If Run in Human Lab

Yes

CBC/BIOCHEMISTRY/URINALYSIS

- Low serum sodium concentration
- Other abnormalities depend on the underlying cause.

OTHER LABORATORY TESTS

- Fractional excretion of sodium—a single urine sample can be used for sodium and creatinine measurements, which are compared with serum sodium and creatinine concentrations determined at the same time ($[Na_u^+/Na_s^+]/[Cr_u/Cr_s]$); suspect renal disease if >1%
- Plasma osmolality—should be low with hyponatremia; if in the normal or high range, rule out renal failure and causes of pseudohyponatremia.

IMAGING

N/A

DIAGNOSTIC PROCEDURES

N/A

TREATMENT

Therapy depends on the severity of hyponatremia and the underlying disorder.

MEDICATIONS

DRUGS OF CHOICE

- Correct acute clinical hyponatremia rapidly and chronic hyponatremia (≅48 hours) gradually.
- Moderate hyponatremia (122—132 mEq/L)—treatment probably not critical, but depends on clinical signs
- Treat severe hyponatremia; therapy depends on the acuteness of the disorder.
- Acute clinical hyponatremia—elevate serum sodium to 125 mEq/L over 6 hours, then gradually increase to normal. The amount of Na^+ needed to elevate serum Na^+ to a concentration of 125 mEq/L = (125 − measured serum Na^+ [mEq/L] × 0.67 × BW [kg]). Isotonic or hypertonic (3%) saline is suggested for states of volume contraction.

SODIUM, HYPONATREMIA

- Chronic hyponatremia—not well defined in horses; appropriate fluid would be 0.45% NaCl in 2.5% dextrose; use the formula above to calculate the amount of Na^+ needed.
- Sodium bicarbonate—if indicated for concurrent, severe metabolic acidosis; calculate the dosage carefully to avoid correcting serum sodium too rapidly
- DMSO and NSAIDs (e.g., phenylbutazone, flunixin meglumine) can be used for treatment of cerebral ischemia and inflammation.
- Corticosteroids may be used with caution for cerebral edema.
- Mannitol can be used to reduce cerebral edema in cases of acute clinical hyponatremia if serum sodium concentrations are concurrently normalized, but it is not recommended with suspected cerebral hemorrhage or chronic hyponatremia.

CONTRAINDICATIONS
N/A

PRECAUTIONS
Rapid correction of serum sodium in cases of chronic hyponatremia has led to osmotic cerebral demyelination in humans, but this has not been reported in horses.

POSSIBLE INTERACTIONS
N/A

ALTERNATIVE DRUGS
N/A

FOLLOW-UP

PATIENT MONITORING
Frequently measure serum electrolytes, urine output, and BW

POSSIBLE COMPLICATIONS
Depend on the underlying disorder

MISCELLANEOUS

ASSOCIATED CONDITIONS
Other acid–base and electrolyte abnormalities often are associated.

AGE-RELATED FACTORS
N/A

ZOONOTIC POTENTIAL
N/A

PREGNANCY
N/A

SYNONYMS
N/A

SEE ALSO
N/A

ABBREVIATIONS
- ADH = antidiuretic syndrome
- BW = body weight
- DMSO = dimethyl sulfoxide
- GI = gastrointestinal

Suggested Reading

Carlson GP. Clinical chemistry tests. In: Smith BP, ed. Large animal internal medicine. St. Louis: Mosby, 1996.

Johnson PJ. Electrolyte and acid-base disturbances in the horse. Vet Clin North Am Equine Pract 1995;11:491–514.

Schmall LM. Fluid and electrolyte therapy. In: Robinson NE, ed. Current therapy in equine medicine 4. Philadelphia: WB Saunders, 1997.

Authors Wendy S. Sprague and E. Duane Lassen

Consulting Editor Claire B. Andreasen

SOLANUM SPP. (NIGHTSHADE) TOXICOSIS

BASICS

OVERVIEW

- Numerous *Solanum* spp. (nightshade family) are potentially toxic to animals—*S. nigrum* (black nightshade), *S. dulcamera* (bittersweet nightshade), *S. carolinense* (horse nettle), *S. rostratum* (buffalo burr), *S. tuberosum* (potato), and others
- Plants in this genus are widely distributed.
- Toxicity is attributed primarily to tropane alkaloids and steroidal glycoalkaloids (e.g., solanine), but few equine data are available.
- Anticholinergic, muscarinic, and GI irritant effects have been described in intoxicated animals.
- Muscarinic effects may result from cholinesterase inhibition, but this has not been verified clinically.
- GI irritation is believed to result from a saponin-like effect of the steroidal glycoalkaloids.
- Documented cases of equine intoxication are rare, and those in the literature do not provide significant information concerning pathophysiologic effects.

SIGNALMENT

No known breed, age, or sex predispositions

SIGNS

- GI signs predominate—anorexia, nausea, salivation, colic, and diarrhea with or without blood.
- Nervous system signs—apathy, drowsiness, trembling, progressive weakness or paralysis, recumbency, and coma

CAUSES AND RISK FACTORS

- Contamination of hay with *Solanum* spp.
- Unavailability of alternative desirable forage
- Access to old potatoes or potato refuse
- Toxicity varies with environment, plant part ingested, and time of year.
- Unripe berries contain the highest glycoalkaloid concentration, which declines with maturity.
- Green portions of potato contain the highest toxin concentration.

DIAGNOSIS

DIFFERENTIAL DIAGNOSIS

- Establishing the diagnosis relies on evidence of consumption of *Solanum* spp.
- Other causes of colic—lack of exposure to *Solanum* spp.

CBC/BIOCHEMISTRY/URINALYSIS

N/A

OTHER LABORATORY TESTS

N/A

IMAGING

N/A

DIAGNOSTIC PROCEDURES

N/A

PATHOLOGIC FINDINGS

- Evidence of plant in the stomach
- Grossly, there may be evidence of GI irritation and diarrhea with or without hemorrhage.
- Histopathologically, there is congestion, inflammation, hemorrhage, and ulceration of the GI mucosa.

TREATMENT

- Remove animal from source of exposure.
- If soon after ingestion, consider GI decontamination.
- Symptomatic and supportive care

MEDICATIONS

DRUGS

- AC (2–5 g/kg PO in water slurry [1 g of AC in 5 mL or water])
- One dose of cathartic (70% sorbitol at 3 mL/kg PO or sodium or magnesium sulfate at 250 mg/kg PO, the latter two being administered in a water slurry) with AC if no diarrhea or ileus
- NSAIDs—flunixin meglumine (0.1 mg/kg IV or IM as necessary)

CONTRAINDICATIONS/POSSIBLE INTERACTIONS

N/A

SOLANUM SPP. (NIGHTSHADE) TOXICOSIS

FOLLOW-UP

PATIENT MONITORING

N/A

PREVENTION/AVOIDANCE

- Limit or prevent access to *Solanum* spp.
- Do not feed potatoes or potato refuse.

POSSIBLE COMPLICATIONS

N/A

EXPECTED COURSE AND PROGNOSIS

- With early intervention and appropriate symptomatic and supportive care, prospects for recovery are good.
- With severe clinical signs, prognosis is guarded.

MISCELLANEOUS

ASSOCIATED CONDITIONS

N/A

AGE-RELATED FACTORS

N/A

ZOONOTIC POTENTIAL

N/A

PREGNANCY

Congenital craniofacial malformations have been induced in fetuses of pregnant laboratory animals fed *Solanum* spp. glycoalkaloids. The significance of this finding for horses is unknown, but prevent pregnant mares from ingesting any *Solanum* spp.

SEE ALSO

N/A

ABBREVIATIONS

- AC = activated charcoal
- GI = gastrointestinal

Suggested Reading

Dalvi RR, Bowie WC. Toxicology of solanine: an overview. Vet Hum Toxicol 1983;25:13–15.

Author Robert H. Poppenga
Consulting Editor Robert H. Poppenga

SORBITOL DEHYDROGENASE (SDH)/IDITOL DEHYDROGENASE (IDH)

BASICS

DEFINITION

- SDH catalyzes the reversible oxidation of D-sorbitol to D-fructose with the help of NAD.
- Although present at high concentration in hepatocytes and testes, SDH is a liver-specific enzyme, with essentially all serum activity attributed to hepatocytes.
- Because of the low ALT activity in hepatocytes of horses and other large animals, SDH is the enzyme of choice for detection of recent and ongoing hepatocellular damage/necrosis.
- Reported equine values for SDH range from 1.9–6.8 U/L.

PATHOPHYSIOLOGY

- SDH is an "injury" enzyme; it escapes to the circulation when the cytoplasmic cell membrane is injured.
- The magnitude of the elevation generally is proportional to the number of hepatocytes affected, not to the severity of a particular insult. For example, an insult producing sublethal damage to many hepatocytes (e.g., diffuse hepatitis) may cause higher serum SDH levels than an insult producing lethal damage to few hepatocytes (e.g., localized abscess).
- SDH is a specific indicator of acute and ongoing hepatocellular damage because of its short half-life (a few hours) and tissue specificity.
- Activity of SDH may increase within 4 hours of a single episode of hepatocellular injury and return to the reference range within 2–3 days. In contrast, AST (also an "injury" enzyme) takes longer to peak after injury and has a half-life of several days.
- Differences in the appearance rates and half-lives of AST and SDH allow clinicians to better understand the chronology of an insult and to determine if it is ongoing.
- After hepatocellular injury, SDH increases quickly, before AST. Elevated SDH, with normal or increased AST, indicates acute or ongoing hepatocellular injury.
- If serial serum chemistries reveal continuously or progressively elevated SDH activity, ongoing hepatocellular damage is likely.
- During treatment of hepatic disease, the enzymes can be used to monitor cessation of the insult. If, after documenting recent hepatocellular injury, serial serum chemistries reveal elevated AST and progressively decreasing or normal SDH activity, cessation of the original insult is likely.

SYSTEM AFFECTED

Hepatic

SIGNALMENT

- Foals that are 2–4 weeks old may have slightly higher SDH activity compared with normal adult horses.
- Parturient mares receiving tetanus antitoxin appear to have an increased incidence of serum hepatitis, but this may simply reflect the higher incidence of antitoxin administration in this population.

SIGNS

Historical Findings

Vary with the primary disease process or insult.

Physical Examination Findings

- Vary according to the primary cause.
- Typically, horses with liver disorders may exhibit jaundice, neurologic deficits, and many other nonspecific signs—anorexia, abdominal pain, weight loss, and fever
- Horses also may present with no significant clinical signs.
- Clinical signs of hepatic failure generally do not appear until 75% of the hepatic functional mass is lost.

CAUSES

- Degenerative conditions—cirrhosis; choleliths
- Anomaly, congenital diseases—biliary atresia
- Metabolic diseases—shock, hypovolemia, hypoxia caused by severe anemia or during anesthesia, and severe GI disease
- Neoplastic or nutritional diseases—primary neoplasia, metastatic neoplasia, leukemias, and hepatic lipidosis
- Infectious and immune-mediated disease—hepatitis of various causes (e.g., viral, bacterial, protozoal, fungal, parasitic), serum sickness, amyloidosis, endotoxemia, and chronic active hepatitis
- Toxic or trauma—pyrrolizidine alkaloid–containing plants, cottonseed, castor, oaks, alsike clover, fungal toxins (e.g., aflatoxins, cyclopiazonic acid, fumonisin, phalloidin [mushrooms], rubratoxins), and blue-green algae and chemical compounds/elements (e.g., ethanol, chlorinated hydrocarbons, carbon tetrachloride, monensin, copper, iron, petroleum and its products, phosphorus).

RISK FACTORS

- Familial disease, exposure to infected animals, overweight and miniature poines, poor nutrition, or exposure to toxic compound or plants; these vary according to the specific disease.
- The anesthetic halothane is metabolized by the liver, and prolonged anesthesia has been associated with transiently increased SDH activity.
- Hypoxia during halothane anesthesia results in significantly greater evidence for hepatocellular injury than with similar hypoxia during isoflurane anesthesia.

SORBITOL DEHYDROGENASE (SDH)/IDITOL DEHYDROGENASE (IDH)

DIAGNOSIS

DIFFERENTIAL DIAGNOSIS

- The differential diagnosis list should follow that given under *Causes.*
- Complete history, physical examination, diagnostic imaging, and laboratory tests help to narrow the list to the most likely causes.
- Microscopy of fine-needle aspirates and formalin-fixed tissue biopsy specimens; bacterial, viral or fungal culture; immunologic testing; and toxicologic testing of tissue, blood, or feed may establish a definitive diagnosis.

LABORATORY FINDINGS

Drugs that May Alter Lab Results

As outlined above, a multitude of compounds may produce hepatocellular damage and lead to increased SDH; none are known to directly interfere with laboratory measurement of SDH.

Disorders that May Alter Laboratory Results

- Unlike other enzymes (e.g., AST), SDH is unstable at room temperature or when refrigerated and may lose as much as 25% of its activity during freezing after 1 week.
- If the serum or plasma sample is not analyzed within 8–12 hours, storage in a freezer is recommended.

Valid If Run in Human Lab?

Yes, if properly submitted

CBC/BIOCHEMISTRY/URINALYSIS

CBC

- Erythrocytes—liver disease may cause nonregenerative anemia and morphologic changes (e.g., acanthocytes, target cells, nonspecific poikilocytosis, normochromic microcytosis in portosystemic vascular shunts); severe anemia of any cause may cause cellular damage due to tissue hypoxia.
- Leukocytes—leukocytosis or leukopenia may be seen with inflammatory diseases and leukemias; morphologic changes of the leukocytes also may be seen (e.g., neutrophil toxicity in inflammation; neoplastic cells).
- Platelets—quantitative decreases and increases may be seen with a variety of systemic diseases that affect the liver.

Serum/Plasma Biochemistry Profile

- Various parameters may be abnormal, with the direction and magnitude of the change depending on the primary causes, severity of the disease, and other concurrent diseases or factors.
- Glucose—increased in diabetes mellitus and glucocorticoid influence (e.g., exogenous, endogenous); decreased in end-stage liver disease and sepsis/endotoxemia
- BUN—decreased in liver insufficiency and end-stage liver disease because of decreased conversion of ammonia to urea
- Albumin—decreased in end-stage liver disease because of decreased production; minimally to mildly decreased in inflammation
- Globulins—generally increased in end-stage liver disease
- AST—increased with skeletal muscle and hepatocellular injury
- ALP—increased with concurrent cholestatic disease
- GGT—increased with cholestatic disease or hepatocellular injury
- Conjugated bilirubin—increased in cholestatic disease
- Unconjugated bilirubin—increased with anorexia and prehepatic cholestasis (i.e., massive in vivo hemolysis)
- Cholesterol—may be increased with cholestasis and decreased with hepatic insufficiency; generally, cholesterol is within the reference range during liver disease.
- Triglycerides—may be increased in associatation with hepatic lipidosis.

Urinalysis

Bilirubinuria—conjugated bilirubin, detected by the commonly used "dip-stick" and the diazo tablet methods, indicates cholestatic disease and should not be elevated if only hepatocellular injury is present.

SORBITOL DEHYDROGENASE (SDH)/IDITOL DEHYDROGENASE (IDH)

OTHER LABORATORY TESTS

SBAs

- Very sensitive test for hepatobiliary disease, but not very specific for the type of disease and may be elevated with cell injury, cholestasis, or hepatic insufficiency/decreased functional mass. Specificity for the latter condition is greatly increased when SBAs are elevated with normal or minimally elevated markers for hepatocellular injury (i.e., SDH, AST, GGT) and cholestasis (i.e., ALP, GGT, conjugated bilirubin).
- The main advantage of SBAs compared with plasma ammonia (i.e., a more specific test for hepatic insufficiency/decreased functional mass) is that immediate analysis of the sample is not necessary.

Plasma Ammonia Levels

- Hepatic insufficiency/decreased functional mass is indicated by increased fasting or challenged levels of ammonia.
- A sensitive and specific test, because it is not affected by other factors (e.g., cholestasis); however, ammonia measurement requires special handling, which limits its general availability.
- Consult the reference laboratory for specific requirements.

Sulfobromophthalein and Indocyanine Green Dye Clearance

- Decreases in clearance of these dyes indicate hepatic insufficiency.
- These tests have largely been replaced by serum ammonia and SBAs.

Coagulation Tests and Fibrinogen

- The liver manufactures many coagulation factors, and significant decreases in liver function may lead to deficiencies in these factors and to coagulation abnormalities.
- Commonly used tests—APTT and PT; decreases in these parameters are seen when <30% of the activity of the factors is present.

Serologic Tests

May help in detecting an infectious cause.

Toxicology

- Analysis of tissue biopsy material, feed, ingesta, serum/plasma, or other body fluids may indicate presence of a toxin.
- Contact the reference laboratory regarding sample selection and submission.

Bacterial, Fungal or Viral Culture

- May establish a definitive diagnosis regarding the infectious agent involved and help to guide treatment.
- Request bacterial antibiotic sensitivity to determine appropriate antibiotic therapy.
- Contact the reference laboratory regarding sample selection and submission.

IMAGING

Ultrasonography

- Limited by the position and size of the liver.
- Evaluate size, echogenicity, shape, and position.
- Useful in obtaining biopsy material for cytology, histopathology, and microbiology.

Radionucleotide Imaging

- Reveals information regarding liver architecture and function.
- Expensive and available only at selected institutions.

DIAGNOSTIC PROCEDURES

- Aspiration cytology and histopathology of formalin-fixed tissue
- Cytology has the advantages of simplicity, quicker turnaround, better individual cellular detail, and better recognition of individual infectious organisms.
- Histopathology has the advantage of permitting examination of the tissue architecture and distribution of the lesion.
- The success of these procedures depends on the quality of the sample submitted, the area sampled, and the disease process itself—some hepatic diseases do not have significant microscopic alterations.

SORBITOL DEHYDROGENASE (SDH)/IDITOL DEHYDROGENASE (IDH)

TREATMENT

• Depends on the primary disease process and secondary complications.
• Choice of fluids depends on the primary cause of the disease and any metabolic imbalances (e.g., acid–base disturbances) present.

MEDICATIONS

DRUGS OF CHOICE

Depend on the primary cause of the disease and any complicating factors present.

CONTRAINDICATIONS

N/A

PRECAUTIONS

With suspected hepatic insufficiency, assess the relative safety/risk of performing invasive procedures (e.g., fine-needle aspiration, tissue biopsy, laparoscopy, surgery) in light of the coagulation panel results.

POSSIBLE INTERACTIONS

N/A

ALTERNATIVE DRUGS

N/A

FOLLOW UP

PATIENT MONITORING

Serial serum biochemical analyses to monitor progression or improvement of the disease process (see *Pathophysiology*)

POSSIBLE COMPLICATIONS

• With primary disease of infectious origin, take precautions not to contaminate the facilities and to infect other horses in the clinic or stables.
• Establish appropriate quarantine/isolation and disinfection procedures.

MISCELLANEOUS

ASSOCIATED CONDITIONS

N/A

AGE-RELATED FACTORS

See *Signalment.*

ZOONOTIC POTENTIAL

Salmonellosis

PREGNANCY

See *Signalment.*

SYNONYMS

IDH

SEE ALSO

See *Causes.*

ABBREVIATIONS

• ALT = alanine aminotransferase
• APTT = activated partial thromboplastin time
• AST = aspartate aminotransferase
• GGT = γ-glutamyltransferase
• GI = gastrointestinal
• SBA = serum bile acids
• PT = prothrombin time

Suggested Reading

Barton HM, Morris DD. In: Reed SM, Bayly WM, eds. Equine internal medicine. Philadelphia: WB Saunders, 1998.
Kramer JW, Hoffmann WE. In: Kaneko JJ, Harvey JW, Bruss ML, eds. Clinical biochemistry of domestic animals. 5th ed. San Diego: Academic Press, 1997.
Meyer DJ, Harvey JW, In: Veterinary laboratory medicine: interpretation and diagnosis. 2nd ed. Philadelphia: WB Saunders, 1998.
Tennant BD. In: Kaneko JJ, Harvey JW, Bruss ML, eds. Clinical biochemistry of domestic animals. 5th ed. San Diego: Academic Press, 1997.

Authors Armando R. Irizarry-Rovira and John A. Christian
Consulting Editor Claire B. Andreasen

SORGHUM SPP. TOXICOSIS

BASICS

OVERVIEW

- *Sorghum vulgare* var. *sudanense* (i.e., sudangrass or hybrid sudangrass) causes ataxia, cystitis, and teratogenesis in horses.
- Grazing of sudan pastures and ingestion of freshly cut hay are associated with these syndromes, but feeding of cured hay is not.
- Generally, intoxication occurs during periods of high rainfall and rapidly growing plants.
- Fertilization has no effect on toxicity.
- The toxin is believed to be a lathyrogenic agent—β-cyanoalanine
- Onset of clinical signs is after weeks to months (average, 8 weeks) of grazing a sudan pasture.
- Geographically, sudangrass most commonly is used as forage in the southwestern and central U.S.
- Ingestion of *Sorghum* spp. also is associated with cyanide and nitrate toxicoses (see *Cyanide Toxicosis* and *Nitrate Toxicosis*).

SIGNALMENT

Sorghum cystitis—ataxia is more common in mares but can occur in geldings or stallions; all ages are susceptible

SIGNS

- Posterior ataxia and incoordination
- Forced movement enhances ataxia.
- Fall when backed up
- Recumbency
- Constant urine dribbling from full bladder
- Urine scalding
- Cystitis
- Frequent opening and closing of the vulva—winking
- Mares may appear to be in constant estrus
- Fetal malformations (e.g., extreme flexion of joint, ankylosis) when mares graze sudan pastures between days 20–50 of gestation

CAUSES AND RISK FACTORS

Grazing sudan grass is the primary risk.

DIAGNOSIS

DIFFERENTIAL DIAGNOSIS

- Trauma—history; physical examination; sudden onset of clinical signs
- Neuritis of the cauda equina—automimmune neuritis (CSF evaluation, serum P2 antibody, and cranial nerve involvement)
- Spinal abscess—CSF evaluation; CBC
- Neoplasia—physical examination; imaging
- EHV-1 myeloencephalitis—signs; CSF evaluation; serology
- EPM—signs; CSF evaluation; *S. neurona* antibodies in CSF; response to treatment
- Rabies—postmortem examination; FA test

CBC/BIOCHEMISTRY/URINALYSIS

- Leukocytosis
- Lymphocytosis
- Sediment—large numbers of RBCs, WBCs, epithelial cells, bacteria, hyaline casts, and granular casts
- Normal pH and specific gravity
- Proteinuria

OTHER LABORATORY TESTS

Urine bacterial cultures generally isolate opportunistic bacteria—*Escherichia coli, Proteus vulgaris, Staphylococcus* spp., *Pseudomonas aeruginosa,* or *Corynebacterium* spp.

IMAGING

N/A

DIAGNOSTIC PROCEDURES

N/A

PATHOLOGIC FINDINGS

Gross Findings

- Cystitis with marked bladder wall thickening
- Full bladder
- Hyperemic ureters
- Hyperemic urethra
- Vaginal hyperemia
- Ulcerations of the bladder mucosa
- External abrasions from falling
- Areas of urine scalded skin
- Pyelonephritis

Histopathologic Findings

- Necrotizing cystitis
- Pyelonephritis
- Inflammation of the ureters, urethra, bladder, and vagina
- Axonal degeneration of the spinal cord and cerebellum
- Myelomalacia of the spinal cord and cerebellum

TREATMENT

- Treatment can be performed on an outpatient basis
- Generally, treatment is unsuccessful in horses that exhibit incoordination or urine dribbling.
- Temporary cure of cystitis/pyelonephritis can be achieved, but recurrence is common 2-3 weeks after therapy is stopped.
- Prevent further exposure by removing horses from access to sudan.
- Treat urine-scalded areas.
- Base antimicrobial treatment of cystitis/pyelonephritis on culture and sensitivity tests.

MEDICATIONS

DRUGS
Choose antibiotics based on culture and sensitivity tests.

CONTRAINDICATIONS/POSSIBLE INTERACTIONS
Avoid use of potentially nephrotoxic antibiotics.

FOLLOW-UP

PATIENT MONITORING
Monitor urine for evidence of bacteria/cystitis twice weekly both during and after antibiotic therapy.

PREVENTION/AVOIDANCE
Avoid exposure to sudangrass pastures.

POSSIBLE COMPLICATIONS
With severe GI ulceration and necrosis, scarring and strictures are possible.

EXPECTED COURSE AND PROGNOSIS
- Recovery of clinically affected horses is extremely rare.
- Horses that continue to have recurrent cystitis should not be used for work or riding because of residual nervous system damage.
- Horses may still be used for breeding, but cystitis, vaginitis, or urethritis can complicate breeding efforts.

MISCELLANEOUS

ASSOCIATED CONDITIONS
N/A

AGE-RELATED FACTORS
N/A

ZOONOTIC POTENTIAL
N/A

PREGNANCY
Fetal malformations (e.g., extreme flexion of joints, ankylosis) when mares graze sudan between days 20–50 of gestation

SEE ALSO
- Cyanide toxicosis
- Nitrate toxicosis

ABBREVIATIONS
- CSF = cerebrospinal fluid
- EHV = equine herpes virus
- EPM = equine protozoal myelitis
- FA = fluorescent antibody
- GI = gastrointestinal

Suggested Reading

George LW. Sorghum toxicity. In: Smith BP, ed. Large animal internal medicine. St. Louis: Mosby–Year Book, 1996:1164–1166.

Author Jeffery O. Hall

Consulting Editor Robert H. Poppenga

SPIDER ENVENOMATION

BASICS

OVERVIEW

• Localized dermatitis and pain at the spider bite in both foals and adults may result from spider envenomation.
• Horses are reportedly very sensitive to black widow (*Lactrodectus mactans* or *hesperus*) spider bites, with resultant hypertension, pain, and muscle spasms 15 minutes to 6 hours after envenomation.

SIGNALMENT

N/A

SIGNS

• Acute dermatitis characterized by heat, swelling, and pain at the bite.
• Subcutaneous edema and pain at the bite are the main clinical signs because of the small quantity of venom from spiders.
• Brown recluse (*Loxosceles reclusa*) spiders produce venom that commonly results in dermal necrosis in small animals; however, this has not been reported in horses.
• Although uncommon in horses, black widow spider bites may result in colic if the bite is in the lower extremities and in muscle spasms on the upper body if the bite is in upper extremities.
• Generalized hypertension and pain in areas of regional lymph nodes and extremities may be seen.
• Most black widow spider bites produce symptoms that peak in 3–4 hours.

CAUSES AND RISK FACTORS

• Garbage, old newspapers, old tarpaulins, and discarded furniture or farm equipment are good spider habitats.
• Spiders also may be found on the underside of ledges, rocks, and plants, or wherever a web might be strung.

DIAGNOSIS

DIFFERENTIAL DIAGNOSIS

• A localized abscess might be confused with a spider bite; actually observing a spider on the horse probably is the only way to associate a bite wound with a spider.
• Colic resulting from other causes can be confused with *Lactrodectus* spp. envenomation.

CBC/BIOCHEMISTRY/URINALYSIS

N/A

OTHER LABORATORY TESTS

N/A

IMAGING

N/A

DIAGNOSTIC PROCEDURES

N/A

TREATMENT

• Supportive and symptomatic
• Ice packs applied to the bite area may be beneficial.

MEDICATIONS

DRUGS

• Systemic glucocorticoids or antihistamines may be useful.
• Dapsone (1 mg/kg BID for 10 days) has been used for brown recluse spider envenomation.
• A black widow antivenin exists but should be used only if necessary, because it is of equine origin. If used, dilute in 50–100 mL of saline (one vial/horse) and administer IV.

CONTRAINDICATIONS/POSSIBLE INTERACTIONS

Watch the animal closely for signs of anaphylaxis if antivenin is administered.

FOLLOW-UP

PATIENT MONITORING
N/A

PREVENTION/AVOIDANCE
Clean-up potential spider habitats.

POSSIBLE COMPLICATIONS
N/A

EXPECTED COURSE AND PROGNOSIS
Recovery from a spider bite generally is within 7–14 days.

MISCELLANEOUS

ASSOCIATED CONDITIONS
N/A

AGE-RELATED FACTORS
N/A

ZOONOTIC POTENTIAL
N/A

PREGNANCY
N/A

SEE ALSO
N/A

Suggested Reading

Moriello KA, DeBoer DJ, Semrad SD. Spider bites. In: Reed SM, Bayly WM, eds. Equine internal medicine. Philadelphia: WB Saunders, 1998:550.

Author Eric L. Stair
Consulting Editor Robert H. Poppenga

SPINAL CORD TRAUMA

BASICS

DEFINITION
Trauma to the spine or associated soft tissues resulting in primary damage to the spinal cord

PATHOPHYSIOLOGY
- After a traumatic insult to the spinal cord, a cycle of cellular events occurs, including membrane disruption, ischemia, hypoxia, edema, and hemorrhage.
- The severity of these events depends on the type and extent of the initial injury.
- After trauma, changes in the spinal cord are most pronounced in the gray matter, which most likely relates to the high vascular-cell content and increased metabolic requirements for oxygen and glucose by the nerve-cell bodies in the gray matter.
- After initial injury, hemorrhage is followed by an inflammatory reaction and increased circulation time.
- Impaired blood supply to the spinal cord results in ischemia and necrotic changes in the cord.
- Initial edema and hemorrhage in the gray matter progress outward to include central necrosis, white-matter edema, and demyelination of the entire spinal cord. Mediators of this process include vasoactive monoamines, calcium, iron, copper, certain prostaglandins, and endogenous opioids. Initial hemorrhage causing hypoxia results in a shift toward anaerobic metabolism, furthering the process. Additionally, with hypoxia, inhibition of the Na^+/K^+-ATPase–dependent cell pump occurs, which is an important mechanism in development of cord edema. Damage is worse in the large myelinated motor and proprioceptive fibers compared with the nonmyelinated nociceptive fibers, therefore; ataxia and loss of proprioception and motor function occur before loss of deep pain.

SYSTEMS AFFECTED
- Musculoskeletal—spine fracture(s); postural gait abnormalities due to disruption of motor pathways; other lacerations/fractures from the traumatic episode
- Nervous—disruption of neural pathways, resulting in changes in respiratory rate and rhythm and in neurologic test results
- Respiratory—respiratory depression can occur with high cervical (C1 to C2) trauma.

GENETICS
N/A

INCIDENCE/PREVALENCE
N/A

SIGNALMENT

Species
Equine

Breed Predilections
N/A

Mean Age Range
N/A

Predominant Sex
N/A

SIGNS

Historical Findings
- Ascertain any known trauma or physical evidence of trauma to the horse or its environment.
- May have gait changes, inability to rise, or recumbency.

Physical Examination Findings
Direct the initial evaluation toward identification and stabilization of life-threatening problems—open skull fractures, airway obstruction, hemorrhage, cardiovascular collapse, pneumothorax, and other fractures

Neurologic Examination Findings
- Neurologic deficits may range from inapparent to recumbency.
- If ataxia, weakness, spasticity, or hypermetria are present without cranial nerve signs and dementia, the lesion is localized to below the foramen magnum.
- Lesions in the cervical spinal cord (C1 to C6) manifest as ataxia, weakness, and spasticity (i.e., hyperreflexia) in all four limbs, with the rear limbs being more affected.
- Lesions in the cranial intumescence (C6 to T2) manifest as profound weakness with hyporeflexia in the front limbs and hyperreflexia to normoreflexia in the rear limbs.
- Lesions from T3 to L3 manifest as mild ataxia with normal front limbs and weakness or spasticity in the rear limbs.
- Lesions in the caudal intumescence (L4 to S2) manifest as profound weakness, ataxia, and hyporeflexia in the rear limbs, with normal front limbs. These horses may assume a dog-sitting posture.
- Trauma to the peripheral nerves of the cauda equina (>S2) manifests as tail weakness, bladder atony, and perianal hypalgesia with normal gait.

CAUSES
Head trauma

RISK FACTORS
- Young age
- Fractious behavior
- Unsafe environment

DIAGNOSIS

DIFFERENTIAL DIAGNOSIS

Other Spinal Cord Disorders:

- Infection—equine herpes myeloencephalitis; bacterial meningitis
- Inflammation—polyneuritis equi
- Neoplasia
- Degenerative disease—equine degenerative myeloencephalopathy
- Parasitic diseases—equine protozoal myeloencephalitis; aberrant parasitic migration
- Spinal cord infarct
- Developmental disease—cervical vertebral stenotic myelopathy

CBC/BIOCHEMISTRY/URINALYSIS

- Changes in any of these tests may reflect changes in other organ systems secondary to the effects of trauma or due to other underlying disease processes.
- No specific changes in any of these tests for spinal cord trauma.

OTHER LABORATORY TESTS

N/A

IMAGING

- Spinal radiography may reveal fractures, luxations, and subluxations. Radiographs of other areas (e.g., long bones, chest) with evidence of trauma is warranted.
- CT or magnetic resonance imaging of the head and neck may reveal fractures, hemorrhage, or foreign bodies.
- Scintigraphy is useful in establishing the diagnosis of nondisplaced and occult fractures and of soft-tissue lesions, especially of the pelvic region.

DIAGNOSTIC PROCEDURES

- CSF analysis in cases of trauma may show xanthochromia, with mild to moderate increases in protein.
- In acute or chronic cases, CSF may be normal.
- A cisternal CSF tap is contraindicated if increased ICP is suspected due to the possibility of brain herniation.
- Nerve conduction velocities and electromyography can be used to thoroughly evaluate the lower motor neuron unit and can aid with lesion localization.

PATHOLOGIC FINDINGS

Gross and histopathologic findings may include vertebral fractures, spinal cord laceration/foreign body, hemorrhage, edema, and evidence of hypoxia.

TREATMENT

APPROPRIATE HEALTH CARE

Usually requires intensive inpatient care, often on an emergency basis.

NURSING CARE

- Treat shock first, because neurologic status may improve once shock is corrected.
- Adhere to the ABCs of trauma management.
- Monitor oxygenation with pulse oximetry, and provide supplemental oxygen as necessary.
- Institute fluid therapy to avoid hypotension.
- Overzealous administration of crystalloids (shock doses [40–90 mL/kg per hour) may exacerbate increased ICP. Possibly, use of colloids (e.g., hetastarch, dextran 70, or hypertonic saline) is preferable to restore normal blood volume while preventing increases in ICP. Use of colloids is contraindicated if hemorrhage is ongoing.
- Hypertonic saline (4–6 mL/kg IV over 15 minutes) is the preferred fluid choice in horses with spinal cord trauma and shock. Isotonic fluids then may be used for maintenance requirements (60 mL/kg per day).
- In recumbent horses, physical therapy is critical to prevent myositis, decubital sores, and hypostatic pulmonary congestion. Lubricate the eyes, and turn the horse every 2–4 hours.
- Use deep bedding.
- Hydro/massage therapy and therapeutic ultrasound are useful to maintain circulation to the large muscle groups.
- Ensure normothermia, and especially, avoid hyperthermia.

ACTIVITY

- Restricted, with strict stall confinement
- Once the horse is stable, begin controlled exercise as physical therapy/rehabilitation.

SPINAL CORD TRAUMA

DIET

- Allow access to food and water if the horse's mental status allows.
- Provide supplemental tube feedings or parenteral nutrition if the horse is unable/ unwilling to eat and drink.
- Adequate nutrition must be maintained to provide for the increased metabolic demands of the recovery period.

CLIENT EDUCATION

- The true neurologic status may not be evident for several days, and intensive and potentially costly care may be required.
- Full recovery may take months, and residual deficits may persist.
- An ataxic horse is a potential danger to humans.

SURGICAL CONSIDERATIONS

Consider intervention for displaced vertebral body fractures or subluxations and for retrieval of foreign bodies; however, the practicality of this in the horse is suspect.

MEDICATIONS

DRUGS OF CHOICE

- Reduce inflammation with corticosteroids.
- Dexamethasone (0.1–0.25 mg/kg IV q6–24h) may be used for 24–48 hours.
- Currently, high-dose methylprednisolone treatment (30 mg/kg IV followed by 12.5 mg/kg IV 2 and 6 hours after the original loading dose) within 8 hours of the traumatic insult is the steroid treatment of choice after spinal cord trauma in humans. Studies of its efficacy in horses with spinal cord trauma have not been performed, however, and such treatment would be potentially cost-prohibitive.
- Dimethyl sulfoxide (1 g/kg IV as a 10%–20% solution BID) for 3 days may help to improve blood flow and decrease edema.
- Spinal cord edema may be treated with 20% mannitol (0.25–2.0 mg/kg IV over 20 minutes) or glycerol (1 g/kg PO QID) once the horse is adequately hydrated.
- Furosemide (1–3 mg/kg IV up to four times daily) also may decrease edema and interacts synergistically with mannitol.
- Use of broad-spectrum antimicrobials (trimethoprim-sulfa [30 mg/kg]) is warranted if open fractures are present and for treating secondary complications of recumbent horses—pneumonia; decubital sores
- Management of pain should be undertaken with appropriate medications—phenylbutazone (2.2–4.4 mg/kg IV or PO BID); ketoprofen (2.2 mg/kg IV or IM QID); butorphanol (0.1 mg/kg IV or IM PRN)
- Thiamine (1 g IM QID for 5 days) may be administered to aid breakdown of lactic acid and for its action as a necessary coenzyme in neural energy pathways.
- Selenium (0.055 mg/kg IM weekly) may be of use for its antioxidant effects.
- Sedate recumbent horses that are thrashing and a potential hazard to themselves and humans with xylazine (0.3–1 mg/kg IV or IM) or detomidine (0.02–0.04 mg/kg IV or IM).

CONTRAINDICATIONS

Drugs that may increase ICP (e.g., ketamine) or cause hypertension.

PRECAUTIONS

- Avoid overzealous fluid administration, which may cause hypertension.
- Hypertonic saline may increase ICP due to its high salt content.
- Hypertonic saline and mannitol may worsen neurologic signs if used when intracranial hemorrhage is ongoing.
- Corticosteroids may increase the possibility of laminitis.
- Ulcer disease may occur with the use of NSAIDs.

POSSIBLE INTERACTIONS

N/A

ALTERNATIVE DRUGS

N/A

SPINAL CORD TRAUMA

FOLLOW-UP

PATIENT MONITORING

- Evaluate progress with serial neurologic examinations.
- Perform examinations several times a day initially, and then taper the frequency based on stability of the horse.

PREVENTION/AVOIDANCE

- Keep the area in which horses are housed free of clutter.
- Tranquilize fractious horses as necessary to perform procedures.

POSSIBLE COMPLICATIONS

- Problems associated with recumbent horses—myositis, decubital sores, corneal lacerations, hypostatic pulmonary congestion leading to pneumonia, or fecal and urine scalding
- Malnutrition, seizures, respiratory abnormalities, and death

EXPECTED COURSE AND PROGNOSIS

- The best prognosis is in horses with minimal injury that is identified early and for which prompt treatment is sought.
- Horses that show rapid improvement with stabilization of signs have a better prognosis.

MISCELLANEOUS

ASSOCIATED CONDITIONS

N/A

AGE-RELATED FACTORS

N/A

ZOONOTIC POTENTIAL

N/A

PREGNANCY

N/A

SYNONYMS

- Spinal trauma
- Traumatic spinal cord injury

SEE ALSO

- Recumbency
- Weakness
- Ataxia

ABBREVIATIONS

- CSF = cerebrospinal fluid
- ICP = intracranial pressure

Suggested Reading

Matthews HK. Spinal cord, vertebral, and intracranial trauma. In: Reed SM, Bayly WM, eds. Equine internal medicine. Philadelphia: WB Saunders, 1998:457–466.

Rucker NC. Management of spinal cord trauma. Prog Vet Neurol 1990;1:397–412.

Author Hilary K. Matthews

Consulting Editor Joseph J. Bertone

SPLENOMEGALY

BASICS

OVERVIEW

• Abnormally enlarged spleen
• Hypersplenism—characterized by splenomegaly, decrease in one or more cellular elements in the blood, and reversal by splenectomy
• Difficult to diagnosis due to marked individual animal variation in size.
• Pathophysiology depends on the underlying disease process.
• The spleen is a large, reticuloendothelial organ where blood percolates through ill-defined spaces, allowing exposure to endothelial and lymphoid cells. It filters unwanted elements from the blood, presents antigen as a major secondary lymph organ, provides hematopoietic and lymphoreticular cells through extramedullary hematopoiesis, and functions as a reserve pool for RBCs and WBCs.
• Acute splenitis—reticuloendothelial hyperplasia and infiltration of RBCs and WBCs in response primarily to blood-borne pathogens; cellular infiltrates depend on the type of offending agent and vary from mononuclear to neutrophilic.
• Hemolytic anemia—stasis of blood hyperplasia of reticuloendothelial system as macrophages increase in number and size, and giant cell formation with marked hemosiderin accumulation
• Venous congestion—venous drainage impeded by obstruction of hepatic or splenic veins and right-sided heart failure
• Infiltrative disease—accumulations of neoplastic cells or intracellular accumulations of abnormal lipids, resulting in increased splenic mass and size
• Infarction—often chronic, with necrotic cellular debris mixed with recent accumulations of erythrocytes, pigment, and organizing connective tissue; acute hematoma results in pooling of blood, with capsular thickening.

SIGNALMENT

N/A

SIGNS

Historical Findings

Vary with the underlying cause

Physical Examination Findings

• Abdominal discomfort
• Caudal and ventral displacement of the left kidney and a palpable border of the spleen within the pelvic inlet
• Pale mucous membranes, depression, anorexia, weight loss, tachypnea, tachycardia, and increased rectal temperature
• Ventral edema and edema of the peripheral limbs associated with the underlying cause

CAUSES AND RISK FACTORS

Congestive States

• Portal or splenic vascular occlusion secondary to parasites
• Right-sided congestive heart failure

Hemic/Lymphatic/Immune

• Disseminated intravascular coagulation
• Immune-mediated hemolytic anemia
• Immune-mediated thrombocytopenia
• Purpura hemorrhagica

Infectious

• Abscess
• Nonspecific blood-borne infections
• EIAV
• *Ehrlichia equi*
• *Salmonella sp.*
• Babesiosis
• Trypanosomiasis
• Anthrax
• Echinococcosis

Neoplastic

• Melanoma
• Lymphoma
• Leukemia

Idiopathic

• Primary splenomegaly
• Splenic infarction
• Splenic hematoma

Risk Factors

Residence in an area with a high incidence of equine blood-borne pathogens

DIAGNOSIS

DIFFERENTIAL DIAGNOSIS

• Primary intestinal lesion—complete work-up for abdominal pain indicated (i.e., abdominal auscultation, rectal examination, nasogastric intubation, and abdominocentesis); exploratory celiotomy when indicated by progression of disease, lack of response to analgesia, and palpable displacement
• Nephrosplenic entrapment—rectal examination; detection of large intestine along left abdominal wall with ultrasound
• Gastric distension—nasogastric intubation
• Hepatomegaly—evaluation of liver indices, abdominal ultrasound, and liver biopsy
• Abdominal abscess—CBC for increased WBC, fibrinogen, and total plasma protein; abdominocentesis for high WBC and elevated protein concentration; cytology for inflammation; culture for bacteria; and rectal examination for abdominal mass
• Abdominal tumor—sonography of all abdominal organs; work-up similar to that for abdominal abscess

CBC/BIOCHEMISTRY/URINALYSIS

• Highly variable
• Anemia
• Other abnormalities depend on the underlying cause—thrombocytopenia, leukopenia, neutropenia, lymphopenia, hyperfibrinogenemia, increased hepatic enzyme activity, and hematuria

OTHER LABORATORY TESTS

• Abdominocentesis—consistent blood contamination
• Coggins test for equine infectious anemia
• Serology for infectious agents
• Blood culture
• Fecal culture

IMAGING

• Ultrasonography to assess splenic size, detect infiltrative disease, and allow for guided biopsy
• Located on the left abdominal wall along the greater curvature of the stomach; cranial angle of dorsal extremity abuts the left kidney and seventeenth thoracic vertebrae. Apex position highly variable—usually at the ninth to eleventh rib and 4–5 inches dorsal to the costal arch; can be on the right side of the ventral midline when enlarged.
• Size—highly variable; average weight, 1 kg; average length, 50 cm; and average width, 20–25 cm
• Enlarged spleens can also be imaged transrectally
• Thoracic radiography
• Echocardiography

DIAGNOSTIC PROCEDURES

• Splenic aspiration
• Splenic biopsy and culture

TREATMENT

• Level of care depends on severity of the primary underlying disease process.
• Specific treatment recommendations for underlying disease
• Supportive care
• Splenectomy

MEDICATIONS

DRUG

• Choice depends on the underlying disease process.
• Antimicrobials
• Antiparasitics
• Anti-inflammatories

CONTRAINDICATIONS/POSSIBLE INTERACTIONS

N/A

FOLLOW-UP

PATIENT MONITORING

• Monitor splenic size by rectal palpation or sonography.
• Monitor primary disease process as indicated.

POSSIBLE COMPLICATIONS

Splenic rupture

MISCELLANEOUS

ASSOCIATED CONDITIONS

N/A

AGE-RELATED FACTORS

N/A

ZOONOTIC POTENTIAL

N/A

PREGNANCY

N/A

SEE ALSO

• Anemia
• Babesiosis
• EIAV
• Neoplasia
• Thrombocytopenia
• Trypanosomiasis

ABBREVIATION

• EIAV = equine infectious anemia virus

Suggested Reading

Jubb RVFK, Kennedy PC, Palmer N, eds. Pathology of domestic animals. 4th ed. San Diego: Academic Press, 1998.

Author Maureen T. Long
Consulting Editor Debra C. Sellon

STAPHYLOCOCCAL INFECTIONS

BASICS

DEFINITION

Infections caused by Staphylococci, which are gram-positive, facultatively anaerobic bacteria.

PATHOPHYSIOLOGY

Although *Staphylococcus* spp. are ubiquitous in nature, their preferred habitats include the skin, dermal glands, and mucous membranes of mammals and birds. The mouth, upper respiratory tract, genitourinary tract, intestinal tract, mammary glands, and blood of these hosts are also occasional sites. Strains of staphylococci are classified into two basic groups based on their ability to coagulate plasma. More than 30 coagulase-negative strains (CoNS) have been identified. CoNS species are a major component of the normal flora of humans, and until recently were not considered to be pathogenic. Now, CoNS are the most common cause of catheter-associated infection and bacteremia in human patients. Four coagulase-positive strains have been identified—*S. aureus, S. hyicus, S. intermedius,* and *S. xylosus. Staphylococcus hyicus* is primarily a problem in swine and *S. intermedius* is generally considered a canine pathogen, but both have been cultured from skin lesions of equines. *Staphylococcus aureus* (SA) is the most common secondary invader of skin lesions and wounds in many species. It is a very effective opportunist, producing numerous toxins and enzymes that encourage survival. SA also has a significant ability to acquire or develop resistance to antimicrobials and antiseptics. It is a prevalent member of the normal flora of humans and is commonly associated with post-operative and nosocomial infection in hospitalized humans. A wide range of infections is associated with SA in humans, including dermatoses, wound and incisional infections, invasive infections (bacteremia, pneumonia, phlebitis, osteomyelitis, endocarditis, meningitis, etc.), and toxin-associated syndromes. In human medicine, antibiotic resistance of all microbes has increased in direct proportion to the use of antibiotics. SA strains resistant to all antibiotics except vancomycin are now widespread in humans. Resistance to methicillin (methicillin-resistant SA, or MRSA) and other classes of antibiotics has been identified in strains of SA from equines at several veterinary schools in the last few years. Although these strains are still susceptible to some antibiotics, these drugs are frequently quite costly or are not acceptable for systemic use. Because SA is not a prevalent member of the normal flora of the equine, it is theorized that these equine isolates probably originated in humans. If veterinary medicine follows the human example, antibiotic resistance to the remaining sensitive classes of drugs will gradually develop if control measures are not instituted.

SYSTEMS AFFECTED

Staphylococcus aureus, and occasionally *S. intermedius* or *S. hyicus,* are frequently cultured from skin lesions of horses, especially folliculitis or furunculosis and granulomatous masses known as *pseudomycetoma* or *botryomycosis.* Traumatic wounds and post-operative incisional infections are also frequent sites of secondary infection with SA. It is the most commonly isolated organism in cases of cellulitis of the lower limb and iatrogenic septic arthritis. Nosocomial infection has been identified in a series of cases in at least two veterinary schools and a breeding facility in Japan. Most cases involved secondary infection of wounds or surgical incisions, but also included thrombophlebitis, respiratory sites, and metritis.

INCIDENCE/PREVALENCE

Not established

SIGNALMENT

No breed, sex, or age is predisposed to infection with staphylococci.

SIGNS

Historical Findings

Weather changes and some seasons or climates may be associated with some dermatoses. Previous antibiotic or other therapies may have been given with skin and wound infections. Sometimes there is no history of a wound, or an injury can be very difficult to find in some cases of cellulitis.

Physical Examination Findings

The first sign of folliculitis or furunculosis may be raised tufts of hair; early lesions often are more easily palpated than seen. Papules and pustules of varying sizes eventually develop; these rupture and become small ulcers or erosions with variable amounts of crusts and exudate. The lesions may be painful, but patients are not usually pruritic or febrile. Tail pyoderma and pastern dermatitis are cases of folliculitis/furunculosis specific to these areas. Isolated masses that are actually clusters of firm nodules with purulent cores containing white granules are seen with pseudomycetoma. These are usually located in subcutaneous tissue of the face or limbs, but may occur in any organ. The stump of the spermatic cord has been affected in geldings. Acute swelling of a limb and severe lameness is seen with cellulitis; patients are often febrile and may be depressed and tachycardic. Ulceration and skin slough are common. Signs of post-operative incisional or wound infection with staphylococci include heat, pain, swelling, redness, and drainage that begins as serous but becomes purulent. Local cellulitis, abscessation, and dissemination to other organs can follow.

STAPHYLOCOCCAL INFECTIONS

CAUSES AND RISK FACTORS

Disruption of normal skin defenses must be present to develop staphylococcal dermatoses. Minor trauma or maceration from water, sweat, abrasions, cuts, punctures, insect bites, rubbing, scratching, topical medications, tack, or harness may be involved. Poor grooming practices, poor sanitation, lack of dry housing, and exposure to fomites may also predispose to staph infections of the skin. Lack of aseptic techniques in performing surgery or handling wounds provides exposure for wounds and surgical sites. Immunocompromise, antibiotic therapy, or exposure to human carriers or environments contaminated with strains of MRSA may predispose to infection with resistant staphylococci. The presence of an IV catheter predisposes to thrombophlebitis.

DIAGNOSIS

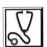

DIFFERENTIAL DIAGNOSIS

Dermatoses

- Dermatophilosis
- Corynebacterial abscessation/folliculitis
- Allergic dermatitis
- Dermatomycosis
- Pemphigus foliaceous

Pseudomycetoma

- Eosinophilic granuloma
- Pythiosis
- Habronemiasis
- Sarcoid

Cellulitis

- Vasculitides
- Lymphangitis

CBC/BIOCHEMISTRY/URINALYSIS

May be normal or may show a leukocytosis and hyperfibrinogenemia; anemia with chronic infection. Other changes correspond to areas affected.

OTHER LABORATORY TESTS

N/A

DIAGNOSTIC PROCEDURES

Microscopic examination of impression smears of crusts or exudate may identify *Dermatophilus congolensis.* Skin scrapings and fungal cultures are useful for dermatophytes. Histopathology is very useful for severe acute or chronic skin conditions and mass lesions. Gram staining and microbiologic culture of exudate or tissues should be performed whenever bacterial infection is suspect. Species identification should be requested for staphylococci. Antibiotic sensitivity testing should be performed to identify local trends. Methicillin or oxacillin should be included to rule in/out MRSA. Histopathologic analysis of biopsies may be useful in cellulitis cases to identify the presence of vasculitis. Other tests may be useful for invasive infections (e.g., tracheal wash for pneumonia, ultrasound and blood culture for thrombophlebitis, abdominocentesis for peritonitis).

IMAGING

Ultrasound and radiographs of areas with wounds or cellulitis may identify a primary lesion, foreign bodies, or damage to deeper tissues and bone. Ultrasound is very useful to determine the extent of thrombophlebitis.

TREATMENT

Improvement or change in management or the horse's environment that may predispose to skin damage is necessary for resolution of staphylococcal infections, especially dermatoses of the limbs. Shelter with dry, clean bedding is essential for healing of pastern dermatitis. Mild cases of folliculitis may resolve spontaneously or with improved grooming and hygiene. Local therapy is very important for dermatoses and cellulitis. Clipping, bathing with povidone–iodine, chlorhexidine, or benzoyl peroxide shampoos, and drying affected areas may be all the therapy necessary for localized dermatitis. Some cases of pastern dermatitis may have large areas with thick crust and exudate that is difficult to remove. Initial cleaning followed by generous application of antibiotic ointment under a soft bandage for a few days may soften the area and allow more thorough removal. Mupirocin ointment has recently been reported to be efficacious against staph infections with pastern dermatitis. Complete surgical removal and specific antibiotic therapy for several weeks are necessary for resolution of the masses seen with pseudomycetoma. Aggressive intervention is necessary in cellulitis cases. Frequent hydrotherapy for swelling, and debridement and lavage of ulcerated or sloughed areas may be needed initially. Bandaging of limbs is important to decrease damage to soft tissues, which can result in permanent scarring and

STAPHYLOCOCCAL INFECTIONS

thickening of limbs. Limbs should remain bandaged several weeks to months beyond resolution of inflammation and major swelling to discourage recurrent filling of the limb and permanent thickening of the areas involved. Skin grafts may be necessary in cases with severe skin slough. Wound and incisional infections must be opened, drained, and undergo debridement when necessary.

MEDICATIONS

Staphylococci found in skin infections may still be sensitive to a wide range of antibiotics. Those found in wounds and invasive infections are usually resistant to penicillin and some are resistant to multiple antibiotics. Broad-spectrum antibiotic therapy such as penicillin and an aminoglycoside or trimethoprim–sulfonamide should be instituted initially in severe dermatoses, pseudomycetoma, cellulitis, and wound infections. Results of culture and sensitivity should guide further therapy. Because staphylococci can be associated with significant tissue damage, exudate, and abscessation, drugs that maintain activity in such environments may be more effective. Although MRSA strains identified in horses may still be sensitive to several antibiotics, only a few of these are feasible for use; others are quite costly. Sensitivity to trimethoprim–sulfonamide combinations, erythromycin, ceftiofur, and gentocin is quite variable. Most are sensitive to amikacin, enrofloxacin, and sometimes chloramphenicol. Rifampin is very effective but cannot be used alone, as resistance develops quickly. Vancomycin is effective, but this drug is not without side effects and is very expensive. NSAIDs should be used for their anti-inflammatory and analgesic effects. Regional nerve blocks or epidurals may be helpful in cellulitis cases if weight bearing is limited.

CONTRAINDICATIONS/POSSIBLE INTERACTIONS

Rifampin is a potent inducer of microsomal enzymes of the liver, whereas erythromycin inhibits these systems. Serum levels of other drugs given concurrently may be affected. Enrofloxacin has been associated with cartilage damage in young foals. Renal function should be monitored in patients treated with aminoglycosides. Allergic sensitivities to some topical therapies may be seen in some horses.

FOLLOW-UP

PATIENT MONITORING

Temperature should be monitored in patients with wound or invasive infections or cellulitis. Persistent fever or fever spikes are indicative of inadequate response to therapy or dissemination of infection. Biopsy of recurrent dermatoses is indicated if initial therapy is not effective.

POSSIBLE COMPLICATIONS

Bone sequestra and laminitis in the affected or contralateral limb has been seen in cases of severe cellulitis. Complications following invasive infection with MRSA depend on the site affected. Thrombophlebitis has been associated with bacteremia and dissemination to other sites, including the lung, spinal cord and meninges, and liver.

PREVENTION/AVOIDANCE

Regular grooming/cleaning of the haircoat and skin may help prevent some dermatoses. A gentle touch and the use of nonabrasive equipment may be helpful. Access to dry areas in the winter and regular cleaning of stalls or sheds/open barns where horses congregate can prevent pastern dermatitis. Thorough handwashing has been shown to prevent transmission of staphylococci in humans. Masks and gloves may be necessary for caretakers with colonization by resistant SA. Cellulitis might be prevented by regular examination of limbs for minor injuries and appropriate first aid.

EXPECTED COURSE AND PROGNOSIS

Prognosis is good for dermatoses and superficial wound infection, but is guarded for cellulitis and invasive infections, especially if MRSA is present.

MISCELLANEOUS

ZOONOTIC POTENTIAL

Humans are susceptible to colonization with staphylococcal organisms from contact with horses. Colonization does not necessarily result in infection.

SEE ALSO

Septic arthritis

ABBREVIATIONS

- CoNS = coagulase-negative staphylococci
- MRSA = methicillin resistant *Staphylococcus aureus*
- SA = *Staphylococcus aureus*

Suggested Reading

Panlilio AL, Culver DH, et al. Methicillin-resistant staphylococcus aureus in US hospitals, 1975–1991. Infect Contrl Hosp Epidem 1992;13:582-586.

Adams, JG. Nosocomial infection with MRSA in veterinary patients. Proc ACVIM. May 1998:185-187.

Archer GL. *Staphylococcus aureus:* a well-armed pathogen. Clin Inf Dis 1998;26:1179-1181.

Scott DW. Staphylococcal skin diseases. In: Robinson NE, ed. Current therapy in equine medicine III. Philadelphia, WB Saunders, 1992:701-702.

Markel MD. Cellulitis associated with coagulase-positive staphylococci in racehorses: nine cases (1975–1984). JAVMA 1986;189:1600-1603.

Scott DW. Bacterial pseudomycosis (botryomycosis) in the horse. Eq Prac 1988;10:15-19.

Evans AG. Diagnostic approach to equine skin disease. Comp Cont Ed Pract Vet 1986;8:652-661.

Fadok VA. An overview of equine dermatoses characterized by scaling and crusting. In: VA Fadok, ed. Vet Clin N Am Eq Prac Derm 1995;11:43-51.

Rosenkrantz WS. Systemic/topical therapy. In: VA Fadok, ed. Vet Clin N Am Eq Prac Derm 1995;11:127-146.

Author Jennifer Adams

Consulting Editor Corinne R. Sweeney

STATIONARY NIGHT BLINDNESS

BASICS

OVERVIEW

• A disease of the outer or middle retina that is present at birth and persists throughout life
• Rod photoreceptors, which are responsible for vision at low levels of light (i.e., scotopic vision) are affected more severely than cone photoreceptors, which allow vision in daylight (i.e., photopic vision).
• Organ system—ophthalmic

SIGNALMENT

• Breed—Appaloosa, but also Thoroughbred, Paso Fino, and Standardbred
• No known sex-predilection
• Age—present at birth and persists throughout life

SIGNS

• Visual impairment in dim light with generally normal vision in daylight; behavioral uneasiness and unpredictability occurring at night despite normal ophthalmoscopic examination.
• Foals may appear disoriented, stare off into space, and have a bilateral dorsomedial strabismus.
• Owners may report repeated injuries during the evening hours.
• Poor day or photopic vision can occur in a few cases.
• In mild cases, the disease is not observable until weaning, when the mare's guidance no longer is available. Some foals appear clumsy, and a vision problem is not suspected until 1 year of age.
• If visual disturbance is not obvious in normal lighting, observe the horse in a dark area.

CAUSES AND RISK FACTORS

Congenital, sex-linked recessive trait in Appaloosas

DIAGNOSIS

DIFFERENTIAL DIAGNOSIS

Rule out other congenital and acquired blinding disorders of the retina, optic nerve, and brain—colobomas, retinal detachments, and chorioretinitis; in the latter diseases, visual impairment is not limited to dim light.

CBC/BIOCHEMISTRY/URINALYSIS

N/A

OTHER LABORATORY TESTS

N/A

IMAGING

N/A

DIAGNOSTIC PROCEDURES

• Ophthalmoscopy—the ocular fundi appear normal.
• Electroretinography is required for a definitive diagnosis. Decreased b-wave amplitude and a large, negative, monotonic a-wave potential in the scotopic flash ERG confirm the presence of night blindness. The photopic flash ERG shows reduced amplitude and increased implicit b-wave time.

PATHOLOGIC FINDINGS

Histologically, the affected retina is normal; subtle microphthalmos may occur.

STATIONARY NIGHT BLINDNESS

TREATMENT

None.

MEDICATIONS

DRUGS

N/A

CONTRAINDICATIONS/POSSIBLE INTERACTIONS

N/A

FOLLOW-UP

PREVENTION/AVOIDANCE

Do not use affected horses for breeding.

POSSIBLE COMPLICATIONS

In a very few cases, progression to poor photopic or day vision

EXPECTED COURSE AND PROGNOSIS

- The disease rarely progresses.
- Horses can undergo training and perform well during the day.

MISCELLANEOUS

SEE ALSO

- Chorioretinitis
- Ocular problems in the neonate—congenital, inherited, and acquired
- Optic neuropathy
- Progressive retinal atrophy
- Retinal detachment

ABBREVIATION

- ERG = electroretinogram

Suggested Reading

Brooks DE. Equine ophthalmology. In: Gelatt KN, ed. Veterinary ophthalmology. 3rd ed. Philadelphia: Lippincott Williams & Wilkins, 1999.

Author Andras M. Komaromy
Consulting Editor Dennis E. Brooks

STREPTOCOCCUS EQUI INFECTION

BASICS

DEFINITION
Streptococcus equi infection (strangles) is an acute upper respiratory tract infection characterized by fever, lethargy, purulent rhinitis, and regional lymph node abscessation.

PATHOPHYSIOLOGY
Streptococcus equi is inhaled or ingested after direct contact with mucopurulent discharge from infected horses or contaminated equipment. It adheres to the epithelial cells of the buccal and nasal mucosa. Eventually it spreads to the regional lymph nodes, such as the submandibular, submaxillary, and retropharyngeal lymph nodes. The M protein is important for adherence of the organism to the epithelium and also protects from ingestion by polymorphonuclear leukocytes. The hyaluronic acid capsule is important in the pathogenicity by repelling phagocytic cells due to its strong negative charge. Carrier horses are responsible for maintaining the infection in affected herds. These carriers are asymptomatic, and the organism is often isolated from their guttural pouches.

SYSTEMS AFFECTED
Upper Respiratory Tract
Rhinitis

Lymphatics
• Lymphadenopathy • Lymph node abscessation, potentially in many sites, including the abdomen

INCIDENCE/PREVALENCE
Streptococcus equi occurs worldwide.

SIGNALMENT
Streptococcus equi can occur in any age group, although those between the ages of 1 and 5 years are predisposed. There is no breed or sex predilection.

SIGNS
Historical Findings
• Depression • Anorexia • Fever • Nasal discharge • Cough • Submandibular lymph node enlargement • Dyspnea (occasionally)
Also, some horses may stand with neck stretched and be reluctant to swallow.

Physical Examination Findings
Findings on physical examination are characterized by serous to mucopurulent nasal discharge and lymphadenopathy of the submaxillary, submandibular, or retropharyngeal lymph nodes. Acutely, the lymph nodes are firm, but then become fluctuant as liquefaction and suppuration develop. Eventually they rupture and drain. With excessive lymphadenopathy and abscessation, respiratory obstruction and dyspnea can occur.

CAUSES
The causative bacteria are *Streptococcus equi,* a gram-positive cocci.

RISK FACTORS
Young animals in crowded conditions.

DIAGNOSIS

DIFFERENTIAL DIAGNOSIS
Other causes of nasal discharge include:
• Influenza • EHV-1 and EHV-4
• Rhinovirus • Other viruses (adenovirus, reovirus, ehv-2) • Pharyngitis • Chronic pharyngeal lymphoid hyperplasia • Nasal/paranasal sinus infection/cysts/polpys/tumors
• Early bacterial pneumonia/pleuirits • Guttural pouch infection/mycosis • Overflow of nasolacrimal ducts • Chronic obstructive pulmonary disease
Other causes of fever would include any disease that causes inflammation.
Other causes of lymphadenopathy and abscessation include:
• Lymphoma • Upper respiratory tract infection • *C. pseudotuberculosis* lymphadenitis • Bacterial endocarditis
• Ulcerative/epizootic/sporadic lymphadenitis • Glanders • Plasma cell myeloma
• Tuberculosis • Hemolytic–uremic-like syndrome
The diagnosis of strangles is based on the classic clinical signs, especially lymphadenopathy with abscessation and rupture. Confirmation is by isolation of *S. equi* from nasal or lymph node discharge. If it looks like strangles, then treat it like strangles.

CBC/BIOCHEMISTRY/URINALYSIS
A neutrophilic leukocytosis, hyperfibrinogenemia, and possibly an anemia of chronic disease. Serum biochemistry and urinalysis are normal. Any abnormalities may indicate complications.

OTHER LABORATORY TESTS
Streptococcus equi can be isolated from cultures of draining lymph nodes or nasal and pharyngeal swabs. The lymph node culture yields a higher isolation rate. Also, aspirate or biopsy from lymph nodes may isolate the organism.

IMAGING
Typically not performed in uncomplicated cases of strangles, although may be useful in cases of severe lymphadenopathy that result in respiratory obstruction or complicated/atypical strangles. In these cases, radiographs of the skull or laryngeal region may be helpful to assess the extent of the lymphadenopathy. Endoscopy of the upper respiratory tract or guttural pouches may also be useful. In cases of complicated strangles, ultrasound, radiographs, and echocardiography of the appropriate system may assist in the diagnosis.

PATHOLOGIC FINDINGS
Hyperplastic lymph nodes with increased numbers of neutrophils, monocytes, and macrophages, which are all due to antigenic stimulation. Also, gram-positive cocci are present. Nasal lesions are characterized by edematous, hyperemic, and occasionally ulcerated mucosa with a variable amount of creamy yellow exudate. In cases of complicated strangles the pathologic findings are variable, depending on the organ system involved.

TREATMENT

APPROPRIATE HEALTH CARE
Horses affected or suspected of being affected should be quarantined immediately. Treatment of horses with strangles depends on the stage of the disease in each individual. Typically the disease has been characterized with four stages, which include horses with early clinical signs, horses with regional lymph node abscessation, horses exposed to strangles, and horses with complications. Horses with early clinical signs often are febrile, anorexic, depressed, and have purulent nasal discharge. The progression of the disease, including submaxillary, submandibular, and retropharyngeal lymph node abscessation, can be arrested with the appropriate antimicrobial treatment. This may be an effective way of controlling outbreaks in stables with horses that show early clinical signs. However, if the horse remains exposed to infected horses, there is a high probability of relapse following cessation of therapy. Protective immune responses are poor in antimicrobially treated horses; thus they are susceptible to infection on future exposure.
Horses with regional lymph node abscessation generally require therapy aimed at enhancing maturation and drainage of the abscesses. Recommended procedures include isolation of the sick horse, local application of hot packs and poultices to the abscess, and if needed, lancing of the abscess to allow for better drainage. Once an abscess begins to drain, it should be flushed regularly. Most veterinarians would agree that antimicrobial therapy slows the progression of lymph node abscessation, and therefore is not beneficial at this time.
Horses with advanced signs, such as prolonged fever, anorexia, depression, lethargy, or dyspnea, warrant systemic antimicrobial treatment. Rarely do affected horses require intensive supportive therapy.

Horses that have been exposed to *S. equi* can be treated with antimicrobials in the hopes of preventing "seeding" of the pharyngeal lymph nodes. Ideally, therapy should be continued until the affected horses are isolated. If the horse is still exposed when the antimicrobials are discontinued, infection may then develop. Horses that develop complications from *S. equi* must receive therapy directed at treatment of the specific problem. Usually, these horses require high levels of antimicrobials.

NURSING CARE

Minimal unless respiratory obstruction or complications occur. In those cases with lymph node abscessation, regular hot packing, poulticing, or flushing may be required.

ACTIVITY

Usually limited because the horse should be quarantined.

CLIENT EDUCATION

Usually responds well to treatment, although complications due to spread of the organism can occur.

SURGICAL CONSIDERATIONS

An abscessed lymph node may need to be lanced to allow for proper drainage, especially if it is causing respiratory obstruction.

MEDICATIONS

DRUG(S) OF CHOICE

Penicillin provides adequate gram-positive coverage. Dose: 22,000–44,000 IU/kg IM q12h of procaine penicillin or IV q6h of aqueous potassium penicillin.

Lanced or draining abscessed lymph nodes can be flushed with 2% iodine solution.

NSAIDs, such as flunixin meglumine, may be required to reduce pain and fever.

Horses with complications may need additional drug therapy directed at the specific problem.

ALTERNATIVE DRUGS

Most antimicrobials that provide good gram-positive coverage could theoretically be administered.

FOLLOW-UP

PATIENT MONITORING

In cases of uncomplicated strangles, response to therapy can be noted by resolution of clinical signs. Temperature, attitude, and appetite must be noted several times a day. Leukocyte response and fibrinogen can be monitored every 3–4 days, but generally this is not needed.

In cases of complicated strangles, patient monitoring depends on the severity of the disease and the system affected.

PREVENTION/AVOIDANCE

Non-immunologic strategies of control include the following recommendations: Isolation of new horses for 2–3 weeks, with close observation for signs of strangles or any disease. Temperature should be monitored at least twice daily. Affected horses or horses suspected of being affected should be quarantined immediately, with isolation of all equipment and tools, that were in contact with these animals. People who care for the infected horses should avoid any contact with healthy horses. Those horses that were in contact with the affected horses should be observed closely for signs of disease and have their temperatures monitored. The appropriate disinfectants, including phenols, iodophores, and chlorhexidine compounds, should be used to destroy the *S. equi* organism.

Several vaccines are available but do not guarantee the prevention of strangles. The level of immunity stimulated by these vaccines is lower than that produced during recovery from the disease because of failure to provide local protection. Natural infection causes a rise in both systemic and local antibodies, whereas vaccine only causes a rise in systemic antibodies. Currently, the following systemic vaccines are available: Equibac II (a killed suspension of *S. equi* in aluminum hydroxide gel), Strepvax (concentrated M-protein extract of *S. equi*), and Strepquard (purified M-protein extract of *S. equi*). These vaccines tend to cause injection-site reactions; therefore, routine administration is not performed unless there is a persistent endemic problem on the farm. An intranasal vaccine (Pinnacle, -IN) contains a live strain of *S. equi* that is antigenic, but has low pathogenicity.

POSSIBLE COMPLICATIONS

In the majority of the horses with strangles, the disease runs its course and the horse recovers uneventfully. Complications have been reported in about 20% of the cases.

Atypical or bastard strangles results when *S. equi* metastasize to other lymph nodes or body systems. These abscesses can occur anywhere in the body, but more common locations include the lungs, mesentery, liver, spleen, kidney, and brain. Retropharyngeal lymph node abscessation can occur, and horses may present in respiratory distress due to upper respiratory tract obstruction. These cases may require a tracheostomy. Also, laryngeal hemiplegia may be noted as a result of the involvement of the recurrent laryngeal nerve. Suppurative necrotic bronchopneumonia can result from either aspiration of pus from the upper respiratory tract or metastatic spread to the lungs. Guttural pouch empyema is a result of pus from an abscessed lymph node draining into the guttural pouch. Other clinical signs include laryngeal hemiplegia, facial nerve palsy, and Horner's syndrome. Myocarditis can result from myocardial abscesses and endocarditis. *Purpura hemorrhagica* is an aseptic vasculitis reported in mature horses after second natural exposure to infection or after vaccination of animals that previously had strangles. Clinical signs vary from mild to life-threatening. Typical signs include pitting edema of dependent areas of the head, trunk, and extremities and petechiation and ecchymoses of mucous membranes. Therapy consists of antimicrobials, corticosteriods, and supportive care. Septicemia and the development of infectious arthritis, pneumonia, and encephalitis are also possible sequellae.

EXPECTED COURSE AND PROGNOSIS

Prognosis is good for full recovery in cases of uncomplicated strangles. The course of the disease depends on the phase of the infection.

MISCELLANEOUS

AGE-RELATED FACTORS

Horses between the ages of 1 and 5 years are immunologically naïve; therefore, they are most prone to developing the disease. Older horses have probably been exposed to the disease; therefore, they have an immune response.

Suggested Reading

Sweeney CR. Strangles: *Streptococcus equi* infection in horses. Eq Vet Educ 1996;8:317-322.

Sweeney CR, Benson CE, Whitlock RH, Meirs D, Whitehead S, Barningham S. *Streptococcus equi* infection in horses—part I. Comp Cont Educ Pract Vet 1987;9:689-694.

Sweeney CR, Benson CE, Whitlock RH, Meirs D, Whitehead S, Barningham S. *Streptococcus equi* infection in horses—part II. Comp Cont Educ Pract Vet 1987;9:845-852.

Author Bonnie S. Barr

Consulting Editor Corinne R. Sweeney

SUPERFICIAL CORNEAL EROSIONS WITH ANTERIOR STROMAL SEQUESTRATION

BASICS

OVERVIEW
• Injuries of the corneal epithelium that do not penetrate the basement membrane and that can progress to deeper ulcers once the basement membrane is injured
• Superficial erosions commonly are associated with protein deposits in the anterior stroma.
• Organ system—ophthalmic

SIGNALMENT
All ages and breeds

SIGNS
• Chronic, superficial corneal erosions have an opalescent, grayish color; display faint retention of fluorescein dye; and may have thin, undulating, acellular stromal surface membranes.
• Erosions are surrounded by a loose lip of migrating, nonattached epithelium; corneal vascularization; and crystalline stromal deposits.
• Slight uveitis

CAUSES AND RISK FACTORS
• Unknown
• Possible primary corneal disease with chronic secondary irritation, such as secondary to acute corneal ulceration from rubbing of a silicone, subpalpebral lavage system

DIAGNOSIS

DIFFERENTIAL DIAGNOSIS
• Lid abnormalities—distichiasis, trichiasis, and entropion; neuroparalytic and neurotrophic keratitis; keratoconjunctivitis sicca; corneal dystrophies; and corneal foreign bodies
• Inappropriate topical corticosteroid therapy causing delayed corneal healing

CBC/BIOCHEMISTRY/URINALYSIS
N/A

OTHER LABORATORY TESTS
Rule out infectious causes (bacterial or fungal) with corneal scrapings for cytology and culture.

IMAGING
N/A

DIAGNOSTIC PROCEDURES
N/A

PATHOLOGIC FINDINGS
• Ulceration with a thin membrane of altered corneal stroma, representing corneal stromal sequestration
• Lack of epithelial migration or attachment onto the ulcerated surface

TREATMENT
• Epithelial debridement of the loose lip of epithelium
• Superficial grid keratotomy for debridement of ulcers and disruption of superficial membrane
• Postoperative—temporary partial tarsorrhaphy to prevent trauma to ulcers from blepharospasm
• Contact lenses act as bandages.

SUPERFICIAL CORNEAL EROSIONS WITH ANTERIOR STROMAL SEQUESTRATION

MEDICATIONS

DRUGS

- Topical serum q4h
- Topical polysulfated glycosaminoglycans—Adequan™ (diluted with artificial tears solution to 50mg/mL TID)
- Topical broad-spectrum antibiotics—chloramphenicol, bacitracin-neomycin-polymyxin

CONTRAINDICATIONS/POSSIBLE INTERACTIONS

- Topical gentamicin may slow corneal healing.
- Use solutions and not ointments.

FOLLOW-UP

EXPECTED COURSE AND PROGNOSIS

- Lavage system–induced ulcers are notoriously slow to heal.
- Infection is a risk due to epithelial loss.
- Scarring of the cornea may result.

MISCELLANEOUS

ASSOCIATED CONDITIONS

- Infection
- Uveitis

AGE-RELATED FACTORS

N/A

ZOONOTIC POTENTIAL

N/A

PREGNANCY

N/A

SEE ALSO

- Burdock pappus bristle keratopathy
- Calcific band keratopathy
- Corneal laceration
- Corneal stromal abscessation
- Corneal ulceration
- Eosinophilic keratitis
- ERU
- Glaucoma
- Herpes keratitis
- Keratomycosis
- Limbal keratopathy
- Nonulcerative keratouveitis

ABBREVIATION

- ERU = equine recurrent uveitis

Suggested Reading

Brooks DE. Equine ophthalmology. In: Gelatt KN, ed. Veterinary ophthalmology. 3rd ed. Philadelphia: Lippincott Williams & Wilkins, 1999.

Author Andras M. Komaromy
Consulting Editor Dennis E. Brooks

SYNCHRONOUS DIAPHRAGMATIC FLUTTER (SDF)

BASICS

OVERVIEW

- A contraction of the diaphragm that is synchronous with the heartbeat
- Also known as "thumps"
- Results from hyperexcitability of the phrenic nerve secondary to fluid and electrolyte imbalance; the electric impulse generated from atrial depolarization stimulates the phrenic nerve and causes diaphragmatic contraction.
- Commonly observed in endurance horses exercising in hot, humid conditions.

SIGNALMENT

Any breed, age, or sex

SIGNS

Historical Findings

- Often a recent history of prolonged exercise accompanied by intense sweating
- Also associated with GI disease, lactation tetany, transportation, and trauma

Physical Examination Findings

- Pathognomonic sign—a spasmodic contraction of the flank that is synchronous with the first heart sound.
- Flank movements are associated with diaphragmatic contractions and are independent of the normal respiratory cycle.
- Flank twitching may not occur with every heartbeat, but when it does, it is always associated with atrial depolarization.
- Strong contractions may produce a thumping noise, which has led to name "thumps."

CAUSES AND RISK FACTORS

- Electrolyte and acid–base imbalances may increase phrenic nerve excitability. The equine phrenic nerve runs over the right atrium, allowing it to produce an action potential when stimulated by atrial depolarization. In addition, physical irritation of the nerve through the pericardium may induce SDF.
- Hypocalcemia, hypokalemia, and alkalosis, either individually or in combination, have been associated with SDF. Excessive sweating, GI disturbances, transportation, lactation tetany, furosemide therapy, urethral obstruction, and hypoparathyroidism may cause these electrolytic abnormalities. Equine sweat is hypertonic and may lead to substantial amounts of lost electrolytes, particularly sodium, chloride, potassium, and calcium.
- Hypocalcemia increases the excitability of nerve and muscle cells by lowering the depolarization threshold.
- Hypokalemia increases the resting membrane potential of cells and results in increased nerve excitability.
- Alkalosis, which often is accompanied by hypokalemia, increases albumin binding of calcium and results in a decreased ionized calcium concentration.

DIAGNOSIS

DIFFERENTIAL DIAGNOSIS

- Rather than a disease, SDF is a clinical manifestation of deranged electrolyte levels and acid–base status; therefore, many diseases may be associated.
- Hiccups and nonsynchronous diaphragmatic flutter have been observed, but in these cases, diaphragmatic twitching is not synchronous with cardiac contraction.
- Forceful contractions of the abdominal muscles may accompany severe respiratory disease (e.g., heaves, pneumonia). Affected horses present with obvious signs of respiratory disease, however, and each abdominal contraction is associated with expiration, not with a heartbeat.

CBC/BIOCHEMISTRY/URINALYSIS

- Hypocalcemia, hypokalemia, and alkalosis are the most common metabolic abnormalities.
- Serum ionized calcium concentration is more accurate than total calcium concentration to diagnose hypocalcemia.

OTHER LABORATORY TESTS

Blood gas analyses help to assess acid–base status.

IMAGING

N/A

DIAGNOSTIC PROCEDURES

The diagnosis can be confirmed by simultaneously recording the electrocardiogram and the diaphragmatic contractions, either manually or with electromyography or phonocardiography.

PATHOLOGIC FINDINGS

Lesions relate to the primary associated disease, not to SDF itself.

SYNCHRONOUS DIAPHRAGMATIC FLUTTER (SDF)

TREATMENT

Aimed at the underlying condition.

MEDICATIONS

DRUGS

- Oral or parenteral administration of balanced electrolyte solutions is beneficial and often sufficient to correct electrolytic abnormalities.
- Hypocalcemia may be corrected by IV infusion of 20% calcium-borogluconate solution.
- Administration of isotonic-saline solution helps to correct metabolic alkalosis and hypokalemia.
- Cases in horses with excessive sweating may be corrected by oral or parenteral administration of solutions containing sodium, chloride, potassium, and calcium.

CONTRAINDICATIONS/POSSIBLE INTERACTIONS

Excessive administration of alkalinizing solutions (e.g., bicarbonate) may worsen clinical signs by decreasing available free calcium.

FOLLOW-UP

PATIENT MONITORING

Monitor electrolytes, acid–base status, and clinical signs.

PREVENTION/AVOIDANCE

- When large electrolyte losses are anticipated (e.g., endurance ride), administer electrolytes before, during, and after losses occured.
- Avoid excessive calcium supplementation as a prophylactic measure, because it reduces parathyroid hormone secretion and may impair rapid mobilization of calcium from bone when needed.

POSSIBLE COMPLICATIONS

Electrolyte abnormalities may lead to ileus, muscle weakness, and cardiac arrhythmia.

EXPECTED COURSE AND PROGNOSIS

SDF is not life-threatening; in most cases, it is a transient condition that resolves either spontaneously or in response to treatment of the underlying problem.

MISCELLANEOUS

ASSOCIATED CONDITIONS

- Prolonged exercise in hot, humid conditions
- Lactation
- GI disturbances

AGE-RELATED FACTORS

N/A

ZOONOTIC POTENTIAL

N/A

PREGNANCY

N/A

SEE ALSO

Hypocalcemia

ABBREVIATION

- GI = gastrointestinal

Suggested Reading

Mansmann RA, Carlson GP, White NA, Milne DW. Synchronous diaphragmatic flutter in horses. J Am Vet Med Assoc 1974; 165:265–270.

Author Laurent Couëtil
Consulting Editor Michel Levy

SYNOVIAL FLUID

BASICS

DEFINITION

- A dialysate of plasma with the addition of hyaluronan (i.e., hyaluronic acid) and certain glycoproteins
- Normal joint fluid is light yellow, clear, and free of particulate material and viscous, producing a strand $\cong$2.5 cm in length.
- Leukocyte counts usually are done manually using a hemocytometer, but they also may be done using electronic cell counters.
- Smears from normal synovial fluid have low cellularity (<500 cells/μL), consisting primarily of a mixture of small lymphocytes, macrophages, and synovial lining cells. The ratio of lymphocytes, macrophages, and synovial lining cells is variable and generally not of diagnostic significance. Many labs report all these cells collectively as mononuclear cells.
- One consistent feature of normal synovial fluid is that neutrophils should comprise <10% of the cells present. Also, few (if any) erythrocytes should be present.
- Normal synovial fluid yields a finely granular, pink background and has good mucin clot production.
- Normal values for equine synovial fluid protein vary between author and method. Upper limits of normal, as reported by various authors, generally range from 1–3 g/dL.

PATHOPHYSIOLOGY

- Synovial fluid has two functions—to provide nutrients to the avascular articular cartilage; and to act as a lubricant, limiting wear on synovial surfaces.
- Synovial fluid evaluation alone generally does not establish a specific diagnosis, but it reflects the degree and type of inflammation of the synovial lining—synovitis.
- Damage to articular cartilage often is not reflected in routine synovial fluid analysis.
- The paramount benefit of synovial fluid evaluation is detecting the presence of septic arthritis. The many causes of degenerative and traumatic joint injury cannot be differentiated based on synovial fluid evaluation.
- Gross appearance is insensitive and should not be used alone. Samples with similar gross appearance may have marked differences in cell counts and mucin clot results.

SYSTEM AFFECTED

Musculoskeletal

SIGNALMENT

Any horse

SIGNS

Historical Findings

Lameness

Physical Examination Findings

- Lameness
- Swollen joints
- Pain
- Fever

CAUSES

Degenerative/Traumatic Joint Disease

- Many conditions result in traumatic or degenerative joint injury. Associated inflammation is variable and often mild. These conditions sometimes are referred to as nonpurulent or nonsuppurative inflammation.
- Synovial fluid usually is clear, unless there is associated hemorrhage, in which case it may be red tinged.
- Viscosity may be decreased proportionately to the amount of effusion.
- Cell counts vary from normal to moderately increased, usually being <10,000 cells/μL and consisting of >90% mononuclear cells.
- Macrophages may be large and vacuolated, sometimes containing phagocytosed debris.
- Amount of inflammation can be mild, and synovial fluid results may be essentially normal.
- Low-grade degenerative changes cannot be ruled out based on normal synovial fluid analysis results.
- An increased percentage of neutrophils (>10%) may occur in some cases of acute trauma or with hemorrhage into the joint that adds peripheral blood neutrophils to the joint fluid. These conditions must not be confused with sepsis. The total nucleated cell count (and absolute number of neutrophils) generally is much less than typically seen with septic arthritis.
- Traumatic injury usually is associated with a mild (<5,000 cells/μL), predominantly mononuclear cell response, but neutrophilic responses with cell counts up to 30,000 cells/μL have been reported. These can be difficult to differentiate from septic responses, but cell counts of <50,000 cells/μL are unusual in untreated cases of septic arthritis. Also, the cell count with traumatic injury generally declines rapidly.
- Cartilage fragments may be seen in synovial fluid associated with trauma or degenerative joint disease, but this finding is uncommon.

Resolving Synovial Disease or Chronic Synovitis

- Joint disease that is resolving, especially from previous joint sepsis, may appear similar to traumatic or degenerative joint disease.
- There often is a mononuclear component with very vacuolated macrophages and variable numbers of synovial cells and lymphocytes.
- Neutrophils usually are <10% of the cell component.
- Cell counts are within normal limits to slightly increased.
- Chronic synovitis may have a predominance of macrophages/monocytes or lymphocytes.
- Lymphocytic synovial fluid reflects lymphocytic inflammation within the synovial membrane and, rarely, may have plasma cells.
- Lymphocytic synovitis has been attributed to proliferative synovitis and infectious agents.

Septic Arthritis

- A clinical emergency that causes marked changes in synovial fluid.
- Routine synovial fluid examination usually provides sufficient information to establish a presumptive diagnosis.
- Depending on the cell count, fluid color may range from a slightly cloudy, dark yellow to an opaque cream. Red to red-brown is common with inflammation-induced hemorrhage.
- Flocculent material may be apparent.
- Fluid viscosity is markedly reduced, and mucin clot tests generally are poor.
- The most significant finding is a markedly elevated nucleated cell count (usually $>50,000$ cells/μL) consisting predominantly of neutrophils (usually $>90\%$).
- Total protein concentrations also are markedly elevated, typically >4.0 g/dL.
- Bacteria are more numerous in the synovial lining than in the fluid.
- In many, if not most, cases, bacteria are not seen on cytologic examination. Lack of identifiable bacteria, however, should not diminish consideration of sepsis in fluids with markedly elevated neutrophil counts ($>50,000$ cells/μL).
- Many times, neutrophils do not show marked degenerative changes with septic arthritis. Lack of degenerative changes, however, should not diminish consideration of sepsis.

RISK FACTORS

- Septic arthritis—failure of passive transfer in neonates
- Performance horses

DIAGNOSIS

DIFFERENTIAL DIAGNOSIS

See *Causes.*

LABORATORY FINDINGS

General

- Place samples in an EDTA tube for the most important parameters—cell counts, cytology, and protein concentration
- If only a small amount (<0.25 mL) of fluid can be retrieved, make and submit air-dried direct smears.
- Placing extremely small quantities of fluid in an EDTA tube results in excessive dilution of the sample and, possibly, in a falsely increased total protein concentration (if determined by refractometry) resulting from EDTA as a solute.

Physical Characteristics

- Color, clarity, and an estimate of viscosity are noted.
- Viscosity may be estimated by placing a drop of synovial fluid between the thumb and forefinger, slowly pulling the fingers apart, and evaluating the strand length before breaking. Alternatively, strand length before breaking can be noted as synovial fluid is expelled through the tip of a needle.
- Normal synovial fluid may gel on standing, appearing to have clotted, but will return to a liquid state on warming and agitation.

Leukocyte Count (WBC)

- Cell counts often are too low to be accurately determined with an electronic cell counter.
- Leukocyte counts are subject to sources of analytic error and must not be interpreted too strictly when comparing serial counts.
- Markedly exudative samples (e.g., from septic joints) with dramatically elevated leukocyte counts ($>50,000$ cells/μL) often contain numerous cell clumps that preclude an accurate cell count.
- Fluctuations of up to 70,000 cells/μL within a 24-hour period have been reported in studies of septic arthritis. This probably represents a combination of true changes in cell concentration as well as analytic variation.
- Samples of low cellularity are subject to a different source of error. In samples with normal viscosity, cell counts may be falsely low, because the sample fails to mix evenly with the diluent. A greater-than-twofold increase in nucleated cell count has been reported by treating samples with hyaluronidase before enumeration. Despite these difficulties, samples with normal, mildly elevated, and markedly elevated cells counts can be reliably differentiated.
- If a diluent system is used (e.g., Unopette system) along with a hemocytometer, avoid use of a product containing acetic acid as a diluent, because acetic acid causes precipitation of the mucin in synovial fluid.

Erythrocyte Count

- Erythrocyte counts are obtained from electronic cells counters or hemocytometers if a diluent that does not lyse erythrocytes is used.
- Erythrocytes indicate contamination during sample collection or hemorrhage secondary to hemostatic abnormalities, traumatic injury, or inflammatory disease.
- Marked blood contamination increases the nucleated cell count and alters the differential leukocyte count, usually increasing the percentage of neutrophils.

Cytology

- Along with nucleated cell count, probably the most diagnostically important parameter of synovial fluid evaluation
- With a limited sample, direct smears, from which the cell count could be estimated, should be made first.
- Blood contamination, in additional to adding RBCs, can add various leukocytes in proportions typical of peripheral blood (i.e. predominantly neutrophils). Therefore, blood contamination can increase the percentage of neutrophils observed. The person examining the slide should give a subjective assessment regarding whether any increase in the percentage of neutrophils could be explained by blood contamination.
- A predominance of neutrophils, rather than of mononuclear cells, indicates inflammation of the synovial lining.
- In most species, neutrophilic inflammation is seen with septic and immune-mediated joint diseases.
- Because immune-mediated arthritis has not been well documented in horses, the main consideration for neutrophilic inflammation is septic arthritis, but traumatic injury and chemical synovitis must be considered.
- Erythrocytes indicate blood contamination during sample collection or hemorrhage from hemostatic defects, trauma, or inflammatory disease. Differentiating these conditions based on cytology is difficult. Macrophages containing phagocytized RBCs (i.e., erythrophagocytosis) indicate intra-articular hemorrhage if the slides were made soon after collection. Phagocytosis of erythrocytes by macrophages can occur in vitro during prolonged transport (i.e., several hours). Platelets or platelet clumps suggest blood contamination during sample collection.
- Usually the person collecting the sample can best differentiate contamination from hemorrhage. With true hemorrhage, the fluid is uniformly discolored. With blood contamination, fluid may be initially clear and then mix with blood or be initially blood tinged and then clear.

SYNOVIAL FLUID

Mucin Clot Test

- Performed as a measure of synovial fluid viscosity.
- Results are subjectively graded as good, fair, or poor.
- EDTA can cause some degree of depolymerization of hyaluronan and may reduce the quality of the mucin clot.
- Assesses the degree of polymerization of hyaluronan. Dilution of hyaluronan in synovial effusions often results in a fair to poor mucin clot.
- Increases in synovial fluid leukocyte counts may result in degradation of hyaluronan and cause a poor mucin clot.

Total Protein Concentration

- Some laboratories measure protein concentration using a dye-binding method; others use refractometric readings as estimates of protein concentrations.
- Protein measurements may help to indicate the presence of inflammation but are not useful in differentiating between types of inflammation.
- EDTA solution used in liquid EDTA tubes has a very high refractive index. Refractometric estimates of protein concentration can be markedly elevated (>4 g/dL) if an inadequate amount of sample is added to a large EDTA tube, thus insufficiently diluting the anticoagulant with sample.
- Increased protein concentrations are seen with synovial inflammation. Concentrations of >2.5 g/dL probably are abnormal.
- Nonseptic inflammatory conditions usually result in protein levels of <4.0 g/dL.

Drugs That May Alter Lab Results

- Previous therapeutic procedures must be considered.
- Intra-articular injections can produce a high leukocyte count and neutrophil percentage, but the magnitude generally is lower than that seen with septic arthritis.
- Injection of sterile saline produces cell counts of up to 30,000 cells/μL, with neutrophils being the predominant cell type ($\cong$70%).
- Injection of chemicals irritating to the synovial membrane can result in higher counts.
- Intra-articular corticosteroid injections can cause a neutrophilia (upto 98% neutrophils), with cell counts near 20,000 cells/μL.
- With inflammation caused by intra-articular injection, cell counts and neutrophil percentages decline significantly by 3–4 days after the injection.
- Previous intra-articular injections of corticosteroids may delay the onset of changes in synovial fluid with septic arthritis; however, the typical changes still occur.

Disorders That May Alter Lab Results

N/A

Valid If Run in Human Lab?

Yes, if familiar with synovial fluid analysis

CBC/BIOCHEMISTRY/URINALYSIS

Dependent on the underlying disease

OTHER LABORATORY TESTS

- Evaluation of hyaluronan content, serum enzymes and isoenzymes (i.e., creatine kinase, lactate dehydrogenase), glucose, and cartilage fragments have been suggested, but none has gained wide usage.
- Bacterial culture and sensitivity of purulent samples

IMAGING

Radiography, ultrasonography, and nuclear scintigraphy may be useful for establishing a diagnosis.

DIAGNOSTIC PROCEDURES

N/A

TREATMENT

Directed at the underlying cause.

MEDICATIONS

DRUGS OF CHOICE

Specific for the underlying cause.

CONTRAINDICATIONS

N/A

PRECAUTIONS
Samples must be collected aseptically.

POSSIBLE INTERACTIONS
N/A

ALTERNATIVE DRUGS
N/A

FOLLOW-UP

PATIENT MONITORING
Dependent on the underlying disease.

POSSIBLE COMPLICATIONS
N/A

MISCELLANEOUS

ASSOCIATED CONDITIONS
Laminitis

AGE-RELATED FACTORS
Neonates with failure of passive transfer can develop septicemia, including septic joints.

ZOONOTIC POTENTIAL
N/A

PREGNANCY
N/A

SYNONYMS
Joint fluid

SEE ALSO
Related musculoskeletal topics.

Suggested Reading

Mahaffey EA. Synovial fluid. In: Cowell RL, Tyler RD, eds. Cytology and hematology of the horse. 1st ed. Goleta, CA: American Veterinary Publications, 1992:153–161.

Trotter GW, McIlwraith CW. Clinical features and diagnosis of equine joint disease. In: McIlwraith CW, Trotter GW, eds. Joint disease of the horse. Philadelphia: WB Saunders, 1996:137–141.

Tulamo R, Bramlage L, Gabel A. Sequential clinical and synovial fluid changes associated with acute infectious arthritis in the horse. Equine Vet J 1989;21:325–331.

Authors James Meinkoth and Rick L. Cowell
Consulting Editor Claire B. Andreasen

SYSTEMIC LUPUS ERYTHEMATOSUS (SLE)

BASICS

OVERVIEW

- A rare, multisystemic disorder associated with production of autoantibodies that are reactive with nuclear, cytoplasmic, and cell membrane antigens
- Cause unknown
- Clinical manifestations relate to deposition of immune complexes and initiation of an inflammatory response and to direct cytotoxic effects of autoantibodies against membrane-bound antigens.
- Common sites of immune complex deposition—synovial membrane, glomerular basement membrane, skin, and blood vessels
- Systems affected—skin, hemic/lymphatic/immune, musculoskeletal, and renal/urologic

SIGNALMENT

No known breed, age, or sex predilections

SIGNS

- No pathognomonic signs, but clinical manifestations usually reflect multisystem involvement.
- Predominant clinical signs—anorexia, weight loss, fever, generalized alopecia and seborrheic dermatitis, and lymphadenopathy
- Additional signs—oral ulceration, petechial hemorrhages, pale mucous membranes, hemoglobinuria, peripheral edema, and generalized stiffness associated with polyarthropathy
- If untreated, the condition has a remitting and relapsing course, but with gradual deterioration over 4–6 weeks.

CAUSES AND RISK FACTORS

Unknown cause but a suspected immunologic basis

DIAGNOSIS

- No established criteria for diagnosis in horses
- Based on criteria for other species, definitive diagnosis requires a positive ANA test and the presence of two or more of the following: dermatitis, lymphadenopathy, hemolytic anemia, polyarthropathy, and proteinuria.

DIFFERENTIAL DIAGNOSIS

- Extensive differential diagnosis because of the varied clinical manifestations
- Skin diseases, including drug eruption, pemphigus foliaceus, pemphigus erythematosus, bullous pemphigoid, equine exfoliative dermatitis and stomatitis, idiopathic vasculitis, and severe dermatophilosus should be considered when cutaneous manifestations predominate. These skin conditions are differentiated from SLE by lack of evidence for multisystem involvement and distinctive dermatohistopathologic and immunologic findings.
- In the absence of cutaneous manifestations, consider equine infectious anemia and other causes of thrombocytopenia and hemolytic anemia.

CBC/BIOCHEMISTRY/URINALYSIS

- Leukocytosis with neutrophilia
- Nonregenerative or hemolytic anemia
- Thrombocytopenia is possible.
- Serum biochemistry results vary depending on the organ systems affected.
- Urinalysis may reveal moderate proteinuria (glomerulonephritis) and hemoglobinuria (hemolytic anemia).

OTHER LABORATORY TESTS

- Serum ANA, which is considered the most specific and sensitive serologic test, is usually positive; however, a positive test may be seen in a variety of disease states and during treatment with certain drugs (e.g., penicillin, tetracyclines, sulfonamides).
- Direct Coombs' test may be positive depending on previous treatment with glucocorticoids.
- LE cell test results in serum or synovial fluid are variable; this test lacks sensitivity and specificity in the diagnosis of SLE.
- Serum electrophoresis demonstrates increased β- and γ-globulins.

IMAGING

N/A

DIAGNOSTIC PROCEDURES

- Skin biopsies for histology and immunologic testing should be taken from patients with skin lesions—moderate to severe lymphocytic dermatitis with predilection for damage to the basement membrane zone of the epidermis and pilosebaceous structures (interface dermatitis). Immunologic testing of skin sections reveals linear deposition of immunoglobulins at the basement membrane zones of the epidermis and hair follicles.
- Arthrocentesis is indicated in patients with evidence of arthropathy. Analysis of synovial fluid may show mild increases in mononuclear and nondegenerate neutrophil numbers and low viscosity.
- Bacterial cultures of blood, urine, and synovial fluid are negative.

SYSTEMIC LUPUS ERYTHEMATOSUS (SLE)

PATHOLOGIC FINDINGS

- Interface dermatitis with moderate infiltration by mononuclear cells, hydropic degeneration of basilar epithelial cells, and focal thickening of the basement membrane zone. Immunologic staining demonstrates linear deposition of immunoglobulins at the basement membrane zone ("lupus band").
- Membranous glomerulonephritis; immunologic staining may show immunoglobulin deposition in the basement membrane.
- Polyarthritis characterized by fibrin exudation, synoviocyte hyperplasia, and lymphocyte infiltration.

TREATMENT

- Hospitalize patients for initial medical therapy.
- Lower limbs may require support bandages if edema is present.

MEDICATIONS

DRUGS

- Dexamethasone at 0.1–0.2 mg/kg per day IV or IM, or prednisone at 1–2 mg/kg PO q12h. If clinical improvement is seen, the steroid dosage may be gradually decreased.
- Other immunomodulatory drugs (e.g., azathioprine at 3 mg/kg per day PO), either alone or in combination with glucocorticoids, may be required in refractory cases or those requiring high maintenance doses of glucocorticoids.
- NSAIDs q12h or q24h for pain relief in horses with polyarthropathy—phenylbutazone at 2.2—4.4 mg/kg PO, flunixin meglumine at 1.1 mg/kg IV or IM, or ketoprofen at 1–2 mg/kg IV.

CONTRAINDICATIONS/POSSIBLE INTERACTIONS

- Do not give aspirin to patients with thrombocytopenia.
- Concurrent use of corticosteroids and NSAIDs may increase risk of GI ulceration.

FOLLOW-UP

- Monitor rectal temperature, hematocrit, BUN, creatinine, urine protein, ANA titer, and skin lesions at regular intervals during treatment period.
- The disease course is unpredictable but usually chronic and progressive, with periods of exacerbation and remission.
- ANA titer is *not* a useful indicator of disease progression.
- Based on reported equine cases, the prognosis is guarded to poor.

MISCELLANEOUS

ASSOCIATED CONDITIONS

N/A

AGE-RELATED FACTORS

N/A

ZOONOTIC POTENTIAL

N/A

PREGNANCY

N/A

SEE ALSO

- Anemia, immune-mediated
- Thrombocytopenia

ABBREVIATIONS

- ANA = antinuclear antibody
- GI = gastrointestinal
- LE = lupus erythematosus

Suggested Reading

Geor RJ, Clark EG, Haines DM, Napier PG. Systemic lupus erythematosus in a filly. J Am Vet Med Assoc 1990;197:1489–1492.

Author Raymond J. Geor
Consulting Editor Debra C. Sellon

THYROXINE (T_3) AND TRIIODOTHYRONINE (T_4) DETERMINATION

BASICS

DEFINITION

- T_3 and T_4 are the hormones produced by the thyroid gland.
- Once excreted into the circulation, >99% is bound to circulating proteins (primarily albumin).
- Protein-bound thyroxine acts as a reservoir to maintain a steady supply of free T_4, which diffuses into cells, where it is deiodinated to form T_3.
- Increased amounts of T_3 and T_4 in the circulation lead to hyperthyroidism, whereas decreased amounts results in hypothyroidism. Both are pathologic conditions

PATHOPHYSIOLOGY

- The net effect of hypothyroidism is decreased basal metabolic rate and decreased ability to respond to metabolic demands.
- In utero, thyroid hormones are necessary for proper bone, pulmonary, and nervous system development. Foals born with congenital hypothyroidism often have limb deformities caused by incomplete development of the carpal and tarsal bones, other skeletal deformities, and they often are weak, with inadequate respiration.
- Hyperthyroidism caused by either an overdose of exogenous hormone or a secreting thyroid tumor produces an increased metabolic rate that manifests as weight loss and behavioral changes.

SYSTEM AFFECTED

Endocrine/Metabolic

- The endocrine system is primarily affected by abnormal T_3 and T_4; however, because thyroid hormones have such widespread effects, many other body systems are affected as well.
- Energy metabolism is altered by hypothyroidism, and affected horses secrete less-than-normal amounts of insulin and have increased serum cholesterol.

Musculoskeletal

- In foals with congenital hypothyroidism, the musculoskeletal system is dramatically affected.
- Affected foals are born with underdeveloped tarsal and carpal bones, prognathism, ruptured common digital extensor tendons, and forelimb contracture.
- Affected foals often are weak and need assistance to stand.
- Adult horses have an increased incidence of myositis and muscle abnormalities.

Behavioral

- Horses with abnormal thyroid levels may have altered behavior.
- Increased aggression and lethargy have been attributed to hypothyroidism.
- Nervousness and pacing have been attributed to hyperthyroidism.

Cardiovascular

- Thyroidectomized horses have decreased cardiac output, which results in exercise intolerance.
- Immature respiratory tract and respiratory insufficiency have been reported in hypothyroid foals.

SIGNALMENT

- No sex or breed predilections for abnormal T_3/T_4 levels
- Hypothyroidism can occur at any age and exist in utero, with the foal showing characteristic signs at birth.
- Iatrogenic hyperthyroidism generally occurs in adults.
- Disease caused by thyroid tumors occurs in old horses (>10 years).

SIGNS

- Common clinical signs in foals born with congenital hypothyroidism—prognathism, ruptured common digital extensor tendon, forelimb contracture, retarded ossification and crushing of the carpal and tarsal bones, weakness, and poor suckle reflex
- Less common clinical signs in foals born with congenital hypothyroidism—goiter, angular limb deformities, respiratory distress, abdominal hernia, poor muscle development, and osteoporosis
- Hypothermia and bradycardia are consistent findings in adults with hypothyroidism.
- Other signs in adults associated with hypothyroidism—myositis, anhydrosis, laminitis, infertility, agalactia, poor hair coat, and poor growth
- Horses with experimentally induced hypothyroidism—edema of the distal limbs and coarsened features
- The horse described with hyperthyroidism exhibited a thyroid tumor, weight loss, pacing, and nervousness.

CAUSES

- Many factors can lead to decreased blood thyroid hormone levels.
- Certain drugs, including phenylbutazone, iodine-containing compounds, corticosteroids, and sulfa drugs, may cause low serum levels.
- Ingestion of endophyte-containing fescue, high or low iodine levels, or high carbohydrate diets can decrease circulating hormone levels.
- In most instances of hypothyroidism in adults, the cause is unknown.
- Iodine deficiency can cause hypothyroidism in horses, but this is extremely rare.
- Iodine deficiency or excess in the diets of broodmares can cause hypothyroidism in their foals; ingestion of endophyte infected fescue also can result in congenital hypothyroidism.
- Training can decrease thyroid hormone levels. Some racehorses even have no detectable T_4 in their blood yet exhibit no signs of thyroid deficiency.
- Rarely, thyroid tumors cause hypo- or hyperthyroidism in adults. In most instances, thyroid tumors are clinically silent. Debilitated horses or those with other severe diseases often have T_4 and T_3 levels < the reference ranges, which is termed *euthyroid sick syndrome*.
- Foals have increased thyroid hormone levels compared to old horses.
- Very cold weather also can lead to higher thyroid hormone levels.

RISK FACTORS

- Primarily dietary
- Excess or inadequate iodine or ingestion of other goitrogens can lead to hypothyroidism.
- In old horse populations, thyroid tumor is a risk factor for thyroid abnormalities.

DIAGNOSIS

DIFFERENTIAL DIAGNOSIS

- The primary differential diagnosis for adults with suspected hypothyroidism is a pituitary tumor (i.e., equine Cushing's disease), but these horses may have euthyroid sick syndrome. This can be ruled out by provocative testing with either TSH or TRH. A history of administration of a drug that decreases thyroid hormone values can explain abnormally low T_3 and T_4 levels not caused by true disease. A history of overadministration of an exogenous thyroid supplement can explain abnormally high T_3 and T_4 levels.
- Differentials for foals with congenital hypothyroidism include fescue toxicosis, prematurity, angular limb deformities, and sepsis. Dietary history rules out abnormal iodine in the dam's diet. Physical examination and CBC should rule in sepsis or prematurity/dysmaturity without hypothyroidism.

LABORATORY FINDINGS

Drugs that May Alter Laboratory Results

N/A

Disorders that May Alter Laboratory Results

N/A

Valid If Run in Human Laboratory?

Laboratory determination of T_3, free T_3, T_4, and free T_4 is valid. Human thyroid values commonly are higher than equine, though, so use equine reference ranges to interpret results.

CBC/BIOCHEMISTRY URINALYSIS

Hypothyroid horses may exhibit anemia, leukopenia, and hypercholesterolemia.

THYROXINE (T_3) AND TRIIODOTHYRONINE (T_4) DETERMINATION

OTHER LABORATORY TESTS

To confirm the diagnosis of hypothyroidism, consider provocative testing with a TRH or TSH response test. TSH is currently not available, but for a TRH stimulation test, give 1 mg IV of TRH. Collect blood for T_3 and T_4 determination 0, 2, and 4 hours later. One expects to see baseline T_3 and T_4 in the reference range, the T_3 double at 2 hours, and T_4 to double at 4 hours.

IMAGING

Ultrasonography

- Imaging rarely is useful in diagnosing hypothyroidism.
- An enlarged thyroid gland caused by tumor or goiter could be seen via ultrasound.

Radiography

An enlarged thyroid gland caused by tumor or goiter might be seen as increased soft-tissue density on radiographs of the throat-latch area.

DIAGNOSTIC PROCEDURES

A fine-needle aspiration or biopsy may assist with assessing the thyroid gland.

TREATMENT

APPROPRIATE HEALTH CARE

- Foals with congenital hypothyroidism may require inpatient medical management if the disease is severe.
- All other horses with abnormal T_3 and T_4 levels can be treated on an outpatient basis.

NURSING CARE

- Foals may need assistance standing and milk administered via nasogastric tube if they are too weak to suckle.
- Foals may need mechanical ventilation if they cannot respirate on their own.
- Animals with poor hair coat may need blanketing, and cold temperatures should be avoided.

ACTIVITY

Limit activity in foals with musculoskeletal deformities—incomplete ossification of the carpal or tarsal bones

DIET

- Examine the diet of any horse with hypothyroidism and the dams of foals born with hypothyroidism to ensure the proper amount of iodine is being fed.
- Pregnant mares should not receive endophyte-infected fescue hay, particularly during their last months of gestation.

CLIENT EDUCATION

- Prognosis for soundness is poor in most foals suffering from congenital hypothyroidism and should be discussed with owners before initiating expensive treatments.
- Adult horses with hypothyroidism respond well to exogenous replacement hormone, and their prognosis is generally good.
- Horses with hyperthyroidism should have their dose of thyroid supplement decreased.
- Animals that are euthyroid despite low blood T_3 and T_4 levels do not require supplementation.

SURGICAL CONSIDERATIONS

If the cause of increased or decreased T_3 and T_4 concentrations is a tumor of the thyroid gland, surgical removal of the affected thyroid lobe should be curative.

MEDICATIONS

DRUGS OF CHOICE

For decreased T_3 and T_4 levels caused by hypothyroidism, replacement therapy with thyroxine—20 μg/kg maintains T_4 and T_3 levels in the normal range for 24 hours; this constitutes a dose of 10 mg in a 1000-pound horse.

CONTRAINDICATIONS

With low resting T_3 and T_4 values because of some other severe disease (e.g., euthyroid sick syndrome), thyroid replacement therapies may cause further deterioration of the horse's condition. Thus, perform provocative testing to establish the diagnosis of hypothyroidism.

PRECAUTIONS

Exogenous thyroid hormone causes down-regulation and, potentially, atrophy of the thyroid gland; gradually discontinue the hormone supplement over the course of several weeks.

POSSIBLE INTERACTIONS

N/A

ALTERNATIVE DRUGS

Other sources of thyroid hormone replacement—iodinated casein (5.0 g/day) and concentrated bovine thyroid extract (10 g/day).

FOLLOW-UP

PATIENT MONITORING

- Monitor horses on thyroid supplement by measuring serum T_4 and T_3 levels every 30–60 days. If the serum level is low, increase the dosage it reaches the normal range; if the serum level is too high or in the higher end of the normal range, decrease the dosage and retested in 30–60 days.
- Reconsidering the original diagnosis if the patient fails to respond clinically after 6 weeks of therapy.

POSSIBLE COMPLICATIONS

N/A

MISCELLANEOUS

ASSOCIATED CONDITIONS

- Angular limb deformities, hypognathism, weakness, and respiratory distress often are associated with congenital hypothyroidism.
- Infertility and myositis have been associated with hypothyroidism in adults.
- Phenylbutazone is associated with low T_3 and T_4 levels.
- Euthyroid sick syndrome is associated with debilitating disease—equine Cushing's disease

AGE-RELATED FACTORS

- Higher T_3 and T_4 levels are normal in neonatal foals. Levels are highest at birth (10× adult levels), then decrease rapidly in the first weeks of life to adult levels.
- Resting T_3 and T_4 levels decline gradually over the life of a horse, and levels in old horses may be lower than those in younger animals.

ZOONOTIC POTENTIAL

N/A

PREGNANCY

N/A

SYNONYMS

N/A

SEE ALSO

- Hyperthyroidism
- Hypothyroidism
- TRH and TSH stimulation tests

ABBREVIATIONS

- TRH = thyroid-releasing hormone
- TSH = thyroid-stimulating hormone

Suggested Reading

Allen AL, Doige CE, Fretz PB, et al. Congenital hypothyroidism, dysmaturity, and musculoskeletal lesions in Western Canadian foals. Proc AAEP 1993;39:207–208.

Messer NT. Clinical and diagnostic features of thyroid disease in horses. Proc ACVIM 1993;11:649–651.

Sojka JE. Factors which affect serum T_3 and T_4 levels in the horse. Equine Pract 1993;15:15–19.

Sojka JE. Hypothyroidism in horses. Compend Contin Educ Pract Vet 1995;17:845–852.

Author

Consulting Editor Michel Levy

TAXUS SPP. (YEW) TOXICOSIS

BASICS

OVERVIEW

- Extremely toxic evergreen shrub causing sudden death in horses when ingested.
- American yew or ground hemlock (*Taxus canadensis*), Japanese yew (*T. cuspidata*), English yew (*T. baccata*), and Western or Pacific yew (*T. brevifolia*) are all toxic.
- Several species of yew commonly are planted as ornamental shrubs or hedges throughout most of the U.S. They are woody perennials with flat, 0.5–1-inch evergreen leaves, lighter green on the underside and broader than pine needles, with a prominent midvein. Leaves are arranged in opposite pairs along the twigs. The aril is pea-sized, fleshy, and bright scarlet when mature, forming a cup around a black seed.
- Ground hemlock grows ≤5 feet tall, but Western yew can reach 75 feet.
- Foliage is toxic to horses at 0.1% of body weight; 100–200 g of fresh yew may kill a horse.
- The whole plant is considered toxic, except for the flesh of the red aril.
- The alkaloids taxine A and B are found in most *Taxus* spp.; taxine inhibits depolarization in the heart by interfering with calcium and sodium currents.

SIGNALMENT

- May affect all horses.
- Horses readily eat yew, even with other forage present.

SIGNS

- Horses often are found dead.
- Occasionally, trembling, muscle weakness, dyspnea, jugular pulsation and distention and collapse are observed up to 2 days after ingestion.

CAUSES AND RISK FACTORS

- Many horses are accidentally poisoned when yew trimmings are thrown into pastures or ornamental yew is planted within browsing reach.

DIAGNOSIS

DIFFERENTIAL

Other causes of sudden death (see *Malicious Intoxication*)

CBC/BIOCHEMISTRY/URINALYSIS

N/A

OTHER LABORATORY TESTS

Stomach contents may be examined microscopically for *Taxus* spp. needle fragments and analyzed chemically for *Taxus* spp. alkaloids.

IMAGING

N/A

DIAGNOSTIC PROCEDURES

N/A

PATHOLOGIC FINDINGS

- Most commonly, no lesions are observed at necropsy.
- Rarely, hemorrhagic areas on the right myocardium and right atrium are seen, along with pulmonary congestion and edema.

TREATMENT

- First aid usually is impractical, because affected animals die quickly.
- Prevent other animals from being exposed.
- Decontaminate using AC and a cathartic.
- Maintain body fluid and electrolyte balance.
- Treat cardiac dysrhythmias.

TAXUS SPP. (YEW) TOXICOSIS

MEDICATIONS

DRUGS

• AC (2–5 g/kg PO in water slurry [1 g of AC in 5 mL of water])
• One dose of cathartic PO (70% sorbitol at 3 mL/kg or sodium or magnesium sulfate at 250 mg/kg in water) with AC if no diarrhea or ileus.
• Atropine (0.1–0.2 mg/kg IM) has been recommended to combat the cardiodepressant effect of taxine, but it must be given early in the course of toxicosis.

CONTRAINDICATIONS/POSSIBLE INTERACTIONS

Avoid stressing affected horses.

FOLLOW-UP

PATIENT MONITORING

Monitor cardiovascular function—arrhythmia, bradycardia, and heart block may be observed.

PREVENTION/AVOIDANCE

• Never allow yew plants or trimmings within reach of horses.
• Yew is toxic even when dry; thus, hay containing yew is never safe in any amount.

EXPECTED COURSE AND PROGNOSIS

• Extremely guarded prognosis early in the condition; if the horse survives for 72 hours with minimal clinical signs, then recovery is likely.
• No permanent cardiac damage

MISCELLANEOUS

ASSOCIATED CONDITIONS

N/A

AGE-RELATED FACTORS

N/A

ZOONOTIC POTENTIAL

N/A

PREGNANCY

Because taxine may be excreted in the milk, remove foals from nursing mares that have been exposed until the mare recovers fully.

SEE ALSO

N/A

ABBREVIATION

AC = activated charcoal

Suggested Reading

Parkinson N. Yew poisoning in horses. Can Vet J 1996;37:687.

Author Anita M. Kore
Consulting Editor Robert H. Poppenga

TEMPOROHYOID/PETROUS TEMPORAL BONE OSTEOARTHROPATHY AND OTITIS INTERNA

BASICS

DEFINITION

PATHOPHYSIOLOGY

Otitis Media and Interna

- Horses develop otitis media/interna most commonly as foals but rarely compared to other species.
- Presumably, otitis media occurs by extension of an infection of the pharynx, guttural pouch, or external ear or by hematogenous spread from other sites.

Temporohyoid/Petrous Temporal Bone Osteoarthropathy

- Extensive subperiosteal bone proliferation of the petrous temporal and stylohyoid bone, often with bony fusion of the temporohyoid arthrosis
- Clinical signs relate to stricture of the external ear canal and obliteration of the lumen of the tympanic bulla.
- The process often extends into the vestibular labyrinths and facial canal, which relates to the signs of peripheral vestibular and facial nerve dysfunction. In addition, the vagus and hypoglossal nerves can be involved.
- The proliferation may be extensive enough to involve adjacent areas of the medulla, with other cranial nerve and brainstem involvement as well as clinical signs.
- Controversy exists regarding the initiating insult.
- Initial publications indicated the bone reaction was secondary to chronic middle ear infection or guttural pouch disease. However, histopathology of these lesions often does not indicate osteomyelitis or an infectious process.
- Another scenario may be that osteochondroarthrosis of the temporohyoid joint precedes other changes, and that involvement of the osseous bulla and proximal stylohyoid bone occurs by extension of the degenerative joint disease. Subsequently, as the stylohyoid bone is moved during vocalization, prehension, and so on, fractures of the petrosal bone occur, until the horse is decompensated. Infection of the fracture site may lead to secondary otitis media or otitis interna and leptomeningitis.

SYSTEMS AFFECTED

CNS

SIGNALMENT

Otitis Media and Interna

Foals most commonly are affected.

Temporohyoid/Petrous Temporal Bone Osteoarthropathy

The diagnosis has been made in 2-year-old horses but more commonly is seen in those older than 12 years.

SIGNS

Otitis Media and Interna

Historical Findings:

- The disease often is acute, with no specific historical features evident.
- Foals may be under treatment for other infectious conditions.

Physical Examination Findings:

- Acute signs of vestibular disease are common.
- Headshaking may be seen.
- Pyrexia may be evident.
- Concurrent ipsilateral facial paralysis occurs with extension of the suppurative process into the adjacent facial canal or internal acoustic meatus that houses the facial nerve.
- Dysphagia, facial muscle atrophy, and corneal ulceration also can occur.

Temporohyoid/Petrous Temporal Bone Osteoarthropathy

Historical Findings:

- The disease often is acute, with no specific historical features evident.

Physical Examination Findings:

- Acute signs of vestibular disease and facial nerve paralysis are common.
- Signs associated with either cranial nerve can be present without the other. For some unknown reason, signs most commonly are unilaterally on the right side, but left-sided and bilateral disease also is seen.
- Horses may present with acute, severe vestibular disease (i.e., circling, lateralized, or recumbent) or with more mild signs (i.e., mild head tilt).
- Signs of facial nerve paralysis with drooping ears, lips, and palpebral dysfunction are common.
- Dysphagia, facial muscle atrophy, and corneal ulceration also can occur.

CAUSES

See *Pathophysiology.*

RISK FACTORS

None identified

DIAGNOSIS

DIFFERENTIAL DIAGNOSIS

- Trauma
- Equine protozoal myeloencephalitis

CBC/BIOCHEMISTRY/URINALYSIS

No specific abnormalities

OTHER LABORATORY TESTS

N/A

IMAGING

Otitis Media and Interna

- Often, no changes are evident early in the disease.
- In more chronic cases, sclerosis of the petrous temporal bone may be identified.

Temporohyoid/Petrous Temporal Bone Osteoarthropathy

- Radiographic changes and endoscopic findings are consistent.
- Ventrodorsal radiography can be performed on standing horses, and anesthesia is unnecessary in most cases.
- See *Pathophysiology.*

DIAGNOSTIC PROCEDURES

Otoscopy may be useful.

Otitis Media and Interna

- Clinical signs, especially in light of treatment for another infectious disease, are diagnostic.
- Deep ear examination may indicate purulent debris extending from the eardrum.

Temporohyoid/Petrous Temporal Bone Osteoarthropathy

- Endoscopic and radiographic changes usually are extensive by the time neurologic abnormalities are evident.
- Clinical signs, demonstration of a bony thickening of the stylohyoid bone at endoscopy, and radiographic changes are diagnostic.
- Deep ear examination may indicate purulent debris extending from the eardrum.

TEMPOROHYOID/PETROUS TEMPORAL BONE OSTEOARTHROPATHY AND OTITIS INTERNA

TREATMENT

OTITIS MEDIA AND INTERNA

Supportive care and appropriate antimicrobial therapy

TEMPOROHYOID/PETROUS TEMPORAL BONE OSTEOARTHROPATHY

- As with most peripheral vestibular syndromes, signs of vestibular dysfunction will improve regardless of therapy.
- Supportive care is essential.
- A partial tarsorrhaphy may be necessary to manage palpebral dysfunction.
- Removal of a section of the affected stylohyoid bone has been recommended to reduce stresses on the ankylosed temporohyoid joint and, possibly, to reduce the number of subsequent attacks.
- Vestibular function will improve, but even with surgery, facial and other cranial nerve disorders often remain constant, with only slight improvement over time.

MEDICATIONS

DRUGS OF CHOICE

Antimicrobials may be administered when infection is evident.

CONTRAINDICATIONS

N/A

PRECAUTIONS

The acute nature of the fracture and subsequent vestibular disease can make these horses dangerous to riders. It is recommended that these horses not be ridden. (I personally witnessed a horse that was apparently normal that was down in seconds; no warning period occurred.)

POSSIBLE INTERACTIONS

N/A

ALTERNATIVE DRUGS

N/A

FOLLOW-UP

PATIENT MONITORING

N/A

POSSIBLE COMPLICATIONS

- Uveitis and ocular rupture have been seen in a few horses.
- Weight loss can be seen when dysphagia is evident.

EXPECTED COURSE AND PROGNOSIS

Fair prognosis for long-term resolution, even with surgery.

MISCELLANEOUS

ASSOCIATED CONDITIONS

N/A

AGE-RELATED FACTORS

N/A

ZOONOTIC POTENTIAL

N/A

PREGNANCY

N/A

SYNONYMS

N/A

SEE ALSO

N/A

Suggested Reading

Blythe LL. Otitis media and interna and temporohyoid osteo-arthropathy. Vet Clin North Am Equine Pract 1997;13:21–42.

Blythe LL, et al. Prophylactic partial stylohyoidostectomy for horses with osteoarthropathy of the temporohyoid joint. J Equine Vet Sci 1994;14:32–37.

De Lahunta A. Comparative cerebellar disease in domestic animals. Compend Contin Educ Pract Vet 1980;11:8–19.

Power HT, et al. Facial and vestibulocochlear nerve disease in six horses. J Am Vet Med Assoc 1983;183:1076–1080.

Author Joseph J. Bertone

Consulting Editor Joseph J. Bertone

TENESMUS

BASICS

OVERVIEW

- An involuntary straining to evacuate the rectum or bladder, with passage of little fecal matter or urine
- Constant stimulation of the sacral nerves by inflammation or physical pressure gives the horse a continual sensation of the need to defecate or urinate, which leads to repeated attempts to evacuate the bowel or bladder as long as the stimulation remains unrelieved by the attempts.
- Stimulation may result from intrinsic disease of the organ involved (e.g., rectal inflammation); therefore, tenesmus may be seen with diarrhea.
- Stimulation also may result from physical pressure on the organ from within (e.g., rectal stimulation by constipated feces) or from without (e.g., rectal stimulation by a pararectal abscess).
- May lead to rectal or uterine/bladder prolapse (in females only).

SIGNALMENT

N/A

SIGNS

- Repeated attempts to defecate or urinate
- Sometimes a visibly prolapsed rectum, uterus, or bladder (mares) secondary to tenesmus

CAUSES AND RISK FACTORS

- Internal pressure of the rectum—constipation or foreign body
- External pressure on the rectum—pararectal abscess or neoplasm
- Inflammation of the rectum—proctitis/diarrhea or rectal tear
- Inflammation of the urethra—lower urinary tract infection
- Urinary tract obstruction—cystic/urethral calculi
- Inflammation of the vagina—vaginitis
- Direct stimulation of the nervous system—hepatic encephalopathy or damaged nerves caused by rabies
- Parturition/dystocia

DIAGNOSIS

DIFFERENTIAL DIAGNOSIS

- Inflammation of the colon or rectum
- Rectal tears, strictures, polyps, neoplasms, or small colon intussusceptions
- Pararectal abscess
- Meconium impaction or uroperitoneum (i.e., ruptured bladder or urachus) in foals
- Vaginitis or retained placenta
- Urolithiasis or lower urinary tract infection
- Neurologic disorders involving sacral nerves or CNS disorder—hepatic encephalopathy, rabies, or others
- Oak (acorn) poisoning, Psilocybe (magic mushroom) poisoning, or lolitrem B toxicity

CBC/BIOCHEMISTRY/URINALYSIS

- Urinalysis may be abnormal with urinary tract involvement.
- CBC may show neutropenia and thrombocytopenia (caused by endotoxemia) with a rectal tear, retained placenta or intussusception
- CBC may show neutrophilia in cases of inflammation.
- Biochemistry may demonstrate elevated globulins with pararectal abscess.
- Biochemistry may demonstrate liver failure in cases of hepatic encephalopathy; bile salts and blood ammonia also may be elevated.
- Hyponatremia and hypochloremia may occur with uroperitoneum and in foals with meconium impaction if repeated enemas with water have been administered previously.
- Hyperkalemia occurs in cases of uroperitoneum as well.

OTHER LABORATORY TESTS

- Peritoneal tap for uroperitoneum and rectal tears
- Urinary gallic acid equivalent concentration in acorn poisoning

IMAGING

- Abdominal radiography for meconium impaction
- Abdominal ultrasonography for uroperitoneum, intussusception, and pararectal abscess
- Bladder ultrasonography for urolithiasis or neoplasia

DIAGNOSTIC PROCEDURES

- Manual vaginal and rectal examination
- Rectal endoscopy for tears, polyps, neoplasia, strictures, or intussusception
- Vaginoscopy or endoscopy of vaginitis
- Endoscopy of the urethra and bladder for lower urinary tract problems
- Rectal biopsy for proctitis, polyps, or neoplasia

TREATMENT

- Depends on the inciting cause; eliminating the cause relieves the symptom of tenesmus.
- Rectal or uterine/bladder prolapse—reduction of the prolapse is required. Temporary relief from tenesmus can be obtained with caudal epidural (i.e., regional) anesthetic. A caudal epidural also is required before attempting to reduce a prolapse or for surgery of the perineal area. Addition of xylazine in the epidural injection can reduce the dose of local anesthetic required to avoid postepidural hindlimb ataxia.
- Rectal stricture—add laxatives and stool softeners to the diet.
- If rectal prolapse has occurred, prevent recumbency until the prolapse has been reduced to minimize tissue trauma.

MEDICATIONS

DRUGS

No specific medication; treatment depends on the inciting cause.

CONTRAINDICATIONS/POSSIBLE INTERACTIONS

N/A

FOLLOW UP

PATIENT MONITORING

- Depends on the inciting cause
- Rectal prolapse can reoccur.

PREVENTION/AVOIDANCE

N/A

POSSIBLE COMPLICATIONS

- Repeated attempts to evacuate the bowel or bladder may lead to rectal or uterine/bladder prolapse (in females only).
- Rectal prolapse may reoccur after correction if feces are not softened enough.

EXPECTED COURSE AND PROGNOSIS

Prognosis depends on the cause.

MISCELLANEOUS

ASSOCIATED CONDITIONS

- Rectal prolapse
- Uterine or bladder prolapse (in females only)

AGE RELATED FACTORS

- Meconium impaction in neonatal foals
- Ruptured bladder in neonatal foals and parturient mares
- Hamartomatous polyp in neonatal foal
- Urolithiasis in young adults
- Bladder neoplasia in old individuals

ZOONOTIC POTENTIAL

N/A

PREGNANCY

Dystocia

SYNONYMS

- Urgency (human)
- Straining to defecate; dyschezia (though commonly meant to convey pain)
- Straining to urinate; strangury; dysuria (though commonly meant to convey pain)

SEE ALSO

- Dystocia
- Hepatic encephalopathy
- Inflammation of the colon or rectum; colitis; proctitis
- Intussusception
- Meconium impaction
- Rabies
- Rectal prolapse
- Rectal tears or strictures
- Retained placenta
- Ruptured bladder; uroperitoneum
- Urolithiasis or lower urinary tract infection
- Vaginitis
- Other neurologic disorder involving sacral nerves

Suggested Reading

Colbourne CM, Bolton JB, Yovich JV, Genovese L. Hamartomatous polyp causing intestinal obstruction and tenesmus in a neonatal foal. Aust Equine Vet 1996;14(2):78–80.

Jones J. 'Magic mushroom' (Psilocybe) poisoning in a colt. Vet Rec 1990;127:603.

Laverty S, Pascoe JR, Ling GV, LaVoie JP, Ruby AL. Urolithiasis in 68 horses. Vet Surg 1992;21:56–62.

Munday BL, Monkhouse IM, Gallagher RT. Intoxication of horses by lolitrem B in ryegrass seed cleanings. Aust Vet J 1985;62:207.

Author Gail Abells Sutton

Consulting Editor Henry Stämpfli

TERATOMA

BASICS

DEFINITION
• Germ cell tumor of the gonad.
• Mostly well-differentiated and benign, but can become malignant and metastasize into the abdominal cavity.
• Other types—dysgerminoma (female); seminoma (male).
• Characterized by multiple tissue types within the tumor.
• Contain somatic structures derived from all embryonic germ cell layers—ectoderm (hair, teeth); neuroectoderm (nerves, melanocytes); endoderm (salivary gland, lung); mesoderm (fibrous, adipose, bone, muscle); nervous and adipose tissue (nearly always present).

PATHOPHYSIOLOGY
Generally a benign, incidental finding.

SYSTEMS AFFECTED
• Reproductive—gonad.
• Rarely a systemic affect, unless metastasis occurs.

GENETICS
See *Causes.*

INCIDENCE/PREVALENCE
N/A

SIGNALMENT
• Horses of any age may display signs because of teratoma—colic.
• Young males—usual presenting age, 1–2 years.
• Cryptorchid testes—presence in the fetus prevents testicular descent.
• Females—discovered during routine reproductive examination.

SIGNS
• Effects from physical presence of a teratoma $\leq$25 cm in diameter.
• Has been associated with small colon torsion in a foal, colic in mares, and testicular cyst formation.
• Females—palpably abnormal ovarian mass.
• Males—scrotal mass; most often a cryptorchid testicle; may decrease spermatogenesis or induce tubular atrophy of adjacent testicular tissue.

CAUSES
Congenital

RISK FACTORS
• May be concurrent with other gonadal neoplasia—carcinoma; granulosa cell tumor.
• Most are well-differentiated and benign.

DIAGNOSIS

DIFFERENTIAL DIAGNOSIS
• Females—ovarian hematoma; granulosa cell tumor; dysgerminoma; carcinoma; fibroma; abscess.
• Males—seminoma; Sertoli cell tumor; interstitial cell tumor; carcinoma; testicular hematoma; fibroma.

CBC/BIOCHEMISTRY/URINALYSIS
N/A

OTHER LABORATORY TESTS
N/A

IMAGING
Ultrasonography:
• Couple with transrectal palpation.
• Abnormal paraovarian mass—solid; multilocular.

DIAGNOSTIC PROCEDURES
N/A

PATHOLOGIC FINDINGS
• Histopathologic findings—multiple tissue types within neoplasm (adipose, bone, cartilage, hair, nervous elements, and teeth).
• Gross findings—solid, cystic multilocular form; yellow-white.

TERATOMA

TREATMENT

APPROPRIATE HEALTH CARE
Surgical removal.

NURSING CARE
N/A

ACTIVITY
N/A

DIET
N/A

CLIENT EDUCATION
N/A

SURGICAL CONSIDERATIONS
May necessitate concurrent gonadectomy.

MEDICATIONS

DRUGS OF CHOICE
N/A

CONTRAINDICATIONS
N/A

PRECAUTIONS
N/A

POSSIBLE INTERACTIONS
N/A

ALTERNATIVE DRUGS
N/A

FOLLOW-UP

PATIENT MONITORING
N/A

PREVENTION/AVOIDANCE
N/A

POSSIBLE COMPLICATIONS
N/A

EXPECTED COURSE AND PROGNOSIS
N/A

MISCELLANEOUS

ASSOCIATED CONDITIONS
N/A

AGE-RELATED FACTORS
N/A

ZOONOTIC POTENTIAL
N/A

PREGNANCY
N/A

SYNONYMS
N/A

SEE ALSO
Large ovary syndrome

Suggested Reading

Buergelt CD. Color atlas of reproductive pathology of the domestic animals. St. Louis: Mosby—Year Book, 1997:55–56, 106–107.

Jubb KVC, Kennedy PC, Palmer N. Pathology of the domestic animals. 4th ed. San Diego: Academic Press, 1993;3:368, 510.

Author Peter R. Morresey
Consulting Editor Carla L. Carleton

TETANUS

BASICS

DEFINITION
Tetanus is a disease caused by exotoxins produced by *Clostridium tetani.* It is characterized by muscular rigidity (tetany) and can lead to death by respiratory arrest or convulsions. Vaccination tends to increase survival in affected animals.

PATHOPHYSIOLOGY
Clostridium tetani is ubiquitous in the environment (soil or feces) and has world-wide distribution. Puncture wounds are the most common site of infection, but any potentially contaminated anaerobic site, such as an injection, can lead to development of the disease.

When the bacterium is inoculated into an anaerobic environment, the spores germinate into the vegetative form. Necrotic tissue, infection of a wound with other bacteria, and foreign bodies can increase sporulation.

Three main exotoxins are produced by the vegetative form and are thought to be the major pathogenic components. These are tetanolysin, tetanospasmin, and a nonspasmogenic toxin. Tetanolysin increases local tissue necrosis, thereby enhancing sporulation and spread of infection. Tetanospasmin is a lipoprotein that spreads hematogenously to the central nervous system, where it migrates along the axons of motoneurons to presynaptic inhibitory interneuron cells. It is thought that the toxin inhibits the release of glycine and gamma-aminobutyric acid (GABA), which would result in disinhibition of motoneurons and cause the clinical sign of tetany. The nonspasmogenic exotoxin most likely causes excessive stimulation of the sympathatic nervous system.

SYSTEM(S) AFFECTED
- Neuromuscular
- Other systems can become involved as complications occur, such as aspiration pneumonia or decubital ulcers.

GENETICS
N/A

INCIDENCE/PREVALENCE
- Worldwide distribution
- Horses as a species tend to be more sensitive to tetanus
- Horses often live in unsafe environments with a high degree of fecal contamination that can increase the incidence of the disease. However, overall, as management of horses has improved, the case numbers have declined.

SIGNALMENT
Nonspecific, but more common in horses not vaccinated.

SIGNS

General Comments
Initial signs may be variable and can include colic, vague stiffness, and lameness.

Historical Findings
History of a puncture wound within the previous 2–4 weeks, most commonly of the foot (note the incubation period is variable).

Physical Examination Findings
- Stiff, stilted gait
- Generalized muscular rigidity, particularly of the antigravity muscles, leading to a characteristic "sawhorse" stance
- Opisthotonos
- Lips are often pulled back into a grimace and the jaws are commonly clenched (hence the name *lockjaw*).
- Prolapse of the nictitating membrane
- Hyperesthesia—signs of muscular spasms can be exacerbated by sudden noise, light, or tactile stimulation.
- As the muscular tetany progresses, there may be fever and sweating.
- Dysphasia leading to oral accumulation of saliva and/or aspiration pneumonia
- As the respiratory muscles become involved, hypoxia can develop and can progress to respiratory arrest.

CAUSE
Exotoxins produced by *C. tetani,* a spore-forming anaerobic gram-positive bacterium.

RISK FACTORS
- Wounds or injection sites that are likely to set up an anaerobic condition.
- Unsafe and/or dirty environments with fecal contamination.
- Animals that are not protected by vaccination.

DIAGNOSIS

DIFFERENTIAL DIAGNOSIS
Other causes of tetany and/or convulsions include:
- Metabolic disturbances, such as hypocalcemia (lactation or transport), hypomagnesemia, and hyperkalemia (HYPP)
- Exertional rhabdomyolysis
- Rabies
- Toxins, such as strychnine or organochlorines
- Other causes of stiff gait or lameness
- Laminitis
- Any of a number of common musculoskeletal problems that affect the horse, such as foot abscess or osteoarthrosis

CBC/BIOCHEMISTRY/URINALYSIS
- Non-specific
- Stress leukogram
- If secondary problems have occurred, results of complete blood count may reveal an inflammatory process.
- Results of the serum biochemistry profile and urinalysis typically are normal, but they may reveal evidence of dehydration.

OTHER LABORATORY TESTS
- Culture of any suspected site of bacterial inoculation
- Care should be taken to minimize exposure to oxygen of any samples obtained

IMAGING
Because it can sometimes be difficult to find the source of infection, ultrasonography of any soft-tissue regions that exhibit local heat or swelling may be useful, especially when shadowing suggestive of entrapped gas is noted.

OTHER DIAGNOSTIC PROCEDURES
N/A

PATHOLOGIC FINDINGS
Non-specific other than if the site of infection is identified and *C. tetani* is cultured.

TREATMENT

APPROPRIATE HEALTH CARE
- Must be able to provide a quiet environment
- Transport to a hospital setting can exacerbate clinical signs; however, intensive care may be required. Transport of affected animals can be facilitated by placing cotton in the ears and providing sedation.

NURSING CARE
- Deeply bedded, quiet, dark stall
- Pack ears with cotton
- Consider the use of external support, such as a sling, if the patient is unable to stand
- Avoid contact or activities that stimulate the patient
- Maintain hydration, which may require intravenous infusion of a balanced polyionic fluid
- Fluids and nutrients can be given via stomach tube, but the placement of the tube can cause severe exacerbation of clinical signs. A stomach tube should only be placed in the very early phase of the disease, with the horse heavily sedated. It should be left in place.

ACTIVITY
Restrict activity; the horse should be confined in a dark, quiet stall away from all other horses and activity, and should be disturbed as little as possible.

DIET

- Allow easy access to feed and water, such as a hay net.
- If the animal is not eating or is dysphagic, providing nutritional support may require supplementation via nasogastric intubation (use caution, as this may elicit further muscle spasm and therefore be of limited usefulness) or parenteral nutrition (can be extremely costly in the adult, full-size horse).

CLIENT EDUCATION

Inform clients that properly administered vaccination decreases the risk of disease significantly. Also, suggest that when wounds are noted, it may be prudent to seek advice regarding tetanus prophylaxis and wound care.

SURGICAL CONSIDERATION

If the site of infection is located, surgical debridement of the area is recommended, as *C. tetani* grows under anaerobic conditions. Local infusion with penicillin G may also be considered. These actions will decrease the local spread of infection.

MEDICATIONS

DRUG(S) OF CHOICE

- Penicillin G, −20,000–50,000 IU/kg potassium or sodium penicillin G IV 3–4 times daily or procaine penicillin IM BID
- Sedation to help provide muscle relaxation, such as phenothiazine tranquilizers (promazine, −0.5–1 mg/kg; or acetylpromazine, −0.05–0.1 mg/kg q4–6h)
- Tetanus antitoxin is used to bind exotoxin before the toxin reaches the central nervous system. It can be used locally at the site of infection or given parenterally. There are a wide range of recommended dosages (100–1000 IU/kg).
- Tetanus toxoid may be given as a "booster" if the history indicates previous vaccinations against tetanus.

CONTRAINDICATIONS

Guaifenesin has been recommended to reduce muscular spasms, but this drug inhibits reflex muscle activities.

PRECAUTIONS

- Administration of tetanus antitoxin has been classically associated with acute hepatic necrosis (Theiler's disease, serum hepatitis).
- Intrathecal administration of tetanus antitoxin has been recommended, but complications of this procedure included seizures and infection without clear evidence of significant efficacy.

POSSIBLE INTERACTIONS

Tetanus antitoxin and tetanus toxoid should not be mixed in the same syringe and should be administered at sites distant from each other to be the most effective.

ALTERNATIVE DRUGS

Diazepam, −0.01–0.4 mg/kg q2–4h is effective at producing good muscular relaxation, but due to short duration of action, can become cost prohibitive.

FOLLOW-UP

PATIENT MONITORING

Physical examination and administration of a second dose of tetanus toxoid 1–2 months after initial treatment.

PREVENTION/AVOIDANCE

- Vaccination with an initial series of two tetanus toxoid inoculations 3–4 weeks apart, followed by an annual booster vaccination.
- Avoid potentially hazardous environments.
- Keep fecal contamination to a minimum.
- Clean wounds thoroughly when initially noted, especially puncture wounds, and administer a tetanus toxoid inoculation if the animal has not been vaccinated within the previous 6 months.
- If the wound becomes infected, provide drainage and keep open to the air.

POSSIBLE COMPLICATIONS

- Aspiration pneumonia
- Decubital ulcers and abrasions
- Residual stiff gait or lameness

EXPECTED COURSE AND PROGNOSIS

The prognosis depends on the severity of the clinical signs and the speed of development of the disease. Rapid onset of clinical signs typically carries a more guarded prognosis, as does prolonged recumbency. Mortality rates reportedly range from 50% to 75%.

MISCELLANEOUS

ASSOCIATED CONDITIONS

N/A

AGE-RELATED FACTORS

Foals born to mares not receiving tetanus prophylaxis should receive tetanus antitoxin at birth, followed by vaccination with a series of tetanus toxoid inoculations at 2 and 3 months of age.

ZOONOTIC POTENTIAL

N/A

PREGNANCY

Pregnant mares should be vaccinated with tetanus toxoid inoculation 4–6 weeks prior to breeding.

SYNONYMS

Lockjaw

SEE ALSO

N/A

ABBREVIATIONS

- *C. tetani* = *Clostridium tetani*
- GABA = gamma-aminobutyric acid
- HYPP = hyperkalemic periodic paralysis

Suggested Reading

George LW. Tetanus. In Smith BP, ed. Large animal internal medicine. 2nd ed. St. Louis: Mosby, 1996:1150-1154.

Green SL, et al. Tetanus in the horse: a review of 20 cases (1970 to 1990). J Vet Intern Med 1994;8:128-132.

Kowalski JJ. Anaerobic infections. In: Reed SM Bayly WM, ed. Equine internal medicine. Philadelphia: WB Saunders, 1998:78-80.

Author Peggy S. Marsh
Consulting Editor Corinne R. Sweeney

TETANUS

BASICS

DEFINITION

A neuromuscular blockade disorder associated with tetanospasmin, a potent exotoxin of *Clostridium tetani*

PATHOPHYSIOLOGY

Tetanus

- Most commonly, *C. tetani* infects patients through wound contamination.
- Disease results when relatively anaerobic conditions are present in necrotic, poorly perfused tissues.
- Infection by other pyogenic organisms may be supportive. This is a common scenario in deep puncture wounds.
- The new environment favors spore germination, bacterial proliferation, and toxin elaboration. However, castration sites, endometritis and retained placenta, use of contaminated hypodermic needles, and omphalophlebitis have been associated with tetanus.
- Spores are viable in tissues for many months. Germination may occur long after a wound has healed if a new injury induces a renewed, favorable environment.
- The incubation period usually is 1–3 weeks but may range from several days to several months.

Tetanospasmin

- A water-soluble protein that is produced locally and is distributed to the CNS hematogenously and by passage along peripheral nerves.
- Toxin is irreversibly captured by gangliosides within synaptic membranes localized in the ventral horn gray matter of the spinal cord and brainstem, blocking the release of inhibitory neurotransmitters. The result is that ambient stimulation (i.e., low-level environmental background) stimulates reflex action that normally is inhibited by descending inhibitory motor tracts or by inhibitory interneurons. The result is muscular tetanus, with unrelenting contraction of muscle.
- Peripherally, tetanospasmin is associated with sympathetic nervous system stimulation, neuromuscular blockade, and catecholamine and adrenocorticoid metabolic alterations.
- Progression and severity of clinical signs relate to the rate of toxin elaboration, total dose of toxin, and the affected animal's size, age, and vaccination status.

SYSTEMS AFFECTED

Primarily the neuromuscular system, with the respiratory, urinary, GI, and other systems secondarily involved.

SIGNALMENT

No specific signalment

SIGNS

Historical Findings

- Trauma and lack of vaccination is common.
- Puncture wounds are typical.
- Other historical scenarios include recent foaling, omphalophlebitis, and other pyogenic conditions.

Physical Examination Findings

- The rate of progress and severity of clinical signs relate to the rate of toxin elaboration, total dose of toxin, and the affected animal's size, age, and vaccination status.
- Signs reflect spasticity of striated and smooth muscle.
- The earliest clinical signs often occur in the locale associated with the infectious focus.
- Early generalized clinical signs include overreaction to ambient external stimuli and a stiff gait, with reluctance to forage off the ground.
- Trismus (i.e., masticatory muscle spasm, lockjaw) may cause difficulty in prehension and eating.
- An anxious facial expression (e.g., retracted lips, flared nostrils, erect ears) occurs in association with facial muscular spasm.
- Ocular muscle spasm is associated with eyeball retraction and third-eyelid prolapse.
- Facial stimulation or loud noises are associated with more extensive facial and cervical muscle spasm.
- Clinical signs progress, with worsening extensor rigidity of the neck, limbs, and tail—sawhorse stance
- Paraspinal muscle spasm results in ventral (generalized) or lateral (early, when signs may be asymmetric) arching of the neck and back.
- Inability to posture appropriately can be associated with urine and fecal retention.
- Spasticity of pharyngeal muscles can result in regurgitation or aspiration of feed.
- Abdominal pain may be an early sign or complication. This may be associated with hyperreactive sympathetic function.
- If affected horses fall, they have great difficulty regaining posture.
- Muscle spasms may be severe enough to induce bone fractures.
- Death occurs secondary to asphyxia.
- If horses survive, signs stabilize within 7 days. Recovery is slow and gradual, however, and can take 6 weeks. This period is shorter in horses younger than 1 year.
- Recovery usually is complete, but recovered animals are not protected from further episodes.

CAUSES

C. tetani

- A slender, motile, Gram-positive bacillus that requires anaerobic conditions for growth and replication.
- Most commonly in spore form, and common in the intestinal tract and feces of animals and in organic material–rich soils.
- Spores are resistant to most environmental extremes, chemical disinfectants, and antimicrobial drugs, but they can be destroyed by heating to 115°C for 20 minutes.

RISK FACTORS

- Lack of protective vaccination
- Untreated wounds
- Retained placenta

DIAGNOSIS

DIFFERENTIAL DIAGNOSIS

Hypocalcemic tetani

CBC/BIOCHEMISTRY/URINALYSIS

No associated abnormalities

OTHER LABORATORY TESTS

N/A

IMAGING

N/A

DIAGNOSTIC PROCEDURES

- Clinical signs and historical features are nearly pathognomonic.
- A definitive diagnosis can be established by culture and demonstration of toxin.

PATHOLOGIC FINDINGS

None from the primary disease, but secondary findings may be evident—pneumonia; trauma

TREATMENT

NURSING CARE

- Good nursing care is essential to tetanus management.
- Enteral feeding and fluid management may be necessary. Animals often will continue to eat and drink, but monitoring is essential.
- Placement of an indwelling IV catheter minimizes the stress of blood sampling and drug administration and can be used for parenteral nutrition when indicated.
- Manual rectal evacuation and bladder catheterization may be necessary.
- Some animals may need to be placed in a sling.

CONTROL OF MUSCLE SPASM

- Place the affected horse in a quiet, calm, still, dark, and breeze-free environment.
- Place cotton balls in the horse's ears, possibly under an ear fly net, to reduce acoustic stimulation.
- Acetylpromazine (0.05–0.1 mg/kg IV or IM q6–8h) provides mild muscle relaxation and sedation yet leaves the horse in a standing position.

NEUTRALIZATION OF UNBOUND TOXIN

- Attempted with IV, IM, or SC homologous TAT.
- TAT does not cross the blood–brain barrier or combine with toxin in retrograde axonal transport.
- Circulating levels of toxin usually are low, so large TAT doses often are unwarranted. A dose of 5,000–10,000 U should be sufficient.
- Larger doses may be administered before wound debridement, because further toxin absorption can occur during manipulation.
- Natural disease does not induce protective immunity. Therefore, administer tetanus toxoid at a separate site.
- Intrathecal (subarachnoid) administration of TAT has been used with variable success. The principle for administration via this route is the ability to circumvent the blood–CSF barrier and inactivate unbound toxin. In humans, progress of the disease is arrested, and survival rates improve. However, severe, adverse events (e.g., seizures) can occur. This therapy must be given early in the disease to be effective; 1,000–5000 IU of homologous TAT at the cisternal or lumbosacral site after slow removal of an equivalent volume of CSF are recommended. The addition of 20–100 mg of prednisone succinate has been recommended in human patients, but its use has not been reported in horses.

INHIBITION OF TOXIN ELABORATION

- Accomplished using antimicrobial therapy and wound debridement.
- Increased doses of sodium or potassium penicillin (40,000–200,000 U/kg IV q6h for the first 2–4 days) have been suggested to destroy the vegetative organism in poorly perfused necrotic tissue. These high doses should generate some concern of diarrhea in hospital conditions.
- There is concern that early debridement of wounds may be associated with increased toxin elaboration. Administer TAT before debridement, and perform tissue manipulation carefully and unaggressively until the animal is medicated and stabilized.

LONG-TERM NURSING CARE

The goal is to maintain the horse until the toxin–ganglioside complexes are gradually replaced by unaltered gangliosides.

MEDICATIONS

DRUGS OF CHOICE

See *Treatment.*

CONTRAINDICATIONS

N/A

PRECAUTIONS

N/A

POSSIBLE INTERACTIONS

N/A

ALTERNATIVE DRUGS

N/A

FOLLOW-UP

PATIENT MONITORING

N/A

PREVENTION/AVOIDANCE

Vaccination programs are effective.

POSSIBLE COMPLICATIONS

- Trauma associated with recumbency and muscle spasm is common.
- Decubital ulcers, rhabdomyolysis, bone fracture, muscle or tendon rupture, and pneumonia can occur.

EXPECTED COURSE AND PROGNOSIS

- Fair prognosis in horses that remain standing.
- Horses in lateral recumbency are less likely to recover.

MISCELLANEOUS

ASSOCIATED CONDITIONS

N/A

AGE-RELATED FACTORS

N/A

ZOONOTIC POTENTIAL

N/A

PREGNANCY

N/A

SYNONYMS

N/A

SEE ALSO

N/A

ABBREVIATIONS

- CSF = cerebrospinal fluid
- GI = gastrointestinal
- TAT = tetanus antitoxin

Suggested Reading

Green SL, et al. Tetanus in the horse: a review of 20 cases (1970–1990). J Vet Intern Med 1994;8:128–130.

Muylle E, et al. Treatment of tetanus in the horse by injection of tetanus antitoxin into the subarachnoid space. J Am Vet Med Assoc 1975;167:47–48.

Sanders RKM, et al. Intrathecal antitetanus serum (horse) in the treatment of tetanus. Lancet 1977;1:974–977.

Author Joseph J. Bertone

Consulting Editor Joseph J. Bertone

TETRALOGY OF FALLOT

BASICS

DEFINITION

A group of congenital defects that includes a VSD, overriding aorta, right ventricular outflow tract obstruction, and right ventricular hypertrophy

PATHOPHYSIOLOGY

- Blood shunts from right to left in affected horses.
- The overriding aorta, right ventricular outflow tract obstruction, and VSD result in blood from the right ventricle shunting out the aorta during systole, creating the right-to left-shunt.
- Some shunting of blood between the right and left ventricle also occurs during systole and diastole.
- A pressure overload of the right ventricle occurs secondary to the right ventricular outflow tract obstruction, resulting in right ventricular hypertrophy.
- Size of the VSD and severity of the right ventricular outflow tract obstruction are the primary determinants for the severity of clinical signs.
- Horses with severe right ventricular outflow tract obstruction have marked resting arterial hypoxemia caused by the large right-to-left shunt.

SYSTEM AFFECTED

Cardiovascular

GENETICS

Not yet determined in horses

INCIDENCE/PREVALENCE

- Low prevalence in the equine population
- Reported in <5% of congenital cardiac disease in horses.

SIGNALMENT

- Murmurs are detectable at birth.
- Diagnosed most frequently in neonates, foals, and young horses.

SIGNS

General Comments

Usually detected during routine auscultation postpartum or because the foal is unthrifty.

Historical Findings

- Unthrifty youngster that has grown poorly
- Exercise intolerance
- Congestive heart failure

Physical Examination Findings

- Grade 3–6/6 coarse, band- or ejection-shaped, pansystolic murmur with PMI in the pulmonic valve area
- Grade 3–6/6 coarse, band-shaped, pansystolic murmur with PMI in the tricuspid valve area; this murmur usually is one grade softer than that found in the pulmonic valve area.
- Tachycardia
- Cyanotic mucous membranes—rare at rest; more likely after exercise

CAUSES

- Congenital malformation of the interventricular septum, right ventricular outflow tract, pulmonic valve, or pulmonary artery
- Aortic malalignment

RISK FACTORS

N/A

DIAGNOSIS

DIFFERENTIAL DIAGNOSIS

- VSD with pulmonic stenosis—no cyanosis; differentiate echocardiographically.
- Outflow tract VSD—foal not stunted; no cyanosis; differentiate echocardiographically.
- Pulmonic stenosis—rare; no cyanosis present; differentiate echocardiographically.
- Tricuspid regurgitation—murmur has PMI over the tricuspid valve area; foal not stunted; no cyanosis present; differentiate echocardiographically.

CBC/BIOCHEMISTRY/URINALYSIS

Polycythemia may be present but rarely is reported.

OTHER LABORATORY TESTS

N/A

IMAGING

Electrocardiography

A right-axis shift may be detected associated with right ventricular hypertrophy.

Echocardiography

- VSD usually is in the membranous and perimembranous portion of the interventricular septum, immediately beneath the septal leaflet of the tricuspid valve and right or noncoronary leaflet of the aortic valve.
- The aorta overrides the interventricular septum and may appear dextraposed.
- The pulmonary artery and pulmonic valves usually are hypoplastic, but valvular pulmonic stenosis also occurs.
- Poststenotic dilatation of the pulmonary artery may be present.
- The right ventricle is enlarged, and the right ventricular free wall and moderator band are thickened.
- Contrast echocardiography reveals shunting of blood from the right ventricle to the aorta; some blood flow from the right to the left ventricle also may be detected.
- Pulsed-wave or color-flow Doppler reveals the right ventricular outflow tract obstruction with its high-velocity turbulent jet in the pulmonary artery and shunting of blood from the right ventricle out the aorta. The pressures between the two ventricles are similar; thus, little shunting usually occurs through the VSD.

Thoracic Radiography

Decreased pulmonary vascularity and cardiac enlargement may be detected.

DIAGNOSTIC PROCEDURES

- Right-sided cardiac catheterization can be performed to directly measure right atrial, right ventricular, and pulmonary arterial and aortic pressures and to sample blood for oxygen content.
- Elevated right ventricular pressure and decreased oxygen saturation of blood obtained from the left ventricle, aorta, and peripheral arteries in affected horses
- The catheter also may be guided through the VSD to sample blood from the left ventricle and to measure left ventricular pressure.

TETRALOGY OF FALLOT

PATHOLOGIC FINDINGS

- VSD, overriding aorta, and cause of the right ventricular outflow tract obstruction are detected.
- In most horses, the pulmonary artery and pulmonic valve are hypoplastic.
- Poststenotic dilatation may be detected in the main pulmonary artery.
- Jet lesions may be detected along the VSD margins and around the outflow tract obstruction.
- The right ventricular free wall and moderator band are thicker than normal and hypertrophied.
- Congestive heart failure—ventral and peripheral edema, pleural effusion, pericardial effusion, and chronic hepatic congestion may be detected.

TREATMENT

APPROPRIATE HEALTH CARE

- Affected horses usually develop congestive heart failure by 2 years of age.
- Affected horses should be humanely destroyed once clinical signs of congestive heart failure develop or at diagnosis.

NURSING CARE

N/A

ACTIVITY

Affected horses are not safe to use for athletic performance and should not be broken to ride or drive.

DIET

N/A

CLIENT EDUCATION

- Do not use affected horses for any type of athletic work.
- Do not breed affected horses.
- If humane destruction is not chosen at diagnosis, closely monitor the horse for exercise intolerance, respiratory distress, venous distention, jugular pulsations, or ventral edema that, if detected, should prompt euthanasia.

SURGICAL CONSIDERATIONS

Surgical repair of the defect is not practical and does not result in an equine athlete.

MEDICATIONS

DRUGS OF CHOICE

N/A

CONTRAINDICATIONS

N/A

PRECAUTIONS

N/A

POSSIBLE INTERACTIONS

N/A

ALTERNATIVE DRUGS

N/A

FOLLOW-UP

PATIENT MONITORING

N/A

PREVENTION/AVOIDANCE

N/A

POSSIBLE COMPLICATIONS

N/A

EXPECTED COURSE AND PROGNOSIS

- All affected horses have a grave prognosis for life.
- Foals with large VSDs (>4 cm) and severe right ventricular outflow tract obstruction are likely to develop congestive heart failure during the first year of life; foals with less severe right ventricular outflow tract obstruction may survive slightly longer.
- The oldest reported horse with the condition was 3 years old.

MISCELLANEOUS

ASSOCIATED CONDITIONS

- Tricuspid regurgitation can develop in horses with significant right ventricular volume and pressure overload secondary to stretching of the tricuspid annulus.
- Aortic regurgitation can develop in horses with large aortic roots and aortic valve prolapse. The aortic valve leaflet lacks the support from the interventricular septum and prolapses into the defect, resulting in aortic regurgitation.
- Patent ductus arteriosus also may be present in some horses, which is a condition known as Pentalogy of Fallot.

AGE-RELATED FACTORS

Young horses are more likely to be diagnosed.

ZOONOTIC POTENTIAL

N/A

PREGNANCY

Do not breed affected horses.

SYNONYMS

N/A

SEE ALSO

- Congestive heart failure—right sided
- Pulmonic stenosis
- Systolic murmurs
- VSD

ABBREVIATIONS

- PMI = point of maximal intensity
- VSD = ventricular septal defect

Suggested Reading

Cargile J, Lombard C, Wilson JH, Buergelt CD. Tetralogy of Fallot and segmental uterine aplasia in a three-year-old Morgan filly. Cornell Vet 1991;81:411–418.

Marr CM. Cardiac murmurs: congenital heart disease. In: Marr CM, ed. Cardiology of the horse. Philadelphia: WB Saunders, 1999:210–232.

Reef VB. Cardiovascular disease in the equine neonate. Vet Clin North Am Equine Pract 1985;1:117–129.

Reef VB. Cardiovascular ultrasonography. In: Reef VB, ed. Equine diagnostic ultrasound. Philadelphia: WB Saunders, 1998:215–272.

Reef VB. Echocardiographic findings in horses with congenital cardiac disease. Compend Contin Educ Pract Vet 1991;13:109–117.

Author Virginia B. Reef
Consulting Editor N/A

THORACIC TRAUMA

BASICS

DEFINITION

• May be penetrating or blunt.
• Penetrating trauma usually results from collision with an object.
• Blunt trauma occurs in neonatal foals at parturition.
• Pneumothorax, internal (i.e., hemothorax) or external hemorrhage, shock, fractured ribs and foreign bodies may be associated problems.

PATHOPHYSIOLOGY

• The pleural cavity is formed by the opposing parietal and pulmonary pleurae, which normally are separated by a thin film of serous fluid.
• Pneumothorax (i.e., air in the pleural cavity) causes varying degrees of lung collapse, mechanical inability to inflate the lung, and inadequate ventilation.
• Open pneumothorax occurs when air can enter and leave the pleural cavity during respiration through a wound.
• Tension pneumothorax occurs with an influx of air on inspiration without an equivalent volume efflux on expiration, causing a build up of pressure, either progressive or acute, in the pleural cavity. The lungs collapse and, eventually, also may be compressed, leading to a severe and often life-threatening ventilatory compromise.
• Fractured ribs cause pain and may lead to hypoventilation; the latter, when combined with pulmonary contusions, can lead to pneumonia.
• Hemothorax displaces the pulmonary lobes and reduces ventilatory ability; subsequently, a fibrous layer may cover the lung surface and decrease pulmonary compliance.
• A penetrating injury combined with hemothorax carries a risk of septic pleuritis.
• Large vessel or cardiac injury can cause shock.
• Transdiaphragmatic perforation can cause viscus rupture and septic peritonitis.

SYSTEMS AFFECTED

• Respiratory—pneumothorax, rib fracture, and pulmonary parenchymal contusions or laceration
• Cardiovascular—cardiac tamponade or laceration, great vessel, and intercostal artery or pulmonary parenchymal vessel injury
• GI—foreign-body penetration of the abdominal cavity, causing intestinal or abdominal organ injury

GENETICS

N/A

INCIDENCE/PREVALENCE

• Penetrating trauma is rare.
• Blunt trauma occurs in 20% of newborn foals at birth but is clinically important in a much smaller percentage.

SIGNALMENT

• Neonatal foals are predisposed to rib fracture.
• No sex or breed predilections

SIGNS

Historical Findings

• History of penetrating or blunt trauma
• Tachypnea or increased respiratory effort
• Colic
• Foals may be lethargic and lie in a sternal position.

Physical Examination Findings

• Cyanotic or pale mucous membranes
• Absence of lung sounds dorsally on thoracic auscultation and increased resonance on percussion—indicative of pneumothorax
• Reduced lung sounds ventrally and decreased resonance on percussion—suggestive of hemothorax
• Inspection and palpation of the thoracic cage may permit detection of a penetrating wound, edema, or fractured ribs associated with birth trauma.
• Subcutaneous emphysema usually is palpated with penetrating thoracic wounds.
• When neonatal foals are carefully placed in dorsal recumbency, anterior thoracic cage asymmetry, caused by fractured ribs or costochondral dislocation, at the site of birth trauma may be observed.

CAUSES

• Collision with an object, particularly fences, is the most common cause of penetrating thoracic wounds.
• Birth trauma in foals occurs resulting from compression of the thorax during passage through the dam's pelvis. Fractured ribs caused by birth trauma may lacerate the pulmonary lobes, causing pneumothorax; the heart, causing sudden death or hemothorax; or the diaphragm, causing diaphragmatic hernia.

RISK FACTORS

• Free-roaming horses
• Newborn foals from primiparous mares
• Dystocia

DIAGNOSIS

Because these horses may suffer from polytrauma, an approach consisting of first look, shock and emergency treatment, recheck, and then diagnosis is suitable.

DIFFERENTIAL DIAGNOSIS

• Pain can cause rapid shallow breathing.
• Diaphragmatic hernia
• Pleural effusion or pneumonia

CBC/BIOCHEMISTRY/URINALYSIS

• CBC—stress leukogram and leukocytosis if secondary bacterial infection; anemia caused by blood loss
• Serum chemistry—hypoproteinemia indicating blood loss

OTHER LABORATORY TESTS

Arterial blood gas analysis may reveal hypoxemia, hypo- or hypercapnia, respiratory alkalosis, or respiratory or metabolic acidosis depending on the magnitude of pneumothorax and hemothorax and ability of the animal to compensate.

IMAGING

Thoracic Radiography

• Performed when the horse is stabilized
• Retraction of lung margins from the thoracic wall, with varying degrees of lung collapse, will be evident; radiopaque foreign objects, fluid in the thorax, fractured ribs, or diaphragmatic hernia also may be seen.

Echocardiography

• The air resulting from a pneumothorax appears similar to a normal, aerated lung.
• Fluid/gas interfaces permit recognition of pneumothorax.
• Fluid may result from hemothorax or pleural septic effusion.
• Foreign bodies or fractured ribs may be detected.
• Diaphragmatic hernia may be diagnosed based on visualization of bowel loops in the thoracic cavity.
• Abdominal fluid may indicate hemoperitoneum caused by diaphragmatic perforation and abdominal organ damage or peritonitis caused by viscus trauma.

DIAGNOSTIC PROCEDURES

• Thoracocentesis confirms a diagnosis of pneumothorax or hemothorax and should be performed as a therapeutic measure in dyspneic animals.
• Thoracoscopy to evaluate pulmonary pathology and to detect nonradiopaque foreign bodies
• Abdominal paracentesis when abdominal cavity perforation is suspected

PATHOLOGIC FINDINGS

• Hemothorax
• Rib fracture
• Pulmonary contusion or laceration
• Cardiac tamponade or laceration
• Diaphragmatic laceration
• Intestinal or abdominal organ injury
• Septic pleuritis or peritonitis
• Extrathoracic trauma

THORACIC TRAUMA

TREATMENT

APPROPRIATE HEALTH CARE

- Emergency care and continuous surveillance for severe cases.
- Inpatient care until stabilized
- Respiratory function should be monitored carefully.

NURSING CARE

- Administer oxygen by nasopharyngeal insufflation (10–15 L/min) for dyspneic and hypoxemic patients.
- Control of external hemorrhage and shock treatment with IV fluids (hypertonic/isotonic) during in the acute period; however, remember the contused lung is extremely sensitive to overload with IV crystalloid solutions, which should be used sparingly.
- Temporarily close penetrating wounds with sterile antibiotic ointment and gauze; suture after the patient is stabilized.
- Decompress the pleural cavity when clinical signs are observed at rest and the wound is sealed. Perform thoracocentesis using a large-gauge needle or teat cannula attached to a three-way stop cock, extension set, and 60-mL syringe . The site for aseptic air evacuation is the dorsal thoracic cavity, just in front of the twelfth to fifteenth ribs, to avoid the intercostal blood vessels along the caudal surface of the latter.
- For severe or active pneumothorax, place a thoracostomy tube in the pleural cavity, and attach to a Heimlich valve or continuous-suction apparatus in cases with rapid reaccumulation of air. Evacuation pressures $\leq$20 cm H_2O should be used, and the air should be removed from the thorax slowly to avoid re-expansion pulmonary edema (i.e., a complication of rapidly reinflating a lung after a period of collapse secondary to pneumothorax, hemothorax, or pleural effusion).
- Positive-pressure ventilation and decompression of the pneumothorax before surgery
- When clinical signs caused by pneumothorax are minimal at rest, the pneumothorax will gradually resorb if the animal is confined.
- Drain a hemothorax in the presence of a penetrating thoracic wound, because the blood may serve as a medium for bacterial growth. Evacuation of a hemothorax also prevents development of a fibrinous layer around the lung, which impedes pulmonary expansion.
- Fractured ribs usually are not stabilized, but rough edges may be rongeured and fragments removed.
- Debride and close wounds primarily when possible.
- Confine foals with fractured ribs for 2–3 weeks, and if possible, avoid manipulation of these foals to prevent exacerbating injuries by the fractured ribs.
- Blood or plasma transfusions should be considered if hemorrhage has caused severe blood loss.
- IV fluid therapy for patients in cardiovascular shock.

ACTIVITY

Box stall rest until all associated problems resolve

DIET

N/A

CLIENT EDUCATION

Discuss clinical signs of pneumothorax, and advise immediate return with recurrence.

SURGICAL CONSIDERATIONS

Suture wounds whenever possible to rapidly achieve an air-tight seal.

MEDICATIONS

DRUGS OF CHOICE

- Broad-spectrum antibiotics for patients with wounds.
- Analgesics to avoid splinting and hypoventilation because of pain from fractured ribs.

CONTRAINDICATIONS

Avoid drugs such as xylazine or opioids, because they may reduce PaO_2.

PRECAUTIONS

N/A

POSSIBLE INTERACTIONS

Check for signs of hypoventilation—increased $PaCO_2$, decreased PaO_2.

ALTERNATIVE DRUGS

N/A

FOLLOW UP

PATIENT MONITORING

- Respiratory rate and effort, mucous membrane color, heart rate and pulse quality, auscultation, and measurement of PCV and total solids during the first 24–48 hours.
- Serial blood gas analyses reveal effectiveness of ventilation.
- Radiography can be repeated at 48 hours.

PREVENTION/AVOIDANCE

Appropriate restraint to avoid further trauma.

POSSIBLE COMPLICATIONS

- Recurrence of pneumothorax or hemothorax
- Pyothorax
- Bacterial pneumonia in young foals
- Septic peritonitis and shock when intestinal viscus penetration has occurred.

EXPECTED COURSE AND PROGNOSIS

- Full recovery if the injury is not severe and does not involve the great vessels or abdominal cavity
- Complications addressed above may alter the expected course.

MISCELLANEOUS

ASSOCIATED CONDITIONS

- Fractured ribs
- Diaphragmatic hernia
- Ruptured trachea
- Thoracic and abdominal organ lacerations
- Other complications of trauma

AGE-RELATED FACTORS

N/A

ZOONOTIC POTENTIAL

N/A

PREGNANCY

N/A

SYNONYMS

N/A

SEE ALSO

- Diaphragmatic hernia
- Expiratory dyspnea
- Inspiratory dyspnea
- Pleuropneumonia
- Pneumothorax

ABBREVIATIONS

- GI = gastrointestinal
- PCV = packed cell volume

Suggested Reading

Holcombe SJ, Laverty S. Thoracic trauma. Auer Equine Surg, 2nd ed. Philadelphia: WB Saunders, 1999, 382–385.

Jean DA, Laverty S, Halley J, Hannigan D, Leveillé R. Thoracic trauma in newborn foals. Equine Vet J 1999;31(2)149–152.

Laverty S. Thoracic trauma. Current therapy in equine medicine 4. Philadelphia: WB Saunders, 1997, 463–465.

Laverty S, Lavoie JP, Pascoe JR, Ducharme N. Penetrating wounds of the thorax in 15 horses. Equine Vet J 1996:220–224.

Author Sheila Laverty

Consulting Editor Jean-Pierre Lavoie

THROMBOCYTOPENIA

BASICS

DEFINITION

• A peripheral platelet count <the lower limit of normal
• Defined by most laboratories in the horse as a peripheral platelet count <100,000 cells/μL.

PATHOPHYSIOLOGY

• Platelets are anucleate fragments produced by bone marrow megakaryocytes with a life span in the bloodstream of 4–5 days.
• Normally, peripheral platelet counts remain stable, because platelet production is equivalent to platelet removal from the circulation.
• Low numbers of circulating platelets can result from decreased production, increased destruction, sequestration, or increased utilization.
• Decreased platelet production most often results from generalized bone marrow disease secondary to an infiltrative process (e.g., myelofibrosis or myeloproliferative disease) or toxin (e.g., phenylbutazone or chloramphenicol). In these horses, all bone marrow cell lines (i.e., leukocytes, erythrocytes, and platelets) usually are decreased in the peripheral circulation.
• Increased platelet destruction usually results from immune-mediated processes—production of true antiplatelet antibodies (autoimmune thrombocytopenia), immune complex disease, drug-related antibodies that cross-react or nonspecifically adhere to platelets, or alteration of platelet surface antigens to enhance antibody attachment.
• Platelets may be sequestered in a large spleen or areas of abnormal vasculature (e.g., hemangiosarcoma).
• The most common cause in horses admitted to referral hospitals is increased utilization of platelets during DIC; transient, mild thrombocytopenia also may occur as platelets are utilized after trauma or hemorrhage.

SYSTEMS AFFECTED

• With a platelet count <30,000 cells/μL, hemorrhage can occur into any organ system.
• Hemorrhage most commonly is observed in the skin, respiratory, GI, and renal/urologic systems.

SIGNALMENT

• May be more common in Standardbreds
• Neonatal alloimmune thrombocytopenia has been recognized in newborn foals and may be more common in mule foals

SIGNS

General Comments

• Clinical bleeding rarely is observed in horses with platelet counts >30,000 cells/μL.
• Most horses with clinical signs have platelet counts <10,000 cells/μL.

Historical Findings

Spontaneous and inappropriate bleeding from mucous membranes, skin, nasal cavity, urinary tract, and GI tract

Physical Examination Findings

• Petechial and ecchymotic hemorrhages of mucosal membranes
• Prolonged bleeding after venipuncture
• Epistaxis, melena, or hyphema

CAUSES

Increased Utilization

• DIC
• Vasculitis
• Excessive hemorrhage or trauma
• Hemangiosarcoma or hemangioma
• Hemolytic uremic syndrome
• Thrombosis

Increased Destruction

• Primary IMTP—autoimmune or idiopathic thrombocytopenia
• Secondary IMTP—secondary to neoplasia, bacterial or viral infection, or drugs
• Drug- or toxin-induced platelet damage
• Snake bites

Decreased Production

• Hereditary defects
• Myelophthisis
• Myeloproliferative disease
• Myelosuppressive drugs or toxins
• Idiopathic pancytopenia

Increased Sequestration

Splenomegaly

Miscellaneous

• EIA
• Equine granulocytic ehrlichiosis (*Ehrlichia equi*)
• Acute viral diseases

RISK FACTORS

• Potentially, any drug may result in IMTP, but heparin and myelosuppressive drugs are specifically incriminated
• Viral or bacterial infections
• Neoplasia
• Autoimmune or immune-mediated disorders

DIAGNOSIS

DIFFERENTIAL DIAGNOSIS

• An underlying GI disorder or gram-negative infection and clinical signs of endotoxemia strongly suggest DIC; in these horses, many clotting parameters are often abnormal—prolonged PT and APTT, increased FDPs, and decreased plasma ATIII
• Evidence of recent hemorrhage, trauma, or exposure to vitamin K antagonists suggests increased utilization.
• Splenomegaly and mild thrombocytopenia suggest sequestration.
• History of treatment with drugs may indicate secondary IMTP.
• With neoplasia, consider secondary IMTP.
• EIA and equine granulocytic ehrlichiosis can be confirmed by appropriate serologic testing.
• Consider primary/idiopathic IMTP by exclusion of other causes.
• Concurrent neutropenia and anemia suggest a primary bone marrow production deficit.

CBC/BIOCHEMISTRY/URINALYSIS

• With anemia and leukopenia, consider decreased production.
• Inclusion bodies in granulocytes indicate equine granulocytic ehrlichiosis.
• Inflammation, toxic changes, or left shift may indicate endotoxemia/DIC; a coagulation profile is indicated.
• Poor venipuncture technique can result in clumping or activation of platelets, leading to a falsely low platelet count. Clumping may occur in samples collected into EDTA, resulting in EDTA-dependent pseudothrombocytopenia. Blood smears should be visually evaluated for platelet clumping before automated platelet counts are reported.
• Equine platelets are smaller than human platelets. Check with the laboratory to ensure their equipment is accurately calibrated to detect equine platelets; if not, request a manual platelet count.
• Endotoxemia may produce in vivo platelet activation and clumping of platelets with a falsely low platelet count.

THROMBOCYTOPENIA

OTHER LABORATORY TESTS

- Coggins test to rule out EIA
- Serum titers to rule out equine granulocytic ehrlichiosis
- Coagulation profile (e.g., PT, APTT, FDPs, or ATIII).
- Normal clotting times rule out DIC and exposure to vitamin K antagonists.

IMAGING

- Abdominal ultrasonography may be indicated to identify splenomegaly, hepatomegaly, internal hemorrhage, and neoplasia.
- Thoracic radiography may be useful to detect thoracic disease—pleuropneumonia, abscess, or neoplasia.

DIAGNOSTIC PROCEDURES

- Bone marrow evaluation is indicated to rule out primary bone marrow disease.
- Bone marrow core biopsy is preferable to bone marrow aspiration to evaluate megakaryocyte numbers
- Core biopsy specimens may be obtained from the sternum or wing of the ilium.

TREATMENT

APPROPRIATE HEALTH CARE

- Treat patients with severe thrombocytopenia on an inpatient basis until stabilized; once stabilized, treat on an outpatient basis.

NURSING CARE

- Restrict the number of invasive diagnostic procedures to minimize bleeding; apply extended pressure after venipuncture.
- With life-threatening hemorrhage, transfuse fresh whole blood or platelet-rich plasma.
- Discontinue any current medication being administered to horses with suspected IMTP.

ACTIVITY

Restrict activity if thrombocytopenia is severe to minimize the risk of excessive hemorrhage.

MEDICATIONS

DRUGS OF CHOICE

- IMTP—initial administration of dexamethasone (0.1 mg/kg IV or IM twice daily, gradually tapering to once daily); if long-term maintenance therapy is required, alternate-day oral or parenteral administration of the lowest effective dose of dexamethasone or prednisolone is indicated.
- Refractory IMTP—azathioprine (3 mg/kg PO once daily).
- DIC—heparin (see *Disseminated Intravascular Coagulation*).
- Rickettsial disease (*E. equi*)—oxytetracycline (7 mg/kg IV once or twice daily)

CONTRAINDICATIONS

NSAIDs that interfere with platelet function, especially aspirin

PRECAUTIONS

N/A

POSSIBLE INTERACTIONS

N/A

ALTERNATIVE DRUGS

N/A

FOLLOW-UP

PATIENT MONITORING

- Monitor extent of bleeding closely.
- Daily platelet counts until patient is stabilized, then weekly platelet counts until count returns to the normal range
- Repeated clotting profiles if DIC suspected

POSSIBLE COMPLICATIONS

Excessive hemorrhage

EXPECTED COURSE AND PROGNOSIS

- Very variable, depending on the inciting cause
- Some patients with IMTP respond to corticosteroid therapy in 6–7 days and can be off medication within 15 days. Others respond much more slowly, and others require maintenance therapy. Some do not respond at all.
- Prognosis varies with the underlying cause
- Response to therapy is a useful prognostic indicator.

MISCELLANEOUS

ASSOCIATED CONDITIONS

- Immune-mediated hemolytic anemia
- Bacterial, viral, or fungal infection
- Neoplasia

AGE-RELATED FACTORS

Young foals tend to have higher platelet counts than adult horses, especially males.

ZOONOTIC POTENTIAL

N/A

PREGNANCY

N/A

SYNONYMS

N/A

SEE ALSO

- Coagulation defects, acquired/induced
- Coagulation defects, inherited
- DIC
- EIA
- Equine granulocytic ehrlichiosis
- Myeloproliferative diseases
- Pancytopenia (aplastic anemia)
- Petechia/ecchymoses/bruising

ABBREVIATIONS

- APTT = activated partial thromboplastin time
- ATIII = antithrombin III
- DIC = disseminated intravascular coagulation
- EIA = equine infectious anemia
- FDPs = fibrin degradation products
- GI = gastrointestinal
- IMTP = immune-mediated thrombocytopenia
- PT = prothrombin time

Suggested Reading

Sellon DC, Grindem CB. Quantitative platelet abnormalities in horses. Comp Contin Educ Pract Vet 1994; 16:1335–1346.

Sellon DC, Levine J, Millikin E, Palmer K, Grindem C, Covington P. Thrombocytopenia in horses: 35 cases (1989–1994). J Vet Intern Med 1996;10:127–132.

Author Janene K. Kingston

Consulting Editor Debra C. Sellon

THROMBOCYTOSIS

BASICS

OVERVIEW

• Platelet count exceeds the upper limit of the reference range; at Washington State University, the reference range in horses is 100,000–350,000 platelets/μL.
• Most frequently occurs because of increased platelet production in response to a chronic infectious or inflammatory disease. Increased interleukin 6 production as part of the acute-phase inflammatory response may stimulate increased bone marrow platelet production.
• Primary thrombocytosis results from primary overproduction of platelets by the bone marrow (myeloproliferative disorder).
• Usually no systemic effects
• Usually no thrombosis, but an increased tendency to thrombosis may be present with very high platelet counts (>1,000,000 cells/μL). If thrombosis occurs, it may lead to organ dysfunction and associated clinical signs.
• Coagulation usually is normal; bleeding may occur in patients with concurrent platelet functional defects.

SIGNALMENT

Young male horses normally have higher platelet counts.

SIGNS

Usually no signs directly attributable to thrombocytosis

Historical Findings

Relate to the primary underlying disease process and may reflect a primary infectious or inflammatory disorder (e.g. fever, depression, inappetance, exercise intolerance)

Physical Examination Findings

Reflect the primary underlying disease process and vary accordingly

CAUSES AND RISK FACTORS

Primary Thrombocytosis

Essential thrombocythemia—primary bone marrow production excess

Secondary (Reactive) Thrombocytosis

• Chronic infection or inflammation—pleuropneumonia, peritonitis, abscesses, septic arthritis, and septicemia
• Chronic GI inflammation—chronic colitis, protein-losing enteropathy, and hepatitis
• Neoplasia—any form of marrow or nonmarrow neoplasia, including lymphosarcoma, adenocarcinoma, and leiomyosarcoma
• Rebound after an episode of hemorrhage or thrombocytopenia
• Immune-mediated hemolysis or other forms of hemolysis, including neonatal isoerythrolysis
• Corticosteroid therapy
• Iron deficiency
• Trauma—fractures and soft-tissue trauma
• Excitement—mobilization of splenic platelet reserves

DIAGNOSIS

DIFFERENTIAL DIAGNOSIS

• Colic and diarrhea—consider chronic GI inflammation or neoplasia
• Fever—consider chronic infectious or inflammatory disease, including pleuropneumonia, peritonitis, internal abscessation, septic arthritis, and septicemia
• Chronic blood loss—consider iron deficiency
• Trauma—consider bone fracture or soft-tissue injury
• Lameness—consider septic arthritis, bone fracture, or soft-tissue injury
• Drug therapy—consider thrombocytosis associated with corticosteroid administration
• Excitement during blood collection—consider transient splenic contraction
• Abdominal or thoracic mass—consider abscess or neoplasia
• Pleural effusion—consider pleuropneumonia or neoplasia
• Peritoneal effusion—consider pleuropneumonia or neoplasia

CBC/BIOCHEMISTRY/URINALYSIS

• Inappropriate sample collection or handling—traumatic venipuncture, long periods of time between sample collection and processing, and use of EDTA as an anticoagulant may result in a decreased platelet count because of in vitro platelet clumping.
• Endotoxemia—may produce in vivo platelet activation and clumping, with a resultant decrease in the platelet count.
• Observe feathered edge of a stained blood smear—if platelet clumping is apparent, collect a new sample in sodium citrate and recount. Equine platelets are smaller than human platelets. Confirm with the laboratory that their automated cell counters are calibrated to detect these smaller platelets; if not, request a manual count.
• Leukocytosis, neutrophilia, or left shift—consider chronic infectious or inflammatory disorder
• Hyperfibrinogenemia—consider chronic infectious or inflammatory disorder
• Microcytic, hypochromic anemia—consider iron deficiency
• Anemia with hemoglobinemia/hemoglobinuria—consider immune-mediated hemolysis
• Neutrophilia, lymphopenia, and eosinopenia—consider previous corticosteroid administration
• Extremely high platelet count (>750,000 cells/μL)—consider primary myeloproliferative disorder
• Circulatory blast or other abnormal cells—consider myeloproliferative disorder
• Hypoproteinemia or hypoalbuminemia—consider chronic GI inflammatory disorder or chronic peritonitis/pleuropneumonia
• Increased hepatocellular enzymes—consider hepatic disease

OTHER LABORATORY TESTS

• Serum iron, serum ferritin, and bone marrow iron stores should be decreased with iron deficiency anemia.
• Total iron-binding capacity should be increased, and percentage saturation transferrin typically decreased, with iron deficiency anemia.

THROMBOCYTOSIS

IMAGING

- Thoracic radiography or ultrasonography to detect pleuropneumonia, abscess, or neoplasia
- Abdominal ultrasonography to detect peritonitis, abscess, or neoplasia

DIAGNOSTIC PROCEDURES

- Bone marrow core biopsy or aspiration to detect myeloproliferative disorder
- Endoscopy to detect GI disorders (e.g., gastric ulcers)
- Abdominocentesis to detect peritonitis or neoplasia
- Thoracocentesis to detect pleuropneumonia or neoplasia
- Arthrocentesis to detect septic arthritis
- Xylose or glucose absorption tests to detect inflammatory small intestinal disease
- Biopsy or aspiration of any external or internal mass to confirm abscesses or neoplasia

TREATMENT

- Specific treatment to decrease the platelet count usually not indicated or needed
- Treat the underlying disease process.

MEDICATIONS

DRUGS

- Treat the underlying disease process.
- With extremely high platelet counts or evidence of increased tendency to thrombosis, consider aspirin therapy.

CONTRAINDICATIONS/POSSIBLE INTERACTIONS

With evidence of abnormal platelet function, avoid NSAIDs, especially aspirin.

FOLLOW-UP

PATIENT MONITORING

- Monitor CBC and platelet count as needed.
- Monitor the underlying disease process as needed; thrombocytosis should resolve as the underlying disease process resolves.

POSSIBLE COMPLICATIONS

- Thrombosis with extremely high platelet counts, possibly increasing the risk of laminitis or organ dysfunction.
- Hemorrhage if platelet function is impaired.

MISCELLANEOUS

ASSOCIATED CONDITIONS

N/A

AGE-RELATED FACTORS

Young male horses are more likely to be affected.

ZOONOTIC POTENTIAL

N/A

PREGNANCY

N/A

SEE ALSO

Thrombocytopenia

ABBREVIATION

- GI = gastrointestinal

Suggested Reading

Sellon DC, Levine JF, Palmer K, et al. Thrombocytosis in 24 horses (1989–1994). J Vet Intern Med 1997;11:24–29.

Author Debra C. Sellon
Consulting Editor Debra C. Sellon

THYROID TUMORS

BASICS

OVERVIEW
• Thyroid adenoma, adenocarcinoma, and C-cell (i.e., parafollicular) tumors have been reported in horses.
• Adenomatous change is quite common in old horses.
• In one postmortem survey of 100 horses, 34 had normal thyroids, 20 hyperplastic changes, 9 colloid tumors and 37 adenomas.
• Tumors usually are incidental findings and not associated with clinical signs.

SIGNALMENT
• Most common in horses >10 years
• No reported sex or breed predilections
• No known genetic basis

SIGNS
• Typically no associated clinical signs; rather, thyroid tumors are detected at physical examination by palpation of an enlarged thyroid gland.
• Signs more commonly are associated with adenocarcinoma and C-cell tumors and associated with either hypothyroidism or hyperthyroidism.
• The most frequently reported physical sign is weight loss.
• Other associated signs—nervousness, work intolerance, respiratory embarrassment, and cold intolerance.
• Behavioral disturbances—pacing and difficulty when being handled
• Tachypnea and tachycardia also may be present.

CAUSES AND RISK FACTORS
• No known risk factors
• Hypertrophy and adenomatous change may be a common occurrence in old horses.

DIAGNOSIS

DIFFERENTIAL DIAGNOSIS
• The diagnosis usually is established by a combination of physical examination and diagnostic tests.
• Suspect thyroid adenoma in any old horse with an enlarged thyroid gland.
• Diagnostic differentials—goiters without neoplasia, retropharyngeal lymph node enlargement, hematoma, and enlarged guttural pouches

CBC/BIOCHEMISTRY/URINALYSIS
Generally normal

OTHER LABORATORY TESTS
• Serum T_4 and T_3 levels may be increased or decreased if the tumors lead to hypo- or hyperthyroidism.
• In one horse described with hyperthyroidism from an adenocarcinoma, free T_4 concentrations were quite elevated above the normal range, but total T_4 levels were not increased.
• In horses with hypothyroidism, serum T_3 and T_4 concentrations are below the reference range.

IMAGING
• A tumor may be imaged via ultrasonography as one or more nodules within the thyroid gland.
• If the tumor is so large that the entire gland is enlarged, this may be seen on radiographs of the cervical region as a soft-tissue density.

DIAGNOSTIC PROCEDURES
• Fine-needle aspiration allows identification of the tumor as being of thyroid origin but often does not allow differentiation between adenoma and adenocarcinoma.
• Biopsy of the thyroid gland mass provides a definitive diagnosis.

PATHOLOGIC FINDINGS
• Most tumors are adenomas.
• Other tumor types occur infrequently.

TREATMENT
• With a discrete, noninvasive thyroid tumor, surgical removal of the affected thyroid lobe should be curative, but with metastatic disease, the prognosis is poor.
• C-cell tumors and adenocarcinomas spread slowly, and surgical removal generally is curative.

THYROID TUMORS

MEDICATIONS

DRUGS

- Use of antithyroid drugs has not been reported in horses but can be considered if local invasion or metastasis precludes complete surgical removal.
- If bilateral tumors occur and the complete gland is removed, thyroxine supplement (20 μg/kg) is indicated.
- Calcium supplementation is not necessary, because horses have parathyroid tissue spread diffusely in the cervical area.

CONTRAINDICATIONS/POSSIBLE INTERACTIONS

N/A

FOLLOW-UP

- Anesthetic complications have been reported after tumor removal; thus, surgery on hyperthyroid horses should be done in a controlled setting in which monitoring equipment and emergency treatments are available.
- Once the tumor is removed, any clinical signs should gradually resolve.

MISCELLANEOUS

ASSOCIATED CONDITIONS

N/A

AGE-RELATED FACTORS

Affected horses tend to be old (>10 years).

ZOONOTIC POTENTIAL

N/A

PREGNANCY

N/A

SEE ALSO

- Hyperthyroidism
- Hypothyroidism

ABBREVIATIONS

- T_3 = triiodothyronine
- T_4 = thyroxine

Suggested Reading

Held JP, Shaftoe S, Rose ML, et al. Work intolerance in a horse with thyroid carcinoma. J Am Vet Med Assoc 1985;197:1187–1189.

Author Janice Sojka
Consulting Editor Michel Levy

TOXIC HEPATOPATHY

BASICS

OVERVIEW

Many toxins that cause liver disease (i.e., toxic hepatopathy) in horses; however, most do not cause liver failure and, therefore, likely go until a chemistry panel is performed.

SIGNALMENT

- Any age, breed or gender
- Ferrous fumarate (i.e., acute iron poisoning) was common when a previously commercially available product was administered PO to foals before colostrum nursing.
- Adult horses in the western U.S. and eastern Canada often are fed alfalfa hay including pyrrolizidine alkaloid–containing plants.
- A presumed genetic disorder causing liver disease may occur in selected breeding lines of Morgans.

SIGNS

- Mostly those of hepatoencephalopathy—head pressing, circling, blindness, maniacal behavior or depression, and excessive yawning
- Photosensitization may occur on white-haired parts of the body or mucus membranes.
- Icterus and discolored urine may be noted.
- Weight loss has occurred in a few cases of chronic poisoning.

CAUSES AND RISK FACTORS

- The causes and risk factors are numerous.
- Pyrrolizidine alkaloid–containing plants usually are ingested when mixed in "first-cutting" alfalfa hay—*Senecio* sp. (i.e., groundsel and ragwort) and *Amsinckia intermedia* (i.e., fiddleneck) are common in eastern Canada.
- Iron toxicosis generally results from overzealous iron administration PO. In newborn foals, even small amounts of iron given PO before colostrum may be fatal; in adults, large amounts of iron PO are necessary to produce toxicity.
- Mycotoxins may cause hepatic failure—*Fusarium moniliformis* in horses fed moldy corn, and *Aspergillus flavus* rarely in horses fed peanuts or other sources; most horses with *Fusarium* poisoning have leukoencephalomalacia rather than hepatic failure.
- Pasture-associated hepatopathy may occur in horses grazing on alsike clover (northeastern U.S. and Canada) or Klein grass (southwestern U.S.).

DIAGNOSIS

DIFFERENTIAL DIAGNOSIS

- The differential for hepatoencephalopathy includes encephalopathies, encephalitis, or selected metabolic disorders (e.g., severe acidosis).
- These disorders generally involve no increase in hepatic enzymes and certainly no abnormalities in liver function tests (e.g., direct bilirubin).

CBC/BIOCHEMISTRY/URINALYSIS

- CBC abnormalities most often involve neutrophilia with toxic changes.
- Liver enzymes, both hepatocellular (i.e., AST, SDH) and biliary enzymes (i.e., GGT), are markedly elevated in acute toxic hepatopathy. In chronic toxicities (e.g., pyrrolizidine alkaloid poisoning), enzymes may not be markedly elevated, although GGT remains elevated in most cases, even with chronic fibrosis.
- Serum bile acids remain elevated in all cases.
- BUN and fibrinogen generally are abnormally low.
- Albumin, because of its long half-life, may remain.
- Both conjugated and unconjugated bilirubin are increased, with the greatest increase involving unconjugated bilirubin.
- Urine may be discolored (dark brown to orange), and when shaken, the foam may appear green.
- Urine dipstick examination usually is positive for bilirubin.

TOXIC HEPATOPATHY

OTHER LABORATORY TESTS

• Prothrombin and partial thromboplastin times are prolonged.
• Blood ammonia may be high or normal.
• Urinary and/or hepatic concentrations of specific toxins may be found.
• Serum ferritin and measurement of hepatic iron may help to confirm the diagnosis of iron hepatopathy.

IMAGING

Ultrasonography is the procedure of choice.

DIAGNOSTIC PROCEDURES

Liver biopsy is most commonly performed for microscopic diagnosis of either hepatocellular necrosis (e.g., acute iron poisoning), periportal or diffuse fibrosis from chronic toxicosis, and/or megalocytosis (e.g., pyrrolizidine alkaloids).

TREATMENT

• Some horses may need hospitalization, especially with hepatoencephalopathy, to control abnormal behavior and supply supportive therapy (see *Icterus*).
• Avoid activity, sunlight, and high-protein feeds.

MEDICATIONS

DRUGS

• Xylazine (0.2–0.4 mg/kg IV) may be required to control maniacal behavior.
• IV fluids should be continuous for horses with hepatic failure, anorexia, and neurologic signs—acetated Ringer solution (20–40 mEq KCl/L) and dextrose (50 g/L).
• Neomycin (l0 g/500 kg) should be given PO mixed in molasses via syringe q8h for 2 days in cases of hepatoencephalopathy.

CONTRAINDICATIONS/POSSIBLE INTERACTIONS

N/A

FOLLOW-UP

• Fee a moderate-protein/high-energy feed.
• Avoid stress.
• Monitor serum enzymes and bile acids for progression of hepatic disease.
• Prognosis depends on toxin, degree of fibrosis, and progression of disease.
• All cases with moderate to extreme fibrosis have a guarded to poor prognosis for life >1 year.

MISCELLANEOUS

ASSOCIATED CONDITIONS

N/A

AGE-RELATED FACTORS

N/A

ZOONOTIC POTENTIAL

N/A

PREGNANCY

N/A

SEE ALSO

• Icterus
• Photosensitization

ABBREVIATIONS

• AST = aspartate aminotransferase
• GGT = γ-glutamyltransferase
• SDH = sorbitol dehydrogenase

Suggested Reading

Pearson EG. Pyrrolizidine alkaloid toxicosis. In: Robinson NE, ed. Current therapy in equine medicine 4. Philadelphia: WB Saunders, 1997:222–223.

Author Thomas J. Divers
Consulting Editor Michel Levy

TOXIC HEPATOPATHY

BASICS

OVERVIEW
• Many toxins cause liver disease (i.e., toxic hepatopathy) in horses.
• Fortunately, most toxins do not cause liver failure and, therefore, likely go unnoticed unless a chemistry panel is performed.

SIGNALMENT
• Any age, breed or gender
• Ferrous fumarate (i.e., acute iron poisoning) was common when a previously available commercial product was administered orally to foals before colostrum nursing.
• Adult horses in the western United States and eastern Canada often are fed alfalfa hay containing pyrrolizidine alkaloid–containing plants.
• A presumed genetic disorder causing liver disease may occur in selected breeding lines of Morgans.

SIGNS
• Mostly those of hepatoencephalopathy (e.g., head-pressing, circling, blindness, maniacal behavior, depression) with excessive yawning
• Photosensitization may occur on white-haired body parts or mucus membranes.
• Icterus and discolored urine may be noted.
• Weight loss may occur in some cases of chronic poisoning.

CAUSES AND RISK FACTORS
Numerous, but the most common include:

Pyrrolizidine Alkaloid–Containing Plants
• Usually ingested when mixed in "first cutting" alfalfa hay.
• *Senecio* sp. (i.e., groundsel and ragwort) and *Amsinckia intermedia* (i.e., fiddleneck) are common in eastern Canada.

Iron Toxicosis
• Generally a result of overzealous oral iron administration
• In newborn foals, even small amounts of iron given orally before colostrum may be fatal.
• In adult horses, large amounts of iron given orally are necessary to produce toxicity.

Mycotoxins
• May cause hepatic failure in horses.
• *Fusarium moniliformis* in horses fed moldy corn.
• *Aspergillus flavus* (rarely) in horses fed peanuts or other sources
• Most horses with *Fusarium* sp. poisoning have leukoencephalomalacia rather than hepatic failure.

Pasture-Associated Hepatopathy
May occur in horses grazing on alsike clover (northeastern U.S. and Canada) or klein grass (southwestern U.S.).

DIAGNOSIS

DIFFERENTIAL DIAGNOSIS
• Encephalopathies, encephalitis, or selected metabolic disorders—severe acidosis
• These disorders generally have no increase in hepatic enzymes and certainly no abnormalities in liver function test—direct bilirubin.

CBC/BIOCHEMISTRY/URINALYSIS
• CBC abnormalities most often are neutrophilia with toxic changes.
• Liver enzymes, both hepatocellular (i.e., AST, SDH) and biliary (i.e., GGT), are markedly elevated in acute toxic hepatopathy.
• In chronic toxicities (e.g. pyrrolizidine alkaloid poisoning), enzymes may not be markedly elevated, but GGT remains elevated in most cases, even with chronic fibrosis.
• Serum bile acids remain elevated in all cases.
• BUN and fibrinogen generally are abnormally low.
• Albumin, because of its long half-life in the horse, may remain in normal range.
• Both conjugated and unconjugated bilirubin are increased, with the greatest rise occurring in unconjugated bilirubin.
• Urine may be discolored (i.e., dark brown to orange), and when shaken, the foam may appear green.
• Urine dipstick examination usually is positive for bilirubin.

OTHER LABORATORY TESTS
• Prothrombin and partial thromboplastin times are prolonged.
• Blood ammonia may be high or normal.
• Urinary and hepatic concentrations of specific toxins may be found.
• Serum ferritin and measurement of hepatic iron may help to confirm the diagnosis of iron hepatopathy.

IMAGING
N/A

DIAGNOSTIC PROCEDURES

Liver biopsy most commonly is performed for microscopic diagnosis of either hepatocellular necrosis (e.g., acute iron poisoning), periportal or diffuse fibrosis from the chronic toxicosis, or megalocytosis (e.g., pyrrolizidine alkaloids).

TREATMENT

- Some horses may need to be hospitalized, especially those with hepatoencephalopathy, to control the abnormal behavior and to supply supportive therapy.
- Avoid activity, sunlight, and high-protein feeds.

MEDICATIONS

DRUGS

- Xylazine (0.2–0.4 mg/kg IV) may be required to control maniacal behavior.
- IV fluids—acetated Ringer with KCl (20–40 mEq/L) and dextrose (50 g/liver) should be continuous for horses with hepatic failure, anorexia, and neurologic signs.
- Neomycin (10 g per 500 kg PO q8h) should be given mixed in molasses via syringe for 2 days for hepatoencephalopathy.

CONTRAINDICATIONS/POSSIBLE INTERACTIONS

N/A

FOLLOW-UP

- Feed horses a moderate-protein/high-energy feed.
- Avoid stress.
- Monitor serum enzymes and bile acids for progression of disease.
- Prognosis depends on toxin, degree of fibrosis, and progression of disease. All cases with moderate to extreme fibrosis have a guarded to poor prognosis for survival of >2 years.

MISCELLANEOUS

ASSOCIATED CONDITIONS

N/A

AGE-RELATED FACTORS

N/A

ZOONOTIC POTENTIAL

N/A

PREGNANCY

N/A

SEE ALSO

N/A

ABBREVIATIONS

- AST = aspartate aminotransferase
- GGT = γ-glutamyltransferase
- SDH = sorbitol dehydrogenase

Suggested Reading

Pearson EG. Pyrrolizidine alkaloid toxicosis. In: Robinson NE, ed. Current Therapy in Equine Medicine 4. Philadelphia: WB Saunders, 1997:222–223.

Author Thomas J. Divers
Consulting Editor Joseph J. Bertone

TRAILER LOADING/UNLOADING PROBLEMS

BASICS

DEFINITION

- Two general types
- The most common is the horse that hesitates or refuses to enter or exit a trailer or van. The problem can range from mild hesitation, in which the horse takes more than 60 seconds to begin to enter or exit the trailer, to complete refusal to approach or exit the trailer. In some horses this refusal includes fearful, active escape or aggressive behaviors.
- The other extreme is the horse that enters or exits the trailer too rapidly, creating a safety problem for itself and its handlers.

PATHOPHYSIOLOGY

Most cases are not caused by disease; however, impaired vision, impaired balance, or musculoskeletal pain in the back or hindquarters may contribute.

SYSTEMS AFFECTED

- Behavioral—signs range from balking to severe fear responses, with the corresponding involvement of other organ systems.
- Cardiovascular—signs may be consistent with sympathetic stimulation (e.g., tachycardia and vasodilation).
- Endocrine/metabolic—sympathetic stimulation, increases in ACTH and cortisol concentrations, perspiration, and defecation
- Respiratory—increased respiration rate

SIGNALMENT

Any age, sex, or breed

SIGNS

Historical Findings

The horse may be unfamiliar with the trailer or van or with the loading/unloading process, or it may have had an unpleasant experience or injury involving a trailer.

Physical Examination Findings

N/A

CAUSES

- Horses are innately claustrophobic about small, dark, and enclosed areas.
- Unpleasant experiences and injuries involving trailering can create an aversion to the trailer or van.
- Trailers that are too small or poorly designed or inexperienced handlers and drivers can contribute to the problem.

RISK FACTORS

Small or poorly designed trailers as well as poor trailer-driving skills (e.g., sudden accelerations and decelerations or sharp turns).

DIAGNOSIS

DIFFERENTIAL DIAGNOSIS

- Trailer loading/unloading problems usually are behavioral in nature.
- Evaluated for normal vision, balance, and kinesis (ruling out confounding conditions, e.g., spinal ataxia, equine protozoal myelitis, myositis, lameness, etc.); if no abnormalities are found, the problem probably is behavioral.

CBC/BIOCHEMISTRY/URINALYSIS

N/A

OTHER LABORATORY TESTS

N/A

IMAGING

N/A

DIAGNOSTIC PROCEDURES

N/A

TREATMENT

GENERAL COMMENTS

- Trailer loading should be incorporated into every horse's regular training or handling program; during these training times, resistant behavior can be corrected and fearful behavior modified.
- Horses with severe fear or aggression during loading/unloading or with a long, confirmed history of trailering problems should be retrained by a professional trainer.
- Tranquilizers may alleviate loading/unloading problems temporarily but are not an effective, permanent therapy.

MILD PROBLEMS

- Modify the trailer to make it appear more open and less threatening.
- Use rubber mats to make the floors nonslip and less noisy.
- Open doors and windows, use interior lights, or place the trailer where the interior is illuminated.
- Remove the interior partition, or swing it to one side and secure it.
- Change to a step-up or ramp-type trailer, depending on the horse's preference.
- Use a trailer with larger interior dimensions, or try an open stock trailer.
- Use an existing fence or alleyway to limit the horse's movement away from the trailer.
- Make sure the footing in the loading area is nonslip (grass or packed soil is preferable to pavement) and that the ramp, if used, is covered with a nonslip surface.
- Keep the loading ramp level, or minimize the step-up height by parking the trailer on a slight hill.
- Load a quiet horse before the reluctant horse.

TRAILER LOADING/UNLOADING PROBLEMS

TRAINING

- Training a horse to load/unload both willingly and readily is time-consuming and should not be attempted unless the handlers are willing to commit that time.
- Horses that will not load usually do not lead readily and willingly and do not respect their handler as a dominant "leader."
- Teach the horse to willingly walk beside (not behind) the handler by using negative reinforcement techniques. Control the horse with a well-fitting halter and a 10-foot cotton lead. Use a 4-foot whip to tap the horse atop of its rump near the tailhead to encourage active forward movement. Use the whip as negative reinforcer (e.g., tap with just enough intensity to make the horse move forward energetically, and stop using the whip immediately when the horse does so).
- Once the horse leads willingly, take it around the trailer and, finally, approach the trailer entrance. Allow the horse time to investigate the trailer.
- Using the whip, ask the horse to approach the trailer one step at a time. Stay at the horse's side during loading; standing in front of the horse and pulling on the lead is counterproductive.
- If the horse turns away from the trailer, reinforce the leading lesson in a small circle with enough intensity the horse learns it must work if not facing the trailer opening.
- Once the horse willingly faces the trailer opening, encourage it to step forward and into the trailer using the same negative reinforcement technique. When the horse steps into the trailer with one or both front feet, reward it immediately by removing the negative reinforcer and by praising and stroking. Allow or even encourage the horse to back out of the trailer at this point, because the horse also must learn to unload and that the trailer is not a trap.
- After the horse willingly loads and unloads with its front feet, use the negative reinforcer to encourage the horse to put its back feet in the trailer. Remove the negative reinforcer and praise and stroke for any steps into the trailer. Again, allow the horse to place a hind foot in the trailer and to back out repeatedly before asking the horse to load fully.
- Repeat this process numerous times on this day and on following days; repetition of the loading/unloading process teaches the horse this is a nonthreatening routine.
- The horse can be given a food reward after it enters the trailer fully; however, a food reward before this point usually prolongs the training process.

SAFETY ISSUES

- Never stand in front of the horse and pull on the lead or try to pulley the horse into the trailer; the horse may pull back and fall over backward or leap atop the handler.
- Never tie the horse in the trailer until fully loaded and the trailer doors are securely shut. A tied horse that tries to back out of a trailer usually panics, hits its head on the trailer, and may break its legs if they slip under the back of the trailer.
- Always untie the horse and remove butt bars or chains before opening the trailer doors.
- Never get between the horse and the trailer. The handler should always have an escape route. Use the "escape door" in the trailer to access the horse after it is securely loaded, not to escape from a frantic horse; the escape door should be closed during loading/unloading to prevent a frightened horse from using it.
- Never allow the lead rope to become wrapped around the handler.
- Use protective equipment for the handler (e.g., boots and gloves) and for the horse (e.g., leg wraps, bell boots, and head bumper).
- Never load a horse in a light-weight trailer that is not coupled to the tow vehicle, because the trailer could tip or roll with the horse.

MEDICATIONS

DRUGS OF CHOICE

N/A

CONTRAINDICATIONS

N/A

PRECAUTIONS

N/A

ALTERNATIVE DRUGS

N/A

FOLLOW-UP

PATIENT MONITORING

Consult the owner in 2–4 weeks to determine if retraining was attempted and successful; if the problem has not improved, advise the owners to contact a professional trainer for assistance.

POSSIBLE COMPLICATIONS

N/A

MISCELLANEOUS

ASSOCIATED CONDITIONS

Poor hauling behavior—scrambling, kicking, or excessive movement in trailers or vans

AGE-RELATED FACTORS

N/A

ZOONOTIC POTENTIAL

N/A

PREGNANCY

N/A

SYNONYMS

N/A

SEE ALSO

- Fears and phobias
- Scrambling in trailer

Suggested Reading

N/A

Author Cynthia A. McCall
Consulting Editor Daniel Q. Estep

TRAUMA-ASSOCIATED BLINDNESS

BASICS

DEFINITION

Head injuries associated with optic nerve or optic nuclei damage that have minimal other signs

PATHOPHYSIOLOGY

- Injuries to the back of the head can be associated with blindness.
- When blindness occurs, it often is associated with unilateral or bilateral optic nerve rupture.
- Occasionally, blind horses with caudal head trauma can recover their sight within a few days. In these cases, blindness may have resulted from occipital cortical (i.e., optic cortex) edema or other pathology that resolves.
- Optic nerves can possibly be traumatized but not completely ruptured.

SYSTEMS AFFECTED

CNS and other traumatized tissues

SIGNALMENT

No specific signalment

SIGNS

Historical Findings

Recent trauma, especially when the horse rolled backward or received pol trauma

Physical Examination Findings

- Lack of or sluggish pupillary light reflexes and menace response are indicative.
- Degree of other CNS signs depends on the extent of damage.
- Pupils often are widely dilated in bilateral optic nerve rupture.
- Within 2–6 weeks, generalized retinal degeneration and optic nerve atrophy in the affected eye(s)

CAUSES

Trauma, most often to the back of the head

RISK FACTORS

N/A

DIAGNOSIS

DIFFERENTIAL DIAGNOSIS

N/A

CBC/BIOCHEMISTRY/URINALYSIS

No specific abnormalities

OTHER LABORATORY TESTS

N/A

IMAGING

Skull radiography may indicate trauma, but if blindness is the only abnormality, no changes likely will be evident.

DIAGNOSTIC PROCEDURES

Physical examination findings consistent with blindness and recent trauma, most commonly to the back of the head

PATHOLOGIC FINDINGS

Optic nerve rupture

TREATMENT

Unless the injury extends to other CNS tissues, no specific treatment is indicated.

MEDICATIONS

DRUGS OF CHOICE

N/A

CONTRAINDICATIONS

N/A

TRAUMA-ASSOCIATED BLINDNESS

PRECAUTIONS
N/A

POSSIBLE INTERACTIONS
N/A

ALTERNATIVE DRUGS
N/A

FOLLOW-UP

PATIENT MONITORING
Observe the animal for several days; this allows cortical edema to resolve under the circumstances that this is the only abnormality.

POSSIBLE COMPLICATIONS
N/A

EXPECTED COURSE AND PROGNOSIS
No recovery if the nerves are ruptured

MISCELLANEOUS

ASSOCIATED CONDITIONS
N/A

AGE-RELATED FACTORS
N/A

ZOONOTIC POTENTIAL
N/A

PREGNANCY
N/A

SYNONYMS
N/A

SEE ALSO
N/A

Suggested Reading

Martin L, et al. Four cases of traumatic optic nerve blindness in the horse. Equine Vet J 1986;18:133–137.

Author Joseph J. Bertone
Consulting Editor Joseph J. Bertone

TRAINING PROBLEMS

BASICS

DEFINITION

• Behaviors that interfere with training or previously acquired trained responses
• These behaviors may be normal, species-typical behaviors, learned behaviors, the result of pathophysiologies, or some combination of these causes.
• Species-typical behaviors are characteristic of a species, manifest in response to environmental stimuli and opportunity, and are influenced by hormonal states, experience, learning, and physiologic condition of the animal. Courtship behaviors, intermale fighting, and nipping/head wrestling by stallions are species-typical behaviors that interfere with some training goals and safe management practices; shying at a novel object is an adaptive response to a potentially harmful stimulus.
• A training problem may be the manifestation of any one of several different causes; therefore, trying to answer definitively an inquiry based on a few descriptive (and potentially inaccurate) sentences often is counter-productive. For example, bucking under saddle may be a predator defense response, reaction to pain, or even play. Difficulties bridling may be a result of the horse anticipating pain because its ear was previously twisted or it currently has a painful pathology.
• A trainer's response to a problem behavior can profoundly affect the horse not only in the context of the problem but in other, later situations. Whipping a stallion whenever he neighs at another horse or has an erection while in training, for example, may (or may not) stop these unwanted behaviors; however, he later may not maintain an erection during a desired breeding situation and be aggressive when approached by people.

PATHOPHYSIOLOGY

• Watch the horse outside the training situation. If the problem also is apparent there, a physiologic cause is likely.
• If unwanted behaviors arise only during training sessions, the training methods should be carefully examined. If those methods adhere to sound principles of learning and the horse is not subject to abusive techniques, pathophysiologic conditions are likely.
• Pathophysiologic conditions also occur in horses being trained or ridden with inappropriate techniques. In the latter case, addressing the problem is more complex and requires the co-operation of open-minded, competent, and experienced rider/trainer/owners.

SYSTEMS AFFECTED

• Behavioral—species-typical responses and learned behaviors
• Any physiologic systems—musculoskeletal, endocrine, ophthalmic, nervous, etc.

SIGNALMENT

Any age, sex, or breed

SIGNS

Historical Findings

• Behavior signs (particularly those related to fear, pain, conflict, or discomfort) can be the same whether the cause is pathophysiologic or aversive training techniques.
• Common signs of discomfort—wringing or whipping of the tail, champing or fussing with the bit, tossing the head, bucking, head shyness, pinning back of ears, aggression, and evasive behaviors
• Common signs of conflict—pawing, yawning, closing the eyes, and repeatedly engaging in previously reinforced behaviors
• Common signs of fear or anxiety—pacing or attempts to pace, defecation, neighing, and defense responses

Physical Examination Findings

Should be unremarkable unless an underlying pathology is present.

CAUSES

• Behavioral problems during training can be normal, species-typical behaviors elicited by environmental stimuli, the result of pathophysiologies or inappropriate training techniques, or some combination of these causes.
• Dental problems—sharp edges on molars, caps on molars, or normal wolf-teeth. Contact of the bit or pressure from the halter on these structures can elicit bit champing, head tossing, and sometimes, bucking. If the pathology is unilateral, the horse's response may be very specific because of how the rider holds the reins (e.g., the horse only reacts when asked to take the left lead or only tosses his head when the halter is used to turn the head in one direction).
• Skeletal and muscular problems—most often, pain in the spinal column, back, hip, or stifle, but can occur in other locations; bucks under saddle; wrings or whips tail while being ridden.
• Endocrine problems—cystic ovaries (mares that buck only when asked to canter (i.e., weight of the rider shifts back), hypothyroidism (lethargy, slow to respond, seems unable to learn simple tasks), hyperthyroidism (agitated or jittery, runs fences, difficulty standing still), and diabetes (lethargic, will not stand square or still for prolonged periods of time because of frequent attempts to stretch out so they can urinate).
• Infection, parasites, or foreign body in ears—head shy, pin ears when reach for head, and resists the bridle being put on.
• Vision problems—shying (also when not in training situations; more likely to occur in unfamiliar environments), stopping at jumps, or refusing to traverse obstacles that were previously traversed. These same behaviors can be exhibited by horses that have experienced traumatic or punitive events in these circumstances or by naive horses fearful of novel items.
• Common inappropriate training techniques—being too harsh, inconsistency, not allowing the horse to distinguish between training cues, inadvertently rewarding the wrong behaviors, or random and inappropriately timed aversive stimuli. Training problems frequently arise from the trainer/rider giving a signal the horse does not understand; punishment can further compound the problem.
• Common species-typical behaviors—defensive responses to novel or fearful stimuli; social behaviors (e.g., greeting behaviors, separation distress responses, courtship behaviors, intermale aggression or displays).

RISK FACTORS

• Horses born and raised in a uniform, restricted environment or that are rarely handled as they mature are predisposed to fear when put in training situations, especially if transferred to a novel environment. Anxiety and fear interfere with learning processes, and fearful reactions often are met with punitive techniques, which usually makes the situation worse or causes additional problems.
• Trainers who base their training philosophies on "showing the horse who is the boss," "teaching the horse a lesson," and beliefs that horses "are trying to get away with something" or are "willfully disobedient." Rider/trainers with such philosophies are less likely to analyze situations critically for the precise stimuli eliciting the undesirable behaviors and are more likely to use punitive techniques.
• Physical correction of undesirable behaviors is not always contraindicated; negative reinforcement or punishment can be used appropriately and effectively. Aversive stimuli, however, always carry the risk of inducing anxiety and eliciting aggression. Trainers who rely predominantly on punitive procedures are more likely to produce fearful horses that, consequently, perform suboptimally. These horse may be apprehensive in paddocks and deplete energy reserves as they fret during prerace procedures, and they often wring or whip their tails (i.e., behaviors selected against in show rings). Occasionally, these horses become so fearful and defensively aggressive they become unusable.

TRAINING PROBLEMS

DIAGNOSIS

DIFFERENTIAL DIAGNOSIS

- Similar presenting signs can result from environmental, emotional, or pathologic disorders; therefore, a thorough physical examination is necessary.
- Other diagnostic strategies—watching the horse outside the training situation and changing tack, environment, and trainers.
- Detailed behavior history and observation of the problem, sometimes using videotapes

CBC/BIOCHEMISTY/URINALYSIS

Depending on the presenting signs

OTHER LABORATORY TESTS

Depending on the presenting signs

IMAGING

Depending on the presenting signs

DIAGNOSTIC PROCEDURES

Depending on the presenting signs

TREATMENT

- Training problems may persist after correction of the identified pathophysiologies. The horse may be conditioned to respond to cues that signal impending discomfort and continue to behave as before. The horse anticipates pain and reacts as in the past. The trainer must develop a training strategy to address this learned response. Allowing extinction to occur is one option; however, avoidance responses take a long time to extinguish. Another approach is identifying all stimuli associated with the conditioned response (e.g., bucking and tossing of the head when signaled to canter), removing as many of these as possible, and adding new, different stimuli to be associated with cantering. For example, use a hackamore, bosal, or head restraint that has not already been associated with bucking and tossing of the head; use a different saddle, or even a bareback pad; ask for a canter in a different location (e.g., on a trail instead of in a ring); and temporarily, without signaling for a canter, let the horse move into a canter with other horses on a trail. Because the signals to canter are not presented and the source of pain is gone, the horse does not buck when it moves into the canter. Gradually (ideally, one at a time), the stimuli once associated with bucking and tossing of head can be reintroduced.
- Veterinarians and owners should realize that many trainers now use humane training techniques exclusively and adhere to sound learning principles. Numerous successful trainers have written books, produced videos, and hold clinics clearly demonstrating that relaxed, championship horses can be trained with consistent, nonpunitive techniques.
- Training problems exist primarily because the horse does not understand what the trainer wants, the horse is frightened or ill, or because of interfering social behaviors of the horse. Training problems are not caused by the horse "trying to get away with something."
- Social responses (e.g., greeting behaviors, stallion displays, separation distress, fearful behaviors) are species-typical behaviors that must be addressed for most horses to be useful. Some can be addressed by allowing the horse more exposure to other horses and unfamiliar environments before concentrating on training. Separating stablemates for, initially, very short periods and then progressively longer periods of time may ameliorate separation distress responses. Overtraining in an optimum environment can facilitate competing, acceptable responses by the horse when introduced to other situations. Managing the environment is an important variable in preventing and treating training problems.
- Analyze problems, and look for the underlying reason why a behavior occurred—when Pat Parelli was asked what he does when a horse bites him, he answered, "I'd say dang and rub my arm. Then I'd get smarter."

MEDICATIONS

DRUGS OF CHOICE

No drugs are approved by the FDA for use with equine training problems.

CONTRAINDICATIONS

- Major and minor tranquilizers sometimes are used to control excited horses. Such drugs may reduce anxiety and fear of conditioned stimuli, but the animal still may react to an unconditioned stimulus (e.g., pain) with an unconditional response of kicking or attempts to flee.
- Benzodiazepines can reduce fear, but animals, including horses, often become aggressive while under the influence of these drugs.

PRECAUTIONS

N/A

POSSIBLE INTERACTIONS

N/A

ALTERNATIVE DRUGS

N/A

FOLLOW-UP

PATIENT MONITORING

Request the owner call every week with a progress report, or contact the owner at least every 2 weeks, to identify problems with the treatment program and to allow prompt correction of problems.

POSSIBLE COMPLICATIONS

N/A

MISCELLANEOUS

ASSOCIATED CONDITIONS

N/A

AGE-RELATED FACTORS

N/A

ZOONOTIC POTENTIAL

N/A

PREGNANCY

N/A

SYNONYMS

N/A

SEE ALSO

Fears and phobias

Suggested Reading

Borchelt PL, Voith VL. Punishment. In: Voith VL, Borchelt PL, eds. Readings in companion animal behavior. Trenton, NJ: Veterinary Learning Systems, 1996:72–80.

Hunt R. Think harmony with horses. Brunday, ID: Give-It-A-Go Books, 1978.

Parelli P. Savey-Up: The Official Parelli Natural Horse-Man-Ship Newsletter 1998;1:1–4.

Voith VL. Principles of learning. Vet Clin North Am Equine Pract 1986;2:485–506.

Voith VL, Borchelt PL. Fears and phobias in companion animals. In: Voith VL, Borchelt PL, eds. Readings in companion animal behavior. Trenton, NJ: Veterinary Learning Systems, 1996:140–152.

Author Victoria L. Voith
Consulting Editor Daniel Q. Estep

TRAUMATIC OPTIC NEUROPATHY

BASICS

OVERVIEW

- Commonly results from falling over backward and traumatizing the occipital crest.
- Tearing of the dural covering of the optic nerve or direct compression of the optic nerve associated with hemorrhage or fractures of the basisphenoid bone
- During the early stages, the optic disc may appear normal or edematous with hyperemia. Disc material may extrude into the vitreous, and rapid development of optic nerve atrophy is noted.
- Organ system—ophthalmic

SIGNALMENT

N/A

SIGNS

- Sudden blindness after head trauma
- Dilated pupil
- Most often bilateral
- No signs of eye pain

CAUSES AND RISK FACTORS

Skull trauma

DIAGNOSIS

DIFFERENTIAL DIAGNOSIS

- Exudative optic neuritis
- Ischemic retinopathy
- Retinal detachment
- Equine recurrent uveitis

CBC/BIOCHEMISTRY/URINALYSIS

N/A

OTHER LABORATORY TESTS

N/A

IMAGING

N/A

DIAGNOSTIC PROCEDURES

N/A

TREATMENT

MEDICATIONS

DRUGS

Immediate and aggressive parenteral nonsteroidal (flunixin meglumine, 1.0 mg/kg IV SID) or steroidal (prednisolone, 1.0 mg/kg IM SID) anti-inflammatory therapy (or both) may help to preserve some vision.

CONTRAINDICATIONS/POSSIBLE INTERACTIONS

N/A

TRAUMATIC OPTIC NEUROPATHY

FOLLOW-UP

PATIENT MONITORING

Acutely blind horses are anxious and dangerous.

EXPECTED COURSE AND PROGNOSIS

Poor prognosis for return of vision

MISCELLANEOUS

ASSOCIATED CONDITIONS

N/A

AGE-RELATED FACTORS

N/A

ZOONOTIC POTENTIAL

N/A

PREGNANCY

N/A

SEE ALSO

- Equine recurrent uveitis
- Exudative optic neuritis
- Ischemic optic neuropathy
- Retinal detachment

Suggested Reading

Brooks DE. Equine ophthalmology, In: Gelatt KN, ed. Veterinary ophthalmology. 3rd ed. Philadelphia: Lippincott Williams & Wilkins, 1999.

Author Maria Källberg
Consulting Editor Dennis E. Brooks

TREMORGENIC MYCOTOXIN TOXICOSES

BASICS

OVERVIEW

• Several mycotoxins cause equine neurologic disease—fumonisins, swainsonine, slaframine, lolitrems, and paspalitrems.
• Those considered to be "tremorgens" are the lolitrems (lolitrems A,B, C, and D) produced by *Acremonium lolii* and causing perennial ryegrass (*Lolium perenne*) staggers and paspalitrems (paspalinine, paspalitrem A and B) produced by *Claviceps paspali* and causing dallis grass or paspalum staggers (associated with dallis grass [*Paspalum dilatatum*] and bahia grass [*Bahia oppositifolia*]).
• A tremorgenic disease associated with ingestion of Bermuda grass (*Cynodon dactylon*) is believed to result from a mycotoxin, but a specific tremorgen has not been isolated.
• *Acremonium lolii* is an endophytic fungus of ryegrass and propagates via seed.
• *Claviceps paspali* is a soil fungus that invades dallis and bahia grass under favorable environmental conditions.
• Tremorgens are believed to competitively inhibit CNS postsynaptic GABA receptors and, therefore, chloride influx; GABA-receptor antagonism leads to increased nerve discharge and neurologic signs.
• Annual ryegrass toxicosis, whose clinical presentation is similar to that of tremorgenic mycotoxins, can result when the bacterium *Clavibacter toxicus* is carried into annual ryegrass seedheads by the nematode *Anguina funesta. Clavibacter toxicus* produces the neurotoxin corynetoxin, a glycolipid that inhibits the synthesis of lipid-linked oligosaccharides and blocks protein glycosylation.

SIGNALMENT

No breed, sex, or age predispositions

SIGNS

Perennial Ryegrass Staggers

• Signs can occur 5–10 days after grazing highly toxic pastures.
• Initial signs include head tremors and muscle fasciculations of the neck and legs, which progress to include head nodding and swaying while standing.
• Animals that are excited or forced to move develop dysmetria and leg stiffening, leading to collapse and tetanic spasms; if left alone, animals recover in a few minutes and walk away with a relatively normal gait.
• Affected animals rarely die unless they injure or entrap themselves during a tetanic spasm.
• Affected animals may lose weight and are difficult to handle or move because of inducible spasms.

Paspalum Staggers

Signs are identical to those of perennial ryegrass staggers but often less severe.

Annual Ryegrass Staggers

Signs are similar to those of perennial ryegrass staggers.

CAUSES AND RISK FACTORS

Perennial Ryegrass Staggers

• Pastures must be predominantly perennial ryegrass for toxicosis to occur.
• Incidence is greater during the late summer and fall and on ryegrass pastures that have been heavily grazed.
• Environmental temperatures generally > than 23°C
• Frequency of intoxication relates to the degree of fungal infection of the ryegrass. Infection rates <25% are associated with sporadic outbreaks, whereas rates >90% are associated with large outbreaks.

Paspalum Staggers

Toxin production is greatest during a wet period following seed head formation.

Annual Ryegrass Staggers

• Toxin concentration increases in seedheads during the summer and is greatest as the plant dries and seeds ripen.
• Annual ryegrass occurs in patches, and alterations in grazing patterns may predispose to ingestion.
• Newly introduced animals may ingest more ryegrass.

DIAGNOSIS

DIFFERENTIAL DIAGNOSIS

Other plant intoxications such as locoism (*Astragalus* spp.) and white snakeroot (*Eupatorium rugosum*)—evidence of plant consumption; characteristic histopathologic lesions; detection of tremetol in white snakeroot toxicosis

CBC/BIOCHEMISTRY/URINALYSIS

N/A

OTHER LABORATORY TESTS

Perennial Ryegrass Staggers

• Positive identification of perennial ryegrass
• Microscopic detection of fungus in ryegrass
• Mouse bioassay of methanol extracts from ryegrass to produce characteristic clinical signs
• Detection of lolitrems in ryegrass—concentrations of lolitrem B >2 ppm are associated with effects in sheep and cattle.

Paspalum Staggers

• Positive identification of dallis or bahia grass and associated fungal sclerotia on grass seedheads
• Detection of tremorgen

Annual Ryegrass Staggers
- Positive identification of annual ryegrass
- Identification of galls associated with nematode infestation
- ELISA for detection of corynetoxin

IMAGING
N/A

DIAGNOSTIC PROCEDURES
N/A

PATHOLOGIC FINDINGS
- Gross and histopathologic lesions generally are absent.
- Animals with chronic ryegrass staggers may have loss of Purkinje cells in the cerebellum, which is believed to be secondary to hypoxia and hypoglycemia.
- Histopathologic changes associated with annual ryegrass staggers include cerebellar, hepatic, and splenic hemorrhages that may be secondary to endothelial cell damage.

TREATMENT
Remove animals from affected grass pastures.

MEDICATIONS

DRUGS
N/A

CONTRAINDICATIONS/POSSIBLE INTERACTIONS
N/A

FOLLOW-UP

PATIENT MONITORING
Attempt to prevent self-injury during tetanic spasms.

PREVENTION/AVOIDANCE
Perennial Ryegrass Staggers
- Reduce overgrazing of pastures.
- Remove animals from pastures during critical periods—late summer and fall for endophyte-infested ryegrass pastures
- Use endophyte-free ryegrass seed (**CAUTION:** their use is associated with poor stands of grass).
- Use fungicides—reduces seed viability

Paspalum Staggers
Mow pastures to remove toxic seed heads.

Annual Ryegrass Staggers
- Break nematode life cycle by killing ryegrass for two to three growing seasons
- Integrated control measures—herbicide use in the spring, seeding pastures with legumes, burning infested pastures in the early autumn, applying herbicides to selectively kill ryegrass during the summer, and heavy winter grazing

POSSIBLE COMPLICATIONS
- Traumatic injury
- Bloating or drowning during tetanic spasm

EXPECTED COURSE AND PROGNOSIS
- Once removed from affected pastures, animals generally recover within several weeks without treatment.
- Degenerative CNS lesions associated with chronic perennial ryegrass staggers likely prevent full recovery.

MISCELLANEOUS

ASSOCIATED CONDITIONS
N/A

AGE-RELATED FACTORS
N/A

ZOONOTIC POTENTIAL
N/A

PREGNANCY
N/A

SEE ALSO
N/A

ABBREVIATIONS
- ELISA = enzyme-linked immunoadsorbent assay
- GABA = γ-aminobutyric acid

Suggested Reading

Plumlee KH, Galey FD. Neurotoxic mycotoxins: a review of fungal toxins that cause neurologic disease in large animals. J Vet Intern Med 1994;8:49–54.

Author Robert H. Poppenga
Consulting Editor Robert H. Poppenga

TRH AND TSH STIMULATION TESTS

BASICS

DEFINITION

• TRH and TSH stimulation tests are performed to evaluate the ability of the thyroid gland to secrete T_3 and T_4. No increase in blood T_3 and T_4 levels after TRH or TSH administration indicates hypothyroidism. TRH also may used as a screening test in horses with suspected pituitary tumors; increased cortisol after administration of TRH indicates a pars intermedia tumor of the pituitary gland—equine Cushing's syndrome
• TRH test to evaluate thyroid function—Give TRH (1 mg IV), and measure T_3 and T_4 levels at 0, 2, and 4 hours. Normally, the baseline T_3 and T_4 are in the reference range, the T_3 concentration doubles at 2 hours, and the T_4 concentration doubles at 4 hours.
• The TSH test (5 IU IV) is performed in the same manner, with the same expected end points.
• TRH test to evaluate pituitary function—Give TRH (1 mg IV), and measure blood cortisol at 0, 15, 30, 60, 120, and 180 minutes. Normally, the cortisol concentration does not change; an increased concentration suggests a pars intermedia tumor.

PATHOPHYSIOLOGY

• Thyroid hormone levels in blood are regulated by the thyroid-pituitary-hypothalamic axis. Endogenous TRH is released from the hypothalamus and travels to the pituitary gland. The pituitary gland then secretes TSH into the circulation, which stimulates release of T_4 and T_3 from the thyroid gland.
• When exogenous TSH is given, the thyroid gland's ability to secrete hormone is tested.
• When TRH is given, the pituitary gland's ability to respond to this by secreting TSH, and then the thyroid gland's ability to respond to the endogenous TSH is tested.
• In equine medicine, test selection is based primarily on availability of the reagents. Presently, TSH is not available for clinical use; however, TRH is labeled for use in human medicine and, although quite expensive, can be obtained.
• Why pituitary tumor cells respond inappropriately to TRH is not completely understood. Tumor cells are hypothesized to have an alteration in the receptor/adenylate cyclase system that allows for a paradoxic response to specific and nonspecific challenges.

SYSTEM AFFECTED

• The endocrine system is primarily affected by abnormal TSH or TRH stimulation tests—decreased thyroid hormone response to the stimulation test is diagnostic of hypothyroidism; increased cortisol in response to TRH is suggestive, although not diagnostic, of a pars intermedia tumor of the pituitary gland (i.e., equine Cushing's syndrome).

SIGNALMENT

• No sex or breed predilections.
• Hypothyroidism can occur at any age.
• Abnormal response caused by a thyroid or pituitary tumor tends to occur in old horses (>8 years).

SIGNS

• Signs associated with an abnormal TRH/TSH stimulation test are those of hypothyroidism or equine Cushing's syndrome.
• Clinical signs of congenital hypothyroidism in foals—prognathism, ruptured common digital extensor tendon, forelimb contracture, retarded ossification, crushing of the carpal and tarsal bones, weakness, and poor suckle reflex
• Less common signs of congenital hypothyroidism is foals—goiter, angular limb deformities, respiratory distress, abdominal hernia, poor muscle development, and osteoporosis
• Hypothermia and bradycardia are consistent findings in adults with hypothyroidism. Other signs include myositis, anhydrosis, laminitis, infertility, agalactia, poor hair coat, and poor growth.
• Clinical signs of equine Cushing's syndrome include hirsutism and failure to shed a winter coat; also common are abnormal fat distribution, pendulous abdomen, weight loss, polyuria and polydipsia, laminitis, and chronic infections

CAUSES

• The primary cause for lack of response in a TSH/TRH stimulation test is primary hypothyroidism. Many factors can cause low resting T_3 and T_4 levels in blood, but unless the horse is truly hypothyroid, the gland responds normally to exogenous stimulating hormones. When it does not, hypothyroidism is diagnosed.
• The primary cause for increased cortisol after TRH administration is stress response. Increased cortisol also may result from an inappropriate response of a pituitary tumor to TRH.

RISK FACTORS

• Known risk factors for thyroid abnormalities are primarily dietary. Intake of excess or inadequate iodine or ingestion of other goitrogens can lead to hypothyroidism.
• In old populations, thyroid tumor is a risk factor for development of thyroid abnormalities.
• Pituitary tumor is a risk factor for development of abnormal cortisol secretion in response to TRH.

DIAGNOSIS

DIFFERENTIAL DIAGNOSIS

• The primary differential diagnosis for increased cortisol after TRH administration is stress response. Psychic stress from handling, receiving injections, and blood sample collections result in increased blood cortisol.
• Stress response can be differentiated from pituitary tumor by more specific tests for that condition—endogenous ACTH assay or dexamethasone suppression test.

LABORATORY FINDINGS

Drugs that May Alter Lab Results

N/A

Disorders that May Alter Lab Results

N/A

Valid If Run in a Human Lab

Laboratory determination of T_3, free T_3, T_4, and free T_4 is valid if run in a human laboratory. Human thyroid hormone concentrations are higher than equine, though, so use equine reference ranges to interpret results.

CBC/BIOCHEMISTRY/URINALYSIS

• Hypothyroidism—anemia, leukopenia, and hypercholesterolemia
• Equine Cushing's syndrome—stress response with a mature neutrophilia, lymphopenia, and eosinopenia; possibly increased blood glucose and glucosuria

OTHER LABORATORY TESTS

Pituitary function—endogenous ACTH determination, dexamethasone suppression testing, and insulin response test; if results are consistent with equine Cushing's syndrome, this would support a positive TRH test.

IMAGING

• Ultrasonography—rarely useful in hypothyroidism, but an enlarged thyroid gland caused by tumor or goiter could be visualized.
• Radiography—an enlarged thyroid gland caused by tumor or goiter might be seen as an increased soft-tissue density in the throat-latch area.
• Increased pituitary gland size may be visualized with specialized modalities—CT or venous contrast

DIAGNOSTIC PROCEDURES

Fine-needle aspiration or biopsy may assist in assessing the thyroid gland.

TRH AND TSH STIMULATION TESTS

TREATMENT

APPROPRIATE HEALTH CARE

- Foals with congenital hypothyroidism may require inpatient medical management with severe disease.
- All other horses with abnormal TRH/TSH tests can be treated as outpatients.

NURSING CARE

- Foals may need assistance standing and milk administered via nasogastric tube if they are too weak to suckle.
- Foals may need mechanical ventilation if they cannot breathe on their own.
- Animals with poor hair coat may need blanketing.
- Horses with laminitis need corrective hoof trimming and shoeing.

ACTIVITY

- Limit activity of foals with musculoskeletal deformities—incomplete ossification of the carpal or tarsal bones
- Limit activity of horses with laminitis.

DIET

- Examine the diet of any horse with hypothyroidism and of dams with foals born having hypothyroidism to ensure the proper amount of iodine is being fed.
- Pregnant mares should not receive endophyte-infected fescue hay, particularly during the last months of gestation.
- Horses with laminitis generally benefit from a low-carbohydrate, high-fiber diet—grass hay

CLIENT EDUCATION

- The prognosis for soundness is poor in most foals with congenital hypothyroidism and, thus, should be discussed with owners before expensive treatments begin.
- Adult horses with hypothyroidism respond well to exogenous replacement hormone; their prognosis generally is good.
- Horses with Cushing's syndrome may be managed via medication and nursing care, but their prognosis is quite variable. Some do well for several years; others are refractory to treatment. Owners need to understand that treatment of Cushing's syndrome is palliative and required for life.

SURGICAL CONSIDERATIONS

If the abnormal TRH/TSH response test results from a tumor of the thyroid gland, surgical removal of the affected thyroid lobe should be curative.

MEDICATIONS

DRUGS OF CHOICE

- For decreased T_3 and T_4 caused by hypothyroidism, replacement therapy with T_4 is the drug of choice—20 μg/mL maintains T_4 and T_3 levels in the normal range for 24 hours; this constitutes a dose of 10 mg in a 1000-pound horse.
- The two agents most commonly used to alter symptoms of Cushing's syndrome are cyproheptadine (0.25–1.2 mg/kg PO SID) and pergolide (0.75–2 mg/day).

CONTRAINDICATIONS

If the horse has low resting T_3 and T_4 values because of some other severe disease (e.g., euthyroid sick syndrome), thyroid replacement therapies may cause further deterioration; thus, perform provocative testing before administering medication in any horse with suspected hypothyroidism that is debilitated or exhibits signs of any other disease.

PRECAUTIONS

- Exogenous thyroid hormone causes down regulation and, potentially, atrophy of the thyroid gland; thus, discontinue the supplement gradually over the course of several weeks.
- Horses that receive overdoses of cyproheptadine or pergolide may exhibit lethargy and ataxia.

POSSIBLE INTERACTIONS

N/A

ALTERNATIVE DRUGS

Other sources of thyroid hormone supplement are iodinated casein (5.0 g/day) and concentrated bovine thyroid extract (10 g/day).

FOLLOW-UP

PATIENT MONITORING

- Monitor horses on thyroid supplement by retesting serum T_4 and T_3 levels every 30–60 days. If the serum level is low, increase the dosage until the normal range is achieved; if the serum level is too high or on the higher end of the normal range, decrease the dosage and re-test the horse.
- Failure to respond clinically after 6 weeks of therapy should prompt reconsideration of the original diagnosis of thyroid disease.
- Retest horses with Cushing's syndrome every 6–12 weeks by endogenous ACTH determination or dexamethasone response test. Abnormal results indicate the need for an increased dose or a change in medication.

MISCELLANEOUS

ASSOCIATED CONDITIONS

- Angular limb deformities, hypognathism, weakness, and respiratory distress often are associated with congenital hypothyroidism.
- Infertility, skin problems, and myositis have been associated with hypothyroidism in adults.
- Hirsutism, chronic infections, and laminitis are commonly associated with equine Cushing's syndrome.

AGE-RELATED FACTORS

- On the first day of life, foals have little T_3 response to TRH/TSH administration; thus, only a T_4 response should be evaluated in neonatal foals.

ZOONOTIC POTENTIAL

N/A

PREGNANCY

N/A

SYNONYMS

N/A

SEE ALSO

- ACTH
- Hypothyroidism
- Pituitary tumors
- T_3
- T_4

ABBREVIATIONS

- TRH = thyroid-releasing hormone
- TSH = thyroid-stimulating hormone
- T_3 = triiodothyronine
- T_4 = thyroxine

Suggested Reading

Beech J, Garcia M. Hormonal response to thryotropin-releasing hormone in healthy horses and in horses with pituitary adenoma. Am J Vet Res 1985;46:1941–1943.

Morris DD, Garcia M. Thyroid stimulating hormone response test in healthy horses and effects of phenylbutazone on equine thyroid hormones. Am J Vet Res 1983;44:503–507.

Oliver JW, Held JP. Thyrotropin stimulation test: a new perspective on value of monitoring triiodothyronine. J Am Vet Med Assoc 1985;187:931–934.

Sojka JE. Hypothyroidism in horses. Compend Contin Educ Pract Vet 1995;17:845–852.

Author JE Sojka

Consulting Editor Michel Levy

TRICUSPID REGURGITATION

BASICS

DEFINITION

• When the tricuspid valve becomes insufficient, allowing blood to leak backward into the right atrium during systole, which creates a systolic murmur with its PMI in the tricuspid valve area
• The murmur radiates toward the right heart base dorsally or cranially.
• Occasionally, the murmur can be auscultated in the left second to third intercostal space.

PATHOPHYSIOLOGY

• Tricuspid leaflets do not form a seal between the right atrium and ventricle.
• During systole, blood regurgitates into the right atrium, causing increased right atrial pressure and right atrial and ventricular volume overload.
• As the regurgitation becomes more severe, further increases in right atrial pressure produce increased central venous pressure, hepatic congestion, and right-sided congestive heart failure.

SYSTEM AFFECTED

Cardiovascular

GENETICS

N/A

INCIDENCE/PREVALENCE

Reported more frequently in Thoroughbreds, particularly National Hunt horses, and in Standardbred racehorses.

SIGNALMENT

N/A

SIGNS

General Comments

Usually an incidental finding during routine auscultation unless the horse is in congestive heart failure

Historical Findings

• Poor performance
• Sometimes congestive heart failure

Physical Examination Findings

• Grade 2–6/6, band-shaped to crescendo holosystolic murmur with PMI in the tricuspid valve area radiating to the right heart base
• Other, less common findings—atrial fibrillation, accentuated third heart sound, jugular pulsations, generalized venous distention, and ventral edema

CAUSES

• Physiologic tricuspid regurgitation
• Degenerative changes of the tricuspid leaflets
• Pulmonary hypertension
• Nonvegetative valvulitis
• Ruptured chordae tendineae
• Bacterial endocarditis
• Congenital malformation

RISK FACTORS

N/A

DIAGNOSIS

DIFFERENTIAL DIAGNOSIS

VSD—relative pulmonic stenosis murmur; differentiate echocardiographically.

CBC/BIOCHEMISTRY/URINALYSIS

Possible neutrophilic leukocytosis and hyperfibrinogenemia with bacterial endocarditis

OTHER LABORATORY TESTS

• Elevated cardiac isoenzymes may be present (e.g., cardiac troponin I, CK-MB, HBDH, LDH 1 and 2) with concurrent myocarditis or other myocardial disease
• Positive blood culture may be obtained in horses with bacterial endocarditis.

IMAGING

Electrocardiography

• Atrial premature depolarizations may be present in horses with right atrial enlargement.
• Atrial fibrillation often is present in horses with tricuspid regurgitation and significant right atrial enlargement.

Echocardiography

• Most affected horses have normal tricuspid valve leaflets.
• Diffuse thickening of the free edge of the leaflet is more common than nodular thickening of the leaflet's free edge.
• Prolapse of a tricuspid leaflet into the right atrium frequently is detected in affected horses.
• Ruptured chordae tendineae, flail tricuspid leaflet, or bacterial endocarditis infrequently are detected.
• Right atrium—enlarged and dilated, with a rounded appearance
• Right ventricle—enlarged and dilated, with a rounded apex and thinning of the right ventricular free wall and interventricular septum
• A pattern of right ventricular volume overload, including paradoxic septal motion, in severe cases
• Dilatation of the cranial and caudal vena cava and hepatic veins in severe cases
• Pulsed-wave or color-flow Doppler reveals a jet (or jets) of tricuspid regurgitation in the right atrium. In most horses with mild to moderate regurgitation, the jet is directed toward the aortic root. The size and extent of the jet is a good method of semiquantitating severity, as is the strength of the regurgitation signal.

Thoracic Radiography

Cardiac enlargement may be detected, with increased contact between the heart and the sternum.

DIAGNOSTIC PROCEDURES

Cardiac Catheterization

Right-sided catheterization may reveal elevated right atrial and central venous pressures, with normal oxygen saturation of the blood from the right atrium and central veins.

Continuous 24-Hour Holter Monitoring

Useful in horses with suspected atrial or ventricular premature depolarizations

Ultrasonography

• Perform in cases with a thrombosed jugular vein.
• Detection of a cavitated thrombus is consistent with septic jugular vein thrombophlebitis.
• Obtain an aspirate of the cavitation area aseptically under ultrasonographic guidance, and submit for culture and sensitivity.

PATHOLOGIC FINDINGS

• Most horses have relatively normal-appearing tricuspid valve leaflets at postmortem examination.
• Focal or diffuse thickening or distortion of one or more tricuspid leaflets may be present.
• Ruptured chordae tendineae, flail tricuspid leaflets, bacterial endocarditis, or congenital malformations of the tricuspid valve are infrequent.
• Jet lesions may be detected in the right atrium.
• Right atrial enlargement and thinning of the atrial myocardium in cases with significant regurgitation
• Right ventricular enlargement and thinning of the right ventricular free wall and interventricular septum in horses with significant regurgitation
• Dilatation of the cranial and caudal vena cava and hepatic veins in horses with severe regurgitation.
• Pale areas may be seen in the atrial myocardium, with areas of atrial fibrosis detected histopathologically.
• Inflammatory cell infiltrate has been documented in affected horses with myocarditis.
• Myocardial necrosis occasionally is detected in affected horses with primary myocardial disease.
• In horses with congestive heart failure, ventral and peripheral edema, pleural effusion, pericardial effusion, chronic hepatic congestion, and occasionally, ascites may be detected.

TRICUSPID REGURGITATION

TREATMENT

APPROPRIATE HEALTH CARE

• Most affected horses require no treatment and can be monitored on an outpatient basis.
• Treat horses with severe regurgitation and congestive heart failure for congestive heart failure with positive inotropic drugs, vasodilators, and diuretics on an inpatient basis, if possible, and monitor response to therapy.

NURSING CARE

N/A

ACTIVITY

• Affected horses with tricuspid regurgitation are safe to continue in full athletic work until the regurgitation becomes severe or the horse develops exercise intolerance or congestive heart failure.
• Horses with significant right ventricular dysfunction and exercise intolerance are no longer safe to ride.

DIET

N/A

CLIENT EDUCATION

• Monitor the cardiac rhythm regularly; any irregularities other than second-degree AV block should prompt ECG.
• Carefully monitor for exercise intolerance, jugular or generalized venous distention, jugular pulses, ventral edema, prolonged recovery after exercise, or increased resting heart rate; if detected, perform a cardiac re-examination.

SURGICAL CONSIDERATIONS

N/A

MEDICATIONS

DRUGS OF CHOICE

Treat affected horses in congestive heart failure with digoxin, furosemide, and vasodilators.

CONTRAINDICATIONS

N/A

PRECAUTIONS

N/A

POSSIBLE INTERACTIONS

N/A

ALTERNATIVE DRUGS

N/A

FOLLOW-UP

PATIENT MONITORING

• Frequently monitor cardiac rhythm and respiratory system.
• Annual echocardiographic re-examinations are recommended in moderate to severe cases.

PREVENTION/AVOIDANCE

N/A

POSSIBLE COMPLICATIONS

Chronic cases—atrial fibrillation; congestive heart failure

EXPECTED COURSE AND PROGNOSIS

• Many affected horses have normal performance and life expectancy.
• Prognosis for horses with tricuspid valve prolapse and mild regurgitation is excellent, and in many, the amount of regurgitation remains unchanged for years.
• Progression of regurgitation associated with degenerative valve disease usually is slow. If regurgitation is mild, these horses have a good to excellent prognosis.
• Horses with ruptured chordae tendineae, flail tricuspid valve leaflets, or bacterial endocarditis have a more guarded prognosis, because the regurgitation usually becomes more severe and may result in a shortened performance and life expectancy.
• Affected horses with congestive heart failure usually have severe underlying valvular heart and myocardial disease and a guarded to grave prognosis for life.
• Most affected horses being treated for congestive heart failure respond to supportive therapy and improve. Such improvement usually is short lived, however. Most horses of these horses are euthanized within 2–6 months of initiating treatment.

MISCELLANEOUS

ASSOCIATED CONDITIONS

Mitral regurgitation

AGE-RELATED FACTORS

Old horses are more likely to be affected.

ZOONOTIC POTENTIAL

N/A

PREGNANCY

• Affected mares should not experience any problems with the pregnancy unless regurgitation is moderate to severe.
• The volume expansion of late pregnancy places an additional load on the already volume-loaded heart, which may precipitate congestive heart failure in mares with severe regurgitation.
• Pregnant mares with congestive heart failure should be treated for the underlying cardiac disease with positive inotropic drugs and diuretics.
• ACE inhibitors are contraindicated because of potential adverse effects on the fetus.

SYNONYMS

Tricuspid insufficiency

SEE ALSO

• Atrial fibrillation
• Bacterial endocarditis
• Congestive heart failure—right sided
• Mitral regurgitation
• Systolic murmurs

ABBREVIATIONS

• ACE = angiotensin-converting enzyme
• AV = atrioventricular
• CK-MB = MB isoenzyme of creatine kinase
• HBDH = α-hydroxybutyrate dehydrogenase
• LDH = lactate dehydrogenase
• PMI = point of maximal intensity
• VSD = ventricular septal defect

Suggested Reading

Blissitt KJ, Bonagura JD. Colour flow Doppler echocardiography in horses with cardiac murmurs. Equine Vet J 1995;19(Suppl):82–85.
Gardner SY, Reef VB, Spencer PA. Ultrasonographic evaluation of 46 horses with jugular vein thrombophlebitis: 1985–1988. J Am Vet Med Assoc 1991;199:370–373.
Marr CM, Reef VB. Physiological valvular regurgitation in clinically normal young racehorses: prevalence and two-dimensional characteristics. Equine Vet J 1995;19(Suppl):56–62.
Patteson MW, Cripps PJ. A survey of cardiac auscultatory findings in horses. Equine Vet J 1993;25:409–416.
Reef VB. Heart murmurs in horses: determining their significance with echocardiography. Equine Vet J 1995;19(Suppl):71–80.
Reef VB. Cardiovascular ultrasonography. In: Reef VB, ed. Equine diagnostic ultrasound. Philadelphia: WB Saunders, 1998:215–272.

Author Virginia B. Reef
Consulting Editor N/A

TRIFOLIUM SP. (ALSIKE CLOVER) TOXICOSIS

BASICS

OVERVIEW

• *Trifolium hybridum* (alsike clover) has been implicated as the cause of equine hepatic failure and neurologic impairment.
• Clinical manifestations of intoxication are acute and neurologic or chronic and cachectic.
• Postmortem histopathologic lesions consistently are found in the liver and include biliary fibrosis and marked bile duct proliferation.
• Occurrence of the two syndromes is associated with ingestion of alsike clover, but a specific toxin has not been identified.
• Photosensitization can occur in conjunction with both syndromes but is uncommon.
• Morbidity varies, but mortality is high.
• A reversible alsike clover–induced photosensitization has been described and is considered by some to be unrelated to the other two syndromes.

SIGNALMENT

• When both syndromes are considered together, there are no apparent breed, age, or sex predispositions; however, a retrospective study of alsike clover–associated disease suggested the nervous form occurs more commonly in old female horses.
• Not all horses in an exposed group develop clinical signs.

SIGNS

• Acute and neurologic—alternating depression and excitement, head pressing, aimless walking, inco-ordination, yawning and grinding of teeth, coma, and death.
• Chronic and cachectic—variable appetite, progressive loss of body condition, weakness, sluggishness, dry and rough haircoat, icterus, yawning, head pressing, and periodic excitement preceding sudden death
• Photosensitization—skin erythema and swelling, pruritus, exudation of serum, hair matting, skin exfoliation, lacrimation, conjunctivitis, photophobia, and keratitis

CAUSES AND RISK FACTORS

• The disease is associated with ingestion of alsike clover–containing pasture or hay.
• Alsike clover is believed to be less palatable than other forages, and horses on pasture may eat less if alternative plants are available.
• The ability of horses to avoid alsike clover in hay is less than that on pasture; thus, horses fed alsike clover–containing hay may ingest more of the plant.

DIAGNOSIS

DIFFERENTIAL DIAGNOSIS

• Ingestion of plants containing pyrrolizidine alkaloids—evidence of consumption; characteristic histopathologic lesions
• Locoism (*Astragalus* spp.)—evidence of consumption; characteristic histopathologic lesions
• *Equisetum arvense* (horsetail) or *Pteridium aquilinum* (bracken fern)—evidence of consumption; response to thiamine administration
• Fumonisin mycotoxins—detection in feed; characteristic gross and histopathologic brain lesions
• Rabies—fluorescent antibody test on brain tissue
• EPM—CSF evaluation; characteristic histopathologic lesions; response to treatment
• Viral encephalitides—CSF evaluation; serology; histologic evaluation of brain
• Brain abscesses or meningitis—clinical signs; CSF evaluation; gross or histopathologic examination
• Narcolepsy—EEG; response to drug administration
• Other causes of liver disease, with or without hepatoencephalopathy

CBC/BIOCHEMISTRY/URINALYSIS

Clinicopathologic changes have not been described in most suspected cases, but one had elevated serum SD and AP and blood ammonia concentrations.

OTHER LABORATORY TESTS

• CSF—normal
• Serology—normal

IMAGING

Ultrasonography—enlarged and irregular liver

DIAGNOSTIC PROCEDURES

Liver biopsy can be useful in differentiating alsike clover toxicosis from other liver diseases.

PATHOLOGIC FINDINGS

Gross Findings

• Enlarged and irregular liver
• Some fibrosis may be evident.
• Icterus is variable.

Histopathologic Findings

• Hepatic lesions include fibrosis of portal triads and around proliferating biliary epithelium.
• Inflammatory changes—uncommon

TREATMENT

• Treat photosensitivity by preventing sun exposure.
• Remove animal from the source of exposure to the plant.
• Treatment of the hepatic and nervous syndromes commonly is unrewarding.
• Symptomatic and supportive care including sedation for nervous syndrome, balanced electrolyte fluid administration, correction of hypoglycemia if present, and treatment of liver failure and hyperammonemia
• If the animal is eating, small meals given frequently are suggested.
• Diet should provide adequate energy and limited protein, primarily as branched-chain amino acids.

TRIFOLIUM SP. (ALSIKE CLOVER) TOXICOSIS

MEDICATIONS

DRUGS

- Sedation—xylazine (0.3–0.5 mg/kg IV as needed)
- Hyperammonemia—neomycin (20–30 mg/kg PO QID) or lactulose (90–120 mL PO TID–QID)
- Energy provision—continuous 5% or 10% dextrose drip (2 or 1 mL/kg per hour IV, respectively)

CONTRAINDICATIONS/POSSIBLE INTERACTIONS

- Diazepam is contraindicated in hepatoencephalopathy.
- Use care when administering drugs requiring hepatic metabolism for activity or elimination.

FOLLOW-UP

PATIENT MONITORING

Monitor hepatic function.

PREVENTION/AVOIDANCE

Because the conditions under which animals are intoxicated are poorly defined, the only specific recommendation is to prevent horses from ingesting alsike clover.

POSSIBLE COMPLICATIONS

N/A

EXPECTED COURSE AND PROGNOSIS

- Recovery from hepatic and neurologic syndromes is unlikely.
- Recovery from uncomplicated photosensitization is expected with appropriate treatment.

MISCELLANEOUS

ASSOCIATED CONDITIONS

N/A

AGE-RELATED FACTORS

N/A

ZOONOTIC POTENTIAL

N/A

PREGNANCY

N/A

SEE ALSO

N/A

ABBREVIATIONS

- AP = alkaline phosphatase
- CSF = cerebrospinal fluid
- EPM = equine protozoal myelitis
- SD = sorbitol dehydrogenase

Suggested Reading

Nation PN. Hepatic disease in Alberta horses: a retrospective study of "alsike clover poisoning" (1973–1988). Can Vet J 1991;32:602–607.

Author Robert H. Poppenga

Consulting Editor Robert H. Poppenga

TRYPANOSOMIASIS

BASICS

OVERVIEW

- Blood-borne parasitic disease of subtropical and tropical climates caused by several species of trypanosomes
- Depending on the species, found in Africa, Asia, South and Central America
- Infection of hemic/lymphatic/immune system with secondary involvement of hepatobiliary, nervous, ophthalmic, renal, and reproductive systems
- Depending on species, direct infection of reproductive tract

SIGNALMENT

- For vector-transmitted disease, no known sex, age, or breed predilection
- Horses, mules, and donkeys susceptible
- More severe disease in horses
- With dourine or venereally transmitted trypanosomiasis, donkeys are considered to be the reservoir. Light horse breeds are more severely affected than draft breeds; indigenous breeds also experience less disease.
- Females experience less mortality than males.

SIGNS

- Depending on species of parasite, the severity of signs varies.
- Cyclic parasitemia 3–4 weeks after exposure
- Acute and chronic infection
- Anorexia, depression, pyrexia, urticaria, peripheral edema, mucosal hemorrhage, mucous membrane pallor, icterus, lymphadenopathy, splenomegaly, weight loss, weakness, ataxia, recumbency, and death
- Ophthalmic signs—edema, hyperemia, and petechiation of the conjunctiva from direct intraocular infection
- Dourine—initial swelling of genitalia, with progression to typical signs of trypanosomiasis; CNS signs are common, with facial paralysis a frequent sign; ocular lesions include photophobia, keratitis, and corneal opacity.

CAUSES AND RISK FACTORS

- *Trypanosoma evansi* (surra, mal de caderas)—primary host-adapted species, ranging from acute to chronic forms
- *T. equinum*—name for *T. evansi* in the New World
- *T. vivax*—moderate to severe disease
- *T. congolenses*—mild, peripheral edema
- *T. brucei*—peripheral and scrotal edema; relapse with infection in the CNS is common despite treatment.
- *T. equiperdum* (dourine, maladie du coit)—venereally transmitted, resulting in clinical signs similar to vector-transmitted disease
- Subtropical and tropical location
- Exposure to vectors (tsetse fly, tabanids, vampire bats) is a risk factor.

DIAGNOSIS

DIFFERENTIAL DIAGNOSIS

- Equine infectious anemia virus (EIAV)
- Babesiosis (piroplasmosis)
- Leptospirosis
- Immune-mediated hemolytic anemia
- Purpura hemorrhagica
- Toxins causing Heinz-body hemolytic anemia
- Dourine—vesicular exanthema and equine herpesvirus 3

CBC/BIOCHEMISTRY/URINALYSIS

- Decreased PCV (extravascular hemolysis)
- Decreased erythrocyte count
- Decreased hemoglobin
- Leukopenia, neutropenia, lymphocytosis, and monocytosis
- Thrombocytopenia
- Metabolic acidosis
- Hyperbilirubinemia
- Hyperproteinemia (inconsistent, depending on A:G ratio), hypergammaglobulinemia, and hypoalbuminemia
- Increased BUN

OTHER LABORATORY TESTS

- Serology for other infectious diseases
- Crystal violet or new methylene blue stain of red blood cell smears for Heinz-body inclusions
- Clotting profile

TRYPANOSOMIASIS

IMAGING
N/A

DIAGNOSTIC PROCEDURES
- Thick/thin Giemsa- or Leish-stained direct blood smears
- Hematocrit centrifuge technique for detection of trypanosomes
- Mouse inoculation
- Antigen ELISA
- *T. equiperdum*—ELISA and complement fixation

TREATMENT
- Supportive care
- Blood transfusion
- Intravenous fluids

MEDICATIONS
- NSAIDs
- Suramin, quinapyramine—short period of prophylaxis also conferred
- Quinapyramine salt available as long-term prophylaxis
- Diminazene (Berenil®) has higher toxicity in horses
- Melarsomine dichlorhydrate recommended for CNS infection

FOLLOW-UP

PATIENT MONITORING
- Because chronic disease and reinfection can occur, monitoring of appetite, weight, temperature, and PCV is recommended.
- Reinfection is common.

PREVENTION/AVOIDANCE
- Prophylaxis recommended through use of quinapyramine salt
- Combination treatment with suramine and diminazene
- Elimination of trypanosomes from resident mammalian population through segregation, quarantine, and prophylaxis
- Vector control is recommended in theory but is difficult in practice.

MISCELLANEOUS

ASSOCIATED CONDITIONS
N/A

AGE-RELATED FACTORS
N/A

ZOONOTIC POTENTIAL
No documented evidence that trypanosomes of domestic animals cause infection in humans

PREGNANCY
Trypanosomes cause abortion.

SEE ALSO
- Anemia
- Babesiosis
- Equine infectious anemia

ABBREVIATIONS
- A:G = albumin:globulin ratio
- ELISA = enzyme-linked immunosorbent assay
- PCV = packed cell volume

Author Maureen T. Long
Consulting Editor Debra C. Sellon

TUBERCULOSIS

BASICS

OVERVIEW

Tuberculosis is a rare infection in the horse. Most cases are related to infection with *Mycobacterium bovis,* although some reported cases have been caused by *M. avium*-complex. No specific syndromes have been described.

SIGNALMENT

There is no apparent age or breed predilection.

SIGNS

Signs are variable, and relate to the system or systems involved. The infections are chronic and slowly progressive. An intermittent fever may be recorded. Weight loss is a common feature. In primary pulmonary cases varying degrees of dyspnea may be present, and in some cases cough and nasal discharge may also be present. Involvement of cervical vertebrae has been described, and neurologic signs consistent with a cervical spinal cord lesion have been observed. In some horses with granulomatous enteritis, *M. avium* has been identified in the feces or the intestinal tissues. These latter horses have clinical signs of malabsorption or protein-losing enteropathy or both.

CAUSES AND RISK FACTORS

No specific risk factors have been identified. Cases are too rare and sporadic to establish any particular pattern.

DIAGNOSIS

DIFFERENTIAL DIAGNOSIS

As the infection can occur in almost any site, tuberculosis can be considered as a differential diagnosis in almost any chronic progressive disease of the horse. It is, however, rare, and therefore should be low on the list for most of these syndromes.

CBC/BIOCHEMISRY/URINALYSIS

There are no specific clinical pathology data typical for this disease in horses. Hematology may be consistent with a chronic inflammatory process, (i.e., neutrophilia, hyperfibrinogenemia, and anemia). Other laboratory values may be changed depending on the organ system(s) involved.

OTHER LABORATORY TESTS

Results of tuberculin testing in horses are variable and the tests are considered to be unreliable for diagnostic purposes. Many false positives occur, and the tuberculin may induce an anaphylactic response. Identification of the organisms in aspirates or biopsies using acid-fast staining is strongly supportive of a diagnosis of equine tuberculosis.

IMAGING

Depending on the region of the body affected, radiography or ultrasonography or both may demonstrate the nature and extent of the infection. For example, miliary lesions have been described in the lung, and these provide a very suggestive radiographic image.

DIAGNOSTIC PROCEDURES

Biopsies of affected organs may be indicated to determine the nature of the lesions, and collection of exudate (e.g., by transtracheal aspiration or bronchoalveolar lavage), is indicated in specific cases.

PATHOLOGIC FINDINGS

Multiple lesions are often present in a variety of organs, particularly lymph nodes and spleen. Involvment of bone is said to be more frequent in horses than cattle. Lesions tend to be firm in all tissues, and may appear to be neoplastic. Histopathologic evaluation is needed to confirm the diagnosis.

TREATMENT

There is no effective treatment for equine tuberculosis.

MEDICATIONS

DRUG(S) OF CHOICE

There does not appear to be any reports of successful treatment of confirmed cases of equine tuberculosis. Drugs used in other species (isoniazid, rifampin, streptomycin, etc.) could be considered, but there are no guidelines for their use in the horse for this condition. Based on experiences in human medicine it would be expected that therapy, if attempted in an equine case, would have to be given for several months or even a year or more.

CONTRAINDICATIONS/POSSIBLE INTERACTIONS

N/A

FOLLOW-UP

N/A

EXPECTED COURSE AND PROGNOSIS

As therapy is not usually a viable option, the prognosis for established cases is hopeless, and a recommendation for euthanasia would be appropriate.

MISCELLANEOUS

ZOONOTIC POTENTIAL

This is a potential zoonosis, particularly to immunocompromised persons. If a confirmed case is to be kept alive, either to attempt treatment or for other reasons (e.g., for an affected mare to foal), then specific cautions should be issued to the owner and handlers. It would be prudent to seek permission to advise appropriate health-care workers of the situation.

Suggested Reading

No review of the subject is available.

Author Christopher M. Brown
Consulting Editor Corinne R. Sweeney

TYZZER'S DISEASE

BASICS

OVERVIEW

• An uncommon, peracute, and usually fatal hepatic failure in young foals caused by infection with *Clostridium piliformis* (formerly *Bacillus piliformis*), which leads to multifocal coagulative necrosis of the liver and inflammation

SIGNALMENT

Foals between 7–42 days of age are affected in a sporadic nature.

SIGNS

• Foals are usually found dead, with little or no history of disease.
• Living foals usually are severely depressed to comatose and may exhibit signs of hepatic encephalopathy.
• Mucous membranes may be icteric.

CAUSES AND RISK FACTORS

• *C. piliformis*—a gram-negative, spore-forming, obligate intracellular bacterium. Culture is difficult by routine bacteriologic methods, and the endospores are resistant to heat up to 60°C and to many disinfectants.
• A monoclonal antibody inhibition assay has been developed; in one equine series, at least 22% tested positive for equine isolate of *C. piliformis* and 14% for the rat isolate, which suggests that inapparent infection may be relatively common.
• Route of transmission in the horse is unknown, and occurrence of clinical disease in foals is sporadic.
• No predisposing factors noted
• Mares with high inhibition on the assay appear to pass this antibody onto their foals in their colostrum.

DIAGNOSIS

DIFFERENTIAL DIAGNOSIS

Icterus/hepatic failure—equine herpes virus-1 infection, septicemia, and neonatal isoerythrolysis, all of which usually are present at or soon after birth whereas Tyzzer's disease occurs in foals $\geq$1 week in age

CBC/BIOCHEMISTRY/URINALYSIS

• Neutropenia is the most common WBC abnormality in living affected foals.
• Severe hypoglycemia
• Elevated liver enzymes—AST, GGT, and LDH
• Elevated bilirubin with both elevated direct and indirect components.

OTHER LABORATORY TESTS

A metabolic acidosis has been reported.

IMAGING

Ultrasonography—hepatic enlargement and possible increased vascular pattern.

DIAGNOSTIC PROCEDURES

N/A

PATHOLOGIC FINDINGS

• Nearly all foals die without preliminary signs.
• Gross findings—hepatomegaly and icterus; small, white/gray spots on the liver surface in some cases.
• Histologic findings—multifocal areas of hepatic necrosis; long, slender, bacterial rods on the periphery of necrosis with a Warthin-Starry stain.

TREATMENT

If the foal is alive, correct the hypoglycemia with a bolus of 15–20% glucose and correction of the metabolic acidosis with bicarbonate therapy; these foals are in extremis and require intensive fluid therapy.

MEDICATIONS

DRUGS

• In vitro culture suggests a sensitivity to penicillin (22,000 IU/kg IV QID), tetracycline (11 mg/kg IV BID), erythromycin (25 mg/kg PO QID), and streptomycin.
• Prophylactic use of antibiotics in foals on problem farms has been reported to reduce the incidence of this disease.

CONTRAINDICATIONS/POSSIBLE INTERACTIONS

Sulfonamide drugs, either alone or in conjunction with corticosteroids, may induce this disease in rodents and rabbits that are inapparent carriers.

TYZZER'S DISEASE

FOLLOW-UP

PATIENT MONITORING

Monitor glucose and acid–base status frequently during the course of disease.

EXPECTED COURSE AND PROGNOSIS

- Grave prognosis
- Foals usually are found dead or die soon after.

MISCELLANEOUS

ZOONOTIC POTENTIAL

C. piliformis causes the disease in cattle, dogs, rodents, rabbits, raccoons, and marsupials, whether the disease is contagious from animal to animal is unknown.

SEE ALSO

- Neonatal isoerythrolysis
- Septicemia

ABBREVIATIONS

- AST = aspartate aminotransferase
- GGT = γ-glutamyltransferase
- LDG = lactate dehydrogenase

Suggested Reading

Chanter N. Infection of horses by Tyzzer's bacillus. Equine Vet J 1995;27:1–3.

Hook RR, Riley LK, Franklin CL, Besch-Williford C. Seroanalysis of Tyzzer's disease in horses: implications that multiple trains can infect equidae. Equine Vet J 1995;27:8–12.

Humber KA, Sweeney RW, Saik JE, Hansen TO. Clinical and clinicopathologic findings in two foals infected with *Bacillus piliformis.* J Am Vet Med Assoc 1988;193:1425–1428.

Peek SF, Byars TD, Rueve E. Neonatal hepatic failure in a Thoroughbred foal: successful treatment of a case of presumptive Tyzzer's disease. Equine Vet Educ 1994;6:307–309.

Turk MAM, Gallina AM, Perryman LE. *Bacillus piliformis* infection (Tyzzer's disease) in foals in Northwestern United States: a retrospective study of 21 cases. J Am Vet Med Assoc 1981;178:279–281.

Author Mary Rose Paradis

Consulting Editor Mary Rose Paradis

ULCERATIVE KERATOMYCOSIS (EXPANDED)

BASICS

DEFINITION
• Manifests clinically as ulcerative keratitis, stromal abscessation, and iris prolapse.
• Ulcerative keratitis—a disruption of the corneal epithelium, with varying amounts of stromal loss, that may have concurrent bacterial and/or fungal infection
• Ulcers infected with fungi range from minor, corneal epithelial abrasions/erosions to superficial plaques to extremely deep, severe interstitial keratitis.

PATHOPHYSIOLOGY
• Fungi are normal inhabitants of the equine conjunctival microflora, but they can become pathogenic after corneal injury.
• Fungal organisms are ubiquitous in the equine environment, but regional geographic differences undoubtedly exist to account for the variation in fungal species particular to specific regions.
• Exposure to vegetative material (e.g., hay, grasses, shavings, straw) and dust may influence exposure to fungi.
• Commonly begins with corneal trauma resulting in an epithelial defect and stromal invasion by the commensal fungal organism or seeding of fungi from a foreign body of plant origin; stromal destruction results from the release of proteases and other enzymes from the fungi, leukocytes, and keratocytes.
• Fungi appear to have an affinity for Descemet's membrane, with hyphae being frequently found deep in the equine cornea; deeper corneal invasion by the fungi can lead to sterile or infectious endophthalmitis.

SYSTEM AFFECTED
Ophthalmic

GENETICS
NA

INCIDENCE/PREVALENCE
Much more common and aggressive in warm climates

SIGNALMENT
All ages and breeds

SIGNS
• Clinical signs—miosis, blepharospasm, epiphora, and photophobia
• Slight droopiness of the upper lid eyelashes may be a subtle sign of corneal ulceration.

CAUSES
Septate filamentous fungi, including several species common to the equine eye—*Fusarium, Aspergillus, and Penicillium*

RISK FACTORS
• Horses may be more susceptible to fungal corneal invasion and infection because of the large surface area and prominence of the equine eye and some weakness in the corneal immune system.
• Topical antibiotic or corticosteroid therapy of a noninfected corneal ulcer may predispose to fungal invasion and colonization.

DIAGNOSIS

DIFFERENTIAL DIAGNOSIS
Ocular pain also may be found with bacterial corneal ulcers, uveitis, conjunctivitis, glaucoma, blepharitis and dacryocystitis.

CBC/BIOCHEMISTRY/URINALYSIS
N/A

OTHER LABORATORY TESTS
N/A

IMAGING
N/A

DIAGNOSTIC PROCEDURES
The diagnosis is established by finding fungal hyphae, mold, or yeast during cytologic examination of a corneal scraping, culture of the corneal lesion, or surgical histopathologic examination of a keratectomy specimen.

PATHOLOGIC FINDINGS
• Fungi show a marked affinity for the deep corneal stroma and Descemet's membrane.
• Hyphae often are found with neutrophils in the stroma but rarely free in the anterior chamber.

TREATMENT

APPROPRIATE HEALTH CARE
N/A

NURSING CARE
N/A

ACTIVITY
• Horses with keratomycosis and secondary uveitis should be stall-rested until the condition is healed.
• Intraocular hemorrhage and increased severity of uveitis are sequela to overexertion.

DIET
Should be consistent with the training level.

CLIENT EDUCATION
• Ulcerative keratomycosis is a serious, sight-threatening disease in the horse.
• Long-duration exposure to antifungal drugs is required for complete fungal destruction and resolution of clinical signs.

SURGICAL CONSIDERATIONS
• Combined medical and surgical therapy is indicated if ulcers are extremely deep, are not responding to medical treatment, or worsen despite medical treatment.
• Surgeries for keratomycosis—conjunctival pedicle grafts, bridge grafts, hood grafts, island grafts, and full-thickness penetrating keratoplasty.
• Surgery may leave the horse with a larger scar, but bulbar conjunctival grafts usually prevent corneal rupture and allow for physical support, regional blood supply, and supply of endogenous antiproteases to the ulcer site.

ULCERATIVE KERATOMYCOSIS (EXPANDED)

MEDICATIONS

DRUGS OF CHOICE

- Director treatment against the fungi and the corneal and intraocular inflammatory responses that occur after fungal replication and hyphal death.
- Miconazole (1%) has been used successfully and frequently as a topical antifungal agent. The IV form is preferred, but the vaginal product also may be used.
- Natamycin is employed topically in horses and is very effective against *Fusarium* and *Aspergillus* sp.
- Amphotericin B (1.5 mg/mL) may be administered topically.
- Silver sulfadiazine is a topical antimicrobial agent with both antifungal and antibacterial activity that is believed to be fungicidal and is used in equine eyes.
- Dilute (1:50) povidone-iodine is effective topically against *Fusarium* isolates.
- Topical itraconazole and fluconazole are being used successfully.
- Topical antifungal therapy—miconazole, amphotericin B, or natamycin three to four times during the first few days; this treatment frequency was determined empirically as the intensity of iridocyclitis often was noted to magnify dramatically on the day after topical miconazole administration at treatment frequencies higher than this.
- Sudden death of stromal fungi caused by initiation of antifungal drug therapy can result in acute iridocyclitis; in this case, topical antifungal medications are increased to six times per day on subsequent days.
- Iridocyclitis is present whenever a horse has a corneal ulcer and can intensify after hyphal death following antifungal therapy. Flunixin meglumine (1 mg/kg IV, IM, or PO BID) is the most frequently used NSAID in horses for systemic treatment of iridocyclitis and also may reduce the speed of corneal vascularization.
- Atropine sulfate (1%), a parasympatholytic agent, is used in all cases for its mydriatic and cycloplegic effects to dilate the pupil and to diminish ciliary body muscle spasms associated with the axon reflex uveitis that occurs with equine corneal ulceration. It may be administered q4h until the pupil is dilated, after which the frequency of administration is reduced.

CONTRAINDICATIONS

Administer topical atropine cautiously, because it may predispose some horses to colic.

PRECAUTIONS

N/A

POSSIBLE INTERACTIONS

N/A

ALTERNATIVE DRUGS

N/A

FOLLOW-UP

PATIENT MONITORING

- Protect the horse from self-trauma with hard or soft cup hoods.
- Monitor for colic and persistent signs of eye pain.

PREVENTION/AVOIDANCE

N/A

POSSIBLE COMPLICATIONS

- Persistent pain
- Uveitis
- Endophthalmitis
- Blindness

EXPECTED COURSE AND PROGNOSIS

- Vision after keratomycosis may be retained in as few as 50% of eyes if treatment is not aggressive.
- Aggressive medical and surgical therapy should result in positive visual outcome and ocular survival in >90% of eyes. Therapy is quite prolonged, however, and corneal scarring may be prominent.
- Enucleation may be necessary in horses that become blind and continue to experience ocular pain.

MISCELLANEOUS

ASSOCIATED CONDITIONS

Severe uveitis

AGE-RELATED FACTORS

N/A

ZOONOTIC POTENTIAL

N/A

PREGNANCY

N/A

SYNONYMS

N/A

SEE ALSO

Corneal ulcers

Suggested Reading

Andrew SE, Brooks DE: Equine ulcerative keratomycosis: visual outcome and ocular in 39 cases (1987–1996). Equine Vet J 1998; 30:109–116.

Brooks DE: Equine ophthalmology. In Gelatt KN, ed. Veterinary ophthalmology. 3rd ed. Philadelphia: Lippincott Williams & Wilkins, 1999.

Author Dennis E. Brooks
Consulting Editor Dennis E. Brooks

URINALYSIS

BASICS

DEFINITION

Evaluation of selected urinary parameters via dipstick (e.g., protein, glucose, ketones, pH, blood/Hb/Mb, bilirubin, urobilinogen), refractometry or osmometry (e.g., specific gravity, osmolality), or microscopy of sediment.

PATHOPHYSIOLOGY

- Blood is filtered by glomeruli in the kidneys, and the filtrate passes through renal tubules, in which components of the filtrate are reabsorbed, electrolytes are excreted into the filtrate, or both.
- The urinary bladder stores urine for elimination through the urethra.
- Abnormalities in various organ systems can produce changes in urinary parameters via changes in the filtrate presented to glomeruli.
- Abnormalities of the kidney, ureters, bladder, urethra, reproductive tract, or external urogenital structures are likely to result in altered urinary parameters, depending on the method of urine collection.

SYSTEMS AFFECTED

- Dependent on the parameter and the underlying disorder
- Myoglobinuria or hemoglobinuria can cause damage to renal tubules.

SIGNALMENT

- Dependent on the abnormality and its underlying cause
- Most abnormalities in urinary parameters carry no age, sex, or breed predispositions.

SIGNS

Dependent on the abnormality.

CAUSES

See *Disorders That May Alter Lab Results.*

Dipstick analysis

- Positive for protein—hematuria (accompanied by RBCs), inflammation (accompanied by WBCs), renal disease (particularly glomerular, which usually is unaccompanied by bacteria, WBCs, RBCs, or casts), and causes not directly related to the urinary system (e.g., fever, cardiac disease, neurologic disease, shock, exertion, paraproteinemias).
- Positive for glucose—hyperglycemia above the renal threshold (serum glucose, 160–180 mg/dL; consider hyperadrenocorticism, stress, catecholamine release, glucose-containing IV fluid administration, diabetes mellitus); defective renal tubular reabsorption (rare)
- Positive for ketones—increased serum acetone or acetoacetate above the tubular reabsorption capacity (resulting from excessive fat degradation or carbohydrate metabolism perturbance; consider diabetes mellitus, starvation, low carbohydrate/high fat diet)
- Increased pH—alkaline urine is normal in horses.
- Decreased pH—after strenuous exertion, prolonged fasting/anorexia, and metabolic acidosis
- Positive "blood"—hemoglobinuria (consider hemolysis intravascularly or hemorrhage in urogenital tracts with subsequent artifactual RBC lysis), myoglobinuria (i.e., muscle disease), or hematuria (i.e., hemorrhage somewhere within the urogenital tracts). Differentiate by centrifugation (Hb and Mb do not clear but RBCs from hemorrhage clear from supernatant), examination of plasma after centrifugation of whole blood (Hb binds in blood to haptoglobin until haptoglobin is saturated; thus, hemoglobinuria is accompanied by hemoglobinemia [i.e., red plasma]; Mb is not retained in blood, and plasma is normal in color), and examination of sediment (intact RBCs are present in urine with hemorrhage but not with hemoglobinuria because of hemoglobinemia or with myoglobinuria).
- See also *Differential Diagnosis* and *Other Laboratory Tests.*
- Positive bilirubin—increased conjugated bilirubin in serum; consider bile flow obstruction and hemolysis.
- Positive urobilinogen—patent bile duct (a negative urobilinogen does not indicate the bile duct is not patent); may increase in hemolysis.
- Nitrites—unreliable for assessing the presence or absence of bacteria.

Specific Gravity/Osmolality

- Dipstick specific gravity pads are completely unreliable for nonhuman specimens.
- Osmolality is the best determinant of urine particle concentration, but specific gravity by refractometry is acceptable.
- Random specific gravity values of <1.025 are meaningless alone.
- Specific gravity of ≥ 1.025 indicates adequate concentrating ability.
- Specific gravity of <1.008 (i.e., hyposthenuria) indicates ability to dilute urine.

• Persistent hyposthenuria, or an osmolality less than that of serum, suggests abnormal ADH release (i.e., diabetes insipidus) or renal response (i.e., nephrogenic diabetes insipidus), medullary washout, chronic sodium depletion, chronic liver disease, or psychogenic polydipsia.
• With dehydration or with increased BUN and creatinine, specific gravity of <1.1018–1.020 suggests renal compromise–acute or chronic renal failure

Changes in Sediment

• Bacteria—contaminants; sepsis
• Fungi—usually contaminants
• Crystals—normal, especially calcium carbonate, urolithiasis, hyperammonemia if ammonium biurate
• Increased RBCs (>5 cells/HPF)—hematuria (e.g., trauma, inflammation, neoplasia, coagulopathy)
• Increased WBCs (>5–8 cells/HPF)—inflammation (e.g., trauma, sepsis, urethral habronemiasis)
• Epithelial cells—normal, unless bizarre/numerous (i.e., neoplasia) or renal tubular cells (i.e., tubular damage)
• Casts—a few may be normal or pathologic alteration in renal tubules; hyaline indicates mucoprotein; granular indicates mucoprotein, debris; epithelial indicates epithelial cells; RBC indicates hemorrhage/inflammation; WBC indicates inflammation; waxy indicates chronic tubular disease; absence of casts does not rule out renal tubular disease.

RISK FACTORS

Dependent on the underlying cause

DIAGNOSIS

DIFFERENTIAL DIAGNOSIS

• Dependent on the parameter affected
• Positive blood—muscle pain, reluctance to move, and history of recent exercise suggest muscle necrosis and myoglobinuria; signs of anemia, history of red maple leaf ingestion, snake bite, bacterial infection, and heavy metal exposure suggest intravascular hemolysis and hemoglobinuria.
• Stranguria, fever, and palpably abnormal kidneys or ureters suggest infectious urinary tract infection.
• Significant weight loss may indicate anorexia or starvation and frequently accompanies chronic renal failure.
• Polyuria/polydipsia is compatible with endocrine imbalance, psychogenic polydipsia, and renal failure.
• Hirsutism may suggest endocrine imbalance—hyperadrenocorticism.

LABORATORY FINDINGS

Drugs That May Alter Lab Results

• Xylazine—transiently increased urine volume, decreased osmolality/specific gravity, and glucosuria
• Diuretics, corticosteroids, and fluid administration—increased urine volume, decreased osmolality/specific gravity, and altered electrolyte excretion

Disorders That May Alter Lab Results

• Hot weather, exertion, food and water intake, salt supplementation, and water deprivation
• Alkaline urine—falsely positive protein; verify with chemical methods (e.g., sulfosalicylic acid precipitation).
• Ascorbic acid, lactose, galactose, pentose, ascorbic acid, conjugated gluconates, and salicylates—altered glucose results, depending on the method used
• Hyposthenuria—lysis of RBCs in hemorrhage, causing hemoglobinuria without hemoglobinemia
• Discolored urine—affects interpretation of all dipstick color reactions.
• Delayed analysis—affects ketones, bilirubin, urobilinogen, pH, and sediment (e.g., crystals, bacteria, cells)
• Exposure to light—false-negative bilirubin
• Microbial peroxidase; oxidizing contaminants—false-positive blood

Valid If Run in Human Lab?

Yes, except for dipstick analysis of nitrite, WBC, or specific gravity.

CBC/BIOCHEMISTRY/URINALYSIS

CBC

• Inflammatory leukogram or increased fibrinogen with proteinuria, hematuria, or pyuria suggest sepsis, particularly pyelonephritis, but may be absent in lower urinary tract infections.
• Anemia may accompany chronic urinary tract hemorrhage—neoplasia; inflammation

URINALYSIS

• Anemia with or without morphologic changes in erythrocytes and hemoglobinemia producing red plasma indicate that positive blood on a urine dipstick results from hemoglobinuria secondary to intravascular hemolysis.

Biochemistry

• Increases in serum CK and AST as well as absence of discolored plasma indicate positive blood on urine dipstick is caused by Mb from muscle necrosis.
• Decreased serum albumin occurs in severe proteinuria caused by glomerular loss—glomerulonephritis; amyloidosis
• Glucosuria is not likely to result from a tubular defect when preceded or accompanied by hyperglycemia of >160–180 mg/dL.
• Low serum chloride or high anion gap may suggest metabolic acidosis when urine pH is low; blood gas evaluation is more definitive.
• Increases in serum bilirubin generally occur with increases in urine bilirubin; increased GGT activity indicates cholestasis as the cause.
• Increased BUN or creatinine with concentrated urine indicate dehydration; with a specific gravity of <1.018–1.020, consider acute or chronic renal failure.
• Hypercalcemia frequently accompanies chronic renal failure in horses.

OTHER LABORATORY TESTS

• Distinguishing hemoglobinuria from myoglobinuria—addition of saturated ammonium sulfate solution to urine results in precipitation of Hb but not Mb; spectrophotometric tests that distinguish Hb from Mb can be done by commercial labs.
• To determine the significance of proteinuria, urine protein:urine creatinine ratios are recommended. A ratio of <0.5 is normal, of 1–3 suggests tubular disease, and of >3 suggests glomerular disease.
• Wright- or Gram-stained sediment as well as quantitative urine culture and sensitivity are indicated when significant WBCs or bacteria are seen in fresh urine sediment.
• Cytologic evaluation of Wright-stained sediment is recommended when numerous or bizarre epithelial cells are seen in urine sediment.
• Urine chemistry tests (e.g., electrolytes, creatinine) in conjunction with serum/plasma chemistry and fractional excretion—with azotemia, urinary sodium of <20 mEq/L and urine:plasma creatinine ratio of >20 suggest a prerenal cause; urinary sodium of ≥20 mEq/L and urine:plasma creatinine ratio of ≤20 suggest renal compromise.
• Water-deprivation tests (**NOTE**: contraindicated when BUN and serum/plasma creatinine are increased; monitor patients carefully during test) to determine whether the kidneys can concentrate urine to a specific gravity of ≥1.025; lack of concentration during abrupt deprivation suggests diabetes insipidus, renal failure, or medullary washout. If urine is concentrated after gradual deprivation, suspect medullary washout—hyperadrenocorticism; psychogenic polydipsia
• In hemoglobinuria, thoroughly evaluate RBC morphology and consider Coombs' testing to determine the cause of hemolysis—toxic; immune mediated
• ACTH determination or stimulation tests are indicated for hyposthenuria/isosthenuria or glucosuria and hyperglycemia to assess for hyperadrenocorticism.

IMAGING

• Ultrasonography of the bladder, ureters, or kidneys to localize lesions
• IV pyelography of foals with suspected pyelonephritis

DIAGNOSTIC PROCEDURES

• Commonly employed—palpation of ureters, kidneys, and bladder to localize lesions
• Rarely required—ultrasound-guided renal biopsy if indicated (suspected glomerular disease, i.e., glomerulonephritis or amyloidosis); bladder endoscopy or biopsy to assess for cystoliths or tumors

TREATMENT

• Urinalysis is an essential part of diagnostic workup that enhances hematology, serum chemistry, history, and physical findings, but urinalysis should not be used alone as a diagnostic tool. Therefore, urinalysis findings generally do not require treatment in and of themselves.
• Exceptions are hemoglobinuria and myoglobinuria, which require immediate therapy because of their potential for causing permanent damage to renal tubules.
• The mainstay of this acute therapy is administration of IV fluids.

URINALYSIS

MEDICATIONS

DRUGS OF CHOICE
N/A

CONTRAINDICATIONS
N/A

PRECAUTIONS
With hemoglobinuria, patients are anemic. Therefore, use IV fluids with care, and monitor the hematocrit during therapy to avoid exacerbating the anemia.

POSSIBLE INTERACTIONS
N/A

ALTERNATIVE DRUGS
N/A

FOLLOW UP

PATIENT MONITORING
Dependent on the parameter affected and the underlying cause

POSSIBLE COMPLICATIONS
- Hemoglobinuria or myoglobinuria can result in permanent damage to the renal tubules.
- Uncorrected dehydration can result in permanent renal compromise.
- Uroliths/cystoliths can result in urethral obstruction.

MISCELLANEOUS

AGE-RELATED FACTORS
- Colostrum intake results in transiently increased urinary protein in horses <2 days old.
- Neonatal foals typically have acidic urine—pH of <7
- Urine of normal suckling foals has low specific gravity. Sources differ regarding whether this results from a less-developed concentrating ability or from the large fluid intake of suckling foals.
- Serum creatinine of neonates, particularly premature foals, can be higher than adult reference intervals, making evaluation of renal function challenging.

ZOONOTIC POTENTIAL
N/A

PREGNANCY
N/A

SYNONYMS
N/A

SEE ALSO
- BUN
- CK
- Creatinine
- Hemolysis
- Polyuria/polydipsia
- Renal failure
- Urine chemistry

ABBREVATIONS
- ADH = antidiuretic hormone
- AST = aspartate aminotransferase
- CK = creatine kinase
- GGT = γ-glutamyltransferase
- Hb = hemoglobin
- HPF = high-power field
- Mb = myoglobin

Suggested Reading

Carlson GP. Clinical chemistry tests. In: Smith BP, ed. Large animal internal medicine. St. Louis: Mosby, 1996.

Divers TJ. Diseases of the renal system. In: Smith BP, ed. Large animal internal medicine. St. Louis: Mosby, 1996.

Duncan JR, Prasse KW, Mahaffey EA. Urinary system. In: Veterinary laboratory medicine. 3rd ed. Ames: Iowa State University Press, 1994.

Seanor JW, Byars TD, Boutcher JK. Renal disease associated with colic in horses. Mod Vet Pract 1984;65(5):A26–A29.

Trim CM, Hanson RR. Effects of xylazine on renal function and plasma glucose in ponies. Vet Rec 1986;118:65–67.

Author Ellen W. Evans

Consulting Editor Claire B. Andreasen

URINARY TRACT INFECTION (UTI)

BASICS

DEFINITION

• Two categories—those affecting the upper urinary tract (i.e., kidneys, ureters), and those affecting the lower urinary tract (i.e., bladder, urethra)
• Most commonly caused by bacteria, but protozoal (*Klossiella equi*) and other parasitic infections (e.g., *Strongylus vulgaris, Halicephalobus gingivalis* [*deletrix*], and *Dioctophyma renale*) also occur.

PATHOPHYSIOLOGY

Upper UTI

• Recognized infrequently
• Often a serious, potentially life-threatening problem
• Most commonly ascending infections that develop due to stasis of urine flow and vesiculoureteral reflux (as with bladder paralysis) or damage to renal parenchyma (as with polycystic disease or NSAID toxicity and medullary crest necrosis)
• Less commonly a result of neonatal septicemia (*Actinobacillus equuili* and other organisms), but other clinical problems usually are more serious than the renal disease.

Lower UTI

• Usually a consequence of anatomic or functional causes of abnormal urine flow, especially bladder paralysis
• Frequently accompanied by urolithiasis and partial obstruction.
• Except for single large cystoliths (predisposing affected horses), it often is difficult to determine if nephroliths, ureteroliths, multiple small cystoliths, and urethroliths are a predisposing cause or a consequence of UTI.

Parasitic Infection

• Although rare, *H. gingivalis* infection often is life-threatening due to CNS involvement. Only the female parasite has been identified in equine tissues, and large granulotamous lesions full of the rhabditiform nematodes usually are found in the kidneys. Renal involvement typically is inapparent.
• *D. renale* is a large, bright-red nematode, and the female may reach 100 cm in length. Typical hosts are carnivorous species, but horses occasionally ingest the intermediate host (i.e., annelid worm) while grazing or drinking from natural water sources. Once localized in the kidney, the parasite may live from 1–3 years. Eggs are shed in the urine. The renal parenchyma is completely destroyed, and death of the parasite leads to shrinking of the host kidney into a fibrous mass.
• Occasionally, hydronephrosis or renal hemorrhage may be serious complications of parasitic infection.
• In contrast to infection with nematodes, infection with *K. equi*, a coccidian parasite, appears common, but clinical disease associated with this coccidial infection has not been reported. Thus, *K. equi* infection is considered an incidental finding.

SYSTEMS AFFECTED

• Renal/urologic—infection and failure (with bilateral upper UTI)
• Nervous—with *H. gingivalis* infection

GENETICS

No inherited diseases predisposing to UTI are documented, but developmental anomalies leading to altered urine flow increase risk.

INCIDENCE/PREVALENCE

• Bacterial UTIs are uncommon.
• Occasional "outbreaks" of cystitis have been described in association with eating hybrids of *Sorgum* sp. (e.g., Johnson grass, Sudan grass) in the southwestern United States, but UTIs in affected horses likely were a complication of sublethal intoxication that resulted bladder paralysis.
• Another outbreak of "cystitis," manifested by hematuria more than UTI or incontinence, was described in Western Australia. Affected horses were on range pasture. Although not proven, a fungal toxin was suspected, because sporidesmin, a toxin produced by *Pithomyces chartarum*, was known to cause bladder lesions in sheep and cattle.
• Clinically significant renal nematode infections are rare, despite necropsy surveys revealing that up to 20% of equine kidneys have evidence of *Strongylus vulgaris* migration.
• *K. equi* infection of equine kidneys occurs worldwide; one necropsy survey found the protozoa in 12% of horses examined.

SIGNALMENT

Breed Predilections

None documented

Mean Age and Range

• Foals <30 days of age are at greater risk for septic nephritis associated with septicemia.
• Critically ill neonates receiving broad-spectrum antibiotic treatment may develop ascending UTI with *Candida* sp.

URINARY TRACT INFECTION (UTI)

Predominant Sex

• A shorter urethra increases risk of UTI in females of most species, but UTI is also rare in mares.
• Injury to the lower urinary tract during breeding and parturition increase risk of bladder paresis and UTI, especially after dystocia.

SIGNS

Historical Findings

• Horses with upper UTI usually present with weight loss or fever of undetermined origin.
• Less commonly, hematuria or pyuria may be observed.
• Occasionally, recurrent colic may be reported when upper tract obstruction accompanies UTI.
• With lower UTI, dysuria (e.g., pollakiuria, stranguria, hematuria) are common presenting complaints. Urinary incontinence also may be observed with either bladder paresis or pollakiuria.

Physical Examination Findings

Upper UTI:
• Depression, lethargy, fever, partial anorexia, intermittent colic, and mild dehydration
• Rectal examination may reveal enlarged ureters and kidneys.
• Occasionally, obstructing ureteroliths can be palpated.
Lower UTI:
• In addition to dysuria, affected horses may have urine scalding, but general health usually is good.
• Rectal examination usually reveals a thickened bladder wall; cystoliths or other bladder masses also may be detected.
• Assess for bladder paresis (i.e., large atonic bladder with incontinence produced by compressing bladder) versus the small bladder that usually accompanies pollakiuria.

CAUSES

Upper UTI

• Ascending infections with bladder paralysis and vesiculoureteral reflux or obstructive disease may be caused by a variety of bacteria—*Escherichia coli, Proteus mirabilis, Klebsiella* sp., *Staphylococcus* sp., *Enterobacter* sp., *Corynebacterium* sp., and *Pseudomonas aeruginosa.*
• Mixed infections are not uncommon.
• Less commonly, a hematogenous infection with septicemia occurs—*Rhodococcus equi, Actinobacillus equuili,* and other Gram-negative bacteria

Lower UTI

• Ascending infections usually develop from anatomic or functional causes of abnormal urine flow, especially bladder paralysis.
• Organisms are similar to those isolated from upper UTIs.
• With instrumentation of the urinary tract (e.g., indwelling bladder catheters, ureteral stents), UTI with *Enterococcus* sp. (formerly *Streptococcus faecalis*) may develop.
• Infection with *Candida* sp. may develop in recumbent neonatal foals receiving broad-spectrum antibacterial therapy.

RISK FACTORS

• Vesiculoureteral reflux is an important predisposing problem for ascending upper UTI that may develop with bladder paresis or partial obstruction.
• Anatomic or functional causes of abnormal urine flow, especially bladder paralysis, also are important for development of lower UTI.
• Use of indwelling catheters is a significant risk factor, but routine instrumentation of the urinary tract (e.g., bladder catheterization, cystoscopy) carries a relatively low risk.

DIAGNOSIS

DIFFERENTIAL DIAGNOSIS

• Upper UTI—disease processes that may lead to depression, lethargy, partial anorexia, weight loss, fever, recurrent colic, or hematuria
• Lower UTI—normal estrus activity in mares, ectopic ureter, and other causes of dysuria (e.g., urolithiasis, neoplasia)

CBC/BIOCHEMISTRY/URINALYSIS

• Usually normal PCV, normal WBC count, or leukocytosis with upper UTI; platelets usually normal
• Azotemia usually is not present unless bilateral pyelonephritis results in chronic renal failure.
• Urine specific gravity—usually normal (>1.020) unless UTI is associated with chronic renal failure and isosthenuria (specific gravity, 1.008–1.014)
• Urinalysis generally reveals microscopic or macroscopic hematuria and pyuria; bacteria may be detected on sediment examination.

OTHER LABORATORY TESTS

• Perform quantitative urine culture in all suspected cases; recovery of >10,000 CFU/mL is diagnostic.
• Consider bacterial culture of the center of uroliths accompanying UTIs after surgical removal, because many will have positive results despite negative urine culture results.

URINARY TRACT INFECTION (UTI)

IMAGING

Transabdominal Ultrasonography

• Kidneys may be shrunken or enlarged, with loss of detail of the corticomedullary junction or areas of decreased echogenicity with pyelonephritis.
• Nephroliths (diameter, >1 cm) should be readily detected.
• Useful for evaluation of the left kidney, ureters, and bladder

Urethroscopy/Cystoscopy

Useful to assess uroepithelial damage, patency of the ureteral orifices, and urine flow from each side of the upper urinary tract

Nuclear Scintigraphy

May provide semiquantitative information about relative perfusion and function of each kidney.

DIAGNOSTIC PROCEDURES

• Urine collection—for urinalysis and quantitative urine culture
• Ureteral catheterization—can be performed during cystoscopy (or by a manual transurethral approach in mares) to collect urine from each side of the upper urinary tract when unilateral pyelonephritis is suspected.

PATHOLOGIC FINDINGS

• With pyelonephritis, mild to marked deformation of normal renal architecture may be detected, with complete replacement by abscess formation in severe cases of unilateral infection.
• Nephroliths, ureteroliths, and ureteral dilation commonly accompany pyelonephritis.
• Lower UTI—generally thickened bladder wall and inflamed mucosa, with areas of erosion/ulceration and adhesion of crystalloid material

TREATMENT

APPROPRIATE HEALTH CARE

• Assess for predisposing causes; institute appropriate antimicrobial therapy.
• Surgical correction of anatomic defects or removal of uroliths that may accompany UTI

NURSING CARE

• Regular cleaning of perineum and hind limbs to minimize skin irritation from incontinence
• Application of petrolatum to scalded areas

DIET

Salt supplementation (sodium chloride [1 oz. PO BID–QID]) to increase urine flow

CLIENT EDUCATION

• Primary UTIs are rare; further diagnostic evaluation is needed to rule out predisposing causes.
• With bladder paralysis, the prognosis for elimination of UTI is guarded to poor.

MEDICATIONS

DRUGS OF CHOICE

• Trimethoprim/sulfonamide combinations (20–40 mg/kg PO q12h—sulfadiazine may be preferred over sulfamethoxazole, because the former is excreted largely unchanged in urine but the latter is metabolized largely to inactive products before urinary excretion.
• Procaine penicillin G (22,000 IU/kg IM q12h) and sodium ampicillin (10–20 mg/kg IV or IM q6–8h) are effective for upper or lower UTI caused by susceptible *Corynebacterium* sp., *Streptococcus* sp., and some *Staphylococcus* sp. Many isolates of the Enterobacteriaceae family demonstrate resistance to ampicillin in vitro, but this drug is highly concentrated in urine. Thus, many organisms that are resistant in vitro may be killed in the urine of treated animals.
• Reserve gentamicin (6.6 mg/kg IV q24h) and amikacin (15 mg/kg IV q24h) for lower UTI caused by highly resistant organisms or acute, life-threatening upper UTI caused by Gram-negative organisms.
• Ceftiofur (4.4 mg/kg IV or IM q12h) or enrofloxacin (2.5 mg/kg PO q12h) when urinary pathogens demonstrate resistance to trimethoprim/sulfonamide combinations and penicillin.
• NSAIDs—phenylbutazone (2.2 mg/kg PO q12–24h) or flunixin meglumine (0.5–1.0 mg/kg PO q12–24h) may be useful adjunctive treatment with pollakiuria or apparent pain during urination.

CONTRAINDICATIONS

N/A

PRECAUTIONS

• Enrofloxacin—consider potential cartilage damage in young horses; discuss with owner before pursuing treatment.
• NSAIDs—avoid or used sparingly in cases of upper UTI with azotemia.

POSSIBLE INTERACTIONS
N/A

ALTERNATIVE DRUGS
N/A

FOLLOW-UP

PATIENT MONITORING
- Institute antibiotic treatment for at least 1 week for simple (i.e., no apparent underlying cause) lower UTI; follow-up should include another quantitative urine culture the week after treatment is discontinued.
- Institute antibiotic treatment for 4–6 weeks for upper UTI; follow-up should include a quantitative urine culture during the week after treatment is discontinued.
- Assess renal function of patients with azotemia consequent to bilateral pyelonephritis at regular intervals (i.e., monthly or longer) during the early stages of chronic renal failure.
- Discontinuation of broad-spectrum antibiotics usually is all that is required for resolution of lower UTI caused by *Candida* sp. in neonates.

PREVENTION/AVOIDANCE
Salt supplementation may increase urine flow and decrease risk of recurrence.

POSSIBLE COMPLICATIONS
- Urolithiasis
- Chronic renal failure

EXPECTED COURSE AND PROGNOSIS
- Favorable prognosis for recovery from simple lower UTI
- Guarded prognosis for recovery in patients with upper UTI and recurrent lower UTI
- Guarded long term prognosis in patients with bilateral pyelonephritis accompanied by azotemia; affected horses typically progress to chronic renal failure.

MISCELLANEOUS

ASSOCIATED CONDITIONS
- Urolithiasis
- Bladder paralysis
- Chronic renal failure

AGE-RELATED FACTORS
- Foals <30 days of age are at greatest risk for septic nephritis associated with septicemia.
- Sick neonates receiving broad-spectrum antibiotic treatment are predisposed to ascending UTI with *Candida* sp.

ZOONOTIC POTENTIAL
N/A

PREGNANCY
Postpartum mares are at risk of urethral and bladder trauma leading to urethral sphincter incontinence and bladder paralysis.

SYNONYMS
- Cystitis
- Pyelonephritis

SEE ALSO
- Chronic renal failure
- Urolithiasis
- Bladder paralysis and incontinence

ABBREVIATIONS
- CFU = colony-forming unit
- PCV = packed cell volume

Suggested Reading

Divers TJ. Urinary tract infections. In: Smith BP, ed. Large animal internal medicine. 2nd ed. St. Louis: Mosby, 1995:962–965.

Divers TJ, Byars TD, Murch O, Sigel CW. Experimental induction of *Proteus mirabilis* cystitis in the pony and evaluation of therapy with trimethoprim-sulfadiazine. Am J Vet Res 1981;42:1203–1205.

Schott HC. Urinary tract infections. In: Reed SM, Bayly WM, eds. Equine internal medicine. Philadelphia: WB Saunders, 1998:875–880.

Author Harold C. Schott II
Consulting Editor Harold C. Schott II

URINE POOLING/UROVAGINA

BASICS

OVERVIEW

• Reflux of urine from the urethral orifice into the vagina.
• Once in the vagina, urine may enter the uterus when the cervix relaxes during estrus or after irritation (and relaxation) of the cervix.
• May cause infertility and permanent endometrial, cervical, or vaginal damage.
• Caused by an altered position of the urethral orifice relative to the vulval opening and vestibular sphincter that results in incomplete voiding and retention of urine within the vestibule and vagina.
• Inherited predisposition for vulvar conformation and, thus, the location of the urethral orifice.
• Possible tendency for soft-tissue supporting structures of the vestibule to decrease with age.

SIGNALMENT

• All breeds.
• Most common in breeds with less muscle in the perineal area.
• Greater problem in old pluriparous mares.
• Females.

SIGNS

• Few to no outward signs.
• Sole complaint may be infertility.
• Mares bred multiple cycles that remain open/barren.
• On dismount, stallion may have urine evident on the glans and shaft of the penis.
• Transrectal examination may disclose fluid within the uterus.
• Vaginal examination may disclose urine in the vagina.
• Speculum examination may reveal increased hyperemia and ulcers (from urine scalding) of the vaginal wall and external cervical os.

CAUSES AND RISK FACTORS

• With increasing age, vulvar conformation often worsens.
• Frequently described as an elevation of the vulvar commissure.
• Frequently coupled with elevations of the vestibule, which raises the caudal urethral opening and permit urine to reflux into the cranial vagina.
• Inherited conformational traits.
• Multiparous mares.

DIAGNOSIS

DIFFERENTIAL DIAGNOSIS

Vaginitis or, possibly, pneumovagina.

CBC/BIOCHEMISTRY/URINALYSIS

N/A

OTHER LABORATORY TESTS

N/A

IMAGING

N/A

DIAGNOSTIC PROCEDURES

N/A

PATHOLOGIC FINDINGS

• Urine in the uterus and or vagina accompanied by severe inflammation of the uterus and vagina from the urine.
• Relative dorsal displacement of the external urethral os and downward slant (i.e., caudocranial) of the *vagina to the cervix.*
• Careful examination of the spatial relationship of the urethral opening to the ventral vulvar commissure, vestibular sphincter, and vagina.

TREATMENT

GENERAL COMMENTS

• No systemic signs; no systemic therapy.
• Flushing the uterus and vagina before insemination may increase the likelihood of conception but does not prevent subsequent urine accumulation and pregnancy loss. The condition (i.e., angulation) becomes more extreme as the uterus increases in weight later during gestation, pulling the vestibule further forward and ventrally.
• If poor vulvar/vestibular conformation is secondary to loss of vaginal fat (e.g., mare that is cachectic, thin, poor conditioning), urine pooling may be a slight problem and may resolve itself if the mare gains weight, which may increase the amount of fat within the pelvic cavity and elevate the vestibular floor in relationship to the ventral vulvar opening. This is considered to be a temporary solution, however, because the condition most likely will recur with age, parity, or subsequent weight loss.

SURGICAL CONSIDERATIONS

Surgical repair is only permanent means of correction.

Pouret

Correction of vulvar conformation by transection of the perineal body, allowing the vulva to lie more posterior and ventral, with subsequent movement of the urethral orifice posteriorly, which reduces the possibility of urine pooling.

URINE POOLING/UROVAGINA

Urethral Extension

- Posterior relocation of the urethral orifice by undermining strips of the vaginal wall, folding the mucosa medially, and suturing it to extend the urethra to be longer than it initially was.
- Serves to move the external urethral opening closer to the vulvae, permitting urine to exit without reflux.

Monin Vaginoplasty

- Ventral tissue dam of, or immediately cranial to, the vestibular sphincter—limited success.
- The dam is to reduce the likelihood of urine entering the vagina.
- This procedure is usually torn at the time of delivery, and surgery must be performed again after delivery to again correct the urine pooling.

MEDICATIONS

DRUGS

N/A

CONTRAINDICATIONS/POSSIBLE INTERACTIONS

N/A

FOLLOW-UP

PATIENT MONITORING

Examine mares after treatment to determine success of the approach used.

PREVENTION/AVOIDANCE

No specific way to prevent this condition.

POSSIBLE COMPLICATIONS

- Infertility
- Vaginitis

EXPECTED COURSE AND PROGNOSIS

- Early recognition and treatment may assist in avoiding permanent damage to the vagina and endometrium.
- Without surgical correction, mares continue to pool urine.
- As the condition progresses, more *irritation and urine accumulation* in the vagina and uterus occurs.

MISCELLANEOUS

ASSOCIATED CONDITIONS

- Thin mares may be more predisposed to urine pooling.
- Usually most severe when the mare is in estrus and vestibular tissues are relaxed.
- Increased inflammation and fibrosis of the endometrium.

AGE-RELATED FACTORS

Old mares have a higher occurrence of this condition.

ZOONOTIC POTENTIAL

N/A

PREGNANCY

May observe infertility or loss of pregnancy because of urine pooling.

SYNONYMS

Vesicovaginal reflux.

Suggested Reading

McKinnon AO, Beldon JO. Urethral extension technique to correct urine pooling (vesicovaginal reflux) in mares. J Am Vet Med Assoc 1988;192:647–650.

Shires GM, Kaneps AJ. A practical and simple surgical technique for repair of urine pooling in the mare. Proc AAEP 1986;51–56.

Author Walter R. Threlfall

Consulting Editor Carla L. Carleton

UROLITHIASIS

BASICS

DEFINITION

- A calculus or stone in any portion of the urinary tract
- Anatomically divided into nephrolithiasis, ureterolithiasis, cystolithiasis, and urethrolithiasis, which may occur separately or together.
- Accumulation of a large mass of urine sediment in the ventral aspect of the bladder of horses with bladder paresis is termed sabulous urolithiasis.

PATHOPHYSIOLOGY

- Despite the large amount of calcium carbonate crystals in normal equine urine, urolithiasis is rare in this species compared to small animals.
- The low incidence likely relates to lubricating mucus produced by glands in the renal pelvis and proximal ureter that protects the uroepithelium.
- Urolith formation usually requires damage to the renal parenchyma or the uroepithelium of the ureters, bladder or urethra.
- Calcium carbonate crystals readily adhere to damaged uroepithelium; such areas may provide a nidus for subsequent stone formation.
- Developmental anomalies, ascending or hematogenous infection, acute tubular necrosis due to nephrotoxic or ischemic injury, or neoplasms can produce areas of parenchymal damage that may serve as a nidus for stone formation. In particular, renal medullary crest necrosis due to use of NSAIDs is a risk factor for developing stones in and adjacent to the renal pelvis.
- Ureterolithiasis most commonly is due to passage of small nephroliths into the ureters.
- Cystolithiasis may develop spontaneously or be associated with damage to the bladder uroepithelium.
- Most spontaneously occurring bladder stones are disc-shaped, mildly spiculated, and porous.
- Porosity is due to stone formation by sedimentation of concentric layers of calcium carbonate crystal aggregates on the surface of the growing stone.
- Porosity makes these cystoliths relatively easy to fragment during removal. Less commonly, equine cystoliths are more dense concretions that can develop with greater phosphate content of the precipitating mineral.
- In horses with bladder paresis, sedimentation of normal urine crystals can lead to formation of a sabulous urolith in the ventral aspect of the bladder. Unlike cystoliths, this mass usually is indentable with firm digital pressure and often can be removed with aggressive lavage and bladder manipulation via rectal palpation.
- Urethroliths may develop at sites of damaged uroepithelium (e.g., site of a previous perineal urethrotomy) but more commonly result from passage of small nephroliths, ureteroliths, or cystoliths into the urethra.

SYSTEM AFFECTED

Renal/urologic—stone formation, infection, and occasionally, postrenal failure or bladder rupture (with obstructive disease)

GENETICS

No inherited diseases predisposing horses to urolithiasis are documented.

INCIDENCE/PREVALENCE

- Urolithiasis is uncommon and reported to be responsible for 0.11% of equine admissions to 22 veterinary teaching hospitals, accounting for $\cong$8% of all urinary tract disorders.
- In the same study, cystoliths were most common (60% of all urinary stones) followed by urethroliths (24%), nephroliths (12%), and ureteroliths (4%); $\cong$10% of affected horses had multiple calculi at different levels of the urinary tract.

SIGNALMENT

Breed Predilections

None documented

Mean Age and Range

Generally a disease of adult horses (mean age $\cong$10 years). However, the age range is wide, and horses $<$1 year have been affected with stones at all levels of the urinary tract.

Predominant Sex

- $\cong$75% of all reports are in male horses—intact as well as geldings
- A longer urethra increases risk of cystolithiasis and urethrolithiasis in males, but risk of nephrolithiasis, ureterolithiasis, and sabulous urolithiasis (with bladder paresis) is similar in both sexes.

SIGNS

Historical Findings

- Horses afflicted with nephroliths and ureteroliths usually are presented for weight loss or fever of undetermined origin.
- Unilateral upper tract stones may be incidental findings at necropsy.
- Less commonly, hematuria or pyuria may be observed.
- Occasionally, recurrent colic may be reported when upper tract obstruction accompanies lithiasis.
- With cystolithiasis, lower urinary tract signs (e.g., pollakiuria, stranguria, hematuria) predominate, and hematuria after exercise is common.
- Urinary incontinence may be observed and usually is the primary complaint with sabulous urolithiasis—bladder paresis
- Urethrolithiasis may cause severe renal colic signs when obstruction is complete, and bladder rupture can be a complication.

UROLITHIASIS

Physical Examination Findings

- Depression, lethargy, fever, partial anorexia, intermittent colic, and mild dehydration may be found with nephroliths and ureteroliths.
- Rectal examination may reveal enlarged, turgid ureters, and obstructing ureteroliths occasionally can be palpated.
- In addition to dysuria, horses with bladder stones may have urine scalding, but general health usually is good.
- Rectal examination usually reveals a thickened bladder wall; cystoliths in the bladder are usually palpable if the bladder is not distended.
- During rectal examination, assess for bladder paresis (i.e., large atonic bladder with incontinence produced by compressing bladder) versus the small bladder that usually accompanies pollakiuria.
- In addition to renal colic, a markedly enlarged bladder usually can be palpated per rectum in horses with obstructive urethroliths.
- A distended, sometimes pulsating urethra may be found below the anus, and careful palpation may allow location of the obstructing stone.
- Repeated obstruction with urethroliths provides support for upper tract disease as a source of ureteroliths.

CAUSES

Nephrolithiasis and Ureterolithiasis

- Renal parenchymal damage due to developmental anomalies, ascending or hematogenous infection, acute tubular necrosis, or neoplasia serves as a nidus for development of calcium carbonate stones.
- Renal medullary crest necrosis with NSAID use is a risk factor for development of stones in and adjacent to the renal pelvis.
- Ureterolithiasis usually results from passage of small nephroliths into the ureters.

Cystolithiasis

- High-calcium diets (i.e., legume hays) may lead to increased risk of spontaneous bladder stone formation.
- Ascending infections and anatomic or functional causes of abnormal urine flow may lead to calcium carbonate stone formation.
- Sabulous cystolithiasis develops as a consequence of bladder paralysis.

Urethrolithiasis

Damage to urethral mucosa or passage of small cystoliths into the urethra.

RISK FACTORS

- Although poorly documented, high-calcium diets (e.g., alfalfa and other legume hays) likely are a risk factor for calculi at all levels of the urinary tract.
- An area of damaged uroepithelium usually is needed to serve as a nidus for initiation of stone formation.

DIAGNOSIS

DIFFERENTIAL DIAGNOSIS

- Upper tract lithiasis—broad list of disease processes that may lead to depression, lethargy, partial anorexia, weight loss, fever, recurrent colic, or hematuria
- Lower tract lithiasis—normal estrus activity in mares and other causes of hematuria or dysuria (e.g., urinary tract infection, neoplasia)

CBC/BIOCHEMISTRY/URINALYSIS

- Normal to low PCV (with more severe hematuria), normal WBC count or leukocytosis with concurrent upper tract infection, and normal to mildly decreased platelets (with hematuria)
- Azotemia usually is not present unless lower tract obstruction develops (i.e., postrenal azotemia) or bilateral nephrolithiasis/ ureterolithiasis is associated with chronic renal failure.
- Urine specific gravity—usually normal (>1.020) unless lithiasis is associated with chronic renal failure and isosthenuria (specific gravity, 1.008–1.014)
- Urinalysis generally reveals microscopic or macroscopic hematuria and pyuria; bacteria may be detected on sediment examination with concurrent urinary tract infection.

OTHER LABORATORY TESTS

- Perform quantitative urine culture in all cases of suspected urolithiasis to assess for concurrent urinary tract infection.
- Consider bacterial culture of the urolith center after surgical removal, because many will have positive culture results despite negative urine culture results

IMAGING

Transabdominal Ultrasonography

- Nephroliths (diameter >1 cm) should be readily detected.
- Dilation of the renal pelvis and proximal ureter may be detected with obstructive ureterolithiasis.
- Useful in evaluating the left kidney, ureters, bladder, and proximal urethra.

Urethroscopy/Cystoscopy

- To confirm cystolithiasis and urethrolithiasis
- To assess uroepithelial damage and urine flow from each side of the upper urinary tract

DIAGNOSTIC PROCEDURES

Urine collection—for urinalysis and quantitative urine culture

PATHOLOGIC FINDINGS

- Nephroliths and ureteroliths may be incidental findings at necropsy if they were not producing bilateral obstructive disease.
- When accompanying chronic renal failure, nephroliths typically are found in small, irregularly shaped kidneys, but nephroliths and ureteroliths occasionally may produce hydronephrosis when obstruction is complete.
- Cystolithiasis is accompanied by bladder-wall thickening.
- Extensive mucosal damage accompanies cystolithiasis and urethrolithiasis.

TREATMENT

APPROPRIATE HEALTH CARE

- Appropriate antimicrobial therapy for prophylaxis or treatment of urinary tract infection
- Dietary modification, salt supplementation, and medication with urinary acidifying agents may be useful to prevent recurrence.
- With sabulous urolithiasis, the primary problem of bladder paralysis should be the focus of attention.

UROLITHIASIS

NURSING CARE

- Regular cleaning of the perineum and hind limbs to minimize skin irritation from incontinence or after perineal urethrotomy; application of petrolatum to scalded areas
- Horses with obstructive urethrolithiasis may benefit from temporary placement of an indwelling bladder catheter for the first few days after perineal urethrotomy if bladder distension was prolonged (>24 hours) or incomplete emptying is detected via rectal palpation.

ACTIVITY

N/A

DIET

- Decrease dietary calcium intake by providing grass rather than legume hay.
- Oral electrolyte supplementation—sodium chloride (1 oz.) can be administered in concentrate feed or as an oral slurry/paste BID–QID to encourage increased drinking and urine output (to decrease risk of further urolith formation).
- Use of urinary acidifying agents may be considered.

CLIENT EDUCATION

- Urolithiasis may recur in as many as 40% of affected horses.
- Avoid use of NSAIDs in horses with upper tract lithiasis.
- With sabulous urolithiasis, prognosis for recovery is guarded to poor because of underlying bladder paralysis.

SURGICAL CONSIDERATIONS

- Nephrotomy for removal of obstructing nephroliths or possible unilateral nephrectomy for nephroliths accompanied by pyelonephritis and limited function of the affected kidney
- Elective surgical removal of cystoliths via cystotomy, pararectal approach, or perineal urethrotomy; manual removal of small cystoliths may be accomplished in mares.
- Possible emergency perineal urethrotomy for relief of urethral obstruction or bladder repair if obstruction leads to bladder rupture—after initial stabilization of electrolyte (i.e., hyperkalemia with uroperitoneum) and acid–base alterations
- Electrohydraulic or laser lithotripsy is the treatment of choice for ureteroliths and may be the preferred treatment for cystoliths and urethroliths when equipment is available.
- Placement of an indwelling bladder catheter and aggressive lavage and rectal manipulation of the bladder may obviate cystotomy in cases with sabulous urolithiasis.

MEDICATIONS

DRUGS OF CHOICE

- Appropriate antibiotic agents for prophylaxis or treatment of urinary tract infection—see *Urinary Tract Infection.*
- Urinary acidifying agents may be used in an attempt to decrease urine pH and, thereby, the amount of calcium carbonate crystals in urine—ammonium chloride (50–200 mg/kg per day PO) and ammonium sulfate (200–300 mg/kg per day PO), but these are rather unpalatable.
- Developing an anionic diet (i.e., low cation–anion balance) will also reduce urine pH—requires testing of hay and addition of necessary supplements
- Changing from alfalfa to grass hay likely will decrease the amount of calcium carbonate crystals in urine more than addition of a urinary acidifying agent to a legume-based diet will.

CONTRAINDICATIONS

N/A

PRECAUTIONS

Evalute horses with recurrent urethral obstruction for upper tract lithiasis and infection; these problems may be the source of the recurrent urethroliths.

POSSIBLE INTERACTIONS

N/A

ALTERNATIVE DRUGS

N/A

UROLITHIASIS

FOLLOW-UP

PATIENT MONITORING

- Assess clinical status of patients managed surgically at least twice daily during the initial 2–4 days after surgery, emphasizing urine output and signs of dysuria.
- Assess renal function of patients with nephrolithiasis or ureterolithiasis at regular intervals (monthly or longer) during the early stages of chronic renal failure.
- In patients with recurrent cystolithiasis or urethrolithiasis, carefully examine the entire urinary tract for predisposing causes—anatomic defects or pyelonephritis

PREVENTION/AVOIDANCE

- Dietary modifications
- Use of urinary acidifying agents

POSSIBLE COMPLICATIONS

- Recurrent urolithiasis
- Chronic renal failure
- Bladder rupture and uroperitoneum
- Urethral stricture

EXPECTED COURSE AND PROGNOSIS

- Prognosis for recovery after surgical correction of cystolithiasis and urethrolithiasis generally is favorable, unless the problem is recurrent.
- Issue a guarded long term prognosis for patients with recurrent cystolithiasis and urethrolithiasis.
- Issue a guarded long term prognosis for patients with nephrolithiasis or ureterolithiasis; these problems usually are accompanied by loss of renal function and, when lithiasis is bilateral, eventual progression to chronic renal failure.

MISCELLANEOUS

ASSOCIATED CONDITIONS

- Renal colic—with obstructive disease
- Urinary tract infection
- Bladder paralysis
- Chronic renal failure

AGE-RELATED FACTORS

N/A

ZOONOTIC POTENTIAL

N/A

PREGNANCY

Postpartum mares may be at greater risk of developing bladder paralysis, especially after dystocia.

SYNONYMS

- Lithiasis
- Calculus formation
- Urinary tract stones

SEE ALSO

- Chronic renal failure
- Urinary tract infection
- Bladder paralysis and incontinence

ABBREVIATIONS

PCV = packed cell volume

Suggested Reading

Holt PE, Mair TS. Ten cases of bladder paralysis associated with sabulous urolithiasis in horses. Vet Rec 1990;127:108–110.

Laverty S, Pascoe JR, Ling GV, Lavoie JP, Ruby AL. Urolithiasis in 68 horses. Vet Surg 1992;21:56–62.

Mair TS, Holt PE. The etiology and treatment of equine urolithiasis. Equine Vet Educ 1994;6:189–192.

Neumann RD, Ruby AL, Ling GV, Schiffman P, Johnson DL. Ultrastructure and mineral composition of urinary calculi from horses. Am J Vet Res 1994;55:1357–1367.

Schott HC. Obstructive disease of the urinary tract. In: Reed SM, Bayly WM, eds. Equine internal medicine. Philadelphia: WB Saunders, 1998:880–890.

Author Harold C. Schott II
Consulting Editor Harold C. Schott II

UROPERITONEUM

BASICS

DEFINITION

Free urine in the abdomen

PATHOPHYSIOLOGY

- In neonatal foals, most often results from rupture of the urinary bladder or urachus and, more rarely, from ureteral or urethral tears.
- Urine is partially composed of water, urea nitrogen, and creatinine and has a high concentration of potassium and low amounts of sodium and chloride.
- When urine accumulates in the abdomen, urea nitrogen and electrolytes equilibrate rapidly with the levels in the blood, which generally results in azotemia, hypochloremia, hyponatremia, and hyperkalemia. This abnormality is compounded by mare's milk being low in sodium and chloride and high in potassium.
- Creatinine, a larger molecule, diffuses poorly across the peritoneum and, therefore, may not be reflected by a rise in peripheral blood levels.
- Urine leakage results from a ruptured bladder, usually at birth, but clinical signs may not be evident for 2–4 days, when the foal's clinical pathologic abnormalities develop.
- Hyperkalemia is the most life-threatening abnormality and may be responsible for bradycardia, atrial standstill, and cardiac arrest, if not corrected.
- As urine accumulates in the abdomen and progressive distention of the abdomen occurs, the foal's ventilation may be impaired.

SYSTEMS AFFECTED

Urinary

- Primary system involved.
- Rupture of the urinary bladder most frequently occurs along its dorsal surface in neonatal foals.
- Urachal perforations generally occur secondary to omphalophlebitis and at the cranial tip of the bladder.

GI

Abdominal discomfort, ileus, gastric reflux, and loss of appetite result from an inflamed peritoneum.

Cardiovascular

Myocardial depression, ventricular fibrillation, third-degree AV block, atrial standstill, and cardiac arrest can occur secondary to hyperkalemia.

Respiratory

Tachypnea and increased intrathoracic pressure results from compression of the thorax from abdominal distension.

Nervous

Depression

GENETICS

N/A

INCIDENCE/PREVALENCE

Sporadic event; population-based data for estimation of incidence not available

SIGNALMENT

- Any breed of foal
- Some studies suggest a predilection for males, but others find no difference.

SIGNS

Historical Findings

- Foals appear normal at birth.
- Clinical signs usually are observed during the first 24–72 hours of life but may manifest as late as 3–4 weeks.

Physical Examination Findings

- Frequent posturing to urinate, but with no or little urine production
- Progressive abdominal distention—may be able to ballot a fluid wave
- Progressive depression and loss of appetite
- Mild to moderate colic
- Bradycardia or tachycardia
- Tachypnea; pleural effusion
- Scrotal hernia or fluid accumulation
- Progressive dehydration

CAUSES

- The common temporal association of onset of clinical signs within the first 3–4 days of life and presence of hemorrhage and necrosis around the bladder rupture site suggest that high intra-abdominal pressure during parturition plays a role.
- A higher frequency in male foals has been attributed to their narrower pelvis, longer urethra, and greater urethral tone, which could result in higher intravesicular pressures with compression. This does not, however, explain ruptured bladders in females.
- A developmental defect of the bladder wall also has been postulated.
- Ascending infection of the umbilical structures can result in ischemia and necrosis of the tissue, leading to urachal tears and uroperitoneum.
- Foals with omphalophlebitis often are septic; the most common organism isolated from these foals is *Escherichia coli.*
- Spontaneous rupture has been reported in association with cystitis and trauma. Iatrogenic rupture with urinary catheters also is possible, and ureteral and urethral rupture has been reported as well.

RISK FACTORS

- Male gender
- Age <4 days
- Septicemia
- Prematurity
- Abdominal trauma

UROPERITONEUM

DIAGNOSIS

DIFFERENTIAL DIAGNOSIS

- Meconium impaction can be differentiated from a ruptured bladder by body posture. Foals that strain to urinate usually assume a stance that is base-wide, with ventroflexion of the back, whereas foals with meconium retention arch their backs dorsally.
- Colic for other reasons must be ruled out.
- Foals with ruptured urachus have signs identical to those with ruptured bladder or have subcutaneous, abdominal wall swelling if the rupture is retroperitoneal.
- Urethral obstruction caused by a persistent frenulum and twist may cause increased bladder pressure, which then leads to bladder rupture.

CBC/BIOCHEMISTRY/URINALYSIS

- Important laboratory abnormalities include elevated serum creatinine and potassium and decreased serum sodium and chloride.
- Electrolyte shifts may be less pronounced in septicemic foals not fed milk or milk products.

OTHER LABORATORY TESTS

- Blood gas analysis may be normal or show metabolic acidosis.
- Abdominocentesis yields copious amounts of clear, yellow-tinged fluid. Creatinine concentration of abdominal fluid is at least twice that of serum. Peritonitis rarely is evident in uncomplicated cases.

IMAGING

Abdominal Radiography

- Shows loss of detail.
- Standing thoracic films may reveal a ventral fluid line.
- Contrast cystography (10% solution of water-soluble iodine media) can confirm bladder rupture.

Abdominal Ultrasonography

- Reveals greatly increased abdominal fluid.
- May delineate edges of the bladder or urachal tear.
- Pleural effusion may be visualized.

DIAGNOSTIC PROCEDURES

- If other modes of imaging are not available, new methylene blue can be instilled via urinary catheter and detected in peritoneal fluid if a rupture is present.
- Electrocardiography shows broad QRS complexes and very tall T waves; arrhythmias also may be present—atrial standstill; heart blocks

PATHOLOGIC FINDINGS

- At necropsy, the abdomen is filled with urine, and a tear is found in the bladder wall. Typically, the tear is on the dorsal or dorsocranial margin of the bladder, and the area around the tear frequently is necrotic and hemorrhagic. Other areas of hemorrhage may be present as well.
- Urachal ruptures are associated with omphalophlebitis.
- Retroperitoneal urine accumulation and edema are found with ureteral ruptures.

TREATMENT

APPROPRIATE HEALTH CARE

- Immediate referral to a surgical facility
- Surgery as soon as the patient is stabilized.

NURSING CARE

- If possible, stabilize the foal before transportation and absolutely before general anesthesia and surgery. Rehydrate the foal, with consideration of acid–base and electrolyte disturbances. Typically, saline or saline with dextrose is employed, and bicarbonate may be added if warranted by severity of the acidosis. If abdominal distension is severe and compromising the respiratory and cardiovascular systems, the abdomen can be slowly drained via a teat cannula or catheter.
- If hyperkalemia is marked and unresponsive to saline and dextrose infusion, regular insulin (0.1–0.2 U/kg SC or IV) may be administered if a continuous dextrose drip is used concurrently and blood glucose levels are closely monitored.
- With only a small tear or a rupture secondary to other major diseases precluding safe anesthesia, a urinary bladder catheter may be employed to facilitate bladder emptying until the leak seals or surgery can be performed. After the foal is stabilized, the bladder is repaired via abdominal celiotomy using standard surgical techniques.

UROPERITONEUM

ACTIVITY

• Restrict to a box stall before surgery and for at least 7 days after surgery.
• Limited handwalking until the abdominal sutures are removed, then small paddock turnout until the abdominal wall is fully healed.

DIET

• Allow the foal to nurse until shortly before general anesthesia.
• The foal may resume nursing after it is fully recovered from the effects of anesthesia.

CLIENT EDUCATION

• Discuss care of the abdominal incision and exercise restrictions with the client.
• Observe the foal closely for signs of urine leakage, suggesting failure of the repair.

SURGICAL CONSIDERATIONS

• Stabilize the foal before anesthesia to prevent death because of cardiac arrhythmias.
• Place a urethral catheter before surgical preparation of the abdomen.
• Thoroughly inspect the bladder and urachus, because more than one leak may be present.
• Resect or oversew necrotic areas.
• Laparoscopic repair is also feasible after abdominal drainage.

MEDICATIONS

DRUGS OF CHOICE

Consider broad-spectrum antibiotics perioperatively or if other signs warrant their use.

CONTRAINDICATIONS

Avoid potassium administration because of hyperkalemia—potassium penicillin

PRECAUTIONS

Use aminoglycosides and NSAIDs cautiously in neonates with dehydration and azotemia.

POSSIBLE INTERACTIONS

N/A

ALTERNATIVE DRUGS

Sodium penicillin, ampicillin, or third-generation cephalosporins can be used instead of potassium penicillin for antibiotic coverage.

FOLLOW UP

PATIENT MONITORING

• Before surgery, the foal's abdominal circumference can be monitored with a girth or measuring tape.
• Serial serum potassium determinations every 1–2 hours can be useful for ascertaining when anesthesia is safer. Ideally, serum potassium concentrations should be <6 before induction of anesthesia.
• Postoperatively, record the foal's urinary output.
• Use of a urinary catheter is controversial because of the risk of ascending infection.

PREVENTION/AVOIDANCE

N/A

POSSIBLE COMPLICATIONS

• Affected foals may die from effects of the progressive uroabdomen or electrolyte abnormalities or from additive effects of anesthesia.
• The bladder may rerupture or leak after surgical repair.
• Peritonitis can develop, particularly if cystitis or septicemia were present preoperatively.
• Incisional complications (e.g., dehiscence, hernia formation) may occur infrequently.
• Intra-abdominal adhesions have been reported.

EXPECTED COURSE AND PROGNOSIS

• If the condition is recognized early in an otherwise healthy foal and that foal is stabilized before induction of anesthesia, the prognosis with surgery is excellent, with a success rate of as high as 95%.
• In the septicemic or premature foals, the prognosis is only fair, because complications are more commonly observed.

MISCELLANEOUS

ASSOCIATED CONDITIONS

N/A

AGE-RELATED FACTORS

Prognosis is more guarded in premature foals, which tend to have multiple organ system dysfunction.

ZOONOTIC POTENTIAL

N/A

PREGNANCY

N/A

SYNONYM

Cystorrhea

SEE ALSO

• Acute abdominal pain
• Meconium impaction
• Patent urachus

ABBREVIATIONS

• AV = atrioventricular
• GI = gastrointestinal

Suggested Reading

Behr MJ, Hackett RP, Bentinch-Smith J, Hillman RB, Jing JM, Tennant BC. Metabolic abnormalities associated with rupture of the urinary bladder in neonatal foals. J Am Vet Med Assoc 1982;178:263–266.

Kablack KA. Uroperitoneum in the septic equine neonate: retrospective study of 31 cases, 1988–1997. Proc Dorothy R. Havemeyer Foundation Neonatal Septicemia Workshop 1998;2:27–28.

Richardson DW, Kohn CW. Uroperitoneum in the foal. J Am Vet Med Assoc 1983;182:267–271.

Hackett RP. Rupture of the urinary bladder in neonatal foals. Compend Contin Educ 1984;6:488–494.

Wilson DA. Surgery of the equine urinary bladder and urethra. In: Wolfe DF, Moll HD, eds. Large animal urogenital surgery. Baltimore: Williams & Wilkins, 1999:63–69.

Author Julia H. Wilson
Consulting Editor Mary Rose Paradis

UTERINE INERTIA

BASICS

OVERVIEW

Primary Uterine Inertia

• Lack of myometrial contractions.
• May result in retention of fetal membranes.
• May result from failure of the myometrium to respond to hormonal stimulation; lack of hormonal release; or deficiency of hormonal receptors for oxytocin, estrogen, and/or $PGF_2\alpha$.
• Associated/related conditions—lack of exercise, overconditioning, chronic illnesses, twinning, uterine disease, and aging.

Secondary Uterine Inertia

• Usually follows prolonged labor without expulsion of the fetus and exhaustion of the myometrium.
• More common than primary uterine inertia.
• The exact mechanisms responsible for secondary uterine inertia are understandable, because exhaustion of the muscle fibers occurs with prolonged labor.
• Incidence of $<1\%$ of foaling mares.
• To increase the likelihood of delivering a live fetus, assist mares with uterine inertia once the condition is diagnosed.

SIGNALMENT

• All breeds.
• All females of breeding age.

SIGNS

• Mares in dystocia frequently are affected.
• Often a history of prolonged labor, then an absence of the signs of labor.

CAUSES AND RISK FACTORS

• The major cause is dystocia.
• Lack of exercise has been incriminated repeatedly as a cause.
• Benefits observed in fit mares—less fatigue with/during delivery, shortened time for parturition, and improved body tone and abdominal strength.
• Overconditioning—overweight.
• Restricted exercise during pregnancy.
• Old mares
• Mares in dystocia.

DIAGNOSIS

DIFFERENTIAL DIAGNOSIS

Dystocia from any cause.

CBC/BIOCHEMISTRY/URINALYSIS

N/A

OTHER LABORATORY TESTS

N/A

IMAGING

N/A

DIAGNOSTIC PROCEDURES

Assess the effectiveness of uterine contractions—observe the mare's expulsive efforts, and examine the uterus to determine if purposeful contractions are occurring.

PATHOLOGIC FINDINGS

None specific.

TREATMENT

• At the time when secondary uterine inertia is diagnosed, no correction is possible before the dystocia is resolved.
• With primary uterine inertia, first assist with the delivery of the fetus, then administer oxytocin. If oxytocin is administered before the fetus has been delivered, it will cause the uterus to contract around the fetus and compound problems with delivery.
• Foaling mares need assistance if normal delivery times for stages I and II are exceeded. The window of time for successful delivery (i.e., live foal) is very short in the mare.

MEDICATIONS

DRUGS

After removal of the fetus, oxytocin (10 IU IM) is the hormone of choice.

CONTRAINDICATIONS/POSSIBLE INTERACTIONS

- Avoid high doses of oxytocin, which are unnecessary and may cause excessive and uterine prolapse.
- $PGF_2\alpha$ enhances uterine contractions, but the clinical significance of these contractions has been questioned.
- Do not attempt correction of uterine inertia before the fetus is delivered, and only then treat with low doses (10 U IM) of oxytocin.

FOLLOW-UP

PATIENT MONITORING

Postpartum uterine examinations—determine if involution is proceeding normally after oxytocin administration; determine if fetal membranes have all passed.

PREVENTION/AVOIDANCE

- Exercise and proper nutrition play important roles in preventing primary uterine inertia.
- Secondary uterine inertia occurs most often but may be impossible to prevent unless parturition is observed and assistance is rendered as soon as dystocia is observed.

POSSIBLE COMPLICATIONS

- RFM
- Delayed uterine involution.
- Both RFM and delayed uterine involution may result in uterine infection and/or inflammation, which can delay rebreeding or result in infertility.

EXPECTED COURSE AND PROGNOSIS

- Excellent prognosis with proper treatment.
- May be warranted to skip breeding on foal heat.
- Reserve making the final decision regarding foal-heat breeding until examination of the uterus near/at the time of breeding, because some mares recover quickly.

MISCELLANEOUS

ASSOCIATED CONDITIONS

- Dystocia can cause secondary uterine inertia.
- RFM can occur after uterine inertia.

AGE-RELATED FACTORS

Incidence increases with age.

ZOONOTIC POTENTIAL

N/A

PREGNANCY

Occurs only at parturition and shortly thereafter.

ABBREVIATION

RFM = retained fetal membranes

Suggested Reading

Roberts SJ. Veterinary obstetrics and genital diseases (theriogenology). 3rd ed. Woodstock, VT: published by the author; 1986:347–352.

Author Walter R. Threlfall

Consulting Editor Carla L. Carleton

UTERINE TORSION

BASICS

DEFINITION

Torsion or twisting of the uterus at its body that sometimes extends caudally to involve the cervix.

PATHOPHYSIOLOGY

- Lengthening of the broad ligament, which permits the uterus additional leeway to twist on itself, is of primary importance.
- This lengthening may result from repeated stretching during previous gestations, rapid movement of the fetus, or falling and turning of the mare faster than the speed with which the fetus and uterus can rotate.

SYSTEM AFFECTED

Reproductive

GENETICS

- No hereditary predisposition has been linked to uterine torsion.
- If the supporting tissue (i.e., broad ligament) is longer in some animals because of genetics, however, this would support that theory of hereditary predisposition.

INCIDENCE/PREVALENCE

- This condition occurs infrequently and at anytime during the last 6 months of pregnancy.
- The later in gestation that uterine torsion occurs, the more serious the consequences can be.

SIGNALMENT

- Females; all breeds.
- Most affected are mares with deeper bodies or larger abdomens.
- All mares of breeding age.
- Increased occurrence in pluripara.

SIGNS

General Comments

The mare exhibits a variety of clinical signs, depending on the stage of gestation when torsion occurs.

Historical Findings

May present with signs of slight to mild colic, inappetent, depression, or general decrease or increase in activity, sweating, and increased urinations.

Physical Examination Findings

- Depending on stage of gestation, the mare may exhibit tense abdomen, increased heart rate on auscultation, and increased respiratory rate.
- Transrectal palpation reveals twisting of the broad ligament and body of the uterus and/or cervix.
- Vaginal examinations are less valuable in mares (compared with cows), because involvement of the vagina in the torsion is uncommon.
- At term, mares fail to show signs of labor, because the fetus is unable to enter the pelvic canal and cervix (i.e. absence of Ferguson reflex). Therefore, fetal death may occur from placental separation without the owner's knowledge.

CAUSES

- Cause unknown.
- There appears to be a relationship to relaxation or decrease of the suspensory nature of the broad ligament.
- Fetal movement plus the possibility of the mare falling or rolling can add to the probability of developing uterine torsion.

RISK FACTORS

- Dam with a large abdomen.
- Multiple pregnancies.
- Primipara may be affected.

DIAGNOSIS

DIFFERENTIAL DIAGNOSIS

- Intestinal colic—rule out by transrectal palpation and determining that the broad ligament twists to the left or right.
- Normal labor—rule out by the absence of membrane rupture, release of chorioallantoic fluid, and so on.

CBC/BIOCHEMISTRY/URINALYSIS

N/A

OTHER LABORATORY TESTS

N/A

IMAGING

Transabdominal ultrasonography—may help to determine viability of the fetus.

DIAGNOSTIC PROCEDURES

N/A

PATHOLOGIC FINDINGS

- The uterus is turned CW or CCW, with increased tension on the broad ligament, and the uterine wall may have increased tone.
- CCW torsion is more common than CW torsion.

TREATMENT

APPROPRIATE HEALTH CARE

- Accurate diagnosis is important to correct torsion before the fetus dies.
- If left untreated, a torsion of $> 180°$ compromises the blood supply to the fetus and uterus, and fetal death may occur, especially if the mare is near term.

Rolling

- Usually not indicated, unless sufficient help is available and the mare is not near term (<9 months of gestation).
- Mare must be anesthetized, and multiple people are necessary to rapidly roll the mare in the direction of the torsion.
- Lay the mare down on the side toward which the torsion is turning (i.e., CW torsion, on the right side; CCW torsion, on the left side), then roll the mare over on its back.
- Contraindications as the mare approaches term pregnancy—uterine artery rupture or uterine wall tears
- Assistance is required after the procedure until the mare recovers from anesthesia and rises to its feet.

Laparotomy

- Excellent technique, because minimal assistance is necessary and repositioning is very successful, especially before 9 months.
- As the mare approaches term, additional help may be required, including the possibility of a second incision to allow a second surgeon to work from the opposite flank.
- If one incision is to be used, make it to allow the surgeon to pull the ventral aspect of the uterus into proper position. It is easier to pull the uterus than it is to push the uterus and fetus.
- If an additional incision is necessary , the second surgeon can pull the dorsal aspect as the primary surgeon applies traction to the ventral aspect of the uterus.

UTERINE TORSION

Cesarean Section

- Can be performed in cases of uterine torsion, but correcting the torsion before incising the uterus, thus making it easier to extract the fetus and to suture the uterus, is preferable.
- Usually only necessary when the fetus is at term and delivery must be immediate or if the fetus is dead and vaginal delivery is not possible.
- Usually not necessary, because most torsions occur before the onset of labor.

NURSING CARE

Implement care in bedding changes in the stall, cross-tying, or other managerial options that may discourage the mare from rolling in the stall.

ACTIVITY

- After correction of the torsion, stall rest the mare.
- Hand walk the mare until parturition, if possible.
- Prevent the mare from running or having the opportunity to roll.

DIET

- Permit access to free-choice hay.
- Quality is not as important as quantity to keep the abdomen as full as possible.

CLIENT EDUCATION

Remind owners that as with any condition of pregnant mares, subtle changes in the mare's demeanor or behavior may indicate abnormal gestation and that immediate assistance should be sought.

SURGICAL CONSIDERATIONS

- A grid incision usually fails to provide sufficient area for manipulation, and incision of the abdominal muscles is necessary.
- A hand is moved ventrally under the uterus, and a hock or other extremity is grasped and then pulled toward the incision.
- At first, the uterus will be difficult to move, but as it begins returning to its normal position, movement will become easier. Once the uterus passes the halfway point, it will easily move the remainder of the distance.
- If one person cannot return the uterus to its normal position, a second incision can be made on the opposite side, and both surgeons can pull the uterus to its normal position.

MEDICATIONS

DRUGS OF CHOICE

- IV Xylazine, followed 5–10 minutes later with IV morphine or detomidine
- Infiltrate the area for incision with 2% carbocaine, to effect.

CONTRAINDICATIONS

N/A

PRECAUTIONS

- Confirm the diagnosis as rapidly as possible, especially if the mare is near term, to save the fetus.
- Administration of the previously mentioned agents should not be detrimental to fetal viability at any stage of gestation.

POSSIBLE INTERACTIONS

N/A

ALTERNATIVE DRUGS

N/A

FOLLOW-UP

PATIENT MONITORING

- Frequent after correction of uterine torsion.
- Close, daily observation and transrectal examination of the uterus at 1–2-week intervals until it appears that recurrence is not likely.
- For mares at term and in labor, recurrence of this condition after delivery has not been reported.

PREVENTION/AVOIDANCE

- Limiting exercise is one possible method to reduce the likelihood of the mare falling or rolling, but this rarely is indicated or warranted.
- Limited exercise also creates other problems—an increase in difficult deliveries because of lack of exercise.
- Free-choice hay is advisable and also may reduce the occurrence of abdominal colic.

POSSIBLE COMPLICATIONS

Uterine torsion can result in prolonged delivery and fetal death.

EXPECTED COURSE AND PROGNOSIS

Correction before term requires follow-up examinations, because recurrence is possible.

MISCELLANEOUS

ASSOCIATED CONDITIONS

N/A

AGE-RELATED FACTORS

Old mares may have increased occurrence because of previous broad ligament stretching.

ZOONOTIC POTENTIAL

N/A

PREGNANCY

Only occurs in pregnant animals.

SYNONYMS

N/A

SEE ALSO

- Dystocia
- Premature placental separation
- Stages of normal parturition

ABBREVIATIONS

- CW = clockwise
- CCW = counterclockwise

Suggested Reading

Guthrie RG. Rolling for correction of uterine torsion in a mare. J Am Vet Med Assoc 1982;181:66–67.

Perkins NR, Robertson JT, Colon LA. Uterine torsion and uterine tear in a mare. J Am Vet Med Assoc 1992;201:92–94.

Vaughan JT. Equine urogenital systems. In: Morrow DA, ed. Current therapy in theriogenology 2. Philadelphia: WB Saunders, 1986:756–775.

Wichtel JJ, Reinertson EL, Clark TL. Nonsurgical treatment of uterine torsion in seven mares. J Am Vet Med Assoc 1988; 193:337–338.

Youngquist RS. Equine obstetrics. In: Morrow DA, ed. Current therapy in theriogenology 2. Philadelphia: WB Saunders, 1986:699.

Author Walter R. Threlfall

Consulting Editor Carla L. Carleton

VACCINATION PROTOCOLS

INTRODUCTION

Numerous factors must be considered when determining the need for vaccination of horses. The efficacy of the vaccine must be weighed against the risk and consequences of infection and the adverse effects and cost of the vaccine. Once it has been determined that vaccination is necessary, the timing of the primary series may be influenced by the effect of passively acquired maternal antibodies on the foal's response to vaccination. The timing of subsequent vaccination is influenced by the duration of immunity provided by the vaccine and time of anticipated risk of exposure, if it can be estimated. The guidelines that follow have evolved with the consideration of these factors.

RABIES

Because rabies is a fatal zoonosis, all horses residing in endemic areas should be vaccinated. Vaccine manufactures recommend primary vaccination at 3 months of age, followed by a second dose at 1 year of age and annual vaccination thereafter. Vaccination is safe, but recent reports of rabies in vaccinated horses suggest that efficacy should be more closely evaluated. It is the only inactivated equine vaccine that does not require two closely spaced primary vaccinations.

TETANUS

Due to the sensitivity of the horse to tetanus toxin and frequency of this pathogen in the environment, all horses should be vaccinated beginning at 3 months of age, with an initial series of two doses of toxoid 4 weeks apart. Thereafter, yearly boosters are adequate. Vaccination is safe and effective. Although vaccination confers long-lasting immunity, it is an accepted practice to booster horses that incur lacerations more than 6 months since the last vaccination. Tetanus toxoid should be given to brood mares 4–6 weeks prior to the anticipated foaling date.

Unvaccinated horses or horses with an uncertain vaccination history should receive tetanus anti-toxin and tetanus toxoid if wounded. Vaccination should be given at separate sites. Foals born to unvaccinated mares should receive tetanus anti-toxin shortly after birth. Tetanus anti-toxin is rarely associated with fatal acute hepatic necrosis.

ENCEPHALOMYELITIS

In North America, eastern equine encephalitis (EEE) is restricted to the eastern and southeastern United States, and although western equine encephalitis (WEE) occurs primarily in the western United States and western Canada, cases of WEE have been reported on the east coast. Fortunately, all commercially available encephalomyelitis vaccines are inactivated and provide protection to both EEE and WEE. Venezuelan equine encephalitis (VEE) has not been reported in the United States since the early 1970s, but due to the presence of the disease in Mexico, horses residing in states on the Mexican border are frequently vaccinated.

The vaccines are safe and effective and should be given in the spring prior to the emergence of the insect vector in cool climates. In warm climates, where the vector is present throughout the year, biannual vaccination is appropriate. Pregnant mares should be vaccinated 4–6 weeks prior to the anticipated foaling date. Foals that receive adequate colostral antibody are protected for the first 6 months of life, and thus may not need to receive the primary immunization series until the following spring in climates without year-round vector exposure. There is debate about the effect of passive transfer of maternal antibodies on the efficacy of vaccination. Until a consensus is achieved, the manufacturer's recommendation should be followed.

RHINOPNEUMONITIS

Vaccination against equine herpesviruses 1 (EHV-1) and 4 (EHV-4) provides a short-lived and incomplete protection against abortion and respiratory disease. Both modified-live and inactivated vaccines are available. Vaccines are specifically labeled for protection against either respiratory disease or abortion. Although many practitioners initiate the primary immunization series for foals at 3 months, there is evidence that foals do not mount good humoral responses to vaccination. Therefore, foals should receive an additional booster 6 months later. Alternately, the initial series may be delayed until 6 months of age. Vaccination against rhinopneumonitis depends on the risk of infection, need for protection, and use of the horse. For example, valuable performance horses in which the inability to compete due to rhinopneumonitis is costly, and in which potential viral exposure is frequent, should be vaccinated every 3 months to maintain protective immunity. Conversely, some owners may wish to accept the low risk of infection in horses that are not frequently exposed to other horses rather than perform frequent vaccinations.

To aid in the prevention of abortion, brood mares should be vaccinated against EHV-1 during the fifth, seventh, and ninth months of gestation. Furthermore, vaccination against EHV-1 and -4 4–6 weeks prior to foaling increases colostral antibodies that are necessary to protect the foal from these common respiratory diseases.

INFLUENZA

Influenza and rhinopneumonitis are two of the most common causes of upper respiratory tract disease. As with rhinopneumonitis, vaccination for influenza provides immunity that is short in duration and incomplete in protection. However, due to the ubiquitous nature of this pathogen and the explosive nature of outbreaks, regular vaccination is especially beneficial for horses entering high-risk environments, such as shows, training centers, and breeding farms. In this author's experience, muscle soreness is more common in horses vaccinated frequently, and thus vaccination should be avoided immediately prior to competition.

Commercially available vaccines are inactivated products and are given by intramuscular injection. Manufacturers generally recommend a primary series of two doses 3–6 weeks apart; however, a three-dose series may provide a higher antibody titer and longer immunity. Vaccination of brood mares 4–6 weeks prior to the anticipated foaling date enables passive transfer of colostral antibodies to the foal. Timing of foal vaccinations is controversial. Although manufacturers suggest initiation of the primary series anytime after 3 months of age, there is evidence that maternal antibodies interfere with vaccination before 6 months of age. More research is needed to define appropriate vaccination protocols for foals with adequate maternal antibodies. Vaccination of foals born to unvaccinated mares can be initiated at 1 month of age.

BOTULISM

Clostridium botulinum produces several different toxins. In North America, horses are most frequently affected by type B. Types A and C also occur in the United States, but they are rare compared to type B. Although all three forms cause severe neuromuscular paralysis, the currently available toxoid only protects against type B. Vaccination of brood mares is especially important due to the frequent occurrence of toxicoinfectious botulism in foals. Ideally, unvaccinated brood mares in endemic areas should receive an initial series of three vaccinations each 1 month apart, with the final dose 4 weeks prior to the anticipated foaling date. Thereafter, a single yearly booster is given 4 weeks prior to foaling. Foals should receive three vaccinations at monthly intervals beginning at 3 months of age. On farms where botulism is common, vaccination of foals may begin earlier because maternal antibodies do not appear to interfere with vaccination. Vaccination is effective and is not associated with side effects; thus, it is highly recommended for horses in endemic areas.

POTOMAC HORSE FEVER

Potomac horse fever (PHF) is caused by *Ehrlichia risticii* and is characterized by fever, diarrhea, depression, anorexia, laminitis, colic, and death. Although the disease has been documented in most of the United States, recent evidence suggests *E. risticii* inhabits fluke-infested snails, thus explaining the association of the disease with streams and seasonal occurrence. Vaccination is generally limited to areas with a high prevalence. Unfortunately, there are several concerns about the efficacy of vaccination. First, the duration of immunity is short and protection incomplete. The latter problem may be due to heterogeneity of the organism. In spite of these shortcomings, the vaccine is safe and should be given prior to the disease season. In the eastern and midwestern United States, PHF occurs from mid-summer to fall, and in California it occurs from fall to spring. Due to the short duration of immunity, revaccination may be necessary 3–4 months later. Brood mares are vaccinated 4–6 weeks prior to the anticipated foaling date. It is recommended that foals in endemic areas receive three doses 1 month apart, beginning at 4 months of age.

STRANGLES

Whole-cell bacteria and M-protein extract vaccines are available in the United States. Two or three doses are given at 2- to 4-week intervals followed by yearly boosters. Mares should be vaccinated with an approved product 4–6 weeks prior to the anticipated foaling date because foals suckling these mares are frequently resistant to infection until weaned. Vaccination of foals should begin earlier than 4 months of age because young foals do not mount a good response to vaccination.

A modified live intranasal vaccine (Pinnacle I.N., Fort Dodge Animal Health, Fort Dodge, IA) has become available that has the advantage of promoting the mucosal secretory antibody that is important in preventing infection.

Due to occasional muscle soreness and incomplete protection associated with the intramuscular products, vaccination is generally limited to horses at risk. Horses residing on farms with previous outbreaks or horses entering these farms are candidates for vaccination. Although vaccination is not indicated for horses already infected, uninfected horses may benefit from vaccination during an outbreak. *Purpura hemorrhagica* is a rare adverse reaction to vaccination.

EQUINE VIRAL ARTERITIS

Equine viral arteritis (EVA) is characterized by abortion in mares and severe respiratory disease in neonates. In adult horses, clinical signs include fever, anorexia, limb and ventral edema, and nasal and ocular discharge. The virus is frequently spread by aerosolized respiratory secretions during outbreaks of respiratory disease. Chronically infected carrier stallions act as a reservoir for the virus, and may infect mares by the venereal route.

A modified-live vaccine is available in the United States and has been effective at controlling outbreaks of respiratory disease, protecting mares that are to be bred to infected stallions, and preventing stallions from becoming chronically infected. Some states have developed programs aimed at controlling spread of the virus, and state or USDA officials should be consulted prior to vaccination. Recommendations include vaccination of at-risk breeding stallions 3 weeks prior to the breeding season. Mares to be bred to infected stallions should be vaccinated not less than 3 weeks prior to breeding. Pregnant mares should not be vaccinated. Foals should not be vaccinated prior to 6 months of age as maternal antibodies may interfere with the development of an effective antibody response. Owners should be aware that seropositive horses may be ineligible for export to some countries.

Suggested Reading

Wilson WD. Equine vaccination and infectious disease control. In: Smith BP, ed. Large Animal Internal Medicine. 2nd ed. St. Louis: Mosby, 1996.

Author Mark T. Donaldson, VMD
Consulting Editor Corinne R. Sweeney, DVM

VAGINAL PROLAPSE

BASICS

OVERVIEW

- Displacement of all or part of the vaginal wall posteriorly through the vulvae.
- Predisposing factors thought to be involved—relaxation of the vaginal wall, such as occurs postpartum; relaxation of the vulvar lips, permitting protrusion of the vaginal wall; secondary to increased abdominal pressure, which places additional pressure on the vaginal wall; a previous dystocia that may have damaged the perineal area, including the vagina and vulva.

SIGNALMENT

- All breeds.
- All females of breeding age.

SIGNS

- The vaginal wall protrudes through the vulvae.
- The vaginal wall may become damaged and permit paravaginal fat to protrude through the prolapsed wall.
- This protruded fat may cause additional straining and further prolapse.
- The protruding tissue has a characteristic pink to red color, depending on the length of time it has been outside the body.
- Differentiating the vagina from the bladder, intestines, uterus, cervix and vestibule is essential before initiating treatment.

CAUSES AND RISK FACTORS

Generally secondary to other abnormalities that initially predispose mares to everting part of the vaginal wall; this may cause straining and additional tissue protrusion and injury.

DIAGNOSIS

DIFFERENTIAL DIAGNOSIS

Must differentiate from:

- Eversion of the bladder, uterus, or cervix.
- Vaginal tears through which paravaginal fat or intestines may be protruding.
- Eversion of the vestibular wall.

CBC/BIOCHEMISTRY/URINALYSIS

N/A

OTHER LABORATORY TESTS

N/A

IMAGING

N/A

DIAGNOSTIC PROCEDURES

Careful visual and digital examination to differentiate the vaginal wall from other prolapsed tissues.

PATHOLOGIC FINDINGS

Protrusion of the vaginal wall through the vestibule and vulvar lips.

TREATMENT

- Reduction of prolapse (i.e., returning tissues to their normal anatomic location) and termination of subsequent expulsive efforts are critical to permanent resolution.
- Reduction of inflammation, if present, also is advisable.
- No restriction of activity, unless the activity increases abdominal pressure.
- Any protrusion of tissue through the vulvar lips requires immediate attention.
- Caslick's vulvoplasty may help to prevent further vaginal irritation and, thus, decrease the likelihood of additional straining and tissue damage. This surgery, however, does not prevent recurrent prolapse from straining.

MEDICATIONS

DRUGS

- Epidural anesthetic may be indicated to reduce straining.
- Application of local, nonirritating antibiotics may aid in recovery.

CONTRAINDICATIONS/POSSIBLE INTERACTIONS

N/A

FOLLOW-UP

PATIENT MONITORING

At re-examination, careful and gentle assessment of previously affected tissues to prevent renewed irritation and reinitiation of straining.

PREVENTION/AVOIDANCE

- Treat any conditions (e.g., vaginal damage or irritation) that may initiate straining and result in eventual prolapse of the vaginal wall.
- Initiating treatment of prolapsed vaginal tissue as quickly as possible, once recognized, is critical to limit tissue trauma.

POSSIBLE COMPLICATIONS

Infections and abscessation of/within the vagina.

EXPECTED COURSE AND PROGNOSIS

- Rapid recovery if the inciting cause is removed.
- Satisfactory recovery if further damage can be avoided.

MISCELLANEOUS

ASSOCIATED CONDITIONS

N/A

AGE-RELATED FACTORS

N/A

ZOONOTIC POTENTIAL

N/A

PREGNANCY

Usually occurs after parturition.

SEE ALSO

- Dystocia
- Postpartum period
- Vaginitis

Suggested Reading

Cox JE. In: Surgery of the reproductive tract in large animals. Liverpool: Liverpool University Press, 1987:127–143.

Author Walter R. Threlfall

Consulting Editor Carla L. Carleton

VAGINITIS AND VAGINAL DISCHARGE

BASICS

OVERVIEW
- Inflammation of the vagina.
- Can be infectious or solely inflammatory in nature.
- One must first establish whether vulval discharge originates from the vagina, vestibule, or urethra.
- Pneumovagina—one of the major causes of vestibular and vaginal inflammation; caused by abnormal vulval conformation.
- Also may occur in fillies or mares in training or racing because of incomplete vulvar development.
- Breed differences—increased incidence in mares with poor body condition (i.e., little fat) or less muscle around/in the perineal area (e.g., contrast Thoroughbreds and Standardbreds with Quarter Horses).
- Possible inheritance of poor vulval conformation, which results in vaginitis.
- Prevalence increases with age
- Vulval discharge can occur but only infrequently is an obvious/external sign.

SIGNALMENT
- All breeds.
- All females of breeding age.
- Occurs more often in old mares.

SIGNS

Normal Discharge
- Urine, especially the characteristic appearance of calcium carbonate crystals that may accumulate at/on the ventral vulval commissure during estrus.
- This occurs secondary to frequent urination and evacuation of sediment common in equine urine, especially during estrus.

Abnormal Discharge
- Can be of mucoid or fluid consistency, and may be odiferous.
- Color can range from white to yellow to brown.
- **NOTE:** mares may have vaginitis with no external discharge.

Historical Findings
- Infertility
- Periodic discharge throughout the cycle.

Physical Examination Findings

When Secondary to Infection or Inflammation, May Be:
- Discharge on the tail and perineum.
- Fluid in the vagina or uterus.

CAUSES AND RISK FACTORS
- Poor vulval conformation.
- Trauma at parturition.
- Vaginal breeding injury.
- Pneumovagina.
- Multiparous broodmares are highest risk
- Less frequent in young maidens (not broodmares).

DIAGNOSIS

DIFFERENTIAL DIAGNOSIS
- Uterine disease/infection.
- Urinary tract infection.

CBC/BIOCHEMISTRY/URINALYSIS
N/A

OTHER LABORATORY TESTS
N/A

IMAGING
N/A

DIAGNOSTIC PROCEDURES
Careful speculum examination per vagina is the best means to establish a definitive diagnosis.

PATHOLOGIC FINDINGS
- Hyperemia of the vaginal mucosa.
- Fluid accumulation may be observed.
- Abrasions, ulcerations, and lacerations may be present—recent or chronic with adhesions or fibrin deposition.
- Vulvar discharge does not always accompany vaginitis.
- Large amounts of discharge may be adhered to the tail or attract flies during summer months.
- Discharge may be evident only when the mare is more excitable—being ridden or otherwise worked.

VAGINITIS AND VAGINAL DISCHARGE

TREATMENT

• Exact cause must be determined before treatment is initiated.
• If only vaginitis (i.e., not secondary to injury), treatment need only halt additional contamination, and the inflammation should subside.
• Systemic antibiotics have no value.
• Local therapy if antibiotics are indicated and used.
• Caslick's vulvoplasty to repair deficits in vulval conformation, if present.

MEDICATIONS

DRUGS

If indicated after vulvoplasty, nonirritating, local application of antibiotics may reduce the mare's discomfort. This usually is not necessary, however, because inflammation decreases rapidly once the source of irritation is resolved.

CONTRAINDICATIONS/POSSIBLE INTERACTIONS

N/A

FOLLOW-UP

PATIENT MONITORING

Re-examination 1–2 weeks after vulvoplasty

PREVENTION/AVOIDANCE

Caslick's vulvoplasty or other cosmetic repair of vulvae:
• Mares born with poor vulvar conformation have an increased likelihood of vaginitis—breed or individual mare predisposition.
• Postpartum, if injured at foaling.

POSSIBLE COMPLICATIONS

If left untreated, may result in infertility, endometrial damage, and/or vaginal adhesions.

EXPECTED COURSE AND PROGNOSIS

If treated early in the course of disease, excellent resolution and normal fertility.

MISCELLANEOUS

ASSOCIATED CONDITIONS

Linked with chronic vaginitis and uterine contamination:
• Metritis
• Endometritis
• Pyometra

AGE-RELATED FACTORS

Conformation problems and/or damage to the caudal genital tract increase with age and parity.

ZOONOTIC POTENTIAL

N/A

PREGNANCY

May prevent pregnancy or cause abortion.

SEE ALSO

• Caslick's vulvoplasty
• Dystocia
• Endometritis
• Metritis
• Pneumouterus
• Pneumovagina
• Vulvar conformation

Suggested Reading

Ricketts SW. Vaginal discharge in the mare. In: Boden E, ed. Equine practice. Philadelphia: Bailliere Tindall, 1991:1–26.

Author Walter R. Threlfall
Consulting Editor Carla L. Carleton

VENTRICULAR SEPTAL DEFECT (VSD)

BASICS

DEFINITION

• A congenital defect (i.e., hole) in the interventricular septum resulting in communication between the right and left ventricles
• Can be located in any portion of the interventricular septum—membranous (most common) or muscular

PATHOPHYSIOLOGY

• Blood shunts from the higher-pressure left ventricle to the lower-pressure right ventricle, creating primarily a left atrial and ventricular volume overload and, to a lesser degree, a right ventricular volume overload.
• Size and location of the VSD determines severity of the volume overload and the degree of involvement by the right ventricle.
• With a large, membranous VSD, the left ventricular and atrial volume overload is severe. Over time, stretching of the mitral annulus occurs, and mitral regurgitation develops. As the mitral regurgitation becomes more severe, increases in left atrial pressure cause increased pulmonary venous pressure, increased pulmonary capillary pressure, pulmonary edema, pulmonary hypertension, and clinical signs of left-sided congestive heart failure. As pulmonary hypertension becomes more severe, clinical signs of right-sided congestive heart failure appear.
• With a large, muscular VSD, the left atrial and ventricular volume overload and right ventricular volume overload are severe, and clinical signs of right-sided heart failure may predominate.

SYSTEM AFFECTED

Cardiovascular

GENETICS

Not yet determined in horses, but likely to be heritable.

INCIDENCE/PREVALENCE

• Welsh Mountain ponies are reported to be at significantly higher risk than Thoroughbreds.
• Standardbreds also appear to be more frequently affected than Thoroughbreds.

SIGNALMENT

• Murmurs are detectable at birth.
• Diagnosed most frequently in neonates, foals, and young horses, but may be found at any age if careful auscultation has not been performed.

SIGNS

General Comments

Usually an incidental finding

Historical Findings

• Medium to large VSDs—poor performance
• Large VSDs—congestive heart failure

Physical Examination Findings

• Grade 3–6/6, coarse, band-shaped, pansystolic murmur with PMI in the tricuspid valve area; membranous defect has loudest murmur here.
• Grade 3–6/6, coarse, band- or ejection-shaped, holosystolic or pansystolic murmur with PMI in the pulmonic valve area; outflow defect has loudest murmur here.
• Other, less common findings—accentuated third heart sound, grade 1–6/6 holodiastolic decrescendo murmur with PMI in aortic valve area, and atrial fibrillation

CAUSES

Congenital malformation of the interventricular septum

RISK FACTORS

N/A

DIAGNOSIS

DIFFERENTIAL DIAGNOSIS

• Tricuspid regurgitation—no relative pulmonic stenosis murmur; differentiate echocardiographically.
• VSD with pulmonic stenosis—loudest murmur usually in the pulmonic valve area; differentiate echocardiographically.
• Tetralogy of Fallot—foals are often stunted and may be tachycardic and hypoxemic; loudest murmur usually in the pulmonic valve area; differentiate echocardiographically.

CBC/BIOCHEMISTRY/URINALYSIS

N/A

OTHER LABORATORY TESTS

N/A

IMAGING

Electrocardiography

Atrial premature depolarizations or atrial fibrillation may be present in horses with left atrial enlargement.

Echocardiography

• The most common location for a VSD is the membranous portion of the interventricular septum, immediately beneath the septal leaflet of the tricuspid valve and right or noncoronary leaflet of the aortic valve.
• Outflow VSD is less common and more difficult to detect echocardiographically, because it is ventral to the aortic and pulmonic valves and difficult to detect in the long axis.
• Muscular VSD in other portions of the interventricular septum is less common, but if suspected, the entire ventricular septum should be examined.
• Left atrium and ventricle—enlarged, dilated, and rounded in appearance
• Left ventricular free wall and interventricular septum—thinner than normal; pattern of left ventricular volume overload if the ventricle is coping well with the left-to-right shunt
• Normal or decreased fractional shortening in horses with left ventricular enlargement is consistent with myocardial dysfunction.
• Pulmonary artery dilatation in horses with a large shunt fraction
• Pulsed-wave or color-flow Doppler reveals the shunt from left to right through the VSD.
• Hemodynamic significance can be determined from the peak velocity of the shunt through the VSD—a peak velocity >4 m/sec is consistent with a restrictive defect and a shunt of lesser hemodynamic significance; a peak shunt velocity ≤ 3 m/sec indicates a very hemodynamically significant shunt and a large VSD.
• A jet of mitral regurgitation may be present with a large VSD and marked left atrial and ventricular volume overload.

Thoracic Radiography

• An enlarged cardiac silhouette and increased pulmonary vascularity should be detected in horses with a large VSD.
• Pulmonary edema may be present in affected horses with congestive heart failure.

DIAGNOSTIC PROCEDURES

Cardiac Catheterization

• Right-sided catheterization can be performed to directly measure right atrial, right ventricular, and pulmonary arterial pressures and to sample blood for oxygen content.
• Elevated right ventricular pressure should be detected with an increased oxygen saturation of blood obtained from the right ventricle and pulmonary artery if the shunt is left to right.

Continuous 24-Hour Holter Monitoring

Useful in the diagnosis of suspected atrial premature depolarizations

PATHOLOGIC FINDINGS

• Most frequently found in the membranous septum underneath the septal leaflet of the tricuspid valve and the right or noncoronary leaflet of the aortic valve, but also can be present in any portion of the interventricular septum.
• Associated jet lesions along the margins of the defect and on the adjacent right ventricular endocardium
• Left atrial and ventricular enlargement and thinning of the left atrial and ventricular myocardium and interventricular septum in horses with a significant shunt.
• Right ventricular enlargement and thinning of the right ventricular free wall in horses with a VSD that is large or in a muscular location
• Pulmonary artery dilatation in horses with a large shunt fraction and in those with pulmonary hypertension

VENTRICULAR SEPTAL DEFECT (VSD)

TREATMENT

APPROPRIATE HEALTH CARE

- Most affected horses require no treatment and can be monitored on an outpatient basis.
- Monitor horses with hemodynamically significant shunts on an annual basis.
- Affected horses with congestive heart failure can be treated for congestive heart failure with positive inotropic drugs, vasodilators, and diuretics on an inpatient basis, if possible. Monitor response to therapy. Consider humane destruction if congestive heart failure develops, however, because only short-term, symptomatic improvement can be expected.

NURSING CARE

N/A

ACTIVITY

- Affected horses are safe to continue in full athletic work until significant mitral regurgitation or atrial fibrillation develops.
- Horses with small VSDs can have unrestricted activity and may be able to compete reasonably successfully at upper levels of athletic competition.
- Monitor horses with hemodynamically significant VSDs echocardiographically on an annual basis to ensure they are safe to ride and compete. These horses can be used for lower-level athletic work but are unlikely to compete successfully at upper levels.
- Horses with significant pulmonary artery dilatation are no longer safe to ride.
- Affected horses that develop atrial fibrillation often decompensate and are no longer safe to use for athletic performance.

DIET

N/A

CLIENT EDUCATION

- Regularly monitor cardiac rhythm; any irregularities other than second-degree AV block should prompt ECG.
- Carefully monitor for exercise intolerance, respiratory distress, prolonged recovery after exercise, increased resting respiratory or heart rate, or cough; if detected, perform a cardiac re-examination.
- Because the defect most likely is heritable, do not breed affected horses.

SURGICAL CONSIDERATIONS

- Closure of the VSD would be possible with transvenous umbrella catheters if the umbrella diameter was large enough to close the defect.
- Surgical closure would require rib resection for the thoracotomy and cardiac bypass, however, which are not financially feasible or practical for obtaining an equine athlete.

MEDICATIONS

DRUGS OF CHOICE

N/A

CONTRAINDICATIONS

N/A

PRECAUTIONS

N/A

POSSIBLE INTERACTIONS

N/A

ALTERNATIVE DRUGS

N/A

FOLLOW-UP

PATIENT MONITORING

- Frequently monitor cardiac rate rhythm and respiratory rate and effort.
- With defects >2.5 cm in two mutually perpendicular planes or peak shunt velocity >4 m/sec, annual echocardiographic re-examinations are recommended.

PREVENTION/AVOIDANCE

N/A

POSSIBLE COMPLICATIONS

Large VSD—atrial fibrillation; congestive heart failure

EXPECTED COURSE AND PROGNOSIS

- Horses with small, membranous VSDs (≤ 2.5 cm) that are restrictive (peak shunt velocity, >4 m/sec) should have normal performance and life expectancy. Horses with small VSDs can even race successfully, although not at the top levels.
- Progression of mitral regurgitation in horses with moderate VSDs usually is slow. These horses have normal life expectancy, but usually perform successfully only at lower levels of athletic competition.
- Horses with large VSDs (>4 cm) that are hemodynamically significant (peak flow velocity, ≤ 3 m/sec) have a guarded prognosis, because they usually have shortened performance and life expectancy.
- Affected horses with congestive heart failure and mitral regurgitation have a guarded to grave prognosis for life. Most affected horses being treated for congestive heart failure respond to supportive therapy and transiently improve, but once congestive heart failure develops, euthanasia of the horse is recommended.

MISCELLANEOUS

ASSOCIATED CONDITIONS

- Aortic regurgitation can develop in horses with VSDs and aortic valve prolapse. The aortic valve lacks the support normally provided by the interventricular septum and prolapses into the defect, resulting in aortic regurgitation.
- Mitral regurgitation can develop in horses with significant left atrial and ventricular volume overload secondary to stretching of the mitral annulus, further contributing to left atrial and ventricular volume overload.

AGE-RELATED FACTORS

Young horses are more likely to be diagnosed.

ZOONOTIC POTENTIAL

N/A

PREGNANCY

Do not breed affected horses because of the possibly heritable nature of these defects.

SYNONYMS

Septal defect

SEE ALSO

- Congestive heart failure—left sided
- Systolic murmurs

ABBREVIATIONS

- AV = atrioventricular
- PMI = point of maximal intensity

Suggested Reading

Pipers FS, Reef V, Wilson J. Echocardiographic detection of ventricular septal defects in large animals. J Am Vet Med Assoc 1985;187:810–816.

Reef VB. Cardiovascular ultrasonography. In: Reef VB, ed. Equine diagnostic ultrasound. Philadelphia: WB Saunders, 1998:215–272.

Reef VB. Echocardiographic evaluation of ventricular septal defects in horses. Equine Vet J 1995;19(Suppl):86–95.

Reef VB. Echocardiographic findings in horses with congenital cardiac disease. Compend Contin Educ Pract Vet 1991;13:109–117.

Reef VB. Heart murmurs in horses: determining their significance with echocardiography. Equine Vet J 1995;19(Suppl):71–80.

Author Virginia B. Reef
Consulting Editors N/A

VERMINOUS MENINGOENCEPHALOMYELITIS

BASICS

DEFINITION
Meningoencephalomyelitis associated with, most often, aberrant migration of parasitic organisms of other organ systems

PATHOPHYSIOLOGY
- Aberrant migration of parasitic organisms of other organ systems
- Also speculated that disintegration of a verminous thrombus can result in an embolic shower associated with infarction.

SYSTEMS AFFECTED
CNS and other specific tissues associated with the more common parasitic migration pattern

SIGNALMENT
Not specific

SIGNS
- Historical and physical examination signs are associated with the migratory pattern in each specific case.
- Signs often progress with further migration and inflammation.
- Any CNS defect(s) can occur.
- Suspect verminous involvement in any case of acute CNS disease without history of trauma or intracarotid injection.

CAUSES
Many parasites have been implicated and identified—*Strongylus vulgaris, Micronema deletrix, Hypoderma* sp., *Setaria* sp., and others

RISK FACTORS
Horses under good deworming management schemes

DIAGNOSIS

DIFFERENTIAL DIAGNOSIS
Any CNS dysfunction

CBC/BIOCHEMISTRY/URINALYSIS
No specific findings

OTHER LABORATORY TESTS
N/A

IMAGING
N/A

DIAGNOSTIC PROCEDURES
- Most commonly, the diagnosis is established histopathologically based on necropsy specimens.
- Any number of eosinophils in cerebral spinal fluid is highly suggestive, but inflammatory or hemorrhagic cytologic findings are more common—xanthochromia; elevated protein concentration; RBCs

PATHOLOGIC FINDINGS
Parasitic lesions with typical eosinophilic and other inflammatory infiltrates

TREATMENT
N/A

MEDICATIONS

DRUGS OF CHOICE
- Anti-inflammatory therapy may be useful—flunixin meglumine (1.1 mg/kg q12–24h); dexamethasone (0.05–0.1 mg/kg q6–24h)
- Administer suggested larvicidal doses of antiparasitic drugs.
- Treat suspect horses with fenbendazole (60 mg/kg, given once).
- Avermectins may be useful.

VERMINOUS MENINGOENCEPHALOMYELITIS

CONTRAINDICATIONS

Avermectins:

- Avermectins function by GABA inhibition, which may be a safety and efficacy concern.
- The concern is distribution of these drugs across the blood–brain barrier and CNS GABA inhibition.
- For these drugs to be larvicidal in the CNS, they must reach concentrations that induce GABA inhibition in the CNS.

PRECAUTIONS

N/A

POSSIBLE INTERACTIONS

N/A

ALTERNATIVE DRUGS

N/A

FOLLOW-UP

PATIENT MONITORING

As needed in patient support

POSSIBLE COMPLICATIONS

Trauma associated with the neurologic deficits

MISCELLANEOUS

ASSOCIATED CONDITIONS

N/A

AGE-RELATED FACTORS

N/A

ZOONOTIC POTENTIAL

N/A

PREGNANCY

N/A

SYNONYMS

N/A

ABBREVIATIONS

GABA = γ-aminobutyric acid

Suggested Reading

Lester G. Parasitic encephalomyelitis in horses. Compend Contin Educ Pract Vet 1992;14:1624–1630.

Author Joseph J. Bertone
Consulting Editor Joseph J. Bertone

VESICULAR STOMATITIS

BASICS

OVERVIEW

Vesicular stomatitis—an acute, highly contagious viral disease of horses, sheep, cattle, swine, goats, camelids, wildlife, and humans—is caused by a Lyssavirus in the family of Rhabdoviridae, causing ulceration of the mucous membranes and mucocutaneous junctions of the dermis.

SIGNALMENT

Any age, sex, or breed of animal can be affected.

SIGNS

- Vesicles and/or ulcers on the oral cavity, coronary bands, and, less commonly, on the teats, external genitalia, and udders of horses
- Fever is rarely documented, and if found is seen only in the initial phase of the disease
- Salivation
- Anorexia
- Weight loss
- Lameness secondary to coronitis
- Laminitis and sloughing of the hoof may occur rarely, secondary to the coronitis
- Ulcers may also be present in the nasal turbinates or nasopharynx
- Epistaxis
- Nasal edema
- Laryngitis and/or pharyngitis

CAUSES AND RISK FACTORS

Because the mode of transmission is not known, risk factors cannot be definitively identified. High morbidity has been noted in animals grazing in wooded pastures in the summer and fall; thus, virus-infected insects and plants may be a reservoir of the virus.

DIAGNOSIS

DIFFERENTIAL DIAGNOSIS

- Bullous pemphigoid—this disease can be differentiated by histologic examination of the skin and course of disease; only one animal will be affected and horse will not recover within 2 weeks.
- Candidiasis can be differentiated by histologic examination of the skin.
- Non-steroidal anti-inflammatory drug toxicosis can be differentiated by physical examination; ulcerations are within the oral cavity, not at the mucocutanous junction, and no other mucous membranes or areas of skin are affected.
- Blister beetle toxicosis is usually accompanied by dark urine.
- Oral ulcers secondary to organophosphate paste dewormer administration can be differentiated by a detailed history, and ulcerations are found only within the oral cavity.

CBC/BIOCHEMISTRY/URINALYSIS

CBC and biochemistry results are often normal, although a stress leukogram may be present. If patient is anorexic or dysphagic, then electrolyte abnormalities and dehydration with hemoconcentration may be present.

OTHER LABORATORY TESTS

The ideal diagnostic test is virus isolation from saliva, fluid obtained from a recently ruptured vesicle, or epithelial tissue. Other diagnostic tests available are virus isolation from tissue culture, electron microscopy, fluorescent antibody tests on serum or tissues, and virus neutralization.

IMAGING

N/A

DIAGNOSTIC PROCEDURES

Biopsy and histologic examination of the skin, including an intact vesicle or recently ruptured vesicle, may be useful in differentiating between other immune-mediated bacterial and fungal skin diseases. A sample can also be submitted for virus isolation.

PATHOLOGIC FINDINGS

Biopsy of recently ruptured vesicles or lesions show non-specific neutrophilic dermatitis, edema, epidermal necrosis, and reticular degeneration.

TREATMENT

Supportive care, such as soft mashes for feed or nasogastric feedings if oral ulcerations are causing reluctance to swallow, are suggested. Analgesics and corrective shoeing may be necessary for severe coronitis, which may lead to laminitis or hoof deformities. Antiseptic mouth rinses, such as iodine or potassium permanganate, may be helpful.

VESICULAR STOMATITIS

MEDICATIONS

Recent studies suggest recombinant equine interferon-beta-1 given at a dose of 0.3–1.0 μg/kg IM every 2 days may be useful as a prophylactic treatment for animals at high risk, or animals showing the initial signs of the disease. Oral or intravenous phenylbutazone or flunixin meglumine may be indicated if coronitis is severely painful.

FOLLOW-UP

EXPECTED COURSE AND PROGNOSIS

Vesicular stomatitis is a self-limiting disease. Ulcers heal in 1–5 weeks; however, hoof deformities may need attention for several months or years. Depigmentation of the skin may occur where ulceration had been present. Prognosis is good unless there was severe laminitis. Immunity to re-infection is, at most, 6 months in duration, and there is no effective cross-protection between the different strains of virus, of which there are at least two.

EPIDEMIOLOGY/PREVENTION

Reports of vesicular stomatitis range from northern South America and extend through Central America to southern North America. It is endemic is certain areas of Peru, Ecuador, Colombia, Venezuela, Central America, Mexico, and the southeastern United States. The virus is transmitted from animal to animal via aerosol and secretions, but is not absorbed through intact skin, only through wounds and mucous membranes. Affected animals are highly infectious for the first 48–72 hr that clinical signs are present and should be isolated from all other livestock. All communal drinking and eating areas should be cleaned and insect elimination measures should be undertaken. A vaccine was developed for use in horses during the 1995 outbreak, but its efficacy is unknown.

COMPLICATIONS

- Laminitis
- Gastrointestinal impaction secondary to dehydration and anorexia

MISCELLANEOUS

ZOONOTIC POTENTIAL

Because vesicular stomatitis is transmissible to humans, protective face shields, eyewear, and gloves should be worn when treating these animals. In humans, vesicular stomatitis is characterized by an influenza-like illness, with rarely any vesicle or ulcer development of the skin or mucous membranes.

Public Health

Vesicular stomatitis is a reportable disease in the United States due to its identical clinical appearance to hoof and mouth disease in ruminants.

PREGNANCY

No known effects on pregnancy are documented.

Suggested Reading

Green SL. Vesicular stomatitis in the horse. Vet Clin North Am Eq Pract 1993;9(2):349-353.

Scott DW. Viral diseases. In Scott DW: Large animal dermatology. Philadelphia: WB Saunders, 1988.

Marquardt J, Marquardt G, Deegan E. Therapeutic indications of recombinant equine interferon-beta1. Eq Pract 1996;18(8):15-17.

Bridges VE, McCluskey BJ, Salman MD, Hurd HS, Dick J. Review of 1995 vesicular stomatitis outbreak in the western United States. J Am Vet Med Assoc 1997;211(5):556-560.

Author Brett Dolente
Editor Corinne R. Sweeney

VICIA VILLOSA (HAIRY VETCH) TOXICOSIS

BASICS

OVERVIEW
- A systemic granulomatous disease described in horses grazing green *Vicia villosa* (hairy vetch) and hypothesized to result from an unknown immunogen
- Other *Vicia* spp. (e.g., *V. dasycarpa, V. benghelensis*) also have been implicated.
- *Vicia* spp. are legumes found throughout temperate regions of the U.S. and used as pasturage, hay, and silage
- No reports of disease in animals fed hay or silage
- Low morbidity

SIGNALMENT
No reported breed, age, or sex predispositions

SIGNS
- Listlessness
- Welts on the skin
- Alopecia
- Dermatitis
- Skin peeling around the nares
- Lymphadenomegaly
- Dependent-limb edema
- Low-grade, persistent fever
- Wasting
- Diarrhea

CAUSES AND RISK FACTORS
- The specific phytochemical responsible is unknown.
- The condition is hypothesized to be a type IV hypersensitivity reaction.
- Associated with ingestion of the green plant.
- Outbreaks are more common at the peak of plant growth during the spring.
- Not all individuals grazing hairy vetch are affected, so unknown factors (e.g., growth stage of plant, dietary or environmental factors, individual susceptibility) may be involved.

DIAGNOSIS

DIFFERENTIAL DIAGNOSIS
- Systemic granulomatous disease caused by other unidentified causes—no known exposure to *Vicia* spp.
- Dermatophytosis—negative fungal cultures
- Bacterial dermatitis—negative cultures for dermatopathogens
- Pemphigus foliaceus—skin biopsy
- Drug eruption—history of recent drug administration
- Chronic urticaria—skin lesions pit with pressure.

CBC/BIOCHEMISTRY/URINALYSIS
- Lymphocytosis
- Hyperproteinemia

OTHER LABORATORY TESTS
N/A

IMAGING
N/A

DIAGNOSTIC PROCEDURES
Skin biopsy

PATHOLOGIC FINDINGS

Gross Findings
- Thickened skin with scaling and alopecia
- Paleness of organs—heart, kidney, adrenal and lymphoid tissues
- Lymphadenomegaly

Histopathologic Findings
- Cellular infiltrations of monocytes, lymphocytes, plasma cells, eosinophils and multinucleated giant cells in multiple organs
- Lesions are especially prominent perivascularly.

VICIA VILLOSA (HAIRY VETCH) TOXICOSIS

TREATMENT

- Generally unrewarding
- Anti-inflammatories

MEDICATIONS

DRUGS

Glucocorticoids—prednisone or prednisolone (2.2–4.4 mg/kg) or dexamethasone (0.1–0.2 mg/kg PO SID)

CONTRAINDICATIONS/POSSIBLE INTERACTIONS

N/A

FOLLOW-UP

PATIENT MONITORING

N/A

PREVENTION/AVOIDANCE

Avoid reintroduction to pastures containing *Vicia* spp.

POSSIBLE COMPLICATIONS

N/A

EXPECTED COURSE AND PROGNOSIS

Mortality is high in affected animals.

MISCELLANEOUS

ASSOCIATED CONDITIONS

N/A

AGE-RELATED FACTORS

N/A

ZOONOTIC POTENTIAL

N/A

PREGNANCY

N/A

SEE ALSO

N/A

Suggested Reading

Woods LW, Johnson B, Hietala SK, Galey FD, Gillen D. Systemic granulomatous disease in a horse grazing pasture containing hairy vetch (*Vicia* sp.). J Vet Diagn Invest 1992;4:356–360.

Author Robert H. Poppenga
Consulting Editor Robert H. Poppenga

VIRAL ARTERITIS

BASICS

DEFINITION

Equine viral arteritis (EVA) is a disease characterized by panvasculitis leading to edema, hemorrhage, and abortion in mares; respiratory disease and edema in other adults; and severe illness or death in the neonate.

PATHOPHYSIOLOGY

EVA is an arterivirus. It is a small, enveloped, positive-stranded RNA virus. The virion is resistant to freezing, drying, and long storage at −70° C, although it is reliably destroyed by a 1:32 dilution of commercially available sodium hypoclorite solution. Virus can be isolated from the urine for up to 3 weeks postinfection. There is only one recognized serotype of EVA, the Bucyrus strain, although there is evidence of antigenic variation among different isolates and variation in the degree of clinical signs produced by various isolates.

Infection with EVA can occur in horses of any age or use due to its highly contagious nature and its spread by direct contact with infected horses and their body secretions, including urine and milk. The disease classically has high morbidity and low mortality in adults. The mortality in known infected neonates is much greater than previously suspected. The incidence of infection, determined by seroconversion, varies considerably by population and geographic location. The chief mode of transmission among racehorse populations appears to be through nasal droplet spray. Transmission at breeding farms is generally via the venereal route.

The carrier of the virus is the intact male. Seronegative mares bred to either short- or long-term carrier stallions, shedding the virus in their semen, serve as a primary source of virus spread. Carrier stallions harbor the virus in their accessory sex glands, and the carrier-state is testosterone dependent. Virus may be present in frozen or cooled semen from carrier stallions.

Seropositive mares bred to a carrier stallion may also shed virus for a short period of time. Abortion due to EVA infection is thought to occur secondary to myometrial necrosis and edema, resulting in failure to the uteroplacental unit, although there is evidence of direct infection of the placenta.

Foals born to seropositive dams acquire passive immunity through the colostrum and become seronegative after passive immunity wanes. Foals may also acquire the virus through colostrum and milk; at least two foals are thought to have acquired a fatal form of the disease in this manner.

Experimental innoculation of animals by nasal challenge have shown that the virus first replicates within bronchoalveolar macrophages of the lung and then appears in the bronchial lymph nodes. The virus is then spread throughout the body via the circulation. Vascular lesions develop associated with virus present in tunica media myocytes and within the endothelium. Arterial damage may persist for weeks after infection. The kidney is a site of virus localization, as is the placenta, bronchiolar epithelium, thymic tissue, and enterocytes in foals.

SYSTEMS AFFECTED

- Whole body, excepting CNS.
- Predominant systems affected by age group: respiratory system in young horses, respiratory system in foals, and urogenital system in pregnant broodmares and intact males.

GENETICS

N/A

SIGNALMENT

- Horses of any age or breed can develop EVA, although Standardbreds have the highest seroconversion rates in United States.
- Foals in the immediate perinatal period, young horses in race training, and broodmares at farms with a carrier stallion have the highest rates of incidence.

SIGNS

General Comments

EVA infection can present a wide range of signs, from clinically silent and recognizable only by seroconversion to acute-onset severe disease resulting in abortion and neonatal death.

Historical Findings

- In the case of abortion and neonatal death, the history will include possible exposure by residing on a farm where a carrier stallion is present.
- There may also be history of a seronegative mare returning to the farm after being bred by a carrier stallion.
- Young horses in training may have history of being associated with an outbreak of respiratory disease ranging from mild to severe.
- Neonates born to seronegative mares or that have failure of passive transfer of maternal antibody when born to seropositive mares seem to be at greatest risk.

Physical Examination Findings

- Young adults and broodmares that develop clinical signs typically are febrile for 5–9 days.
- Distal limb edema, particularly of the hindlimbs, may be present, as may edema in other sites, including the conjunctiva, periorbital region, scrotum, and prepuce.
- Epiphora and nasal discharge associated with rhinitis and conjunctivitis may be observed.
- An urticarial skin rash may be present.
- Cough, lethargy, anorexia, lameness, and exercise intolerance have been reported during outbreaks.
- Abortion and stillbirth are seen in pregnant mares.
- Sudden death, although rarely reported in adults, may occur with particularly virulent isolates.
- Foals may be born normal or weak, and may also have edema and lethargy. They may present with sudden death or go through a period resembling hypoxic ischemic asphyxia syndrome before progressing to respiratory failure and death, although foals with EVA perinatal infection have been known to survive for more than 2 weeks prior to death.

DIAGNOSIS

DIFFERENTIAL DIAGNOSIS

In young adults, differential diagnoses for EVA include all other infectious causes of respiratory disease, including but not limited to:

- Equine influenza
- Equine herpes-virus, types 1 and 4
- Equine rhinovirus
- Equine infectious anemia
- Equine adenovirus
- Morbillivirus

Differentials for edema due to vasculitis include:

- Equine infectious anemia
- Equine erlichiosis
- Purpura hemorrhagica

The primary differential in an abortion storm is equine herpes-virus type 1. Differentials for affected neonates include:

- Equine herpes-virus type 1
- Bacterial sepsis
- Hypoxic ischemic asphyxial insult

CBC/BIOCHEMISTRY/URINALYSIS

- CBC may demonstrate lymphopenia and thrombocytopenia, although these are variable and non-specific findings.
- Serum biochemistry analysis is non-diagnositic.
- Urinalysis may reveal renal tubular inflammation with or without casts.

OTHER LABORATORY TESTS

Virus Isolation

Can be diagnostic antemortem. Acute cases have positive virus isolation from nasopharyngeal swabs or buffy coats from EDTA or citrated whole blood samples. Virus can be isolated from the urine in more chronic cases. EVA is isolated from the placenta or fetal tissues in the case of abortion, although maternal blood and urine may also be submitted.

VIRAL ARTERITIS

Serology

Complement fixation (CF) and virus neutralization (VN) tests can be used. CF is best in acute cases and will show a rise in titer 2–4 weeks after infection. This titer becomes undetectable after about 8 months. VN titers develop along with CF titers, peak at 2–4 months, and remain increased for years.

DIAGNOSTIC PROCEDURES

Immunohistochemistry

Immunoperoxidase histochemistry performed on post-mortem or biopsy tissues can provide an accurate diagnosis in cases where EVA is supected but has not been confirmed or as an adjunct to virus isolation and serology.

PATHOLOGIC FINDINGS

- Aborted and stillborn fetuses seldom have gross or histologic lesions, although EVA antigen may be identified in the fetus and/or placenta by immunoperoxidase histochemistry.
- Adults and foals that die of fulminant EVA infection have a broncho-interstitial pneumonia. The lungs are heavy, wet, and congested grossly. The pneumonia is characterized by hypertrophy and hyperplasia of type II pneumocytes and the presence of eosinophilic laminar to granular material scattered within the alveolar lumen. Histologically, the pneumonia may appear similar to morbillivirus infection in adults. Lymphocytic arteritis and periarteritis with varying degrees of tunica media fibrinoid necrosis may also be observed.
- Some infected foals are also reported to have pronounced gastointestinal lesions.
- Renal tubular epithelial necrosis and interstitial nephritis is present in most chronic cases.
- Areas of edema are characterized by a lymphocytic vasculitis and perivasculitis.

IMAGING

Thoracic Radiographs

Increased bronchiolar and interstitial pattern with areas of consolidation.

TREATMENT

APPROPRIATE HEALTH CARE

- Most horses with clinical disease recover with only supportive care. Horses may be best managed at home.
- In the case of an outbreak, all affected horses should be kept isolated for a period of 40 days following the appearance of the last case.
- Affected neonates need intensive medical management and should be hospitalized, although kept isolated from the rest of the hospital population, particularly pregnant mares.

NURSING CARE

- Nursing care is minimal for adults.
- Animals should be encouraged to eat and have stalls with good ventilation.
- Hydrotherapy and support wraps may benefit those patients with distal limb edema.
- Affected foals require intensive nursing, including intravenous fluid administration, frequent turning, feeding by nasogastric tube or by intravenous total parenteral nutrition, and respiratory management, up to and including assisted ventilation.

ACTIVITY

- Activity should be minimal.
- Racehorses should be out of training until they are no longer shedding virus, a period of about 40 days.
- Handwalking is permissible, and may benefit those with edema, but contact with other horses should be minimal while the horse continues to shed virus.
- Acutely affected colts and stallions should have a prolonged period of sexual rest to decrease their chance of being chronic carriers.
- Affected foals are incapable of activity.

DIET

No dietary changes are required.

CLIENT EDUCATION

- Owners of affected foals should be informed of the poor prognosis for survival.
- Owners of affected colts and stallions should be informed of the risk of their horse becoming a carrier.
- All owners should be informed of the potential economic implications of seroconversion to EVA regarding import and export.

SURGICAL CONSIDERATIONS

N/A

MEDICATIONS

DRUG(S) OF CHOICE

- There is no specific treatment for EVA.
- Non-steroidal antiinflammatory drugs may be used to treat fever in adults.
- Affected neonates may be treated with broad-spectrum anti-microbial drugs to combat secondary bacterial infection. Anecdotally, treatment of foals with plasma harvested from a donor with high EVA titers has been attempted.

CONTRAINDICATIONS/PRECAUTIONS/ POSSIBLE INTERACTIONS/ ALTERNATIVE DRUGS

N/A

FOLLOW-UP

PATIENT MONITORING

Patients should be monitored for continued fever and potential secondary bacterial invaders.

CLIENT EDUCATION

It is important that clients be educated regarding control of EVA. Many states have regulations surrounding the use of EVA carrier stallion, notably New York and Kentucky. These programs have significant decreased the incidence of the disease in those states.

PREVENTION/AVOIDANCE

- Vaccination against EVA is available, but is tightly controlled in some states. It is a modified-live vaccine and control programs usually involve vaccination of all non-carrier stallions and seronegative mares served by carrier stallions. Carrier stallions are evaluated periodically by breeding to seronegative mares and performing virus isolation on semen samples.
- Although international rules are loosening, seroconversion of a horse may result in problems regarding import and export to certain countries.

MISCELLANEOUS

ABBREVIATIONS

- CF = complement fixation
- VN = virus neutralization

Suggested Reading

Del Piero F, Wilkins PA, Lopez JW, et al. Equine viral arteritis in newborn foals: clinical, pathological, serological, microbiological and immunohistochemical observations. Equine Vet J, 1997; 29(3):178-185.

Doll ER, Knappenberger RE, Bryans JT. An outbreak of abortion caused by the equine arteritis virus. Cornell Vet, 1957;47:69-75.

McCollum WH, Swerczek TW. Studies on an epizootic of equine viral arteritis in racehorses. Equine Vet J, 1978;2:293-297.

McKenzie J. Equine viral arteritis and trade in horses from the USA. Surveillance, 1990;16:17.

Timoney PJ, McCollum WH. Equine viral arteritis. Vet Clin North Am Equine Pract, 1993;9(2):295-309.

Author Pamela A. Wilkins

Consulting Editor Corinne R. Sweeney

VISION

BASICS

OVERVIEW

The equine eye has developed a number of unique anatomic and physiologic features to suit its special visual needs. Adaptive influences include the horse's role as a prey species, its grazing habits, and the need for arrythmic (diurnal and nocturnal) activity. Important adaptations to avoid predators are a large visual field and an improved detection of motion. However, these adaptations limit the ability to detect fine visual detail.

The horse has a wide total visual field of about 350° due to the extreme lateral globe position, the nasal extension of the retina, and the horizontal shape of the pupil. It has narrow blind spots immediately anterior to the nose and posterior to the tail. A small frontal binocular field of 65–70° develops postnatally. Binocular depth thresholds are comparable to cats and indicate that horses possess stereopsis. Horses are also capable of utilizing monocular depth cues in judging distance.

The horse has 0.6 times the acuity of humans, 1.5 times that of dogs, and 3 times that of cats. That would mean a Snellen acuity of 20/33 (i.e., a horse viewing an object at a distance of 20 feet has approximately the visual acuity of a person viewing the object at 33 feet).

Horses have minimal refractive errors ranging from +3D to −3D. The aphakic equine globe is +9.9D hyperopic. In spite of that, aphakic horses after cataract surgery seem to have relatively normal functional vision. This suggests that horses have a retinal ganglion cell receptor field size several times larger than humans, and means that the enlarged blurred retinal image in the aphakic equine eye could still fall within the retinal ganglion cell receptor field of the horse and not cause significant loss of visual acuity.

The retina of the horse contains both rod and cone photoreceptors, with rods outnumbering cones. Rods are most sensitive to dim light and are useful for motion detection. Cones are most sensitive to bright light, are responsible for color vision, and provide good visual resolution.

Cone density in the retina of the horse is highest in the area centralis, which provides the area of maximal visual acuity. The equine area centralis is divided into two areas: (1) area centralis rotunda—a small, circular region temporal and dorsal to the optic disc, and (2) the visual streak—a horizontal, narrow band above the optic nerve. Changes in head orientation, dynamic accommodation, and the presence of the area centralis aid near vision in horses.

Measurements of equine spectral sensitivity have shown a primary peak at 550 nm (greenish yellow), with a second peak at the far blue end of the color spectrum. The horse thus sees blue and yellow color, but may not see red. The fibrous tapetum of the dorsal fundus enhances night vision but might, by scattering of light, degrade photoreceptor image resolution.

The optic nerve of the horse is unique in that it contains a substantial proportion of axons of large diameter. Large retinal ganglion cells possess large diameter axons and are involved in motion detection, stereopsis, and sensitivity to dim light, suggesting that the horse has strong retinal adaptions for these visual characteristics.

VISION

The equine eye also shows diurnal adaptations, such as the corpora nigra (protects the ventral retina during grazing), occludable pupils, and yellow pigment in the lens (limits transmittance of very short wavelengths, which help protect the photoreceptors in the retina).

SYSTEMS AFFECTED

Ophthalmology.

SIGNALMENT

N/A

SIGNS

N/A

CAUSES AND RISK FACTORS

N/A

DIAGNOSIS

DIFFERENTIAL DIAGNOSIS

N/A

CBC/BIOCHEMISTRY/URINALYSIS

N/A

OTHER LABORATORY TESTS

N/A

IMAGING

N/A

DIAGNOSTIC PROCEDURES

N/A

TREATMENT

N/A

MEDICATIONS

N/A

DRUGS

N/A

CONTRAINDICATIONS/POSSIBLE INTERACTIONS

N/A

FOLLOW-UP

N/A

MISCELLANEOUS

ABBREVIATION

- D = Diopter

Suggested Reading

Veterinary Clinics of North America: Equine Practice, Vol 8, no 3 Dec. pp 451-457, 1992.

Author Maria Källberg
Consulting Editor Dennis E. Brooks

VITAMIN K_3 (MENADIONE) TOXICOSIS

BASICS

OVERVIEW

- Toxicosis associated with empiric use of parenteral vitamin K_3 (i.e., menadione) solutions to prevent epistaxis in race horses or to treat hemorrhage of unknown cause.
- Toxic doses have ranged from 0.5–11 mg/kg.
- Intoxication results from an unknown pathophysiologic mechanism.
- Menadione is an oxidative toxicant capable of causing methemoglobinemia, Heinz bodies, and hemolytic anemia in some species or in vitro.
- Hemoglobinuria has not been noted in most reported equine cases of menadione toxicosis; more likely, menadione or its metabolites are direct, renal tubular toxicants.

SIGNALMENT

- No known breed, age, or sex predilections
- Race horses prone to epistaxis or horses with hemorrhage of unknown cause

SIGNS

- Renal colic within 48 hours of parenteral use of vitamin K_3.
- Signs include arching of the back, backing into a corner of stall and rubbing of the perineum, and abdominal pain manifested by frequent lying down, rising, and viewing of flanks; rolling usually is not a feature.
- Other signs include depression, anorexia, stranguria, and hematuria.
- A mild to moderately enlarged, soft left kidney may be palpated on rectal examination.
- Fever frequently is present.
- Onset time is dose dependent, ranging from 4–48 hours after parenteral administration.
- May progress to chronic renal failure in animals surviving the acute syndrome.

CAUSES AND RISK FACTORS

- Inappropriate use of vitamin K_3—vitamin K_3 should not be used in horses; vitamin K_1 is preferred.
- Oral vitamin K preparations may be safer alternatives.

DIAGNOSIS

DIFFERENTIAL DIAGNOSIS

- Cantharidin toxicosis—detection of beetles in hay; detection of cantharidin in urine
- Red-maple toxicosis—history of ingestion; hemolytic anemia
- Aminoglycoside toxicosis—history of administration
- NSAIDs—history of administration; detection in plasma or urine samples
- Amyloidosis—biopsy
- Immune-mediated glomerulonephritis—urinalysis, serum chemistries, ultrasonography, and biopsy

CBC/BIOCHEMISTRY/URINALYSIS

- Altered serum indices—azotemia, hypercreatinemia, hyponatremia, hypochloremia, hyperkalemia, and hypercalcemia
- Altered urine indices—proteinuria, hematuria, isosthenuria, and multiple casts

OTHER LABORATORY TESTS

Elevated GGT:Cr ratio in urine specimen

IMAGING

Enlarged kidneys on ultrasonography

DIAGNOSTIC PROCEDURES

Kidney biopsy

PATHOLOGIC FINDINGS

- Enlarged and pale kidneys that bulge when sectioned
- Renal tubular nephrosis with dilated tubules containing proteinaceous, cellular debris and granular casts
- More chronic cases may have smaller kidneys with adherent capsules and histologic evidence of interstitial fibrosis and lymphocytic infiltrates

TREATMENT

- Manage acute renal disease with fluid therapy to replace volume deficits and to correct electrolyte abnormalities.
- Provide additional caloric support for anorexic patients.

VITAMIN K_3 (MENADIONE) TOXICOSIS

MEDICATIONS

DRUGS

- Isotonic saline (40–80 mL/kg per day until serum Cr is decreased, then 12–20 mL/kg per day)
- Furosemide (1 mg/kg q2h up to three doses) to promote diuresis if isotonic saline does not.
- Caloric supplementation with IV dextrose or PO gruel
- Multiple B vitamins administered IV may stimulate appetite.

CONTRAINDICATIONS/POSSIBLE INTERACTIONS

N/A

FOLLOW-UP

PATIENT MONITORING

- Monitor renal function.
- Monitor horses surviving the acute syndrome for reappearance of azotemia, hypercreatinemia, and isosthenuria.

PREVENTION/AVOIDANCE

Do not use vitamin K_3 in horses.

POSSIBLE COMPLICATIONS

Acute laminitis and DIC have been seen as terminal consequences of the acute renal syndrome.

EXPECTED COURSE AND PROGNOSIS

N/A

MISCELLANEOUS

ASSOCIATED CONDITIONS

N/A

AGE-RELATED FACTORS

N/A

ZOONOTIC POTENTIAL

N/A

PREGNANCY

N/A

SEE ALSO

- Aminoglycosides
- Renal failure, acute

ABBREVATIONS

- Cr = creatinine
- DIC = disseminated intravascular coagulopathy
- GGT = γ-glutamyltransferase

Suggested Reading

Maxie G, van Dreumel T, McMaster D, et al. Menadione (vitamin K_3) toxicity in six horses. Can Vet J 1992;33:756–757.

Author Dennis J. Blodgett
Consulting Editor Robert H. Poppenga

VULVAR CONFORMATION (VC)

BASICS

DEFINITION

• The quality/grade of VC is determined by the anatomic orientation of the anal sphincter to the vulvae and pubis. This orientation impacts directly on the mare's reproductive health and affects her ability to maintain a healthy uterus and to carry pregnancies to term.
• Good VC implies the dorsal commissure of the vulva is at or below the level of the pubis. This generally is coupled with vulvae that exhibit an effective side-to-side seal and are not slanted cranially, effectively protecting the genital tract from fecal contamination or aspiration of air.
• Fair VC implies the dorsal vulvar commissure is elevated above the floor of the pubis and/or the vulvae slope anteriorly, permitting pneumovagina or fecal contamination of the vestibule.
• Poor VC implies the dorsal vulvar commissure is elevated above the pubis. This usually is accompanied by an obvious anterior slant of the vulvae. Fecal contamination of the vestibule occurs frequently to continually.
• Problems with VC account for a major portion of equine infertility.

PATHOPHYSIOLOGY

Factors predisposing mares to poor VC—breeds/individuals with less muscle in the perineal area; perineal lacerations; being underweight

SYSTEM AFFECTED

Reproductive

GENETICS

• Influences vulvar conformation (mother/daughter) and should be considered when selecting broodmares. This is particularly important if farm-born fillies are to be the source of replacement stock.
• Mares with good VC have fewer reproductive problems.

INCIDENCE/PREVALENCE

• Abnormal VC is extremely common, especially in some breeds—Thoroughbreds; Standardbreds
• More muscular breeds or certain families within breeds have less of a problem with less-than-ideal VC.

SIGNALMENT

• Compromises of VC can occur in all breeds and in any stock of breeding age.
• Incidence of poor VC increases in old, pluriparous mares.

SIGNS

General Comments

• The condition is fairly easy to evaluate. Assessment of each broodmare's VC should be noted on her record at the start of each breeding season.
• Can worsen with age.

Historical Findings

• History of infertility because of failure to conceive or termination of pregnancy
• In addition to endometritis, vaginitis or cervicitis may be present.

Physical Examination Findings

• Less than ideal VC may result in gross/histopathologic changes of the tubular genital tract.
• Transrectal palpation—enlargement of uterine horns, intraluminal fluid accumulation, and aspiration of air (e.g., pneumovagina, pneumouterus); if severe, echogenicities identified at ultrasonography may be caused by fecal aspiration into the uterus.
• Vaginal examination using sterile lubricant and sterile vaginal speculum may reveal inflammation, discharge (e.g., endometritis, cervicitis, vaginitis), urine pooling, and/or adhesions (if chronic).
• Other physical parameters usually are normal.

CAUSES

• Inherited poor VC
• Perineal laceration resulting from abnormal posture or fetal position at parturition
• Fetal extremities pushed dorsally, causing the fetus' feet to tear into the wall of the vagina or vestibule

RISK FACTORS

• No specific risk factors other than pregnancy
• Posterior presentation of a fetus might be linked with an increased incidence of perineal lacerations, but this has not been reported.
• Fetal posture and position can change within minutes of birth, so previous examinations for fetal position and posture have little predictive value.

DIAGNOSIS

DIFFERENTIAL DIAGNOSIS

N/A

CBC/BIOCHEMISTRY/URINALYSIS

N/A

OTHER LABORATORY TESTS

N/A

IMAGING

N/A

DIAGNOSTIC PROCEDURES

• Careful palpation of the vestibule, vagina, and rectum to identify lacerations.
• Rectovaginal fistulas may be small and not readily identified but result in sufficient contamination of the uterus to affect fertility.

PATHOLOGIC FINDINGS

• Partial to full-thickness lacerations of the vestibule and/or vagina
• Aspiration of air into the vagina and/or uterus
• Fecal contamination of the vagina and vestibule, with resulting inflammation of the vestibule, vagina and cervix, and possibly, the endometrium

TREATMENT

APPROPRIATE HEALTH CARE

• Determine that a laceration does not extend into the perineal cavity—rare with perineal laceration or rectovaginal fistula.
• Systemic antibiotics seldom are indicated.
• Local medication also rarely is indicated.
• Repair lacerations before attempting rebreeding.
• Boost with a tetanus toxoid if status is not current or is unknown.

NURSING CARE

N/A

ACTIVITY

Normal activity, no restrictions

DIET

Normal; no restrictions

CLIENT EDUCATION

- Review importance of closely observing foaling.
- Many lacerations occur before a foaling problem is noticed, even with trained attendants.

SURGICAL CONSIDERATIONS

General Comments

- Lacerations are repaired only after the inflammatory reaction of the surrounding tissue has subsided.
- Feces must remain soft after surgery until healing is complete to minimize pressure applied to the repair site, which improves the likelihood of healing and lessens the incidence of dehiscence. This can be achieved early in the spring by placing the mare on pasture before surgery and returning her to pasture immediately after surgery.
- Bran and mineral oil have been used to soften stools but are not as good as green grass with its high moisture content.
- For additional details of these or alternative surgical approaches, see *Suggested Reading.*

Two-Stage Laceration Repair

- Begins with epidural anesthesia and sedation of the mare using agent of choice.
- The tail is wrapped, elevated over the mare, and attached to a support directly above.
- The rectum and vagina/vestibule are emptied of feces and thoroughly but gently cleaned. Minimize irritation that could result in straining after surgery.
- First-stage repair—reconstruction of the perineal body; make an incision into the perineal body ≅ 2–3 cm cranial to the extent of the existing laceration; continue the incision posteriorly along the sides of the existing laceration, in a plane approximating the original location of the perineal body; reflect the vestibular and vaginal mucosa are ventrally by ≅2 cm; use simple interrupted sutures to appose first the perineal body and then the submucosa of the vagina or vestibule; after placing of one or two interrupted sutures, begin a continuous pattern in the most cranial aspect of the reflected mucosal membrane to appose the submucosal surfaces; extend the continuous suture pattern caudally in concert with placement of additional simple interrupted sutures as described.
- Second-stage repair—completed after healing of the first stage; debride the anal sphincter, and suture this structure to re-establish sphincter tone, if possible.

One-Stage Laceration Repair

Similar to the two-stage repair, except that anal sphincter repair is accomplished at the same time as perineal body reconstruction.

MEDICATIONS

DRUGS OF CHOICE

- Systemic antibiotics may be indicated immediately after the laceration to prevent possible systemic involvement.
- The only other medications required would be those used during surgical correction.

CONTRAINDICATIONS

- Depends on the agent used for sedation.
- No specific contraindication of a medication because of this condition.

PRECAUTIONS

N/A

POSSIBLE INTERACTIONS

N/A

ALTERNATIVE DRUGS

Any agent designed for sedation or analgesia can be used during the surgical correction.

FOLLOW-UP

PATIENT MONITORING

- Immediately after a suspected laceration, evacuate feces, and examine the area.
- If a laceration is found, re-examine in ≅2 weeks to evaluate the damaged area for degree (i.e., decrease) of inflammation and presence of epithelial tissue granulation.

PREVENTION/AVOIDANCE

- Predicting which mares will suffer tears is difficult.
- The only sure way to prevent tears is to not breed a mare.

POSSIBLE COMPLICATIONS

- Abscess formation of the laceration is uncommon because of the wide surface area for drainage and granulation from the deeper layers outward.
- Attempting a repair immediately after a tear carries an increased possibility of abscess formation.

EXPECTED COURSE AND PROGNOSIS

- Without surgical correction, mares with third-degree perineal lacerations and recto-vaginal fistulas have a very low probability of conceiving and maintaining a pregnancy to term.
- Perform surgical repair before attempting to rebreed.

MISCELLANEOUS

ASSOCIATED CONDITIONS

N/A

AGE-RELATED FACTORS

N/A

ZOONOTIC POTENTIAL

N/A

PREGNANCY

Only occurs after gestation and parturition.

SYNONYMS

N/A

SEE ALSO

- Dystocia
- Pneumovagina
- Pneumouterus
- Perineal lacerations
- Rectovaginal fistulas

Suggested Reading

Aanes WA. Surgical repair of third degree perineal lacerations and recto-vaginal fistulas in the mare. J Am Vet Med Assoc 1964;144:485–491.

Colbern GT, Aanes WA, Stashak TS. Surgical management of perineal lacerations and recto-vestibular fistulae in the mare: a retrospective study of 47 cases. J Am Vet Med Assoc 1985;186:265–269.

Heinze CD, Allen AR. Repair of third-degree perineal lacerations in the mare. Vet Scope 1966;11:12–15.

Stickle RL, Fessler JF, Adams SB, et al. A single stage technique for repair of recto-vestibular lacerations in the mare. J Vet Surg 1979;8:25–27.

Roberts SJ: Veterinary obstetrics and genital diseases (theriogenology). 3rd ed. Woodstock, VT: published by the author, 1986:609–612.

Author Walter R. Threlfall

Consulting Editor Carla L. Carleton

WEST NILE VIRUS (WNV)

BASICS

OVERVIEW

• A seasonal and sometimes fatal disease of birds, horses, and humans, introduced to the United States through New York in 1999.
• Most infected horses are asymptomatic, but infection can present as a neurologic disease.
• WNV is carried and transmitted by mosquitoes.
• Wild birds are the principal host for WNV.
• The virus is amplified in the bird population through infected mosquitoes.
• Once the virus reaches high enough levels in the mosquito population, it may spill over into the equine population.
• WNV enters the body through the bite of an infected mosquito. It then multiplies and travels in the bloodstream. If it crosses the blood–brain barrier, it leads to meningo-encephalitis and, in some cases, death.
• Crows appear to be extremely susceptible to infection, with extremely high mortality rates.

SIGNALMENT

• Age of horses in the 1999 outbreak—range, 2–30 years; average, 14.5 years
• No breed or gender predilection
• Species affected—horses, humans, and birds; other species can have titers.

SIGNS

• Signs range from asymptomatic through stumbling, ataxia, down, and acute death.
• Nonspecific neurologic sign—no way to diagnose WNV solely based on clinical signs
• Fever tends not to be a presenting sign.
• Course of disease ranges from 24 hours to several weeks.
• Some horses also have tested positive for EPM.

CAUSES AND RISK FACTORS

• Cause—WNV is a member of the genus *Flavivirus*, family *Flaviviridae*; this family also includes St. Louis encephalitis.
• Risk factor—exposure to infected mosquitoes

DIAGNOSIS

DIFFERENTIAL DIAGNOSIS

• Other causes of equine neurologic disease
• EEE, WEE, and VEE
• Rabies
• EPM
• Equine herpes virus
• Poisoning—moldy corn; lead
• Brain abscess
• Equine degenerative myelopathy
• Aberrant strongyles migration
• Wobbler's syndrome
• Head trauma

CBC/BIOCHEMISTRY/URINALYSIS

• Typical of viral infection
• Serum—HI, ELISA, plaque-reduction neutralization (requires BSL-3 lab)
• Need paired serum samples—fourfold rise in titer indicates infection; interpret as with any other titer
• IgM titer is indicative of acute infection

OTHER LABORATORY TESTS

Brain—virus identification/isolation; PCR, Vero cell culture, or mouse inoculation (requires BSL-3 lab)

DIAGNOSTIC PROCEDURES

N/A

TREATMENT

• No specific treatment
• Supportive treatment based on presenting signs

MEDICATIONS

DRUGS

N/A

CONTRAINDICATIONS/POSSIBLE INTERACTIONS

N/A

WEST NILE VIRUS (WNV)

FOLLOW-UP

PREVENTION/AVOIDANCE

- No vaccine
- Control rests with minimization of mosquito-breeding sites. Mosquitoes that carry WNV breed in standing water; thus, eliminate mosquito habitat.
- Recommendations include eliminating containers that collect water; keeping watering devices, especially automatic waterers, clean; improving existing drainage; and maintaining basic sanitation.
- Potential collection sites include discarded tires, unwashed bird baths, clogged rain gutters and drainage ditches, stagnant water buckets and troughs, wheelbarrows, plastic wading pools, unused swimming pools, and any other receptacle that collects water.

EXPECTED COURSE AND PROGNOSIS

- In 1999, 9 of 25 horses that became ill on Long Island, NY, died or were euthanized. The rest recovered, and several more that did not become ill had positive WNV titers.
- Prognosis depends on presenting signs and subsequent course of disease. A mildly affected horse that does not worsen over the next several days has a relatively good prognosis. If a horse initially is only mildly affected but then significantly worsens or is found acutely down, the prognosis is very poor.

MISCELLANEOUS

ASSOCIATED CONDITIONS

N/A

AGE-RELATED FACTORS

N/A

ZOONOTIC POTENTIAL

- Humans are susceptible.
- Only infected mosquitoes can transmit the virus. Horses cannot transmit WNV to other horses or humans, and humans cannot transmit WNV to other humans or horses.
- Humans in areas with WNV-positive mosquitoes, birds, or horses should take measures to protect themselves from mosquitoes.

PREGNANCY

N/A

SEE ALSO

N/A

ABBREVIATIONS

- BSL =
- EEE = eastern encephalitides
- ELISA = enzyme-linked immunoadsorbent assay
- EPM =
- HI =
- PCR = polymerase chain reaction
- VEE = Venezuelan encephalitides
- WEE = western encephalitides

Suggested Reading

Crans WJ. West Nile virus. Power Point Presentation, 2000.

Trock SC. West Nile virus equine summary as of January 18, 2000. In: Proceedings of the West Nile Virus Action Workshop, Tarrytown, NY, January 2000:61.

Authors Jennifer Jacobs Fowler and Susan C. Trock

Consulting Editor Joseph J. Bertone

WHITE MUSCLE DISEASE (WMD)

BASICS

DEFINITION

- Myopathy reported in horses from <1 to $\cong$9 months of age and attributed to vitamin E and selenium deficiency
- Also known as nutritional myodegeneration and Zenker's necrosis.

PATHOPHYSIOLOGY

- GPX is a selenium-containing enzyme that, in concert with vitamin E, protects cells against damage associated with production of superoxide radicals and hydroxyl radicals.
- Superoxide and hydroxyl radicals disrupt cellular structure and function, disrupting cellular membranes and resulting in release of the lysosome contents.
- Loss of cell membrane integrity causes loss of cell osmotic regulation, resulting in cellular swelling and death.
- Damage to protein structure and function results in inactivation of certain enzymes and irreversible conversion of the activities of others.
- Damage to nucleic acids causes mutation and inhibits the ability of cells to reproduce.
- GPX and vitamin E work as endogenous antioxidants, GPX by reducing hydroperoxides to alcohols as part of the recycling of glutathione; GPX also acts within the erythrocyte to prevent formation of methemoglobin by peroxides.
- Vitamin E is free radical scavenger associated with cell membranes.
- Affected foals have higher concentrations of type IIc fibers and lower proportions of types I and IIa fibers than nonaffected foals of similar age.
- Myofibrils are affected early in the disease, with damage to small vessels, connective tissue, and neuromuscular elements occurring later.

SYSTEMS AFFECTED

- Musculoskeletal—all skeletal muscle, including the diaphragm, is affected, resulting in weakness and recumbency; cardiac muscle also may be affected, resulting in sudden death.
- Respiratory—if the diaphragm is affected, the foals may hypoventilate; affected upper airway muscles may result in dysphagia and aspiration pneumonia.

GENETICS

N/A

INCIDENCE/PREVALENCE

Most commonly reported in areas of known selenium-deficient soil.

SIGNALMENT

- Most common in foals <2 months of age, but any age may be affected.
- Usually seen in individuals, but a number of foals may be affected in one location.
- No known breed or sex predilections

SIGNS

- May be peracute to acute. Death may occur rapidly or several hours after exhaustion and circulatory collapse.
- Weakness, stiffness, and lethargy in less severely affected cases. Muscles may be firm and painful on palpation, and affected foals may be recumbent and unable to rise. Dysphagia frequently is reported as the first clinical sign. Aspiration pneumonia may be associated with dysphagia, and tachycardia, dysrhythmias, and respiratory distress are reported with cardiac and diaphragm involvement.
- Myoglobinuria frequently is reported.
- Hypo- or hyperthermia.
- Old foals may be presented with complaints of painful lumps ventrally, over the rump, and associated with the nuchal crest. These lumps result from steatitis.

CAUSES

N/A

RISK FACTORS

The soils of certain regions of the United States are selenium deficient. Grains and forage from these areas typically are low in selenium, and foals from mares fed this feed without selenium supplementation are at higher risk.

DIAGNOSIS

DIFFERENTIAL DIAGNOSIS

- Sudden death
- Septic shock in neonates may result in sudden death, but CK levels generally are normal.
- Trauma sometimes may be differentiated through the history.
- Recumbency, weakness, stiffness, and lethargy
- Septicemia often first presents as lethargy. This generally is seen during the first days of life and is associated with failure of passive transfer of maternal antibodies from colostrum.
- Botulism—affected foals usually are weak, with poor muscle tone, but not stiff.
- Viral or bacterial encephalitides, including EHV-1, may produce a profoundly depressed foal. A pleocytosis usually is present at CSF analysis.
- Spinal cord diseases, including abscess, result in neurologic disease that might mimic WMD. Clinical signs depend on location of the lesion.
- Tetanus presents as a stiff foal. A history of no vaccination of the dam or foal for tetanus may lead one to suspect this disease.
- Cerebellar disease
- Trauma
- Hyperkalemic, periodic paralysis may present with similar signs and should be suspected if the foal is from the "Impressive" Quarterhorse lineage.
- Dysphagia
- Other causes of dysphagia—cleft palate, pharyngeal collapse, arytenoiditis, and pharyngeal cysts; upper airway endoscopy helps to rule out these problems.
- Dyspnea
- Primary pneumonia causes increased rate and effort of respiration. Thoracic radiography aids in establishing this diagnosis.
- Primary cardiac disease, usually from congenital defects, may result in dyspnea. Careful ascultation of the heart helps to detect the presence of murmurs.
- Red urine—myoglobinuria
- Neonatal isoerythrolysis also results in the production of red urine. These animals also are anemic; PCV and TP should differentiate this cause of the red urine from myoglobinuria and hemoglobinuria.

CBC/SERUM BIOCHEMISTRY/URINALYSIS

- CBC reflects secondary infections (e.g., aspiration pneumonia), if present.
- AST and CK are markedly increased during the acute states.
- Severely affected foals may have profound metabolic acidosis and life-threatening hyperkalemia. Hyponatremia and hypochloremia also are reported.
- BUN and creatinine may be increased, initially because of prerenal factors and later associated with acute renal failure.
- Urine tests positive for blood, and specific analysis for myoglobin reveals this to result from myoglobinuria.

OTHER LABORATORY TESTS

- Low GPX, selenium, and vitamin E levels may be found in normal as well as affected animals.
- Reference values vary by laboratory. Samples collected for vitamin E determination should not be in contact with rubber. Additionally, vitamin E levels should be determined on multiple blood samples obtained throughout the day and then pooled.

IMAGING

N/A

DIAGNOSTIC PROCEDURES

- Acetate electrophoresis of urine may demonstrate myoglobinuria.
- Muscle biopsy may aid in establishing the diagnosis.
- Liver biopsy may aid in establishing diagnosis by determination of liver selenium concentration—a concentration <0.160 ppm on a wet-weight basis is considered deficient.

PATHOLOGIC FINDINGS

- Neonatal foals that die peracutely may have few to no macroscopic abnormalities.

WHITE MUSCLE DISEASE (WMD)

• Muscles may appear pale. Streaking, which is representative of muscle fibers undergoing coagulative necrosis next to more normal fibers, may be apparent, but the distribution of changes generally is uniform and symmetric.
• Frequently, all muscle groups of the fore and hind limbs are affected.
• The diaphragm, tongue, muscles of mastication, pharyngeal muscles, and cervical muscles frequently are affected.
• More chronic cases may demonstrate yellow-white streaks in muscle, including that of the heart, representing calcification of the damaged muscle.
• Histologic changes progress from extensive granular and severe hyaline degeneration of muscle fibers to phagocytosis of necrotic tissue, with endomysial thickening, edema, and mononuclear and fibroblast proliferation. The final stages include epimyseal connective tissue proliferation concurrent with evidence of regeneration and continued degeneration.

TREATMENT

APPROPRIATE HEALTH CARE
• Immediately place affected foals in a controlled environment, where their movements are minimized.
• Frequently, cases can be managed at the farm, but hospitalize severely affected foals.

NURSING CARE
• Keep affected foals in quiet, well-bedded, and padded surroundings.
• Use head protection and leg wraps in down foals or those likely to harm themselves.
• Intranasal oxygen supplementation or mechanical ventilation may be warranted in foals with aspiration pneumonia or those with involvement of cardiorespiratory or upper airway muscles.
• Dysphagic, anorexic, depressed, or recumbent patients require IV fluid support to maintain hydration and to address electrolyte and acid–base disturbances.
• Myoglobin is toxic to the kidneys; thus, diuresis is important to decrease these toxic effects.

ACTIVITY
Maintain foals as quietly as possible, and limit activity by stall confinement.

DIET
Foals with evidence of dysphagia may require feeding through an indwelling nasogastric tube to minimize use of swallowing muscles and to decrease the possibility of aspiration pneumonia.

CLIENT EDUCATION
• Inform clients of the strong possibility that severely affected animals will die despite appropriate care.
• Measuring vitamin E and selenium levels of other horses on the farm may be helpful to determine whether a nutritional deficiency exists.

SURGICAL CONSIDERATIONS
N/A

MEDICATIONS

DRUGS OF CHOICE
• Administer deep IM injection of vitamin E and selenium.
• Broad-spectrum antimicrobial therapy of the clinical's choice may be administered as a protective measure against secondary bacterial infection or for aspiration.
• Sedation may be required in hyperesthetic or excitable horses.
• Anti-inflammatory agents may be administered—flunixin meglumine (0.5 mg/kg) or DMSO (1 g/kg IV, diluted as a 15% solution)

CONTRAINDICATIONS
Selenium levels of 200 μg/kg are reported to be toxic.

PRECAUTIONS
• Closely monitor renal function if aminoglycosides are included in antimicrobial therapy. Ideally, obtain peak and trough values, and monitor creatinine daily.
• Injudicious use of NSAIDs may predispose to gastroduodenal ulceration.

POSSIBLE INTERACTIONS
N/A

ALTERNATIVE DRUGS
N/A

FOLLOW-UP

PATIENT MONITORING
• Acute renal failure has been associated with myoglobinuria. Monitor renal function closely, particularly if aminoglycoside therapy is instituted.
• Acid–base and electrolyte abnormalities, particularly hyperkalemia, can be life-threatening. Check potassium levels frequently; rebound hypokalemia can occur with correction of metabolic acidosis.
• Cardiac arrest and respiratory failure may occur at any time, associated either with primary muscle damage or with electrolyte and blood gas abnormalities. Frequent ECG recordings and arterial blood gas analyses may be warranted in certain cases.
• Upper airway collapse may result in acute asphyxiation.

PREVENTION/AVOIDANCE
• Inform clients that other animals on their farm may be affected, either clinically or subclinically.
• Prevention involves supplementation with vitamin E and selenium, preferably daily, either in an oral form or as a feed additive. Fatal reactions have been reported using injectable forms, particularly if used IV. Foals born in areas known to be deficient may benefit from an IM injection at birth.

MISCELLANEOUS

ASSOCIATED CONDITIONS
N/A

AGE-RELATED FACTORS
Usually seen in young animals, from birth to ≅9 months of age.

ZOONOTIC POTENTIAL
N/A

PREGNANCY
If a mare previously produced a foal that developed WMD during the neonatal period, the mare possibly may have been deficient in vitamin E and selenium during pregnancy; monitor these levels during subsequent pregnancies.

SYNONYMS
Nutritional myodegeneration

SEE ALSO
N/A

ABBREVIATION
• AST = aspartate aminotransferase
• CPK = creatine phosphokinase
• CSF = cerebrospinal fluid
• DMSO = dimethyl sulfoxide
• EHV = equine herpes virus
• GPX = glutathione peroxidase
• TP = total protein

Suggested Reading

Dill SG, Rebhun WC. White muscle disease in foals. Compend Contin Educ Pract Vet 1985;7:S627–S632.
Lofstead J. White muscle disease of foals. Vet Clin North Am Equine Pract 1997;13:169–185.
Maylin GA, Rubin DS, Lein DH. Selenium and vitamin E in horses. Cornell Vet 1980;7:272–289.
Perkins G, Valberg SJ, Madigan JM, Carlson GP, Jones SL. Electrolyte disturbances in foals with severe rhabdomyolysis. J Vet Intern Med 1998;12:173–177.

Author Pamela A. Wilkins
Consulting Editor Mary Rose Paradis

INDEX

Note: Page number followed by "t" denote tables

C

D

H

I

O

U

V

W

X

Y

Z

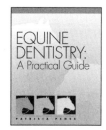